Fundamentals of Toxicologic Pathology

Second edition

"To teach is to learn …" Japanese Proverb

We are profoundly grateful to those individuals responsible for our love of pathology and who mentored us during our careers, including Drs. Gordon Chalmers, Chirukandath Gopinath, Daniel H. Gould, Dwayne W. Hamar, Clive R. Huxtable, Kenneth V.F. Jubb, John M. King, Lennart Krook, Kenneth McEntee, (Niels) Ole Nielsen, Peter Richards, Bruno Schiefer, Neill Sullivan, Reginald Thompson, Mike Tumbleson and Hanspeter Witschi.

We also thank our partners, Vincent F. Hock Jr., Jennifer L. Hoy and Kathleen A. Wallig who have encouraged and supported us during our efforts to complete this revision.

Fundamentals of Toxicologic Pathology

Second edition

Wanda M. Haschek
Department of Pathobiology
College of Veterinary Medicine
University of Illinois
Urbana, Illinois
USA

Colin G. Rousseaux
Department of Pathology and Laboratory Medicine
Faculty of Medicine
University of Ottawa
Ottawa, Ontario
Canada

Matthew A. Wallig
Department of Pathobiology
College of Veterinary Medicine
University of Illinois
Urbana, Illinois
USA

ELSEVIER

AMSTERDAM • BOSTON • HEIDELBERG • LONDON • NEW YORK • OXFORD
PARIS • SAN DIEGO • SAN FRANCISCO • SINGAPORE • SYDNEY • TOKYO
Academic Press is an imprint of Elsevier

Academic Press is an imprint of Elsevier
32 Jamestown Road, London NW1 7BY, UK
30 Corporate Drive, Suite 400, Burlington, MA 01803, USA
525 B Street, Suite 1900, San Diego, California 92101-4495, USA

First edition 2007
Second edition 2010

Notice
No responsibility is assumed by the publisher for any injury and/or damage to persons or property
as a matter of products liability, negligence or otherwise, or from any use or operation of any methods,
products, instructions or ideas contained in the material herein. Because of rapid advances in the medical
sciences, in particular, independent verification of diagnoses and drug dosages should be made

British Library Cataloguing-in-Publication Data
A catalogue record for this book is available from the British Library

Library of Congress Cataloging-in-Publication Data
A catalog record for this book is available from the Library of Congress

ISBN: 978-0-12-370469-6

For information on all Academic Press publications
visit our website at www.elsevierdirect.com

Typeset by Macmillan Publishing Solutions
(www.macmillansolutions.com)

Printed and bound in Canada

10 11 12 13 14 15   10 9 8 7 6 5 4 3 2 1

Contents

CHAPTER 4   NOMENCLATURE: TERMINOLOGY FOR MORPHOLOGIC ALTERATIONS   67

CHAPTER 5   TECHNIQUES IN TOXICOLOGIC PATHOLOGY   81

CHAPTER 6   RESPIRATORY SYSTEM   93

CHAPTER 10   PANCREAS   237

CHAPTER 18   MALE REPRODUCTIVE SYSTEM   553

Preface

"What is toxicologic pathology?" Although the answer to this question is not simple, toxicologic pathology can be defined as a medical science focusing on the study of structural and functional changes in cells, tissues, and organs that are induced by toxicants. The list of toxicant includes drugs, industrial and agricultural chemicals, environmental contaminants, toxins (chemicals of biological origin such as mycotoxins and phycotoxins), and physical agents such as heat and radiation. Toxicologic pathology also includes the investigation of the mechanisms by which these changes are induced and the development of risk assessment and risk management policies based on this information. Therefore, toxicologic pathology relies heavily on disciplines that are included within toxicology (e.g., biochemistry, pharmacodynamics, and risk assessment), those that are prerequisites for pathology (e.g., physiology, microbiology, immunology, and molecular biology), and other associated disciplines. Since most toxicologic pathology is performed in an experimental setting, knowledge of experimental design and biostatistics is essential. In addition, toxicologic pathologists need to be cognizant of newly emerged and emerging scientific areas of study (e.g., genomics and proteomics), and relevant technologies (e.g., tissue microarray analysis and new imaging technologies). Obviously it is too much to expect individuals to have in depth expertise in all of these areas; therefore, there is a critical need for individuals in this discipline to have a broad background in related disciplines as well as strong communication skills and the ability to work in teams, in order to function effectively in solving problems and resolving issues in this field.

Emergence of toxicologic pathology as a discipline was stimulated by the advent of worldwide concerns about the adverse health effects of pollutants and food contaminants, as well as the human and ecological safety of pesticides and pharmaceuticals. The first formalized program in the United States, the cancer bioassay, was originally under the auspices of the National Cancer Institute (NCI) and later transferred to the National Toxicology Program (NTP), both within the National Institute of Health (NIH). With the advent of toxicologic pathology there have been marked advances in understanding the mechanisms of toxicity and the manifestations of toxic effects.

Most toxicologic pathologists are veterinarians who are trained in diagnostic pathology and, ideally, in toxicology and experimental methods. A smaller number of toxicologic pathologists are physicians or biologists with advanced training in pathology. Toxicologic pathologists are employed in industry, academia, government, contract research laboratories or as consultants. Diagnostic and forensic pathologists also need to be familiar with tissue responses to xenobiotics. The ultimate goal of toxicologic pathology is to protect the health of people, animals and the environment.

The purpose of this revision of the *Fundamentals of Toxicologic Pathology* is to update the information presented in the first edition and to broaden the scope of the book to appeal to a wider range of readers interested in toxicologic pathology. The current edition targets toxicology and pathology graduate students and residents as well as pathologists and toxicologists who need an overview of the integration of structure and functional changes to toxic injury. The increased scope of the revised text should appeal to diagnostic and forensic pathologists and toxicologists (both graduate students and professionals) as well as professionals in industry, contract research organizations and government.

Acknowledgments

Our thanks to the authors of the original chapters from the *Handbook of Toxicologic Pathology,* that were used as a basis for this book.

Elizabeth H. Jeffery: Biochemical Basis of Toxicity

Matthew A. Wallig: Morphologic Manifestation of Toxic Cell Injury

Stephen Mastorides and R. R. Maronpot: Carcinogenesis

G.S. Smith, R.L. Hall and R.M. Walker: Applied Clinical Pathology in Preclinical Toxicology Testing

Ronald A. Herbert, James R. Hailey, John C. Seely, Cynthia C. Shakelford, Michael P. Jokinen, Jeffery C. Wolf and Gregory S. Travlos: Nomenclature

Thomas J. Bucci: Basic Techniques

Paul S. Cooke, Richard E. Peterson and Rex A. Hess: Endocrine Disruptors

Wanda M. Haschek, Kenneth A. Voss and Val R. Beasley: Selected Mycotoxins Affecting Animal and Human Health

Sharon M. Gwaltney-Brant: Heavy Metals

Wanda M. Haschek, Hanspeter R. Witschi and Kristen J. Nikula: Respiratory System

Adres J.P. Klein-Szanto and Claudio J. Conti: Skin and Oral Mucosa

T.A. Bertram: Gastrointestinal Tract

Russell C. Cattley and James A. Popp: Liver

Daniel S. Longnecker and Glenn L. Wilson: Pancreas

Kanwar Nasir M. Khan and Carl L. Alden: Kidney

Samuel M. Cohen, Hideaki Wanibuchi and Shoji Fukushima: Lower Urinary Tract

John F. Van Vleet, Victor J. Ferrans and Eugene Herman: Cardiovascular and Skeletal Muscle Systems

J.C. Woodward, J.E. Burkhardt and W. Lee: Bones and Joints

David C. Dorman, Karrie A. Brenneman, Brad Bolon, Adalbert Koestner and Stata Norton: Nervous System

C. Frieke Kuper, Emile de Heer, Henk Van Loveren, Joseph G. Vos, Henk-Jan Schuurman and Magda A.M. Krajnc-Franken: Immune System

V.E. Valli, J.P. McGrath, I. Chu and R.D. Irons: Hematopoietic System

Charles C. Capen, Ronald A. DeLellis and John T. Yarrington: Endocrine System

Dianne M. Creasy and Paul M.D. Foster: Male Reproductive System

Yang-Dar Yuan and George L. Foley: Female Reproductive System

Ronald D. Hood, Colin G. Rousseaux and Patricia M. Blakley: Embryo and Fetus

Principles of Toxicology

THE EFFECT OF THE BODY ON THE CHEMICAL

ABSORPTION

Passage across Membranes

Simple Diffusion

With the process of simple diffusion there is no substrate specificity and no receptor requirements. It involves the entire membrane and depends solely on the lipid–water partition. Polar, or water-soluble, compounds are in equilibrium between ionized and non-ionized forms. The ionized form has such a low lipid–water partition that it is essentially insoluble in lipid membranes, and only the non-ionized portion is available for diffusion across the membrane. Ionization is dependent upon the pK_a of the compound and the acidity of the environment. Due to the volume disparity between aqueous and lipid areas of the cell, diffusion is rate-limited by lipid solubility, increasing with increasing lipid solubility. Once through the membrane the substance re-equilibrates between ionized and non-ionized forms, depending on the pH of the aqueous intracellular environment.

Passage through Pores

Plasma membranes contain pores that allow small, ionized particles to pass through them. Typically the pore size is only 2–7 Å, and only 2% or 3% of the membrane is devoted to these pores. As the pressure rises

1

on one side of the membrane, particles that are almost the same size as the pores (about 100 MW) are forced through these pores. There are larger intercellular pores, or gaps, between the endothelial cells of the capillary walls in most tissues, allowing passage of larger water-soluble compounds from plasma into the extracellular space. The number and size of these interendothelial gaps varies widely: they are absent in the brain due to the tight junctions between cells, ~40 Å in most other tissues and larger (70 or 80 Å) in the renal glomerulus, allowing molecules of less than 69 000 MW to filter into the urine.

Specialized Transport Systems

Substrate-specific carrier proteins allow rapid transport of polar compounds across membranes. Some carrier proteins facilitate diffusion, transporting compounds down a concentration gradient, while others are integrated into an energy-requiring active transport system for transport of substances against a concentration gradient. Xenobiotics bearing structural or charge similarities to nutrients and endogenous substrates can interact with the specific carrier systems, competing with the endogenous substrate for uptake. For example, the active transport system for uracil and other pyrimidine bases is involved in the uptake of the chemotherapeutic agents, 5'-fluorouracil and 5'-bromouracil. Since these systems do not normally function at saturation, this additional uptake usually has little effect on transport of the true substrate.

Absorption Routes

Toxicologically significant routes of absorption are the gastrointestinal tract, the lungs, and the skin. During transport, some chemicals are modified through metabolism and/or binding. Because of this modification, correct modeling of absorption is essential in toxicological evaluations. Although weak acids and neutral compounds can be absorbed by simple diffusion from the acid stomach, the small intestine is the major site for absorption of xenobiotics from the gastrointestinal tract. Because of the large surface area, the rapid blood flow, and the thin alveolar wall, pulmonary absorption is a rapid and effective route of uptake for gases, volatile compounds, and even some small particulates. Ionizable compounds are absorbed rapidly across the alveolar wall by passive diffusion. For compounds that are relatively poorly water soluble, such as ethylene, uptake is limited by blood flow. Metals do not accumulate in the lungs, but pass directly into plasma so that metal absorption is many times greater in the lungs than in the intestine. The skin is an excellent barrier to all but highly lipid-soluble compounds, such as solvents. However, if the keratinized epidermal layer is removed by abrasion or hydrated by soaking the skin for a prolonged period of time, absorption is greatly increased.

DISTRIBUTION

Volume of Distribution

Body water may be divided into three compartments: the vascular, extracellular, and intracellular spaces. To pass from plasma to extracellular fluid, a compound must be either lipid soluble for diffusion across the endothelial membrane, or sufficiently small to pass through an interendothelial pore. To pass on from the extra- to the intracellular space, a compound must either diffuse or pass through the very much smaller pores of the plasma membrane. With no further refinements, the volume of distribution of a compound would be either 3, 12, or 41 liters in the average adult male, depending on whether distribution was limited to the vascular space alone, the vascular and extracellular spaces, or freely diffusible throughout total body water, respectively.

Two factors serve to add complexity to this distribution pattern. First, excretion is continuous, so that after an initial distribution period of a few minutes, even compounds totally confined to the plasma compartment slowly disappear as they are excreted from the body. Second, very few compounds are evenly distributed within each compartment. This simple three-compartment model must therefore be refined to contain multiple compartments depending on: (1) variation in capillary interendothelial pore size, from very large in the liver to almost absent in the brain; (2) presence of transport systems that permit organ-specific concentration of toxic compounds, such as uptake of iodine in the thyroid; and (3) presence of intracellular storage sinks which shift the equilibrium toward the storage organ, for example, the uptake of fluoride, lead, or strontium into the hydroxyapatite lattice of bone.

Barriers to Distribution

Blood–Brain Barrier

The historical concept of an impenetrable blood–brain barrier is no longer valid. Although water-soluble compounds are effectively excluded, lipid-soluble substances can pass freely across this barrier to concentrate in the fatty nervous tissue. Exclusion of polar substances depends on the fact that junctions between the capillary endothelial cells are far tighter in the brain than in the rest of the body, eliminating interendothelial pores. Astrocyte end feet tightly abut the endothelium, so that a compound must pass through, rather than around, two extra cell layers to pass into the cerebrospinal fluid. Furthermore, active transport systems similar to those found in kidney serve to transport organic acids and bases out of the brain. The blood–brain barrier is undeveloped in immature animals, and develops incompletely in certain areas of the brain, such as the olfactory bulbs. Somewhat similar to the blood–brain barrier is the blood–testis barrier, protecting the male gamete from many xenobiotics, but there is no known corresponding barrier protecting the female gamete.

Placental Barrier

Lipid-soluble xenobiotics freely diffuse from maternal to fetal blood, and thus to the fetus. The less lipid-soluble a compound, the more effectively it is excluded by the placenta. This barrier is equally effective from either direction; therefore any fetal metabolism of a xenobiotic to a more polar metabolite would tend to trap the metabolite in the fetus. Fortunately, most drug-metabolizing systems develop after birth, so that this particular event is avoided.

BIOTRANSFORMATION

Biotransformation, or metabolism, of a xenobiotic can dramatically alter its distribution and action, leading to detoxification and excretion, or to bioactivation and toxicity. Compounds that are so physically similar to an endogenous compound that they enter the body via its active transport mechanism may also share its sites for biochemical action and its route of metabolism, leading to eventual catabolism and excretion. For xenobiotics entering by diffusion, several organs, particularly the liver, contain enzymes with very broad substrate specificity that will metabolize a wide variety of lipid-soluble compounds. Biotransformation to a more water-soluble product usually enhances excretion, decreasing the likelihood of accumulation to toxic levels. However, these same enzymes can bioactivate a number of xenobiotics to reactive intermediates, producing cytotoxicity or carcinogenicity.

Biotransformation has traditionally been divided into two phases. Phase I metabolism is degradative, involving oxidative, reductive, and hydrolytic reactions that cleave substrate molecules. Products may be more or less toxic than the parent compound. Phase II metabolism is synthetic, involving conjugation or addition of xenobiotics to endogenous molecules. While traditionally phase II metabolites have been considered as almost invariably nontoxic, exceptions are growing with our increasing knowledge base. Frequently phase

I metabolism produces a suitable site on the metabolized molecule to allow phase II conjugation to occur. For example, benzene is not a substrate for any phase II reaction, but can undergo phase I oxidation to phenol. Phenol can undergo phase II glucuronidation, forming phenol-O-glucuronide, which is excreted.

Phase I Metabolism

Cytochrome P450

The cytochromes P450 (CYP) are a family of enzymes involved in oxidation and reduction of lipid-soluble compounds. In highest concentration in the liver, they are present in most tissues, including kidney, lung, gut, and nasal epithelium. Several CYP are dedicated to specific endogenous metabolic steps, such as kidney mitochondrial 1-a-hydroxylase, which is highly substrate specific and appears to metabolize 25-hydroxycholecalciferol and no xenobiotics. However, the CYP in the hepatic endoplasmic reticulum show far less substrate specificity, catalyzing oxidation or reduction of many chemicals. Furthermore, a single substrate may be metabolized to the same product by several CYP, each with its own kinetic characteristics. In excess of 20 isozymes are now recognized. CYP-dependent oxidation frequently leads to a decrease in the lipid–water partition, decreasing fat storage and increasing the fraction in body water, resulting in an increased rate of urinary excretion. Oxidative attack occurs at N, S, and C bonds, resulting in the insertion of one atom of oxygen. Occasionally, the oxidized products are highly toxic unstable electrophiles. Of the many mechanisms of oxidative attack, N-hydroxylation and aromatic C-oxidation (epoxide formation) are most frequently associated with bioactivation to toxic intermediates. Rather than aiding excretion, this change traps the electrophile inside the cell. Excretion is dependent on further metabolism by epoxide hydration or glutathione (GSH) conjugation. When this does not occur, GSH stores are depleted, covalent binding to cellular components occurs, and excretion is inhibited.

Epoxide Hydrase

Epoxide hydrase (or hydrolase) hydrates epoxide products of CYP oxidation to form the corresponding dihydrodiols. The enzyme most studied is microsomal and forms trans-diols. A cytosolic epoxide hydrase exists which may be more active towards lipid epoxides. Epoxide hydration is associated with detoxification of reactive epoxides, increased water solubility, and increased excretion. For example, epoxide hydrase catalyzes the hydrolysis of the toxic 3,4-epoxide of bromobenzene to an excretable product, 3,4-dihydrodiol. For a few compounds, epoxide hydration is a step towards further metabolism to form a toxic product. Benzo[*a*]pyrene is oxidized by CYP to the 7,8-epoxide. This is hydrated by epoxide hydrase, and the dihydrodiol is further oxidized at the 9,10-position, forming the ultimate carcinogen benzo[*a*]pyrene 7,8-dihydrodiol 9,10-epoxide.

Other Phase I Reactions

Hydrolyzing enzymes are widespread throughout the body, including the plasma, and catalyze the hydrolysis of esters. Classification is ill-defined, due to the wide substrate distribution and overlapping substrate specificity.

A number of nitro and azo compounds undergo an NADPH-dependent reduction that can be inhibited by carbon monoxide, implicating cytochrome P450 in this reaction, although a separate flavin nitroreductase also exists. Carbon tetrachloride and halothane are metabolized, both oxidatively and reductively, by cytochrome P450. In both cases, reduction causes bioactivation to a toxic intermediate, while oxidation is a detoxification step. The oxygen tension in the liver affects the route of metabolism, and reduction is favored as the oxygen tension falls. A number of aldehyde reductases, including alcohol dehydrogenase (named for the reverse reaction), are found throughout the body, and may catalyze reduction of toxic lipid-oxidation products.

There is an FAD-containing mono-oxygenase that is a non-CYP, microsomal system able to oxidize secondary amines and several sulfur compounds, including sulfides, thiols, and thioesters. Another microsomal oxidation system, particularly prevalent in kidney, is prostaglandin synthetase, a glycoprotein with a heme center. This enzyme produces peroxide as a byproduct during synthesis of prostaglandins from arachidonic acid. A number of xenobiotics are co-oxidized during this process by the peroxide. However, the *in vivo* significance of this co-oxidation is unknown at present. There are also at least two other distinct groups of amine oxidases, both widely distributed. The monoamine oxidases are mitochondrial flavoproteins involved primarily in catabolism of monoamine neurotransmitters and several xenobiotic amines. The diamine oxidases are vitamin B6-dependent cytosolic enzymes that preferentially metabolize short chain aliphatic diamines.

Alcohol dehydrogenase is a cytosolic enzyme present in liver and eye which catalyzes the oxidation of a variety of alcohols, including methanol, ethanol, and ethylene glycol. In the reverse direction, it catalyzes the reduction of a number of xenobiotics, including chloral hydrate. There are also large numbers of aldehyde dehydrogenases and oxidases with no metabolic role yet assigned to them.

Phase II Metabolism

Most frequently, products of phase II metabolism are more water soluble, more easily excretable, and less toxic than either parent compounds or phase I metabolites. Typically, conjugation involves the addition of an endogenous compound (e.g., glucuronic acid) to a xenobiotic in a two-step reaction, each step requiring an enzyme. Step 1 is the high-energy activation of either the conjugating agent (e.g., UDP-glucuronic acid formation for glucuronidation), or the xenobiotic (e.g., benzoyl-CoA formation for benzoic acid conjugation to glycine). Step 2 is the synthesis of the conjugate.

Glucuronidation

Glucose is readily available for glucuronidation, while the pool of sulfate or glycine available for conjugation is relatively small. This availability of endogenous substrate serves to increase the importance of glucuronidation relative to sulfation in endogenous and xenobiotic metabolism. The enzymes responsible for glucuronide conjugation, the glucuronosyl transferases, are present in the microsomal fraction of liver and other tissues. N-, O-, and S-glucuronides are formed and excreted into bile and urine.

Glutathione Conjugation

Glutathione (GSH), either spontaneously or with the aid of transferase enzymes, conjugates electrophiles, allaying potential toxicity of reactive metabolites. The resultant conjugate is further metabolized to the cysteinyl conjugate by removal of glutamate and glycine. The cysteinyl conjugate is acetylated, and the product formed, a mercapturic acid, is readily excreted in the urine. The hepatic synthesis of GSH, limited by the availability of cysteine, is frequently slower than conjugation. For this reason, GSH stores can fall during conjugation, leading to a temporary inability to conjugate electrophiles, loss of redox potential, and inability to quench peroxidation via GSH peroxidase. Since GSH levels exhibit a distinct diurnal variation, xenobiotics that only exert their toxicity after GSH has been depleted exhibit greatest potency at approximately 6 pm in rodents, the nadir in their diurnal variation in hepatic GSH levels. Recently, a number of GSH conjugates, including many allylic compounds, have been found to undergo further metabolism to reactive thionocompounds, producing nephrotoxicity.

ENZYME LOCATION IN TOXICITY

When a reactive intermediate is formed during metabolism, often it will exert its toxicity in the immediate vicinity. Many of the xenobiotics which are bioactivated by hepatic CYP cause centrilobular necrosis. The highest concentration of CYP is in the centrilobular region. The centrilobular region is also rich in conjugating enzymes. The oxygen-rich periportal region contains mostly enzymes of intermediary metabolism for plasma protein synthesis, and lipid and carbohydrate metabolism. Necrosis of the periportal region is associated with direct-acting hepatotoxic agents that enter the liver at the portal triad via the portal vein, and do not require bioactivation. Examples are hepatotoxic metals such as iron, manganese, and arsenic, and also phosphorus. Because the biliary tree drains from this region, bile salt damage and hepatic necrosis resulting from accumulation of biliary excretory products during cholestasis is first seen in the periportal region.

The kidney contains many of the same metabolizing enzymes as the liver, but at lower concentration. Also, depending on the route of exposure, the kidney receives a smaller dose of xenobiotic than the liver, because of the first-pass effect. The enzymes for bioactivation are located in the straight portion of the proximal tubule, resulting in necrosis at this site following bioactivation of a xenobiotic. The kidney also contains the enzyme cysteine β-lyase, which deconjugates cysteinyl conjugates formed in liver or kidney, producing reactive sulfur intermediates. This pathway is responsible for the nephrotoxicity of vinyl halides. A similar intestinal pathway exists whereby intestinal microflora deconjugates biliary metabolites of aromatic halides. This is followed by portal uptake of the sulfur metabolite, and transport to the liver for hepatic S-methylation and S-oxidation. The toxicologic consequences of this intestinal pathway have yet to be determined.

EXCRETION

Urinary Excretion

Excretion of xenobiotics into urine depends on filtration without reabsorption, and/or active secretion through the renal tubular epithelial cell. Components greater than 69 000 MW, such as those bound to plasma proteins, are too large to pass through the glomerular filtration apparatus, and therefore are not available for filtration. In addition, active secretory systems catalyze excretion through the proximal tubule cell into the tubular lumen, regardless of plasma protein binding. Since proximal tubule cells contain many of the drug-metabolizing enzymes found in the liver, xenobiotics often undergo metabolism during passage through these cells.

Once filtered, nutrients such as glucose are reabsorbed in the proximal tubule. This is also the site for reabsorption of a number of xenobiotics, leading to recirculation or accumulation in kidney. Both passive and active reabsorption processes exist. There also are at least two separate systems for active secretion in which xenobiotics (or metabolites) might interact, one for organic acids and the other for organic bases. The physiologic role for the acid system is clearance of uric acid and the glucuronide and sulfate conjugates of endogenous compounds, such as steroids. That this is a single carrier-mediated transport system is shown by competition between the various endogenous acids.

Biliary Excretion

Unlike urinary excretion, biliary excretion is relatively independent of hydrostatic pressure. Rather, biliary excretion depends on hepatic concentration of the xenobiotic. Substances passing into the bile have been grouped according to their plasma:bile ratios. Group A, those with a plasma:bile ratio approximating 1.0, are thought to pass into bile passively down a concentration gradient. Substances in Group A are mostly small molecules in equilibrium with total body water. Group B substances, those that are concentrated in the bile, constitute a growing number of compounds known to be actively secreted into the biliary canaliculi. Group C, those with a plasma:bile ratio greater than 1.0, tend to be bulky polar molecules, such as insulin and mannitol, that cannot readily cross membranes. Compounds of less than a certain molecular weight (325 in rats; 500–700 in humans) are thought to be excreted mainly in urine, while larger compounds are excreted into bile. However, this generalization is not accurate for highly polar substances.

As in the kidney, there appear to be two separate carrier-mediated biliary transport systems for excretion of organic acids and bases. A third transport system is responsible for excretion of steroids. Unless biliary metabolites are ionized at intestinal pH, excretion is thwarted by reabsorption, termed enterohepatic recirculation. Glucuronides are often deconjugated by intestinal microflora; this increases lipid solubility, permitting reabsorption and recirculation. This enterohepatic circulation can greatly increase the biological half-life of a xenobiotic, prolonging toxicity by producing chronic exposure.

Glutathione conjugates are excreted into the biliary canaliculi, where *gamma*-glutamyl transpeptidase and a dipeptidase on the luminal surface remove first glutamate and then glycine, leaving the xenobiotic conjugated only to cysteine. All three products are reabsorbed into the liver, from where the cysteinyl conjugate travels to the kidney for acetylation and excretion as a mercapturic acid.

Pulmonary Excretion

The lungs are an important site for absorption and excretion of volatile substances including solvents, alcohols, anesthetic gases, pesticide fumigants, and cyanide. Excretion is passive, and hyperventilation improves excretion of these substances by maximizing the concentration gradient. The Clara cell, present within the bronchiolar epithelial lining, contains an active drug metabolizing system, and therefore can bioactivate certain xenobiotics, causing necrosis. With such a ready source of oxygen for production of free radicals, alveolar cells are particularly susceptible to compounds that produce oxidative stress, such as bleomycin and paraquat.

INTERACTION OF CHEMICAL AND THE BODY

ENZYME INDUCTION AND INHIBITION

Activation, Induction, or Synergism

Interaction of xenobiotics with enzymes at sites other than the substrate-binding site can either increase or decrease enzyme activity. An increase in maximal velocity of an enzyme, with no concomitant increase in the amount of that enzyme, is termed activation and may be caused, for example, by allosteric addition of a cofactor which might aid in bringing substrates into juxtaposition at the site of action of an enzyme. In contrast, chelation and removal of the cofactor could inhibit the enzyme.

While activation/deactivation causes no change in the absolute amount of enzyme, many xenobiotics can cause the induction of enzyme, resulting in increased flux due to increased amount of enzyme. Commonly, xenobiotics cause the increased synthesis of the enzymes specifically involved in their own metabolism. Due to lack of substrate specificity of most drug-metabolizing enzymes, this induction also increases the rate of metabolism of other xenobiotics. While xenobiotics can be grouped according to which of several different isozymes they induce, the mechanism of induction of drug-metabolizing systems remains unknown for all but a select few xenobiotics. A cytosolic carrier has been identified that binds a number of polycyclic hydrocarbons, such as TCDD and 3-methylcholanthrene, traveling with them into the nucleus, where DNA-directed synthesis of new cytochrome P450 occurs. This carrier does not bind phenobarbital, and a search for a cytosolic protein binding to phenobarbital or to any xenobiotic that induces the same CYP enzymes as phenobarbital has been unsuccessful.

Synergism is an increase in the activity or toxicity of two or more components, over and above the added effects of the individual components, regardless of mechanism. Ethanol and carbon tetrachloride, both hepatotoxins, produce unexpectedly severe hepatotoxicity when administered together. Cigarette smoking and occupational carcinogen exposure in miners and steel workers appears to be synergistic with relation to induction of lung cancers. Similar to synergism is potentiation, where the potentiator alone appears to have no adverse effect, but greatly increases the toxicity of another xenobiotic. GSH depletors potentiate the toxic effect of many xenobiotics normally removed harmlessly via GSH conjugation. Diethylmaleate removes GSH by direct binding and buthionine sulfoximine by actual inhibition of GSH synthesis. Both potentiate the toxicities of acetaminophen and bromobenzene. The area of synergism and potentiation of toxicities deserves a great deal of attention if our knowledge of toxicology is to be more than academic, since exposure to a polluted environment seldom consists of exposure to a single chemical.

INHIBITION

A number of xenobiotics can inhibit the normal action of an enzyme by competing as substrates. Often these are not very potent *in vivo* inhibitors, because neither the xenobiotic nor the natural substrate is present at a sufficiently high concentration for the enzyme to become rate-limiting. Conversely, xenobiotics that form a stable substrate–enzyme complex that dissociates only very slowly are potent *in vivo* inhibitors. For example, organophosphate pesticides and related chemical warfare agents form a lasting complex with acetylcholine esterase which, when involving greater than 50% of the enzyme, cause accumulation of the natural substrate, acetylcholine, to toxic levels.

Some xenobiotics, while still interacting at the substrate-binding site, are termed suicide substrates, because they destroy the enzyme during metabolism, effecting a long-lasting noncompetitive inhibition that requires synthesis of new enzyme to reverse the inhibition. Many xenobiotics containing allyl groups, such as allylisopropyl acetamide, are bioactivated to such highly reactive intermediates that, immediately upon formation, they covalently bind to cytochrome P450, causing breakdown of the heme center of the CYP.

Some xenobiotics, termed antimetabolites, successfully replace the normal enzyme substrate, forming an abnormal product that then disturbs metabolism at a later point in intermediary metabolism. Fluoroacetate, galactosamine, and ethionine are examples. A number of antimetabolites have been developed as anticarcinogenic drugs, becoming incorporated into the pathways of purine and pyrimidine biosynthesis. Chemotherapeutic efficacy relies on sensitivity being greatest in cells that are most actively replicating. For example, the antifolate methotrexate, while nonspecifically inhibiting all DNA synthesis, is most toxic to those cells in the logarithmic growth phase, including cells of growing tumors.

DOSE DEPENDENCY AND SITE OF ACTION

Interaction between a toxic agent and an organism depends on the dose arriving at a particular site, and the affinity of the xenobiotic for that site. If a xenobiotic or nutrient interacts with more than one site in the organism, each site will have its own peculiar affinity for the xenobiotic, measurable as the dissociation constant K_d (or K_m if the site is an enzyme). As the dose of a xenobiotic is increased, the xenobiotic interacts with an ever-increasing number of different sites, with ever-decreasing affinities. In the test tube or cell culture, and to a lesser degree even in whole animals, it is possible to reach concentrations seldom reached in the environment. Thus, while the interaction of a biological ligand with very high concentrations of a xenobiotic may be a useful tool for mechanistic studies, it does not necessarily portray the site of toxicity of that same xenobiotic at lower concentrations.

ORGAN SPECIFICITY FOR TOXICITY

Site specificity, as described in the preceding sections, refers to a particular intracellular site, due to specificity of a chemical interaction. Often a xenobiotic interacts at that same subcellular site in several organs, although a particular organ is always the first to exhibit toxicity. This organ specificity, termed the critical organ, is due to a variety of causes. In toxicities causing generalized loss of energy metabolism, such as cyanide inhibition of cytochrome oxidase, the critical organ is the central nervous system (CNS), and death due to respiratory arrest occurs because of the greater oxygen sensitivity of the respiratory center, even though cytochrome oxidase is inhibited in all tissues. Similarly, radiation and the antimetabolites that interfere with purine and pyrimidine metabolism first affect organs undergoing most rapid DNA turnover, such as bone marrow, intestinal mucosa, and actively growing tumors.

SITE-SPECIFIC INTERACTIONS AND TOXICITY

Receptors and Enzymes

The more site-specific a toxic agent, the more likely it is that its action depends on physically mimicking the natural component that interacts at that site. Once at the site, its difference from the natural component produces the characteristic toxic action. A xenobiotic may interact with a receptor, either causing (as an agonist) or preventing (as an antagonist) the effect evoked by the endogenous substrate for this receptor. For example, atropine is a muscarinic antagonist, interacting with the acetylcholine-binding site at nerve terminals, but eliciting no signal. If a xenobiotic is only able to evoke a submaximal response, the term "partial agonist" may be applied.

Direct and Cascade Effects

The initial insult by a toxic xenobiotic may be one or two steps removed from the final physiological change that overwhelms the body. For many chemicals, the initial insult causes a sequence or cascade of effects, for example, by switching on a cAMP-dependent pathway, or causing the slow accumulation of an endogenous metabolite. Thus the normal balance of intermediary metabolism is disrupted. Triglyceride accumulation is a common response to a number of hepatotoxic agents, because of a disruption of the balance between uptake, synthesis, and release of triglycerides. However, individual xenobiotics vary in the mechanisms by which they cause this imbalance. For example, ethanol is thought to inhibit mitochondrial utilization of lipids, hydrazine to increase uptake and synthesis of lipids, and carbon tetrachloride to inhibit release of triglycerides by inhibition of lipoprotein synthesis.

NONSPECIFIC INTERATIONS AND TOXICITY

Electrophiles and Covalent Binding

Xenobiotics that are bioactivated to electrophiles bind to certain tissue macromolecules—lipid, protein, or DNA—depending on the xenobiotic in question. The nucleophile GSH is utilized by the family of GSH S-transferases, enzymes of which have a great affinity for electrophiles. Toxicity appears to ensue only after GSH levels have been depleted by conjugation to less than 20% of normal, and irreversible covalent binding to cellular components has commenced. Loss of GSH *per se* does not appear to be the toxic event, since a number of GSH-depleting agents are relatively nontoxic; rather, covalent binding after depletion would appear to be the culprit. However, the role of covalent binding in the toxicity of electrophiles is controversial, since the extent of covalent binding does not always correlate with toxicity. This has led to the suggestion that, at least for some xenobiotics, covalent binding may play no role in toxicity, while for others toxicity correlates closely with covalent binding. One possible reason for this seeming dichotomy is that covalent binding at a specific site produces toxicity, while concomitant binding at several nonspecific sites is without toxicity. To date, no target protein binding with subsequent inhibition of any specific cellular process has been found to connect covalent binding to cell death. Determination of the site of covalent binding and the specificity or lack thereof is presently an active area of research.

These findings are somewhat in contrast to studies of covalent binding of xenobiotics to DNA, where carcinogenic electrophiles have been found bound to specific sites on DNA. Some studies report generalized binding of a carcinogen to a specific base, and a specific location on that base, followed by site-specific repair of bases at certain sites and not others. The anticarcinogenic action of selenium has been proposed to protect specific bases from accumulating covalently bound material, while other bases continue to exhibit binding, with no carcinogenic outcome. Carcinogenic electrophiles also exhibit a specificity of binding to cellular components. Benzo[a]pyrene incubated with GSH, DNA, and microsomes will bind GSH most avidly, then DNA, and exhibits least affinity for microsomal protein, reflecting the binding pattern that this carcinogen exerts in the whole animal. The basis for this specificity, whether due to the strength of the nucleophilic tissue site, to the lack of hindrance about that site, or to some other characteristic, is presently unknown. Discovery of the basis for this specificity may lead to a method for inhibition of carcinogenesis.

Free Radicals and Lipid Peroxidation

When a xenobiotic is bioactivated to an intermediate that breaks down to a free radical, an available source of hydrogen atoms to quench the radical is the unsaturated lipid of the cell membranes. The lipid radical thus formed by removal of the hydrogen atom readily interacts with oxygen to form a peroxy radical. Quenching of the peroxy radical by a hydrogen atom abstracted from a second unsaturated lipid leaves a lipid peroxide, and produces a new lipid radical, thus propagating lipid peroxidation. Peroxidation may also be initiated by xenobiotics, such as paraquat and menadione, that cycle between oxidized and reduced states, producing an oxygen radical each time it cycles back to the oxidized form. The oxygen radical then initiates peroxidation. Any other sources of partially-reduced oxygen, such as that produced by uncoupling of oxidative phosphorylation, can also initiate peroxidation. Unless removed by catalase or GSH peroxidase, hydrogen peroxide formed as a byproduct of metabolism, or as a result of uncoupling of mixed function oxidation, forms hydroxyl radicals which initiate peroxidation and cause single strand breaks in DNA. Inhibition of peroxidation by GSH peroxidase, catalase, or vitamins C and E can often forestall cytotoxicity and necrosis, and toxicity generally ensues only after GSH depletion.

The precise mechanisms whereby peroxidation causes cytotoxicity and necrosis are controversial. One possibility is that breakdown products of peroxidized lipids, such as 4-hydroxynonenal, are cytolytic and destroy the membrane. Alternatively, radical products of peroxidation may covalently bind to essential cellular components. Another possibility is that peroxidation of the plasma membrane may cause sufficient change in its physical properties that basic functions such as calcium homeostasis are lost. Whatever the cause, cell death appears to be directly preceded by a loss of calcium homeostasis, a massive influx of calcium, a loss of ATP, and an activation of a number of calcium-dependent phospholipases and proteases.

FURTHER READING

Eaton, D.L., and Klaassen, C.D. (2001). Principles of toxicology. In *Casarett and Doull's Toxicology: The Basic Science of Poisons* (Klaasen, C.D. ed.), 6th edn, pp. 11–34. Macmillan, New York, NY.

Lu, F.C. (1985). *Basic Toxicology. Fundamentals, Target Organs, and Risk Assessment*. Hemisphere, Washington, DC.

Pelkonen, O., and Raunio, H. (1997). Metabolic activation of toxins: tissue-specific expression and metabolism in target organs. *Environ. Health Perspect.*, 105(Suppl 4), 767–774.

Pratt, W.B., and Taylor, P. (1990). *Principles of Drug Action: The Basis of Pharmacology*, 3rd edn. Churchill Livingstone Inc., Edinburgh.

Rozman, K.K., and Klaassen, C.D. (2001). Absorption, Distribution and Excretion of Toxicants. In *Casarett and Doull's Toxicology: The Basic Science of Poisons* (Klaasen, C.D. ed.), 6th edn, p. 128. Macmillan, New York, NY.

Timbrell, J.A. (1982). *Principles of Biochemical Toxicology*. Taylor and Francis, London.

Manifestations of Toxic Cell Injury: Cell Injury/ Death and Chemical Carcinogenesis

SECTION I CELL INJURY, CELL DEATH AND SEQUELAE

INTRODUCTION

Whatever the cause of injury to a cell, toxic or otherwise, whatever the biochemical events, simple or complex, that lead to the injury or death of that cell, the pathologist must rely on a visible morphologic change to detect a disruption of homeostasis. This visible manifestation of disrupted function, at the ultrastructural, microscopic or macroscopic levels, is a lesion. The lesion is still the primary means by which a toxicologic pathologist arrives at a diagnosis, one that ideally includes the etiology, as well as a description of the underlying morphologic alterations.

The basic unit of life is the cell; therefore, any morphologic alterations to a tissue as a result of injury must begin with the response of the cell itself to injury. A thorough evaluation and understanding of a lesion must logically begin at the cellular level. The development of a lesion is dependent on a variety of factors which influence how the cell responds to the disruption in homeostasis forced upon it.

Key Cellular Components in Cell Injury

Although damage to any one organelle or structure in a cell can result in injury to the cell as a whole, there are several critical cell systems that are of prime importance in cell injury. It is these structures where disruptions of structure or function will almost always result in injury to, or death of, the cell. These structures are: the plasma membrane—site of osmotic, electrolyte and water regulation, as well as signal transduction; the mitochondrion—site of aerobic respiration; the endoplasmic reticulum—site of much protein synthesis, as well as calcium storage; and the nucleus, where the genetic material of the cell is sequestered, and in which transcription of the genetic code takes place. Accordingly, it is these structures on which toxicologists and pathologists have focused in their studies of the genesis of cell injury and death.

Factors Influencing Injury

Perhaps the most obvious factor influencing lesion development is the severity of the damage itself. If damage to the cell is mild, with rapid recovery, a lesion may never manifest itself morphologically, although a temporary functional disruption may occur or a biochemical alteration may become detectable. On the other hand, the damage may be so severe that tissue structure is obliterated to the point where determining a pathogenesis or etiology is impossible. Another possibility is that the damage is so swift and so profound that not only the cell dies, but also the entire individual is affected and death of the individual occurs before the injury can manifest morphologically. Acute cyanide intoxication is a classic example.

The overall metabolic rate of a cell has a significant effect on lesion development. Cells with high metabolic activity tend to suffer injury more easily and quickly. One need only compare the response of a neuron to that of a fibroblast under conditions of hypoxia to observe the effect of high metabolic demand on a cell's ability to adjust to injury. Metabolically active cells such as neurons, myocardial cells, and renal proximal convoluted tubule epithelium, are absolutely dependent on a continuous oxygen supply for normal function. They need uninterrupted and high concentrations of O_2 for oxidative phosphorylation, to provide the necessary ATP for maintenance of membrane polarity and membrane integrity (neurons), for continual muscular contraction/relaxation and Ca^{2+} transport (myocardium), and for transport of fluids, electrolytes, and metabolites (PCT of kidney). Even small changes in O_2 tension mildly decreasing ATP production will cause serious disruptions of the essential functions of these cell types, with serious consequences for the survival of the individual. By contrast, cells with low metabolic activity, such as fibroblasts and adipocytes, are less affected by low O_2 supply, and can tolerate a very low oxygen environment—hence their prominent role in regeneration and scarring.

Related to this, the degree of specialization can be an important determinant of a response to injury. Some cells, such as the fibroblast, a cell which is quite "plastic" in its adaptability to a variety of conditions and which can assume an assortment of different roles due to its relatively undifferentiated nature, can tolerate almost totally anaerobic conditions and a variety of toxic insults. Retinal rods and cones, on the other hand, which must expend much energy in maintaining their highly specialized membrane structures for trapping photons of light, can only tolerate an absolute minimum of disruption of homeostasis before degeneration or death ensues.

The "metabolic peculiarities" of a particular cell may have a substantial impact on its response to a particular injurious stimulus. The presence of specific receptors on a cell—the *fas* receptor, for example, may induce a cell to undergo apoptotic necrosis (i.e., apoptosis) when a *fas* ligand binds to it, whereas a cell without this receptor will be totally unaffected.

In similar fashion, certain cells may accumulate toxic concentrations of xenobiotics because they have specific uptake systems which allow the cell to "mistakenly" accumulate a substance that it either cannot metabolize or that it bioactivates. Gentamicin toxicity in the proximal convoluted tubular epithelium is an example of this. Gentamicin is taken up by the organic transport system, accumulates in the lysosomes, and eventually interferes with lipid metabolism and lysosomal function, to the point where the lysosomes malfunction and kill the cell. The sensitivity of pancreatic acinar cells to excessive dietary lysine or arginine is another example. Possession of certain phase I metabolizing enzymes, especially certain members of the cytochrome P450 family, may result in bioactivation, rather than detoxification of certain xenobiotics, leading to an enhanced or selective susceptibility to damage by a particular xenobiotic. The presence in the hepatocyte of CYP 2E1 makes it uniquely susceptible to damage by acetaminophen, which is bioactivated to a highly reactive quinone imine by this P450 isozyme.

The "innate" ability of a cell to respond to the injurious stimulus—a high activity of antioxidant enzymes, for example—can have a substantial impact on its ability to handle injury. The hepatocyte, for example, which receives 60% of its blood supply directly from the gastrointestinal tract, can tolerate a high degree of "toxic" insult entering from that source. This is due to its tremendous complement of phase I and phase II detoxification enzymes, as well as its high concentrations of antioxidants such as glutathione, Vitamin E, and Vitamin C. These feature all the hepatocytes to accomplish this within in a relatively oxygen-poor environment. However, a high complement of phase I and phase II detoxification enzymes, while protective under most conditions can be liability as well as an asset in some cases, where phase I- or phase II-mediated bioactivation of a highly lipid-soluble, but otherwise innocuous, compound can result in the production of highly damaging soluble intermediates. Cells lacking high concentrations of endogenous antioxidant or antioxidant enzymes, or lacking the appropriate concentrations and/or combinations of phase I and phase II enzymes, can be especially prone to toxic injury, especially if cells like the hepatocyte or the Clara cell fail to do their job of detoxifying toxins before they reach the general circulation.

Reaction of the Body to Injury

The reaction of surrounding viable tissues to the injured or dead cell has a key role in the morphologic manifestation of toxic cell injury. In some cases, it is the exuberance of the inflammatory cells attracted into the affected area, rather than the injury itself, that leads to the development of an overt lesion. Although in most cases the inflammatory reaction is an essential component in ridding the areas of damaged cells, the inflammatory reaction can be a "two-edged sword," converting a relatively mild injury into a severe one. Much of the severe necrotizing damage in acute toxic pancreatitis, for example, arises not from the release of zymogen granules from dying acinar cells, but rather from the activated neutrophils attracted into the lesion by the released cell contents. Such a reaction is typically associated with the type of cell death that has been termed "oncotic necrosis" or "oncosis," whereas the inflammatory reaction is much more likely to be muted, or even absent, with the type of cell death described as "apoptotic necrosis" or "apoptosis." The differences in response, to be discussed in more detail below, are linked to the leakage of intracellular components out of the cell dying by oncotic necrosis, as well as pro-inflammatory substances produced by the dying cell itself. These substances elicit a response from neutrophils, the "foot soldiers" of the acute inflammatory response. On the other hand, in situations where cells have undergone apoptotic necrosis, with its orderly sequence of disintegration and preservation of membrane integrity, local macrophages, rather than neutrophils attracted from the circulation, ingest and break down the dead cells with no overt inflammatory response.

Adaptation

A cell typically exists within a very narrow range of physiochemical conditions, and it will exert much of its metabolic energy and resources towards maintaining these conditions. This process is termed homeostasis. Ion gradients, intracellular pH and cytosolic osmolarity, for example, are vigorously maintained by the cell, even at the risk of losing its own specialized functions. A cell threatened with a loss of homeostasis will often jettison its specialized structures and cut back on its specialized functions, no matter how important they may be to the rest of the organism, in order to maintain its internal environment. Substantial deviations from homeostasis may lead to the death of the cell, while less substantial deviations can lead to a new level of function or metabolic activity in an attempt to maintain internal environment. A cell dealing with disrupted homeostasis can respond in a variety of ways to maintain itself short of death. This is called adaptation.

Atrophy

One form of adaptation is atrophy, which is a reduction of mass in a cell, tissue, or organ. At the cellular level, atrophy is often a response to decreased demand for the specialized functions of a particular cell. Decreased workload on a skeletal muscle attached to a limb immobilized by a cast will lead to a decrease in content of actin, myosin, and other proteins associated with muscle contraction. This will in turn be reflected as decreased diameters and volumes of myofibers within that muscle (Figure 2.1). Loss of appropriate stimulation needed for specialized function may result in a decrease not only in the metabolic activity of the affected cell, but also a decrease in overall content as well, including loss of organelles. Loss of innervation to a muscle, or lack of hormonal stimulation to an endocrine-dependent tissue such a thyroid follicular cell, will result in a reduction in cell size, if not ultimately the death of the cell itself. A reduction in nutrient or oxygen supply due to inadequate or reduced blood flow will almost certainly result in a reduction in the mass of a cell.

At the most basic level, it can be said that an atrophied cell has undergone catabolism. Ultrastructurally, this is reflected by an overt breakdown of mitochondria, endoplasmic reticulum, microtubules and microfilaments. Typically, there are increased numbers of autophagic vacuoles within the cell. These are often fused with lysosomes. Specialized structures such as cilia, contractile apparatuses, secretory granules, and microvilli may be reduced in number or even absent.

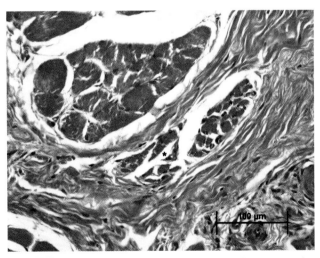

FIGURE 2.1 Atrophy. Skeletal muscle from the tongue of a young horse. The affected muscle (*) atrophied when blood supply to that portion of the tongue was impaired, due to an arterial embolus. Both muscle bundles and individual myofibers are reduced in size, and there is increased space between fibers. Hematoxylin and eosin stain.

In severe cases, loss of specialized structures may be so extensive that the cell may no longer be recognizable phenotypically. In metabolically active cells that have a high turnover of membrane components, lysosomes filled with solid precipitates of partially-degraded complex lipids and lipoproteins may accumulate over time, forming golden brown lipofuscin and ceroid, the "wear and tear" pigments. Histologically, the cell may be obviously reduced in size, have decreased staining affinity, have an altered shape, or be less differentiated in morphology. Grossly, one may only see a reduction in the overall size or mass of the tissue or organ in which the affected cell is found, with perhaps a softer texture or paler color.

Atrophy at the tissue or organ level, however, can reflect more than just a reduction in cellular mass, for a decrease in cell number can also result in a gross reduction in mass. Atrophy in this case is the result of cell death, either by apoptotic necrosis or oncotic necrosis, leaving behind a tissue which may not only be smaller, but which also may have a variety of altered characteristics, depending on the cause of the atrophy. In cases where cell loss occurred via apoptotic necrosis, there may be macrophages, vacuoles, or granules that are in reality phagolysosomes containing portions of the dead cells in various stages of degradation within nearby tissue. Histologically, these granules may appear as hyalin droplets. Inflammation or scarring is not usually present. Grossly, atrophy associated with reduction in cell numbers due to apoptotic necrosis resembles that observed with a simple reduction in cellular mass without cell death.

By contrast, in cases where oncotic necrosis is the cause of the reduction in cell number, there will be some degree of inflammation, often with resultant scarring. In these situations, the reduction in tissue or organ size may be irregular and distorted—depending on the degree of scar tissue present, firmer than normal and grayish or whitish as a reflection of the scarring.

Hypertrophy

Hypertrophy, by definition, is an increase in mass of a cell, tissue, or organ without cellular proliferation. While less commonly encountered in toxicologic pathology than atrophy or other signs of adaptation, it can nevertheless, on occasions, have significant consequences for the overall well-being of the individual. Classically, hypertrophy is a response to increased metabolic demand for a specialized function provided by the particular cell. At the ultrastructural and histological levels, this translates into an increase in the volume of cytoplasm and an increase in the number

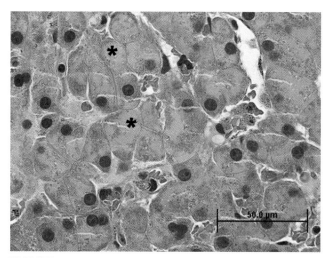

FIGURE 2.2 Pathologic hypertrophy. Liver from a dog with enlarged hepatocytes having increased pale, "waxy" cytoplasm (a*), due to profound increase in smooth endoplasmic reticulum. The animal had been treated for a prolonged period of time with oral phenobarbital to control convulsions. Hematoxylin and eosin stain.

of cell organelles, microfilaments, microtubules, and other specialized structures. Hypertrophy is usually difficult to quantify at the ultrastructural and light microscopic levels without specialized morphometric techniques, but it is usually evident grossly. As with atrophy, weighing an organ and calculating organ to body weight ratios may be the only way to detect subtle forms of hypertrophy. The consequences of hypertrophy are often benign, and merely reflect a physiological response to increased metabolic demand for specialized function. However, there are situations where the increased mass exceeds physiologic limits, and dysfunction of the hypertrophied tissue occurs. Examples of "pathologic" hypertrophy in response to a toxic stimulus do exist, for example, the tremendous hypertrophy of smooth endoplasmic reticulum in the hepatocyte in individuals treated with phenobarbital and other anticonvulsant drugs (Figure 2.2), which in severe cases can lead to loss of other hepatocytic functions.

REVERSIBLE CELL INJURY

Reversible injury is sometimes referred to as degeneration, although this term has been used in the past to describe other conditions, which may not be reflective of injury. Reversible injury is not enough to kill the cell, even if its specialized function in the body is impaired. It must be remembered, however, that although a cell may be reversibly injured, if the loss of its function is one that is vital for the survival of the

individual as a whole, death of the individual may occur even though a single cell has not died. There are two cellular morphologic changes commonly recognized as reflecting reversible injury, although in either case these changes may progress further to those characteristic of cell death. These are cell swelling and fatty change.

Cell Swelling

Cell swelling is an early change that occurs in most types of acute injury, and which may be a prelude to more drastic changes. By light microscopy, the cells in an affected tissue are typically swollen, with compression or displacement of adjacent structures. Staining affinity is often diminished, generally giving the cells a pale or cloudy appearance. Clear spaces or vacuoles may form. These are usually manifestations of dilated endoplasmic reticulum or Golgi. This type of change has, in the past, been termed vacuolar degeneration. Sometimes vacuoles are not present at all in the affected cells; rather, the cytoplasm is diluted and organelles are widely dispersed within the rarefied cytoplasm (Figure 2.3). This change has been termed ballooning degeneration by some. Nuclear changes are often mild or minimal, at least early on, and the nucleus generally occupies a location that is typical for the particular cell type.

Cell swelling occurs when the cell loses its ability to control the movement of ions and water into and out of the cytosol precisely. For the most part, this reflects the influx of sodium and water across the membrane

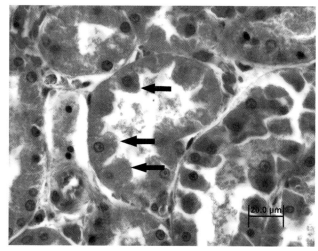

FIGURE 2.3 Cell swelling. Swollen renal tubular epithelial cells from a dog in septic shock. Note the bulging of the apical portions of the cells (arrows), loss of brush border, and elevation of the nuclei from the basal portions of the cells. Hematoxylin and eosin stain.

into the cell, due to altered function or insufficient capacity on the part of membrane Na^+-K^+-ATPases to exchange sodium for potassium at a rate sufficient to maintain water balance. Direct damage to these pumps, inadequate supplies of the essential substrate, ATP, or inability to keep up with the influx of sodium due to direct damage to the plasma membrane itself may also be causes. Vacuoles may form if the Na^+-K^+-ATPases in the endoplasmic reticulum are sufficiently functional to pump at least some of the excess sodium (followed by water) into its lumenal spaces. Contributing to the morphologic changes associated with cell swelling is loss of normal shape, due not only to the influx of water, but also to the influx of calcium into the cell via the diminished capacity or function of the Na^+-Ca^{2+} exchange pumps, which are also dependent on ATP. The dissociation of cytoskeletal elements, and the loss of intercellular connections that result from excessively high free cytosolic calcium levels, lead to additional loss of a shape and a tendency for the cell to assume a spherical shape if anatomically possible.

Cell swelling is not lethal *per se*, and may indicate relatively mild injury; however, cells that are severely injured or lethally injured usually also go through a phase of swelling. Therefore, it must be remembered that lethally injured cells that were fixed in the early stages of death may be interpreted as only being mildly injured, when in fact they are severely damaged. The location of the cell swelling must also be considered when assessing the consequences of cell swelling. Cell swelling in the myocardium secondary to poor vascular perfusion will at some point lead to separation of actin-myosin microfilaments and alter contraction. Ion shifts will also occur that affect depolarization—with serious consequences even if the myocardial cells are reversibly injured. Swelling of astrocytes in the brain during hyperammonemia during liver failure can have tremendous functional consequences, even if no lethal injury has occurred. By contrast, cell swelling in the liver can be quite marked, with few long-term consequences if the injurious stimulus is removed.

Fatty Change

Fatty change is a second manifestation of reversible injury that is often observed in cells that metabolize large quantities of lipids for energy, in particular the liver, but also myocardium and renal tubular cells. Although conditions other than injury can lead to intracellular accumulation of lipid, damage to certain organelles can also lead to fatty change. Direct damage

to membranes in cells with a high flux of triglycerides can lead to excessive build-up of triglyceride within the cytoplasm, due to impaired capability to re-export triglycerides. Hypoxia or damage to mitochondria within a cell can lead to insufficient β-oxidation of triglycerides and accumulation of unmetabolized triglycerides within the damaged mitochondrion, and also within the cytoplasm. Damage to protein synthetic machinery in endoplasmic reticulum by the direct action of toxins or hypoxia can result in decreased synthesis of apoproteins for lipid transport, and decreased synthesis of oxidative enzymes for β-oxidation of fatty acids, with the resultant storage of unmetabolized and/or untransported lipids within the cytoplasm. Swelling of fat-laden cells can progress to the point of occluding blood supply or can simply crowd out other organelles needed for other essential cellular function, leading to cell death.

Ultrastructurally, fatty change is characterized by accumulation of amorphous, moderately electron-dense cytoplasmic inclusions free within the cytosol but often associated with proliferative or mildly dilated endoplasmic reticulum. The inclusions can be small and dispersed—often associated with acute, rapidly developing injury—or quite large, occupying the entire central area of the cell and pushing organelles peripherally. This type of "macrovesicular" fatty change has been linked to more slowly-developing toxic injury. Histologically, lipid-laden cells are swollen and clear, with numerous, clearly defined round spaces (vacuoles) or one large central vacuole compressing cytosol and nucleus around the periphery of the cell (Figure 2.4). Due to conventional processing techniques that wash out triglycerides and other

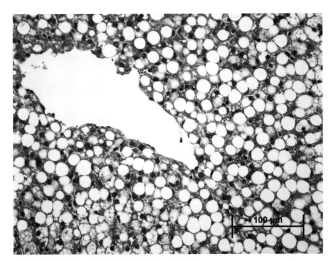

FIGURE 2.4 Fatty change in the liver from a goat with pregnancy toxemia. The vacuoles are large and displace other cellular structures to the periphery of the cell. Hematoxylin and eosin stain.

lipids, frozen sections must be used to preserve the fat in place, followed by special stains like Oil Red O, Sudan black, or osmium tetroxide, to stain lipids orange or black. This is occasionally done to distinguish lipid-filled vacuoles from other types of vacuoles, in particular those filled with water. The gross appearance of fatty liver is a classic lesion in pathology, with its orange or yellow coloration, reticulated pattern and friable, often greasy, texture. Lipid accumulations in non-hepatic tissues are less visible, but can be noted occasionally in the myocardium under conditions of hypoxia, usually in the myocytes bordering an infarctive lesion. This is due to damage to the β-oxidation pathways in the damaged mitochondria. It must be remembered, however, that not all fatty change is due to toxic injury. The kidney, for example, will accumulate triglycerides when there is hyperlipidemia during the course of diabetes mellitus. Macrophages will often accumulate lipids when involved in inflammatory lesions, where large amounts of lipid released from dead or dying cells must be taken up, digested, and metabolized. This a common change when there is degeneration or death of tissue in the CNS, especially in the lipid-rich white matter.

IRREVERSIBLE INJURY

Cell injury is any disruption that results in the loss of a cell's or tissue's ability to maintain homeostasis, normal or adapted; in other words, the cell can no longer regulate its environment within physiologic limits. The "point of no return" at the biochemical level for an injured cell has been much debated and researched over recent years, with the slowly emerging understanding that the mitochondrial permeability transition, leading to leakage of the electron transport chain enzyme cytochrome c into the cytosol, may be the final step in both (oncotic) necrosis and apoptotic necrosis (apoptosis). Determining the "point of no return" morphologically at the ultrastructural and histologic levels is even more difficult, particularly for histologic assessment, and a variety of other considerations must enter into any evaluation of a lesion where a judgement regarding the reversibility of the lesion must be made. This is in large part due to the lag time between the biochemical events leading to injury and the morphologic manifestations of these biochemical disruptions. In the case of ultrastructural change, the lag may be only minutes or hours, but for histologic manifestations to appear, it may be hours, or in some cases days, for a change to become apparent. Grossly, the appearance of a lesion may

be even longer. Because of this lag other lines of evidence—morphological and non-morphological—must be utilized to reach a conclusion. Such things as the presence of an inflammatory reaction, the duration of the injurious stimulus (if known), the clinical signs in the affected individual, clinical pathology changes (if available), even the type of cell involved and the tissue affected, may have to enter into the equation before a conclusion of irreversible injury can be made.

Irreversible injury that leads to death of the cell in the living organism is termed necrosis. If the process is uncontrolled, the result is sometimes termed "oncotic" or "accidental" necrosis or simply "necrosis." If the process of cell death is tightly regulated and orderly, the process has been termed "apoptotic" necrosis or simply "apoptosis." In either case, the cell after death will ultimately be degraded and dissolved, disappearing permanently. In both forms, the exact point of "death" is disputed, but the morphologic changes that precede, or follow, the "point of no return" can be identified, and conclusions drawn as to mechanism or etiology (Table 2.1). It must be emphasized; over and over again, that the term necrosis encompasses not only the actual occurrence of cell death in the living organism, but also the degenerative changes that follow the death process. The degenerative changes that follow death of the cell are often the most important part of identifying lethal cell injury morphologically, especially in cases of oncotic necrosis. Generally, it is these secondary changes that are most obvious grossly, or histologically. It must also be remembered that postmortem autolysis involves similar processes, and that these changes occur in all cells after death of the entire organism. Fortunately, it is the reaction of the surrounding tissues to the dead cells that usually allows the pathologist to distinguish antemortem cell death from the postmortem autolytic changes that follow the death of the individual.

Oncotic Necrosis

The initial ultrastructural changes that occur in oncotic necrosis (Figure 2.5A) are frequently the same as those that follow reversible cell injury; there is typically cell swelling with rarefaction of the cytosol due to the influx of water, dilation of the endoplasmic reticulum, loss or deformation of specialized surface features and rounding of the cell. The ultrastructural changes precede the histologic manifestations of injury by a long interval of hours to days, but they are nevertheless important to be aware of since they give valuable clues to the ultimate morphologic manifestations of lethal injury as observed histologically.

TABLE 2.1   Necrosis versus apoptosis

Characteristic	Necrosis	Apoptosis
Gross changes	Grossly evident with disruption of normal tissue structure and detail, scarring if long term	Minimal or atrophy without scarring
Histologic changes	Whole fields of cells affected	Individual cells scattered throughout the affected tissue
	Hypereosinophilia	Hyperbasophilia or hypereosinophilia
	Loss of cell borders with irregular fragmentation	Formation of round bodies, often within a "halo"
	Irregular chromatin clumping, pyknosis, karyorhexis and/or karyolysis; rupture of nuclear envelope	Chromatin condensation into "caps" or "crescents," within round nuclear bodies; preservation of nuclear envelope
Ultrastructural changes	Swelling and loss of surface structures with "blebbing" and loss of apical portions of cytoplasm	Condensation, followed by rapid "zeiosis" (budding)
	Rarefaction of cytoplasm, followed by condensation after death	Condensation of cytoplasm, followed by rarefaction after ingestion by phagocytes
	Swelling and loss of organellar integrity	Preservation of organellar integrity
	Low amplitude swelling of mitochondria, followed by high amplitude swelling and rupture	Preservation of mitochondrial ultrastructure
	Rupture and degradation of internal and external membranes, with bursting of the cell	Preservation of internal and external membranes, with preservation of membrane around apoptotic bodies
	Irregular clumping and degradation of chromatin; rupture of nuclear envelope	Migration of uniformly-degraded chromatin to margins of nuclear envelope; preservation of nuclear envelope
Sequelae	Release of intracellular enzymes into extracellular millieu	Retention of intracellular enzymes within the apoptotic bodies
	Release of pro-inflammatory cell breakdown products	No release of pro-inflammatory products
	Ingress of neutrophils, followed by macrophages	Ingestion by adjacent cells, or by tissue macrophages
	Active inflammation with scarring	Atrophy with stromal collapse, but *no* scarring

Plasma membrane changes are among the first changes observed after injury, and are characterized by loss of surface specialization with disappearance of microvilli and swelling of cilia swell. Intercellular attachments break down, and the injured cell may detach from neighbors because of separation of gap junctions, dissolution of the terminal web of cytoskeletal filaments, and degradation of maculae densae and zonulae adherentes that are supposed to adhere the affected cell to its neighbors and to its surrounding stroma. Cytoplasmic "blebs" or outpouchings may form on the surfaces of injured cells. These may actually detach from the surface of the swollen cells, and float away into the interstitial space, to eventually lyse and release their contents. As swelling continues, the plasma membrane will ultimately rupture. Portions of partially degraded, insoluble membranes will eventually aggregate into laminated structures termed "myelin whorls."

Mitochondria are perhaps the most dramatically affected organelles during the process of oncotic necrosis, first undergoing a form of swelling termed "low amplitude" swelling, as ATP is progressively depleted. This change is typified by swelling of the outer compartment as water and electrolytes are lost

FIGURE 2.5   Morphologic changes associated with oncotic (A); and apoptotic (B); necrosis in a "prototypical" secretory epithelial cell. (C indicates a cilium, ER represents rough endoplasmic reticulum, G indicates Golgi apparatus, M signifies a mitochondrion, Ma represents a macrophage, MV indicates microvillous brush border, N signifies the nucleus, Ne indicates a neutrophil and S represents the smooth endoplasmic reticulum.) The changes represented in A: (1) Toxic stimulus affecting the entire population of cells; (2) Initial swelling with swelling of microvilli and cilia, low amplitude swelling of mitochondria (*), clumping of chromatin and dilation of endoplasmic reticulum cisternae;

(Continued on next page)

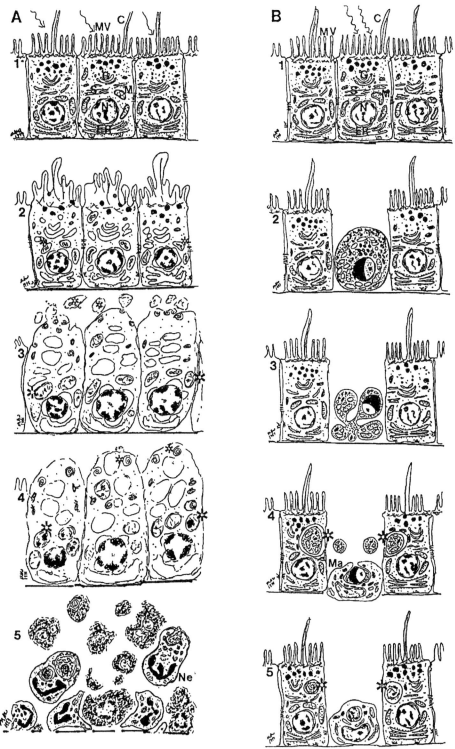

FIGURE 2.5   (3) Continued swelling of cells, with loss of microvilli and cilia, "blebbing" with loss of bits of superficial cytoplasm (*), high amplitude swelling of mitochondria (*), further clumping of chromatin, further dilation of endoplasmic reticulum cisternae and detachment of ribosomes; (4) Rupture of plasma membrane and internal membranes, including the nuclear membrane, further condensation of chromatin, myelin
whorls (*) and flocculent densities within burst mitochondria (*); (5) Condensation of cellular remnants and ingestion of cellular debris by neutrophils. The changes represented in B: (1) Reception of an apoptotic stimulus by a single cell in the population; (2) Abrupt condensation of cytoplasm, shrinkage and rounding of the cell with preservation of organellar morphology and condensation of chromatin into a homogenous cap at
one pole of the nucleus; (3) Budding of the cell into membrane bound bodies containing intact organelles; (4) Ingestion of the apoptotic bodies by
tissue macrophage and adjacent epithelial cells(*); and (5) Digestion of the apoptotic bodies by the macrophage and adjacent epithelial cells (*).

from the inner compartment and pass into the inter-membranous space. The result is early condensation of the inner compartment, but this does not necessarily indicate irreversible injury. Inclusions may form, either due to precipitation of small, very electron-dense calcium phosphate crystals as internal calcium homeostasis is lost, or larger, more electron-dense "flocculent densities," composed of partially degraded protein and membrane elements as they accumulate. On further severity or persistence of the injury, mitochondria will undergo high amplitude swelling, with massive swelling of both inner and outer compartments and large-scale accumulation of precipitated mineral and protein, a sure sign of impending doom for both the organelle and the cell. It is at the point where the inner compartment swells and the outer compartment swells to the point of bursting that the mitochondrial permeability transition, considered by many the biochemical "point of no return" in the process of cell death, occurs. The particles on the inner membrane responsible for ATP production become detached, preventing any further ATP production. The accumulation and precipitation of Ca^{2+} salts is especially prominent if some degree of blood flow is present. Soon after the permeability transition, the outer mitochondrial membrane ruptures. At this point, the swollen mitochondrion may resemble a partially double-walled vacuole containing bits of precipitated membrane.

As mitochondria are undergoing the changes that ultimately lead to the death of the cell, efflux of water into the cytosol continues, and there is dilation and fragmentation of the endoplasmic reticulum in an attempt to eliminate the excessive accumulation of water from the expanding cytosol. Endoplasmic reticulum often dilates so much that it forms water- and ion-filled, electron lucent cisternae which are observable as vacuoles by light microscopy. Eventually, ribosomes detach from the rough endoplasmic reticulum, and protein synthesis is no longer possible. After rupture of the cell membranes (both external and internal), protein degradation begins in earnest, especially after lysosomes begin to release their enzyme contents. At this point, the remnants of cytoplasm become denser and actually shrink. This process of swelling during the process of death, followed by condensation afterwards, is characteristic of oncotic necrosis and in marked contrast to that which occurs in apoptotic necrosis, where the opposite pattern is observed.

Nuclear changes associated with irreversible cell injury leading to oncotic necrosis are manifested morphologically mainly by changes in the morphology of chromatin. Nuclear chromatin clumps along the nuclear membrane and loses the distinction between euchromatin and heterochromatin, because of the drop in pH that typically occurs during the progression of oncotic necrosis. Initially, there may be shrinking and condensation of the nucleus and its chromatin as the swollen cytosol and enlarged perinuclear space impinge on the nucleus, creating the morphologic change known as pyknosis. Eventually the nuclear membrane will break down and rupture, as the nucleus itself swells with dispersion of aggregated bits of chromatin attached to the fragmented membranes. This produces the changes characteristic of karyorhexis. Eventually the entire mass of chromatin, nucleoplasm, and nuclear membrane become sufficiently degraded to fade from view, a morphologic change termed karyolysis.

After the cell is "dead" functionally, lysosomes begin to swell and release enzymes into the cytosol. "Autolysis," as traditionally described, begins at this point. Lysosomal membranes are relatively resistant to damage and degradation, and in most cases of toxic injury release their contents late in the process. The cases where activation of lysosomes is the primary trigger in oncotic necrosis are relatively few, for example in copper toxicity, in which the large amounts of copper that accumulate in lysosomes eventually cause their rupture, with release of enzymes and highly-oxidative forms of copper into the cell. Whatever the situation, after release of lysosomal enzymes, uncontrolled degradation of the cell begins. It is at this point that the cell usually can be identified as "necrotic" by light microscopy.

Once the point of no return in the process of oncotic necrosis has occurred, and release of lysosomal enzymes has occurred, degradation of cell components becomes widespread, and the lesion that is easily recognized as "necrosis" becomes manifest via the light microscope. The morphologic changes are relatively stereotypical, although there are variations between tissues, due to biochemical, functional, and morphologic peculiarities. In most cases, the cytoplasm becomes hypereosinophilic and hyalinized, due to degradation of proteins, releasing reactive groups that can interact with eosin, and due to degradation of normally basophilic ribosomal RNA. Occasionally, eosinophilic or basophilic cytoplasmic granules, representing swollen or mineralized mitochondria, respectively, may be observed. As degradation processes continue, the cytoplasm becomes "moth-eaten" and fragmented. In some tissues, especially where there is a large flux of calcium in and out of the tissue, there may be a very marked degree of calcification. These tissues may be replete with basophilic crystals, giving the tissue a bluish, stippled, fragmented, or even crystalline appearance. As mentioned above, there are nuclear changes that are characteristic of oncotic necrosis—pyknosis, karyorhexis, or karyolysis (Figure 2.6). These changes do not necessarily follow in sequence, and one or all can be observed in a necrotic tissue. The response of surrounding tissues to cells that have undergone oncotic necrosis will be described below.

Gross changes associated with oncotic necrosis are variable and very much depend on the tissue in which the injury occurs, the etiology of the injury, and the response of surrounding tissues. In some cases, affected tissue may be paler than surrounding tissue and somewhat reduced in volume, in particular if blood flow to the affected area has been compromised or cut off completely. If blood supply is still intact or has been restored after the lethal insult, the tissue may be swollen, engorged with blood, darker than normal and soft. On occasion, there is a central pale area surrounded by a zone of red tissue—a vascular response to the dead tissue. The gross and histologic manifestations of oncotic necrosis have been classified into several categories in the past, three of which will be briefly described. With "coagulation necrosis," the general structural organization of the tissue is still discernible, although specific details are lost. Histologically, "shadows" of dead cells can be ascertained. This type of change is most often observed when blood supply is cut off, and inflammatory cells have not had a chance to move in and clean up the dead cells, but it may also be seen in tissues where cells contain few lysosomes and the autodegradation

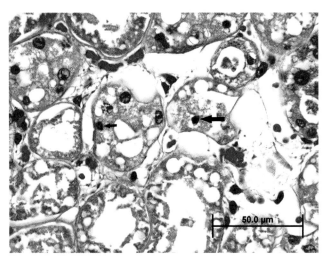

FIGURE 2.6 Oncotic necrosis. Nuclear and cytoplasmic changes in renal tubular epithelium from a cat with lily toxicosis. The entire tubular profile is affected, with loss of cellular detail and fragmentation of cytoplasm. Nuclear changes consistent with pyknosis (large arrow), karyorhexis (small arrow) and karyolysis are present. Hematoxylin and eosin stain.

of dead cells proceeds at a slow pace. Liquefaction necrosis is more often seen in cases where infectious rather than toxic agents have caused the injury. Often there is a severe acute inflammatory response, with large numbers of neutrophils. The neutrophils spill out their degradative enzymes into the affected tissues, creating a lesion that is soft and liquefied. Some tissues, particularly the central nervous system, undergo liquefactive necrosis as a matter of course whenever there is large-scale oncotic necrosis, leading to resultant softening or malacia. Caseous necrosis is confined almost entirely to situations where persistent infectious agents or foreign material are involved. In this case, the necrotic tissue that is whitish, pale yellow or pale green, and pasty.

Apoptotic Necrosis

Apoptotic necrosis is a common type of cell death that has had a variety of names in the past, including "single cell necrosis," "programmed cell death," "cell suicide," "necrobiosis," and "apoptosis," to name just a few. Morphologically, apoptotic necrosis is usually much harder to detect than oncotic necrosis, due its rapid progression once triggered and the rapid disposition of the dead cells via ingestion by adjacent cells or resident macrophages. In addition, only small numbers of cells at any one time undergo this process in most situations. The causes and biochemical events leading to this very orderly and highly regulated form of cell death have been the focus of intense research in the past decade and a half.

Ultrastructurally, apoptotic necrosis has features that are quite distinct from oncotic necrosis (Figure 2.5B). Initial dilation of the endoplasmic reticulum may be observed, but this is indicative of active pumping of ions and water into the cisternae as a prelude to condensation of the cytoplasm. As the cytosol becomes denser and organelles cluster closer together, "zeiosis" or budding off of portions of the cell into spherical membrane-bound fragments frequently occurs. It must be emphasized that the integrity of the plasma membrane is preserved during this process, even after dispersal of the cell fragments. The organelles within the rounded "apoptotic bodies" are well preserved and may even be functional. Most strikingly there is preservation of mitochondrial morphology, and even maintenance of ribosomal attachment to the rough endoplasmic reticulum. Nuclear changes unique to apoptotic necrosis can occur prior to, during, or after the cytoplasmic changes. These changes are characterized by preservation of the nuclear envelope, segregation of the nucleolus from chromatin, and the uniform

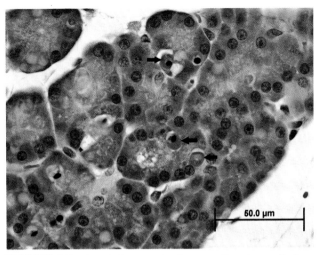

FIGURE 2.7   Apoptotic necrosis of pancreatic acinar cells from a Fischer 344 rat twelve hours after exposure to the phytochemical crambene. Apoptotic bodies (arrows) are present in several acini. Hematoxylin and eosin stain.

condensation of chromatin into crescents or "caps" along the intact nuclear envelope. The nucleus may also undergo zeiosis. It is only after ingestion by adjacent tissue cells or resident macrophages that changes more typical of oncotic necrosis in the affected cells are observed. Thus, in contrast to oncotic necrosis, condensation rather than swelling is the key feature during the death process, followed by swelling only after the apoptotic bodies have been ingested.

When actually observed histologically (Figure 2.7), the changes associated with apoptotic necrosis are unique. The most obvious change is a "rounding-up," shrinkage, and fragmentation of scattered individual cells, rather than loss of whole fields of cells. The rounded-up cells or their fragments are shrunken and condensed, with hyperbasophilia or hypereosinophilia. The bodies are uniformly round in profile and have clearly defined borders. The bodies are almost always surrounded by a clear space or "halo," which in most cases represents a phagocytic vacuole within an adjacent tissue cell or macrophage that has ingested the apoptotic body. Dense condensation of chromatin within an intact nuclear membrane is prominent, with the chromatin forming a "cap" or "crescent" along one edge of the nuclear envelope. The number of cells undergoing apoptotic necrosis observed at any one time in a tissue is relatively low, and only 1–2% of the total cell population may have the characteristic apoptotic morphology, even in a tissue in which widespread and massive apoptotic necrosis is occurring. The rapidity of formation and the rapid degradation of the bodies by adjacent cells or phagocytes are major factors behind the low number of identifiable apoptotic bodies in a histologic section.

Although apoptotic necrosis can be triggered by a huge variety of stimuli, many of them having nothing to do with toxic injury directly, it should be remembered that mild toxic injury, insufficient to lead outright to oncotic necrosis, can nevertheless trigger apoptotic necrosis. This is especially true for toxic insults that injure the genome such that DNA repair systems are overwhelmed, triggering the *p53*-related pathways to initiate the cell death process. It should also be emphasized that mild injury not involving the genome can trigger apoptotic necrosis in cells that are capable of utilizing this pathway, and that apoptotic necrosis is, in some respects, a "preferred" way for a cell to die.

Some investigators have seen sufficient variability in the morphologic manifestations of apoptotic necrosis to further subdivide it into at least two types, based on differences in the sequence of cytosolic and nuclear changes that occur among various cell types. "Type I" apoptotic necrosis, also known as "heterophagic" or "classic" apoptosis, is most commonly seen in cell types with high mitotic activity or the potential for high mitotic activity. In this form, nuclear condensation of chromatin is an early event, and ingestion by resident tissue macrophages a prominent feature. Cells undergoing this type of death also tend to have low lysosomal content, making the apoptotic fragments more stable. In "Type II" apoptosis, condensation of chromatin is often considerably delayed, sometimes until after fragmentation of the entire cell has occurred. Vacuolation can be prominent and internal lysosomal release of enzymes often begins before fragmentation has begun, even though external membrane integrity is preserved. Phagocytosis of the apoptotic fragments by adjacent tissue cells rather than tissue macrophages is a prominent feature of this type.

Apoptotic necrosis of thymocytes is considered to be typical of the Type I form, whereas apoptotic necrosis in the renal tubules caused by okadaic acid is typical of the Type II form of apoptotic necrosis. A mixture of the two types, however, has also been observed, for example in the prostate gland undergoing involution after castration.

It must also be stated that both types of cell death—oncotic and apoptotic—can and do occur simultaneously in an injured tissue, with those cells insufficiently injured to lose control of their osmoregulatory apparatus, energy production or protein synthetic machinery going down the path of orderly, controlled cell death, rather than succumbing to the unregulated and willy-nilly process that typifies oncotic necrosis. More severely injured neighbors in the lesion may not have that option, and die by the oncotic necrosis. Therefore, a combination of both processes may be observed in many cases of toxic cell injury if one looks closely.

Sequelae to Irreversible Cell Injury

The clinico-pathological consequences of cell injury or death are often evident before the animal dies, for cytoplasmic blebs can break off an injured cell and release cytoplasmic enzymes into the interstitial space to eventually find their way into the plasma. A lethally injured cell will also spill its contents into tissue fluids. One may then be able to localize the site where tissue injury may be occurring, based on the type of enzyme or constituent released. In general, free cytosolic enzymes will leak out first from an injured cell, followed by mitochondrial membrane-bound and ultimately lysosomal enzymes, as cell injury becomes progressively more severe. In addition, isoenzymes specific for certain tissues can also be measured to determine the site of injury.

Sequelae to Oncotic Necrosis

An inflammatory response of some sort is an almost universal sequela to oncotic necrosis, although the severity and extent of the injury in a particularly vital tissue may cause death of the affected individual before the response becomes evident. Membrane fragments and partially degraded cellular contents released when the dying cells burst are in large part responsible for eliciting the inflammatory reaction. Lipid fragments released from damaged membranes are especially attractive to neutrophils and macrophages. Endothelial cells in the vicinity of the dying cells, if they themselves are injured or activated by contact with the spilled cellular contents, also release soluble mediators of inflammation, such as interleukin-1. Some lethally-injured cells have the capability of making their own mediators, such as leukotrienes, which then act as chemoattractants for neutrophils. The initial influx of inflammatory cells into an area where there is oncotic necrosis is generally neutrophilic at first, with macrophages becoming prominent later, usually days later. It is the influx of neutrophils that is important from a pathophysiologic viewpoint, since neutrophils are often indiscriminate in the manner in which they scavenge cellular debris and dying cells, often releasing their degradative

enzymes into the extracellular matrix, damaging stroma as well as degrading dead or dying cells. Neutrophils also produce mediators that attract more neutrophils and macrophages to the site of injury.

Damage caused to the supporting stroma of an injured tissue by neutrophils leads to replacement of that tissue by non-functional fibrous scar tissue (Figure 2.8). The scar tissue serves as a "filler" to replace the missing supportive tissues. Fibrous scar tissue, composed predominantly of Type I collagen with little elastin, laminin, Type IV collagen, or other types of stromal proteins that maintain parenchymal tissue cells in proper arrangement, is a poor environment in which to support the growth of new parenchymal tissues. Thus, parenchymal regeneration is frequently incomplete, or even non-existent, when scarring occurs. In general, the amount of scar tissue produced is proportional not only to the initial amount of damage by the toxicant to the parenchyma, but also to a large extent by the degree of inflammation elicited in response to the injury.

There are a variety of factors that determine the degree of inflammation that occurs after toxic injury. The type of tissue affected may predispose it to an exuberant influx of neutrophils. Exocrine pancreas, with its rich supply of proteases, stimulates a dramatic influx of neutrophils when undergoing oncotic necrosis. This in turn causes even more damage, often converting a mild lesion into a fulminating one. Another factor is the extent of damage caused by the toxic insult. A renal infarct, with its extensive loss of

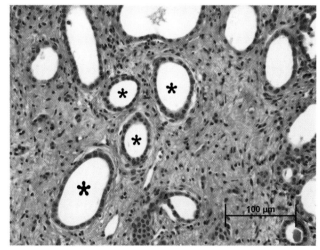

FIGURE 2.8 Extensive fibrosis in the kidney following a bout of severe widespread oncotic necrosis. Tubules (*) are lined by flattened, incompletely-differentiated tubular epithelium that is trapped within the scar tissue. Hematoxylin and eosin stain.

parenchymal tissue, will elicit a more intense inflammatory response than a localized lesion on only part of a nephron. The degree of blood flow to the injured tissue has an important impact on the degree of inflammation. Intact blood flow into an area of oncotic necrosis will lead to a greater influx of inflammatory cells than an ischemic lesion. The extent of damage to supporting stroma by the toxic insult will also have an impact on the degree of inflammation. Damage to epithelium that leaves the basement membrane and underlying stromal tissue intact—for example, a shallow erosive lesion that does not fully penetrate the basement membrane—will elicit far less inflammation than an ulcerative insult that penetrates the basement membrane and damages the underlying stroma. Finally, the response of adjacent cells, especially if these cells are part of the fixed macrophage system, will have a substantial effect on the degree of inflammation that occurs after oncotic necrosis. Activation of Küpffer cells in the liver after a toxic insult to hepatocytes causes much more inflammation and subsequent damage than situations where these cells remain quiescent.

Sequelae to Apoptosis

Perhaps the most distinguishing feature of the sequelae to apoptotic necrosis is the lack of a classic inflammatory response. In uncomplicated apoptotic necrosis, no biologically active substances chemoattractive to neutrophils are generated. Thus, neutrophils are not observed, even when widespread apoptosis is present. There are changes, however, in the membranes of the apoptotic bodies that make them quite attractive to adjacent cells and macrophages. Phosphatidyl serine on the outer membrane of an apoptotic body, everted from the inner side of the cell membrane during the cytoskeletal derangement that occurs during the process of zeiosis, is especially attractive to macrophages, as are the "immature" glycans that are exposed on the surface of an apoptotic cell. Another sequela is that release of intracellular enzymes into surrounding tissue fluids or into the bloodstream is generally minimal and insufficient to trigger an endothelial reaction, meaning that the vascular "gate" of inflammation remains closed.

As might be expected, atrophy is a frequent sequela to apoptosis (Figure 2.9). Although this may be highly unfavorable in the short-term, due to loss of function, the atrophied tissue has the potential to completely regenerate if the apoptotic stimulus is removed. This is because the supporting stroma is intact and unaffected by lytic enzymes from neutrophils and other activated inflammatory cells. The preservation of supporting

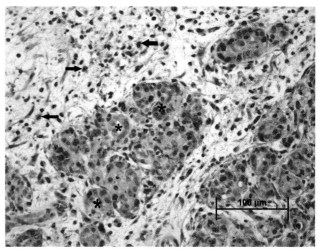

FIGURE 2.9 Atrophy without scarring in the exocrine pancreas of a Fischer 344 rat three days after exposure to the phytochemical crambene. There is extensive loss of acinar cells and atrophy of remaining acinar cells (*), with increased interstitial space, but no inflammation or deposition of collagen. Note the prominence of tissue macrophages (arrows) which are enlarged due to ingestion of apoptotic bodies.

stroma allows for complete regeneration of the tissue if the apoptotic stimulus is removed and trophic stimuli generated. Furthermore, scarring does not take place, and therefore there is no inhibition to regeneration by bands of dense fibrous scar tissue. Finally, since apoptosis affects individual cells, and generally does not completely eliminate every single cell in a tissue, there are usually healthy, undamaged stem cells nearby that can replace the lost cells if the apoptotic stimulus is removed. However, in so-called "permanent" cell populations, where mitosis is no longer an option (e.g., neurons, and retinal rods and cones), apoptotic necrosis may nevertheless result in permanent loss of function.

Hyperplasia

Hyperplasia can be elicited by a variety of means, both physiologic and pathologic, and its occurrence can serve to create a favorable environment for initiated cells to "fix" genetic mutations that can lead to cancer. Hyperplasia in this context will be discussed later in this chapter. In the context of cell injury, however, compensatory hyperplasia can be an important and visible response to cell injury, both reversible and irreversible. This type of hyperplasia occurs when a portion of an organ or tissue is removed or damaged, and the remaining portion undergoes hyperplasia to compensate for the loss and to regenerate the lost tissue. Hyperplasia of this sort can only occur in labile or stable cell populations with the capacity to undergo mitosis. Tissues such as liver or bone marrow are typical examples of tissues that readily undergo such reparative process. The hyperplastic response may result in resolution of the lesion if conditions are appropriate for orderly regeneration—e.g., intact stromal support, adequate vascular supply, and a suitable milieu of hormones or growth factors. However, hyperplasia may also be inappropriately exuberant, unorganized, or even harmful if these factors are not present. Furthermore, the increase in mitotic activity increases the chances that genetic alterations that may have occurred during the toxic insult may propagate those changes within a new cell population.

Metaplasia

Metaplasia, the reversible substitution of one type of fully-differentiated cell for another type within a given tissue can also be a sequela to cell injury under some conditions. In relation to cell injury, metaplasia occurs when there is abnormal stimulation of tissue growth, generally because of faulty wound healing from persistent toxic insult or constant mechanical disruption of the injured area. The metaplastic cells have a selective advantage over normal parenchymal cells in the area under the pressure of persistent toxic insult, but function of the affected tissue will be impaired because the original population of specialized cells has been replaced by less specialized cells. As with hyperplasia, metaplasia can predispose a tissue to neoplastic changes, since alternative biochemical pathways, inactive in the original cell population, are now expressed, possibly predisposing the tissue to further preneoplastic changes if oncogenes happen to be in those pathways.

CONCLUDING COMMENTS

The descriptive information provided in the preceding paragraphs is in many ways "generic" in nature, portraying events as they should occur in all cells that are injured, regardless of the insult that initiated the injury. It is a synopsis of numerous *in vivo* and *in vitro* observations made in countless studies over a large span of years. Yet, even though the morphologic manifestations of cell injury and death are in many ways stereotypical, especially at the ultrastructural level, there are nevertheless many minor (and often major) variations that can occur at all levels— ultrastructurally, histologically and grossly—which

make each situation in which cell injury occurs unique. This is due to a seemingly endless variety of factors that modify or influence the response of the injured cell. Factors external to the cell, such as blood flow (or lack thereof) to the affected tissue, the impact of injury to other organ systems, the nature of the toxicant itself, absorption and distribution of the toxicant, the rate of metabolism and excretion of the toxicant, the innate inflammatory and immune response of the organism as a whole, and a large number of other factors all have an impact on the reaction of the cell to a specific injury and, conversely, the reaction of the rest of the organism to the injured cell. Factors within the cell itself are also key in determining the exact morphologic pattern that will become manifest when the cell is injured or killed. Factors such as the degree of specialization, the function of the cell in the body, the dependence of the cell on oxidative phosphorylation, the degree of membrane turnover, and many, many others discussed here and elsewhere, also contribute to the morphologic pattern of injury that is ultimately viewed and interpreted by the pathologist. The succeeding chapters in this book will deal with many of these factors and situations, from the standpoint of peculiarities unique to each organ system and from the aspect of specific groups of toxicants and their mechanisms of causing injury.

SECTION II CHEMICAL CARCINOGENESIS

OVERVIEW

The purpose of this portion of the chapter is to describe the basic features of a form of toxic cell injury that results not in cell death and its sequelae, but which instead results in disturbed cell growth, ultimately leading to cancer. In many ways, the genesis of cancer—the unregulated, abnormal and autonomous growth of a genetically altered cell population—is initially an adaptive response to injury to the genome. This simplistic viewpoint, however, does not adequately address the highly complex multi-step changes that must occur before a neoplasm develops. Those changes, and the mechanisms thereof, will be discussed briefly below. In this section the terminology associated with carcinogenesis, including nomenclature of neoplasms and other relevant pathology terms, will also be discussed, as will mechanisms and principles currently believed to provide a basis for understanding the processes of chemical carcinogenesis.

In particular, emphasis will be placed on critical molecular and genetic determinants associated with carcinogenesis and modes of action of chemical carcinogens. Finally, several *in vivo* tests for assessing chemical carcinogenesis will be described.

It is estimated that viruses are the cause of 5% of human cancers, 5% are caused by radiation, and the remaining 90% are caused by chemicals. Of the 90% caused by chemicals, tobacco products cause an estimated 30%, the rest are caused by diet, lifestyle, and environmental carcinogens. The importance of chemical products in the etiology of cancer is reflected in the fact that up to 8% of all human cancers are of occupational origin, induced by chemicals known as carcinogens.

The term "carcinogen" is generic. Under specific experimental conditions, where dose and temporal sequence of dosing can be controlled, a given agent may behave as a complete carcinogen or as an incomplete carcinogen. The latter category includes tumor initiators, tumor promoters, and co-carcinogens. However, even complete carcinogens may be without apparent effect when given at sufficiently low doses. Carcinogenesis may be considered a form of toxicity in which cells achieve a different steady state from normal, and do not respond normally to homeostatic mechanisms regulating their growth and differentiation. The constitutive features of cancer include an ability to invade, an ability to metastasize, and autonomous growth. The process of carcinogenesis is usually prolonged, requiring one-third to two-thirds of the lifespan of the affected individual to develop. While perturbations of cellular DNA are essential to carcinogenesis, such perturbations alone are not sufficient to bring about cancer in all cases. In some experimental situations, a few minutes of exposure to a carcinogen are enough to ultimately produce cancer; in other situations—even using the same carcinogen, but at a lower dose—cancer will not result unless there is additional chemical exposure. Simultaneous administration of another agent with a carcinogen may enhance, diminish, or block the carcinogenic process, depending on the agents employed.

Several phenomenological events have been documented during the process of carcinogenesis. To be effective as an initiator of carcinogenesis in the adult, a carcinogen must generally be mitogenic or cytotoxic; typically, on initial exposure, cell death and restorative hyperplasia is induced. This has been clearly shown in the rodent liver. Thus, cell death may play a key role as a rate-limiting step in the initiation of cancer in some tissues. Other carcinogens appear to facilitate the growth of neoplasms by inducing immune suppression in the host. In addition, several environmental, hormonal, and dietary factors are known to affect the progression of transformed cells into malignant neoplasms. Loss of differentiation or changes in patterns of differentiation and gene expression are additional changes that are documented in tissues undergoing neoplastic transformation. Finally, chronological histopathologic study of chemically-induced lesions repeatedly shows that many neoplasms progress from hyperplasia to benign neoplasia, and ultimately to malignant neoplasia. Thus, multiple stages in the evolution of proliferative lesions appear to accompany the carcinogenic process. These observations provide strong empirical evidence that cancer is a multi-step process, and that a cascade of critical events is necessary for malignancy to develop.

NOMENCLATURE OF NEOPLASMS

Most neoplasms are classified histogenetically (cell type of origin) and behaviorally (benign or malignant). The "name" of the neoplasm is based on these categories (Table 2.2). Thus, a benign epithelial neoplasm originating from a gland would have the prefix "adeno-," designating glandular origin, and the suffix "-oma," designating it as benign. The adenoma might be further qualified by a specific tissue of origin, for example, hepatocellular adenoma, pituitary adenoma, or renal tubular adenoma. If this same type of neoplasm has morphologic features resembling finger-like or warty projections, it may be called a papillary adenoma; if it contains cystic spaces, a cystadenoma; and if it contains both, a papillary cystadenoma. Benign mesenchymal neoplasms also utilize the suffix "-oma" in their name, for example, fibroma, meningioma, or hemangioma.

Malignant epithelial neoplasms are generally named carcinomas, and qualified by histogenetic origin. Thus, epidermal carcinomas arise in superficial layers of skin. If they are composed primarily of squamous cells, they will be called squamous cell carcinomas. If they consist mostly of basal cells, they will be called basal cell carcinomas. Malignant mesenchymal neoplasms are called sarcomas, for example fibrosarcoma, osteosarcoma, or leiomyosarcoma.

As with all general rules, there are exceptions. Examples are thymoma, lymphoma, and melanoma. These neoplasms are generally regarded as malignant, despite their benign appearing name. In fact, preferred names for these neoplasms are malignant thymoma, lymphosarcoma, and malignant melanoma. Some neoplasms are composed of mixtures of cells, and are named accordingly, for example, fibroadenoma, adenosquamous carcinoma, or carcinosarcoma.

TABLE 2.2 Selected taxonomy of neoplasms

Tissue	Benign neoplasia[a]	Malignant neoplasia[b]
Epithelium		
Squamous	Squamous cell papilloma	Squamous cell carcinoma
Transitional	Transitional cell papilloma	Transitional cell carcinoma
Glandular	(Tissue of origin) Adenoma	(Tissue of origin) Adenocarcinoma
Liver cell	Hepatocellular adenoma (Hepatoma)	Hepatocellular carcinoma
Islet cell	Islet cell adenoma	Islet cell carcinoma
Connective tissue		
Adult fibrous	Fibroma	Fibrosarcoma
Embryonic fibrous	Myxoma	Myxosarcoma
Cartilage	Chondroma	Chondrosarcoma
Bone	Osteoma	Osteosarcoma
Fat	Lipoma	Liposarcoma
Muscle		
Smooth muscle	Leiomyoma	Leiomyosarcoma
Skeletal muscle	Rhabdomyoma	Rhabdomyosarcoma
Cardiac muscle	Rhabdomyoma	Rhabdomyosarcoma
Endothelium		
Lymph vessels	Lymphangioma	Lymphangiosarcoma
Blood vessels	Hemangioma	Hemagiosarcoma
Lymphoreticular		
Thymus	(not recognized)	Thymoma
Lymph nodes	(not recognized)	Lymphoma/lymphosarcoma
Hematopoietic		Leukemia
Bone marrow	(not recognized)	Granulocytic
		Monocytic
		Erythroleukemia
Neural tissue		
Nerve sheath	Neurolemmoma	Neurogenic sarcoma
Oligodendrocytes	(Oligodendro)glioma	Malignant (Oligodendro)glioma
Astrocytes	Astrocytoma	Malignant astrocytoma
Embryonic cells	(not recognized)	Neuroblastoma

[a] "-oma," benign neoplasm

[b] "Sarcoma," malignant neoplasm of mesenchymal origin; "Carcinoma," malignant neoplasm of epithelial origin

SPECTRUM OF PROLIFERATIVE LESIONS

Quantitative Cell Proliferation (Hyperplasia)

Hyperplasia is characterized by an absolute increase in the number of cells per unit of tissue. It may be diffuse or nodular, and is often accompanied by hypertrophy. Hyperplasia is typically nonprogressive; that is, it is limited in amount and terminates when the stimulus that evoked it has ceased. Different cell types have varying capacities to undergo hyperplasia. Hyperplasia is often classified to provide a basis for appreciating proximate underlying causes.

Physiological Hyperplasia

Physiological hyperplasia is a normal process occurring during development and maturation, for example, bone growth, lymphoid tissue development, or liver growth. Hormonal hyperplasia is brought about by the influence of hormones on specific target tissues, such as the mammary gland in response to prolactin, or the thyroid gland in response to secretion of thyrotrophic hormone by the pituitary gland. Physiological adaptive hyperplasia, which may also be called compensatory, regenerative, or reparative hyperplasia, represents an attempt to repair an injury or disease that has resulting in loss of functional tissue (see Section I above). Tissues undergoing adaptive hyperplasia do not exhibit excessive uncoordinated growth; the proliferative response ceases when the stimulus is removed, or the functional integrity of the tissue has been restored.

Physiological adaptive hyperplasia may play an important role in the pathogenesis of neoplasia; cells undergoing rapid cell division are at greater risk of sustaining a permanent genetic alteration that may result in the initiation or progression of carcinogenesis. Clonal expansion of latent cancer cells may also occur as a result of regenerative or reparative proliferation.

Pathological Hyperplasia

In pathological hyperplasia there are significant abnormalities in organization and cytomorphology. The causes of pathological hyperplasia may be similar to those producing physiological hyperplasia; however, in pathological hyperplasia, a change in intrinsic cell control produces a subpopulation of cells that is less subject to normal tissue regulatory mechanisms. Many forms of pathological hyperplasia result from excessive hormonal stimulation of target cells—for example, adenomatous hyperplasia of the endometrium.

In some instances, pathological hyperplasia may progress to neoplasia. For example, hepatocellular adenoma or carcinoma is closely related to compensatory hyperplasia of hepatic parenchymal cells seen in cirrhotic livers of chronic alcoholics. However, in humans and undoubtedly in animals, the majority of neoplasms develop without any previous reparative proliferation or hyperplasia of the tissues from which they arise. The coexistence of cell repair or hyperplasia with neoplasia, either in space or time, is not proof of a cause and effect relationship between the two.

Qualitative Cell Proliferation

Qualitative changes, such as metaplasia and anaplasia, can occur in hyperplastic cells and represent one of the hallmarks of pathological hyperplasia. However, qualitative changes in the phenotype, or in the association and organization of groups of cells, can also occur in the absence of clear-cut evidence of hyperplasia.

Metaplasia

Metaplasia is the reversible substitution of one type of fully differentiated cell for another within a given tissue; it is seen most commonly in epithelial tissues. For example, squamous metaplasia occurring in an area normally populated by ciliated respiratory epithelium represents a situation in which fully differentiated squamous cells have replaced the ciliated cells.

Metaplastic cells originate from cells capable of undergoing cell division. We generally consider metaplastic cells to originate from "reserve cells" or from basal cells. The causes and regulatory mechanisms associated with metaplasia are unknown. Neoplastic transformation occasionally occurs at a site of metaplasia.

Dysplasia

Abnormal formation or dysplasia of a tissue refers to alteration in its shape, size, and organization. Dysplasia usually affects epithelium, and is generally reversible. This form of qualitative cellular proliferation lacks normal cell-to-cell relationships and orientations. In epithelial tissues, this is manifested as disruption of normal cell layering. Dysplastic cells exhibit nuclear and cytological pleomorphism and increased mitotic activity. Dysplasia may be associated with chronic irritation, may occur together with metaplasia, and is occasionally associated with neoplastic transformation.

Anaplasia

Anaplasia is a qualitative alteration of differentiation. Anaplastic cells are typically poorly differentiated or undifferentiated, and exhibit advanced cellular pleomorphism. In fact, anaplasia and pleomorphism are sometimes incorrectly used as synonyms. Pleomorphism refers to variation in size and shape of cells. Several sizes and shapes of cells are usually present in anaplastic tissue, and true giant cells sometimes form. Anaplastic cells generally have hyperchromatic nuclei, prominent nucleoli, and a nucleus to cytoplasm size ratio that approaches 1:1. There is increased mitotic activity (sometimes with formation of abnormal mitotic figures), loss of cell orientation, and lack of normal organization in the anaplastic tissue. Neoplasms, especially malignant neoplasms, are frequently composed of cells that are pleomorphic and anaplastic. In nonneoplastic tissue, anaplasia may represent the borderline between dysplasia and neoplasia.

Preneoplasia

Preneoplastic lesions are usually indicative of exposure to a carcinogen. Patients or animals with preneoplastic lesions are at increased risk of developing a neoplasm at the tissue site at which preneoplasia is present. Preneoplastic lesions themselves are believed to progress to neoplasia, although unequivocal proof of this is difficult to document. Examples of preneoplasia from human medicine include leukoplakia of the oral cavity or vulva, senile keratosis, and xeroderma pigmentosum. Numerous putative preneoplastic lesions have been identified in laboratory animals, especially in animal models used to study the process of chemical carcinogenesis.

In experimental studies of liver neoplasia using rats exposed to potent hepatocarcinogens, the initial changes detected in liver tissue are foci of cellular alteration. These foci consist of nests or islands of hyperplastic and/or hypertrophic hepatocytes that differ phenotypically from adjacent normal parenchyma. Eventually, the rats develop hepatocellular neoplasms. There are several phenotypically distinct foci of cellular alteration, and the ultimate neoplasms may or may not resemble the foci phenotypically. Because of their consistent production by known hepatocarcinogens, and their temporal relationship with neoplasia, foci of cellular alteration are operationally regarded as preneoplastic lesions.

Neoplastic Cell Proliferation

Benign comes from the Latin word "benignus," and means innocuous. A benign neoplasm is localized and its growth is by expansion, hence it may compress

TABLE 2.3   Comparative features of benign and malignant neoplasms

	Benign	Malignant
General effect on host	Little, usually do not cause death	Almost always kill the host if untreated
Rate of growth	Slow; may stop or regress	More rapid (but slower than "repair" tissue); autonomous; never stop growing or regress
Histologic features	Encapsulated; remain localized at primary site	Infiltrative or invasive into surrounding tissues; metastasize at some point
Mode of growth	Usually grow by expansion, displacing surrounding normal tissue	Invasive; destroy and replace surrounding tissue
Metastasis	Do not metastasize	Most metastasize
Architecture	Encapsulated; have complex stroma and adequate blood supply	Not encapsulated; usually poorly developed stroma; may be necrotic at center
Damage to host	Most without lethal significance	Always ultimately lethal unless removed or destroyed *in situ*
Injury to host	Usually negligible, but may become very large and compress or obstruct vital tissue	Can kill host directly by destruction of vital tissue
Radiation sensitivity	Radiation sensitivity near that of normal parent tissue	Radiation sensitivity increases in rough proportion to malignancy; often treated with radiation
Behavior in tissue	Cells are cohesive and inhibited by mutual contact	Cells do not cohere; frequently not inhibited by mutual contact
Resemblance to normal tissue	Cells and architecture resemble tissue of origin	Cells atypical and pleomorphic; disorganized with bizarre architecture
Mitotic figures	Mitotic figures are rare and normal	Mitotic figures may be numerous and abnormal in polarity and configuration
Shape of nucleus	Normal and regular; usual staining affinity	Irregular; nucleus frequently hyperchromatic
Size of nucleus	Normal; ratio of nucleus to cytoplasm near normal	Frequently large; nucleus-to-cytoplasmic ratio increased
Nucleolus	Not conspicuous	Hyperchromatic and larger than normal

adjacent normal tissues. Benign neoplasms ordinarily grow very slowly, and they are not life threatening unless they interfere with normal function of the organ in which they are located. Characteristic features of benign neoplasia are listed in Table 2.2. Controversy regarding the significance of benign neoplasia with respect to development of malignancy is similar to that associated with preneoplastic lesions. In chemical carcinogenicity tests using rodents, carcinogens frequently produce both benign and malignant neoplasms, and morphologic evidence exists that the benign lesions progress to malignancy in some instances.

Malignant comes from the Latin word "malignus," and means malicious. Malignant neoplasms grow rapidly, and are locally invasive. Areas of necrosis seen in some malignant neoplasms presumably result when growth is so rapid that the neoplastic tissue outgrows the existing blood supply. Malignant growth is disorganized, and as such may spread by extension into adjacent organs or by metastasis to distant sites via the blood and lymphatic systems. Characteristics of benign versus malignant neoplasms are listed in Table 2.3.

Diagnostic Distinction between Preneoplasia, Benign Neoplasia, and Malignant Neoplasia

Given the presence of specific hallmarks of malignancy (e.g., anaplasia, local invasiveness, and metastasis), there is usually little difficulty in obtaining consistent and concordant agreement among pathologists regarding diagnosis of malignant neoplasms. More serious problems arise with benign proliferative lesions. Small lesions are especially difficult, because very little tissue mass is available for examination in a search for characteristic features that form the basis for diagnosis. A circular lesion consisting of 75 to 100 cells may be a preneoplastic change or, alternatively, a benign or a malignant neoplasm that has just started to grow. At this stage, even a true malignant neoplasm may not demonstrate features of local invasiveness. The name given to such a lesion becomes largely a matter of judgement by the pathologist.

Another problem associated with evaluation of proliferative lesions, particularly in rodent chemical carcinogenicity studies, is the consistent categorization of lesions, especially those that have some features of both benign and malignant neoplasia. Even with well-defined diagnostic criteria, specific lesions are always found that fall between two adjacent diagnostic categories. There is no easy resolution to this problem. Communicating such problems to the other scientists and administrators who use such carcinogenicity data is always difficult. In situations where

the borderline between hyperplasia and neoplasia is not distinct, a consistently applied size criterion may be helpful. However, it should be used as a last resort in categorizing a given proliferative lesion, and not as a convenience.

STEPS IN THE NEOPLASTIC PROCESS

Multi-step models of carcinogenesis have proven useful for defining events in the neoplastic process; they form the cornerstone for current hypotheses of the biological mechanisms of carcinogenesis. Oncology research, however, has generated a lexicon that may cause confusion. Practical and generally accepted definitions of commonly used terms are presented in Table 2.3.

Initiation

During the initiation phase a normal cell undergoes an irreversible genetic change, characterized by an intrinsic capacity for autonomous growth. This capacity for autonomous growth remains latent for weeks, months, or years, during which time the initiated cell may be phenotypically indistinguishable from other parenchymal cells in that tissue. Without exception, initiation implies alteration of cellular DNA at one or more sites in the genome. Such alteration by definition is a mutational event that is hereditary.

Metabolic activation of a carcinogen to its chemically reactive products, and their subsequent reaction with cellular targets (e.g., DNA bases), occurs within a few hours of exposure. Most tissues have the ability to repair this damage over a period of days or weeks. Currently accepted dogma suggests that chemically damaged DNA, if not first repaired by normal cellular processes, is converted to a stable biological lesion (mutation, chromosomal rearrangement, and so forth) during DNA replication. Thus, if a round of cell replication occurs before the DNA damage is repaired, the lesion in the DNA is said to be "fixed." This phenomenon may explain the high frequency of neoplasms in proliferating tissue, because of the intrinsically high rate of cell turnover. In contrast to initiation, conversion of an initiated cell to a fully malignant neoplasm is usually prolonged, lasting months in animals and years in humans.

There are several salient characteristics of initiation (Table 2.4). It can occur following a single exposure to a known carcinogen. The changes produced by the initiator may be latent for weeks or months, and are considered irreversible. The interval between initiation

TABLE 2.4   General characteristics of initiators and promoters of neoplasia

Initiators/initiation

Irreversible

Additive

Initiated cells cannot be identified

"Pure" initiation does not result in neoplasia unless promoter is subsequently applied

Number of initiated cells dependent on dose

No measurable threshold dose

No measurable maximal response

Are considered carcinogens

Must be administered before promoter

Only one exposure may be sufficient to initiate

Electrophile production and covalent binding to DNA

Usually mutagenic

Promoters/promotion

Reversible

Nonadditive

Not capable of initiation

Modulated by diet, hormones, environment, and related factors

Measurable threshold dose

Measurable maximal response

Not considered carcinogens, but co-carcinogens

Must be administered after the initiator

Prolonged exposure usually required

No electrophile production and no covalent binding to DNA

Usually not mutagenic

and promotion may be as long as one year in mouse skin-painting studies and still yield skin neoplasms. Initiation is additive and yield of neoplasms is dose-dependent. Increasing the dose of initiator increases the incidence and multiplicity of resulting neoplasms, and shortens the latency to manifestation of these neoplasms. Since the initiating event must be "fixed" by a round of cell proliferation, it becomes obvious that initiation is dependent on the cell cycle. Finally, there is no readily measurable threshold dose for maximum and minimum response to initiators. Unrealistically large numbers of animals would be required to demonstrate minimum responses, and confluence of multiple neoplasms following high doses precludes accurate quantification of the neoplastic response.

The majority of known carcinogens has both initiating and promoting activity and can thus induce neoplasms rapidly and in high yield when given repeatedly. When given at sufficiently low single doses, a complete carcinogen may act instead as a "pure" initiator requiring subsequent promotion for the detection of any resultant neoplasms. Under such circumstances, the agent can be operationally regarded as an "incomplete carcinogen."

Promotion

Promotion is classically considered that portion of the multi-step carcinogenic process in which specific agents, known as promoters, enhance the development of neoplasms from a background of initiated cells (Table 2.4). A promoter is typically given at some time after chemically-induced or fortuitous initiation, and the doses of the promoting agent are insufficient to produce cancer without prior initiation. Promoters include agents such as drugs, plant products, and hormones that do not directly interact with host cellular DNA (i.e., are not genotoxic), but somehow influence the expression of genetic information encoded by cellular DNA.

Promoters appear to have relatively high tissue specificity. Thus, phenobarbital functions as a promoter for rodent liver neoplasia, but not for urinary bladder neoplasia. Tumor promotion may be modulated by several factors, such as age, sex, diet, and hormone balance. The increased rate of breast cancer in women following a Western lifestyle has implicated an important role for meat and fat consumption in breast cancer development. The role of a high-fat diet in promotion of mammary cancer in rats exposed to the mammary carcinogen dimethylbenzanthracene (DMBA) has been documented. Most promoters cause hyperplasia or trigger inflammation, which in itself may trigger proliferation.

Progression

Progression is that part of the multi-step neoplastic process associated with the development of an initiated cell into a biologically malignant cell population. Progression is frequently used to signify the stages whereby a benign proliferation becomes malignant, or where a neoplasm develops from a low grade to a high grade of malignancy. During progression, neoplasms show progressively increased invasiveness, develop the ability to metastasize, and have alterations in biochemical, metabolic, and morphologic characteristics.

The most plausible mechanism of progression invokes the notion that during the process of tumor growth there is selection that favors enhanced growth of a subpopulation of neoplastic cells. In support of this mechanism is the observation of increased phenotypic heterogeneity in malignant versus benign neoplastic neoplasms. Presumably a variety of sub-populations arise, with subsequent emergence of a subpopulation with more malignant biological characteristics. Distinction between tumor promotion and tumor progression is not readily discernible in the routine histopathologic evaluation of neoplasms, especially in the early stages of progression.

HYPOTHESES OF MODE OF ACTION OF CHEMICAL CARCINOGENS

Overview

Four principal hypotheses, not necessarily mutually exclusive, have been proposed to explain the development of cancer: the mutational genetic hypothesis; the nonmutational genetic hypothesis; the epigenetic hypothesis; and the viral hypothesis. According to the mutational genetic hypothesis, malignant transformation results from small structural molecular perturbations of cellular DNA. An example of such a perturbation is a point mutation. For the nonmutational genetic hypothesis, large structural genomic changes (e.g., structural chromosomal alterations) that are not true mutations are postulated to cause neoplastic transformation. In the epigenetic hypothesis of carcinogenesis, changes in intracellular regulatory processes controlling cell proliferation and differentiation, *not* structural alterations in genomic material, result in neoplasia. The viral hypothesis of cancer induction postulates that infection by exogenous DNA or RNA viruses plays a role in malignant transformation. Vertically-transmitted endogenous proviruses that are ubiquitous in the cellular genome may be involved in the neoplastic process, but their potential role is as yet undefined.

Mutational Genetic Hypothesis of Chemical Carcinogenesis

Mutational Events

A critical step in carcinogenesis is structural alteration in the genetic machinery of a somatic cell. This appears to be true whether the active agent is a chemical, ionizing radiation, or a virus. According to the mutational hypothesis, a point mutation is responsible for at least the initial step in the neoplastic process. According to the somatic mutation theory, cancer originates when an otherwise ordinary cell undergoes a mutation; if a large enough population of somatic cells live for a sufficient length of time, gene mutations will occur in some of them. As the mutated cells proliferate,

there is a finite probability that some of them will sustain a second mutation. As the process of successive mutation and proliferation continues, cells will eventually sustain enough genetic alterations to become autonomous, resulting in cancer. Accumulation of successive mutations would be expected to increase, both as a function of age and the degree of cell proliferation. Early occurrence of cancer might be expected to result from exposure to mutagens, or to agents that increase the rate of cell proliferation.

Supporting the mutational hypothesis of cancer causation is the correlation between mutagenicity and carcinogenicity, the correlation between faulty DNA repair mechanisms and some cancers, and the heritable nature of neoplastic transformation. While the correlation between mutagenicity and carcinogenicity is not perfect, many chemical carcinogens are mutagenic either alone or after metabolic activation. Endogenous hereditary defects in mutational repair in the face of exposure to environmental mutagenic factors are known to lead to some cancers. Most notable is the occurrence of carcinomas and melanomas of the skin in xeroderma pigmentosum patients subjected to mutations caused by ultraviolet radiation.

Finally, a large body of experimental data supports the contention that malignant cancer is generally not reversible. Even in initiation/promotion studies, the initial mutational changes constituting initiation may remain latent for weeks or months before being expressed by administration of a promoting agent. This "memory effect" is compatible with a stable somatic mutation.

In the past five years, activated oncogenes have been identified in the DNA of many human neoplasms, as well as in spontaneous and chemically-induced neoplasms in animals. The activated oncogenes are frequently part of the *ras* oncogene family. Activated *ras* oncogenes have been repeatedly shown to differ from their homologous proto-oncogene, by virtue of a single point mutation. In some experimental situations, carcinogen-induced activation of some oncogenes appears to be an early event in the carcinogenic process. While it can be argued that activation of oncogenes may be a necessary event in the genesis of some cancers, it is unlikely that a single point mutation associated with an activated oncogene is sufficient in and of itself for development of all cancers.

Interaction of Genotoxic Chemical Carcinogens with Their Cellular Targets

Nonalkylating Agents

Nonalkylating carcinogens directly substitute for exocyclic amino groups of nucleosides. Examples include nitrous oxide, which causes oxidative deamination, and formaldehyde which forms cross-links within DNA. Formaldehyde also causes hydroxymethyl adducts and, thus, may also act as an alkylating agent.

Alkylating Agents

Alkylating chemical carcinogens either directly interact with cellular genomic material (direct-acting carcinogens), or must first be metabolized by the host to a reactive species (indirect-acting carcinogens). Examples of direct alkylating agents include methylnitrosourea and ethylnitrosourea. Indirect-acting alkylating agents include chemicals such as dimethylnitrosoamine and benzo[*a*]pyrene. For both direct- and indirect-acting agents, the reactive form of the carcinogen is an electron-deficient species (electrophile) that interacts nonenzymatically with electron-rich or nucleophilic molecular sites in the cell. These nucleophilic sites are not limited to DNA, but also include RNA and cellular proteins. Thus, the alkylating reaction is not specific for genomic material or for nucleic acids. The interaction of electrophilic forms of the carcinogen with host cellular material result in the formation of covalent adducts (addition products). Mutations are produced throughout the genome on exposure to the carcinogen. Some of these mutations may be lethal. The nonlethal reactions with cellular targets are the most relevant for carcinogenesis, because initiation occurs when one of these reactions occurs at a critical genomic site.

Nonmutational Genetic Hypothesis of Chemical Carcinogenesis

Chromosomal Aberrations and Neoplasia

Numerical or structural chromosomal abnormalities and alterations are almost universally present in neoplasms, particularly malignant neoplasms. Chromosomal aberrations are found in apparently spontaneous neoplasms, as well as in those induced by chemical carcinogens or by oncogenic viruses. Against a backdrop of apparently random chromosomal aberrations in neoplasms are a few constant karyotypic changes associated with specific neoplasms. Most notable is the association of the Philadelphia chromosome with the lymphoma/leukemia group of human diseases. However, in light of the relatively few constant karyotypic changes associated with specific histogenetic types of neoplasms, and the random nature of the preponderance of chromosomal aberrations observed in neoplasms, it is difficult to establish a cause and effect relationship between specific chromosomal aberrations and cancer.

Gene Amplification

Gene amplification represents a situation where there is an increase in the amount of DNA present in a specific region of a chromosome. Chromosomal aberrations observed in karyotype preparations reflect gene amplification. Assuming the amplified gene is transcriptionally active, an excess of product encoded by the amplified gene would follow. Drug-induced gene amplification is known to result in drug resistance, due to an increase in the amount of gene product. It has been suggested that increased production of normal protein products of amplified proto-oncogenes (e.g., c-*ras*) may contribute to the malignant phenotype. For example, amplification of the proto-oncogene, c-*myc*, in small cell carcinoma of the lung in humans correlates with clinical aggressiveness.

Epigenetic Hypothesis of Chemical Carcinogenesis

The nonmutational genetic or epigenetic hypothesis postulates that a genomic perturbation other than a mutation may lead to cancer. Of the proposed mechanisms listed in the overview, hormonal effects and enhanced cell proliferation will be discussed.

Altered Methylation

Methylation of genes influences the regulation of transcription of genes. Methylation of cytosine residues in DNA is a means of "silencing" genes that are not needed by a particular cell. Methylated genes cannot be transcribed, but must be demethylated first, a relatively laborious and time-consuming process for a cell. The more advanced the state of differentiation in a cell, the more of its genes are methylated and hence inactive. Tissue-specific alterations in methylation patterns have been observed after exposure to chemicals. In general, genes from cancer cells are hypomethylated compared to their normal counterparts, and carcinogens are known to interfere with gene methylation. Unfortunately, the dilemma for researchers is deciding if the hypomethylation of genes is a cause of malignancy, or a consequence of the altered metabolism of the malignant cells.

Blocked Differentiation

One apparent characteristic of transformed cells is a partial or total block of terminal differentiation. The paucity of knowledge relative to normal mechanisms that regulate differentiation makes it difficult to elucidate the potential role of abnormal cell differentiation in the genesis of development of cancer. Despite morphologic evidence for loss of terminal differentiation, experiments have shown that under specific conditions, neoplastic cells retain an intrinsic ability to revert to a normal phenotype, suggesting that additional endogenous or exogenous factors must be present continually to maintain the neoplastic phenotype.

Intercellular Communication

Intercellular communication is known to play an important role in phenotypic expression. In some culture systems, the presence of normal cells in co-culture with malignant cells blocks the expression of abnormal phenotype by the cancerous cells. It has been suggested that the inhibition of cellular communication may be the mode of action of many chemicals that induce neoplasia but do not affect the genome directly. Many tumor-promoting agents inhibit the intercellular communications via gap junctions. This interruption is associated with aberrant expression of the essential gap protein, connexin, and loss of function of cell adhesion molecules.

Hormones

Hormones are chemical messengers that bind to specific cellular receptors and form hormone-receptor complexes that trigger a cellular response. The cellular response is specific, both for the hormone and the target cell. The target cell response to hormone stimulation is typically an increase or decrease in cell division, or an acceleration or deceleration in differentiation.

Just how hormonal interaction with a cell receptor leads to cancer is unknown, but may relate to an increase in cell turnover among cells that already possess latent genetic change. Thus, endogenous hormones may serve to promote already initiated cells. Alternatively, hormonal imbalance could lead to increased proliferation of a sensitive cell population that then undergoes secondary genotoxic damage from any one of several environmentally prevalent genotoxic agents. The two possibilities are not mutually exclusive.

Endogenous hormones are associated with the development of specific neoplasms, and in some cases with the inhibition of carcinogenesis. Hormones or hormone imbalances undoubtedly play a major causative role in cancers of certain hormone-sensitive tissues (ovary, uterus, prostate, testes, and other endocrine organs). However, it is unlikely that they play a major causative role in the development of neoplasia in non-hormone-sensitive tissues.

Cell Proliferation and Apoptosis

Increased cell proliferation, or mitogenesis, can theoretically make an important contribution to the process of carcinogenesis. This can come about in either or both of two ways. First, the enhanced cell turnover can lead to "fixation" of genotoxic damage. A second way in which enhanced mitogenesis can contribute to neoplasia is to stimulate cell division in an already initiated cell, thereby allowing it to expand clonally. With a nongenotoxic mitogen, it is likely that both mechanisms act in a complementary fashion. Whether a mitogen acts by either, or both, mechanisms, cancer "induction" by the mitogen is secondary to the actual inciting event (i.e., damage to the genome). Many situations exist in animal carcinogenicity models where nongenotoxic chemicals given at sufficiently high doses play a causative role in development of neoplasia, simply by enhancing cell proliferation. Examples of agents that may operate through this mechanism include phenobarbital and sodium saccharin.

Current data strongly suggest that cell death may be as essential as cell proliferation in carcinogenesis. The ratio between cell "birth," and counterbalancing cell death, determines the rate of tumor growth. Whereas necrosis can frequently be observed in malignant tumors when the developing cancer outgrows its blood supply, apoptosis is the predominant form of cell death observed in preneoplastic lesions. An increase in apoptosis often parallels the increase in cell proliferation observed in preneoplastic lesions and tumors. It has been reported that the growth of dioxin-promoted preneoplastic liver foci in rat hepatocarcinogenesis is due to inhibition of apoptosis, rather than to enhanced cell proliferation. This occurrence has been observed in other tumors as well, for example in developing basal tumors of the skin. In addition malignant cells, due to their inherent genomic instability, are often more prone to chemically-induced apoptosis than their normal counterparts. An underlying principle of cancer chemotherapy is indeed that selective induction of apoptosis in neoplastic cells, allowing the clinician to use lower doses than would otherwise be needed to kill cells. Indeed, the ability to "escape" apoptosis is a major feature in some cancers, most notably those that are resistance to radiation or chemotherapy. Overexpression of the mitochondrial anti-apoptotic gene, *Bcl-2*, leads to resistance to apoptosis and corresponding resistance to apoptosis-inducing chemotherapeutic agents.

Viral Hypothesis of Carcinogenesis

The viral hypothesis of carcinogenesis has gained steady support, because of the frequency with which

DNA and RNA viruses are isolated from animal neoplasms and human leukemias. However, tumor viruses have subsequently been found to be widespread in healthy animals and humans. Since the probability that retroviruses without transforming genes will transform cells is low, on the order of 10^{-11}, and because relatively few cancers are caused by DNA viruses, it has been argued that viruses may not be a significant natural source of exogenous cancer genes. In fact, it has been proposed that cellular transformation is typically a virus-independent event, and that viral integration occurs during the process of clonal expansion of transformed cells. At any rate, the issue of whether a chemical carcinogen can activate a latent oncogenic virus as its primary mode of inducing neoplasia has been debated, but never resolved.

ONCOGENES AND TUMOR SUPPRESSOR GENES IN CHEMICAL CARCINOGENESIS

Genes and Oncogenes

Up to 10 000 genes are estimated to be present in the mammalian genome. These genes can be placed into two general categories: structural genes and regulatory genes. Structural genes are nucleotide sequences that encode for the various protein products produced by the cell. Regulatory genes, on the other hand, control the activity of structural genes, as well as other regulatory genes, and can be thought of as the switches that initiate, maintain, enhance, block, or stop the functioning or transcription of structural genes. Considering that all nucleated somatic cells contain the entire genetic code for the species, but that only specific genes are transcriptionally active in a given cell type, the proper functioning of regulatory genes is not a trivial matter.

Oncogenes are dominant acting structural genes that encode for protein products capable of transforming the phenotype of a cell. Oncogenes were first identified as the transforming genes of retroviruses. These oncogenes were not necessary for the life cycle of the virus, but were responsible for transforming virally infected cells and producing cancer in the host. It was later learned that the transforming oncogenes were not intrinsic viral genes, but rather normal cellular structural genes captured from eukaryotic organisms previously infected by the retrovirus. The virus assimilated these normal cellular genes by a process called transduction. The transduced oncogene in the viral genome is referred to as a viral oncogene

(abbreviated v-*onc*). The homologous gene in the host genome is called a cellular oncogene (abbreviated c-*onc*), or a proto-oncogene. In capturing the cellular proto-oncogene, the virus lost some of its own structural genes and, consequently, often became incapable of replicating in the absence of helper viruses.

It is now known that proto-oncogenes encode for proteins that are important in cell growth, development, and differentiation. Since cancer is a perturbation of normal cell growth and differentiation, the potential significance of alterations in proto-oncogenes becomes apparent. It is, thus, not surprising that examination of DNA from human and animal tumors has demonstrated the existence of dominant transforming oncogenes, some of which correspond to those responsible for the carcinogenicity of acute transforming retroviruses.

Proto-oncogene Function

Proto-oncogenes have derived their names from the respective retroviral diseases in which their homologs were discovered (Table 2.5). Examples of different proto-oncogenes, their retroviral counterparts, species of origin, and their encoded protein products are presented in Table 2.5. Proto-oncogenes encode intracellular regulatory proteins (e.g., protein kinases), growth factors, and growth factor receptors that occupy specific intracellular and cellular membrane sites. All these are important for cell growth and differentiation. Increased transcription of proto-oncogenes occurs during embryogenesis, during stimulation of cell mitosis by growth factors, and during regeneration of lost tissue. Protein kinase C, for example, controls such diverse functions as cell growth and specialization, metabolism, hormone action, nerve signal transmission, fertilization, and gene activity. Perturbations in expression of proteins caused by inappropriate proto-oncogene activation or enhanced expression could lead to alterations of growth and differentiation and, thus, contribute to neoplasia.

Proto-oncogene Activation

There is increasing evidence that proto-oncogene activation contributes to the neoplastic process. Activation can occur in several ways (see Table 2.5). Retroviral transduction had been shown to result in acquisition of point mutations, deletions, or gene fusions within the coding sequence of the transduced proto-oncogene. This leads not only to abnormal

TABLE 2.5   Example of proto-oncogenes with viral counterparts

Oncogene product and oncogene	Source of name (species of origin)
Tyrosine protein kinase	
src	Rous sarcoma virus (chicken)
abl	Abelson leukemia virus (mouse)
fes	Feline sarcoma virus (cat)
Kinase-related	
raf	3611 murine sarcoma virus (mouse)
mos	Murine sarcoma virus (mouse)
GTP-binding proteins	
H-ras	Harvey sarcoma virus (rat)
K-ras	Kirsten sarcoma virus (rat)
N-ras	Neuroblastoma (human)
Growth factor	
Sis (platelet derived growth factor)	Simian sarcoma virus (monkey)
Growth factor receptor	
erbB (epidermal growth factor receptor)	Avian erythroblastoma virus (chicken)
fms (colony-stimulating factor receptor)	McDounough sarcoma virus (cat)
Nuclear proteins	
c-myc	MC29 myelocytomatosis virus (chicken)
N-myc	Neuroblastoma (human)
myb	Myeloblastosis virus (chicken)
fos	FBJ osteosarcoma virus (mouse)

function, but also to changes in levels and schedules of expression of other encoded protein products. Retroviruses can also affect the expression of proto-oncogenes by a process called insertional mutagenesis. In this situation the retroviral DNA integrates into the host cell DNA adjacent to or within the coding sequence of a proto-oncogene. The powerful retroviral promoters (regulatory genes) then drive transcription of the normal or truncated gene product of the proto-oncogene.

Activation of proto-oncogenes can also occur by mechanisms independent of retroviral involvement. Point mutations and DNA rearrangements, such as translocations or gene amplifications, can result in inappropriate proto-oncogene activation, to altered levels or schedules of expression of the protein product. Examples of activated oncogenes detected in human neoplasms are listed in Table 2.6.

Oncogene Activation in Chemical Carcinogenesis

Activation of proto-oncogenes in spontaneous and chemically-induced neoplasia has received considerable attention in recent years. A variety of activated oncogenes have been documented in rodent neoplasms (Table 2.7). From experimental studies it appears that certain types of oncogenes are activated by carcinogen treatment in the early stages of tumor induction. Other studies of human and rodent neoplasms suggest that oncogene activation is involved later in the carcinogenic process, specifically during tumor progression. While high levels of expression of a single ras oncogene are sufficient to transform cultured rodent cells in some systems, the concerted expression of at least two oncogenes is necessary for transformation in other in vitro culture systems. Furthermore, loss of specific regulatory functions, such as tumor suppressor genes, also appears to be a distinct step in neoplastic transformation. Thus, oncogenes seem to play an important role in chemical carcinogenesis. They may, in fact, be necessary for carcinogenesis, but are not sufficient in and of themselves to cause cancer. This is consistent with a multi-step process of carcinogenesis.

The patterns of oncogene activation in spontaneous versus chemically-induced rodent neoplasms suggest that the molecular lesions associated with chemically-induced cancer are sometimes different from those in spontaneous cancer. Furthermore, the patterns of oncogene activation in several rodent model systems appear to be carcinogen specific, are consistent with known or expected DNA adduct formation, and, in some cases, are similar to patterns of oncogene activation documented in human neoplasms.

The most frequently identified activated oncogenes detected in chemically-induced neoplasms belong to the ras gene family. H-ras, K-ras, and N-ras genes that differ from their proto-oncogene homologs by a single point mutation are located in a specific codon (Table 2.7). These mutations lead to nucleotide mispairing during DNA replication. The altered DNA gives rise to an abnormal protein product that theoretically alters cell growth or differentiation. The mammary carcinogen MNU is very labile, with an estimated biological half-life of a few minutes. Thus, it is likely that the effect produced by this carcinogen occurs as an early event in the carcinogenic process. Since hormone-stimulated cell division in mammary tissue is also necessary for the development of mammary neoplasia in this model, it is unlikely that activation of the H-ras oncogene is sufficient in and of itself for production of mammary neoplasia. Another example of

TABLE 2.6 Mechanisms of oncogene activation

Proto-oncogene	Mechanism of activation	Oncogene
c-onc	Retroviral transduction	v-onc
c-myc	Chromosomal translocation	lg/myc
c-abl	Chromosomal translocation	bcr/abl
N-myc	Gene amplification	DM/HSR
c-myc	Gene amplification	
K-ras	Gene amplification	
c-H-ras	Point mutation	12th, 13th or 61st codon mutation
c-K-ras	Point mutation	12th, 13th or 61st codon mutation
c-N-ras	Point mutation	12th, 13th or 61st codon mutation
myc	Promoter/enhancer insertion	LTR/c-onc
myb	Promoter/enhancer insertion	LTR/common domain
erb B	Promoter/enhancer insertion	
mos	Promoter/enhancer insertion	
int-1	Promoter/enhancer insertion	
int-2	Promoter/enhancer insertion	

TABLE 2.7 Selected examples of activated oncogenes in animal neoplasms

Tumor	Method of induction[a]	Frequency of positives	Oncogenes present[b]
Mouse liver	Spontaneous	17/27	H-ras (5)
			raf (1)
			Unknown (1)
Rat mammary	MNU (single dose)	61/71	H-ras (61)
Mouse liver	VC (single dose)	10/10	H-ras (10)
Rat liver	AFB1 (continuous)	10/11	K-ras (2)
			Unknown (9)
Rat lung	TNM (continuous)	18/19	K-ras (18)
Mouse lung	TNM (continuous)	10/10	K-ras (10)
Mouse skin	DMBA (continuous)	4/4	H-ras (3)
			Unknown (1)
Mouse skin	DMBA + TPA (initiation and promotion)	33/37	H-ras
Rat neuroblastoma	ENU (transplacental)	3/3	neu (3)
Rat schwannoma	MNU (transplacental)	10/13	neu (10)
Mouse skin	Gamma radiation	4/4	K-ras
Rat skin	Ionizing radiation	6/10	H-ras

[a]MNU, N-methyl-N-nitrosourea; VC, vinyl carbamate; TNM, tetranitromethane; DMBA, 7,12-dimethylbenz[a]anthracene; TPA, 12-O-tetradecanoyl phorbol 1,3-acetate; ENU, N-ethyl-N-nitrosourea
[b]Number of neoplasms with the activated oncogene given in parentheses

the H-*ras* oncogene associated with neoplasia is seen in mouse skin carcinomas induced by dimethylbenzanthracene (DMBA), followed by promotion with phorbol ester. In this instance there is a mutation in the 61st codon of the H-*ras* gene. The induction of novel point mutations in this, and other chemically-induced neoplasms, suggests that it may be possible to distinguish between spontaneous and chemically-induced neoplasms on the basis of patterns of oncogene activation.

Tumor Suppressor Genes and Carcinogenesis

In vitro neoplastic transformation and somatic cell fusion studies show that malignant transformation represents a balance between genes that enhance expression and genes that suppress malignancy. Growth suppressing genes, sometimes referred to as tumor suppressor genes, or antioncogenes, may play a critical role in *in vivo* carcinogenesis. Growth suppressor genes are regulatory genes that normally function to limit or suppress normal growth by inhibiting the activity of structural genes responsible for growth. As such, they have a function opposite to that of oncogenes, and effectively oppose the action of oncogenes. While proto-oncogenes have to be activated to influence carcinogenesis, suppressor genes have to be inactivated for the transformed phenotype to be expressed. Inactivation can be achieved by chromosome loss, gene deletion, recombination, gene conversion, or point mutation. Proto-oncogene activation is generally the result of a somatic mutation. Mutant forms of tumor suppressor genes might be present in germ cells, and thus may be hereditary. Recent advances in documenting the molecular biology of retinoblastoma have clearly pointed to the potential significance of tumor suppressor genes in carcinogenesis. It is reasonable to expect that inactivation or loss of growth suppressor genes, such as *p53*, working in concert with activation of oncogenes, and with a variety of endogenous and exogenous stimuli, will be recognized as playing an important part in the complex process of carcinogenesis.

CELL CYCLE AND CARCINOGENESIS

The pivotal role of cell proliferation in all phases of carcinogenesis is inextricably linked to positive and negative cell cycle control mechanisms as influenced by oncogenes, tumor suppressor genes, growth factors, and their cognate receptors, hormones and their receptors, and the action of exogenous agents on cell cycle control. Uncontrolled cell proliferation is the hallmark of neoplasia, and many cancer cells demonstrated damage to genes that regulate their cell cycles directly. The prevailing model of the cell cycle is that of a series of transients at which certain criteria must be met before the cell proceeds to the next phase.

Cyclins and Cdk Proteins

The cell cycle is composed of an S (DNA synthesis) phase and an M (mitotic) phase, separated by two gap phases (G1 and G2). Progression through the cell cycle is tightly controlled by a group of heterodimeric protein kinases, comprising a "cyclin" as a regulatory element and a catalytic subunit known as a "cyclin-dependent kinase" (Cdk). There are many combinations of cyclin/Cdk complexes, and each phase of the cell cycle is characterized by a specific pattern of expression and activity. Five major classes of mammalian cyclins have been described. Cyclins C, D1-3, and E reach their peak of synthesis and activity during the G1 phase and regulate the transition from the G1 to the S phase. However, cyclins A and B102 achieve their maximal levels later in the cycle, during the S and G2 phases, and are regarded as regulators of the transition to mitosis. Depending on the cyclin partner, and therefore the cell cycle stage, different key target molecules are phosphorylated. These events occur in a highly regulated temporal sequence that is maintained through a series of checkpoints, allowing for DNA repair before further progression into the cycle. The cyclin systems are not essential to the workings of the cycle itself, but instead act as "brakes" in the face of cell stress or DNA damage. Abrogation of these checkpoints with agents such as methylxanthine analogs or pentoxifylline increases the cytotoxicity of DNA-damaging agents. The importance of DNA damage in triggering a cell cycle shutdown is obvious.

Retinoblastoma Checkpoint

Two major checkpoints are thought to be particularly important following DNA damage and have been established at the middle to end of G1 (preceding DNA replication) and G2 (preceding chromosome segregation). Loss of the G1 checkpoint dependent on cyclin D1 (degraded at the G1/S transition) and cyclin E (degraded in mid-S phase) is the first. Overexpression of either cyclin D1 or cyclin E with subsequent activation of the cyclin D1 and cyclin E1/Cdk complexes results in entry into the S phase and decreased G1 time. Cyclin D1 is overexpressed in many human cancers, including breast and non-small cell lung carcinomas, sarcomas, melanomas, B-cell lymphomas, and squamous cell carcinomas of the head and neck. Cyclin D1/cdk4 complexes to phosphorylated pRB, the product of the *pRB* retinoblastoma susceptibility gene. pRB exerts a negative regulatory effect on gene expression through complex formation with DNA-binding proteins, including members of the E2F family. In nondividing (G0) cells, pRB is bound to E2F members, leading to repression of transcription. On phosphorylation by cyclin/cdk complexes, pRB dissociates from E2F proteins, leading to transcription of genes promoting S-phase entry. Thus, underphosphorylated pRB maintains cells in G1, while phosphorylation allows exit from G1.

p53 Checkpoint

Another tumor suppressor gene, p53, is necessary for G1 phase arrest after DNA-damage. Mutations at the *p53* locus are the most frequent genetic alterations associated with cancer in humans. The majority of mutations involve several highly conserved regions within the DNA-binding core of the molecule. Lack of p53 permits synthesis of damaged DNA, and increases the incidence of selected types of mutation. This has been shown after exposure to a variety of DNA-damaging etiologies, such as ionizing radiation (strand breaks), alkylation, and UV light (photo-dimers). Wild-type p53 protein is normally kept at very low steady state levels by its relatively short half-life. It becomes stabilized and accumulates in cells undergoing DNA damage, or in those responding to certain forms of stress. After DNA damage, p53 activates the transcription of several "downstream" genes, including p21, a gene that belongs to a family of negative cell cycle regulators that inhibit Cdk proteins. P21 inactivates most cyclins involved in the cell cycle, and as a result pRB remains underphosphorylated, keeping the cell in G1.

The p53 protein also activates the *BAX* gene. Bax and similar gene products act at the mitochondrial membrane to initiate apoptosis. Expression of this gene is a "late function" of p53-induced transcription of certain genes, and occurs when DNA damage is too extensive to repair before progression into the next phase of the cell cycle. Bax expression leads to apoptosis of the damaged cell before replication can occur. The p53 protein regulates its own function, through activation of the *MDM2* gene. The mdm2 zinc finger protein binds to p53 and inhibits its transcriptional activity. The mdm2 protein also binds to and suppresses its function.

The high rate and mutation pattern of p53 and pRB in primary tumors identifies them as prototype tumor suppressor genes. Furthermore, detection of p53 and pRB mutations, and altered expression of their encoded products, appears to be of clinical prognostic significance. It will be essential to further advance our understanding of the intricate molecular mechanisms that govern chemical carcinogenesis by these and other growth-related genes, to allow us to improve strategies for assessing human cancer risk and design effective treatment regimens.

TESTS FOR CARCINOGENIC POTENTIAL OF CHEMICALS

Widespread and routine evaluation of chemicals for their carcinogenic potential began in earnest in the mid-1960s, with the use of a standardized protocol for the bioassay program of the National Cancer Institute (NCI). The original NCI bioassay has evolved to the present-day National Toxicology Program two-year carcinogenicity study. Throughout this period, a variety of alternative *in vivo* and *in vitro* assay schemes have been introduced in the hope of identifying potential carcinogens more quickly and for less money. Some of these alternative testing models have been highly beneficial tools to help explore the processes of carcinogenesis, to identify and quantify the genotoxicity of chemicals, and to identify the specific mechanisms by which given agents produce a carcinogenic response. Testing batteries, tier approaches, and decision-point analyses have been proposed to provide a basis for prioritizing chemicals in the testing queue, and to provide a larger database for risk assessment. These efforts serve to emphasize that there is no ideal test for identifying potential human carcinogens. In general, efforts to supplant the long-term carcinogen bioassay with less costly short-term tests have been frustrated by poor concordance of the latter with the traditional long-term test results. Meanwhile, increasing costs for conducting long-term carcinogenicity studies have resulted in fewer chemicals being tested annually for potential carcinogenicity. Currently, much thought is being given to developing medium-term tests for carcinogenicity, concomitant with analyses of reasonable ways to reduce the cost of the standard long-term rodent carcinogenicity test.

In Vivo Chronic Rodent Carcinogenesis Studies

The current strategy for identifying potential carcinogenicity of chemicals involves systemic (including dermal) exposure of male and female rats and mice to high doses (and fractions thereof) of test chemical over a two-year period (rodent bioassay). At the end of two years, the carcinogenicity of the chemical being studied is assessed by measuring the excess in neoplasm production above background levels, documenting the occurrence of rare neoplasms with negligible background levels, or demonstrating a reduced latency in neoplasm development in exposed animals versus controls. The original NCI bioassay was intended as a screen for carcinogenicity in the rodent. It was not generally intended to be used for risk assessment, determining carcinogenic potency, identifying subtleties of chronic toxicity, determining the mechanism of observed carcinogenic responses, or establishing the pathogenesis of lesions. The implication behind the original NCI bioassay was that, if a chemical was found to cause neoplasms in treated animals, further studies would need to be designed and conducted specifically to determine parameters, such as the mechanism of cancer induction, the nature of the dose response, chemical metabolism, and target organ dosimetry. More definitive testing of positive chemicals identified by the bioassay has generally not occurred. In the absence of such additional relevant data, the bioassay results have out of necessity been used as a basis for human risk assessment and regulation.

In an effort to consciously expand the original NCI bioassay and to make the test results more relevant for the interpretations being applied, considerable evolution has occurred in the design, conduct, and interpretation of long-term rodent carcinogenesis tests conducted under the auspices of the NTP. While the estimated maximum tolerated dose (EMTD) concept has been retained in principle, it is more conservatively applied in setting the high dose. In addition to the high dose or EMTD, at least two additional lower doses are employed in NTP rodent carcinogenicity studies. A conscious effort is made to use human and environmental exposure information to set the low doses. This permits better definition of dose response, and allows better utilization of data for risk assessment.

To more fully characterize the toxicity of chemicals, modifications to the chronic rodent carcinogenicity study protocol have been selectively introduced by the NTP. Interim sacrifices and stop studies are incorporated into the design of many carcinogenicity studies to better define the pathogenesis and biological relevance of the anticipated response. The route of administration of chemicals is chosen to mimic natural routes of human exposure whenever possible. Consequently, corn oil gavage of chemicals is rarely used in contemporary study design. Ancillary studies, such as chemical disposition and metabolism, reproductive toxicity,

teratology, behavioral testing, and immunotoxicity frequently complement contemporary two-year carcinogenicity studies. In addition, a battery of genotoxicity tests is conducted for each chemical. The quality of the pathology evaluation for both neoplastic and nonneoplastic lesions is rigorously peer-reviewed. The final interpretation of study results is likewise subjected to intensive peer review and any carcinogenic response is categorized according to levels of evidence for the presence or absence of carcinogenicity in the study. All of this has resulted in a markedly improved product, but has also resulted in expenditure of more time and money to evaluate each chemical.

There are positive and negative attributes of the contemporary NTP two-year rodent carcinogenicity study. On the positive side, the test as currently performed is a thoroughly conducted and peer-reviewed assessment of carcinogenicity and chronic toxicity for the chemical under study. The study results provide a better basis for risk assessment than previously designed rodent bioassays permitted. All data are published to allow for close scrutiny of the scientific basis for each interpretation. To date, the two-year rodent carcinogenicity study appears to be the single best system for identifying potential carcinogens. Not only has the two-year rodent carcinogenicity test been sufficiently sensitive to identify known human carcinogens, it has also identified carcinogens such as aflatoxin, 4-aminobiphenyl, *bis*(chloromethyl)ether, diethylstibesterol, melphalan, mustard gas, and vinyl chloride, prior to the identification of these compounds as carcinogens in humans. Disadvantages of the chronic rodent carcinogenicity test relate primarily to the high cost of each study, to the long time interval required to obtain results, and to the large number of animals used. The high costs make the studies too expensive to repeat, thereby obviating the principle of reproducibility demanded by good science. However, in 70 "near-replicate" comparisons, good overall reproducibility of positivity, target site, and carcinogenic potency was found by comparing published studies performed in rats, mice, or hamsters. The identification of rodent carcinogens on the basis of repeated exposure to high doses of a chemical has been criticized as unrealistic with respect to most human exposure situations. While cost and lack of evidence of reproducibility remain valid criticisms of the chronic rodent carcinogenicity test, it still remains the best test system for identifying potential human carcinogens.

The maximum tolerated dose (MTD) concept continues to be one of the most debated and controversial issues in toxicology. Studies that are negative for carcinogenicity and conducted with doses below the MTD leave doubt about the adequacy of the chronic rodent carcinogenicity test. One never knows if the animals were sufficiently challenged with the chemical. Studies conducted at or above the MTD may compromise host homeostasis to such a degree that a positive result may have little relevance to human exposure situations. Since it is not always possible to determine the MTD prior to exposure of the animals over much of their lifespan, the real problem lies in how the study results are used in risk assessment. Thus, conclusions regarding carcinogenicity, or lack thereof, as determined in chronic rodent tests must be qualified as occurring under conditions of the specific study in question. The limitations of the particular study should be pointed out as they relate to MTD, the original design and purpose of the study, study conduct, confounding toxicity, and other study conditions. In addition, a standardized approach for describing the reasoning used to make a conclusion about the carcinogenicity of a chemical is desirable. For this purpose categorization of the observed response using levels of evidence is helpful.

Additional *In Vivo* Tests for Carcinogenicity

The carcinogenicity model described here as short-term is probably not quite accurate. When used with potent carcinogens, a preneoplastic or neoplastic response is often observed in a few weeks, hence the designation "short-term." However, for less potent carcinogens, and for noncarcinogens, tests are typically conducted for several months. In the case of the mouse skin-painting model, lifetime studies may sometimes be conducted to assess carcinogenicity. Because of the sharp contrast in the study duration for these so-called short-term *in vivo* test models, relative to truly short-term (days or weeks) *in vitro* test systems, they have more recently been referred to as "medium-term" bioassays for carcinogens, indicating a study shorter than the conventional two-year rodent carcinogenicity study. Short-term or medium-term *in vivo* carcinogenesis animal models consist of an intact animal capable of chemical metabolism (activation and detoxification), complex tissue and hormonal interactions, and possessing repair mechanisms. All of these can influence the ultimate expression of carcinogenic responses to chemical exposure.

Various investigators have proposed specific short-term *in vivo* rodent models to supplant the more costly chronic rodent carcinogenicity studies. In those instances where appropriate validation studies have been conducted, these short-term models have shown unacceptable concordance with results obtained using the

"gold-standard" chronic rodent carcinogenicity test. Few individuals seem to have considered simple questions such as "Why would a short-duration lung tumor assay system be expected to identify chemicals that produce renal cancer in a chronic rodent study?" Despite this unfortunate shortcoming, short-term *in vivo* carcinogenicity models can play an important role in defining chemical carcinogenesis. First, *in vivo* short-term tests are useful in defining the nature of the carcinogenic response observed in a chronic rodent carcinogenicity study. For specific target tissues, they can identify whether a chemical is an initiator or promoter, and they can help define the relative potency of the carcinogen. Second, they can help elucidate the mechanistic basis of carcinogenesis. Third, when used as part of a battery or tier approach to carcinogen testing, they help set priorities for more extensive carcinogenicity testing of chemicals.

A brief description of selected *in vivo* short-term models is provided in the next six sections. These have been selected based on general popularity and recommendations for their use in decision-point judgements, and tier approaches to carcinogen identification.

Strain A Mouse Pulmonary Tumor Test

The Strain A mouse lung tumor model is sensitive for some classes of chemicals, but insensitive for others. Typically, agents are administered to weaning strain A mice by intraperitoneal injection three times a week for eight weeks. Mice are killed 24 weeks after the start of treatment, and lungs are removed and fixed. Results (incidence and multiplicity) based on gross enumeration of lung nodules are compared with untreated and vehicle controls. The sensitivity of a given cohort of mice is assessed, by running a positive urethane control. The strain A pulmonary tumor test system is particularly useful for assessing potency of pulmonary carcinogens and for mechanistic studies of carcinogenesis.

Rat Mammary Neoplasm Test

Single or sometimes multiple doses of agent are given to virgin female Sprague–Dawley rats at about day 55 of age, which corresponds to maximum developmental activity of the mammary tissue. Animals are examined periodically by palpation for detectable masses over the next six to nine months to determine mammary neoplasm incidence and multiplicity. Dimethylbenzanthracene is included as a positive control, and typically results in detectable neoplasms in about two months and a 100% incidence of malignant mammary cancer after nine months. This *in vivo* carcinogenesis model has been particularly useful in assessing the influence of hormonal enhancement of mammary carcinogenesis, and in demonstrating the role of dietary fat in promoting mammary carcinogenesis.

Subcutaneous Injection Test

The subcutaneous injection test consists of administering single or repeated doses of chemical injected subcutaneously into rats or mice. Developing sarcomas are clinically detected at the injection site by palpation, and such data are used to determine time to tumor formation. Since some solid substances and persistent foreign body reactions can cause localized sarcomas in rodents, production of neoplasms at the injection site indicates that further studies are needed. However, production of neoplasms at distant sites is generally regarded as evidence of carcinogenicity.

Mouse Skin-painting Test

The mouse skin-painting model is used contemporarily to determine potential carcinogenicity by repeated application of a chemical to the shaved skin of the back throughout all or most of the lifespan of the mouse. Clinical observation of papillomas and carcinomas in the treated area, with histopathologic confirmation, constitutes the most common endpoint. This test allows for determination of time to neoplasm formation, neoplasm incidence, and neoplasm multiplicity (a measure of potency). In situations in which there is systemic absorption of carcinogens, neoplasms in visceral organs can also be induced. A negative or vehicle control group, as well as a positive control group (e.g., benzo[a]pyrene), are included in the experimental design. The chemical is usually given at the maximum dose (concentration) that does not produce shortening of the lifespan or excessive skin irritation.

The experimental protocol may be modified to permit assessment of the initiating and promoting potential of the chemical under test. Practically all of our current concepts of cancer formation, that is, initiation, co-carcinogenesis, promotion, progression, and more recently stages of promotion, have been derived from mouse skin-painting studies.

In Vivo Rat Liver Neoplasm Model

A variety of treatment protocols have been proposed for *in vivo* rat liver carcinogenesis models. The altered focus model is particularly useful for examining multi-stage hepatocarcinogenesis, and for identifying liver tumor promoters. Examples of treatment protocols include: sequential feeding of carcinogen and promoter; single treatment with a necrogenic dose of carcinogen followed by a proliferative stimulation in the presence of growth suppression (selection model); single treatment with a carcinogen during liver regeneration followed by repeated or continuous administration of a promoter (partial hepatectomy model); production of lipotrope deficiency following exposure to carcinogen; and initiation at birth with subsequent natural proliferation stimulation followed by promotion after weaning (neonatal rat model). A recently proposed test system for detection of hepatocarcinogens involves quantification of the number and size of diethylnitrosamine (DEN)-initiated placental glutathione S-transferase (PGST)-positive foci of cellular alteration in the rat liver.

While known hepatocarcinogens produce PGST and other histochemically identifiable foci, the occurrence of foci of cellular alteration is known to be modulated by a variety of factors, e.g., strain, sex, or diet. Many foci regress or remodel on cessation of treatment, and only a few foci (estimated at between 1 out of 1000 to 1 out of 10 000) progress to actual liver neoplasms. Hence, an observed positive focus response should be qualified in regard to its carcinogenic significance, and indicates the need for further confirmatory testing.

Rat liver neoplasm models have been extremely useful in confirming and extending the observations made in mouse skin-painting models on the mechanisms of carcinogenesis. Liver focus models may be useful in assessing carcinogen potency based upon a quantitative endpoint.

Genetically Altered Mouse Models for Carcinogenicity

Several models that are currently being validated utilize genetically altered transgenic and gene-targeted knockout mice. To produce transgenic mice, oncogenic genes or fusion genes are introduced at the pronucleus state of embryogenesis, resulting in the early development of neoplasia at one or more target tissue sites. Production of gene-targeted knockout mice entails selecting specific genes, such that their function is silenced. A potentially wide array of knockout mice prone to different types of neoplasms will eventually be available. At least three popular models are being studied or utilized for assessing carcinogenic potential of various chemicals. These are the *p53* +/− mouse (in which one *p53* allele has been silenced), the Tg:Ac skin-promoting model (which contains the viral *ras* transgene), and the rasH2 mouse carrying the normal H-*ras* with its endogenous promoter sequence. These three models show promise as adjunct models that yield results in approximately six months. In addition to their potential use in carcinogen identification, genetically altered mice provide a test system to assess how chemical agents may modulate the process of progression of neoplasia.

Additional carcinogenicity models have been developed, including a rat urinary bladder model, a rat pancreatic cancer model, a gastric cancer model, a rat thyroid cancer model, a fish liver neoplasm model, and rat and mouse colon cancer models. Two recently emergent models offer great promise and warrant brief mention. One is the short-term multi-organ test system for carcinogens, in which rats are treated by multiple carcinogens, to cause initiation in several target tissues. This is followed by administration of the test chemical for 12 weeks. Endpoints which lend themselves to quantitation include preneoplastic lesions in the liver, thyroid, lung, forestomach, urinary bladder, and esophagus. The second model is an untested model using transgenic mice. The greatest potential of the various short-term organ-specific animal carcinogenesis models is for understanding the underpinnings of the carcinogenic process.

In Vitro Short-term Tests

It is beyond the scope of this chapter to extensively discuss short-term *in vitro* or *in vivo* models or combined *in vivo–in vitro* models for assessing genotoxicity of chemicals. Such models are discussed in the references cited in the suggested reading list. Endpoints include evidence of a chemical's mutagenic, clastogenic, and cell transformation activity. The utility of these tests as predictors of carcinogenesis has had mixed reviews. Data derived from *in vitro* and *in vivo* tests for genotoxicity are used in tier testing, decision-point analysis, and in the weight-of-evidence method for risk assessment.

CONCLUSION

Cancer is a complex multi-step process associated with a wide array of endogenous and exogenous perturbations. Endogenous factors associated with carcinogenesis include genomic alterations, phenotypic and functional changes in cells, abnormal expression of growth factors, and alterations in cell-to-cell communication. Exogenous events, such as interaction of critical molecular targets with xenobiotic agents and tissue response to mitogenic stimuli, initiate or otherwise serve to drive the cascade of events culminating in cancer development. Operational paradigms, such as the initiation, promotion, and progression scheme, are useful in helping to tease out the underpinnings of

the carcinogenic process. Recent progress in analysis of molecular factors, especially oncogene activation, offers significant opportunities to help unravel the complexities of carcinogenesis.

Among the practical considerations in carcinogenesis is the need for prudent selection of appropriate animal models to identify potential carcinogens. Two-year studies (bioassays) in which rats and mice are repeatedly given chemical agents orally or by inhalation represent the generally accepted method of identifying potential chemical carcinogens. Use of short-term animal models, such as an altered liver focus test in the rat, or use of the Strain A mouse pulmonary tumor model, provide opportunities to explore organ-specific responses following single or limited exposure to chemicals. Any data derived from animal model systems or chronic bioassays should be used as part of the weight-of-evidence for classifying a chemical agent as a carcinogen and as a potential human health risk.

FURTHER READING

PART ONE

Bosman, F.T., Visser, B.C., and van Oeveren, J. (1996). Apoptosis: Pathophysiology of programmed cell death. *Path. Res. Pract.*, 192, 676–683.

Cheville, N.F. (1994). Interpretation of acute cell injury: Degeneration, Chapter 2. In *Ultrastructural Pathology: An Introduction to Interpretation* (Cheville, N. ed.), 1st edn, pp. 51–79. Iowa State University Press, Ames, IA.

Cheville, N.F. (1994). Consequences of acute cell injury: Necrosis, recovery and hypertrophy, Chapter 3. In *Ultrastructural Pathology: An Introduction to Interpretation* (Cheville, N. ed.), 1st edn, pp. 80–123. Iowa State University Press, Ames, IA.

Cokoran, G., Fix, L., Jones, D.P., Moslen, M.T., Nicotera, P., Oberhammer, FA., and Buttyan, R. (1994). Apoptosis: Molecular control point in toxicity. *Toxicol. Appl. Pharmacol.*, 128, 169–181.

Columbano, A. (1995). Cell death: Current difficulties in discriminating apoptosis from necrosis in the context of pathological processes *in vivo*. *J. Cell. Biochem.*, 58, 181–190.

Cotran, R.S., Kumar, V., and Collins, T. (2005). Cellular adaptations, cell injury and cell death, Chapter 1. In *Robbins and Cotran Pathologic Basis of Disease* (Cotran, R.S., Kumar, V., and Collins, T. eds), 7th edn, pp. 3–46. Elsevier, Philadelphia, PA.

Davis, M.A., and Ryan, D.H. (1998). Apoptosis in the kidney. *Toxicol. Pathol.*, 26, 810–825.

Duke, R.C., Witter, R.Z., Nash, P.B., Ding-E Young, J., and Ojcius, D.M. (1994). Cytolysis mediated by ionophores and pore-forming agents: Role of intracellular calcium in apoptosis. *FASEB J.*, 8, 237–246.

Farber, E. (1994). Programmed cell death: Necrosis versus apoptosis. *Mod. Pathol.*, 7, 605–609.

Farber, J.L. (1994). Mechanisms of cell injury by activated oxygen species. *Environ. Health Perspect.*, 102(10), 17–29.

Farber, J.L. (1982). Biology of disease: Membrane injury and calcium homeostasis in the pathogenesis of coagulative necrosis. *Lab. Invest.*, 47, 114–123.

Jones, T.C., Hunt, R.J., and King, N.W. (1996). Introduction: Cells: Death of cells and tissues, Chapter 1. In *Veterinary Pathology* (Jones, T.C., Hunt, R.J., and King, N.W. eds), 6th edn, pp. 1–23. Williams & Wilkins, Baltimore, MD.

Kerr, J.F.R. (1971). Shrinkage necrosis: A distinct mode of cellular death. *J. Pathol.*, 105, 13–20.

Kerr, J.F.R., Wyllie, A.H., and Currie, A.R. (1972). Apoptosis: A basic biological phenomenon with wide-ranging implications in tissue kinetics. *Br. J. Cancer*, 26, 239–257.

King, N.W., and Alroy, J. (1996). Intracellular and extracellular depositions; degenerations, Chapter 2. In *Veterinary Pathology* (Jones, T.C., Hunt, R.J., and King, N.W. eds), 6th edn, pp. 25–56. Williams & Wilkins, Baltimore, MD.

Lemasters, J.J., Nieminen, A.L., Qian, T., Trost, L.C., and Herman, B. (1997). The mitochondrial permeability transition in toxic, hypoxic and reperfusion injury. *Mol. Cell Biochem.*, 174, 159–165.

Levin, S. (1995). Commentary: A toxicologic pathologist's view of apoptosis or I used to call it necrobiosis, but now I'm singing the apoptosis blues. *Toxicol. Pathol.*, 23, 533–539.

Levin, S., Bucci, T.J., Cohen, S.M., Fix, A.S., Hardisty, J.F., LeGrand, E.K., Maronpot, R.R., and Trump, B.F. (1999). The nomenclature of cell death: Recommendations of an *ad hoc* committee of the Society of Toxicologic Pathologists. *Toxic. Pathol.*, 27, 484–490.

Majno, G., and Joris, I. (1995). Apoptosis, oncosis and necrosis: An overview of cell death. *Amer. J. Pathol.*, 146, 3–15.

Searle, J., Kerr, J.F.R., and Bishop, C.J. (1987). Necrosis and apoptosis: Distinct modes of cell death with fundamentally different significance. *Pathol. Ann.*, 17, 229–259.

Trump, B.F., and Berezesky, I. (1998). The reactions of cells to lethal injury: Oncosis and necrosis—The role of calcium. In *When Cells Die* (Lockshin, R.A., Zkeri, Z., and Tilly, J. eds), pp. 57–96. Wiley-Liss, New York, NY.

Weinberg, J.M. (1991). The cell biology of ischemic renal injury. *Kidney Int.*, 39, 476–500.

Wyllie, A.H., Kerr, J.F.R., and Currie, A.R. (1980). Cell death: The significance of apoptosis. *Int. Rev. Cytol.*, 68, 251–306.

Zakeri, Z., Bursch, W., Tenniswood, M., and Lockshin, R.A. (1995). Cell death: Programmed, apoptosis, necrosis, or other?. *Death Differentiation*, 2, 87–96.

PART TWO

Barrett, J.C. (ed.) (1987). Mechanisms of Environmental Carcinogenesis Vols. I and II. CRC Press, Boca Raton, FL.

Borzsonyi, M., Day, N.E., Lapis, K., and Yamasaki, H. (eds) (1984). *Models, Mechanisms, and Etiology of Tumour Promotion.* IARC Scientific Publication $NO56. IARC, Lyon, France.

Iversen, O.H. (ed.) (1988). *Theories of Carcinogenesis.* Hemisphere, New York, NY.

Pimentel, E. (1987). *Hormones, Growth Factors, and Oncogenes.* CRC Press, Boca Raton, FL.

Pito, H.C. III, and Dragon, Y.P. (2001). Chemical carcinogenesis. In *Cassarett and Doull's Toxicology. The Basic Science of Poisons* (Klaassen, C.D. ed.). McGraw-Hill, New York, NY.

Pitot, H.C. (2002). *Fundamentals of Oncology*, 4th edn. Marcel Dekker, New York, NY.

Tannock, I.F., and Hill, R.P. (eds) (2004). *The Basic Science of Oncology*, 4th edn. McGraw-Hill, New York, NY.

Clinical Pathology

INTRODUCTION

Clinical pathology highlights the diagnostic and experimental aspects of *in vivo* pathology. In experimental toxicologic pathology, *in vivo* testing is an integral component of evaluation of the toxicologic potential of therapeutic agents, pesticides, and industrial chemicals. Results of hematology, clinical chemistry, and urinalysis evaluation provide information regarding the overall health status of animals, as well as general metabolic, adaptive, or toxic processes and target organs associated with exposure to toxic agents or test articles, and assist in establishing the mechanisms of toxicity in both diagnostic and experimental settings. In particular, they are necessary to evaluate adverse effects, and toxicologic dose–response relationships in non-clinical toxicology testing. These studies provide a link with clinical and morphologic pathology findings, and information regarding potential xenobiotic (test article)-adverse effects with laboratory tests.

Clinical pathology is an important tool for monitoring the onset, course, and severity of toxic insults. It is important in diagnosing disease states in a diagnostic setting or in non-clinical animal models used for safety assessment. Therefore, clinical pathology helps identify critical endpoints for determining the effects of a poisoning in the diagnostic laboratory, or dose–response changes in the experimental toxicology pathology setting. In toxicologic pathology, valuable information regarding target organ effects can be compared within and across animal species. The importance and relevance of these findings in laboratory animals exposed to a test substance is used for dose selection in chronic studies, and extrapolation to humans for risk assessment and management.

Diagnostic clinical pathology is addressed in a number of standard texts (see Suggested Reading). Many of these texts outline clinical pathology changes associated with many disease states, including poisonings by a toxicant or toxin. These tests also provide data for recommendations or requirements to support experimental study of potential therapeutic agents and other chemicals. These requirements are outlined in guidelines provided by national regulatory agencies, such as the United States Food and Drug Administration (USFDA), the United States Environmental Protection Agency (USEPA), the Canadian Health Protection and Foods Branch (HPFB), Environment Canada (EC), the Pest Management Regulatory Agency (PMRA), the European Agency for the Evaluation of Medicinal Products (EMEA), the Therapeutic Goods Administration (TGA), the Japanese Ministry of Health and Welfare (MHW), and many others. Although globally-recognized clinical pathology testing regulatory guidelines do not exist for experimental studies, a Joint Scientific Committee for International Harmonization of Clinical Pathology Testing, formed in 1992, has published minimum recommendations for clinical pathology testing in laboratory animals used in regulated safety assessment and toxicity studies.

The clinical pathology component of the toxicology study should be designed to meet specific study objectives. The elements that will be required in reporting of clinical pathology results should be fully considered at the time of protocol preparation to ensure these can be addressed. Inclusion of test parameters that have unproven sensitivity or specificity for anticipated toxicities may be worthy of evaluation in an exploratory investigative study, where the objective is to search for a potential marker of a difficult-to-monitor effect, e.g., coronary vasculitis. However, inclusion of unproven tests in definitive preclinical studies is likely to provide data that cannot be interpreted, which may cause

regulatory issues; therefore, such inclusion is not usually recommended.

Judicious study design to permit discriminating interpretation of test results requires knowledge of the characteristics of test parameters in healthy and pathological states, species differences, and causes of spurious or spontaneous variations in test results for a particular parameter and species. Test compound characteristics such as formulation, pharmacology, pharmacokinetics, and anticipated toxicity, which are based on previous experience with the compound or pharmacologic class, should be considered in selecting the species for study, sampling time points, and the parameters to be assessed.

The objective of this chapter is to provide guidance on principles of interpretive clinical pathology in species used in toxicology studies and also touch on domestic animal species of importance in the diagnostic laboratory. The interpretation of clinical pathology findings can be extrapolated from the following discussion; however, it is recommended that the reader consult standard clinical pathology texts for specific domestic animal species not covered in this chapter. This chapter is not intended to provide a comprehensive, detailed description of characteristics of all potential test parameters in each laboratory species.

In order to provide a framework for interpretation of clinical pathology test results, an overview of key features of hematology, plasma and serum clinical chemistry tests, and urinalysis follows. Based on this overview, the design of the clinical pathology component of experimental toxicology studies, and the interpretation and reporting of clinical pathology results are discussed. Finally, the importance of integrating the clinical pathology findings into other study findings in the assessment of overall safety or risk assessment is highlighted.

HEMATOLOGY

Parameters Generally Included in Study Protocols

Potential hematological effects of test articles are identified primarily by evaluation of changes in numbers of red blood cells (RBCs), white blood cells (WBCs), and platelets in peripheral blood, and evaluation of the bone marrow. Although many automated hematology analyzers are capable of flagging abnormal populations of peripheral blood cells and aberrations in cell morphology, treatment-related alterations in cell morphology should be evaluated microscopically.

A representative number of blood smears from control and high dose animals should be examined. Assessment of RBC morphology is particularly important when red cell parameters have been affected by administration of the test article. Function tests of RBCs, WBCs, or platelets are not routinely performed in toxicology studies. Such special investigative studies (e.g., neutrophil adherence, bactericidal ability, or chemotaxis; lymphocyte blastogenesis; *in vitro* and *in vivo* assays of lymphocyte effector functions; bleeding time; platelet aggregation or adhesion; release of platelet adenine nucleotides) can be conducted as required.

Erythron

In addition to changes in red cell number, red cell T parameters (hemoglobin, hematocrit), and red cell indices—mean cell volume (MCV), mean cell hemoglobin (MCH), mean cell hemoglobin concentration (MCHC), red cell distribution width (RDW)—are evaluated. In some studies, platelet indices—mean platelet volume (MPV) and platelet distribution width (PDW)—also are evaluated. Decreases in RBC count, hemoglobin and hematocrit may be proportionate or disproportionate, while increases are generally proportionate. Importantly, interpretation of red cell parameters must be made with knowledge of hydration status.

Several factors affect RBC size and hemoglobin content, in particular the stage of maturity of the cell at time of release from bone marrow. Thus, reticulocytosis usually results in increased MCV and decreased MCHC. Reticulocytes are the immature non-nucleated RBCs that contain residual RNA and mitochondria, which correspond to the polychromatophilic RBCs observed in Wright's stained blood smears. In humans, increased MCV may also occur following administration of folate inhibitors (e.g., methotrexate) that cause megaloblastic changes. RBC agglutination can produce a false increase in MCV. Low MCV may result from iron deficiency (which is an infrequent outcome of toxic insult, but not an uncommon disease process in the clinical setting), or portal systemic shunts in dogs. A true increase in MCHC does not occur, so increased values generally reflect *in vivo* or *in vitro* hemolysis. RDW is a numerical value for the variance of the size distribution curve of the RBCs and is an index of the degree of anisocytosis of RBCs. Thus, reticulocytosis and anemias with microcytosis or macrocytosis usually have increased RDW.

Quantification of reticulocytes in circulation is an index of bone marrow erythropoietic activity and responsiveness. Species differences occur in the number of absolute circulating reticulocytes in healthy animals, with up to approximately 1% in dogs and monkeys, and 5% or more in rats and mice. Usually, reticulocyte numbers are reported as absolute values. Hence, laboratories use flow cytometry to perform reticulocyte counts as a protocol-required test, irrespective of peripheral blood findings.

Leukon

Total WBC count, relative and absolute WBC differential counts, and platelet counts are integral components of most toxicology protocols. Some laboratories also report MPV and, less often, PDW, which is a measure of platelet anisocytosis. Prothrombin time (PT), which measures the extrinsic and common pathways, and activated partial thromboplastin time (APTT), which measures intrinsic and common pathways, are the coagulation tests most commonly performed.

Bone Marrow

Histopathologic examination of bone marrow is routinely performed in most toxicology studies, while cytologic evaluation of bone marrow is generally contingent on the results of peripheral blood hematology and bone marrow histopathology. Some laboratories routinely perform bone marrow differential counts using flow cytometry.

Interpretative Hematology

Understanding the fundamentals and kinetics of production, time in circulation, and fate of cellular blood elements (represented schematically in Figure 3.1) is the key to interpretation of hematology results. The pluripotent stem cell (colony forming unit-spleen or CFU-S) in marrow or spleen can differentiate along lymphoid or hematopoietic lines. Numerous cytokines or glycoproteins comprise the hematopoietic growth factors that stimulate and inhibit hematopoiesis at some level. Some growth factors are promiscuous, e.g., interleukin-3 (IL-3) and granulocyte macrophage colony stimulating factor (GM-CSF), and may affect erythropoiesis, granulopoiesis and megakaryocytopoiesis, while the growth factors erythropoietin and thrombopoietin are more restricted in their targets. Stimuli that increase stem cell input into a particular cell line may decrease the number of early progenitors being directed into other cell lines.

It can be readily appreciated from an awareness of red cell lifespan in different species that anemia due to

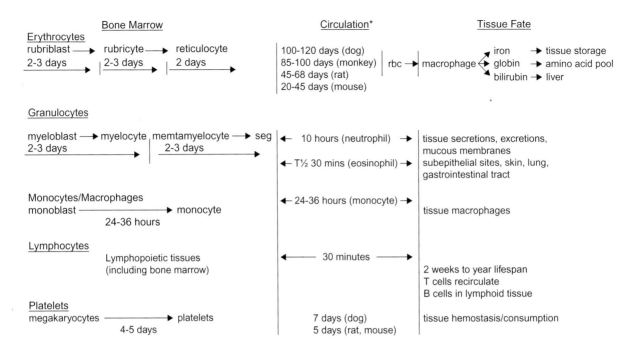

* Values represent approximate time in circulation with exception of eosinophil where value represents T½

FIGURE 3.1   Kinetics of production, approximate time in circulation, and fate of blood cells.

decreased red cell production induced by a test article would take longer to become evident in the dog compared with the rat. As a corollary example, if the RBC count in a monkey is 3.1×10^{12}/L after two weeks of test article treatment, compared with 5.9×10^{12}/L pretest (reference range $5.2–7.8 \times 10^{12}$/L), then decreased erythropoiesis can be ruled out as the primary mechanism underlying the effect. Therefore, the etiology and pathogenesis of the developing anemia is either hemorrhagic or hemolytic in nature. Also, based on circulating lifespan, it can be anticipated that agents causing direct injury to pluripotent hematopoietic stem cells or their stromal microenvironment (e.g., irradiation, chemicals, chemotherapeutics, antimetabolites, or cytotoxic agents) will manifest effects on peripheral blood granulocyte, platelet and reticulocyte counts earlier than on RBC counts.

Causes of Increases in Red Cells, Leukocytes, and Platelets

Increased numbers of blood cellular elements may occur for a number of reasons, depending on the cell line involved. Increased production of marrow progenitors with concomitant increases in peripheral blood occurs following administration of biotechnology-derived growth or colony-stimulating factors in most common laboratory animal species, even though most of these manufactured products are human proteins.

Increased tissue requirements for one or more of the blood cellular elements (e.g., following hemolysis, hemorrhage, or tissue inflammation) stimulate an increase in bone marrow production of specific cell lines that have been lost or utilized.

During a regenerative response, the bone marrow is typically hypercellular. Increased bone marrow release of reticulocytes and segmented neutrophils from the neutrophil storage pool occurs relatively soon (i.e., within hours) following onset of a stimulus. When demand exceeds the normal homeostatic rate of production, the release of less mature, larger cells such as nucleated RBCs, neutrophil bands, metamyelocytes, and large platelets ("shift" or giant platelets) may maintain an approximation of normal numbers of cells of a particular series in peripheral blood. Release of immature cells is termed a "left shift," and indicates increased demand of the given cell type in the peripheral blood or tissues. In the case of neutrophils and platelets, moderate or marked increases in counts may be observed once marrow and the spleen, especially in rodents, accelerate production and release new cells. If the demand for cells is overwhelming, the number of circulating cells will be reduced. Some toxicants (e.g., heavy metals) can cause RBCs to be released from the bone marrow.

Proportionate increases in red cell numbers, hemoglobin, or hematocrit generally reflect hemoconcentration and dehydration, which may also increase serum total protein and albumin concentrations, as well as serum blood urea nitrogen (BUN) and creatine, and urine specific gravity.

Increased peripheral blood leukocytes may reflect physiologic-, pathologic-, or xenobiotic-induced effects. Physiologic neutrophilia occurs in response to fear, excitement, or exercise, and is a mild (up to a two-fold increase), short lived (10–20 minutes) increase reflecting an epinephrine-mediated mobilization of neutrophils from the marginal pool to the circulating pool. Exogenous or endogenous corticosteroids seen in acute disease or stress induce a mild to moderate neutrophilia (generally $<25 \times 10^9$/L in dogs) accompanied by lymphopenia, eosinopenia, and occasionally monocytosis. The neutrophilia is typically seen without a left shift, and is due to increased bone marrow release of neutrophils and decreased migration of neutrophils from circulation to tissues, reflecting a shift of cells from the marginal to the circulating pool.

Inflammation occurs in response to several chemical mediators released in conjunction with tissue injury, infectious agents, or both. Cytokines and growth factors affect neutrophil proliferation, maturation, bone marrow release into blood, and tissue migration. The number of neutrophils in blood reflects the balance between the rate of tissue emigration and bone marrow release. Both total blood and circulating neutrophil pools are increased in inflammation, and a left shift may or may not be present. Mild or long-standing inflammation may not produce a left shift. When the tissue demand for neutrophils depletes the marrow storage pool of segmented neutrophils in severe inflammation, the bone marrow releases larger, less mature, neutrophils in the form of bands, metamyelocytes, and possibly earlier precursors to peripheral blood. Severe inflammation may result in white blood cell (WBC) counts in the range of 30–60×10^9/L or greater (e.g., 100×10^9/L) in dogs. The neutrophilia of inflammation is frequently accompanied by lymphopenia and eosinopenia in the dog, whereas monocytosis is an inconsistent finding. WBC counts seldom extend beyond 30–40×10^9/L in rodents or monkeys with inflammation. However, chronic lesions in older rats and mice (e.g., purulent heel sores) may be associated with WBC counts $>50 \times 10^9$/L. Lymphocytosis often contributes to the leukocytosis seen accompanying inflammation in rodents. Neutrophilia may also occur in association with hemorrhage or hemolysis. Here, a left shift and monocytosis are frequently associated with a significant hemolytic anemia.

Myeloproliferative, and more commonly lymphoproliferative disorders, are expected background findings in rats and mice on long-term toxicity studies. Myeloproliferative disorders are relatively uncommon in non-rodents, except for cats (e.g., infected with feline leukemia virus).

Increased platelet counts are occasionally observed in toxicology studies. Primary thrombocytosis, an unusual finding, is an anticipated effect when the test article is a hematopoietic growth factor such as thrombopoietin. Reactive or secondary thrombocytosis may occur secondary to catecholamine-induced splenic contraction, or to generalized bone marrow stimulation as in hemolytic anemia, blood loss or inflammation.

In addition, increased platelet production may be reflected in the presence of younger, larger platelets, called "shift platelets," which may cause increased MPV, although changes in MPV are inconsistently present. Also, a rebound thrombocytosis may follow thrombocytopenia, due to reversible inhibition of platelet production by chemotherapeutic agents.

Causes of Decreases in Red Cells, Leukocytes, and Platelets

Anemia is characterized by a hemoglobin concentration below the lower reference limit, and is broadly classified as regenerative or non-regenerative, according to the presence or absence of reticulocytosis. The term "anemia" connotes an adverse effect, and its judicious use depends on the extent of the decrease in hemoglobin. In anemic animals, decreases in RBC count and hematocrit that approximate the proportionate decrease in hemoglobin are typically observed. Decreases in red cell parameters may be caused by hemorrhage, hemolysis, or decreased marrow production. Anemia caused by decreased bone marrow production will be "non-regenerative," due to lack of production of immature RBCs. Release of immature red cells from the bone marrow or spleen via extramedullary hematopoiesis is a typical response to hemorrhage or hemolysis. Erythropoiesis will be evident from changes in RBC parameters, including increased MCV and RDW and decreased MCHC. These parameters reflect increased production and release of reticulocytes that are larger in size and have decreased hemoglobin content compared to mature RBCs. Cytologic examination of peripheral blood will show marked anisocytosis and polychromasia in the RBC population, and when the demand is extensive, nucleated RBCs can also be observed. An absolute increase in reticulocytes indicates a responsive marrow, and that the cause of anemia arises from changes outside the bone marrow, such as hemolysis or hemorrhage. This response is referred to as a regenerative anemia.

In responsive situations, reticulocytosis is observable about 48 to 72 hours following onset of anemia,

TABLE 3.1   General causes and characteristics of anemia

Parameter	Anemia			
	Decreased production	Acute blood loss	Chronic blood loss	Hemolysis
Reticulocytosis	−	+ + +	+	+ + +
Polychromasia	−	+ + +	+	+ + +
NRBC	−	+ + +	+	+ + +
MCV	Normal	↑	Normal or ↓	↓ (Extravascular) or ↑ (Intravascular)
MCHC	Normal	↓	↓	Normal or ↓
Marrow cellularity	↓	↑	Variable	↑
Serum protein	Normal	↓	Normal or ↓	Normal or ↑
Hyperbilirubinuria	−	−	−	N (Extravascular) or + (Intravascular)
Hyperbilirubinemia	−	−	−	+
Hemoglobinemia	−	−	−	N (Extravascular) or + (Intravascular)

with maximum reticulocytosis occurring about seven days post-onset. Hyperbilirubinemia, hemogolbinemia, and hemoglobinuria (the latter two with intravascular hemolysis only) may be associated with hemolytic anemia but not with anemia of decreased production or blood loss. In anemia due to decreased production or chronic blood loss, MCV is normal or decreased. Typical features of anemias of varying etiology and pathogenesis are summarized in Table 3.1.

Interpretation of the findings from hematology evaluations needs to reflect the dynamic processes involved. For example, some of the features of anemia secondary to hemorrhage may resemble those of hemolytic anemia early in the process when the bone marrow may be responsive. However, with continued hemorrhage, particularly in external hemorrhage, excessive iron loss may occur, bone marrow reserves become depleted, and the marrow fails to respond adequately. It should be noted that chronic external hemorrhage is often an occult process, and additional tests for blood in feces or urine may be needed to uncover the source of blood loss. The most common hematology findings in non-clinical toxicology studies are mildly decreased red cell parameters, usually within 10–15% of concurrent control values, without a corresponding increase in absolute reticulocyte count. These findings are often seen in animals with mild reductions in food consumption, body weight or weight gain, sometimes accompanied by mildly decreased serum total protein and albumin. All clinical and clinical pathology findings must be considered together to determine the underlying mechanism causing the effects.

In situations where an experimental procedure directly suppresses bone marrow progenitors, the time to onset of peripheral blood abnormality, and time to recovery following withdrawal of the inciting agent, depends on the bone marrow series and progenitor stage affected. Abnormalities in blood cell numbers and/or morphology can indicate toxic effects.

In health, there is a large reserve of mature neutrophils present in the marrow storage pool. However, neutrophils granulocytes in peripheral blood have a short half-life of about four to eight hours. Thus, suppression of granulopoiesis results in a rapid drop in neutrophil numbers within five to seven days. Removal of exposure to the agent causing bone marrow suppression generally results in rapid recovery, with return to approximate normal neutrophil numbers within about 72 hours. A number of drugs, such as phenothiazine derivatives and clozapine, are associated with the development of agranulocytosis. The response of granulocytes to toxic injury, mechanisms underlying drug-induced hematotoxicity via immunogenicity, accumulation of toxic metabolites, and generation of toxic metabolites within neutrophils are thought to play an important part in the development of agranulocytosis and neutropenia, in addition to toxic granulation.

The effect of bone marrow suppression has similar effects on thrombocytes. Because the lifespan of platelets in peripheral blood is relatively short (~10 days in dogs, five days in rats and mice), agents that impair thrombopoiesis result in the lowering of blood platelet counts within a relatively short time frame. Recovery of blood platelet numbers is rapid following removal of the offending agent, as platelet production

TABLE 3.2   Hematology data (mean +/− SEM): 4-week rat study

Group parameter	Control	Low dose	Mid dose	High dose
Platelets (10^9/L)	1153 ± 42	937 ± 38[a]	829 ± 17[a]	789 ± 36[a]
MPV (fL)	6.2 ± 0.1	6.6 ± 0.1	7.1 ± 0.1[a]	7.1 ± 0.2[a]

[a]Significantly different (p < 0.01) from control
MPV = mean platelet volume

time from megakaryocytes is short (around four to five days). In the example provided in Table 3.2, dose-related decreases in group mean platelet counts occurred in treated rats following four weeks administration of a xenobiotic. While further investigations are necessary to establish the cause and pathogenesis of the effect, the increased MPV seen in treated groups is suggestive of marrow responsiveness. The response of thrombocytes to toxic injury and the toxicologic implications of modulation of platelet function by a large number of xenobiotics have been implicated in immune-mediated platelet destruction in humans.

Impairment of bone marrow erythropoiesis takes longer to cause anemia, due to the comparatively longer red cell lifespan. Recovery following agent removal will start to be observed in peripheral blood within a week, because time of development from a committed stem cell to reticulocyte is about four to five days. However, recovery to circulating red cell numbers approximating pretest values may take several weeks, depending on the degree of anemia caused by the inciting agent. Since hypoxia stimulates the bone marrow to respond, a rapid response may not occur in cases of mild anemia.

While follow-up investigative studies may be conducted to explore mechanisms of treatment related anemia, neutropenia, or thrombocytopenia (e.g., ^{51}Cr RBC survival, erythropoietin quantification, or ^{111}indium platelet mean lifespan determination), definitive identification of the underlying pathological process is seldom accomplished. Protein electrophoresis, immunoglobulin quantification, and antineutrophil or antimegakaryocye antibody tests may provide added information to help define the pathogenesis and etiology. A frequently asked question following identification of treatment related thrombocytopenia in animal studies is whether platelet function has been altered. To address this question, a number of *ex vivo* evaluations can be performed, such as platelet aggregation, platelet adhesion, and clot retraction. Bleeding time, while a nonspecific and relatively crude test, can be used to investigate whether treatment-related effects on platelet numbers have *in vivo* functional relevance.

A decrease in blood lymphocyte counts in toxicity studies may reflect direct (e.g., chemotherapeutic or immunosuppressive agents), or indirect effects (e.g., inanition or stress). However, the distinction of direct from indirect causes of decreased counts is frequently difficult. Correlation of hematological findings with histopathological changes seen in lymphoid organs may clarify the situation. Total blood lymphocyte counts may remain within the reference range, despite changes in lymphocyte subsets. Similarly, some immunosuppressive drugs may interfere with T-cell function without causing overt toxicity to lymphocytes. It should be noted, however, that treatment-related changes in eosinophil counts rarely occur in toxicology studies, and basophils are seldom identified in laboratory animal species other than the rabbit. In the diagnostic setting, eosinophilia is most commonly associated with parasitism and allergic diseases.

In comparison with the diagnostic setting, changes in the morphology of blood cells occur relatively infrequently in toxicology studies. However, a representative number of blood smears from control and treated animals should be screened for altered cell morphology. Examples of treatment-related morphologic changes reported in animal studies are Heinz bodies seen in Heinz body hemolytic anemia, spherocytosis in immune mediated hemolytic anemia, schistocytosis associated with vasculitis or disseminated intravascular coagulation, and megaloblastoid red cell and neutrophil precursors associated with folate inhibitors. Parasitic diseases of erythrocytes also occur. *Plasmodium* sp organisms are often observed in blood films from cynomolgus and rhesus monkeys, and while the infections are typically asymptomatic, they do have the potential to confound hematological data interpretation.

Bone Marrow Evaluation

Bone marrow from sections of femur or sternum is generally included in the list of protocol-required tissues for histopathologic evaluation. Smears of bone marrow should be evaluated for cytological changes in situations of unexplained reductions in RBC, WBC, or platelet counts, or to investigate potential hematopoietic or non-hematopoietic neoplasia, marrow infiltrative disease, or osteomyelitis. There is limited scientific merit in performing manual differential counts on bone marrow samples from animals with a normal peripheral blood profile.

Cytological marrow evaluations include cellularity of erythroid, myeloid, lymphoid, histiocytic, and megakaryocytic hematopoietic cell lines; maturation and progression of cells within cell lines; proportion of fat cells; ratio of myeloid to nucleated erythroid cells (M/E ratio); morphology of cells; and estimation of the amount of iron present. In healthy animals about 80–90% of erythroid cells should be rubricytes and metarubricytes, and about 80% of the myeloid series should be in the maturation pool, i.e., segmented neutrophils, bands, and metamyelocytes.

Interpretation of the M/E ratio requires knowledge of the peripheral blood cell counts. An increased or decreased M/E ratio is reflective of changes in the erythroid compartment when the WBC count is normal. When the M/E ratio is high and the WBC count is normal, the anemia is likely due to erythroid hypoplasia. On the other hand, if both the M/E ratio and the WBC count are high, anemia cannot be attributed to decreased erythropoiesis with certainty, as granulocytic hyperplasia alone may be responsible for the high M/E ratio. Iron in the bone marrow is absent or reduced in iron deficiency anemia, but the marrow iron may be increased in anemia of chronic disease. Iron stores in cats cannot be estimated by microscopy.

Coagulation Tests

The intrinsic and extrinsic coagulation pathways are routinely evaluated by the activated partial thromboplastin time (APTT) and one stage prothrombin time (OSTP or PT), respectively. These assays are relatively insensitive and nonspecific, as activity of a single clotting factor must be reduced to about 30% of normal before meaningful prolongation of times occurs. However, small, statistically-significant differences between the mean values for control and treated animals for these assays are occasionally observed in toxicology studies. Although usually not biologically meaningful, interpretation of these small differences requires consideration of many factors, including, but not limited to, the pharmacologic activity of the test article, potential correlative clinical observations (e.g., retinal hemorrhage or melena), potential correlative histopathological findings (especially vascular or hepatic findings), the presence or absence of similar findings in earlier studies with the test article, and the possibility that the differences may be spurious due to iatrogenic effects during blood collection. For example, it may be more difficult to acquire

high quality blood specimens from treated animals that are smaller, in poor health, or dehydrated.

APTT and PT are insensitive measures of liver function. While the liver synthesizes most clotting factors, the large liver functional reserve means that severe liver pathology is generally required before coagulation times are affected. In the absence of obvious mechanisms for treatment-related, clinically-relevant prolongation in APTT or PT, abnormal test results can be followed by determinations of specific clotting factor activities and plasma fibrinogen concentration. Examples of disease processes that cause prolongation of APTT and PT include disseminated intravascular coagulation, decreased absorption of vitamin K, vitamin K antagonism, and liver failure.

CLINICAL CHEMISTRY

Clinical chemistry tests are routinely performed in the diagnostic setting and in toxicology studies. These tests generate information regarding metabolism of carbohydrates, lipids and proteins, and the integrity of urinary, hepatobiliary, musculoskeletal, cardiovascular, and gastrointestinal systems. Unfortunately, routinely performed clinical chemistry tests are poor indicators of central nervous system (CNS) toxicity.

Blood gas analyses may be part of a diagnostic work-up, but they are not generally a component of non-clinical toxicology protocols. When included, blood gas results may provide some relatively nonspecific information regarding respiratory and gastrointestinal systems in particular. Other gastrointestinal, pancreatic, or endocrine function tests may be conducted as a follow-up to determine the significance and relevance of initial clinical and clinical pathological findings, or to define test article effects on body systems or specific organs more accurately.

In assessing the significance of clinical chemistry and clinical pathology results in general, it is important that individual parameters are not evaluated in isolation, but rather in concert with other study findings. Thus, inspection for associations between test parameters is necessary for accurate interpretation. Common causes of increases and decreases in blood biochemistry parameters measured in non-clinical toxicology studies are indicated in Figure 3.2.

Cholesterol, Triglycerides, and Glucose

Changes in cholesterol, triglycerides, or glucose are typically reflective of general metabolic events, rather than serving as indicators of specific target organ

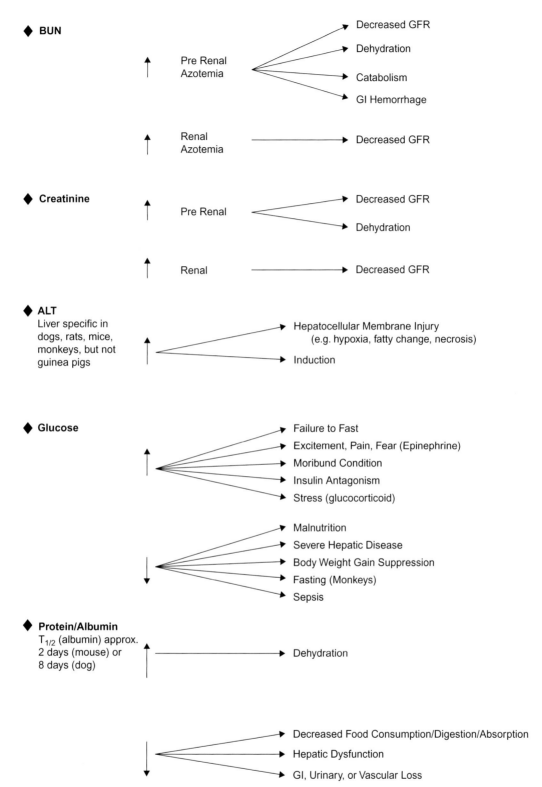

FIGURE 3.2 Some factors commonly affecting clinical pathology results in toxicology studies (GFR = glomerular filtration rate, GI = gastrointestinal).

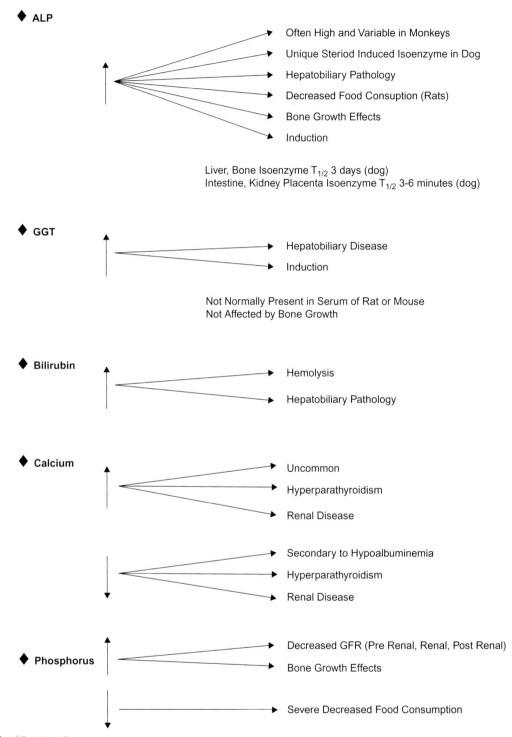

◆ ALP
→ Often High and Variable in Monkeys
→ Unique Steriod Induced Isoenzyme in Dog
→ Hepatobiliary Pathology
→ Decreased Food Consuption (Rats)
→ Bone Growth Effects
→ Induction

Liver, Bone Isoenzyme $T_{1/2}$ 3 days (dog)
Intestine, Kidney Placenta Isoenzyme $T_{1/2}$ 3-6 minutes (dog)

◆ GGT
→ Hepatobiliary Disease
→ Induction

Not Normally Present in Serum of Rat or Mouse
Not Affected by Bone Growth

◆ Bilirubin
→ Hemolysis
→ Hepatobiliary Pathology

◆ Calcium
→ Uncommon
→ Hyperparathyroidism
→ Renal Disease

→ Secondary to Hypoalbuminemia
→ Hyperparathyroidism
→ Renal Disease

◆ Phosphorus
→ Decreased GFR (Pre Renal, Renal, Post Renal)
→ Bone Growth Effects

→ Severe Decreased Food Consumption

FIGURE 3.2   (Continued)

toxicity, although cholesterol may be the pharma-cologic target of hypolipidemic agents leading to extremely low serum cholesterol concentrations at dose levels used in toxicology studies.

Cholesterol and triglycerides are derived from die-tary intake and endogenous synthesis, particularly by the liver. They are components of chylomicrons, and are eliminated via the hepatobiliary system. Cholesterol is required for the synthesis of bile acids, corticosteroids, and sex steroids. Triglycerides are a source of energy. Mild or moderate increases or decreases in serum cholesterol or triglyceride

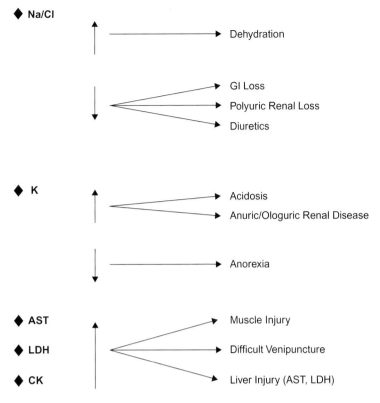

FIGURE 3.2   (Continued)

concentrations are relatively frequent findings in toxicology studies, although the exact mechanisms involved are often unknown. Several factors may be involved, including food consumption, body weight, physical activity, liver function, and hormone balance.

Serum glucose concentration depends on intestinal absorption, hepatic production, and tissue uptake of glucose. Several hormones affect homeostasis of glucose, most importantly the glucose-reducing action of insulin and the glucose-elevating action of glucagon. The maintenance of blood glucose concentrations occurs via hepatic glycogenolysis, glycolysis, and gluconeogenesis. In addition, corticosteroids, catecholamines, and growth hormone are insulin antagonists, and interfere with insulin's action on cells. Common causes of increased glucose concentrations in toxicology studies include non-fasting samples, samples from moribund animals, catecholamine release, as well as stress and glucocorticoids. In contrast, *in vitro* glycolysis, decreased food consumption, malabsorption, and hepatic disease may lead to decreased blood glucose concentrations.

Serum Proteins

The total serum protein (TP) concentration includes the total of specific proteins in plasma with the exception of those that are consumed in clot formation, such as fibrinogen and the clotting factors. Plasma protein is about 3–5 g/L greater than serum protein. Hydration status of the animal should be considered when interpreting protein changes. Hypoproteinemia, as with anemia, can be masked by dehydration. It is important to remember that hematologic and serum chemistry values will be falsely elevated in dehydrated animals. Albumin and globulins are increased proportionately in simple dehydration.

Albumin accounts for 35–50% of total serum protein concentration in animals, and for about 75% of plasma colloidal activity. Synthesis occurs in the liver. There is a direct correlation between albumin turnover and body size. For example, plasma albumin half-life is two and eight days in the mouse and dog, respectively. Occurrence of hypoalbuminemia following seven days of administration of a test compound in the rat could reflect decreased assimilation of albumin, e.g., decreased food consumption, digestion or absorption, or hepatic pathology. However, other underlying causes, such as gastrointestinal, urinary, or vascular loss of albumin would be more likely causes of hypoalbuminemia in this time frame in the dog. Albumin is considered a negative acute phase protein, and may decrease during acute inflammatory conditions.

Globulins constitute a number of heterogeneous proteins, including coagulation factors, transport proteins, mediators of inflammation, and immunoglobulins. Electrophoretic separation will identify α, β, and γ fractions. Electrophoresis, sometimes used in the diagnostic setting, is not generally included in most non-clinical toxicology protocols, but may identify fractions affected in hyper- or hypoglobulinemia. The liver synthesizes most globulins. Immunoglobulins are synthesized by B-lymphocytes and plasma cells, and are generally found in the γ fraction of the electrophoretogram, although they may extend into the β region. The most frequent causes of hyperglobulinemia are dehydration or a polyclonal gammopathy secondary to antigenic stimulation. Increased acute phase proteins, such as alpha$_2$-macroglobulin, haptoglobulin and ceruloplasmin, are frequently part of the increased total globulins in the general response to inflammation.

The albumin:globulin (A/G) ratio reflects whether changes in protein concentrations involve changes in either albumin or globulin, or both. Thus, if albumin is selectively lost through a protein losing nephropathy or is not produced, as in hepatic disease, then the A/G ratio will be low. However, if there is a concomitant loss or failure to synthesize globulins, as occurs in hemorrhage, enteropathy, exudation, and malassimilation, then panhypoproteinemia and a normal A/G ratio may occur.

Indicators of Hepatic Integrity and Function

The most commonly affected target organs of xenobiotic administration in non-clinical toxicology studies are the liver and kidneys, frequently reflecting test article tissue distribution, metabolism, and excretion patterns. The metabolic, synthetic, and excretory roles of the liver, and the enzymes required to perform these functions, result in the potential for numerous biochemical alterations in response to perturbations due to xenobiotic administration.

As the liver has large functional reserves, it is possible that a significant loss of functional tissue may occur with minimal or no detectable change in routine laboratory tests. Alterations in clinical chemistry parameters may be associated with hepatocellular injury, decreased hepatic functional mass, cholestasis, altered hepatic blood flow, enzyme induction, or altered Küpffer cell activity. Clinical chemistry abnormalities may be due to one or a combination of these events. While no single test is supreme in all situations, the pattern of findings in a selected battery of tests may indicate the location and severity of liver lesions.

Enzymes are not indicators of liver function *per se*, but rather several are indicators of cellular degeneration or necrosis and increased membrane permeability. For this reason it is incorrect to call the release of enzymes in the blood "liver function tests." The utility of an enzyme depends on a number of factors, including liver specificity, intrahepatic location, concentration gradient between the cell and serum, serum half-life, *in vitro* stability, as well as ease, accuracy, and cost of measurement.

Enzymes associated with hepatocellular integrity most commonly measured in the diagnostic setting and in non-clinical toxicology studies are alanine aminotransferase (ALT) and aspartate aminotransferase (AST). ALT is generally regarded as liver specific in dogs, nonhuman primates, rats, mice, and hamsters. Guinea pigs have low hepatocellular ALT activity, and ALT is an insensitive indicator of liver injury in this species. Increased ALT is pragmatically regarded as a specific enzyme indicator of hepatocellular injury in most species used in non-clinical toxicology studies.

Hepatocellular ALT activity is about 10 000 times greater than in serum under normal circumstances. Serum ALT activity increases within 12 hours, peaks in 1–2 days, and has a half-life of about 60 hours in dogs following toxic insult to hepatocytes. ALT activity may be misleadingly low several days after occurrence of massive liver necrosis, due to an exhausted coenzyme supply. Manual restraint methods in mice that involve grasping the abdomen may lead to increased ALT activities, presumably due to mechanical trauma to the liver. Routine handling of male C3H/HeJ mice has been reported to cause a five-fold increase in ALT activity, which suggests there is a potential for handling to affect serum enzyme activities in mice. This elevation emphasizes the importance of the use of concurrent controls handled in a similar manner in toxicology studies (Table 3.3).

Serum AST activity may be increased in hepatocellular injury; however, this is nonspecific as AST also has high activity in muscle. Cytosolic and mitochondrial AST isoenzymes exist. Serum AST activity tends to parallel serum ALT activity in liver injury. AST is present in red blood cells, and therefore hemolysis may increase its concentration in serum. The serum half-life of AST is about 12 hours in dogs. Serum ALT or AST activities may increase within hours of injury. In general, the magnitude of the increase in AST concentrations correlates with the number of affected hepatocytes, and is not an indicator of the severity or reversibility of the lesion on a pathologic basis.

Other enzymes that may be elevated due to hepatocellular injury include lactate dehydrogenase (LDH), sorbitol dehydrogenase (SDH), ornithine

TABLE 3.3 Effect of gavage dosing on plasma enzyme activities (mean ± SE) in female B6C3F1 mice

Enzyme activity	Single dose[a] (n = 6)		Seven daily doses[a] (n = 8)	
(U/L)	Not gavaged	Gavaged	Not gavaged	Gavaged
ALT	31 ± 3	81 ± 27[b]	50 ± 14	157 ± 59
AST	89 ± 16	164 ± 65	101 ± 26	377 ± 156
LDH	227 ± 14	254 ± 60	241 ± 24	475 ± 122
CK	356 ± 116	281 ± 66	181 ± 30	669 ± 233

[a]0.5% methylcellulose at 5 mL/kg body weight

[b]Significantly (p < 0.05) different from not gavaged mice

carbamoyltransferase (OCT), glutamate dehydrogenase (GDH), isocitrate dehydrogenase, and arginase. LDH is not liver specific and is used more as an indicator of muscle injury. The other named enzymes are considered liver specific; however, they are not frequently included in study protocols. SDH is very useful in horses and cattle. GDH is located in mitochondria, and consequently determination of serum GDH activity has promise as an indicator of necrosis. Theoretically, determination of GDH activity should provide data complementary to cytosolic ALT and AST cytosolic and mitochondrial isoenzymes. However, GDH is not a sensitive predictor of hepatocellular injury in some models of hepatotoxicity.

Serum albumin, cholesterol, glucose, and bilirubin are parameters commonly measured in toxicology studies that may be affected by liver function. As urea synthesis depends on hepatic uptake of ammonia absorbed from the gastrointestinal tract and subsequent liver urea cycle synthesis, liver dysfunction may lead to low BUN concentrations. However, low BUN is seldom observed in toxicology studies. Clotting factors, bile acids, and α and β globulins may also be affected by decreased hepatic functional mass. Measures of hepatic function may not be detectably altered until more than one half of the hepatocellular mass is dysfunctional or non-functional.

Cholestasis may develop due to intrahepatic biliary flow obstruction secondary to hepatocellular swelling or extrahepatic obstruction. Cholestasis may also reflect an abnormal secretory activity by hepatocytes (i.e., alterations in uptake, conjugation, and secretion), although this is rarely identified in non-clinical toxicology. Increased serum and urine bilirubin, serum bile acids and increased serum alkaline phosphatase (ALP), and gamma glutamyl transferase (GGT) activities are indicators of cholestasis. Leucine aminopeptidase and 5-nucleotidase may be increased in cholestasis, but are seldom used in toxicology protocols. The mechanism underlying increased production of ALP and GGT in cholestasis is uncertain, but may involve bile acid-stimulated synthesis. Unconjugated hyperbilirubinemia is uncommon in toxicity studies compared to diagnostic cases; its occurrence is usually due to marked hemolysis. Periportal and extrahepatic lesions generally cause greater conjugated hyperbilirubinemia than centrilobular lesions. It should be noted that serum concentration of bile acids is a relatively sensitive measure of hepatobiliary function, but is not routinely used.

ALP is a sensitive indicator of cholestasis in the dog but lacks specificity. The increased alkaline phosphatase activity may reflect the hepatic isoenzyme, but other isoenzymes, particularly bone and a glucocorticoid-induced enzyme in dogs, should also be considered as potential sources of increased ALP activity. The bone isoenzyme contributes significantly to serum activities in young growing animals, and thus ALP activities are noticeably higher in young animals. This higher activity is seen in rats, typically at about six weeks of age at study initiation. The serum half-life is about three days for liver and bone isoenzymes in dogs. The short half-life of about 3–6 minutes for intestine, kidney, and placental isoenzymes makes it unlikely that any increase in serum ALP activity will be due to these isoenzymes in dogs. However, the gastrointestinal isoenzyme contributes to serum activity in the rat to a greater extent than the liver isoenzyme. Serum GGT may be less sensitive than ALP in hepatobiliary disease in some species; however, serum activity is not affected by bone growth. Serum GGT activity in rats and mice is generally too low to be quantified in "normal" animals.

The time course of increases in hepatobiliary enzymes and serum bilirubin concentrations in a monkey with drug-induced multifocal hepatocellular necrosis and deposition of crystalline occlusions in bile canaliculi and within hepatocytes is demonstrated in Figure 3.3.

Increased serum activities of ALT, AST, ALP, and GGT may reflect enzyme induction by administered

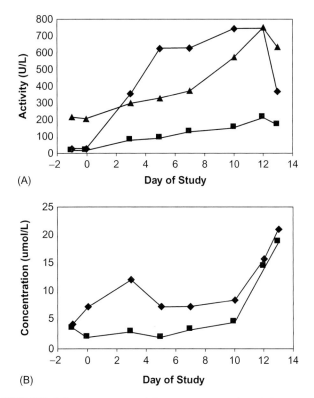

FIGURE 3.3   Time course of changes in serum clinical chemistry parameters in a monkey following daily xenobiotic administration. (a) Increased ALT (◆), AST(■), and ALP(▲) activities following daily xenobiotic administration. Moderate to marked increase in ALT by Day 3. Maximum values for each parameter occurred on Day 12. (b) Moderate increases in total (and direct) bilirubin on Days 12 and 13 following daily xenobiotic administration.

xenobiotics, rather than due to hepatobiliary injury, as can be seen after corticosteroids or anticonvulsant therapy. Most inducible enzymes are membrane associated. Increased serum enzyme activity may occur days following the inciting action, and several days to weeks may be required before peak activity is reached, so the distinction between induction and leakage may be difficult, as some xenobiotics cause both. Altered hepatic blood flow can result in hypoxia, with resultant increased hepatocellular membrane permeability and increased serum enzyme activities.

Indicators of Renal Function

Serum urea nitrogen, or blood urea nitrogen (BUN) and creatinine are used in conjunction with urine specific gravity or osmolality to evaluate renal function. BUN and creatinine are relatively insensitive to small amounts of damage to the kidney. However, the commonly quoted paradigm that damage to 75% of nephrons is required prior to an increase in BUN is not accurate in well-controlled toxicity studies, particularly in rat studies where the group size and narrow range of BUN values of untreated control rats facilitates detection of relatively small but relevant increases in group mean BUN values secondary to renal insult. By the time 75% of nephrons are non-functional, renal concentrating ability is usually impaired and urine is isothenuric with a specific gravity similar to glomerular fluid within the approximate range of 1.008 to 1.012. "Normal" BUN values do not necessarily exclude renal pathology or test article related renal effects.

Serum creatinine concentrations tend to parallel changes in BUN with renal toxicity. Creatinine diffuses throughout body water at a slower rate than urea, and takes about four hours to equilibrate; therefore, serum creatinine concentration changes more slowly compared with BUN. Endogenous creatinine clearance may be used as a measure of glomerular filtration rate (GFR).

Other potential alterations in chemistry in renal disease include: non-regenerative anemia; hyperphosphatemia reflecting decreased GFR; hyperkalemia (acute disease only); metabolic acidosis due to uremic acids; serum calcium alterations; hyponatremia and hypochloremia through urinary loss due to tubular failure; and hypoproteinemia and hypoalbuminemia in glomerular disease.

There are a number of non-renal causes for elevations in serum concentrations of BUN and creatinine. Urea concentrations can vary with hydration status, diet, gastrointestinal hemorrhage, or protein catabolism. Serum creatinine concentration is influenced by muscle mass, but is relatively independent of dietary influences and protein catabolism compared with BUN. The BUN to creatinine ratio, while not definitive, can be of value in the differential diagnosis of azotemia. Thus, in renal azotemia, BUN and creatinine can be anticipated to increase proportionately, while in prerenal azotemia, BUN may increase disproportionately.

Electrolytes

While reference ranges for sodium, potassium, and chloride electrolytes are fairly wide, the range of results in a well-controlled study is generally quite narrow. Often the reasons for small, statistically significant differences in these parameters between treated groups and controls in toxicity studies are not apparent.

Sodium (Na^+) is the major cation in serum, and the major determinant of extracellular fluid volume. Hypernatremia   generally   indicates   dehydration, although hyponatremia may occur with gastrointestinal or renal loss or hypoadrenocorticism, which is rare in toxicology studies but can be seen more commonly in the diagnostic setting.

Potassium (K^+) is the major intracellular cation, and is maintained within narrow limits because of its critical role in neuromuscular and cardiac excitability. Serum potassium is a relatively poor indicator of total body potassium, because of shifts between intra- and extracellular compartments. Increased serum potassium may occur with acidosis, due to exchange of extracellular fluid hydrogen ions for intracellular K^+ ions.

Chloride (Cl^-) is the major anion in serum. Hyperchloremia may occur secondary to secretory diarrhea or to dehydration. Vomiting may cause hypochloremia in conjunction with normal Na^+ concentrations, as chloride in the form of hydrochloric acid may be lost in excess of sodium.

Calcium and Inorganic Phosphate

Serum concentrations of calcium (Ca^{2+}) and inorganic phosphate (PO_4^{2-}) are affected by parathyroid hormone, calcitonin, and vitamin D, and represent a balance between intestinal absorption, bone formation, and urinary excretion. About 50% of serum Ca^{2+} is in ionized form, which is biologically active in neuromuscular function, bone formation, coagulation, and other physiologic processes. About 40% of serum Ca^{2+} is bound to albumin. The remaining serum Ca^{2+} is bound to anions such as citrate and phosphate. Mild hypocalcemia, secondary to hypoalbuminemia, is a common finding in toxicology studies. As ionized calcium is unaffected, signs of hypocalcemia do not occur in these studies. Hypercalcemia is uncommon in toxicology studies, but can be seen in some forms of cancer.

Hypophosphatemia may be secondary to inanition. Serum inorganic phosphorus concentrations are high in young animals. Hyperphosphatemia may occur in prerenal, renal, or post-renal azotemia, reflecting reduced GFR.

Enzymes of Muscle Origin

Increased serum activities of creatine kinase (CK), LDH, and AST occur with degenerative or necrotizing muscle injury. CK is located primarily in the cytosol. Three isoenzymes exist: CK_1 (BB) present in brain and cerebrospinal fluid (CSF); CK_2 (MB) primarily present in cardiac muscle; and CK_3 (MM) present in skeletal and cardiac muscle. Most serum CK originates from

muscle. CK is generally the most sensitive indicator of skeletal or cardiac muscle injury, with peak activity reached within about 6–12 hours. CK has a relatively short half-life of about 2–4 hours, and thus activity rapidly returns to normal following cessation of myodegeneration or necrosis. Persistent elevation indicates active muscle injury. Intramuscular injection can also elevate CK. Serum activity in healthy dogs varies with age, with pups having higher activity than adults.

Muscle, liver, and hemolyzed red blood cells are the major sources of serum LDH activity. Five isoenzymes exist, and LDH_1 (H_4) is the principal isoenzyme in cardiac muscle and kidney, whereas LDH_5 (M_4) is the principal isoenzyme in skeletal muscle and red blood cells. All tissues contain various amounts of the five LDH isoenzymes. Liver and muscle are considered the main sources of LDH. Maximal LDH activity is reached about 48–72 hours post-injury. AST may also increase with muscle damage, but AST is present in almost all tissues, and hence is nonspecific. AST activity increases more slowly than LDH levels after muscle damage.

Interpretation of relatively small changes in CK, LDH, and AST should be made with caution, as these parameters can be quite variable in healthy animals, particularly with regard to serum CK and LDH activities in nonhuman primates. Description of changes should also be made with the perspective that CK, for example, has the potential to increase over a hundredfold in generalized myopathies.

Quantification of CK or LDH isoenzymes is of no interpretive benefit in treated animals with mild increases in total serum activities, particularly if values are within or approximate the reference range, because the proportions of CK and LDH isoenzymes are variable in healthy animals. Also, there is little scientific merit in using CK or LDH isoenzyme determinations to assess myocardial toxicity at the end of a subchronic study, because the amount of tissue damage necessary to produce a clear difference between control and treated animals would likely lead to the early demise of the treated animals.

MICROSOMAL ENZYME INDUCTION

The laboratory determination of induction potential in animals is frequently conducted as a component of the safety evaluation of new drug candidates and other chemicals. The primary purpose of conducting microsomal evaluations in non-clinical safety evaluations is to determine whether hepatic microsomal induction has occurred. Conversely, such an evaluation may also detect inhibition of cytochrome P450 enzymes. While evaluation of microsomal induction would not generally be considered as part of the scope of clinical pathology evaluation, induction does have implications for the interpretation of clinical pathology results. The advantage in conducting microsomal evaluations within toxicology studies lies in the potential wealth of other data, including clinical and anatomic pathology evaluations, for purposes of correlation and comparison.

Most drugs and other xenobiotics, as well as many endogenous compounds, must be biotransformed or metabolized to more water-soluble forms before they can be eliminated from the body via two groups of reactions called phase I and phase II reactions, which often occur sequentially. Phase I metabolism consists of hydrolysis, reduction, and oxidation. This generally results in introducing or exposing a functional group, such as -OH, -NH$_2$, -SH, or -COOH. Phase II reactions which are frequently, but not always, preceded by a phase I reaction, consist of conjugation with glucuronide, sulfate, glutathione, or an amino acid, and acylation and methylation. This generally confers the bulk of any increase in water solubility to a compound.

The majority of the phase I reactions are catalyzed by the cytochrome P450 enzymes, a superfamily of heme-containing enzymes which are located in the smooth endoplasmic reticulum of many different cell types. Quantitatively, the highest cytochrome P450 concentrations, and hence most of the metabolism by cytochrome P450, occur in the liver. The subcellular component of homogenized tissue that corresponds to the smooth endoplasmic reticulum after ultracentrifugation at $100\,000 \times g$ or greater is termed the microsomal fraction.

Total cytochrome P450 content, and a variety of associated mixed function oxidase enzyme activities with degrees of specificity for the major isoenzyme forms, as well as phase II enzyme activity, can be measured relatively easily by spectrophotometric or fluorometric methods. Mixed function oxidase activities can also be determined by HPLC for a variety of substrates, such as testosterone, which although more labor intensive, provides better sensitivity and specificity. Induction or inhibition by test drugs based on mixed function oxidase activities can also be confirmed by determination of specific isoenzyme concentrations by gel electrophoresis, western blots, or ELISA.

Microsomal induction can occur, but is not commonly examined in diagnostic pathology; however, data generated in such experiments can be used to account for otherwise unexplained liver weight increases, as well as increases in serum GGT, ALT, AST, and ALP. Increased GGT activity has been used as an indirect index of hepatic enzyme induction with some compounds.

The potent and protypical inducer, phenobarbital, induces the levels and activities of multiple cytochrome P450 isoenzymes and increases GGT activity in rat liver at the same time. Phenobarbital also causes an increase in liver weight attributable to hepatocellular hypertrophy, due largely to proliferation of smooth endoplasmic reticulum and hyperplasia, and it is these associated phenomena that may be at least partly responsible for mild increases in liver enzyme markers. However, many inducers do not cause an elevation in GGT, even in the presence of increased liver weight, and therefore an absence of an increase in GGT does not necessarily mean the absence of induction.

Microsomal enzyme induction can also explain decreases in plasma or serum drug levels with repeated dosing, a phenomenon that can occur in toxicology studies as a consequence of auto induction by the test compound. This phenomenon needs to be distinguished from other causes of decreased exposure with repeated dosing, such as reduced absorption or increased excretion. In some cases even a chemical that is not metabolized can induce microsomal enzymes.

Knowledge of microsomal induction is useful in interpreting thyroid changes and alterations in thyroid hormone levels. Hepatic microsomal enzymes are important in thyroid hormone metabolism, since glucuronidation is the rate-limiting step in the biliary excretion of T$_4$ and sulfation of excretion of T$_3$. Induction of these phase II pathways, and glucuronidation in particular, by a wide variety of different chemicals can cause chronic stimulation of the thyroid gland through increased levels of thyroid-stimulating hormone (TSH). This chronic stimulation can cause changes in thyroid weight, thyroid morphologic alterations, and ultimately lead to increased tumor incidence of follicular cells. Rats are more susceptible to these hormone perturbations than nonhuman primates and humans, because rat plasma T$_4$ has a short half-life and is not tightly bound to thyroxin binding protein.

URINALYSIS

Urinalysis, usually consisting of the evaluation of physicochemical properties of the urine and sediment examination, has the potential to provide a specific evaluation of the urogenital tract, as well as information concerning systemic changes. While urinalysis is often included in non-clinical toxicology study protocols, sediment examination is more common in diagnostic cases. However, urinalysis is not used optimally in most toxicology studies, because of technical difficulties surrounding sample collection in laboratory species. Thus, urine samples are frequently taken at a single time point, such as at necropsy, rather than collected over a timed period, and determinations are made without reference to urine volume. Sample contamination may also be an issue, due to collection techniques.

In experimental toxicologic pathology, urinary electrolyte excretion determinations, particularly evident in Japanese toxicity studies, and urinary enzyme activities for the identification of renal tubular toxicity, are incorporated in some toxicity study protocols or in special investigations of potential nephrotoxins. If there are no treatment-related microscopic findings in a representative number of high dose animals, there is generally no justification for expending effort in evaluating microscopic sediment from animals in middle- and low-dose groups in toxicity studies. Over-interpretation of results of urine electrolyte excretion, including fractional clearance, should be guarded against in view of the variability among animals, and the relative lack of experience of most laboratories in performing and interpreting these investigations. Numerous studies have evaluated urinary enzymes, including β-microglobulin, ALP, GGT, LDH, lysozyme, and acid phosphatase, as specific indicators of segmental nephron injury. In addition, protein levels and protein:creatinine ratios can be examined.

Variation between laboratories makes comparison of results impossible, due to lack of standardization of methodologies. Urinary enzyme quantification may be useful in investigations designed to examine specific questions regarding nephrotoxic; however, there is no conclusive evidence to indicate that a particular enzyme or enzyme profile is superior over others as a screening tool for nephrotoxicity in general. The scientific value of conducting urinalysis, in terms of knowledge gained for labor invested, is frequently the subject of question. It is recommended that conduct of urinalysis in toxicity studies be performed under the same guiding principles as for other clinical laboratory parameters. That is, in general toxicity studies where the potential toxicity of the test article is unknown, the urinalysis component of the protocol should be efficiently designed to establish a minimum database of results which can be used as a platform for designing appropriate urinalyses in subsequent studies as required. In initial repeat dose, subacute studies, urinalysis can be used effectively to screen for

overt changes such as hematuria, pyuria, glucosuria, bilirubinuria, presence of casts, or abnormal crystalluria, as well as providing general information regarding hydration and concentrating ability via specific gravity or osmolality, acid base balance via pH, and energy balance via ketone evaluation of the animal at that point in time. In subsequent studies, such as a subchronic or special investigative study, more targeted urine determinations, such as metabolite identification and quantification, characterization of abnormal crystalluria, electrolyte fractional excretion or enzymuria determination may be added to the protocol as indicated.

INTERPRETATION OF CLINICAL PATHOLOGY RESULTS

The two fundamental questions to answer when evaluating an apparent difference between clinical pathology test results, between treated and control animals, or between post-treatment and pretest values are: "Is it real?" and "Is it bad?" The first question encompasses all the considerations that go towards deciding whether the numerical changes seen truly reflect a biological effect of treatment procedures or the test article. Since concurrent controls are not available in diagnostic pathology cases, it is important to have defensible reference standard ranges.

The answer to the question as to whether it is bad is more difficult to answer. A large number of factors have the potential to influence the interpretation of clinical pathology results. It is essential that these be taken into consideration in determining whether changes in parameters are artifacts, or real and treatment-related, or incidental. Therefore a judgement of the degree of health risk needs to be made with a knowledge of: test results in concurrent control animals and pretest values in non-rodent studies; reference ranges for the species, and the laboratory performing the analyses; variations due to artifact and limitations of analytical methodologies; appropriateness of individual tests; effects of site on sample collection; effects of species, sex and age on parameters; study design effects; statistical analysis; and biological significance.

The interpretation of a biological significant effect should be made not only on the basis of change in a parameter in isolation, but rather with a broader knowledge of clinical observations, anatomical pathology findings, other clinical pathology results—hematology, biochemistry, urinalysis—and other information as may be available, such as pharmacologic activity of test article; absorption, metabolism, distribution, excretion of test compound; toxicokinetics; liver microsomal enzyme studies; previous experience with compound or analogs; and previous experience with pharmacologic class of compound.

Potential Effects of Factors Unrelated to Test Article Treatment

Artifacts

Result artifacts may arise from a variety of causes, including improper collection techniques (e.g., clumping of platelets causes a false reduction in platelet counts, which can occur following tail bleeding in rodents); orbital sinus collection using a glass pipette, which can activate the coagulation cascade; improper specimen handling and storage (e.g., inadequate filling of collection tube); holding EDTA samples for more than four hours which leads to high MPV values in dogs and degradation of WBCs; instability of certain enzymes such as CK; hemolysis, which causes artificial decreases in RBC count and spurious increases in serum AST, LDH, inorganic phosphorus and, in some species, potassium; dilution or evaporation errors, where the anticoagulant affects cell morphology; and assay interference (e.g., factitious increases in creatinine due to cephalosporins, tetracycline interference with glucose, and interference in cases of lipemia).

Physiological Influences

Test parameters vary with respect to physiological factors in both diagnostic and experimental clinical pathology. Age is associated with typical changes with maturation of young animals of most species such as decreased reticulocytes, MCV, ALP, inorganic phosphorus, and increased RBC count, Hct, Hb, total serum protein and serum globulin concentration. Gender differences can be observed in several species (e.g., ALP, Hct, and WBC values tend to be higher in male rats). Excitement can result in alterations due to endogenous catecholamine release. Stress affects CBC and glucose results, Hct and WBC are increased in post-exercise samples of some species. Reference ranges can vary markedly in different strains of laboratory animals.

Procedural Influences

Examples of procedural or study design effects include diet with influences on glucose, cholesterol, BUN, and protein concentrations; fasting versus feeding prior to sample collection, where overnight fasting of rats may result in increased RBC, Hb, and Hct, and decreased WBC, serum glucose, BUN, ALT, and ALP; decreased food consumption or feed restriction where rats show decreased WBC and platelet counts, decreased triglycerides, cholesterol, total protein, ALT and ALP, increased serum bilirubin, and electrolyte derangements; restraint and handling methodologies where ALT and AST in nonhuman primates and mice are influenced; anesthetic effects can alter Hb and RBC counts, and increased AST and CK have been associated with ketamine administration in nonhuman primates; site of sample collection where tail samples show reduced platelet counts, total protein, and albumin compared to samples from the right ventricle of rats; repeat bleeding causes increased CK, LDH, and AST activities due to local tissue injury and anemia secondary to iatrogenic blood loss. Other aspects of study design that may affect test results include time of day of sampling, and order of sampling within a study. Therefore, failure to randomize experimental units and sample collection times can lead to differences among groups for several analytes, including glucose, AST, LDH, platelet count, Na^+, K^+, and Cl^-.

Species Differences

Species differences in clinical pathology parameters may influence the interpretation of results. For example, absolute neutrophil counts are low in healthy rats and mice ($\leq 3.0 \times 10^9/L$ and often $\leq 1.0 \times 10^9/L$) compared to dogs ($3-10.5 \times 10^9/L$). Platelet counts are higher in rats and mice (e.g., $\geq 700 \times 10^9/L$, and often $\geq 1000 \times 10^9/L$) than non-rodents ($\sim 180-450 \times 10^9/L$ in dogs and nonhuman primates).

Immature granulocytes described as ring form or "donut" cells are present in the marrow, and occasionally in the circulation of rats, mice, and hamsters. Rabbit neutrophils, called heterophils, contain many large primary granules, whereas their eosinophils have larger, more rounded granules.

Kurloff bodies are present as cytoplasmic inclusions in mononuclear cells, believed to be T-lymphocytes, in guinea pigs. These bodies occur in less than 5% of circulating white blood cells, are more common in females, especially during the first three months of life, and increase during pregnancy. Subclinical malarial infection (*Plasmodium* sp) occurs in imported cynomolgus and rhesus monkeys, which may occasionally result in an acute hemolytic anemia typical of the disease. Lymphocytes are commonly higher in bone marrow of rats and mice compared with non-rodents—up to 25% of nucleated cell count. In the rat and mouse, unlike in other laboratory and domestic species, the spleen normally contributes to hematopoiesis. Estrus-induced bone marrow hypoplasia occurs in ferrets, where an initial increase in platelet and white blood cell count is followed by pancytopenia.

APTT is several times longer in mice than for most other laboratory species, up to 110 seconds for mice versus 12–20 seconds in other species. Factor VII deficiency, present in some laboratory-bred beagles, may result in prolongation of prothrombin times and a tendency to bruising. Factor VII concentration is low in guinea pigs, giving a relatively prolonged prothrombin time (50–100 seconds) in this species. Thrombin time may also be relatively prolonged in guinea pigs.

ALP is more sensitive to cholestasis in the dog than in the rat, because the dog has a unique steroid-induced ALP isoenzyme that is synthesized in the liver. Changes in serum activity of ALP may be reflective of changes in the intestinal isoenzyme rather than the hepatobiliary isoenzyme, and may increase or decrease secondary to decreased food intake in rats. CK, LDH, and ALP tend to be higher and more variable in nonhuman primates than for other species, therefore serum GGT may be of more value in diagnosis of hepatobiliary disease in monkeys than in other species. Serum GGT activity is generally undetectable in rodents, but may increase secondary to hepatobiliary toxins or following microsomal enzyme induction. GGT is detectable in guinea pigs, rabbits, and dogs.

Bilirubinuria is a common finding in dogs and ferrets, as the threshold for bilirubin excretion is low compared with other species. Thus, serum bilirubin may be relatively slow to increase in cholestasis in these species. ALT is insensitive and nonspecific as a marker for hepatocellular injury in guinea pigs, reflecting low concentrations in the liver and high concentrations in other tissues, such as muscle. Also, ALT has higher mitochondrial concentration compared to its cytosolic distribution in guinea pigs. Subclinical enzootic hepatitis A infection in cynomolgus and rhesus monkeys causes ALT increases, thus potentially confounding interpretation of ALT changes during toxicology studies. This increased activity correlates with seroconversion to the virus.

Rats, mice, and nonhuman primates have high red blood cell K^+ concentrations; hence, hemolysis will give spuriously high serum K^+ concentrations in addition to LDH, AST, and, to a lesser degree, PO_4 and bilirubin concentrations. Red blood cell K^+ concentrations are relatively low in most breeds of dogs and in ferrets. Total serum Ca^{2+} is higher in rabbits (up to 4 mmol/L), compared to other species. This high serum Ca^{2+} leads to technical difficulties when performing coagulation tests.

Serum cholesterol may be high in healthy hamsters, and LDH and CK are increased in Syrian hamsters with hereditary myopathy. For an unknown reason, unmodified routine methods yield falsely elevated concentrations of albumin in rabbits as compared to electrophoretic values. Total serum protein, albumin, and globulin concentrations tend to be higher in nonhuman primates than other laboratory species. In addition, serum electrolyte values may be higher and more variable in unanesthetized monkeys (e.g., $Na^+ \leq 170$ mmol/L, and $Cl^- \geq 125$ mmol/L).

Spontaneously Occurring Disease

Clinical pathology is used to help attain a definitive diagnosis in the diagnostic setting. Specific disease processes and conditions alter the clinical pathology parameters in such a manner that a diagnosis can be made. In experimental toxicologic pathology, awareness of spontaneously-occurring syndromes in the species under study is necessary. When such occurrences influence post-treatment values, determination of treatment effects can be confounded. For example, the clinical pathological features of necrotizing polyarteritis or "beagle pain syndrome" can complicate interpretation of toxicity studies. Affected dogs typically demonstrate pain, fever, stiff gait, neutrophilia, decreased red cell parameters, decreased albumin, increased α-2-globulins, thrombocytosis, and necrotizing arteritis and periarteritis. This idiopathic syndrome is considered to be a latent condition, the expression of which can be precipitated in predisposed dogs by experimental treatment.

Another example is the occurrence of a spontaneous wasting syndrome in marmosets. The characteristics of this syndrome are poor weight gain or weight loss, muscle atrophy, alopecia, diarrhea, and colitis. Here the clinical pathological features are macrocytic normochromic anemia, hypoproteinemia, hypoalbuminemia, increased serum AST and ALP, and thrombocytosis. Additionally, proteinuria is a common finding in control rats and mice, especially males, and severity increases with age and development of chronic progressive nephropathy.

Comparators: Concurrent Controls, Reference Ranges

Relevant comparators for interpreting clinical pathology results in toxicology studies are appropriately matched concurrent control animals. However, reference ranges provide an ancillary comparator database for consideration in overall interpretation of test results, and are critical to making a diagnosis in the diagnostic laboratory.

Reference ranges are generally constructed statistically to include the range of values found in 95% of a population of healthy individuals. There are many points for consideration when using reference ranges, and over-reliance on reference ranges may lead to potential misinterpretation of results. For example, it can be anticipated that 1 out of 20 results for a specific test from a group of "normal" animals will be outside the historical reference range. In addition, reference ranges set cut-off points that may result in high false positive or false negative rates.

Results within the reference range for a parameter or group of parameters associated with an organ do not ensure that the organ and its functional or metabolic processes are normal. Unfortunately, animals with severe organ pathology may still have clinical pathology values within the reference range. For example, liver enzymes may be within the reference range in dogs with cirrhosis, white blood cells may be within the reference range in leukemia in rodents, and serum potassium concentrations may be within the reference range despite body and intracellular depletion. The performance of a reference range depends on the population and conditions from which the reference range was derived, as well as the temporal relationship of when the analyses of data constituting the reference range were generated, compared to test study data.

Development of in-house reference ranges is essential, as many variables affect test results, and reference ranges for a certain species of a particular age and sex will only be truly appropriate for the in-house laboratory and the conditions under which the test values were derived. Most variables affecting test results are physiological, procedural, or due to artifacts.

Statistical Analyses

In experimental toxicologic pathology, the first stage in the analysis of continuous data should be to check for homogeneity of variances, as equality of variances in a set of samples is an important precondition for several statistical tests, including ANOVA and t-tests. The information from this preliminary test dictates whether parametric or nonparametric tests should be used.

Most laboratories assume that the variances in their data are homogeneous, and use parametric statistical tests. Clinical pathology data sets frequently do not display a Gaussian distribution, and the skewed distribution may produce too many statistically-significant results in the ANOVA and t-tests. There are so many differences in the variance patterns from one test to another that attempting to use one or two statistical approaches to accurately determine the toxicologic significance of the results of the panel of 30 to 40 clinical pathology tests commonly used would be difficult. Trend tests are useful; however, the use of multiple doses in safety assessment studies results in many borderline differences that are difficult to interpret. Thus, statistical analysis should not be regarded as the ultimate decision-making tool in determination of treatment-related effects, but rather should be used to aid pattern recognition. Final decisions on the biological significance of clinical pathology results must be based on sound biomedical judgement.

In many toxicologic pathology studies, treatment-related changes in clinical pathology test parameters are clearly evident as statistically-significant, dose-related effects. However, interpretive challenges occur when test results in treated animals differ from concurrent controls not in a dose-related manner, particularly when the changes were unanticipated based on previous studies conducted with the test compound or analogs, or with agents of the same pharmacologic class, and when changes are not accompanied by corroborative morphologic pathology findings.

Direct Versus Indirect Effects

Direct and indirect effect of exposure to toxic substances affects both the diagnostic and experimental wings of toxicologic pathology. Once it is established that the change relates to treatment, or accidental poisoning, the importance of the change and relevance to exposure of the intended population or population at risk needs to be established. Thus, it is essential to determine whether the change is due to primary effects of the substance in question, or is a secondary effect. For example, a number of changes in clinical pathology parameters can be expected to occur secondary to decreased food consumption and body weight gain suppression or body weight loss, in rodent studies and domestic animals. Such changes may include hemoconcentration, lymphopenia, decreased platelet count, total protein, globulin, cholesterol, triglyceride, inorganic phosphorus, ALT, ALP, increased bilirubin, and electrolyte derangements. Also, a fatal fasting syndrome can occur in monkeys secondary to anorexia for any reason. This syndrome is characterized by uremia, fatty change of liver and proximal convoluted renal tubules, tubular atrophy, and pancreatic necrosis. Results of samples collected from animals *in extremis* must be interpreted with caution, as multiple and severe derangements in clinical pathology parameters may relate to the moribund state, rather than directly to toxicity.

Pharmacologic Versus Toxic Effects

It is unlikely that the separation of pharmacologic versus toxic effects will be needed in diagnostic pathology, as cause of death definition is the goal. However, treatment-related effects might reflect pharmacologic activity rather than toxic effects of test article administration. For example, decreased serum globulin concentrations occur in rodents administered antibiotics, likely reflecting the effects of altered microbial populations on antigenic stimulation and immune response.

Biological Importance of Treatment-related Effects

Judgement is required in determining whether a treatment-related change is important in the assessment of potential toxicity of a compound, or a suspect toxin or toxicant is the cause of death in the diagnostic setting. For example, changes in analytes such as MCV, cholesterol, and triglycerides caused by high doses of test articles may reflect altered metabolic or adaptive changes, but may not be important regarding potential toxicity compared to changes such as compound related neutropenia, thrombocytopenia, or increased ALT. Factors for consideration include whether the test result indicates that the animal's health is compromised clinically or biologically, correlation between clinical, clinical pathological, and pathological findings, as well as the magnitude of the change.

An essential component of the interpretation of test results is to communicate the severity of treatment-related changes. This is generally done in comparison to concurrent control, pretest, or reference range values. To simply use qualifiers such as "minimal, mild, moderate, or marked" is inadequate, as these terms are subjective according to individual experience. More instructive is to add a tangible perspective wherever appropriate, such as stating the numerical change with respect to reference standards among groups, or by provision of the actual value for the treated animal or group mean and the appropriate comparator.

There are several aspects that should be considered when interpreting the potential toxicologic importance of clinical pathologic findings. Knowledge of the characteristics of the test parameter is essential in arriving at an accurate perspective. The inherent analytical error must be taken into account. For example,

inherent error is approximately 5% in automated WBC counts; therefore, attempting to interpret very small changes in WBC counts is of no merit. Thus, interpretation of leukocyte numerical changes should focus primarily on absolute counts, and less so on relative differential counts.

Understanding of the extent of biological variation in the parameter in health is important. As BUN concentrations and reference ranges in young, fasted, untreated control rats fall into a narrow span, relatively small differences within a group mean values between treated and control values may be of biological significance. In contrast, wild-caught and purpose-bred nonhuman primates have wide reference ranges for serum CK and LDH activities, and undue importance should not be attributed to mild to moderate changes in these parameters.

Temporal and kinetic characteristics of the parameter must be considered in result interpretation. For example, due to the relatively long RBC survival time in all species, significant decreases in RBC counts in short-term studies, or in acute disease processes, should not be attributed to impaired bone marrow production, but rather to potential blood loss or hemolytic processes. However, over the same time, neutropenia could be a reflection of impaired neutrophil production, in view of the short half-life of circulating neutrophils. Similarly, since albumin has a half-life of about eight days in the dog, hypoalbuminemia in a short-term study is not likely due to decreased food intake or decreased liver synthesis, but should be interpreted as indicative of albumin loss from the body (e.g., acute external hemorrhage, gastrointestinal or urinary loss, or less commonly, vascular loss).

Knowledge of the characteristics of the parameter in the species tested is important: for example, moderate changes in ALP may be of no toxicological relevance in monkeys due to the inherent variability of this parameter in this species. Also, information regarding a subpopulation of cells may be important; absolute lymphocyte counts may be within the reference range even though a subpopulation, such as CD4 lymphocytes, is absent.

Interpretation of changes in a particular parameter should be made with knowledge of values of other analytes that may be pathophysiologically linked. For example, attribution of increased serum ALP concentrations in young dogs to either bone growth or treatment-related hepatobiliary effects would be influenced by evaluation of serum GGT, bilirubin, ALT, and urine bilirubin values. Values for RBC count, serum creatinine, total protein, albumin, globulin, and urinalysis will influence attribution of increased BUN to prerenal, renal, or post-renal causes. Investigation of the etiology and pathogenesis of hyperbilirubinemia will include critical evaluation of RBC count, hemoglobin, ALP, GGT, ALT, and urine bilirubin determination.

Knowledge of the pharmacokinetic or toxicokinetic characteristics of the test material in the test species may help place clinical pathology findings in perspective. If administration of a xenobiotic leads to induction of its own metabolism, this could explain why some abnormalities noted early in a study may return to approximate concurrent control or pretest values later in the study. There may also be associated increases in serum activities of inducible enzymes, such as ALP and GGT. Failure to elucidate dose-related increases in clinical pathology test parameters may reflect erratic, non-dose-related absorption of test compound, or saturation of absorption beyond a threshold dose.

REPORTING OF CLINICAL PATHOLOGY FINDINGS

The clinical pathology section of a toxicology study report should clearly identify treatment-related changes and their relationship to dose and gender, as well as their severity and potential reversibility (where applicable). There should be a distinction between biologically-relevant and statistically-significant findings, with identification of background changes and a justification as to why these are not considered treatment-related.

Appropriate use of terminology is important in accurate conveyance of the nature of findings. For example, terms such as pancytopenia, leucopenia, neutropenia, lymphopenia, and anemia must be used accurately, as these terms imply severity of effects. Such terminology should not be used to describe relatively mild decreases with concurrent controls or pretest values that may be statistically significant, but remain within or very near the reference range for the species. These changes are best described factually as decreases compared with concurrent controls and appropriate quantifiers used. It is recommended that use of the term "significant" be restricted to description of statistically significant results.

Reports should not be a simple listing of results and statistically-significant changes, the importance of which is left up to the reader to determine. Therefore, wherever possible, the clinical pathology component of the diagnostic or experimental report should support the overall reporting of the potential toxicity or effects of the test article in the experimental situation, or the suspected exposure that led to the request for diagnostic pathology.

SUMMARY

Clinical pathology relates to descriptive, functional and time-related changes in parameters assessed when the animal is alive. As a diagnostic tool, clinical pathology is often core to effecting diagnoses. The role of clinical pathology in the evaluation of the toxicologic potential of therapeutic agents, pesticides, and industrial chemicals in laboratory animals also occurs during the live phase of non-clinical evaluation, and relies on hematology, clinical chemistry, and urinalysis. Numerous factors (e.g., artifacts, physiologic and procedural effects, spontaneously occurring syndromes, and species differences) have the potential to influence the interpretation of clinical pathology results, both in the diagnostic and experimental settings, and it is essential that these be considered prior to determining what changes reflect a specific disease entity or effects induced by a test article during non-clinical evaluation.

In the experimental situation, the most important and relevant comparators for interpreting results are findings in matched, concurrent control animals. Statistical analysis should be used to aid pattern recognition, but interpretation of the toxicologic importance and relevance of findings must be based on sound biomedical judgement. The associations between clinical pathology parameters, and correlations of clinical pathology results with other study findings (e.g., clinical signs, microsomal enzyme analyses, anatomic pathology, and toxicokinetics), are essential for accurate interpretation of clinical pathology results. Treatment-related effects should be distinguished as direct (primary) or indirect (secondary), and toxic or pharmacologic, and the severity of the effects, dose relationships, and relevance to overall animal health addressed. Clinical pathology results integrated with other study findings often provide important information regarding mechanisms of toxicity, dose–response relationships of target organ effects across different laboratory animal species, as well as the importance and relevance of study findings to humans or animal species potentially exposed to the test article.

FURTHER READING

Boone, L., Meyer, D., Cusick, P., Ennulat, D., Bolliger, A.P., Everds, N., Meador, V., Elliott, G., Honor, D., Bounous, D., and Jordan, H. (2005). Selection and interpretation of clinical pathology indicators of hepatic injury in preclinical studies. *Vet. Clin. Pathol.,* 34, 182–188.

Feldman, B.F., Zinkl, J.G., and Jain, N.C. (2000). *Schalm's Veterinary Hematology*, 5th edn. Lippincott Williams & Wilkins, Baltimore, MD.

Foster, J.R. (2005). Spontaneous and drug-induced hepatic pathology of the laboratory beagle dog, the cynomolgus macaque and the marmoset. *Toxicol. Pathol.*, 33, 63–74.

Hall, R.L., and Everds, N.E. (2003). Factors affecting the interpretation of canine and nonhuman primate clinical pathology. *Toxicol. Pathol.*, 31(Suppl), 6–10.

Harvey, J.W. (2001). *Atlas of Veterinary Hematology. Blood and Bone Marrow of Domestic Animals.* W. B. Saunders Co., Philadelphia, PA.

Latimer, K.S., Maheffey, E.A., and Prasse, K.W. (2003). *Duncan and Prasse's Veterinary Laboratory Medicine Clinical Pathology*, 4th edn. Iowa State Press, Ames, IA.

Loeb, W.F., and Quimby, F.W. (eds) (1999). *The Clinical Chemistry of Laboratory Animals*, 2nd edn. Taylor & Francis, Philadelphia PA.

Lumsden, J.H. (1998). "Normal" or reference values: questions and comments. *Vet. Clin. Pathol.*, 27, 102–106.

Solter, P.F. (2005). Clinical pathology approaches to hepatic injury. *Toxicol. Pathol.*, 33, 9–16.

Stockham, S.L., and Scott, M.A. (2002). *Fundamentals of Veterinary Clinical Pathology.* Iowa State Press, Ames, IA.

Thrall, M.A., Baker, D.C., Campbell, T.W., DeNicola, D., Fettman, M.J., Lassen, E.D., Rebar, A., and Weiser, G. (2004). *Veterinary Hematology and Clinical Chemistry.* Lippincott Williams & Wilkins, Baltimore, MD.

Weingand, K. et al (1996). Harmonization of animal clinical pathology testing in toxicity and safety studies. *Fund. Appl. Toxicol.*, 29, 198–201.

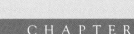

CHAPTER

4

Nomenclature: Terminology for Morphologic Alterations

INTRODUCTION

What is in a name? A name is a word, or set of words, by which a person, animal, place, or thing is known, addressed, or referred to. The word pathology originated as an English word in the early seventeenth century. Pathology is defined as a medical science that deals with all aspects of disease, with special reference to the structural or functional changes that result from the disease processes. Pathology includes evaluation of tissue from the living (antemortem/biopsy which is also called surgical pathology), as well as from the dead (postmortem/necropsy/autopsy) to identify the disease process and its cause. The major subspecialties of pathology are anatomical, pertaining primarily to the gross and microscopic study of tissues and organs, and clinical, pertaining primarily to the study of fluids (blood, urine, etc.) obtained from the living patient.

The anatomic pathologist evaluates, interprets, and names macroscopic (gross) and microscopic (histologic)

structural (morphologic) changes, so as to define the disease process, as well as its site, severity, and duration. The name given to the change or lesion is called a diagnosis, referred to as a morphologic diagnosis. A morphologic diagnosis is not the only type of diagnosis given by the pathologist. Other forms of diagnoses include etiologic diagnosis, which names the cause or agent, and definitive diagnosis, which names the disease.

Morphologic changes seen by the pathologist are rarely pathognomonic; a term that indicates that the morphologic diagnosis has only one etiology. Because identical lesions can arise as a common endpoint for a number of causes, usually a differential diagnosis list is created naming all possible causes of the altered morphology, with the most likely given as the tentative etiologic diagnosis. In fact, to make a definitive diagnosis, most altered morphology must take other findings, e.g., clinical signs, clinical pathology, and microbiology results, into consideration in order to establish the most likely cause.

Further subspecialization of anatomic pathology into diagnostic and toxicologic pathology is common in veterinary medicine, although the principles remain the same. Diagnostic pathology uses an approach aimed at determining the definitive diagnosis through establishing a morphologic, etiologic, and then a definitive diagnosis. Toxicologic pathology can be defined as the evaluation of morphologic changes for evidence of toxic injury. In most cases, toxicologic pathology occurs in an experimental setting, following exposure *a priori* to potentially toxic agents (commonly called test articles) at concentrations that cause tissue alterations. The pathologist in the diagnostic setting must work from a somewhat different perspective, since dose response, and often just plain dose information, are not available. In this instance the pathologist must rely more heavily on history, clinical signs, ancillary tests, and circumstantial data to arrive at an etiologic diagnosis. Nevertheless, in both cases reliable pathology data are essential for interpretation of the toxic effects, and potential risk, and for understanding the biological mechanisms by which toxicologic lesions develop and differences occur in species responses.

In most experimental studies, laboratory species, previously exposed to known concentrations of a test article, are examined *postmortem* for non-neoplastic and neoplastic changes. The changes occurring in treated groups are compared against those occurring in control groups, and against each other, to determine whether or not the test article induces a morphologic effect, and if an effect is observed, to establish the dose response and a no observed (adverse) effect level (NOAEL). Morphologic alterations in such studies may be directly or indirectly related to administration of the test substance. Concurrent disease or confounding variables other than the experimental exposure must also be taken into account.

The findings from a toxicologic pathology study frequently form the basis of regulatory decisions concerning hazard identification and dose response assessment following exposure to many socially and economically important drugs and chemicals. Regulatory agencies often base their decisions regarding the potential toxicity and carcinogenicity of a test article primarily on increases in site-specific effects in animals; these data are used in risk assessment. The toxicologic pathologist in the experimental setting provides information identifying the hazard and the dose response to the test article; the regulator determines the exposure and hence estimates the risk of these findings in humans.

Because histopathological diagnoses are based on subjective observations, the diagnostic or morphologic terminology used to classify lesions is crucial for analysis and interpretation of the data derived from animal toxicological studies. Communication of histopathological findings is embodied within the terminology of diagnoses, as errors or inconsistencies in the terminology used for specific structural changes could significantly affect hazard identification and risk assessment. Diagnostic terminology, or nomenclature, should therefore be as precise, unambiguous, and clear as possible, in both the diagnostic and experimental situations, if an accurate picture of the important morphologic changes is to be made. In particular, regulatory toxicology requires mutually-exclusive variables, each diagnosis should not overlap with another, e.g., all benign tumors should not include a malignant tumor and *vice versa*. For this reason, it is essential to minimize the overlap in nomenclature defining different disease processes, so that mathematical comparison can be made.

BASIC TERMINOLOGY

Most terms used in pathology are derived from classical Greek, and secondarily from Latin roots. A list of classical sites, prefixes, and suffixes can be found in Tables 4.1, 4.2, and 4.3. Using these roots, the approach to making a diagnosis is hierarchical and permits much flexibility and complexity in the range of diagnostic terminology used. A diagnosis is made by sequentially designating the topography (Table 4.1), including as many as three hierarchical terms: (1) organ; (2) site within an organ; and, if necessary (3) a sub site of increasing specificity within sites. The disease process includes morphologic terms, which are used to describe the major pathologic processes or abnormalities occurring in an organ or tissue. Qualifiers specify distribution, duration, character, and severity, and are applied in conjunction with morphologies to further define or characterize the abnormalities.

TERMINOLOGY ISSUES

Since diagnostic pathology addresses individual or small groups of animals, there is typically more flexibility in defining and naming the disease process in each case. Rodent toxicity and carcinogenicity studies, on the other hand, have complex designs and incorporate large numbers of animals. They require statistical comparisons among treatment groups; hence, standardized nomenclature is necessary to make these

TABLE 4.1 Anatomical sites

Root	Site	Uses
Abdomen	probably from abdo, to conceal	abdominal
Acetabulum	small vinegar cup; acetum—vinegar, i.e., acetic acid	acetabulum (receives the head of the femur)
Acr, Acro, Acromion	extremity; topmost shoulder (Gr) akros + omos; acropolis	acromium of the scapula
Adi, Adipose	fat (adeps)	adipose tissue
Amnion	fetal membrane (Gr)	amniotic cavity
Ampulla	narrow-necked jar (ampora) (ampla + bulla—full + vase)	aeminal ampulla
Andro	male (Gr)	androgenous
Angi	vessel	angiomatous, angioplasty
Ankle	angle or corner (angulus)	ankle, hock
Anus	ring (L), the Roman word anus means old woman, from the skin being wrinkled	anululus, anus
Aorte	raise (Gr aeiro), lift something up in order to carry it; some think it comes from aer + tepeo—to keep air, since the Greeks believed Aa contained air; also may be from a sheath which carried a knife with a large, curved handle called an aorta	aorta, aortic
Arcuatus	bow-shaped (arcus)	arcuate vessels of the kidney
Areola	little area; area referred to the open space of a Roman stadium; areola of the breast is probably a corruption of aureolus (golden)	mammary areolae (nipples)
Artery	to keep air (arteria; Gr aer + terein)	arterial wall
Arthron	a joint	arthrology, arthritis
Arthron, Articular, Articulus, Artis	joint (Gr)	articular cartilage, articulated joint
Atrium	entrance hall or open court forming the principal room of an ancient Roman house with no windows and a fireplace in the center; probably from ater (black), due to sooty walls; in the cadaver the altered blood discolors the walls of this chamber	cardiac atria
Auris, Auricular	ear, ear-shaped	auricular cartilage
Axon	axle (Gr)	neuronal axons
Brachium	arm (Gr brachion)	brachial
Bronchus	moisten (Gr breichen), windpipe; Plato thought drinks passed through here (rather than the esophagus), accounting for its moistness	bronchial
Bucca (Bukka)	cheek	buccal cavity
Capillary	hair-like (capillus—hair from capitis + pilus—hair of the head)	capillary bed
Carcino	a crab or cancer	carcinoma, carcinogenic
Cardiac	of the heart (Gr kardia)	cardiac failure
Cauda	tail (cadere—to fall)	caudal lobe, cauda equina
Cava, Caverna, Cavus	hollow, cave as in cavity	vena cava
Cele	a swelling	hydrocele, hematocele, mucocele, cystocele, meningocele, encephalocele
Cephalos, Ceps, Cipital, Capitis	(Gr kephale), caput, capitalis—head	cephalos, ceps = head (Gr kephale); caput, capitalis
Cervix	cervicis—neck	cervix
Chondros	(Gr for granule), cartilage	chondrocyte, endochondral bone
Cochlea	snail (Gr kokhlos—land snail)	cochlea (inner ear)
Colon	large intestine (Gr kolon possibly from koilos—hollow, for it is often found empty during dissection)	colonoscopy

(Continued)

TABLE 4.1   (*Continued*)

Root	Site	Uses
Commisura	a joining together, commit	
Concha	shell	nasal turbinates or conchae
Condyle	knob (Gr kondylos—knuckle)	femoral condyle
Coronary	pertaining to a wreath or crown	coronary arteries
Cortex	rind, bark of tree or any outer covering	adrenal cortex
Costa, Costae	rib(s)	costo-chondral junction
Coxa	hip	coxofemoral joint
Crani	head	cranium, cranial (towards the head)
Cranio	skull (Gr)	cranial fracture
Cubitus	tip of finger to elbow	decubital ulcers
Cyte	cell (Gr kutos)	hepatocyte
Dens, Dentis	tooth, dens also called odontoid process	dental caries
Dermis, Derma	skin (Gr)	dermatitis, dermis, epidermis, dermatology
Diaphragm	between partition/fence, to barricade (Gr dia—completely, phrassein—enclose)	diaphragmatic hernia
Digitus	finger, toe	digital trauma
Dorsum, Dorsal	back	dorsal fin
Ductus	leading	ductus arteriosus
Duodenum	twelve each, 12 finger widths (duo + decem—two and ten) duodenum = twelve each	duodenal ulcer
Dura mater	hard mother, "tough mama"	subdural hemorrhage
Encephalon	brain; enkephalos—brain or simply "in the head"; cephalos—head Gr	encephalitis
Entero	intestine (Gr)	enteritis
Esophagus	esophagus	esophageal obstruction
Fasces	bands	muscle fascia
Femur	thigh, of thigh	femoral artery
Fibula	pin for holding clothes together (Gr perone)	fracture of the fibula
Foramen, Foramina	hole/s (foro—I pierce)	foramen ovale
Ganglion	swelling under the skin (Gr)	autonomic nervous system ganglia
Gaster, Gastro	stomach, belly-shaped (Gr)	gastric carcinoma
Gland (Glans), Glandula	little acorn; originally used for mesenteric lymph nodes	pineal gland
Glans	a pellet of lead or clay that was slung at the enemy	glans penis
Glossa/Glottis	tongue (Gr), lingua	glositis
Hem, Hemato	blood (Gr)	hemorrhage
Hepatic	relating to the liver (hepatis)	hepatitis
Histo	tissue (Gr)	histopathology
Humerus, Humeri	shoulder(s), bone of the arm or upper extremity	humeral fracture
Ileum	twist (Gr eilo), ilium means flank	ileal mucosal atrophy
Incus	anvil	middle ear bone
Infundibulum	funnel	infundibulum of mamillary body or oviduct
Inguen, Inguinis	Groin, abdominal	inguinal hernia
Ischium, Sciatic	Gr ischion—hip, ischys—strength; pronounced iskium or ishium	wing of the ischium

TABLE 4.1 *(Continued)*

Root	Site	Uses
Jejunus	hungry, wanting, empty; jejune is that part of the intestine that was usually found to be empty by early anatomists.	jejunum (small intestine)
Kera, Cera	kera—horn (Gr), as in keratin	keratitis (inflammation of the cornea) triceratops = three-horned face
Labium, Labia	lip(s) curved edge of a vessel was called a labium	labial erosion
Larynx	gullet (Gr larungao—to scream)	laryngitis
Ligamentum	bandage (ligare—to bind bone to bone in anatomy); ligaments connect bone to bone	ligaments
Lingua	tongue (Gr glossa/glottis)	sublingual dosing
Lumbus	loin, lower back	lumbar puncture
Lympha	pure spring water	lymphatic system
Mamma, Mammillary	breast, of the breast	mammillary body
Mandibula, Mando	chew, jaw	mandible
Maxilla	maxilla	maxillary osteomalacia
Mediastinum	servant, drudge	mediastinal lymphoma
Meninx, Meninges	membrane(s) (Gr)	meningitis
Mesentery	around intestine (Gr mes + enteron)	mesenteric tear
Metra	uterus (perimetrium, myometrium, endometrium)	pyometra
Mitos	thread	mitosis
Mitral	resembling a miter (mitra) a two-peaked hat, such as the Pope wears	mitral valve
Myelon	marrow, spinal cord (Gr); myelencephalon becomes the medulla oblongata	myelitis
Myo	muscle	myocarditis
Nasus	nose—nasus, rhin—nose	nasal obstruction
Navel	center of the hub of a wheel (Middle English nave), umbilicus—navel	navel
Nephro	kidney (Gr), renalis—kidney	nephrology
Neuron	nerve, sinew	neuronal degeneration
Occiput	lower back of head (occipio—I begin or commence); may be from the fact that the back of the head usually comes out first in birth	occipital swelling
Ocular	eye	ocular discharge
Oculus	eye; optic, ophthalmos—eye (Gr)	ocular discharge
Oo, Ovum	egg	oophoritis
Orkhis	testis (Gr), orchiectomy—remove a testis, also spelled orchidectomy; orchid plant so named because the shape of its root suggests a testis	orchitis
Os, Oris	mouth	oral administration
Os, Ossis (Osteo)	bone	osseous metaplasia
Oto	ear (Gr)	otolith (ear stone) otitis media
Palpebra	eyelid (palpitare—to move quickly, pant, as in palpitate)	palpebral fissure
Pancreas	all flesh (Gr pas + kreas)	pancreatitis
Ped, Pes	foot (pes, pedis), pod—foot (Gr)	podiatry
Peritoneum	encircling stretch (Gr peri + teino)	peritonitis
Pharynx, Pharyngeal	throat (Gr pharanx—cleft, chasm); Greeks used pharynx for larynx	pharyngitis
Phleb	vein (Gr)	phlebotomy

(Continued)

TABLE 4.1   (*Continued*)

Root	Site	Uses
Phrenic	diaphragm or mind (Gr phren, phrenos), as in frenzy; in Homer phren referred to the heart region, uncertain exactly how it became associated with the diaphragm	phrenic nerve
Pia mater	pious mother (pius—tender, affectionate, devout, faithful); protective covering around brain and spinal cord—the most faithful layer of the CNS	inflammation of the pia mater
Pleura	side, rib (Gr)	pleurisy
Pneumo	lung, air (Gr), pulmonarius—lung	pneumonia
Popliteal	behind knee (poples, poplitis—ham), a ham is the thigh cut of meat	popliteal lymph node
Prostates	to stand before, one on the front rank (Gr pro + istanai), the organ that stands before the bladder; NOT the same word as prostrate, to lay flat, from the Latin prosternere	prostatic hyperplasia
Pulmonarius	lung, pneumo—lung, air (Gr)	pulmonary edema
Pyo	pus (Gr)	pyogenic infection
Sarco	flesh (Gr sarkos)	sarcoma
Seminalis, Semen	Seed	seminal vesicles
Septum, Septa	wall(s), paries, parietes—wall(s) (Gr)	nasal septum
Soma	body (Gr)	somatotropin
Splanchnic	supplying the viscera (Gr splanchnikos—entrail, viscus)	splanchnic circulation
Steno	narrow (Gr)	aortic stenosis
Stroma	framework (bed)	connective tissue stroma
Synovia	"together egg" (Gr syn—together; L ovum—egg); presumably referred to the egg-white-like nature of synovial (joint) fluid, but Paracelsus used it in a general way, so his original meaning is obscure	synovitis
Theca	enclosed, envelope, sheath	ovarian thecal cells
Thorax	piece of armour that protected the chest and abdomen (Gr); Plato restricted the term only to the chest region, which Galen followed	pneumothorax
Thymus	thyme (Gr thymos); possibly from thyme being burned as incense during sacrificial burnings of the gland; or it is related to thymos, as in vital force or sensibility, the heart used to be regarded as the seat of sensibility, and this gland overlies it	thymic involution
Thyroid	large shield shape (Gr thyreos)	thyroiditis
Tibia	musical pipe, such as one bar on a pan flute, if a tibia is broken at one end it resembles a musical pipe, shin-bone is probably from skin bone, from the fact that the tibia is easily palpable	tibial chondrodysplasia
Trachea	rough (Gr trachea); Aristotle thought the aortic artery carried air, and named them smooth aortic artery and the trachea a rough artery	tracheotomy
Urachus	urine holder (ur + echo)	part of the fetal urinary system that closes perinatally
Vagus	wandering, as in vagrant; early anatomists were struck by the fact that it "wanders" to many organs	vagal indigestion
Vas, Vasa	vessel; a vascular organ is one that has a profuse blood supply	vasa vasorum
Ventricle	little belly (ventriculus, venter)	ventricular arrhythmia
Vertebra, Vertebrae	joint(s), something turnable, vertere to turn, as in revert, invert, divert, subvert, convert, introvert, extrovert, advert, and other perversions of "to turn"	vertebral fracture
Viscera	organ, entrails (viscus), thick and gooey stuff that oozes out, as opposed to flows	visceral lesion

TABLE 4.2 Common prefixes

a(d)- ... towards	a(n)- ... without	ab- ... from
ab(s)- ... away from	ad- ... towards	allo- ... other, another
ambi- ... both	amphi- ... on both sides, around	ana- ... up to, back, again, movement from
aniso- ... different, unequal	ante- ... before, forwards	anti- ... against, opposite
ap-, apo- ... from, back, again	bi(s)- ... twice, double	bio- ... life
brachy- ... short	cata- ... down	circum- ... around
con- ... together	contra- ... against	cyte- ... cell
de- ... from, away from, down from	deca- ... ten	di(s)- ... two
dia- ... through, complete	di(a)s ... separation	diplo- ... double
dolicho- ... long	dur- ... hard, firm	dys- ... bad, abnormal
e-, ec- ... out, from out of	ecto- ... outside, external	ek- ... out
em- ... in	en- ... into	endo- ... into
ent- ... within	epi- ... on, up, against, high	eso- ... I will carry
eu- ... well, abundant, prosperous	eury- ... broad, wide	ex-, exo- ... out, from out of
extra- ... outside, beyond, in addition	haplo- ... single	hapto- ... bind to
hemi- ... half	hept- ... seven	hetero- ... different
hex- ... six	homo- ... same	hyper- ... above, excessive
hypo- ... below, deficient	im-, in- ... not	in- ... into, to
infra- ... below, underneath	inter- ... among, between	intra- ... within, inside, during
intro- ... inward, during	iso- ... equal, same	juxta- ... adjacent to
kata- ... down, down from	macro- ... large	magno- ... large
medi- ... middle	mega- ... large	megalo- ... very large
meso- ... middle	meta- ... beyond, between	micro- ... small
neo- ... new	non- ... not	ob- ... before, against
octa- ... eight	octo- ... eight	oligo- ... few
pachy- ... thick	pan- ... all	para- ... beside, to the side of, wrong
pent- ... five	per- ... by, through, throughout	peri- ... around, round-about
pleo- ... more than usual	poly- ... many	post- ... behind, after
pre- ... before, in front, very	pros- ... besides	prox- ... besides
pseudo- ... false, fake	quar(t)- ... four	re, red- ... back, again
retro- ... backwards, behind	semi- ... half	sex- ... six
sept- ... seven	sub- ... under, beneath	super- ... above, in addition, over
supra- ... above, on the upper side	syn- ... together, with	sys- ... together, with
tetra- ... four	thio- ... sulfur	trans- ... across, beyond
tri- ... three	uni- ... one	ultra- ... beyond, besides, over

comparisons possible. Microscopic examination of the tissues is often the most time-consuming phase of such studies. During this lengthy process, several factors can directly influence the diagnostic terminology, and consequently, the quality of the pathology data.

Training

The type of training that the pathologist has received can influence terminology. Most anatomic pathologists are trained in 'a clinical setting, where each animal case is considered unique. In this setting, the primary objective of diagnostic toxicologic pathologists is to identify the cause of disease or death for an individual animal or small group, and communicate the findings in a detailed fashion, so that each disease process is identified and recorded as a separate entity. Absolute consistency in terminology among cases is not a major concern if the pathologist adequately communicates the pathogenesis and definitive diagnosis to the clinician and other pathologists.

TABLE 4.3   Common suffixes

-ase ... fermenter	-ate ... do	-cide ... killer
-c(o)ele ... cavity, hollow	-ectomy ... removal of, cut out	-form ... shaped like
-ia ... got	-iasis ... full of	-ile ... little version
-illa ... little version	-illus ... little version	-in ... stuff
-ism ... theory, characteristic of	-itis ... inflammation	-ity ... makes a noun of quality
-ium ... thing	-ize ... do	-logy ... study of, reasoning about
-megaly ... large	-noid ... mind, spirit	-oid ... resembling, image of
-ogen ... precursor	-ol(e) ... alcohol	-ole ... little version
-oma ... tumor (usually)	-osis ... full of	-ostomy ... "mouth-cut"
-pathy ... disease of, suffering	-penia ... lack	-pexy ... fix in place
-plasty ... re-shaping	-philia ... affection for	-rhage ... burst out
-rhea ... discharge, flowing out	-rhexis ... shredding	-pagus ... Siamese twins
-sis ... idea (makes a noun, typically abstract)	-thrix ... hair	-tomy ... cut
-ule ... little version	-um ... thing (makes a noun, typically concrete)	

The situation is different in an experimental setting, where the emphasis is on identifying changes in relation to a defined treatment group under rigorously controlled conditions, rather than in an individual animal. Specifically, the goal of the experimental toxicologic pathologist is to determine whether there are differences in the incidence and severity of a specific lesion in treated groups when compared to control animals and across doses. Study pathologists must still identify the various tissue lesions, but generally have less freedom in the type and number of diagnoses that they may record; consistency and brevity are essential in the statistical evaluation and interpretation of their findings.

A morphologic diagnosis is a qualitative judgement on the nature of a specific lesion and its apparent or expected biological behavior. Each diagnosis is a subjective observation, the accuracy of which depends on the totality of the pathologists' training and experience, the state of knowledge of the specific disease process, and the generally accepted diagnostic criteria and nomenclature within the profession. The proficiency of the pathologist can influence how lesions are interpreted, and hence the selection of diagnostic terminology.

Because most training occurs in a diagnostic setting and is focused on domestic animals, trainees usually are not exposed to the common background lesions of laboratory animals. Often this leads to selection of inappropriate terminology by the novice experimental toxicologic pathologist evaluating rodent studies. Other common errors committed by novice toxicologic pathologists include the use of multiple morphologic descriptive terms or synonyms for a lesion or disease process; inconsistencies in the designation of topography, sites and subsites; and duplication of diagnoses. Data

generated in such a manner can have dire consequences when reviewed by regulatory agencies.

Multiple Pathologists

The size of some toxicologic pathology studies can require that more than one pathologist is assigned to the study. The practice of using multiple pathologists to evaluate a single study or a series of related studies may cause variation in the diagnostic terminology used within and between studies. Due to the volume and breadth of toxicity and carcinogenicity bioassays, this practice often becomes unavoidable.

Because the training, experience, and abilities of pathologists differ, classification of lesions, the thresholds for lesion diagnosis, or severity grading may differ. This is not unexpected, since the observations are subjective. In addition, philosophical differences between pathologists or individual biases can influence the diagnostic terminology selected and, consequently, the consistency in the pathology data. For example, one pathologist may elect to combine the spectrum of lesions observed under a single diagnostic term, e.g., chronic active inflammation. Another pathologist, however, may choose to diagnose each lesion individually using the diagnostic terms inflammation, fibrosis, squamous metaplasia, regenerative hyperplasia, histiocyte infiltrate, and alveolar proteinosis. Arguments can be made for both approaches.

Problems occur when comparing results between studies, particularly when comparing different studies on the same chemical, or if similar lesions in the rat and mouse studies were diagnosed differently. These problems may be amplified when the lesions are subtle or controversial, or there is disagreement as to the nature of the lesion(s) observed. For example, reactive or regenerative epithelial hyperplasia adjacent to treatment-induced ulceration or an area of inflammation may be recorded by one pathologist and ignored by another, who considers it a component of the spectrum of lesions associated with, and secondary to, ulceration.

Diagnostic Drift

Diagnostic drift is the phenomenon whereby variations in the application of diagnostic terminology or criteria occur during the histopathologic evaluation of a study. The microscopic examination of the tissues in a toxicological study may be performed over an extended period. Diagnostic drift is a result of such extended evaluations. The criteria used for diagnosing lesions are influenced by many qualitative and quantitative factors, and maintaining consistency over the long course of the histopathologic evaluation is sometimes a challenge. The selection of multiple terms, or a variety of modifiers for the same or, morphologically or pathogenically, similar lesions may be the most common form of diagnostic drift.

Terminology may also change as the pathologist realizes the full spectrum of treatment-related effects. This may result in the application of slightly different diagnostic and grading criteria to distinguish between closely related lesions over the course of a microscopic evaluation, e.g., hyperplasia versus early adenoma. Substantial delays between the evaluations of individual dose groups can exacerbate this tendency. In fact, the amount of time between the original examination of the control and high dose tissues, and subsequent examination of tissues from lower dose groups may be enough to allow minor differences to occur within diagnostic criteria for a specific lesion.

Severity grading of lesions is especially susceptible to diagnostic drift, particularly if the lesions are subtle and the treatment groups are known. In other cases, updated information obtained from the literature or from scientific meetings may change the way in which certain lesions are diagnosed during the course of the evaluation. The result of diagnostic drift is inconsistent use of diagnostic terminology, which may falsely create or mask treatment-related effects.

Lesion Complexity

The complexity or composition of morphologic features may affect diagnostic terminology used for classification. In these situations, some pathologists may elect to diagnose each component of the lesion, while others may elect to use a single general term to embrace the spectrum of changes present. This decision is influenced by training, experience, or the objectives of a specific study. In addition, synonymous terms exist for many lesions, and individual pathologists may have preferences or biases for alternative terms, based on their training and experience, e.g., the terms fibrosis, organization, and scarring have the same meaning.

In general, lesions with similar characteristics and pathogenesis at a particular site should be consolidated in as few diagnoses as possible, preferably as a single diagnosis that reflects the biological significance of the pathologic process. Excessive splitting of diagnoses may lead to inconsistency in diagnosis, and the masking of a treatment-related effect. A complex lesion that serves as an illustration is the spontaneous age-related renal disease that occurs in F344 rats. Microscopic features include alterations of the renal tubule, such as degeneration, regeneration, dilatation, and the presence of protein casts, plus other components, such as glomerulonephritis, glomerulosclerosis, interstitial fibrosis, chronic inflammation, and mineralization. Various labels for this syndrome include chronic nephrosis, progressive glomerulonephrosis, glomerular hyalinosis, and spontaneous glomerulosclerosis. The histomorphological appearance of the syndrome may vary among individual animals, depending on the age of the animal and the degree of severity of disease. However, the vast majority of affected rats exhibit similar changes and disease progression. Thus, it has been suggested that the characteristic changes are classified under the single diagnosis of "nephropathy." To diagnose each element of nephropathy separately clutters the data, provides no additional useful information, and causes difficulty in analysis and interpretation. In addition, the danger inherent in such a practice is inconsistent diagnosis. As a caveat, when using a single term, such as nephropathy, to cover a spectrum of changes, it is important to clearly define and characterize the term in the pathology narrative.

Conversely, situations exist in which diagnosing each component of a complex lesion is more appropriate. In general, multiple diagnoses should be used when important information about the pathogenesis or biology of a lesion must be conveyed. For example, squamous cell papillomas in the forestomach of rodents may occur secondary to focal ulceration which is often also accompanied by chronic submucosal inflammation and squamous epithelial hyperplasia. Frequently, some component of the lesion is absent in some tissue sections; primary ulceration and inflammation along with papillomas may be the only lesions observed. In other sections, prominent squamous epithelial hyperplasia may be observed with or without ulceration or papillomas; whereas, in still other sections all lesions may be observed. In this situation, it would be improper to combine the non-neoplastic changes under a single diagnosis of ulceration, because information critical to understanding the pathogenesis of the forestomach papillomas would be lost.

Standardized Nomenclature

Toxicologic pathologists have long recognized the need for a harmonization and standardization of nomenclature and diagnostic criteria among rodent studies conducted at different laboratories throughout the world. The lack of a universally accepted, standardized, system of nomenclature has resulted in confusion, controversy, additional costs and delays in the product review and approval by regulatory agencies.

Recent advances in computer technology have now made possible the usage of computer-based systems to capture pathology data. Well-designed systems can facilitate data recording, generate summary and statistical tables, and improve consistency among in-house pathologists. While computerized systems are inherently efficient, they may also exacerbate the lack of standardization that exists for diagnostic terminology.

Many institutions and laboratories have developed in-house computerized pathology data acquisition systems, or use commercially available systems with unique lexicons of diagnostic terminology. Often these lexicons are not standardized, and may be discordant with established standardized nomenclature systems, such as those used by the Society of Toxicologic Pathologists (STP) or the National Toxicology Program (NTP).

Some systems can be restrictive in the available diagnostic terms, while others are overly flexible, in that they do not limit pathologists to the terms already in the lexicon. Other software may even allow pathologists to build his or her personal diagnostic vocabulary. The availability of an excessively wide range of possible diagnostic terms can be a source of confusion and inconsistency for the experienced and inexperienced pathologist alike, let alone the individual who must evaluate the findings and is not trained in pathology.

Recording Pathology Data

In experimental toxicologic pathology, the pathologic diagnosis is the foundation of data collection. As previously mentioned, a diagnosis is made by sequentially designating topography, disease process, and qualifiers in terms of magnitude, distribution, duration, etc. Qualifiers consist of many terms, which permit a variety of possible combinations and permutations in the final diagnosis. In many recording systems, any variation in topographical, morphologic or qualifier designations may define separate and distinct diagnosis categories when tabulated. It is therefore possible for pathologists to record more than one diagnosis for each type of lesion identified. The result is a lack of independence among variables, with violation of the assumptions used in most statistical analysis.

In some situations it may be best to refrain from using site qualifiers. As an example, for generalized inflammation in hollow organs or tissues that have surface epithelia, e.g., the nose, stomach, gastrointestinal tract, or urinary bladder, the use of qualifiers that indicate specific sites (lumen, epithelium, mucosa, submucosa), may not be appropriate. In such instances, differences in lesion distribution may simply reflect the overall severity of the inflammation.

Similar to site qualifiers, distribution qualifiers are used to indicate an inherent feature of a lesion that has a particular biological significance, or is a reflection of a specific pathogenesis. For example, centrilobular hepatic necrosis rarely has the same pathogenesis as hepatic necrosis that is multifocal and randomly distributed; therefore, it is important to include this type of modifier. Likewise, it may be toxicologically relevant to the interpretation of a study to know whether hyperplasia of the forestomach is focal versus diffuse. Conversely, the use of distribution qualifiers is usually not warranted for common background or age-related lesions. The extent of such lesions is best conveyed by the use of severity grades.

Severity grading is the application of a subjective semi-quantitative score to a lesion or process to denote the extent of tissue involvement, the degree of tissue damage, or a combination of these parameters. Severity grades are not absolute; rather they represent degrees of changes relative to similar lesions in other animals in a study. Systems of severity grading and the subjective score vary in usage among pathologists. The following four-term system of severity grading is frequently used: "1 = minimal, 2 = mild, 3 = moderate or 4 = marked." A fifth category, "5 = severe," is sometimes incorporated to denote histopathological alterations that are especially profound, or perhaps related to the death of the animal.

It is important that pathologists in the experimental setting adequately define the grading criteria so that results are reproducible by the same, or other, pathologists. Severity grades are useful when making dose-related comparisons of qualitative changes, e.g., increases in average severity with increasing dose, or when comparing the relative toxicity of structurally-related compounds. Severity grades are generally reserved for non-neoplastic lesions, whereas neoplasms are considered either present or not present, i.e., quantal. For some non-neoplastic lesions, however, severity grading adds little valuable information. Examples include ocular cataract or cysts of the pituitary, pars distalis.

A few separate rules exist for the terminology applied to neoplasms. For neoplasms, each diagnosis should indicate whether the lesion is primary, i.e., arising within the tissue of origin, or metastatic. By convention, for neoplasms arising at sites distant from the primary, the qualifier "metastatic" is added to the diagnosis, and the site of the primary lesion indicated parenthetically. An example would be: lung—neuroblastoma, metastatic (nose). Also by convention, it is assumed that neoplasms not designated as metastatic are primary. For most neoplasms, the diagnosis should indicate whether the lesion is benign or malignant. While this is usually taken care of by separate terminology, e.g., adenoma versus adenocarcinoma, some neoplasms do not have terminology for malignancy, e.g., neuroendocrine cell tumor (stomach), pheochromocytoma (adrenal medulla).

Diagnoses for neoplasms should not contain site qualifiers that signify a gross or subgross location of the lesion, unless such qualifiers serve to distinguish the histogenesis of one neoplasm from another. For example, the site qualifiers "C-cell" or "follicular cell" should be used to distinguished carcinomas of the thyroid gland. The occurrence of multiple and bilateral neoplasms should be indicated, especially when this occurrence appears to be a treatment-related phenomenon. Examples include: "liver—hepatocellular adenoma, multiple," and "kidney, tubule—adenoma, bilateral." Finally, inflammation and other types of paraneoplastic changes may result from the presence of neoplasms in any given tissue. These secondary lesions are usually not meaningful to the study and, therefore, should not be recorded as diagnoses.

SUGGESTED PRACTICES

Terminology problems originating from training may be addressed by adjusting the manner in which pathologists are trained. Training programs for potential toxicologic pathologists must include a solid foundation in the pathology of common laboratory animals, which should include knowledge of the nature and distribution of common background and toxicant-induced lesions, common tissue-specific responses to toxicants, and the terminology used in diagnostic pathology. In addition, training in experimental design and interpretation is important. For the inexperienced pathologist, histopathologic evaluation should initially be performed in consultation with more experienced pathologists, and laboratories performing and evaluating toxicological studies should have procedures for comprehensive review and mentoring of trainee pathologists. Whenever practical, a pathology peer review should be incorporated into the histopathologic evaluation process.

Subchronic, chronic toxicity or carcinogenicity studies are usually conducted in male and female rats and mice. In the ideal situation, one pathologist should evaluate the control and treated groups of both sexes of the test species, since some chemicals are likely to cause similar effects, and comparisons of effects between the species are inevitable. In situations where this practice is not feasible, good communication among pathologists can maintain consistency. Comparison of lesions among pathologists conducting evaluations is essential, as they must be aware of the exact nature of the lesions observed in all sexes and species. Internal pathology peer reviews conducted before the data are finalized are also highly desirable. By working together, pathologists can lessen the potential for inconsistencies in diagnostic terminology.

Diagnostic drift can be minimized as follows. Initially, it is helpful to examine a few animals from the control group, and from each dose group, to determine the salient treatment-related altered morphology. For example, the various treatment groups can be evaluated in replicates of 5 or 10, starting with the controls and high-dose groups and, subsequently, the mid- and low-doses. It should be emphasized that the pathologist needs to be aware of treatment group and not be "masked" (i.e., not given any information about treatments) for the most efficient and useful study evaluation. From the onset of the histopathologic evaluation, pathologists should establish and use a limited set of diagnostic terms, and clearly define the morphologic criteria used for classifying lesions under the terms utilized. In addition to establishing a diagnostic "dictionary" that is specific to a study, this preliminary evaluation allows the pathologist to set thresholds for severity grading, if grading is needed. The overall goal of this exercise is to facilitate the consistent application of diagnostic terminology and criteria, and also to acquaint the pathologist with the range of lesion severity, further facilitating consistency in diagnostic criteria used for grading of lesions. At the end of the initial evaluation, and at the completion of the histopathologic evaluation, the diagnostic dictionary can be reviewed for duplications in terminology, the use of inappropriate terminology for topography, sites and morphology, and for terminology that is inconsistent with previous studies performed on the same or related compounds. If computerized systems are used to record lesions, pathologists should be completely familiar with the system used, with particular respect to the manner by which the system compiles diagnoses, and sorts and analyses microscopic diagnoses.

To address issues associated with lack of standardized terminology, initiatives have been started to harmonize diagnostic terminology by developing an internationally-recognized system of nomenclature for lesions of laboratory animals. There have been a number of these initiatives in the past, and at present there is a multinational effort to standardize nomenclature on an international basis, "International Harmonization of Nomenclature and Diagnostic Criteria for Lesions in Rats and Mice"—INHAND. Previous initiatives include, but are not limited to, "Standardized System of Nomenclature and Diagnostic Criteria (SSNDC): Guides for Toxicologic Pathology" (available at the Society of Toxicologic Pathology website http://www.toxpath.org/ssndc.asp), and "WHO/IARC: International Classification of Rodent Tumors" created by the International Agency for Research on Cancer (IARC). Information contained in the IARC fascicles has been combined with historical control data from carcinogenicity studies, and entered into an electronic database: the "Registry Nomenclature Information System" (RENI). The specific goal of the present and previous initiatives has been to reduce the confusion created by the plethora of diagnostic terms currently in use, to improve the accuracy and consistency of pathology data generated, and to facilitate the evaluation and interpretation of the results from rodent toxicological studies.

Several published texts are excellent sources of standardized nomenclature. The *Pathology of the Fischer Rat*, Boorman (1990), and the *Pathology of the Mouse*, Maronpot (1999), are authoritative and comprehensive pathology reference texts of both spontaneous and induced lesions observed in the Fischer 344 rat and the B6C3F1. The terminology in these texts is based on the National Toxicology Program (NTP) database of millions of extensively peer-reviewed histopathological slides from more than 500 short- and long-term toxicity and carcinogenicity studies conducted under the auspices of the NTP. The diagnostic categories included in these texts are based on standardized diagnostic criteria for the pathology terminology utilized

by the NTP. The mouse text also contains references to lesions of transgenic mouse strains, and mechanistic considerations. Additional reference texts include *Pathobiology of the Aging Rat*, ILSI Monograph Series, 1992; *Pathobiology of the Aging Mouse*, ILSI Monograph Series, 1996; *Rat Histopathology*, Greaves and Faccini, 1984; and *Mouse Histopathology*, Faccini, Abbott and Paulus, 1990.

Due to the subjective nature of pathology, peer review (PR) should be incorporated into the histopathologic evaluation process whenever practical, so as to verify the accuracy of the toxicologically significant microscopic findings, to ensure that the treatment-related effects are properly identified, to confirm that lesions are diagnosed similarly, and to check that the terminology used is contemporary, i.e., quality assurance (QA)/quality control (QC) of the data.

Pathology PR may be prospective or retrospective. In prospective PR, the general design for the review is included in the study protocol, and the pathology data are not final until the review has been completed. In contrast, retrospective PR is conducted after the pathology data is finalized. Basic protocols have been established, in which the reviews of chronic and subchronic studies are flexible and appropriately based on study results and on the size, duration, complexity, and purpose of each particular experiment.

Many institutions routinely conduct an informal PR of the pathology data. This usually entails a review of the original diagnoses by a second pathologist who is a member of the same institution. Such reviews typically do not have standard operating procedures or study-specific protocols, they are often poorly-documented, and it is the responsibility of the study pathologist to finalize the data. Other institutions perform a more formal and rigorous PR, which involves separate Quality Assessment and Pathology Working Group reviews by pathologists outside the institution. This form of PR promotes a higher level of confidence in the pathology data and result interpretations. It follows standard operating procedures, and requires a study-specific protocol that states the extent of the review and the tissues to be examined.

SUMMARY

Pathology has often been considered an art as well as a science, due to the subjective nature of the observations. Such a consideration is very useful for diagnostic pathology, but can cause significant problems in toxicologic pathology. Discerning differences between control and treatment groups and properly communicating these differences to the scientific community is the essence of toxicologic pathology. The goal for toxicologic pathologists is to report findings in a manner that facilitates comparison of the data among related studies. A systematic approach to the diagnosis and documentation of lesions, and the consistent application of a standardized system of nomenclature, are essential elements for assessing comparative toxicologic effects of different or structurally-related chemicals.

FURTHER READING

Crissman, J.W., Goodman, D.G., Hildebrandt, P.K., Maronpot, R.R., Prater, D.A., Riley, J.H., Seaman, W.J., and Thake, D.C. (2004). Best practices guideline: toxicologic histopathology. *Toxicol. Pathol.*, 32, 126–131.

Dua, P.N., and Jackson, B.A. (1988). Review of pathology data for regulatory purposes. *Toxicol. Pathol.*, 16, 443–450.

Faccini, J.M., Abbott, D.P., and Paulus, G.J.J. (1990). *Mouse Histopathology. A Glossary for Use in Toxicity and Carcinogenicity Studies*. Elsevier, Amsterdam, The Netherlands.

Faccini, J.M., Abbott, D.P., and Paulus, G.J.J. (eds) (1984). *Rat Histopathology. A Glossary for Use in Toxicity and Carcinogenicity Studies*. Elsevier, Amsterdam, The Netherlands.

Haschek, W.M., Rousseaux, C.R., and Wallig, M.A. (eds) (2002). *Handbook of Toxicologic Pathology*, 2nd edn, Academic Press, New York.

Mohr, U. (ed.) International Agency for Research on Cancer (1992). *International Classification of Rodent Tumors Part 1: The Rat. 2. Soft Tissue Tumors and Musculoskeletal System*. IARC Scientific Publications., No. 122.

Society of Toxicologic Pathology. *Standardized System of Nomenclature and Diagnostic Criteria (SSNDC) Guides*. www.toxpath.org/ssndc.asp.

Society of Toxicologic Pathology. *International Harmonization of Rat Nomenclature*. www.toxpath.org/nomen.asp.

Society of Toxicologic Pathology. *International Harmonization of Nomenclature and Diagnostic Criteria for lesions in Rats and Mice (INHAND)*. www.toxpath.org/inhand.asp or www.eurotox-path.org/nomenclaure/index.php.

Society of Toxicologic Pathology. *Bibliography*. www.toxpath.org/bibliography.asp.

Society of Toxicologic Pathology. *Best Practices*. www.toxpath.org/positions.asp.

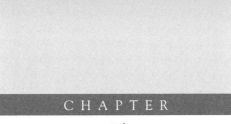

CHAPTER

5

Techniques in Toxicologic Pathology

INTRODUCTION

Toxicologic pathology concerns the effect of potentially noxious products on the body. The question being asked about the product (test substance) usually involves its safety for humans or its efficacy as a medicament, but can also involve exposure to an environmental toxicant under "natural" conditions. The typical context for most toxicologic pathologists in the pharmaceutical and most academic research situations is intentionally controlled exposure of laboratory animals to xenobiotics as surrogates for humans. The animal phase of toxicological studies is very comprehensive in the pharmaceutical setting, and also often less so but nevertheless rigorous in the academic setting. Characterizing the morphologic response of exposed animals is an early but important step among many, to establish the risk to humans who may be exposed to the same test substance or environmental contaminant. As an example, a description of the current US National Toxicology Program (NTP) follows. Like other toxicologic investigations, this program evaluates chemicals for toxic and carcinogenic effects in laboratory

animals. The description, although succinct, indicates clearly the scope of the endeavor:

"Ordinarily, a toxicology and carcinogenesis study of a chemical comprises an integrated approach of toxicological characterization: chemical disposition (absorption, distribution, metabolism, excretion); genetic toxicology (including assays of gene mutations in bacteria and in mammalian cells, chromosome effects and transformation in mammalian cells, and DNA damage and repair); fertility and reproductive assessment (sperm morphology and vaginal cytology); systemic toxicology (14-day and 90–120 day exposures); specific studies as appropriate (immunological, biochemical, neurological, inhalation toxicology, and activated oncogenes); clinical pathology where applicable (hematology, urinalysis, endocrine function, and clinical chemistry); and long-term (two-year) toxicology and carcinogenesis studies. Each study on a chemical usually involves four individual, separate, yet concurrent experiments: male rats, female rats, male mice, and female mice." (Huff et al., 1988)

In the broadest sense of the term, toxicologic pathology, particularly for the pharmaceutical investigator, but also for the academic researcher and diagnostic pathologist, embraces all the elements alluded to in the quotation to varying extents. In the pharmaceutical setting, many short-term studies and longer term investigations are conducted to elucidate the mechanism of action of a test compound, to give some idea of its toxicity, and to identify possible target organs. These studies incorporate standard histopathologic and clinical pathologic techniques. Often specialized techniques, including electron microscopy, immunohistochemistry, autoradiography and quantitative morphometry, are warranted. In academic research, studies may be more targeted, fewer in number, and less extensive in coverage, but more intensely directed toward a specific aspect of mechanism of action or toxicity. In the diagnostic laboratory setting, studies are generally not conducted since diagnosis is the goal, but most of the techniques and many of the principles utilized by the pharmaceutical pathologist are also used by the diagnostic pathologist.

Specific pathology protocols for testing a compound in the pharmaceutical setting vary, depending on the test substance or the sponsoring organization. The design of these protocols is exceedingly important; decisions concerning risk to humans are ultimately based largely on these animal data. Whereas the rationale and procedures involved in risk assessment are beyond the scope of this chapter, some elements of concern to the toxicologic pathologist are germane, namely interspecies extrapolation, and dose extrapolation. To provide the best data for subsequent extrapolations, it is the responsibility of the pathologist to make the most of the controllable aspects of the animal tests.

The first goal of toxicologic pathology for the pathologist in the industrial setting is to establish the precise degree of risk posed to the test animals under the controlled exposure conditions. The process is similar to diagnostic pathology in lesion evaluation, but differs in the manner in which the data are compiled. The focus is on representative response of a treatment cohort, versus individual patients, the objective being to quantify the average response of treated groups compared with untreated ones. There are standardized protocols, peer review procedures, and auspicious review by regulatory agencies.

These distinctive characteristics of toxicologic pathology, especially in pharmaceutical research situations, often require different record keeping than the usual diagnostic description. The differences in records stem from the need to establish quantitative risk to groups of animals exposed to graded doses of the test substance. For example, the volume of morphologic data generated by a two-year study in both sexes of two species of animals is huge. It must be collected in a standardized way, and compiled in a condensed or manageable form.

The most undesirable characteristic of data in toxicologic pathology, short of inaccuracy, is inconsistency.

Most of the factors that influence evaluation of morphologic change (e.g., poor fixation of tissue, postmortem interval) have the undesirable effect of increasing the variability within groups, and subsequently the range of data that the pathologist is forced to accept. This decreases the sensitivity of the methods used. For the diagnostic pathologist these factors can, and often do, substantially impair the attainment of an accurate diagnosis in an individual animal, or even a herd. As one example, when tissue fixation is poor, the pathologist cannot be sufficiently discerning to distinguish early toxic injury from early postmortem autolysis; thus the ability to detect a subtle effect of treatment with or without exposure to a xenobiotic is compromised. Similarly, spontaneous or nonspecific lesions that are similar to lesions associated with a test substance or environmental toxicant compromise evaluation. Vigilance is required to minimize the effect of these complicating factors. Toxicologic pathology requires the art of pathology to be used in conjunction with sound experimental design, methods and analysis in the pharmaceutical and academic situations, and with sound technique, protocols and analysis in the diagnostic setting, where confounding factors abound.

FACTORS INFLUENCING EVALUATION OF ALTERED MORPHOLOGY

Many factors influence the interpretation of the significance of altered morphology. Here factors with special significance to toxicologic pathology are emphasized. All pathologists, including toxicologic pathologists, rely heavily on clinical observation, analyses of blood and body fluids, history (especially in the diagnostic situation) and necropsy findings. Altered morphology is evaluated in the light of everything known about the animal, since the functional significance of the morphologic change can be quite different, depending on the etiology involved. For example, proteinuria associated solely with nephrosis could plausibly be caused by toxicity of a test substance. In contrast, if an animal has a neoplasm of the urinary bladder with hydroureter and hydronephrosis, the proteinuria should be interpreted as secondary to urinary obstruction caused by the neoplasm.

The season of the year and the "occupation" of the animal are examples of factors that are particularly important in other aspects of pathology, but have less influence in toxicologic pathology in the non-diagnostic setting. Cognizance of such variables is essential for comparative purposes in diagnostic pathology. The diagnostic pathologist uses history and variation from the normal population to attain a diagnosis, while by contrast experimental toxicologic pathologists use comparisons of differences among treatment groups of a normal population.

To exaggerate how individual variation can complicate interpretation of bioassay results, a person can imagine a hypothetical bioassay in which all animals in a toxicological study would be histologically perfect. Their tissues would respond only to test substances, and each animal's response would be qualitatively and quantitatively identical. Any morphologic change could, therefore, be attributed directly to exposure to the test substance. In reality, the task is performed with animals that are not identical, even in the pharmaceutical setting using animals of supposedly genetic uniformity. Their responses in the study are various and multifactorial, even under the best of conditions, and these responses may or may not be caused by the test material. The situation is much more challenging in the diagnostic laboratory setting, where the exposed population is far more heterogeneous, the environment is far less controlled, if at all, and dose, as well as duration of exposure to the xenobiotic, is usually unknown.

In the pharmaceutical setting, the routine bioassay is undertaken using two sexes, a minimum of three treatment levels and one control group; usually two species are used. Each treatment group defined by species, sex, and dose is distinct. The pathologist's task is to characterize the background changes, as reflected in the untreated animals, and compare these changes with those found in each of the treated groups of the same species and sex. In effect, each bioassay is an exercise in population statistics. Rather than be concerned with each individual animal for its own sake, the pathologist must regard each animal as a statistical subunit of a set, the treatment group. The focus on representative response of each group necessitates standardization of necropsy and histology procedures, to minimize variation in histologic appearance among animals within or among treatment groups, due to processing or artifact. It necessitates standardized classification of lesions, so the diagnoses can be compared. This is in marked contrast to the diagnostic setting, where the toxicologic pathologist often has to rely on experience, consultation with peers, published texts, earlier cases, and even "educated guesses," to arrive at a reasonable conclusion regarding the cause of the lesion.

Subtle lesions are always difficult to interpret in any setting. Obviously, as lesions produced by the test substance or environmental toxicant become subtler with decreasing dose, they become more difficult to differentiate from background. Experimentally, the dose level at which lesions can no longer be attributed to exposure to the test substance or toxicant is the "No Observable Adverse Effect Level" (NOAEL). Unfortunately, this level is not clearly defined, since background "noise" may interfere with the cut-off point. Identification of this dose has importance for subsequent extrapolation to humans, and it forces the pathologist to wrestle with the threshold between "normal" and "least detectable change." The distinction is made more efficiently when the pathologist reads the slides with knowledge of the animals' treatment (i.e., not "blind"), then later, at least in the research situation, rereads the slides without knowledge of treatment group ("blind"), to confirm the interpretation. Table 5.1 includes some common factors

TABLE 5.1 Factors that influence evaluation of altered morphology

Factors in collection and processing of tissue

Standard operating procedures

Quality of necropsy

Accuracy of organ weights

Fresh versus autolyzed tissue

Type of fixative, adequacy of fixation

Histologic preparation

Factors intrinsic to the animal

Species, strain, sex, age

Spontaneous disease

Physiologic phenomena

Normal histologic variation

Factors related to the environment

Nutrition

Temperature

Illumination

Sound

Factors related to nomenclature

Standardization and consistency

Pathologic process versus component stages

Grading of lesions versus qualifiers

"Blind" reading

Combining of lesions

(other than treatment) that affect the histologic appearance of tissues in toxicologic pathology, or that affect how histologic data are evaluated.

Factors in Collection and Processing of Tissue

Standard Operating Procedures

This section will not contain specific "recipes" for handling tissue, since ample texts and periodical reports exist. Examples are included in the "Further Reading" section. The important message is that the tissue collection procedures selected be codified into institutional Standard Operating Procedures (SOPs), regardless of whether the institution is a large pharmaceutical concern or a small field diagnostic laboratory. Unfailing adherence to well-selected SOPs is the most successful strategy to reduce variability in data; to ensure competently conducted studies or sound, thorough diagnostic investigations; and to preclude the catastrophe of a failed experiment or investigation. There is no substitute, and regulatory agencies or accreditation organizations not only require them for development of new drugs, but also audit their proper and appropriate application.

Quality of the Necropsy

While the necropsy is not an independent factor in interpretation of morphologic change, it is the most critical single procedure in a formal toxicological study. Many authors have emphasized this, but it bears repeating that the animal at the end of the study contains all of the previous effort that went into the study, as well as the results of the study. Similarly, for a diagnostic investigation, the necropsy is the essential procedure necessary not only for the appropriate collection of specimens for analysis, but very often for arriving at a definitive diagnosis. With respect to morphologic evaluation, a dependable standard procedure for necropsy of any species under study is required, to ensure that all gross lesions are identified, so none will be overlooked in subsequent correlations of gross and microscopic lesions; the same SOP should ensure that technicians, pathologists, residents and students carefully collect all required tissues in a standard manner, and that all lesions are described accurately, with uniform terminology and reporting. The trimming of tissues for subsequent processing and embedment is an opportunity to further improve the quality of morphologic evaluation in at least three ways. The trimmer can confirm the prosector's observations and verify tissue accountability; can detect and describe

additional lesions revealed on trimming; and can effect a highly standardized protocol, to provide as far as possible identically-trimmed sets of tissue from each animal. Tight standardization of trimming of tissue blocks is the first step to ensure uniform anatomical and histologic sampling of each tissue, thereby reducing between-animal variation.

Accuracy of Organ Weights

Changes in organ weights, either absolute or relative to body weight, brain weight or other reference, are sensitive indicators of early toxicity, especially under tightly controlled conditions, such as an experimental study. In acute studies there may be no other indicator detected, and weight change reveals the organ as a target (discussed further below). In the case of testes and brain, where early morphologic lesions may not be demonstrable without expensive cytometry, weight change alone may serve as a valid biomarker of toxicity.

Knowledge of organ weights of treated animals versus control or normal animals can be a factor to cause the pathologist to re-evaluate morphologic change. What previously may have been interpreted to be a spectrum of normal variation may now be seen (on re-examination without knowledge of the treatment group) as two separable morphologic manifestations. The value of organ weight data is lost however, if there is not a very rigorous SOP to prepare the organs for weighing. It is essential that fat and adventitia be removed in some highly uniform manner, that blood clots be removed consistently (e.g., from heart chambers), that fluid be blotted uniformly. Small organs lose moisture rapidly under laboratory conditions. For example, a mouse thyroid gland will lose 25% of fresh weight if left uncovered in the laboratory for 15 minutes. Unless these variables are controlled carefully, the time and effort to obtain and use organ weight meaningfully is futile. When small tissues, such as mouse thyroid or adrenal, are to be examined histologically, serious consideration should be given to fixing the organ before trimming and weighing, to reduce morphologic artifacts introduced by the handling and delay incident to obtaining their weight.

Fresh Versus Autolyzed Tissue

No current techniques in pathology can restore autolyzed tissues, and to the extent that autolysis compromises interpretation of tissue changes, all previous investment in that animal is wasted if autolysis is present. Under controlled experimental or study conditions, standard procedure should mandate two or more inspections of the animal colony each day for moribund or dead animals; they should be removed for immediate necropsy when feasible. Bodies should be refrigerated if prompt necropsy is not possible, in order to slow the autolysis process. Nevertheless, even refrigeration has its limits and autolysis will not completely cease—eight hours of refrigeration has been accepted arbitrarily as an upper limit for small rodents, even though small rodents cool quickly after death. Prompt refrigeration pending a delayed necropsy is even more critical, and is often complicated by the sheer size of some larger herbivorous species. Under most "field" conditions in the diagnostic laboratory setting, control over autolysis is usually limited, and sometimes non-existent, even under the best of circumstances. In this case, a thorough knowledge of autolytic change and its manifestations in each particular species under investigation is essential. In general, cells of lymph nodes, renal tubules, and intestinal villus tip are most vulnerable to autolytic change. Autolysis proceeds by degrees, and whereas the pathologist can "read through" mild degrees of autolysis and detect well-developed lesions, the sensitivity of the study is compromised; advanced autolysis seriously compromises the pathologist's ability to detect the presence of toxic effects.

It is also important to realize that all species have their own peculiar patterns of autolytic change, often due to unique anatomic features that alter the general pattern. The heavy wool of sheep, for example, greatly slows cooling after death, even when the animals are quickly refrigerated. The large bacteria-filled rumens, ceca, and/or colons in many herbivorous domestic species make bacterial putrefaction of these organs and adjacent tissues a special challenge. The large size of many of these species adds a further complicating factor, since their sheer mass greatly impedes cooling of internal organs even if the animal is refrigerated immediately after death or necropsied on the spot. Summaries of postmortem autolytic changes and factors which affect such changes are presented in Tables 5.2 and 5.3.

Type of Fixative, Adequacy of Fixation

Failure to achieve adequate fixation of fresh tissues causes the same loss of both data and investment as loss through autolysis. The pathology laboratory may not be able to prevent receipt of autolyzed tissues, but when tissues are fresh upon delivery, exercise of good SOPs for fixation should ensure well-preserved tissue and, with luck, salvage some meaningful morphologic information from not so well-preserved tissue. The purpose of fixation is to stabilize the tissue

to prevent further postmortem change, halt bacterial putrefaction, harden the tissue for processing and imbedding, and preserve the tissue indefinitely if possible. There is perhaps more literature about fixatives and fixation than about most other techniques in pathology. In general, a fixative should be fast acting (i.e., fast penetrating), remain stable (to allow storage of tissue prior to trimming and processing), and produce the least amount of unique artifact in the tissue. Each organization has abundant choice of chemical or physical fixation methods to best suit the objective of each study. A partial listing of fixatives, their general composition, their mechanism of action, their rapidity of fixation and their advantages/disadvantages are laid out in Table 5.4. Fixation by microwave and by vascular perfusion is increasingly used to prepare tissues for specialized examinations. Solutions of formaldehyde in various buffers, most typically "10% neutral buffered formalin," are used universally because of their efficiency, versatility and economy, although formaldehyde's putative carcinogenicity in rats has caused it to be increasingly discredited. Like other procedures in preparation of tissue sections, the specific reagents and techniques used are less important than the uniformity and consistency with which they are employed.

Histologic Preparation

To derive the greatest amount of information from the animal, the pathologist should examine a full set of tissues from each animal, with every organ sectioned in exactly the same, prescribed plane (according to the SOP) across the full face of the embedded tissue block. There should be no artifactual tearing or folding of the section, no extraneous debris or tissue. The sections should be of protocol-prescribed thickness, and be stained uniformly in accordance with the SOP. Any deviation from the highest standard of quality risks compromise of the pathologists' ability to detect or quantify the effects of toxicity. Missing tissues reduce the power of statistical analysis. Sections taken in the wrong plane can lead to faulty interpretation if the pathologist is unaware that a deviation from protocol has occurred. Furthermore, processing artifacts can obscure subtle features necessary for complete interpretation. Variations in stain quality and in tissue thickness interject additional variables that reduce the ability to detect subtle change. Once again, there are many standard procedures that successfully produce high quality sections for various purposes. No single one is advocated; however, slavish adherence to the SOPs should be practiced to minimize even more difficulties with interpretation.

TABLE 5.2   Partial list of organ-specific change associated with postmortem autolysis

Postmortem change	Tissues affected	Mechanism
Bile imbibition	Liver, pancreas, duodenum	Leakage of bile into surrounding tissues, staining them a greenish color
Blood clots in major blood vessels	Major arteries and veins, chambers of the heart	Clotting of stagnant blood after death ("currant jelly" and "chicken fat" clots, with no attachments to vessel walls)
Hemoglobin imbibition	Surfaces of visceral organs	Lysis of red blood cells and leakage of free hemoglobin into tissues, giving them a smudgy red coloration
Livor mortis (hypostatic congestion)	Lungs, intestines, skin	Gravity-dependent settling or pooling of blood in tissues on the "down" side of the animal, giving the appearance of hyperemia or congestion
"Mucoid" sludge, sometimes red-tinged	Lumens of stomach, small intestine, colon	Release of mucus from goblet cells, sloughing of mucosal epithelium, bacterial proliferation giving the appearance of mucopurulent or necropurulent exudate
Pseudomelanosis	Liver, kidney, small intestine, colon, any visceral organ against which intestine abuts	Greenish to green-black deposits of iron sulfide in tissues due to hydrogen sulfide released by putrefactive anaerobic bacteria in the gut
Prolapse through orifices	Rectum, tongue, vagina	Eversion due to gaseous distension of internal organs (see below)
Inhalation of ingesta	Oral cavity, pharynx, trachea, major bronchi	Agonal inspiration of regurgitated rumen or stomach content
Pallor with softening	Skeletal muscle, liver	Postmortem degradation of myoglobin
Emphysema	Lung, Visceral organs	Agonal breathing at time of death (ruminants) Gas produced by putrefactive bacteria (all species)
Minute red streaks	Heart (mainly endocardium and epicardium)	Petechial and echymotic hemorrhages associated with agonal stages of the death process
Rupture of hollow organs	Stomach, small intestine, colon	Secondary to severe tympanites (see below)
Tympanites (gaseous distension of hollow organs)	Mainly GI tract	Gas produced by putrefactive bacteria

TABLE 5.3   Partial list of factors the influence postmortem autolysis

Factor	Impact
Postmortem interval	Autolysis progressive as time between death and necropsy increases, even with cooling
Cause of death	Animals that are febrile or with bacterial sepsis prior to death will autolyze much faster
Condition before death	Obese animals will cool less quickly than emaciated ones
Anatomic factors	High GI microflora content (e.g., rumen, cecum) hastens autolysis
Rate of cooling	Slow rate of cooling enhances autolysis; small animals cool faster than larger ones; heavy hair coats (e.g., wool) slow cooling

TABLE 5.4 Common fixatives used in toxicologic pathology

Fixative	Composition	Fixation/ penetration	Mode of action	Recommended use	Advantages/ disadvantages
Bouin's	Picric acid in ethanol, acetic acid, formaldehyde in water	Relatively slow fixation; good penetration	Precipitates (picric acid) and cross-links proteins (formaldehyde)	Fetal tissues, bone, reproductive tissues, endocrine tissues	Can be explosive if dried out
Glutaraldehyde	Usually glutaraldehyde in 4% formaldehyde or 4% paraformaldehyde in phosphate buffered water	Rapid fixation; poor penetration	Cross-links proteins and alters α-helical structure	Electron microscopy	Best cellular detail/must be kept refrigerated on charcoal, must only fix small pieces of tissue
Michel's	N-ethylmaleimide, potassium citrate, magnesium sulfate in water	Rapid fixation; poor penetration	Cross-links proteins via sulfhydryls	Immunofluorescence	Excellent for antigen preservation/cannot be used to fix tissues for paraffin imbedding and section, must only fix small pieces of tissue
Microwave	Saline solution at 2.45 GHz frequency and 600 Watts output	Rapid on the surface, slow and uneven penetration	Cross-links (via heat) proteins	Generally used in combination with formalin	Best used in combination with aldehyde fixatives/uneven to poor penetration large or dense specimens
10% neutral buffered formalin	4% formaldehyde in phosphate buffered water, pH adjusted to 7	Intermediate fixation, excellent penetration	Cross-links proteins into a matrix gel	All tissues, routine histopathology	Best general purpose fixative; little harm to any tissue/acid hematin precipitates if not buffered, irritant to nose and eyes
Paraformaldehyde	4% paraformaldehyde polymer in phosphate buffered water	Intermediate fixation; excellent penetration	Cross-links proteins into a matrix gel	Used for perfusion fixation or together with glutaraldehyde for electron microscopy	Best fixative for perfusion/must be prepared fresh
Zenker's	Potassium dichromate, mercuric chloride, glacial acetic acid in water	Rapid fixation; intermediate penetration	Precipitates (mercuric chloride) and cross-links (dichromate) proteins	Lymphohematopoietic tissues, eyes	Good nuclear fixation/ requires removal of mercury before staining, tissue shrinkage and hardening, highly toxic

For bioassay pathology, the volume of work virtually dictates maximum use of automated methods. Automated methods have the added advantage of consistency and, increasingly, of computerized documentation of the steps in the procedure. As the equipment becomes more complex, there is an associated requirement that its calibration be carefully performed, monitored, and documented.

The final step in preparing the sections is to ensure that every tissue of every animal is accounted for, and that each animal's identification is correct. An accurate evaluation by the pathologist, attributed to the wrong animal in a treatment group or submitted diagnostic case, is no better than an incorrect evaluation. Quality control procedures, beginning with receipt of the animals, should be devised to detect and resolve errors at the earliest step, and thus limit their effect on the study.

Factors Intrinsic to the Animal

Species, Strain, Sex, and Age

In the pharmaceutical or basic research situation, some overriding considerations may dictate the choice of animal for the study. The relevance of the model to man should be a primary consideration (comparative physiology, pharmacodynamics if known, etc.). There may be regulatory requirements, and logistic and economic feasibility are important additional factors. If the choice of animal is not proscribed by such factors, the animals selected should be the ones that have the most extensive database, together with the lowest incidence of spontaneous disease in the organs of greatest interest. For chronic studies, special consideration should be given to age-dependent diseases, especially neoplasms. The species, strain, sex, and age of the animal influence evaluation of morphologic change, primarily as a function of the prevalence of spontaneous disease, in most applications.

In any situation—pharmaceutical testing, basic research or diagnostic investigation—the animal's age influences the appearance of virtually every tissue. When a change is detected that is dissonant with an animal's chronological age, the change requires special attention. Atrophy of the thymus is expected in aged animals, but the same change in a young animal must be evaluated as a deviation from the norm. Long-term (24-month) bioassays in rodents involve aged animals, and necessitate an in-depth knowledge of aging changes unique to that particular strain or species. Almost by definition, aged populations of all species, including humans, are diverse pathologically. One characteristic of aging populations that must be appreciated is marked individual variation in the expression of multiple aging changes. Furthermore, individual animals usually differ in the age when these changes first appear, with variability in rates of progression and ultimate severity. Thus, when rodents are used in long-term studies, thorough documentation of age-dependent disease is essential, to distinguish those processes from treatment-related changes. Table 5.5 is an abbreviated listing of age-related changes in some domestic animals.

Spontaneous Disease

Infectious Disease

Infectious diseases are serious considerations in all work with animals. In toxicologic pathology in the pharmaceutical research and basic research settings, infectious disease is more a problem for managers of the animal colony than for the pathologist, since epizootic infection in animals under test is a cause to terminate the study. Even in most "clean" studies there will be individual animals that have focal infections, as in infected rat preputial glands or middle ears, for example. These become factors in the evaluation of potential toxic effects, since interactions between infection and the metabolism of the test compound cannot be known with confidence.

TABLE 5.5   Partial list of grossly visible age-related changes in common domestic animals

Lesion	Species affected
Cholesteatoma (cholesterol) granuloma in the choroid plexus of the brain	Horse
Coxo-femoral osteoarthritis	Dogs
Cystic hyperplasia of the gall bladder mucosa	Dogs, cats
Fatty change in marrow of long bones	Most domestic species
Hemomelasma ilei	Horses
Hepatic fatty cysts	Cats
Hepatic telangiectasia	Cattle
Nodular adrenocortical hyperplasia	Dogs, cats
Nodular exocrine pancreatic hyperplasia	Cats, dogs (less commonly)
Nodular hepatic hyperplasia	Dogs
Nodular prostatic hyperplasia	Dogs
Nodular splenic hyperplasia (lymphoid and non-lymphoid)	Dogs
Nodular valvular endocardiosis	Dogs
Par ovarian cysts	Dogs
Pleural fibrosis (multifocal)	Cattle, sheep
Pulmonary anthracosis (carbon deposits in lung and associated lymph nodes)	Dogs, cats
Pulmonary mineralization (multifocal)	Dogs, cats
Splenic siderotic nodules or plaques	Dogs

For the toxicologic pathologist in the diagnostic situation, infectious disease is a constant companion, and a factor that must always be considered in any investigation into potential toxicity. Here, the margin of uncertainty is increased far more than in the more pristine colony situation. In all cases, certain morphologic changes, such as stimulation (or depletion) of the immune system or adrenal gland, may be caused by the infection, the substance under suspicion or investigation, both, or neither. Since random infections tend to vary in severity among individuals, the severity of the condition in the control or comparison animals (e.g., the "healthy" or "unaffected" animals in a herd in the case of a diagnostic case), may not resolve the uncertainty. In addition, the possibility that the infection is a secondary effect of exposure to a toxicant or test substance, rather than a primary occurrence, must always be considered.

Neoplasms and Age-related Non-neoplastic Disease

Except for epizootic infections, the problems posed by spontaneous disease in any situation are difficult to separate from considerations of species, breed or strain, age and sex of the animals, since each genotype has its own distinctive and sometimes dramatically different, disease pattern and phenotypic response. A toxicologic pathologist must be acutely aware of the spontaneous age-related diseases peculiar to the animal species under study or investigation, otherwise misdiagnosis is a real possibility. Compilations of genotype-specific spontaneous neoplastic and non-neoplastic diseases of laboratory or domestic animals of many species, particularly rodents, but also pet animals and food animals, have been published; some examples are listed under "Further Reading." In the research situation, virtually all animals in 24-month bioassays will have some age-dependent changes. Commonly, a test substance will interact with these processes and affect their prevalence, severity or progression. For example, Fischer 344 rats have a high prevalence of mononuclear cell leukemia, and thus exhibit various degrees of change in the liver and spleen associated with that malignancy. This situation renders those organs difficult to evaluate for potential treatment-related changes. Age-related nephropathies result in a variety of morphologic expressions in virtually all species, laboratory raised or domestic. The numerous age-related lesions in all species obviously complicate the pathologists' efforts to detect subtle patterns of treatment-related or toxicant-related microscopic change.

A primary purpose of the two-year study in the research setting is to determine the carcinogenicity of the test substance or environmental contaminant. Cataloging the number of neoplasms in each treatment group is generally straightforward. Determining whether or not there is a treatment-related, biologically meaningful change in the prevalence of neoplasms can be elusive, however. There is often a high frequency of the same neoplasms in untreated animals, making the determination of an increase in treated groups proportionately less sensitive. Occasionally, the untreated animals in a study will have a higher prevalence of a particular neoplasm than other recent controls in the same laboratory, further complicating evaluation of the number of neoplasms in the treated cohorts. Historical values for untreated animals in the same laboratory must then be considered, to gain perspective, although only "recent" history may be relevant.

The magnitude of the problem presented by spontaneous neoplasia can be inferred from frequency data on Fischer 344 rats and B6C3F1 mice in recent two-year dosed-feed bioassays reported by the NTP. Of approximately 900 untreated control rats of each sex, 28% of males and 51% of females had pituitary tumors, 89% of male rats had adenoma of testicular interstitial cells, and 29% (females) and 51% (males) had mononuclear cell leukemia. Overall, 93% of females and 98% of males were tumor bearing, with malignant tumors in 43% and 67% of them, respectively. Of 850 control mice of each sex, 70% of females and 76% of males were tumor bearing at two years; about 40% of these tumors were malignant. Hepatocellular neoplasms were particularly prevalent (32% in females and 51% in males), and lung tumors occurred in 24% of males. Clearly, substantial consideration must be given to the frequency of spontaneous disease in the specific organ systems of interest. A mouse strain with high prevalence of pulmonary tumors early in life would be a poor choice for a carcinogenicity bioassay using inhalation exposure.

Physiologic Phenomena

Most physiologic phenomena have morphologic correlates, however subtle or not so subtle they may be. Two typical examples encountered in toxicologic pathology are hyperplasia of reproductive structures related to pregnancy/lactation, and the increased smooth endoplasmic reticulum in hepatocytes following induction of hepatic mixed function oxidases by certain drugs. These manifestations of a physiological response must be taken into account in any situation—bioassay, research study or diagnostic investigation—and put into the appropriate perspective if the proper conclusions about the toxicant, contaminant, or test substance are to be made. Not only must the physiologic change and its morphologic correlate be recognized and acknowledged, its relevance to the matter at hand must also be decided. This requires a thorough knowledge of the physiology of the species under study. For example, in a bioassay, the physiologic state of the animals in all groups should be similar at the beginning of the study, and should remain similar throughout the period of the study.

In particular, cyclic physiologic phenomena, when they have morphologic expression, must be carefully identified and defined by appropriate measures. One example is the storage of salivary secretions in

TABLE 5.6   Selected physiologic changes reflected grossly in common domestic animals

Physiologic change	Species affected	Mechanism
Distension of the gall bladder	Most species (especially dogs and ruminants)	Lack of recent food intake
Mucus in the gastric lumen	Horse and pig	Mucus production by pyloric epithelium
Mucus in the renal pelvis	Horses	Mucus production by collecting duct epithelium in renal medulla
Pallor of the liver	Lactating animals (especially ruminants)	Fatty liver associated with nursing
Post-prandial hyperemia of stomach and small intestine	Most species (especially horse and pig)	Food intake shortly before death
Prostatic atrophy	Male animals	Castration leading to loss of testosterone

cytoplasmic granules, and their depletion with feeding activity. The size of the salivary acinar cells, and the weight of the salivary glands, can vary as much as four-fold between fasted and recently fed animals. The changes occur in a few hours in rats and mice. In this example, awareness of feeding and killing schedules would influence the interpretation of size disparity in salivary acinar cells among the animals. Table 5.6 is a partial listing of common physiologic changes that can be observed grossly in common domestic species.

Normal Histologic Variation

Differentiating treatment-related morphologic change from non-treatment or non-exposure related abnormal morphology is an important task for the toxicologic pathologist. Simply deciding whether or not a change from normal exists at all is sometimes very difficult. The ability of pathologists using routine qualitative light microscopy to detect changes in the number or size of structures is undoubtedly a function of experience of the pathologist, as well as the condition of the tissue at time of specimen collection. Yet, at best, estimates credit pathologists with the ability to detect only those changes in number or size that deviate 20–30% from "normal." The inherent variation in normal structures becomes a complicating factor in the evaluation of any subtle morphologic change.

Factors Related to the Environment

Nutrition

Many husbandry-related conditions, other than infectious disease or spontaneous age-related lesions, can influence the outcome of toxicity and safety tests, as well as hamper attainment of a diagnosis in the diagnostic laboratory. The effects caused by the situations must be distinguished from specific toxic effects. In most experimental situations, these conditions would influence treated and control groups similarly, so they would have the same generalized manifestation as a spontaneous disease might. A bigger problem occurs when treated groups are handled differently from the controls during life, and are affected because of that difference, or when treated groups behave differently from controls, and their tissues reflect the difference. For example, an unpalatable test substance in the diet may reduce food consumption. This can cause variation in growth, body weight, longevity, and morbidity as a primary effect of nutrition, but reflects only a nonspecific effect of the compound being tested. The high-dose animals will often be most affected, and the changes could mistakenly be attributed to the test substance. Particularly confusing is the fact that caloric restriction, which occurs with food refusal, often results in *increased* longevity and *decreased* age-related morbidity and mortality rates, especially at a 30–50% reduction in dietary intake. Thus, treated animals that reduce their food intake may also outlive those in the control group, and have a lower prevalence of most spontaneous diseases and neoplasms. Furthermore, because of the self-induced restriction, a high-dose group may actually have ingested less of the test compound than the next lower dose group. A corollary to the enhancement of health by caloric restriction is the emerging acknowledgment that the current rates of "spontaneous disease," especially tumors, are becoming epizootic in frequency in rodents, and that the high rates of degenerative disease and of neoplasia are the result of overfeeding.

By contrast, in the field among domestic animal and wild animal populations, where environmental conditions are minimally controlled or not at all, nutritional factors can have substantial impacts on toxicity and the diagnosis of toxicosis. As implied in the earlier paragraph, nutritional status can greatly affect response to toxicant exposure, but in a somewhat different manner. In field situations, where acute toxicosis, rather than long-term toxicity (in the form of carcinogenesis) is the norm, nutritional status can greatly affect metabolism, distribution, and excretion kinetics, since adipose tissue often serves as a reservoir for lipophilic xenobiotics, greatly altering typical absorption-distribution-metabolism-excretion patterns of the substance. Storage of lipophilic toxicants in the adipose stores of an animal might prevent or mask immediate toxicosis, only to have a more chronic form of toxicosis become manifest as the toxicant is released slowly over time. Furthermore, in many cases diets are much less stringently formulated, and concomitant exposure to other xenobiotics in the diet or water supply that could affect response to the suspected toxicant must be taken into account. Therefore, as stated above, a complete history and background related to the exposed animals, as well as knowledge of dietary intakes and nutritional status, are vital to achieving an accurate diagnosis of toxicity.

Temperature, Illumination, and Sound in Laboratory Situations

In the tightly controlled pharmaceutical and research environments, where all potential confounding factors in a study are compensated for as much as possible, even relatively small and transient changes in ambient temperature cause biologically significant change in the body temperature of rodents. Disturbances, such as stormy weather or unaccustomed handling, that last only minutes can cause 1–4 hour body temperature elevations of 1.0–1.5°C in mice. These effects are probably proportionately less profound in larger species. Body temperature is a reliable indicator of metabolic rate, and therefore an important determinant of metabolism of any test substance administered to animals in an experimental study. One example of the temperature effect is the dramatic impact that a 10°C difference in ambient temperature can have on tail length—rats raised in a 20°C environment have tails that are 3 cm shorter than littermates raised at 30°C. Similar observations to these have also been reported in mice.

Excess ambient illumination has been found to have a significant effect on rodents. Excessively high light intensity causes extensive retinal degeneration in rats and mice. If high-dose animals are routinely housed on the upper shelves of cage racks, the degree of degeneration will appear to be dose-related. Another example is with long photoperiods, which cause regression of ovaries, Harderian glands and adrenal glands, and anestrus in rodents, changes which could be attributed erroneously to a test substance.

In a similar manner, extraneous noise causes biologically significant change in body temperatures of rats and mice. The auditory spectrum of rats and mice, unlike most other laboratory animals, is quite different from that of humans. The most sensitive hearing for most species is in the range of 0.5 to 10 kHz. Although mice cannot hear sounds below 1 kHz, they are exquisitely sensitive to sound in the 10–20 kHz range, the upper limit of which is beyond human perception. Therefore, one must be aware that there are sound frequencies, especially ultrasonic ones, which humans cannot hear, but which provoke stressful changes in mice via neuroendocrine stimulation. Many reports exist of adverse effects of sound on diverse species: behavioral and reproductive dysfunctions, changes in tumor susceptibility and immune response, hypertension, electrolyte metabolism, and body temperature. Extraneous sound clearly can be one source of variable outcome in toxicity tests.

There may be many yet-undetermined influences related to the animal colony environment that affect the incidence of neoplasia, other diseases, and physiologic conditions. These influences may contribute to some of the unexplained variations in prevalence data within and among laboratories.

Factors Related to Nomenclature

Nomenclature is a complex and often hotly debated topic, both among pathologists in general and toxicologic pathologists in particular. Many of the issues relate specifically to the toxicologic pathologist in a pharmaceutical locale, but some, especially in relation to standardization and consistency, are also of importance to toxicologic pathologists in basic research and diagnostic settings. Standardization of nomenclature is perhaps the most relevant to all three venues, since effective communication and effective transfer of information among pathologists in various situations depends to a large extent on some standardization of terms and diagnoses. These issues are discussed at length in the preceding chapter.

FURTHER READING

Anonymous. (1986). Editorial. Society of toxicologic pathologists' position paper on blinded slide reading. *Toxicol. Pathol.*, 14, 493–494.

Anonymous. (1998). *Tumor Incidence in Control Animals by Route and Vehicle of Administration.* F344/Nrats. National Institute of Environmental Health Sciences, Research Triangle Park, NC.

Anonymous. (1998). *Tumor Incidence in Control Animals by Route and Vehicle of Administration.* $B_6C_3F_1$ Mice. National Institute of Environmental Health Sciences, Research Triangle Park, NC.

Anver, M.R., and Cohen, B.J. (1979). Lesions associated with aging. In *The Laboratory Rat* (Baker, H.J., Lindsay, J.R., and Weisbroth, S.H. eds), Vol. I. Academic Press, New York, NY.

Boorman, G.A. et al (1985). Quality assurance in pathology for rodent carcinogenicity studies. In *Handbook of Carcinogen Testing* (Milman, H.A., and Weisberger, E.K. eds), pp. 345–357. Noyes, Park Ridge, NJ.

Calabrese, E. (1988). Comparative biology of test species. *Environ. Health Pers.*, 77, 55–62.

Carson, F.L. (1997). *Histotechnology: A Self-Instructional Text*, 2nd edn. American Society of Clinical Pathologists, Chicago, IL.

Clough, G. (1982). Environmental effects on animals used in biomedical research. *Biol. Rev.*, 57, 487–523.

Fieldname, D.B., and Seely, J.C. (eds) (1988). *Necropsy Guide: Rodents and the Rabbit*. CRC Press, Boca Raton, FL.

Gart, J.J. et al (1986). Statistical methods in cancer research. In *The Design and Analysis of Long-Term Animal Experiments*, Vol. III. IARC, Lyon, France.

Hacman, G. (1988). Prevention of cancer: Restriction of nutritional intake (joules). Mini-review. *Comp. Biochem. Physiol.*, 91A, 209–220.

Hopwood, O. et al (1984). Microwave fixation: Its potential for routine techniques, histochemistry, immunocytochemistry and electron microscopy. *Histochem. J.*, 16, 1171–1191.

Luna, L.G. (ed.) (1968). *Manual of Histologic Staining Methods of the Armed Forces Institute of Pathology*, 3rd edn. McGraw-Hill, New York, NY.

McConnell, E.E. et al (1986). Guidelines for combining neoplasms for evaluation of rodent carcinogenesis studies. *JNCI*, 76, 283–289.

Newberne, P.M. (1988). Importance of diet and nutrition in evaluating the safety of drugs. *Human Path.*, 19, 4–6.

Preece, A. (1972). *A Manual for Histologic Technicians*, 3rd edn. Little, Brown, La Jolla, CA.

Roe, F.J.C. (1988). Toxicity testing: Some principles and some pitfalls in histopathological evaluation. *Human Toxicol.*, 7, 405–410.

Rogers, A.E., and Longnecker, M.P. (1988). Dietary and nutritional influences on cancer: A review of epidemiologic and experimental data. *Lab. Invest.*, 59, 727–759.

Seaman, W.J. (1987). *Postmortem Change in the Rat: A Histologic Characterization*. Iowa State University Press, Ames, IA.

Thompson, S.W., and Luna, L.G. (1978). *An Atlas of Artifacts Encountered in the Preparation of Microscopic Tissue Sections*. CC Thomas, Springfield, IL.

United States Food and Drug Administration. (1998). *Guidance for Industry: S1B. Testing for Carcinogenicity of Pharmaceuticals*. Federal Register (63 FR 8983) or http://www.fda.gov/cder/guidance/index.htm

6

Respiratory System

INTRODUCTION

The respiratory system is vulnerable to injury following airborne or hematogenous exposure to toxicants. Susceptibility to these airborne toxicants results from the extensive interface between the respiratory surface and inspired air, the large volume of air passing continuously into the lung, and the concentration of the toxicant present in the air. Susceptibility to injury via the hematogenous route is due to exposure to toxicants present in the extensive pulmonary capillary bed.

The primary functions of the respiratory tract are gas exchange, olfaction, and protection against noxious agents. Exposure to respiratory toxicants can occur in occupational settings (e.g., silica, asbestos, chronic acid fumes); during medical treatment (e.g., bleomycin, cyclophosphamide, X-rays); in self-inflicted injury (e.g., cigarette smoking, ingestion of paraquat, and cocaine use); and during the course of everyday activities, such as inhalation of common air pollutants (e.g., ozone, nitrogen dioxide, sulfur dioxide, diesel exhaust) or ingestion of toxic agents in food (e.g., toxic rapeseed oil in Spain, pyrrolizidine alkaloids in herbal teas). Lung diseases linked to chemical injury range from an acute reversible disease (e.g., metal fume fever following inhalation of zinc), to chronic irreversible diseases (e.g., fibrosis following inhalation of silica or lung cancer caused by cigarette smoking). A variety of defense mechanisms, such as the mucociliary apparatus and the alveolar macrophage system, can prevent contact of the injurious agent with vulnerable tissues of the lower respiratory tract. However, all too frequently these defenses are inadequate, and injury occurs.

The location and type of injury is the result of complex interactions between the agent and the host. Determining factors are the physicochemical characteristics of the agent, severity of insult (dose), and the metabolic capabilities present in the cellular components of the host tissue. The characteristics of the host response and the severity of insult will determine whether the injury is reversible or irreversible, and whether long-term health effects will occur.

STRUCTURE AND CELL BIOLOGY

Macroscopic and Microscopic Anatomy

Although there is considerable variation among species in the macroscopic and microscopic anatomy of the respiratory tract (Tables 6.1 and 6.2), the general principles involved in gas exchange are identical. The respiratory system consists of three parts: a conducting portion, a respiratory region, and a ventilating mechanism. These function to condition the air, provide oxygen from air, and remove CO_2 from the bloodstream. Approximately 40 different cell types are found in the respiratory system, each with a unique morphologic appearance and distinct functional role, as well as an individual response to toxic injury.

TABLE 6.1 Interspecies comparison of pulmonary anatomy

Anatomical characteristics	Mouse, rat, hamster	Dog, cat, Rhesus monkey	Cattle, pigs	Horses	Human
Pleura	Thin	Thin	Thick	Thick	Thick
Secondary lobulation	Absent	Absent	Present	Incomplete	Incomplete
Pulmonary veins	Cardiac muscle in media	Thin, mainly fibrous wall	Thick, smooth muscle in intima	Thin, mainly fibrous wall	Thin, mainly fibrous wall
Cartilage and submucosal glands in intrapulmonary bronchi	Absent	Present	Present	Present	Present
Respiratory bronchioles	Minimal	Extensive	Minimal	Minimal	Minimal

TABLE 6.2 Interspecies comparison of respiratory epithelia[a]

Epithelial types	Mouse	Rat	Dog	Human
Pseudostratified ciliated, with goblet cells and basal cells	Trachea	Trachea, main bronchi; segmental bronchi	Trachea, main bronchi; lobar bronchi; segmental bronchi	Trachea, main bronchi; lobar bronchi; segmental bronchi; subsegmental bronchi
Simple columnar ciliated, with Clara cells	Main bronchi; lobar bronchi; segmental bronchi	Subsegmental bronchi, bronchioles; terminal bronchioles	Peripheral bronchioles; terminal bronchioles	Peripheral bronchioles; terminal bronchioles
Simple cuboidal, mainly Clara cells, occasionally ciliated cells	Subsegmental bronchi; bronchioles; terminal bronchioles	Respiratory bronchioles	Respiratory bronchioles	Respiratory bronchioles

[a]With permission from Reznik-Schuller, H., and Reznik, G. (1979). *Int. Rev. Exp. Pathol.*, 20, 219

The conducting portion of the system includes the nasal cavity and pharynx, associated sinuses, nasopharynx, and the tracheobronchial tree. It serves to warm, moisten, and filter the inspired air. The anatomy and other characteristics of this region, such as cellular heterogeneity, greatly affect the distribution and toxic effects of inhaled substances. The respiratory portion of the system consists of the pulmonary parenchyma, whose major function is gas exchange. The ventilating system includes the thoracic cage and intercostal muscles, diaphragm, and elastic connective tissue of the lung which move air within the respiratory tract.

Nasopharyngeal and Laryngeal Regions (Upper Respiratory Tract)

Overview

The nose is the major route of entry for air and airborne substances into the respiratory system; the nose is the only route of entry for the rat and mouse, since they are obligate nasal breathers. There are significant species differences in the macroscopic and microscopic anatomy of the nasopharyngeal region, as well as in the distribution of the different types of epithelia, and in the types of cells within specific regions.

The mucosa of the nasal cavity consists of four major types of epithelia: stratified squamous, nonciliated transitional, ciliated respiratory and olfactory (Figure 6.1A). In the rat, stratified squamous epithelium lines the vestibule, the ventral meatus, the distal portion of the nasopharynx, and the larynx. A narrow region of nonciliated cuboidal (transitional) epithelium forms a transition between the squamous and ciliated respiratory epithelium, on both the lateral wall of the nasal cavity and the turbinates. Ciliated pseudostratified respiratory epithelium lines the anterior portion of the turbinates, and the proximal portion of the nasopharynx. The olfactory neuroepithelium lines the posterior portion of the turbinates, especially the ethmoturbinates. Respiratory and olfactory epithelia line the nasal septum. A wide variety of sensory nerve endings, associated with the trigeminal nerve, are present in the nasal mucosa. The lymphoid tissue consists of nasal-associated lymphoid tissue (NALT), present as diffuse aggregates of lymphoid cells, and the palatine tonsils.

The laryngeal mucosa has similar types of epithelium. Stratified squamous epithelium is present cranially, while respiratory epithelium is present caudally. A transition zone between the two epithelial types contains intermediate cell types. Seromucous glands

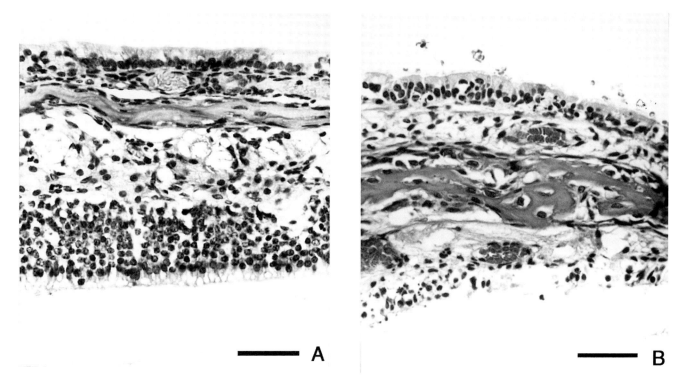

FIGURE 6.1   Nasal cavity, rat. H&E stain. Bar = 40μm. (A) Normal nasal mucosa consisting of respiratory ciliated epithelium (top) and olfactory epithelium with Bowman's glands (bottom). (B) One day after inhalation exposure to 3-methyl furan, the olfactory epithelium (bottom) is undergoing necrosis and sloughing, while the respiratory epithelium (top) is disorganized but relatively normal.

are located at the point of transition from stratified squamous to intermediate epithelium, serving as a marker during histologic sectioning. Microscopic lesions in response to inhaled xenobiotics occur most frequently in this transitional zone of rodent larynx.

Respiratory Mucosa

The respiratory epithelium varies from simple ciliated cuboidal to pseudostratified. It is composed of six different cell types: ciliated cells, nonciliated columnar cells, cuboidal cells, mucous (goblet) cells, brush cells, and basal cells. These cell types are unevenly distributed in the respiratory epithelium, depending on location in the nasal cavity. Intraepithelial axons are present primarily in the basal portion of the epithelium. The underlying lamina propria is very vascular, and contains both serous and mucous-secreting glands, as well as associated nerves.

Olfactory Mucosa

Unique to the nasal cavity, the olfactory neuroepithelium consists of pseudostratified columnar epithelium, basal lamina, and lamina propria. Although the olfactory mucosa is very similar structurally across species, its extent and distribution varies with the degree to which a species uses olfaction. The epithelium consists of basal, neuronal (olfactory), and sustentacular cells, all of which extend to the basal lamina and are distributed uniformly throughout the olfactory epithelium. A narrow dendritic process extends apically from the olfactory bipolar neurons to the luminal surface, ending in an olfactory vesicle. The cytoplasm of the neuronal cell forms a narrow axon distally, which leads through the basement membrane to form nerve bundles that become the olfactory nerve. Undifferentiated basal cells act as stem cells for the neuronal and sustentacular cells.

The underlying lamina propria is poorly vascularized, and contains unmyelinated nerve bundles of the olfactory nerve and myelinated fibers of the trigeminal nerve, as well as serous-secreting Bowman's glands. The glands provide fresh solvent for odorant substances, and a mucous covering for the epithelium.

Transitional Mucosa

The nasal transitional epithelium, separating the squamous and respiratory epithelium, consists of nonciliated epithelial cells. The epithelial cells have microvilli and, in rodents and dogs, abundant smooth endoplasmic reticulum (SER), suggesting a significant role in the metabolism of xenobiotics. The transitional epithelium is a target site of inhaled toxicants, and may be transformed into a secretory epithelium by irritants such as ozone.

Species Differences

Significant anatomical differences exist among species. The most obvious difference is the structure of the turbinate region; this can affect deposition of particles and distribution of inhaled gases in the nasal cavity. The nasal turbinates or scrolls are relatively simple in humans and the higher primates, where the major function of the nose is passage of air, whereas a double scroll is present in rodents, and a complex membranous branched scroll exists in the dog, where the major function is olfaction. Because of these structural differences, inhaled air follows a path through the upper half of the nasal cavity in rodents and dogs, but is confined to the lower two-thirds of the nasal cavity in humans and primates.

Tracheobronchial Region and Bronchioles

Overview

The conducting airways extend from the trachea and bronchi to the respiratory bronchioles, and conduct air to the respiratory portion of the lung where gas exchange takes place. In mammalian species, airways branch in a dichotomous manner, and the majority of bifurcations are asymmetric. With successively greater airway generation number, the summed cross-sectional area increases. The dimensions and geometry of the conducting airways to a large extent determine particle penetration and deposition.

The trachea bifurcates into two primary bronchi which enter the right and left lung. The primary bronchi divide into lobar (or secondary) bronchi which divide again into segmental (or tertiary) bronchi. Segmental bronchi, and the pulmonary parenchyma they ventilate, are known as bronchopulmonary segments. The segmental bronchi undergo further branching and a decrease in diameter to the level of the bronchioles. The bronchioles branch into the terminal bronchioles and, in some species, branch further into well-developed respiratory bronchioles; they finally end at the alveolar ducts.

The tracheobronchial region is lined by respiratory epithelium, similar to that of the nose and nasopharynx. This pseudostratified columnar ciliated epithelium consists primarily of ciliated cells and mucous cells, which play an important role in mucociliary clearance. Serous cells, small granule mucous or intermediate cells, basal cells, and occasional brush and neuroendocrine cells are also present. Serous and mucous glands are variably present within the submucosa. The glands are innervated by both parasympathetic and sympathetic branches of the autonomic nervous system. Hypertrophy and hyperplasia of the mucus-secreting glands, as well as altered secretion (both character and composition), are common responses to inhaled irritants and infection.

Bronchioles no longer have submucosal glands or cartilage. The epithelium becomes simple columnar, with nonciliated bronchiolar epithelial (Clara) cells (Figure 6.2A) replacing mucous cells, and basal cells disappearing. There are species differences in the proportion of ciliated to nonciliated cells. Bronchioles end in alveolar ducts which contain spiral smooth muscle and are lined by alveolar epithelium. Alveoli open into the alveolar ducts. The acinar unit consists of the terminal bronchiole and all the air spaces supplied by it (Figure 6.3). The bronchiole-alveolar duct junction (BADJ) is a vulnerable site for damage by low to moderate concentrations of many inhaled toxicants, both gaseous and particulate.

Airway Cells

Ciliated epithelial cells are cuboidal to tall columnar, with cilia and microvilli extending from the lumenal surface. The ciliary structure is similar in all tissues and species. Ciliated cells are exquisitely sensitive to injury by toxic inhalants such as nitrogen dioxide (NO_2), sulfur dioxide (SO_2), ozone (O_3), hyperoxia, and cigarette smoke. Damage to ciliated epithelial cells may be manifested as ciliostasis, detachment or resorption of cilia, or cell death. The end result is impairment of mucociliary clearance, which can be reversible, or can lead to bronchitis and bronchopneumonia, potentially life-threatening situations.

Mucous (goblet) and serous epithelial cells contribute to the secretion of airway mucus. The mucous cell is columnar; secretory granules eventually fill the cell and protrude at the apical surface to form an apical bleb, creating the classic goblet shape. Serous cells produce a secretion of lower viscosity than that of mucous cells, and may transform into mucous cells after exposure to certain irritants. These cells may replicate by mitosis, or derive from an undifferentiated secretory stem cell. Hypersecretion and mucous cell hyperplasia occur commonly in response to inhaled irritants.

Clara cells are tall, dome-shaped epithelial cells that occur in large numbers in the bronchioles of mammals, but not in birds. Clara cells contain large amounts of SER in rodents, pigs, sheep, and horses, but not in dogs, cats, steer, or primates. Ovoid membrane-bound, electron-dense secretory granules are numerous in most species, but appear to be absent in cats and rare in dogs. Clara cells synthesize, store, and secrete protein components of the extracellular lining of the bronchioles. They are the progenitor cells of bronchiolar ciliated cells and Clara cells, and with continued airway irritation, they can transform into mucus-secreting cells (metaplasia). Clara cells play a major role in the metabolism of xenobiotics by the lung in species with abundant SER, including both phase I and II reactions.

Basal cells are flattened to pyramidal cells that rest on the basement membrane. These cells are considered stem cells for the secretory and ciliated cells,

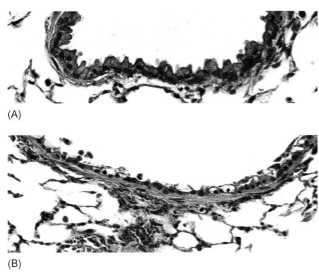

(A)

(B)

FIGURE 6.2 Bronchiole, mouse. H&E stain. (A) Normal bronchiole is lined by dome-shaped, nonciliated Clara cells, with a few interspersed cuboidal ciliated cells. (B) Three days after intraperitoneal injection of chloroform, most of the Clara cells have undergone apoptosis/necrosis and sloughed into the lumen (far left). The remaining cells consist of ciliated cells, some of which are swollen with cytoplasmic clearing (middle, right).

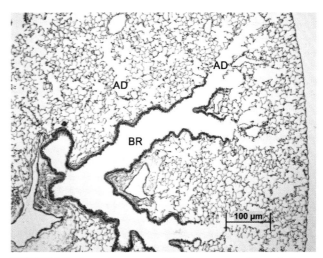

FIGURE 6.3 Lung, intratracheal fixation, mouse. Normal airway distension is retained. Bronchiole (BR) and acinar unit with alveolar ducts (AD), and associated alveoli. The visceral pleura (right) covering the surface is thin. H&E stain.

and may play an important function in anchoring the columnar epithelium to the basement membrane.

Neuroendocrine cells tend to occur singly or in small organized groups contacted by nerves, called neuroepithelial bodies (NEB). Neuroendocrine cells contain active peptides within cytoplasmic granules. The main function of the cell appears to be the monitoring of changes in airway gases or secretions.

Both connective tissue mast cells (located near blood vessels and nerves) and mucosal mast cells are present throughout the respiratory tract, increasing in number from proximal to distal airways. Mast cells are closely associated with immediate hypersensitivity diseases, such as anaphylaxis, allergic asthma, and hay fever.

Lymphoid Tissue

Four major components of lymphoid tissue are found in the respiratory tract: T-lymphocytes, which reside between the epithelial cells of the respiratory mucosa; T- and B-cells, loosely organized in the lamina propria of the mucosa; organized lymphoid tissue lying beneath the epithelium of the nasal cavity, nasopharynx, and bronchi (nasal-associated and bronchus-associated lymphoid tissue; NALT and BALT, respectively); and draining lymph nodes. Small numbers of lymphocytes also reside within the lung interstitium.

The NALT and BALT belong to the mucosa-associated lymphoid tissue (MALT). The organization of these tissues is similar to that of lymph nodes, except that medulla-like areas are absent (see Chapter 15, Immune System). BALT is present in mammals, birds, and reptiles. These lymphoid aggregates are randomly distributed along the bronchial tract, but consistently present at bifurcations. MALT lymphocytes are primarily B-cells, which can switch to IgA-producing B-cells/plasma cells. Secreted IgA is an important part of the local mucosal immune response. The size of these lymphoid nodules varies greatly with immune status of the animal, with hyperplasia occurring following antigenic stimulation.

Species Differences

The number of glands in the tracheal and bronchial submucosa, and the distance that cartilage extends down the airways, varies among species (Table 6.1). Although the basic structure of the respiratory epithelium is the same in all mammals, the location of the various cell types within the epithelia varies with species (Table 6.2). The major species difference in the acinar unit is the presence or absence of respiratory bronchioles (Table 6.1). Humans have a complex acinus, due to the presence of respiratory bronchioles,

whereas most of the common laboratory animals do not. This is an important consideration in the selection of animals for experimental studies, since the junction of the bronchioles with the alveolar ducts (the bronchiole-alveolar duct junction or BADJ; proximal acinus) is the most vulnerable part of the lung for damage by low to moderate concentrations of many inhaled intoxicants, both gaseous and particulate.

Pulmonary Region

Overview

Lobation varies greatly among species: the horse has a single right lobe and a single left lobe; the human has two lobes on the left and three on the right; the monkey, dog, cat, and raccoon have three left lobes and four right lobes; and the mouse, rat, and hamster have a single left lobe and four right lobes. Depending on species, lobes may be divided into bronchopulmonary segments, subsegments, and lobules by interlobular tissue (see Table 6.1). The lobule consists of a lobular bronchiole with its branches and associated structures.

The surface of the lung is covered by visceral pleura and the walls of the pleural cavity by the parietal pleura. Communication between the two pleural cavities (right and left) and pleural thickness (see Table 6.1) is species-dependent. Vessels (pulmonary artery and veins, bronchial artery, and lymph vessels) and nerves enter the lungs with the bronchi at the hilus; the bronchial lymph nodes are also found in this area.

Cells of the Pulmonary Parenchyma

Alveoli arise from the respiratory bronchioles and the alveolar ducts. The alveolar septum or wall consists of three components: epithelium (which lines the alveolus or air space), interstitium, and capillary endothelium. Gas exchange occurs in the alveoli across the thin epithelial lining and adjacent endothelium (air-blood barrier) (Figure 6.4).

The major cell types are the epithelial type I and type II cells, the pulmonary endothelial cells, interstitial cells, and macrophages. Type I cells constitute 8% to 11% of all cells found in the alveolar region, and type II epithelial cells constitute 13% to 16%. Tight junctions are present between epithelial cells. Epithelial cells lie on a continuous basement membrane, as do endothelial cells. In many places, the basement membrane of both cell types is fused, forming an extremely thin air–blood barrier. In other areas, the cells are separated by interstitium that consists of scant connective and elastic tissue and resident interstitial cells, macrophages, lymphocytes, plasma cells, and mast cells.

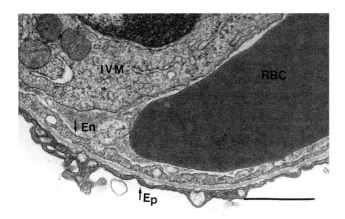

FIGURE 6.4 Lung, alveolar wall, pig. The air–blood barrier consists of fused basement membranes of a type I epithelial cell (Ep) and a capillary endothelial cell (En). The epithelium lines the alveolus and the endothelial cell lines a capillary that contains a red blood cell (RBC) and an intravascular macrophage (IVM). Bar = 1 μm.

Alveolar type I epithelial cells are attenuated, highly-differentiated cells that do not divide; they cover approximately 90% to 95% of the alveolar surface. Since these cells have a large surface area, they are highly susceptible to injury. The main function of the type I cell is the maintenance of a barrier to prevent leakage of fluid and proteins across the alveolar wall into the air spaces, while allowing gases to freely cross the air–blood barrier.

The alveolar type II epithelial cells are cuboidal in shape, located in corners or niches between capillaries, and contain lamellar bodies in which surfactant is stored. The functions of type II cells include the synthesis, storage, and secretion of pulmonary surface-active material; the re-epithelialization of the alveolar wall after lung injury; and transepithelial solute transport to limit the volume of, and perhaps regulate the composition of, alveolar fluid.

The capillaries, which are lined by endothelial cells (30% to 42% of all cells), are of the closed type, without openings or fenestrations. Intercellular junctions between endothelial cells are characterized by zonulae occludens, but are less tight than the epithelial junctions. Therefore, unlike other tissues, the major permeability barrier in the lung is the alveolar epithelium.

Macrophages have been identified in three distinct locations in the lung: the interstitium, alveoli, and capillary lumen. Macrophages present in the alveolar interstitium are derived from bone marrow, can divide, and can either phagocytize particulate material that crosses the alveolar walls or move into the alveolar compartment to become alveolar macrophages. Another macrophage-like cell in the interstitium is the dendritic cell, which is specialized for antigen presentation and accessory function.

Alveolar macrophages (AMs) are derived from the interstitial compartment; however, they do divide and are a self-renewing population of cells. The intravascular macrophage (IVM) is present in humans, pigs, cats, horses, ruminants and marine mammals, but not in rodents or dogs (Figure 6.4). It is a fixed macrophage of the capillary bed, has specialized junctional complexes with adjacent endothelial cells; it is morphologically and, presumably, functionally similar to hepatic Küpffer cells. Intravascular macrophages function similarly to the AM. The IVMs account for some of the species differences that occur in response to pulmonary injury.

Fibroblasts are the major cell type present in the interstitium. Apart from maintaining the structural integrity of the lung and production of collagen and other matrix components, such as fibronectin, fibroblasts produce a variety of enzymes including collagenase, and other factors, such as prostaglandins and plasminogen activator, that may modulate the function of other cell types. Fibroblasts play a major role in disease processes that result in fibrosis.

Blood Vessels, Lymphatics, and Nerves

Blood reaches the lungs through two separate systems, the pulmonary vessels and the bronchial vessels. The pulmonary arterial system differs from other organs in that it is derived from the low-pressure pulmonary arteries, supplying blood for gas exchange in the pulmonary capillaries. It carries high volumes of venous blood from the right heart, and supplies the distal portion of the respiratory bronchioles, the alveolar ducts, alveoli, and pleura. The bronchial system is a high-pressure arterial system derived from the aorta, and carries oxygenated blood to meet the metabolic needs of the larger airways, visceral pleura, and large pulmonary vessels.

The pulmonary arteries differ morphologically from the smaller muscular bronchial arteries. However, because of the reduced pressure, pulmonary arteries and veins may resemble each other fairly closely, especially in large animals. The muscular layer of the pulmonary arteries and veins varies with species (Table 6.1). The pulmonary veins may have an adventitial coating of cardiac muscle arising from the left atrium.

Lymphatics are confined to the extra-alveolar interstitium, i.e., peribronchial, interlobular, and pleural interstitium. Lymph flows centripetally through a subpleural network that is joined by perivascular and peribronchial lymphatics at the hilus. Afferent lymphatic vessels from the lungs drain into the lymph nodes, and then into the thoracic, right, and left lymphatic ducts, and the bloodstream.

The sympathetic and parasympathetic divisions of the autonomic nervous system provide motor (efferent) innervation to the lungs, including bronchial smooth muscle, blood vessels, submucosal glands, and lymphatics. Sensory (afferent) innervation is maintained by way of several types of chemo- and mechano-receptors that respond to inhaled irritants and other stresses.

Physiology and Functional Considerations

The respiratory system has a number of functions, the most important of which is gas exchange, which occurs in the lung. Other functions include protection against noxious agents, removal of vasoactive agents from the blood by endothelial cells, production and release of hormones and mediators, and biotransformation of xenobiotics. Within the nasal cavity, olfaction is a major function of the olfactory epithelium; metabolism of odorants presumably plays an important role in olfaction. Humidification, heating or cooling of the inspired air, as appropriate, are also functions of the nasal mucosa.

Protection of the respiratory system from harmful agents such as particulates, chemical irritants, and infectious agents can occur by both nonspecific and specific defense mechanisms. Nonspecific defenses include particle filtration by the nasal region, adsorption of chemical vapors, reflex responses such as changes in ventilation or coughing, mucociliary clearance, and phagocytosis by alveolar macrophages. Specific defense mechanisms are of immunological nature.

Gas Exchange

The main function of the lung is gas exchange. Three processes are involved: ventilation, perfusion, and diffusion of gases across the air–blood barrier. Ventilation is accomplished by moving air through the upper respiratory tract into the conducting airways, and then into the alveolar zone. Perfusion occurs by blood from the pulmonary artery arising from the right ventricle of the heart. Since the lung receives the entire cardiac output, it may be exposed to substantial amounts of blood-borne toxicants.

In the alveolar zone, O_2 and CO_2 move across the air–blood barrier by diffusion. As a result, venous blood from the right heart gives up its content of CO_2 and becomes enriched with O_2. In order to reach its carrier molecule, the hemoglobin in the red blood cells, O_2 has to cross the pulmonary epithelial cells and their basement membrane; the interstitium; basement membrane and cytoplasm of the capillary endothelial cells; a thin layer of plasma; and finally the membrane of the red blood cells. Carbon dioxide follows the same path, but in the opposite direction. Any process that increases the thickness of any of these consecutive layers may compromise the proper diffusion of O_2 and gas exchange.

Nonspecific Defense Mechanisms

The first line of defense is the nasal region. This convoluted arrangement of turbinates creates a filtering mechanism, so that many particles suspended in the inhaled air will not reach the deeper regions of the respiratory tract. These may, however, injure the nasal mucosa. Similarly, absorption of chemical vapors can protect the lung against some chemicals; however, this in turn may also damage the nasal mucosa.

Reflex responses help to eliminate foreign agents from the respiratory tract. These vary depending on the site of the receptor (i.e., nasal cavity, trachea, or alveoli), and include changes in ventilation, bronchomotor tone, blood pressure, and airway mucus secretion.

Insoluble particles deposited in the conducting airways are primarily cleared by action of the ciliated cells on mucus. Smaller particles may reach the deeper regions of the lung. Foreign particles are generally phagocytized by macrophages, or trapped in the alveolar surface layer. They will then reach the airways, to be transported upward by the mucociliary escalator. Macrophages may also enter the lymphatics or, on occasion, be killed by engulfed particles such as silica. The persistence of such particles may incite the formation of granulomas. Occasionally, particles may migrate directly across the alveolar wall, into the interstitium, and into capillaries or lymphatics. In addition to the macrophage, the polymorphonuclear neutrophil (PMN) is an important phagocytic cell which plays a major role in respiratory defense. Although not a normal resident cell, PMNs are readily recruited from the vascular bed by chemotactic factors secreted by macrophages. This and other important interactions between pulmonary macrophages and PMNs in the lung are illustrated in Figure 6.5. In addition to the role in respiratory defense, these phagocytes, when activated, are key players in injurious processes, especially in the lungs.

The lung also contains antioxidant defense mechanisms, including specific enzymes such as catalase, superoxide dismutase, and glutathione peroxidase, as well as antioxidant substances such as vitamins E and C, and glutathione (GSH). Surfactant also appears to have antioxidant properties. Toxicants can inhibit enzymes, react with oxidant scavengers, or form free radical intermediates that initiate uncontrolled tissue reactions with molecular oxygen, thereby upsetting the

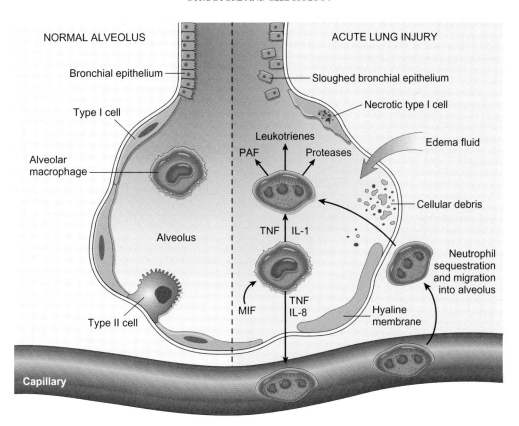

FIGURE 6.5   Interaction between alveolar macrophages and neutrophils in acute lung injury; normal alveolus (left side) compared with injured alveolus. With injury, macrophages release proinflammatory cytokines, such as interleukins 8 and 1 (IL-8, IL-1), and tumor necrosis factor (TNF), which cause neutrophils to sequester in the pulmonary microvasculature with subsequent margination and egress into the alveolar space. Activated neutrophils release leukotrienes, oxidants, proteases, and platelet activating factor (PAF) which contribute to tissue damage, edema, surfactant inactivation and hyaline membrane formation. Macrophage inhibitory factor (MIF) sustains the proinflammatory response until the healing phase starts, with release of macrophage derived fibrogenic factors. (From Hussain and Kumar (2005). In *Robbins and Cotran Pathologic Basis of Disease*, Kumar, V., Abbas, A.K., and Fausto, N. eds, 7th edn. Elsevier Saunders, New York. Figure 15-4, p. 717.)

oxidant–antioxidant *status quo,* and causing tissue damage. Metabolizing enzymes present within the respiratory tissue that can detoxify xenobiotics should also be considered as part of the nonspecific defense mechanism. These are discussed below under "Metabolism of Foreign Compounds."

Specific Defense Mechanisms

The respiratory tract has two immunological compartments that participate in humoral immune responses. The first is the MALT in the upper respiratory tract, with the IgA class of antibodies predominating. IgA acts as an opsonizing antibody to promote uptake and destruction of inhaled particulates by macrophages and neutrophils. IgE can also be synthesized locally, and plays a key role in immediate hypersensitivity responses. The second immunological compartment is in the lower respiratory tract or alveolar region, and is a typical systemic immune response

in which the IgG class of antibodies predominates. The primary site for the generation of antigen-specific B-lymphocytes is the intrathoracic group of lymph nodes from which they are preferentially translocated to the lung. Macrophages and dendritic cells are also an important component of the immune system. They not only function to clear antigen and particulate matter, but also process antigens ("antigen processing cells" or APC) for presentation to lymphocytes for initiation or amplification of immune responses.

Cellular immune responses are presumably also important in respiratory defense reactions; however, relatively little information is available. The active participation of T-cells in immune responses is indicated by the presence of large numbers of natural killer (NK) cells in the lung, and the occurrence of T-cells with the suppressor/cytotoxic phenotype in the lamina propria and within BALT. Inhalation of an antigenic substance can initiate cell-mediated immunity in the lung-associated lymph nodes and deep lungs.

Production and Release of Pharmacological Agents and Mediators

The lung is capable of synthesizing, storing, releasing, removing, degrading, and inactivating a variety of biologically-active substances or mediators. For example, biogenic amines, such as catecholamines, serotonin, and histamine, play an important role in the control of airway and vascular smooth muscle tone, and affect certain epithelial cell functions. The eicosanoids also affect airway and vascular smooth muscle, as well as mucous glands, bronchial epithelial cells, and pulmonary endothelial cells. Conditions associated with pulmonary release of biologically active agents include anaphylaxis, asthma, mechanical stimulation such as hyperventilation, pulmonary thromboembolism, pulmonary edema, and the respiratory distress syndrome.

Xenobiotic Exposure, Metabolism, and Excretion

Routes of Exposure

Xenobiotics may reach the respiratory tract either through inspired air or the bloodstream. Inhalation is a major exposure route, with the respiratory tract being in the first point of contact with airborne toxicants. In humans, approximately 23 000 liters of air per day interact with $70\,m^2$ of respiratory tract surface.

Xenobiotics may enter the bloodstream following ingestion, parenteral administration, or skin absorption. In man, the blood volume circulating through the lung may vary from 6–8 liters per minute, up to 20–30 liters per minute, depending on physical activity. It is the only organ whose capillary bed receives the whole cardiac output.

Deposition, Absorption, Distribution, and Excretion of Inhaled Agents

Deposition (removal of particles from inhaled air by contact with an airway surface) and clearance (physical removal of deposited particles from their initial deposition site) are dependent on physicochemical characteristics of the particle, and biological clearance mechanisms of the respiratory tract. Host characteristics that influence particle deposition include respiratory tract anatomy, and breathing rate and pattern. Retention (= deposition − clearance) is the amount of particles remaining in the respiratory tract at a particular time after exposure. Particles with an aerodynamic diameter greater than 5μm (5 to 30μm) are deposited by impaction, primarily in the nasopharyngeal

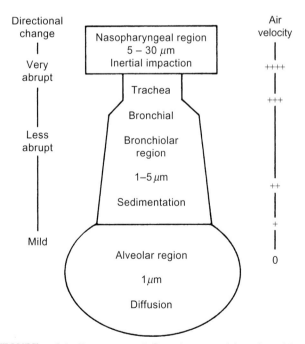

FIGURE 6.6 Parameters influencing particle deposition. (Reproduced with permission from Casarett, L.J. (1972). In *Essays in Toxicology*, Blood, F.R. ed., Vol. 3. Academic Press, New York.)

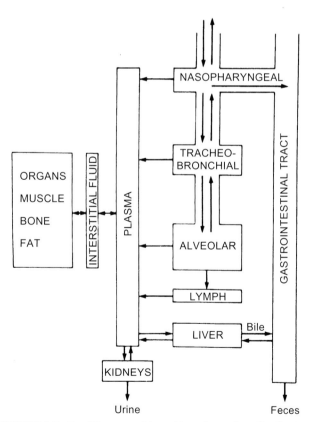

FIGURE 6.7 Possible route of deposition, absorption, distribution, and excretion of inhaled agents. (Reprinted from Inchiosa (1987). In *Inhalation Toxicology*, Salem, H. ed., p. 186, courtesy of Marcel Dekker, Inc.)

region; this region has the highest air velocity and turbulence (Figure 6.6). Impaction may occur deeper on the walls of the tracheobronchial tree under certain circumstances, such as mouth-breathing in humans. Particles 1 to 5 μm in diameter deposit by sedimentation along the tracheobronchial tract; the smallest particles reach the small intrapulmonary airways. For particles 0.1 to 2 μm in diameter, deposition in the conducting airways is usually negligible, compared with deposition in the alveolar zone. However, it must be pointed out that particles of a certain shape and configuration may, because of their aerodynamic properties, also reach the alveolar zone, where they are deposited at the bronchiolar-alveolar junction. Such is the case for asbestos fibers, which can reach 50 μm in length while having a diameter of 0.4 to 1 μm.

Clearance depends on the characteristics of the particle, and its site of deposition in the respiratory tract (Figure 6.7). Removal from the nasopharyngeal region occurs by sneezing, mucociliary transport, nose wiping and blowing, and dissolution (for soluble particles). Transported material may be swallowed, and may potentially serve as an additional source of exposure. Mucociliary transport is the major clearance mechanism in the tracheobronchial region. Other mechanisms include coughing and dissolution (for soluble particles). In the alveolar region, clearance mechanisms include macrophages, interstitial pathways, and dissolution (for soluble and "insoluble" particles). Phagocytosed material is either destroyed or solubilized and absorbed into the circulation. Macrophages containing indigestible material may be cleared by the mucociliary escalator, enter the lymphatics and be deposited in lymph nodes, retained within the lung (e.g., anthracotic pigment), or even destroyed by the ingested material (e.g., silica).

Nonparticulate substances, such as gases and vapors, may potentially be absorbed by respiratory tissue, or pass into the plasma along the entire surface of the respiratory tract. Gas uptake is reversible, dynamic, and saturable. Absorption is mainly by simple diffusion, and is directly related to the lipid solubility of the compound. Since most toxic gases have adequate lipid solubility to cross cell membranes, the rate of diffusion is primarily related to the diffusion coefficient of the gas in aqueous media, and its concentration gradient between the air and plasma. Gases and vapors with higher water solubility, such as SO_2, are removed primarily by the upper respiratory tract, while those with low water solubility may reach the alveoli. Such insoluble gases will enter all regions of the respiratory system, unless they are highly irritant, and cause extensive bronchoconstriction or cessation of respiratory movement. Once the substance enters the bloodstream,

it can be distributed widely in the body. Distribution and excretion of the toxicant would then follow normal toxicokinetics. Translocation of toxicants, such as manganese and mycotoxins, through the olfactory epithelium via the neuronal cells and the olfactory nerves to the brain has been recently described.

Uptake and Accumulation of Blood-borne Toxicants

Preferential accumulation of certain xenobiotics by the lung, such as chlorphentermine, can result in a high tissue to blood concentration ratio (Figure 6.8). This has been shown for a group of compounds that are diverse in both chemical structure and toxicological action (Table 6.3). Many of the compounds are

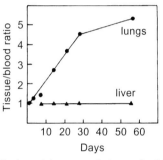

FIGURE 6.8 Preferential accumulation of chlorphentermine by the lung. Tissue accumulation of chlorphentermine following chronic treatment (20 mg/kg ip/day). Ordinate shows the multiples of tissue/blood ratio found one day after a single dose. (Data from Lüllman, H., Lüllman-Rauch, R., and Wasserman, O. (1975). CRC Crit. Rev. Toxicol., 4, 185. With permission.)

TABLE 6.3 Pulmonary accumulation of selected xenobiotics[a]

Xenobiotic	Lung/blood ratio (one hour after injection)	Species
Amphetamine	33	Rat
Chlorphentermine (anorectic drug)	53	Rat
Diphenhydramine (antihistamine)	100	Guinea pig
Clozapine (antipsychotic)	49	Rat
Propanolol (β-adrenergic blocking agent)	125	Rabbit
Paraquat (herbicide)	4	Rat

[a]Modified from: Wilson, A. G. E. (1982). Toxicokinetics of uptake, accumulation and metabolism of chemicals by the lung. In Mechanisms in Respiratory Toxicology, (H. P. Witschi and P. Nettesheim, eds.), Vol. I, pp. 161–185. CRC Press, Boca Raton, Florida

highly lipophilic basic amines, with pK$_a$s in excess of 8, for example, imipramine, propanolol, and amphetamine. For the majority of these compounds, uptake is by diffusion, and accumulation is a result of intracellular binding. Accumulation may occur in a variety of pulmonary cell types including macrophages.

The pulmonary accumulation of basic amphophilic amine drugs, such as chlorphentermine, is the basis of the condition termed drug-induced phospholipidosis. This is characterized by an increase in lung phospholipids and accumulation of the drug and phospholipids within virtually all pulmonary cell types; increased numbers of alveolar macrophages are a prominent feature. The main adverse functional effect of phospholipidosis appears to be at the level of the endothelial cell, resulting in marked alteration of pulmonary clearance of endogenous vasoactive compounds. Pulmonary hypertension has been observed in patients treated with the anorectic drug aminorex.

In contrast to the basic amines, paraquat accumulation by the lung cannot be explained as a consequence of tissue binding. Paraquat is selectively taken up by the lung, due to its structural similarity to the endogenous substrates, diamines and polyamines. It is taken up into alveolar epithelial cells by a receptor-mediated energy-dependent transport system. The strict structural requirements for uptake explain why paraquat is accumulated by the lung (Figure 6.9), but diquat is not.

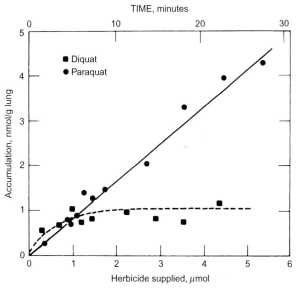

FIGURE 6.9 Preferential uptake of paraquat by the lung. Paraquat and diquat accumulation by the isolated perfused rat lung. The perfusate contained 6.45 μM paraquat or diquat (specific activity 0.8 μCi/mg). Total radioactivity in the lung was determined after various times of perfusion. (Reprinted with permission from Wilson (1982). In *Mechanisms in Respiratory Toxicology*, Witschi, H.P., and Nettesheim, P. eds, Vol. I, p. 176. Copyright CRC Press, Inc. Boca Raton, FL.)

Metabolism of Foreign Compounds

Extrahepatic metabolism is recognized as an important factor in activation and detoxification of foreign compounds and in drug metabolism. The respiratory tract also has this capability to metabolize xenobiotics independent of route of exposure. Examples of bioactivation include the metabolism of the polycyclic aromatic hydrocarbon benzo[α]pyrene to the ultimate carcinogen, benzo[α]pyrene 7,8-dihydrodiol 9,10-epoxide; activation of carbon tetrachloride (CCl$_4$) to the trichloromethyl free radical, and conversion of naphthalene to several reactive naphthalene metabolites.

Most of the major xenobiotic metabolizing enzymes have been identified in the respiratory tract, with the cytochrome P450 enzymes being the most studied. These have highest activity in the olfactory mucosa and the Clara cell. The differences in concentration between liver and various regions of the respiratory tract, and among species, are illustrated in Figure 6.10. Unlike cytochrome P450, aldehyde dehydrogenase activity is found primarily in respiratory mucosa, although a high concentration also occurs in the Clara cell. The toxicity of volatile aldehydes, such as formaldehyde and acetaldehyde, may be modified by this enzyme system.

MECHANISMS OF TOXICITY

Toxic lung damage is an exceedingly complicated series of interlocking and interdependent events. Primary lung injury may be brought about by mechanisms such as metabolism of foreign chemicals to reactive intermediates that are potentially able to interact with intracellular targets, osmotic or cytolytic membrane injury or oxidative damage to cell constituents

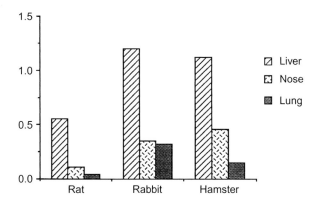

FIGURE 6.10 Comparison of cytochrome P450 enzymes among species and tissues. (Data with permission, from Vainio, H., and Hietanen, E. (1980). In *Concepts in Drug Metabolism*, Jenner, P., and Testa, B. eds, Part A, pp. 25–284. Marcel Dekker, New York.)

mediated through the formation of reactive oxygen species (Table 6.4). Primary lung injury is often amplified through secondary events, such as formation and release of mediators, for example, vasoactive amines and leukotrienes; activation of the kinin and complement cascades; release of lysosomal enzymes; and activation of inflammatory cells. Toxicity may also be directly related to the physicochemical properties of inhaled agents, or their ability to induce immune-mediated responses. Toxicity may also be directly related to the physicochemical properties of inhaled agents or their ability to induce immune mediated responses.

Direct Toxicity

Many agents produce respiratory injury by a direct interaction of the reactive molecule with its cellular target. Examples include oxidant and irritant gases such as oxygen, ozone, phosgene, hydrochloric acid (HCl), and many other fumes and gases. These gases may produce cytolytic changes directly at their site of primary interaction, the exposed cell membrane, or increase the generation and accumulation of reactive oxygen species, and thus trigger cell injury. Injury mediated by oxygen reactive species appears to be an important mechanism in toxic respiratory damage for gases such as oxygen and, perhaps, ozone, ionizing radiation, and bleomycin. In addition, inflammatory cells, particularly macrophages and polymorphonuclear leukocytes, may be recruited into the lung parenchyma. Upon appropriate stimulation, these cells can undergo activation and produce a burst of reactive oxygen species which, in turn, may also damage respiratory cells (see Figure 6.5).

Metabolic Activation

A great deal of information is now available describing the role of metabolic activation of xenobiotics in respiratory toxicity (see section on "Metabolism" above). Three different mechanisms may be involved. In the first scenario, the parent compound itself reaches the respiratory tract, either through the blood following systemic administration, or as an inhalant. The compound then undergoes metabolic activation to the proximate toxin (Figure 6.11A). Interaction with the target is often manifested as covalent binding of the reactive metabolite to cell macromolecules. Activation by microsomal mixed-function oxidases, especially the cytochrome P450 enzymes, is a key element in the process; on the other hand, protective systems such as intracellular levels of GSH and enzymes involved in maintaining reducing equivalents within

the cell are crucial components in protection. Cell types that contain high concentration of cytochrome P450s are particularly important in the detoxification of xenobiotics; however, these cells are vulnerable to injury caused by the reactive metabolites they form. Examples of chemicals that cause respiratory damage following *in situ* metabolic activation include phenacetin, bromobenzene, 4-ipomeanol, butylated hydroxytoluene, CCl$_4$, 3-methylindole, acetaminophen, and 3-methylfuran (Tables 6.4 and 6.5). 3-Methylindole (3MI) is formed in ruminants by bacterial degradation of tryptophan in the rumen, and is also present in cigarette smoke and in the human intestinal tract. 3MI is then absorbed into the circulation, taken up by the lung, and metabolized by the cytochrome P450 enzymes, resulting in toxicity. In cattle, severe damage to alveolar cells results in an acute interstitial pneumonia, which is identical to that caused by

TABLE 6.4 Mechanisms of toxicity to the respiratory system with selected examples

Mechanism	Xenobiotic
Direct toxicity	Oxygen, ozone, phosgene, hydrochloric acid, other fumes and gases
Metabolic activation	
In situ metabolic activation	Acetaminophen, bromobenzene, butylated hydroxytoluene, carbon tetrachloride, 4-ipomeanol, 3-methylfuran, naphthalene
Activation outside the lung	Pyrrolizidine alkaloids (e.g., monocrotaline)
Cyclic reduction/oxidation with production of reactive oxygen species	Paraquat, nitrofurantoin
Immune mediated	
Hypersensitivity reactions	
Type I hypersensitivity	Toluene, diisocyanates, trimellitic anhydride, ozone
Type III hypersensitivity	Trimellitic anhydride, mercury, organic dusts, beryllium
Immune suppression	Oxidant gases, asbestos, tobacco smoke, benzene, toluene, cadmium, zinc, lead
Non-immune secretion of inflammatory mediators can cause hyperreactive airway syndrome	Isocyanates, formaldehyde, trimellitic anhydride, ozone
Xenobiotic interactions through simultaneous or sequential exposure	Oxygen enhances toxicity of paraquat, bleomycin, butylated hydroxytoluene, CdCl$_2$

TABLE 6.5   Specificity of cell damage by selected compounds which undergo *in situ* metabolic activation within the respiratory tract

Compound	Primary cell type affected	Species	Route[a]
Acetaminophen	Olfactory mucosa, transitional epithelium, Clara cell	Rat, mouse	Oral, ip
Bromobenzene	Clara cell	Rat, mouse	ip
Butylated hydroxy-toluene (BHT)	Type I epithelial cell, capillary endothelial cell	Mouse (not rat)	ip
Carbon tetrachloride	Clara cell	Guinea pig	Inhalation
		Rat	ip
4-Ipomeanol	Clara cell (also causes pulmonary edema)	Rat, mouse	ip
3-Methylfuran	Olfactory mucosa, Clara cell	Mouse, rat, hamster	Inhalation
Naphthalene	Clara cell	Mouse, rat	ip, inhalation
Alpha-naphthylthiourea (ANTU)	Capillary endothelial cell	Rat	Oral
Trialkyl phosphoro-thioates	Type I epithelial cell, Clara cell	Rat	Oral, ip
Phenacetin	Olfactory mucosa	Rat	Oral

[a]ip, intraperitoneal

the ingestion of moldy sweet potatoes containing 4-ipomeanol. In mice, both 3MI and 4-ipomeanol cause Clara cell necrosis; 3MI also causes necrosis of olfactory epithelium.

The second mechanism involves uptake of a systemically-administered foreign compound by the liver, or any other organ, where the agent is metabolized to a highly reactive and toxic metabolite(s) (Figure 6.11B). This metabolite(s) may cause liver injury, but also may escape into the circulation via the hepatic veins and inferior vena cava. The next capillary bed encountered is in the lung, and widespread damage may occur. The best-studied examples of chemicals causing this form of lung damage are the pyrrolizidine alkaloids.

The pyrrolizidine alkaloid monocrotaline (MCT) is found in the plant *Crotalaria spectabilis*. Human toxicity has occurred from consuming contaminated grain or herbal teas made from such plants, whereas animal toxicity can occur following grazing on such plants. At high doses, MCT rapidly causes severe liver injury and death. At lower doses, it produces mild liver injury and delayed pulmonary injury, characterized by pulmonary hypertension. MCT is bioactivated in the liver to pyrrolic metabolites by the cytochrome P450 enzyme system. The "putative" reactive metabolite dehydromonocrotaline (MCTP) is toxic to both liver and lung. It is stable enough to reach the lung, which is itself incapable of the bioactivation of MCT. The target cell in the lung is the endothelial cell. Injury is delayed and progressive, both *in vivo* and *in vitro*. The first phase is characterized by vessel leakage, and the later hypertensive phase is characterized by vessel remodeling,

elevated vascular pressure, and hypertrophy of the right heart. *In vitro*, MCTP results in delayed and progressive injury to endothelial cells, and also results in a decrease in their proliferative capability. It has thus been suggested that, *in vivo*, MCTP, in addition to causing endothelial cell injury, also prevents normal repair processes; thus progressive injury takes place.

The third mechanism involves what has been called "futile redox cycling" (Figure 6.11C). It is best exemplified by the pulmonary toxicity of the herbicide paraquat, although other agents, such as nitrofurantoin, may also cause lung damage by a similar mechanism. Paraquat is selectively taken up by pulmonary epithelial cells. It is not metabolized, but undergoes cyclic oxidation and reduction with concomitant production of reactive oxygen species such as superoxide anion, hydrogen peroxide, and hydroxyl free radicals. Direct evidence for the formation of lipid peroxides in paraquat toxicity remains more elusive. This is partly due to the pulmonary antioxidant defense mechanisms, including vitamins C and E, which make it difficult to obtain reliable measurements of peroxidative processes. A second event in paraquat toxicity is excessive oxidation and eventual depletion of cellular reducing equivalents, particularly of NADPH. The extent to which this mechanism contributes to the development of toxic lung damage is unknown.

Immune-mediated Toxicity

Both physical and immunological mechanisms are important in pulmonary defense against chemical and

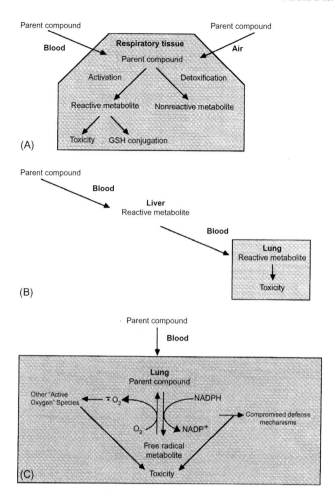

FIGURE 6.11 Mechanisms of respiratory injury involving metabolic activation. (A) *In situ* metabolic activation of parent compound. (B) Activation of parent compound in liver; metabolite produces toxicity in lung. (C) Parent compound undergoes cyclic reduction/oxidation, indirectly inducing toxicity.

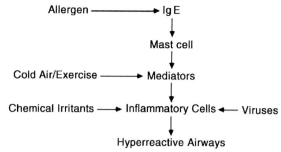

FIGURE 6.12 Immune and nonimmune pathways leading to hyperactive airways. (Modified from Karol and Thorne (1988). In *Toxicology of the Lung*, Gardner, D.E., Crapo, J.D., and Massaro, E.J. eds, from pp. 129. Raven Press, New York.)

infectious agents. However, the immune response may result in an adverse effect if hypersensitivity reactions, immune suppression, or nonimmunological enzymatic injury occur (Table 6.4). Hypersensitivity diseases or allergies are the most common types of immune-mediated respiratory disease caused by inhaled agents. The four types of hypersensitivity reaction are discussed in Chapter 15, Immune System. Type I (anaphylactic), type II (cytotoxic), and type III (Arthus type) are antibody-mediated reactions, whereas type IV (delayed hypersensitivity) is a cell-mediated reaction.

The most common types of hypersensitivity reaction documented in the respiratory tract are types I and III. Exposure to pulmonary sensitizers, either foreign proteins or simple chemicals that act as haptens, at sufficiently high concentrations induces the formation of specific antibodies. Type I hypersensitivity is primarily manifested as rhinitis (inflammation

of the nasal mucosa) or asthma (bronchoconstriction). Initial exposure to the allergen or sensitizer induces production of IgE antibodies, which bind to mast cells and basophils. Subsequent exposure to the allergen triggers mast cell degranulation, with release of vasoactive amines and other mediators (Figure 6.12). Chemicals that produce type I reactions include toluene diisocyanates, trimellitic anhydride, and platinum salts. In domestic species, such as horses and cattle, type I hypersensitivity is manifested as anaphylaxis with severe acute bronchoconstriction and pulmonary edema that is life-threatening. Examples of agents that can induce type I hypersensitivity include vaccines, and antibiotics such as penicillin.

Type III hypersensitivity is manifested as hypersensitivity pneumonitis, also called "extrinsic allergic alveolitis," and results from deposition of antigen–antibody complexes plus complement in the lung, which in turn causes inflammation. Chemicals that produce type III hypersensitivity include trimellitic anhydride, mercury, and organic dusts. Organic dusts, especially fungal antigens, are responsible for occupational disease such as "farmer's lung," as well as chronic obstructive pulmonary disease (COPD) in stabled horses. Type IV hypersensitivity occurs when sensitized T-lymphocytes induce a cell-mediated response after a latent period. An example is the granulomatous reaction induced by beryllium in dogs. However, in rats the granulomas induced by beryllium are considered to be foreign body type granulomas, and beryllium specific T-cells are not found.

Immune suppression has been well-documented in both humans and experimental animals for agents that include oxidant gases (see Chapter 15, Immune System), asbestos, tobacco smoke, benzene, toluene, and metals such as cadmium, zinc, and lead. Toxicants may also enhance normal immune functions. Immune suppression is manifested as altered host resistance to infectious agents or neoplastic cells. Airborne pollutants, such as the photochemical oxidant nitrogen dioxide (NO_2), from gas stoves, increase the incidence of respiratory disease and decrease pulmonary function in young children. This appears to be due to decreased phagocytic function of alveolar macrophages.

Certain chemicals may induce nonimmune-mediated pulmonary disease that mimics immune-mediated disease. Certain chemicals stimulate epithelial irritant receptors that cause secretion of inflammatory mediators without antibody involvement, resulting in a pseudoallergic reaction that resembles immediate or type I hypersensitivity. Such nonspecific airway irritation is called hyper-reactive airway syndrome, and can be stimulated by chemicals such as isocyanates, formaldehyde, trimellitic anhydride, and ozone. The hyper-reactive airway syndrome has been defined as an increased bronchial responsiveness to an inhaled substance that can, depending on dose, produce airway obstruction. Hyper-reactive airways are frequently used as an index of occupational asthma. It should also be noted that viruses and physical stimuli, such as cold air and exercise, may also induce bronchial hyper-reactivity. Finally, interaction of several of these factors may be important in the induction of airway reactivity in any single individual (Figure 6.12).

Toxicity and Responses to Inhaled Particles

Pulmonary toxicity and responses to inhaled particles are influenced by the dose of the material, the amount (mass, number of particles, and surface area) of material in the lung, the toxicity of the particles, and the dynamics of their deposition, retention, and clearance in the lung. There is evidence that, for a given mass of deposited particulate material, ultrafine particles (particles with a diameter less than $0.1\,\mu m$) may be more toxic than larger inhaled particles. The greater toxicity is due to the greater number and surface area of the ultrafine particles, and because of differences in macrophage-mediated clearance and particle interstitialization. For particulate chemicals, metabolism also affects toxicity. Highly soluble particles leave the lung rapidly and the dose is delivered in a pattern that is similar to inhaled gases. In contrast, poorly soluble particles persist in the lung after cessation of exposure, thus delivering a protracted dose to the lung.

After a single inhalation exposure to particles, the amount of particulate material in the lung decreases with time, due to mechanical clearance and/or solubility. However, highly toxic particles, such as silica, are toxic to macrophages and can induce lesions that retard particle clearance. Because of this decrease in clearance, inhalation of toxic particles may result in a greater overall dose (particle mass in the lung × time) compared to inhalation of a relatively non-toxic particle at the same rate to achieve the same initial lung burden. Furthermore, when mixtures are inhaled, physiologic changes and lesions induced by one material may alter deposition and clearance of another material.

Depending on the physicochemical properties of the particle, concentration, duration of exposure, and the species exposed, non-neoplastic parenchymal responses to particles may include infiltrates of alveolar macrophages, inflammation, alveolar epithelial hyperplasia, bronchiolization, and fibrosis. After cessation of exposure, lesions may regress, persist, or progress.

In rats that chronically inhale poorly soluble particles of low acute toxicity, e.g., titanium dioxide, lesions with chronic inflammation, epithelial hyperplasia, and fibrosis often persist or progress after cessation of exposure. Although the amount of particulate material decreases with time after exposure, clearance in these areas with lesions is impaired, so particulate material and a chronic inflammatory response persists. Furthermore, cuboidal epithelial cells and cells with a bronchiolar phenotype that line areas of fibrosis fail to differentiate to type I cells. Thus, a constellation of chronic-active inflammation, alveolar epithelial hyperplasia, bronchiolization, and fibrosis may persist or progress after cessation of exposure. Although in some cases brief exposure results in significant lesions with time, most particulate materials must be inhaled repeatedly to induce lesions in experimental animals. Examples of particles that are generally considered toxic, but that require repeated inhalation exposures to induce significant lesions in experimental animals, include nickel subsulfide, asbestos, and diesel soot.

A number of non-genotoxic, poorly soluble particles, e.g., titanium dioxide, talc, and carbon black induce lesions in rats that are exposed under conditions resulting in overload of macrophage-mediated clearance. Chronic inhalation of these poorly soluble particles by rats can result in pulmonary inflammation, fibrosis, alveolar epithelial hyperplasia, bronchiolization, squamous metaplasia, and squamous cysts. Neoplastic lesions that occur late in life (usually between 24 and 32 months of age) include squamous epitheliomas, bronchiolar-alveolar adenomas, squamous cell carcinomas, and bronchiolar-alveolar adenocarcinomas. In contrast to the rat, mice and hamsters develop less severe lesions, and do not develop lung tumors even though the particle lung burdens are similar to the rat. These findings have raised questions concerning the appropriate use of data from rats, exposed under conditions resulting in clearance overload, for hazard identification in humans.

Xenobiotic Interactions

Toxicological interactions may play a role in the pathogenesis of lung injury. Inhalation of two different aerosols, simultaneously or in sequence, may produce more or less severe lesions than anticipated from the known toxicity of either aerosol alone. It is well known that combination of SO_2 with certain salt aerosols will act synergistically to adversely affect pulmonary function. Concomitant exposure to acidic aerosols and to ozone (at certain specific exposure levels and exposure times) enhances the development of pulmonary fibrosis over that occurring following exposure to either inhalant alone. Of particular importance is the observation that such interactions occur at pollutant levels approximating conditions encountered in the environment. On the other hand, interactions between inhalants occasionally may mitigate toxicity, for example, the neutralization of acidic fumes by ammonia.

Simultaneous exposure to a blood-borne pulmonary toxin and to an inhalant may also greatly enhance the development of untoward effects in the lung. Well-known examples are enhancement of paraquat, bleomycin, or butylated hydroxytoluene (BHT) toxicity by oxygen species. Whether such an interaction accounts for some of the human cases of bleomycin lung damage remains unclear. Finally, it must be pointed out that damaged lung is often much more vulnerable to the toxic effects of a second agent than normal lung. In experimental animals, primary lung injury caused by certain toxic agents, such as inhaled $CdCl_2$, or certain anticancer drugs, can be greatly amplified by subsequent inhalation of oxygen at a concentration (50–70% in the inhaled air) that otherwise would produce little, if any, harmful effect in a normal lung. In humans with diffuse alveolar damage (adult respiratory distress syndrome), oxygen therapy, although necessary, may enhance the later development of fibrotic changes.

Modifying Factors in Toxicity

Factors affecting susceptibility to non-neoplastic and neoplastic pulmonary disease include genetic factors, species differences, age, and nutrition, as well as pre-existing disease, such as asthma. For example, newborn and young rats are usually more resistant to oxygen toxicity than adults. This correlates with their ability to induce superoxide dismutase, catalase, and glutathione peroxidase on exposure to a high concentration of oxygen. In adults, tolerance can be induced by prior exposure to oxygen, which induces the activity of superoxide dismutase. Tolerance cannot be induced in adult hamsters or mice, and they show little increase in superoxide dismutase activity. In addition, a vitamin E-deficient diet can enhance the susceptibility to oxygen toxicity.

Species differences in response to sensory irritants can result in large differences in the actual dose delivered to the respiratory tract. This has been thoroughly studied with formaldehyde. Mice and rats exposed to 15 ppm formaldehyde for six hours, following a similar four-day pretreatment, had an immediate decrease in respiratory rate and minute volume, but no change in tidal volume. The minute volume of mice was decreased to 50% of pre-exposure values, whereas that of rats showed only a 15% decrease. Thus, the nasal cavity of rats received a significantly higher dose of formaldehyde (approximately 75% greater), than that of mice. Histologic lesions and cell proliferation were greater in rats than in mice, thus correlating with the difference in dose received between mice and rats.

RESPONSE TO INJURY

The respiratory tract is continuously exposed to a large variety of potentially injurious agents, both infectious and noninfectious, by way of the airways or bloodstream. As previously described, pulmonary defense depends largely on mucociliary clearance and alveolar macrophage function. If injury does take place, an inflammatory response usually occurs and repair mechanisms are activated. When damage is severe or the agent persists, permanent damage such as fibrosis or emphysema may result. Fortunately, in the majority of cases, the injury is adequately repaired and inflammation is resolved.

General factors that affect tissue response to a toxicant are: the chemical nature of the toxicant; the route of exposure (inhalation or vascular) and exposure duration or regimen; host characteristics such as species, strain, age, and disease state; and tissue and cell susceptibility. Distribution of airway toxicity is dependent on local dosimetry, local defense mechanisms, and cell/tissue sensitivity. Morphologic changes in response to inhaled agents would be expected at the level of the respiratory tract where physiological responses are elicited. This may be restricted to the nasal cavity, the airways, or the pulmonary parenchyma; however, in many cases, several regions of the respiratory tract are affected. Blood-borne agents would be diffusely distributed; however, the distribution of the lesions is highly dependent on tissue and cell susceptibility. For example, acetaminophen causes lesions restricted to the nasal cavity and pulmonary airways, specifically damaging the olfactory and transitional nasal epithelium and Clara cells, all of which contain the high cytochrome P450 activity required for metabolic activation. On the other hand, diffuse alveolar injury occurs in mice following BHT administration, due to selective injury of type I epithelial cells and endothelial cells.

Injury to the respiratory tract is usually manifested as cell degeneration and necrosis. The major non-neoplastic responses elicited by the respiratory tract are listed in Table 6.6. The acute response that follows is characterized by inflammation to remove cellular debris and the inciting agent, as well as by regenerative attempts to restore structural integrity. If this is successful, complete resolution can take place at both the structural and functional levels (Figure 6.13). A more chronic response may be established if injury or subsequent inflammation is severe, if the inciting agent persists within the tissue, or if there are multiple exposures to the agent. Repair processes may still be effective at this point, resulting in resolution of the damage; alternatively chronic irreversible disease may follow. Chronic pulmonary disease is common, due to the widespread practice of cigarette smoking and exposure to airborne pollutants, including particulates. Chronic bronchitis, emphysema, and lung cancer are largely caused by exposure to tobacco smoke.

Chronic bronchitis and emphysema are conditions that are part of "chronic obstructive pulmonary disease" (COPD), which causes dyspnea due to chronic or recurrent obstruction to airflow within the lung. Other disorders that accompany COPD are bronchiectasis, asthma, and bronchiolitis or "small airway disease." The incidence of COPD has increased dramatically over the past few decades, because of the increase in cigarette smoking, environmental pollutants, and other noxious exposures. It now ranks as a major cause of activity-restricting or bed-confining disability in the United States. In veterinary medicine, feline asthma or feline allergic disease and chronic obstructive pulmonary disease of horses fall in this category, but allergens are the inciting cause.

Injury, Regeneration, and Repair

Cell-specific Versus Nonspecific Injury

Exposure of the respiratory tract to a wide variety of agents results in cell injury and death. Injury to individual cells may be reversible, for example, altered mucus production or loss of cilia, or irreversible, leading to cell death. Chemical agents may nonspecifically affect all cells within a region, or may selectively injure a single cell type within that region (Table 6.5).

The most vulnerable cells to injury are the ciliated cells of the respiratory epithelium of larger airways, and the type I epithelial and capillary endothelial cells of the alveolar region. These cells are damaged nonselectively by toxicants, because of their functional and morphologic characteristics, for example, the large surface area presented to inhaled (type I epithelial cell) and blood-borne (endothelial cell) toxicants. Nonspecific injury may also occur when agents are so toxic that all cells in contact with the agent are injured; an example would be aspiration of a caustic solution, which would cause diffuse damage of airway epithelium and associated alveoli.

Susceptibility of other cell types to injury is dependent on the nature of the toxicant, and its interaction

TABLE 6.6   Classification of non-neoplastic alterations to the respiratory system

Alteration	Xenobiotic
Nasal cavity and airways	
Degeneration/necrosis	Acetaminophen, 3-methylfuran
Inflammation	Acetaldehyde, formaldehyde, cigarette smoke, ammonia
Metaplasia/hyperplasia	Acetaldehyde, formaldehyde, cigarette smoke, ammonia
Fibrosis	NO_2, methyl isocyanate
Chronic bronchitis	Chronic exposure to cigarette smoke, irritant gases
Pulmonary parenchyma	
Edema	Phosgene, α-naphthothiourea, endotoxin
Inflammation	Hyperoxia, radiation, bleomycin, paraquat, silica
Fibrosis	Hyperoxia, radiation, bleomycin, paraquat, silica
Emphysema	Smoking, $CdCl_2$

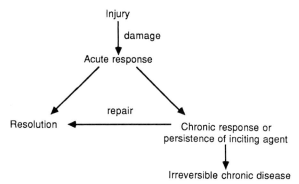

FIGURE 6.13   Possible outcomes following cell or tissue injury.

with the specific cell type because of its unique characteristics. For example, cells and tissues containing a high concentration of cytochrome P450 enzymes, such as the olfactory epithelium and Clara cells, are susceptible to injury by toxicants which require metabolic activation, such as 3-methylfuran, acetaminophen, and 4-ipomeanol.

Cell Proliferation, Regeneration, and Repair Processes

Irrespective of the mechanism of toxicity and cell type affected, initial damage is followed by relatively stereotyped repair processes that include proliferation of stem cells and inflammation. Proliferation of resident cells generally occurs as a regenerative response following cell necrosis; this is an acceleration of the normal cell renewal process by which tissue integrity is maintained. In some situations, cell proliferation can be initiated by the migration of inflammatory cells into the lung. Cell proliferation is also associated with growth of the lung or neoplasia.

Chemical damage to the olfactory epithelium can be repaired by regeneration, if sufficient basal cells survive to initiate this repair process. If injury occurs to the respiratory epithelium, surviving cells spread to cover the denuded basal lamina; this is followed by proliferation of surviving immature secretory cells, stem cells for the respiratory epithelium. Mucous cells may also dedifferentiate, divide and differentiate into ciliated cells, which are incapable of division, or mature secretory cells. Thus, normal epithelium is restored. In the smaller airways, the Clara cell, also a secretory cell, is the stem cell; newly-divided Clara cells differentiate into either mature Clara or ciliated cells.

Injury to the alveolar epithelium is followed by proliferation of type II epithelial cells, whose normal function is surfactant secretion. Newly-divided type II cells can differentiate into type I cells, which are incapable of division, or mature type II cells. Proliferation of type II cells may also follow migration of inflammatory cells from the capillary bed into the alveoli. Injury to capillary endothelium within the lung is repaired by proliferation of remaining endothelial cells or by circulating stem cells. Alveolar macrophage proliferation is also commonly seen in response to injury, due to the release of mediators and various other substances, which results in an influx of polymorphonuclear cells and monocytes into the lung.

Proliferation of fibroblasts located in the walls of the airways and in the pulmonary interstitium frequently follows injury. This proliferation is usually not due to direct injury to the fibroblast, but related to the loss of overlying epithelium and basement membrane,

as well as to the production of mediators and growth factors by alveolar macrophages and inflammatory cells. Excessive fibroblast proliferation and collagen production can lead to fibrosis or "scarring," which compromises normal pulmonary elasticity or compliance and gaseous diffusion.

Under most conditions of injury, proliferation of epithelial cells begins within the first day of injury and peaks over the next few days. Proliferation of other cell types occurs at later times. Inhibition of epithelial cell proliferation can delay or inhibit normal repair, resulting in chronic damage. Remodeling of tissue may occur with chronic injury if repair mechanisms are unable to keep pace. This structural remodeling may be beneficial, or have adverse consequences. In addition, inhibition of cell differentiation, for instance, under conditions of chronic exposure, can result in large numbers of undifferentiated cells. These cells may be less susceptible to the original injury and tolerance may develop. These cells may also play a role in the development of neoplasia.

Thus, mild epithelial or endothelial injury without basement membrane damage, severe inflammation, or persistence of the inciting agent, may be resolved by simple cellular regeneration. With more severe damage, a significant inflammatory component may be elicited which may be followed by tissue destruction or fibrosis. Persistence of the inciting agent within the tissue may lead to the development of granulomatous disease, as observed with beryllium and silica.

Nasopharyngeal and Laryngeal Responses to Injury

Overview

The nasal cavity is susceptible to injury from inhaled agents, due to its anatomic location. Important factors in the pathogenesis of toxicant-induced nasal lesions include airflow, absorption, tissue susceptibility, mucociliary apparatus, and metabolism. The distribution of damage is dependent on regional deposition of inhaled chemicals, and on tissue or cell susceptibility to individual agents. Regional deposition of inhaled chemicals is dependent on airflow and, in the case of particles, on particle characteristics such as size and aerodynamic shape. Species differences in regional airflow play a role in lesion distribution. Nasal uptake of gases is dependent on the partition coefficient of the gas and, in the case of reactive gases, on the rate of reaction. For example, in the dog, nasal uptake is 100% for formaldehyde, 40% to 70% for ozone, and 1% for carbon monoxide (CO). Distribution of nasal lesions is also dependent on cell or tissue susceptibility.

For example, olfactory epithelium is damaged by xenobiotics that require metabolic activation, such as methylbromide, 3-methylfuran, 3-methylindole, carbon tetrachloride, and acetaminophen. This usually occurs irrespective of the route of administration. On the other hand, ciliated cells and perhaps mucous cells are the targets of formaldehyde toxicity.

Substances affecting nasal function may impair mucociliary flow, change nasal airflow resistance, and irritate or damage the nasal mucosa. Damage to the neuronal cells of the olfactory epithelium can result in anosmia (loss of smell). Chemically induced nasal epithelial lesions fall into one or more of the following categories: degeneration and necrosis, inflammation, repair, adaptation, and proliferative lesions including neoplasia (Table 6.6).

Degeneration and necrosis are usually followed by inflammation and cell proliferation to repair damaged epithelium. Excessive proliferation can result in epithelial hyperplasia. Increased cell turnover can potentially predispose to carcinogenesis, since increased DNA synthesis will increase the probability of mutation. Continued low-level toxic exposure may result in adaptive responses, such as squamous metaplasia or mucous cell hyperplasia. The presence of exudate in the nasal cavity is a valuable indication of nasal toxicity, and is readily detected by light microscopy at low magnification (Figure 6.14). However, nasal exudate is also a hallmark of mycoplasma and Sendai virus infections. The relatively stereotyped nature of the response of tissues to injury, independent of etiology, needs to be re-emphasized.

In the larynx the transitional zone between the stratified squamous epithelium cranially to the respiratory epithelium caudally is the most sensitive site for inhaled xenobiotic-induced injury resulting in degeneration, squamous metaplasia, or hyperplasia. Xenobiotics affecting the larynx include tobacco smoke and cobalt sulfate. These lesions must be differentiated from aging changes, thus emphasizing the need for age-matched controls in evaluating xenobiotic induced changes.

Non-neoplastic Lesions

Acute Lesions

In the nasal epithelium, the mildest change may be loss of cilia from ciliated cells or from the olfactory vesicle of neuronal cells, with little change in the underlying or adjacent cells. Similarly, loss of olfactory neuronal cells may be fairly severe, without apparent disruption of the structure of the olfactory epithelium. Acute necrosis and loss of olfactory epithelium may be seen following inhalation or blood-borne exposure to toxicants, requiring metabolic activation by the P450 system, such as 3-methylfuran and acetaminophen, respectively (Figure 6.1B). Once the basement membrane is exposed, cytokines are released, and inflammation takes place. Acetaminophen also causes selective necrosis of nasal transitional epithelium, which is also the target site of ozone toxicity.

More severe lesions, such as segmental loss of basal lamina or ulceration, are most commonly found in regions covered by squamous epithelium. Ulceration may lead to damage of the underlying lamina propria, and even of bone or cartilage. The affected area may be covered by an exudate (rhinitis). Repair may take place or, if repeated exposure occurs, squamous metaplasia of respiratory, or even olfactory, regions may result, occasionally with extensive keratinization.

Chronic Lesions

Chronic non-neoplastic changes of the olfactory mucosa following inhalation of irritant substances such as acrolein, formaldehyde, acetaldehyde, and cigarette smoke, include atrophy of olfactory neuronal cells and replacement of olfactory epithelium by respiratory-like epithelium, with loss of nerve bundles and glands of Bowman. The dorsomedial region of the nasal cavity appears the most vulnerable to these changes. Cessation of exposure may lead to recovery, but the regenerated olfactory epithelium may still appear disorganized and relatively thin. These changes are often accompanied by inflammation of the mucosa or submucosa. Chronic ozone exposure results not only in epithelial hyperplasia and inflammation, but also in atrophy of the turbinates.

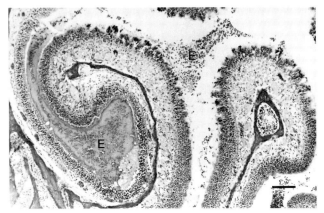

FIGURE 6.14 Nasal cavity; 3-methyl furan, inhalation exposure; mouse. One day after exposure, the olfactory epithelium lining the turbinates is disorganized and sloughing into the lumen. Exudate (E) containing inflammatory cells variably fills the lumen. H&E stain. Bar = 125 μm.

Common changes of the respiratory epithelium following inhalation of irritant substances, such as acetaldehyde, formaldehyde, and cigarette smoke, are hyperplasia and squamous metaplasia of the lining epithelium or submucosal glands. Papillary hyperplasia can progress to papilloma, and nodular hyperplasia to adenocarcinoma. Mucous cell hyperplasia may also occur. The mucus produced by these cells may have an increased concentration of acidic mucous glycoproteins, resulting in altered viscoelastic properties of the mucus, thus affecting airway clearance mechanisms. Stratified squamous metaplasia, with or without keratinization, is also frequently observed, and may also interfere with mucociliary clearance. This change may be reversible following cessation of exposure. If normal repair processes cannot take place because of the severity of damage, fibrosis will occur. Excessive hyperkeratosis, severe inflammatory exudation or fibrosis may lead to obstruction of the nasal cavity and death of the animal.

In summary, chemically-induced injury of the nasal epithelium may be followed by complete repair with restoration of normal epithelium, olfactory epithelial replacement by respiratory-like epithelium, squamous metaplasia, hyperplasia, or fibrosis. In rodents, hyperplastic and metaplastic changes from persistent mucosal injury are considered a prelude to neoplasia.

Incidental Lesions

Incidental lesions that may be found in non-treated animals include small foci of mineralization adjacent to the lamina propria, lymphoid infiltrates in the lamina propria, folding of the respiratory epithelium which sometimes resembles glandular formation, and, in the rat, round to elongated eosinophilic inclusions or hyaline droplets which may be present either intra- or extracellularly. These hyaline droplets vary in size (generally 2 to 10 μm in diameter) and number, can occur in respiratory and olfactory epithelium, as well as submucosal glands, and may increase in number following inhalation of irritants.

Neoplasia

In spite of the rare occurrence of spontaneous nasal tumors in rodents, the nasal cavity is highly sensitive to environmental carcinogens, irrespective of the route of administration, and thus should be examined in all carcinogenicity studies. Grossly these neoplasms appear as gray-white to yellowish infiltrative masses partially occluding the nasal cavity, often with necrotic areas and with destruction of adjacent tissue. These may occasionally extend into the brain or metastasize to other organs. The larynx is also a target site for xenobiotics, and should be routinely examined.

Nasal tumors have been induced experimentally in rodents following inhalation of a variety of important industrial chemicals, such as formaldehyde, acrolein, acetaldehyde, bis(chloromethyl) ether, hexamethylphosphoramide, and vinyl chloride. Obligate nasal breathing and complexity of the nasal turbinates may explain why tumors develop in rodents, but have not been reported in association with exposure to these chemicals in humans. Tumors have also been induced following parenterally-administered chemicals such as nitrosamines. Malignant nasal neoplasms are rare in humans, except for six occupational groups: chromate workers; nickel refiners and workers; mustard gas makers; isopropyl alcohol workers; makers of wooden furniture; and boot and shoe workers. In addition, welders, flamecutters, and solderers have an increased risk of nasal cancer. Animal studies have incriminated certain hexavalent chromium compounds and metallic nickel as carcinogenic agents.

Tumors of the rat nasal cavity have been classified as adenomas, adenocarcinomas and carcinomas of squamous cell, adenosquamous and neuroepithelial (also called olfactory neuroblastoma and esthesioneuroblastoma) type. These mainly arise from the lining epithelium, but may also arise from the submucosal glands. Squamous cell carcinomas and adenocarcinomas have also been reported in the larynx of rats and hamsters. In humans, squamous cell carcinoma is the most common spontaneous tumor (75%), while adenocarcinomas and undifferentiated tumors are less common (10% each). In the dog, adenocarcinoma, squamous cell carcinoma, and undifferentiated carcinoma are equally prevalent.

Airway Response to Injury

Overview

Injury to airways may nonspecifically affect epithelial cells or be limited to a single cell type. Injury may be mild and reversible, with minimal inflammation and complete repair by epithelial regeneration. More severe injury, with nonspecific necrosis or following chronic toxicant exposure, can induce severe inflammation and fibrosis, which is irreversible (Table 6.7). The epithelial lining of the bronchiolar region is exquisitely susceptible to injury by oxidant gases (NO_2, SO_2, and O_3) and toxicants (3-methylindole).

Injury to airway epithelium invariably impairs mucociliary clearance, due to changes in mucus or to injury of ciliated cells. Changes in the ciliated cells may range from ciliostasis or ciliary loss to cell death. An increased rate or amount of mucus secretion is a common response to inhaled toxicants, such as SO_2, O_3, NO_2, and NH_3. Mucus hypersecretion from surface

TABLE 6.7　Selected toxicant-induced pulmonary diseases in domestic animals

Disease	General cause	Specific cause	Source	Species specificity, if any
Interstitial pneumonia (ARDS, most can present as edema at very high exposure levels)	Inhaled toxicants	Oxygen (>50–80%), other irritant gases	Therapeutic application, pollution, silos, manure pits	Horses, pigs, cattle, humans
		Smoke	Fires	Horses, all
	Ingested toxicant or precursors	L-tryptophan converted to 3-methyl indole	Lush green pasture	Ruminants, horses (obstructive disease)
		Perilla ketone	Purple mint (*Perilla frutescens*)	Cattle, horses
			Stink weed, rape, kale (*Brassica* sp)	Cattle
		Furanoterpenoid, 4-ipomeanol	Moldy sweet potatoes (*Fusarium solani*)	Cattle
		Paraquat	Herbicide	Dogs, cats, humans
		Vitamin D toxicity (with mineralization, may be chronic)	Feed, plants (*Solanum malacoxylon*, *Cestrum diurnum*), medications, rodenticide	Pigs, horses, cattle, dogs
	Endogenous metabolic/ toxic condition	Shock, DIC, uremia, pancreatitis		All species
Chronic interstitial pneumonia/fibrosis	Inhaled toxicants	Silicosis (pneumoconiosis, granulomatous)	Soils, mines, quarries	Horses, zoo animals, humans
	Ingested toxicant	Pyrrolizidine alkaloids	Plants (*Crotalaria*, *Senecio* sp, etc.)	Horses, cattle, pigs, sheep, dogs
			Stinkwood (*Zieria arborescens*)	
			Crofton weed (*Eupatorium adenophorum*)	Horses
	Hypersensitivity, type III	Fungal antigens	Organic dusts	Cattle, "farmer's lung" in humans
COPD with alveolar emphysema	Hypersensitivity	Fungal and other antigens	Organic dusts, moldy hay	Horses
Aspiration pneumonia	Aspiration or regurgitation of ingested toxicant or feed material	Low viscosity, volatile hydrocarbons: kerosine, gasoline	Lubricants, degreasers, cleaning fluids, lamp oil, etc.	All species
		Turpentine	Pine oil	Cats
	Gavaged material/feed		Accidental introduction	Horses, pigs, laboratory animals
Edema	Inhaled toxicant, very high concentration of irritant gases	Smoke, hydrogen sulfide, nitrogen oxides, sulfur dioxide, ammonia	Fires, grain silos, manure "pits"	All species
		Teflon, polytetrafluoroethylene	Overheated non-stick cookware	Caged birds
	Ingested toxicant	ANTU, paraquat	Rodenticide, herbicide	All species
		Urea (NH_3)	Feed	Goat
	Hypersensitivity, type I (eosinophils)	Penicillin, vaccination	Therapeutics	Cattle, horses, cats

(Continued)

TABLE 6.7 (*Continued*)

Disease	General cause	Specific cause	Source	Species specificity, if any
	Endogenous toxins	Endotoxin	Some bacteria	Cattle, swine and others with intravascular macrophages
	Exogenous toxins	Venom	Snake	All species
	Secondary, e.g., cardiogenic	Fumonisins	Mycotoxin (corn)	Swine
		Gossypol	Plant toxin (cotton)	Swine, cattle
Neoplasia	Mesothelioma	Asbestos	Mining, milling	Dog, humans

epithelial cells may be stimulated by direct irritation. Hypersecretion and an increase in glycoprotein content from submucosal glands may follow parasympathetic stimulation or parasympathomimetic drugs, such as acetylcholine and pilocarpine. A change in the glyco-protein fraction affects the viscosity of mucus. Excess mucus has an irritant effect on sensory nerve endings, often triggering the cough reflex. Release of acetylcholine from irritated synapses of the autonomic innervation present in the bronchiolar epithelium causes bronchiolar constriction and mucus secretion. Mast cell mediators, as well as prostaglandins and lipoxygenase products, also appear to stimulate mucus secretion.

Morphologically, mucus may be readily observed in airways or submucosal glands of affected animals, whereas in normal animals it is not. In some cases of chronic exposure, increased numbers of mucous cells (hyperplasia) or abnormally located mucous cells (mucous cell metaplasia) may be observed. If these changes persist, they can result in blockage of mucus-producing glands and ducts, airway obstruction, and alveolar injury. Debris can accumulate and incite an inflammatory response. Inflammation, if present, may be confined to the airway wall or may spill over into the lumen. Neutrophils predominate in the early stages of inflammation, whereas mononuclear cells are prominent in later stages. Eosinophils may be associated with allergic conditions.

Injury to epithelium may result in epithelial degeneration, detachment and exfoliation of cells. This loss is normally followed by inflammation and repair. If the basement membrane is not damaged and the injurious agent does not persist, the epithelium will regenerate within a few days by proliferation of immature secretory stem cells or Clara cells in the small airways. Differentiation of these cells is followed by recovery. If basement membrane is damaged, fibroblast precursors may migrate from the ulcerated airway wall into the lumen, particularly when a fibrinous exudate is present. Organization can occur within 7–10 days, resulting in intraluminal fibrosis (bronchiolitis obliterans;

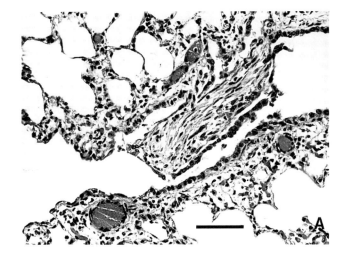

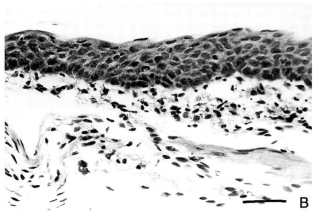

FIGURE 6.15 Airway, coal liquefaction distillate, intratracheal exposure, rat. H&E stain. (A) Bronchiolitis obliterans. Intraluminal fibrosis, characterized by a small polyp, partially occludes the bronchiolar lumen. Bar = 60 μm. (B) Squamous metaplasia. The bronchiolar mucosa is markedly thickened, and consists of stratified squamous epithelium. Bar = 40 μm.

Figure 6.15A). This type of lesion has been reported with highly reactive volatile chemicals, such as methyl isocyanate (MIC), with NO_2 in silofiller's disease, and with diacetyl in microwave-popcorn factory workers. Fibroblast proliferation may also occur in the lamina propria or peribronchially. If severe inflammation is present in addition to basement membrane damage, bronchiectasis (destruction of airway wall with dilation) or abscess formation, following infection, may occur.

If clearance is sufficiently impaired, and spontaneous resolution does not take place, obstruction of airways with concomitant bronchoconstriction and hypoxic vasoconstriction may occur and lead to death from hypoxia, or alveolar injury and emphysema. In the event of continued irritation, squamous metaplasia may occur (Figure 6.15B). Both squamous metaplasia and uncontrolled cell proliferation may potentially be followed by neoplasia.

Cell-specific Injury

Ciliated cells may be selectively damaged by inhaled toxicants; for instance, loss of cilia is a stereotyped response to inhalation of acidogenic gases such as SO_2 and NO_2, while cigarette smoke slows ciliary beat frequency. Ozone selectively damages ciliated cells, causing necrosis which is followed by hyperplasia of nonciliated cuboidal cells. Selective toxicity to the Clara cell is induced by agents that require metabolic activation by the cytochrome P450 enzymes to their putative toxin (see Table 6.5). Damage may be limited to the Clara cells, or may be followed by more extensive pulmonary injury, depending on the specific compound, dose, and species (Figure 6.2B). Examples of selective Clara cell toxins are 4-ipomeanol, naphthalene, 3-methylfuran, CCl_4, and acetaminophen. Necrosis of Clara cells is followed by movement of remaining bronchiolar cells to cover the denuded basement membrane, and rapid proliferation of remaining Clara cells to regenerate normal epithelium. Cell death appears to occur by apoptosis, with little or no associated inflammation.

Selective damage to Clara cells, unrelated to their cytochrome P450 content, has also been reported. This selectivity is presumably related to other unique features of the cell. For instance, methylcyclopentadienyl manganese tricarbonyl (MMT), which is detoxified in the liver by the cytochrome P450 enzymes, causes mitochondrial damage in Clara cells, presumably due to the high oxidative enzyme content of these cells. In addition, some PCB congeners affect Clara cell secretory functions.

Hyper-reactive Airway Disease

Hyper-responsive airways are a possible sequela of bronchiolar injury. It can develop following transient and often innocuous viral infection, from exposure to certain allergens, or exposure to ingested respiratory toxicants. Sustained inhalation of dust particles may also play a role by up-regulating the production of cytokines (interleukin 8, IL-8) and monokine-inducible

protein (MIP-2) by alveolar macrophages, attracting neutrophils into the bronchoalveolar region and causing bronchiolar injury. Airway hyper-responsiveness is characterized by exaggerated bronchoconstriction following exposure to mild stimuli, such as cold air. Typically, increased numbers of mast cells, eosinophils and T-lymphocysts are present in the airway mucosa.

Chronic Obstructive Pulmonary Disease (COPD)

Chronic bronchitis, emphysema, and asthma comprise the clinical entity known as chronic obstructive pulmonary disease. Asthma can be clinically differentiated from chronic bronchitis and emphysema because the obstruction is reversible. Chronic bronchitis and emphysema are difficult to distinguish clinically, but they are distinguished postmortem based on morphologic criteria. A distinction is often made between disease of the larger airways (chronic bronchitis) and disease of bronchioles (bronchiolitis or small airways disease). However, most patients with chronic obstructive lung disease show evidence of both conditions because the etiologic agents, e.g., cigarette smoke, affect the lung at all airway levels. Emphysema also frequently accompanies chronic bronchitis, and contributes to small airway obstruction. In veterinary medicine, feline asthma or feline allergic disease and chronic obstructive pulmonary disease of horses fall in this category.

Asthma

Asthma is recognized clinically as episodic, reversible airway bronchoconstriction. Pathologically, it is a chronic inflammatory disease of airways. Episodic acute inflammation corresponds to clinical exacerbations of asthma. In asthmatics, the control of airway muscle shortening is abnormal. It is thought that chronic inflammation causes the airways of asthmatics to narrow when stimulated, in ways that have minimal effects on non-asthmatics.

Asthma is generally categorized as being intrinsic (idiosyncratic) or extrinsic (Figure 6.16). Intrinsic asthma is initiated by nonimmune mechanisms, and is seen in some patients after ingestion of aspirin, pulmonary (usually viral) infections, cold, inhaled irritants, stress, and exercise. Extrinsic asthma starts as a type I hypersensitivity reaction to an extrinsic antigen, and includes atopic (allergic) and occupational asthma. Allergic or atopic asthma, which is an IgE-mediated sensitivity primarily to inhaled antigens (allergens) which results in bronchoconstriction, is the most common form. Examples of antigens include

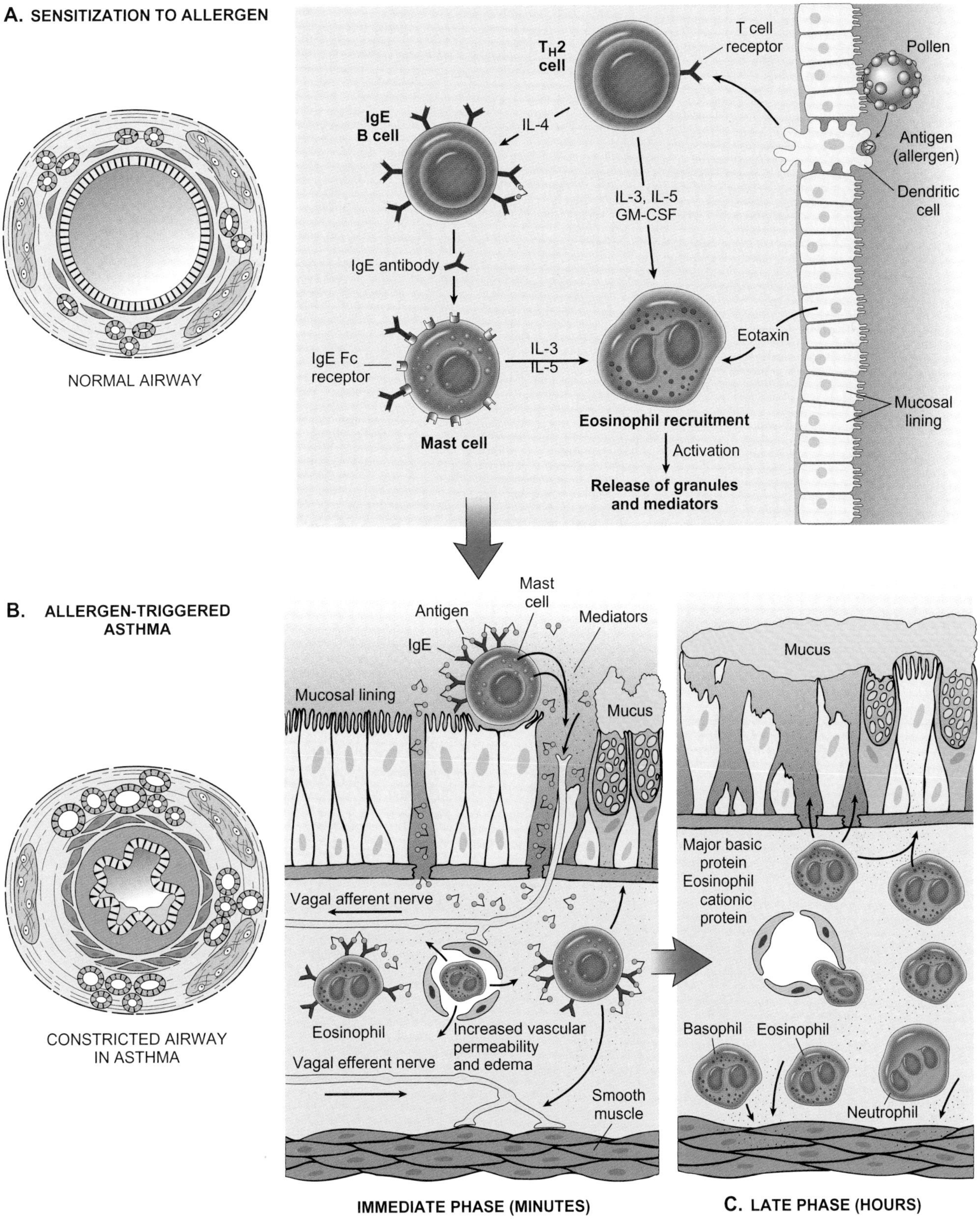

A. SENSITIZATION TO ALLERGEN

NORMAL AIRWAY

T$_H$2 cell

T cell receptor

Pollen

IgE B cell

IL-4

Antigen (allergen)

IgE antibody

IL-3, IL-5 GM-CSF

Dendritic cell

IgE Fc receptor

IL-3 IL-5

Eotaxin

Mast cell

Eosinophil recruitment

Mucosal lining

Activation

Release of granules and mediators

B. ALLERGEN-TRIGGERED ASTHMA

CONSTRICTED AIRWAY IN ASTHMA

Antigen

Mast cell

Mediators

IgE

Mucosal lining

Mucus

Vagal afferent nerve

Eosinophil

Increased vascular permeability and edema

Vagal efferent nerve

Smooth muscle

Mucus

Major basic protein Eosinophil cationic protein

Basophil Eosinophil

Neutrophil

IMMEDIATE PHASE (MINUTES)

C. LATE PHASE (HOURS)

FIGURE 6.16 Allergic asthma. (A) Inhaled allergens (antigen) elicit a T$_H$2-dominated response favoring IgE production and eosinophil recruitment (priming or sensitization). (B) On re-exposure to antigen (Ag), the immediate reaction is triggered by Ag-induced cross-linking of IgE bound to IgE receptors on mast cells in the airways. These cells release preformed mediators that open tight junctions between epithelial cells. Antigen can then enter the mucosa to activate mucosal mast cells and eosinophils, which in turn release additional mediators. Collectively,

dusts, pollens, animal dander, and foods. Initial sensitization (priming) by the antigen induces T-helper lymphocytes that produce interleukin-4 and interleukin-5. These cytokines support Th2 immunity characterized by the production of IgE by B-lymphocytes, increased numbers of mast cells with antigen-specific IgE bound to their receptors, and recruitment of eosinophils. A subsequent exposure to antigen results in an acute response (immediate phase, minutes), and a late phase (hours) reaction. On re-exposure to inhaled antigen, antigen-induced cross-linking of IgE bound to mast cells on the airway surface causes release of preformed mediators that open tight junctions between epithelial cells. Antigen then enters the mucosa and activates mucosal and submucosal mast cells and eosinophils that release additional mediators. These mediators directly, or indirectly through neural reflexes, induce bronchospasm, increased vascular permeability and edema, mucus production, and recruitment of additional inflammatory cells from the blood. The recruitment of neutrophils, eosinophils, basophils, lymphocytes, and monocytes marks the start of the late phase. During the late phase, there is additional mediator release from leukocytes, endothelial cells, and epithelial cells. Endothelins from endothelial and epithelial cells are potent bronchoconstrictors and inducers of airway smooth muscle cell proliferation and fibrosis. Release of eotaxin from airway epithelial cells results in eosinophil recruitment and activation. During this phase, eosinophilic cationic protein and major basic protein released from eosinophils damage the epithelium and cause bronchoconstriction.

Occupational asthma has been associated with exposure to fumes, such as epoxy resins, organic and inorganic dusts such as wood, cotton, and platinum, and gases such as toluene diisocyanate and formaldehyde. The mechanisms underlying occupational asthma may vary according to stimulus. Occupational asthma due to low molecular weight antigens, such as toluene diisocyanate, appears to be IgE-independent and most likely is mediated by CD8+ T-cells, IL-5 secretion, and eosinophils.

The morphologic features of asthma include excess mucus and eosinophils in the bronchial lumen, goblet cell hyperplasia of the surface epithelium, epithelial desquamation, hypertrophy and hyperplasia of the submucosal mucous glands, congestion and edema of the bronchial mucosa, chronic mucosal and submucosal inflammation, collagen deposition below the basement membrane, structural remodeling of airway longitudinal elastic bundles, and hypertrophy and hyperplasia of smooth muscle. The smooth muscle thickening is seen throughout the bronchial tree, but is most pronounced in the segmental airways and terminal bronchioles. The inflammatory cells in the airway walls include eosinophils, lymphocytes, neutrophils, macrophages, and mast cells. Eosinophils are prominent, and may comprise 5% to 50% of the infiltrating cells. This characteristic eosinophilic infiltrate differentiates asthma from other chronic inflammatory conditions of the airway.

In veterinary medicine, feline asthma or feline allergic bronchitis is clinically and pathologically similar to the human disease. Siamese cats appear to be most susceptible, and a similar disease has been reported in dogs. A number of possible allergens have been incriminated including dust, cigarette smoke, and plant and household materials. In stabled horses and ponies, spontaneous chronic obstructive pulmonary disease (COPD, "heaves"), which is characterized by chronic bronchiolitis-emphysema, results in respiratory distress and poor performance. The pathogenesis includes genetic predisposition, the Th2 (allergic) immune response, and hyper-reactive airways to environmental allergens such as fungal antigens in organic dust.

Proliferative Lesions

Squamous metaplasia and hyperplastic lesions occur in the rat trachea, most frequently at the carina, and in the larynx, particularly at the ventral and lateral aspects. The rat larynx appears to be uniquely sensitive to induction of these lesions by various industrial chemicals, pharmaceuticals, and propellants. Papillomas are the main spontaneous neoplasms reported within the airways of rats. Benign neuroendocrine tumors, although uncommon, must be considered when papilloma-like tumors are found.

Pulmonary Parenchymal Response to Injury
Overview

Although it would be of great diagnostic convenience if a characteristic response were elicited by specific agents, the lung responds in a similar way to a wide variety of infectious and toxic agents (Tables 6.6 and 6.7). Viral and chemical agents frequently incite a similar type of interstitial pneumonia, and both need to be considered as differentials for diffuse spontaneous

FIGURE 6.16 (*Continued*) either directly or via neuronal reflexes, the mediators induce bronchospasm, increased vascular permeability, and mucus production, or recruit additional mediator-releasing cells from the blood. (C) The arrival of recruited leukocytes signals the initiation of the late phase of asthma, and a fresh round of mediator release from leukocytes, endothelium, and epithelial cells. Factors, particularly from eosinophils (e.g., major basic protein, eosinophilic cationic protein), also damage the epithelium. (From Hussain and Kumar (2005). In *Robbins and Cotran Pathologic Basis of Disease*, Kumar, V., Abbas, A.K., and Fausto, N. eds, 7th edn. Elsevier Saunders, New York. Fig. 15-11, p. 725.)

pulmonary diseases. Particulates such as silica may incite a granulomatous response similar to that induced by tuberculosis and some mycotic agents. In some cases the etiologic agent can be identified, although methods other than the routine H&E-stained paraffin sections are usually required for detection. The response does vary to some degree, depending on the nature of the agent, and on the severity and persistence of injury, as well as on the particular cell type affected and the reparative processes initiated by the injury.

Endothelial and type I epithelial cells are especially susceptible to toxic injury. When endothelial cells are injured or die, there is an increase in vascular permeability. Platelets may adhere to the exposed basement membrane, resulting in release of vasoactive agents. Complement activation, coagulation, and fibrinolysis may also occur before the basement membrane is repopulated. Increased vascular permeability allows the leakage of fluid into interstitial spaces and lymphatics, and eventually into alveolar spaces. If damage is more severe, edema may be followed by interstitial inflammation.

Epithelial damage is accompanied by the acute exudative phase of inflammation characterized by fibrin, neutrophils, and edema. Type II cells start to proliferate within 12 to 24 hours and, after a few days, may line alveoli; by light microscopy, this appears as a cuboidal epithelial lining. With time, the inflammatory component will consist of increased numbers of mononuclear cells and macrophages. If damage is not too severe and basement membrane is intact, resolution may occur by transformation of type II cells into type I cells and subsidence of the inflammatory component. However, if alveolar epithelium has been denuded and the basement membrane has been damaged, fibroblast precursors move rapidly into the alveolar space and, particularly in the presence of fibrin, will result in intra-alveolar fibrosis. Similarly, fibrosis may be a consequence of severe endothelial cell damage and fibrin deposition. Interstitial fibrosis may occur after distortion of the normal cell–cell contacts by inflammation or edema. Fibroblast proliferation can be noted within 72 hours of initial injury, and fibrosis may be evident in as little as seven days. Atypical type II cells may persist in these areas.

Continued inflammation of the alveolar wall implies persistence of the causative agent or injurious mechanisms, and is an important feature of chronic interstitial pneumonia. The characteristic components of chronic alveolar irritation are proliferation and persistence of type II epithelial cells, interstitial thickening due to fibrosis, and accumulation of mononuclear cells. Intra-alveolar exudate, when present, is usually composed of macrophages. Sustained or recurrent injury to capillary endothelium can lead to progressive vascular remodeling

and chronic pulmonary hypertension (see Chapter 12, Cardiovascular and Skeletal Muscle Systems). Pulmonary hypertension has been reported after ingestion of certain plants or medicines, including the leguminous plant, *Crotolaria spectabilis*, indigenous to the tropics and used medicinally in "bush tea"; the appetite depressant agent, aminorex; and adulterated olive oil.

Edema

Overview

Pulmonary edema can occur as a result of altered hemodynamics or increased permeability of the air–blood barrier. Altered hemodynamics can result from increased capillary hydrostatic pressure due to cardiac failure, acute injury to the nervous system (neurogenic pulmonary edema), or from decreased plasma oncotic levels due to decreased plasma protein levels.

The constituents of the lung that are important in fluid homeostasis are the vascular bed, the endothelial barrier, the interstitial space, lymphatics, the alveolar epithelial barrier, and alveolar surface tension (Figure 6.17). Altered hemodynamics or increased endothelial permeability will result in fluid loss through the moderately leaky endothelium into the adjacent interstitium. Interstitial fluid normally percolates along the interstitium until it reaches the lymphatics that are located adjacent to airways and associated vessels, within interlobular septae (in species that have these), and beneath the pleura. Alveolar fluid clearance across the alveolar epithelium is also a mechanism of fluid removal from the lung. Dilated lymphatics and increased lymph flow are good early indicators of edema. If lymphatic capacity is overwhelmed, interstitial edema will occur. When the capacity of the interstitium is overwhelmed, or if there is damage to alveolar epithelial cells, fluid will leak into the alveoli causing alveolar edema, which interferes with diffusion of gases and results in impaired gas exchange. Because of their tight junctions, alveolar epithelial cells provide a tighter barrier to exudation of fluid than do endothelial cells. Depending on the extent of increased permeability, fibrin and low molecular weight proteins, such as albumin, will accompany the fluid loss. Pleural effusion is a common feature of pulmonary edema in rodents; interstitial fluid passes from the subpleural interstitium into the pleural cavity through stomata in their very thin pleural mesothelium.

The edematous lung is larger and firmer than normal and does not collapse. Fluid oozes from the cut section. The pleura and interlobular septa are thickened by clear fluid (Figure 6.18A). Pleural effusion (hydrothorax) may be present. Froth in the airways, without other findings, may be due to agonal change. These changes are easy to detect in large animals, but

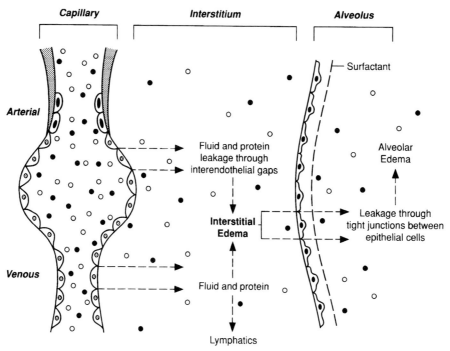

FIGURE 6.17 Pulmonary edema. Interstitial edema occurs when excess fluid enters the interstitium from the pulmonary vasculature. Alveolar edema occurs when interstitial fluid enters the alveolar lumen, either following direct alveolar epithelial damage or following a build-up of interstitial fluid.

more difficult to identify in rodents. Lung wet weight and, more specifically, the wet to dry weight ratio are useful in determining the presence of edema. More sensitive and specific techniques for measuring pulmonary edema are available, in order to discriminate between simple edema and increased blood content (congestion or hemorrhage) or cellular components. On light microscopic examination, early/mild edema is characterized by dilated lymphatics, widening and separation of interstitial tissue (especially perivascularly), and, if alveoli are affected, expansion of the alveolar lumen. This should not be confused with artifacts that can be induced by intratracheal fixation. If the fluid contains protein, it will have a homogeneous eosinophilic appearance on H&E stained sections (Figure 6.18B). Fixation in Zenker's solution precipitates protein, and increases the staining of proteinaceous edema. If fibrin is present, this will appear as pink fibrillar material. Special stains to confirm the presence of fibrin, such as phosphotungstic acid hematoxylin (PTAH), can be used.

Pathogenesis

Permeability edema occurs when there is excessive opening of endothelial gaps or damage to the air–blood barrier (type I epithelial cells or endothelial cells). Changes in capillary permeability may be due directly to endothelial cell injury, or to the effect of cellular or humoral "mediators" of inflammation. Numerous inhaled or circulating toxicants, bacterial toxins, anaphylactic shock, and drugs are believed to cause pulmonary edema by a direct effect on the endothelium or type I epithelial cells. Mediators that alter endothelial permeability may be released from mast cells (histamine) during allergic responses, from aggregated platelets, and from phagocytic cells as they migrate through the endothelium. Since type I epithelial cells are highly vulnerable to toxicants such as NO_2, SO_2, H_2S and 3-methylindole, as well as to free radicals, alveolar edema accompanies many toxic pulmonary diseases.

Pulmonary edema interferes with the respiratory gas-exchange function of the lung. With mild injury, repair processes can result in a return to normal; however, with severe or prolonged injury, inflammation and eventually fibrosis may follow.

Specific Etiologic Agents

The classic example of toxicant-induced pulmonary edema is that induced by α-naphthothiourea (ANTU), a rodenticide. The rat is extremely sensitive to ANTU; massive pulmonary edema and pleural effusion occur as a consequence of endothelial damage to capillaries and venules. Inflammation does not occur. In animals that survive, edema is resolved by 48 hours, without permanent lung damage. Although the mechanism by which ANTU damages the lung is not known, it

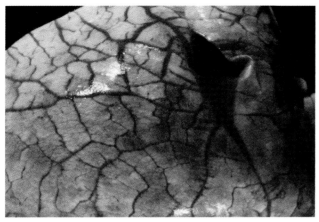

(A)

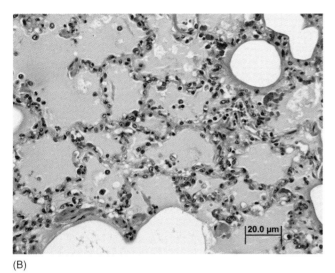

(B)

FIGURE 6.18 Lung, pulmonary edema. (A) Pig, fumonisin B$_1$, dietary exposure. Interlobular septa are widely distended by edema. (B) Cow, pulmonary edema is characterized by transudation of protein-rich fluid that distends the alveoli. A few macrophages and other cells are present within the alveoli. H&E stain.

appears that ANTU is metabolically-activated to a toxic oxidative species.

Many other toxicants also cause edema (Table 6.7). These include bacterial endotoxin, which injures endothelial cells, paraquat which damages epithelial cells (both type I and II), oxygen which damages both endothelial and epithelial cells, and 4-ipomeanol which damages Clara cells. In most cases, pulmonary edema occurs as an acute response, and then resolves or is followed by an inflammatory response. In the case of phosgene and smoke inhalation, the edema is characteristically delayed for one to two days. Delayed edema is also produced by intravenously administered opiates, such as heroin and methadone. These opiates may act through the central nervous system. Delayed onset of severe proteinaceous edema, the "exudative phase" of radiation pneumonitis, occurs after ionizing radiation exposure. Many cardiovascular toxicants ultimately cause pulmonary edema, which may be lethal.

In veterinary medicine, pulmonary edema occurs most commonly as a secondary event following toxicant induced primary cardiotoxicity (see Chapter 12, Cardiovascular and Skeletal Muscle Systems; Table 6.7). An example is the mycotoxin fumonisin B$_1$, which is the causative agent of "porcine pulmonary edema" (PPE). While respiratory distress and death are the primary clinical features, the pathogenesis of the edema is cardiovascular toxicity. Permeability edema, due to epithelial and endothelial or microvascular damage, is seen with a number of gases, including smoke from fires, endotoxemia, drugs, and chemicals such as paraquat. The lung is the target organ for anaphylactic shock in most domestic animals (those with intravascular macrophages); however, the portal-mesenteric vasculature is the primary target in dogs and rodents. Pulmonary edema due to anaphylaxis occurs most commonly in cattle and horses, but also occurs in cats. Systemic anaphylaxis most frequently follows parentral injection of certain drugs, such as penicillin and vaccines, but can also follow oral or inhalation exposure (see Chapter 15, Immune System). Venoms of stinging and biting insects are also important causes of anaphylactic shock. Histologically, pulmonary edema is often accompanied by the presence of eosinophils and bronchoconstriction. Laryngeal and pharyngeal edema has also been reported.

Diffuse endothelial and alveolar damage leading to fulminating edema is termed adult respiratory distress syndrome (ARDS). It is an important condition in humans, characterized by intravascular aggregation of neutrophils; diffuse alveolar damage, permeability edema, and formation of hyaline membranes (see Figure 6.5). The diffuse alveolar damage results from systemic diseases, as well as direct injury to the lung, where macrophages generate overwhelming amounts of cytokines (mainly TNF-α), and neutrophils aggregated in capillaries release destructive enzymes and toxic oxygen metabolites. ARDS can occur due to direct lung injury caused by oxygen toxicity, radiation therapy, inhalation of toxicants and other irritants, such as smoke; or by systemic conditions resulting from shock, pancreatitis, narcotic overdose and other drug reactions. ARDS is difficult to treat and is frequently fatal. This type of lesion also occurs in domestic animals, and is considered to be a very early stage and severe form of interstitial pneumonia.

Inflammation

Overview

Inflammation, also referred to as alveolitis or interstitial pneumonia, results from diffuse or patchy

---

damage to alveolar septa, caused by blood-borne or inhaled toxicants; in humans, the etiology in the majority of cases of interstitial pneumonia is unknown. Inflammation is also a component of pneumoconiosis and other granulomatous diseases; however, once the disease is well-established, the fibrotic component is most prominent.

Pulmonary inflammation is a highly-regulated process that involves a complex interaction of leukocytes that arrive via the circulation and resident leukocytes and pulmonary cells (see Figure 6.5). Once in the lung, imported leukocytes communicate with pulmonary and vascular cells through adhesin and other inflammatory molecules such as the complement system (C3a, C3b, C5a), coagulation factors (Factors V and VII), arachidonic acid metabolites (interleukins, monokines, chemokines), adhesin molecules, enzymes and enzyme inhibitors (elastase, antitrypsin), oxygen metabolites (O_2, OH, H_2O_2), antioxidants (glutathione), and nitric oxide. These and other molecules can initiate, maintain, and resolve the inflammatory process. The pulmonary macrophages are the single most important effector cell and source of cytokines for all stages of pulmonary inflammation. They modulate the recruitment and tracking of circulatory leukocytes in the lung through the secretion of chemokines. Nitric oxide regulates the vascular and bronchial tissue, modulates the production of cytokines, and the recruitment and trafficking of neutrophils in the lung. Uncontrolled production and release of cytokines can result in ARDS, pulmonary fibrosis and asthma.

Interstitial Pneumonia

Interstitial pneumonia (Figure 6.19) can be caused by infectious and chemical agents; it may occur following hyperoxia, ingestion of paraquat, administration of chemotherapeutic drugs such as bleomycin and busulfan, and radiation exposure that damages epithelial and/or endothelial cells, or basement membrane. Pulmonary hypersensitivity reactions can also be manifested as interstitial pneumonia. Since interstitial pneumonia is a diffuse lesion, it can be difficult to identify on gross examination, especially in smaller animals. Failure to collapse to the extent of a normal lung (best identified prior to removal from the thoracic cavity) and firmness on palpation are the key gross features. In most cases it is impossible to determine the causative agent from the histologic changes in the lung; however, in a small percentage of cases, identifying features may be present.

In the acute phase, the capillary endothelial and alveolar epithelial cells are injured, with subsequent flooding of alveoli with serofibrinous exudate. Occasionally, if injury is especially severe, hyaline membranes formed from serum proteins and components of surfactants, line the airspaces. They have a hyaline appearance (eosinophilic, homogenous, and amorphous) on microscopic examination (Figure 6.19). This is followed by leukocytic infiltration of both alveolar lumina and interstitium. In human medicine, this stage of the disease is frequently referred to as acute respiratory distress syndrome (ARDS).

Inhalation of manure ("pit") gases, such as H_2S, and NH_3; NO_2 from silos; and ingestion of paraquat can cause similar injury in humans and animals. Resolution of acute injury occurs by proliferation of stem cells to replace damaged endothelium and epithelium, and by resolution of the inflammatory component. This proliferative stage is characterized by type II cell hyperplasia with thickening of the alveolar wall.

If injury is more severe, or consists of multiple episodes or chronic exposure, inflammation persists and normal regeneration is inhibited. The chronic phase is characterized by intra-alveolar accumulation of various mononuclear cells (mostly macrophages), proliferation and persistence of increased numbers of alveolar type II cells, and interstitial thickening due to accumulations of lymphoid cells, fibroblast proliferation, and collagen deposition. Examples of toxicants causing chronic interstitial pneumonia include paraquat, some chemotherapeutic drugs like bleomycin, and radiation. Once established, fibrosis is irreversible and frequently progressive. Extensive tissue destruction may also occur, resulting in so-called "honeycomb" lung. Honeycomb lung is the end result of severe chronic interstitial lung disease, with both fibrosis and cicatricial ("scar") emphysema as major components.

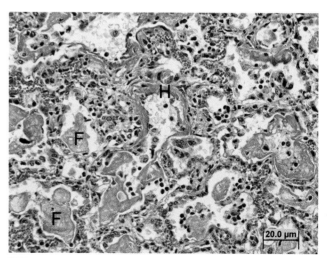

FIGURE 6.19 Lung, interstitial pneumonia, cow. H&E stain. Acute interstitial pneumonia with fibrin (F) deposition, and small numbers of inflammatory cells in the alveoli. Early hyaline (H) membrane formation and proliferation of type II epithelial cells are present.

Interstial Pneumonia in Veterinary Medicine

Interstitial pneumonia is observed in ruminants following ingestion of L-tryptophan, perilla ketone (from the purple mint plant, *Perilla frutescens*), stinkwood (*Zieria arborescens*), rapeseed and kale (*Brassica* species), 4-ipomeanol (produced by sweet potatoes [*Ipomoea batatus*] contaminated by the fungus *Fusarium solani*), in horses and pigs following ingestion of some *Crotalaria* species, and in horses ingesting Crofton weed (*Eupatorium adenophorum*). Chronic granulomatous interstitial pneumonia due to inhalation of silica has been recognized in horses, while hypersensitivity pneumonitis (extrinsic allergic alveolitis) due to fungal allergens, similar to "farmer's lung," occurs in housed dairy cattle. The latter results from a type III hypersensitivity reaction to fungal spores such as *Saccharopolyspora reactivirgula* (*Micropolyspora faeni*), commonly found in moldy hay. In dogs and cats, noninfectious causes of interstitial pneumonia are rarely identified, except for vitamin D toxicity, although paraquat used to be a problem.

L-tryptophan toxicity is a classic example of species-specific toxicity. High concentrations of L-tryptophan occur in lush green pasture, growth that typically occurs in the fall. Following ingestion of the pasture by adult beef cattle, rumenal bacteria convert L-tryptophan to 3-methylindole, which is absorbed into the bloodstream and reaches the lung where it is further metabolized via cytochrome P450 metabolism to the reactive species with release of free radicals, leading to damage to the epithelial cells, including Clara cells. Alteration of the rumenal microflora can modulate toxicity, and young animals do not have the required microflora for this activity. Pulmonary injury results in inflammation characteristic of ARDS with severe edema, hyaline membrane formation and type II cell proliferation. Inflammation is a minor component. Because of the severe respiratory distress, interstitial emphysema is commonly found, hence the clinical name, acute bovine pulmonary emphysema and edema (ABPE). Experimentally, similar pulmonary toxicity is produced in horses given 3-methylindole.

Interstitial pneumonia, characterized primarily by mineralization with little inflammation, may be present with cholecalciferol (vitamin D) toxicity in any species (Figure 6.20). Sources of excess cholecalciferol include feed, due to improper mixing or supplementation, vitamin D-based creams or medications, and certain rodenticides. In large animals, plants that contain the active form of vitamin D_3, 1,25-dihydroxycholecalciferol, such as *Solanum malacoxylon* and *Cestrum diurnum*, can also cause similar toxicity. Persistent hypercalcemia occurs through increased intestinal absorption, renal tubular reabsorption of calcium, and stimulated bone resorption. Soft tissue mineralization can occur throughout the body, but preferential deposition is seen within the kidney, lung, and stomach. In the lung, mineral is deposited along the capillaries of the alveolar walls, within the vasculature, and sometimes within the bronchial submucosa. It may be difficult to visualize the mineralization; however, the alveoli do not collapse normally and have a somewhat angular appearance (Figure 6.20A). Special stains for calcium, such as von Kossa, can be used (Figure 6.20B). Similar changes can occur with uremia, primary parathryroidism, and hypercalcemia of malignancy.

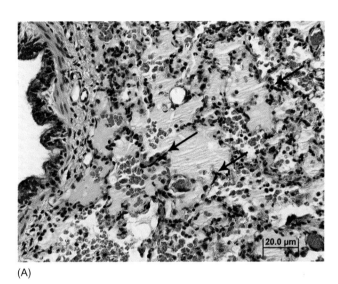

(A)

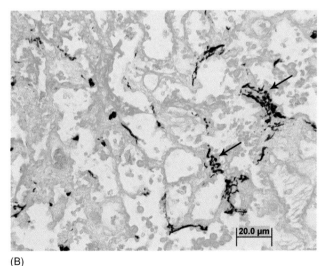

(B)

FIGURE 6.20 Lung, vitamin D_3 toxicity, rodenticide (Quintox) ingestion, dog. (A) Alveolar edema, hemorrhage, and minimal cellular infiltrate. Mineralization is suspected due to the linear appearance of basophilic material (arrows) within the alveolar walls. H&E stain. (B) Pulmonary mineralization. The black staining indicates calcium deposition within the alveolar walls. Von Kossa stain.

As mentioned previously, it may be difficult to determine the etiologic agent for spontaneous interstitial pneumonias based on pulmonary lesions alone. Occasionally the toxicant itself, e.g., particulate material such as silica, or a toxicant-induced effect, such as megalocytosis due to prrolizidine alkaloids, or mineralization due to cholecalciferol toxicity, may be present and assist with establishing the etiology. A good history and information regarding exposure to potential toxicants, including chemicals, plants, drugs and other therapies such as chemotherapeutic agents and oxygen, is essential. In many cases, only a differential list that includes infectious and toxic agents can be generated.

Aspiration bronchopneumonia, a locally extensive, usually anteroventral pneumonia, may occur following ingestion of toxicants such as kerosine, or improper administration of materials intended for ingestion or gavage. The type of tissue response depends on the nature of the material aspirated.

Fibrosis

Overview

The definition of fibrosis is difficult but, for all practical purposes, relates to one or more of the following: an increased amount of collagen; an abnormal location of the deposited collagen; or an abnormality in the nature of the collagen itself. Morphologically, fibrosis is defined as an increase in observable connective tissue at the microscopic level; special stains may be required to demonstrate its presence. Biochemically, fibrosis is defined as an increased amount of collagen, which can be estimated from the hydroxyproline content of the lung, or differences in relative concentration of the different collagen types. Fibrosis can be distributed diffusely or focally throughout the lungs; this will affect the sensitivity of the biochemical and morphologic evaluations. Functionally, there is a reduction in compliance, and an impairment of gaseous diffusion.

Fibrotic lung disease in humans is a heterogeneous group of chronic lung disorders that may be produced by a variety of toxic agents, including inhalation of silica, asbestos, and beryllium; ingested paraquat; and chemotherapeutic drugs or thoracic irradiation. Fibrosis may also be produced in infectious and immune mediated disorders; in many cases, the fibrosis is idiopathic (idiopathic pulmonary fibrosis, IPF). It is possible that IPF is toxic in origin or the result of interaction between several toxicants, or between infectious and toxic agents.

Fibrosis may occur following diffuse alveolar damage, as occurs in interstitial pneumonia, in which case collagen is distributed relatively uniformly throughout

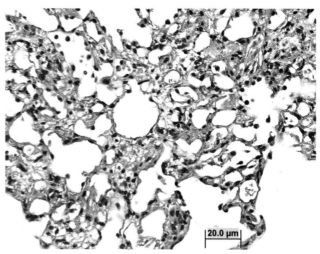

FIGURE 6.21 Lung, butylated hydroxytoluene (BHT), single intraperitoneal exposure, mouse. Interstitial fibrosis. There is loss of normal architecture, and thickening of alveolar walls due to increased collagen. Small numbers of inflammatory cells are present. H&E stain.

the lungs (Figure 6.21). Collagen is deposited within the interstitium of the alveolar walls, and may also be present within the alveolar lumen. Grossly, if the lung is severely affected, it will not collapse when the thoracic cavity is opened, and will be paler and firmer than normal. It is difficult to induce severe pulmonary fibrosis in laboratory animal models.

Fibrosis is also a major component of pneumoconiotic diseases, such as silicosis and asbestosis. In this case, collagen is distributed multifocally throughout the lung as a component of the granulomatous response to inhaled particles (Figure 6.22). Grossly, the lung will contain multiple firm nodules within the parenchyma; nodules may coalesce in severe cases. These may be found on visual examination, but may be more evident on palpation. Pigment may be associated with the lesions, as in coal miners' pneumoconiosis.

Pathogenesis

The development of fibrosis is a very complex process that has been studied extensively both *in vivo* and *in vitro* in numerous experimental models, as well as in humans. Pulmonary fibrosis can occur if there is disruption of the normal repair mechanism following interstitial injury. Such interstitial injury can result from one or more of the following: alteration in number, properties, or differentiation of parenchymal cells; inflammatory and immune responses; modification of connective tissue destruction; or acellular expansion of interstitium by edema fluid.

Most forms of fibrosis are biologically complex, and can be mediated through effector cells of the inflammatory and immune systems, platelets, the

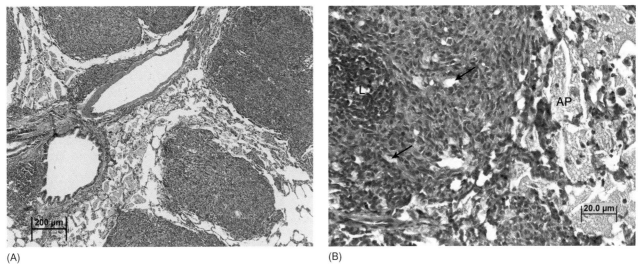

(A)   (B)

FIGURE 6.22   Lung, silicosis, intratracheal exposure, rat. H&E stain. (A) Multiple nodules (granulomas) are scattered within the lung. Alveoli contain dense eosinophilic material (alveolar proteinosis). Bronchus associated lymphoid tissue (BALT) is present to the left of the bronchiole. (B) Granulomatous inflammation is characterized by central aggregates of mononuclear inflammatory cells (L) surrounded by fibroblasts. Clefts represent silica particles (arrows). The alveoli contain granular proteinaceous material (alveolar proteinosis, AP), and an occasional inflammatory cell.

complement cascade, and *in situ* factors. Interaction of these components is exceedingly complex. The macrophage appears to play a central role, although neutrophils, eosinophils, and mast cells may also be involved. However, both neutrophils and macrophages can stimulate, as well as suppress, the fibrotic response, and both contain collagenases.

Specific Etiologic Agents

Experimentally, pulmonary fibrosis has been studied following administration of silica, hyperoxia, radiation, bleomycin, and combinations of agents such as butylated hydroxytoluene (BHT) or bleomycin with oxygen. Ozone, endotoxin and particulate matter induce parenchymal inflammation that can be followed by fibrosis. However, rodents are not considered good models for pulmonary fibrosis in humans.

Fibrosis is also an important component of the pneumoconioses, at least those caused following occupational exposure to mineral dusts, such as asbestos, silica, and beryllium. Inhalation of dust containing crystalline free silica leads to a progressive pulmonary disease characterized by extensive formation of granulomatous lesions and fibrosis throughout the lung parenchyma (Figure 6.22). Silicosis is mostly an occupational disease found in rock miners, sandblasters, stone cutters, and foundry workers, and generally presents decades after exposure. Silica particles that reach the deep lung are phagocytized by alveolar macrophages, and taken up into phagolysosomes. Contrary to many other dusts which may remain within the phagolysosomes, silica has the

potential to destroy lysosomal membranes, resulting in release of digestive enzymes and chemical mediators. These mediators, and other products of destroyed cells, stimulate the migration of additional macrophages to the lesion, and may incite fibroblasts to proliferate and to synthesize increased amounts of collagen. Silica also causes activation and release of mediators by viable macrophages, including interleukin-1, tumor necrosis factor (TNF), fibronectin, lipid mediators, oxygen derived free radicals, and fibrogenic cytokines. The developing silicotic nodules may eventually undergo hyaline degeneration, enlarge slowly, and coalesce into larger lesions. In humans the disease is often associated with tuberculosis.

Coal worker's pneumoconiosis ("black lung") results from the deposition of coal particles in the deep lung. The simple form of the disease (accumulation of pigment with macrophage infiltration) usually does not produce serious symptoms, although the inhaled coal dust may produce chronic bronchitis. The disease usually does not progress once exposure has ceased. Coal miners' pneumoconiosis may become more severe if large amounts of dust are inhaled, or if silica is present in the inhaled coal dust. Anthracosis, the simple accumulation of carbon pigment without a cellular response, is present in coal miners and urban dwellers.

Inhalation of asbestos fibers in mining, milling, and manufacturing operations is another occupational health hazard that may lead to the development of chronic interstitial lung disease (asbestosis). Initially, inflammation develops at the respiratory bronchiolar-alveolar duct junction, a preferred site for deposition of inhaled asbestos fibers. Eventually, diffuse interstitial fibrosis develops. Deposition of iron on deposited fibers gives rise to asbestos bodies, a marker of asbestos exposure. The more important risk following exposure to asbestos is the development of cancer, either from the bronchial epithelium (bronchogenic carcinoma) or from the pleura (malignant mesothelioma). There is a synergistic interaction between asbestos and cigarette smoking in the development of bronchiogenic carcinoma, but not malignant mesothelioma.

Several metals, such as cadmium and beryllium, may also produce interstitial lung disease. Acute beryllium disease is characterized by acute interstitial pneumonia, and is usually associated with accidental exposure to high concentrations of beryllium. Although comparatively rare, it may be rapidly progressive, and has been fatal in 10% to 15% of cases. Chronic beryllium disease is caused by induction of cell-mediated immunity, and is characterized by multiple granulomas in the pulmonary parenchyma. Modern industrial hygiene methods have been successful in eliminating acute, but not chronic, beryllium disease. Beryllium is a known human carcinogen, and beryllium compounds are carcinogenic in rats and monkeys after inhalation or intratracheal instillation. Preliminary studies of materials developed for new technologies, such as carbon nanotubes and microspheres, suggest that they may induce granulomatous inflammation and fibrosis.

Emphysema

Overview

Pulmonary emphysema is defined as abnormal, permanent, enlargement of the airspaces distal to the terminal bronchiole, accompanied by destruction of airspace walls. Emphysema is one of the causes of chronic obstructive pulmonary disease (see airway response to injury). There are two main reasons for the airflow obstruction. The destruction of parenchyma decreases the elastic recoil that is normally used for expiration. In addition, the lumena of small airways, which have lost the structural support and radial tension imparted by normal parenchyma, collapse prematurely during expiration. While pressure–volume curves document decreased elastic recoil and increased compliance, a definitive diagnosis of emphysema requires morphologic assessment.

At autopsy or necropsy, the emphysematous lung is larger than normal, and often does not collapse completely when the thoracic cavity is opened. Airspace wall destruction is recognized microscopically by an increase in the number and size of fenestrations in the alveolar septa, with the alveolar septa appearing as isolated, detached segments in later stages. Fibrosis is not a component of emphysema, but is often present in emphysematous lungs because cigarette smoking, the most common cause of emphysema in humans, also causes bronchiolitis with fibrosis of respiratory bronchioles.

There are two main anatomic types of emphysema, classified according to the distribution of the airspace enlargement within the acinus, panacinar emphysema and centrilobular, sometimes called proximal acinar, emphysema. In panacinar emphysema, the enlargement of airspaces is distributed throughout the acinus and involves the respiratory bronchioles, alveolar ducts, and alveolar sacs. In centrilobular emphysema, the airspace enlargement primarily involves the respiratory bronchioles, with lesser involvement of the alveolar ducts and relative sparing of the alveolar sacs. In humans, approximately 95% of the symptomatic cases of emphysema are centrilobular. Another type of emphysema, irregular emphysema, is primarily associated with fibrous scars, and is sometimes called cicatricial emphysema. Distal acinar emphysema, also called paraseptal emphysema, spares the alveolar ducts. The last two types, irregular and paraseptal emphysema, are not associated with airflow obstruction.

Pathogenesis

The pathogenesis of emphysema is summarized by the protease/antiprotease hypothesis, which states that the susceptibility of the lung parenchyma to proteolytic degradation is determined by the relative balance between elastases and other proteases and their inhibitors. The principal protease activities are derived from inflammatory cells. The principal antiprotease activity in serum and interstitial tissue is α_1-protease inhibitor (PI), but secretory leukoprotease inhibitor in bronchial mucus and α_1-macroglobulin in serum may also be important in lung protection. Lung destruction occurs when protease activity predominates, due to excessive proteases or inhibition of antiproteases. Evidence supporting this theory comes from observations of severe emphysema in patients with α_1-PI deficiency, and experimental models that use inhaled or intratracheally instilled proteases to induce emphysema in animals with anti-protease deficiencies.

Genetic and environmental factors determine the risk for developing chronic obstructive pulmonary disease, including emphysema. Genetic deficiency of α_1-PI is associated with an increased risk for emphysema. Other genes may also influence risk for COPD. Cigarette smoking is the most important risk factor for developing emphysema. Smokers have increased numbers of neutrophils and macrophages in their lungs, and smoking stimulates release of elastase from neutrophils and enhances elastolytic protease activity in macrophages. There is also decreased anti-elastase activity in the lungs of smokers. Another risk factor for emphysema is occupational exposure to a dusty environment, such as in underground coal or gold mining, or exposure to cadmium oxide fumes.

Neoplasia

Lung Cancer in Humans

Lung cancer was a rare disease at the turn of the century. Its incidence had increased after World War I, and by the end of the twentieth century it had become the leading cause of death from cancer in both men and women. The most important risk factor in lung cancer is smoking cigarettes and other inhaled tobacco or plant products. Tobacco use may be responsible for approximately 85% to 90% of all lung cancers. Lung cancer and other tobacco smoke-induced diseases (cardiac disease, pulmonary disease) constitute a public health problem of major proportions.

Lung cancer also is found in non-smokers. One possible risk factor is exposure to environmental tobacco smoke (ETS), a mixture of smoke emanating from the lit end of a cigarette and the smoke exhaled into the surrounding air by active smokers. An additional risk factor is air pollution present in urban areas. Inhalation of common air pollutants, particularly small particles emanating from the combustion of fossil fuels and loaded with carcinogens such as polycyclic aromatic hydrocarbons and nitroarenes, is a risk factor.

In humans, there are four major lung tumor types: squamous cell carcinoma (about 30% of all lung cancers), adenocarcinoma (just over 30%), small cell carcinoma (20 to 25%), and large cell carcinoma (poorly-differentiated carcinomas that do not have features of the three other types). Lung cancer continues to have a notoriously poor prognosis. Most of the tumors appear to originate from the bronchial epithelium, and are often referred to as "bronchial cancer." In laboratory rodents, intratracheal instillation of polycyclic aromatic hydrocarbons has produced such tumors, while inhalation exposure produces lung tumors located much more peripherally, and resembling human bronchiolo-alveolar tumors rather than bronchogenic carcinoma. With the increasing use of molecular techniques, it became apparent that many of the peripherally-located adenomas and adenocarcinomas in animals might represent useful models for human lung cancer. Small cell lung cancer, comprising 30% to 40% of all lung cancers found in smokers,

has not been reproducibly induced in experimental animals.

Pleural mesothelioma is associated with exposure to asbestos and other fibrous materials, although it occasionally occurs in individuals without such known exposure. While the association with asbestos exposure is unequivocal, it is less certain to what extent man-made mineral fibers, widely used in insulating materials, constitute a risk factor. Mesotheliomas have a long latency period, and are invariably fatal. They can be produced in experimental animals by exposing them to fibers via the inhalation route, or by intrapleural or intraperitoneal suspensions of fibers. Fiber size and shape, more so than chemical composition, are important determinants of carcinogenicity.

Lung Cancer in Animals

Spontaneous lung cancers in animals are rare, although certain mouse strains (A/J strain) may have a comparatively high lung tumor rate. Go RENI (http://www.goreni.org/), a standard reference for nomenclature and diagnostic criteria in toxicologic pathology, lists the following classification for neoplasms in mice and rats: bronchoalveolar adenomas, carcinomas (bronchoalveolar, acinar, adenosquamous, and squamous cell), and epitheliomas (rat only; cystic, keratinizing, and non-keratinizing). Most lung tumors found in rodents are found peripherally, originating from the lung parenchyma, including bronchioles. This seems to differentiate lung tumors in rodents from human lung cancer. A second difference is metastasis. While human lung cancer frequently metastasizes to organs such as liver, bone, and brain, distant metastasis is much less frequent from rodent lung cancers, although they are able to invade adjacent tissues, lymphatic and blood vessels. Two rodent lung tumors are described in more detail below, because of their particular significance in toxicology.

Lung Tumors in Mice

The most common spontaneous lung tumor found in mice originates in the peripheral lung from either the type II alveolar epithelial cells or the bronchiolar Clara cells (Figure 6.23). A/J mice or Swiss–Webster mice have a very high spontaneous incidence, with exposure to carcinogens greatly increasing the number of lung tumors per animal, whereas other strains, such as C57Bl, are very resistant and rarely develop lung tumors.

These lung tumors are now accepted to represent a valid model of human adenocarcinoma. Many gene mutations found in human lung adenocarcinoma,

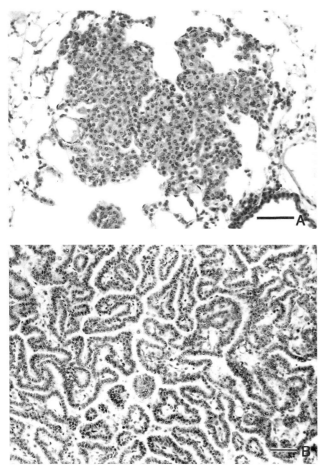

FIGURE 6.23 Lung, bronchiolo-alveolar adenomas, mouse. H&E stain. (A) Adenoma believed to arise from type II epithelial cells. Bar = 40 μm. (B) Adenoma believed to arise from Clara cells. Papillary structures are lined by nonciliated epithelial cells. Bar = 100 μm.

particularly in the ras family of oncogenes, also occur with very high frequency in mouse lung tumors. Alterations in signal transduction pathways and other biochemical parameters in human and mouse tumors are also similar. Thus, lung tumors in mice allow the study of the carcinogenic process from hyperplasia, to adenoma, to carcinoma *in situ*, stages practically inaccessible in man.

Tumors in Rat Lung Exposed to High Concentrations of Particulate Matter

Rats exposed by inhalation to high concentrations of diesel exhaust, oil shale dust, talc, titanium dioxide or carbon black develop adenomas, adenocarcinomas, squamous cell carcinomas, or adenosquamous carcinomas in the peripheral lung. In addition, lesions labeled as keratin cysts, cystic epithelioma or benign keratinizing squamous cell tumors originate from foci of alveolar metaplasia. The tumors consist of whorled

keratin masses surrounded by well-differentiated layers of stratified squamous epithelium. They often arise adjacent to fibrotic foci, and a large bronchiole with hyperplastic epithelium often opens into the lesion. These tumors only develop when the macrophage-mediated clearance mechanism of the lung is overwhelmed, and there is excessive retention of particles in the alveoli ("particle overload"). Excess particulate matter may lead to secondary inflammatory and proliferative lesions, eventually leading to tumors by nongenotoxic mechanisms.

Lung Tumors in Dogs

Dogs have been used fairly widely in inhalation studies, due to their convenient size, cooperative temperament, and similarity to the human in respect to bronchiolar structure and pulmonary deposition of inhaled aerosols. Pulmonary tumors of dogs are also of interest since dogs, as companion animals, are exposed to an environment similar to humans. Bronchiolo-alveolar carcinomas are the most prevalent type of pulmonary neoplasm. Unlike in humans, bronchogenic carcinomas, anaplastic small and large cell carcinomas are infrequent. K-ras mutations (GGT to GGA transitions at codon 12) have been detected, both in spontaneously-occurring and in $^{239}PuO_2$-induced malignant canine lung tumors.

EVALUATION OF TOXICITY

Evaluations of pulmonary function, chest radiographs, cytology of lavage fluid or sputum, as well as morphologic examination of respiratory tissue (biopsy), are all common tests conducted in a clinical setting. Experimentally, respiratory toxicity can be evaluated *in vivo*, *in vitro*, or in combined *in vivo-in vitro* systems. An understanding of the strengths and weaknesses of the various systems or models is critical to this selection. Consideration for whole animal studies include selection of the appropriate routes of exposure for the xenobiotic being studied, species differences in xenobiotic metabolism, and cell susceptibility to toxic injury.

There are many ways in which injury and the response to injury can be characterized and quantitated. A combination of morphology, physiology, and biochemistry is often the most useful way to evaluate toxic lung injury. *In vivo*, acute and chronic respiratory damage can be evaluated by noninvasive and nondestructive respiratory function tests; morphologic methods such as histology, quantitative morphometry, cell kinetics and immunohistochemistry; and biochemical techniques such as analysis of broncho-alveolar lavage fluid and collagen. Similar biochemical and morphologic evaluations can be performed in some *in vitro* systems. Qualitative observations are useful for the characterization of the type and severity of response, while quantitative data allow statistical analyses and descriptive modeling that can be used to extrapolate results beyond the single study and single species.

Methods for Testing

Whole Animal Exposure

Reproduction and study of lung damage caused by blood-borne agents in appropriate animal models usually does not present any special problems or technical difficulties, except where there are marked species differences. To duplicate human inhalation exposure is more demanding, and requires special techniques and equipment. Furthermore, most small rodents are obligatory nose breathers, and many aerosolized noxious agents are filtered out in the upper respiratory passages. When exposed to irritants, rodents may hold their breath, reduce minute ventilation, or simply bury their nose in their fur, thus filtering out airborne pollutants. Inhalation studies are usually satisfactory when exposure is to gases, and when acute or subacute noncarcinogenic lesions are examined.

Inhalation Exposure

Although inhalation is often the most appropriate way to expose experimental animals to airborne toxicants, it is also technically the most demanding. Generation of gases and aerosols, maintaining adequate chamber concentration of the agents examined, and monitoring chamber atmosphere to ensure that the required concentrations of the test agents are maintained require major investments in equipment and personnel. Properly conducted inhalation studies, particularly studies involving long-term exposure, usually require expensive and specialized facilities, and highly-trained personnel.

Inhalation studies may be conducted in a static or dynamic mode. During static exposure, the test agent is introduced into an inhalation chamber only once, at the beginning of the experiment. In a dynamic system, the test agent is mixed with the air that flows through the inhalation chamber, and a constant concentration of the agent within the chamber is maintained throughout the entire experiment. Animals may be exposed to airborne test agents in whole-body chambers or in chambers allowing nose-only

exposure. For whole-body exposures, the animals are placed in chambers containing the test atmosphere. Nose-only exposure is accomplished using specialized inhalation chambers in which animals are kept in small tubes, with only their noses protruding into an inhalation chamber. A specialized version of nose-only exposure is the use of face masks, a technique that usually is only adopted with such animal species as dogs or monkeys. Each method has its own list of advantages and disadvantages.

Intratracheal instillation is an acceptable alternative route of exposure in some cases. With practice, it is possible to repeatedly instill a test chemical under light anesthesia into the trachea, without unduly traumatizing the animal. The major disadvantages are that the test agent, delivered at a high dose rate, becomes unevenly distributed, and the animals must be individually and repeatedly treated. The dose rate to the lung is several orders of magnitude greater than that achieved in experimental, occupational, or environmental inhalation exposures, which greatly confounds interpretation of lung responses.

Comparatively crude measurements used in inhalation toxicology are determinations of LC_{50} and LT_{50}. The LC_{50} is the concentration of a test agent in the inspired air that will cause the death of 50% of experimental animals within a given and predetermined time period. The LT_{50} is the time required for 50% of the animals to die following exposure to a known concentration of the test agent. Newer and more refined measurements, such as the measurement of changes in respiratory rate and depth following exposure to upper respiratory tract irritants, may supplement these crude measurements of toxicity. Quantification of such functional changes often allows direct extrapolation of data from animals to humans, thus creating a scientifically-sound basis for the use of animal data in setting standards for human exposure.

In Vitro Methods

In vitro studies are indispensable tools for characterizing and understanding respiratory tract toxicology. *In vitro* models facilitate the precise application of toxicants, quantification of pathways and kinetics of toxicant interactions, generation of data from specific cells or anatomic compartments, and integration of studies performed at different organizational levels.

Isolated Perfused Lung

Uses of the isolated perfused lung include: study of the metabolic fate of foreign chemicals processed by the lung; characterization of effects on lung function;

characterization of the interactions between lung toxicants and circulating inflammatory cells; and evaluation of the distribution and extent of toxicant-induced cellular perturbations. Lungs from such diverse species as rabbits, rats, and even mice can be used. The toxicant under study can be administered either by the circulatory or ventilatory route.

Major advantages of this system over other *in vitro* systems include the minimal amount of damage caused during preparation, and the maintenance of structural and functional integrity of the lung. Disadvantages include the comparatively short viability of the preparation (about five hours) and the complexity of the methodology. It is not well-suited for examining the effects of toxic agents on lung structure and function.

Tissue Sections and Organ Cultures

Whole lung tissue slices, airway rings, isolated airways, micro-dissected tissue sections and arterial rings or strips have all been used to maintain a degree of structural or organizational integrity of targeted respiratory components. The advantages are the simplicity of the preparation and the maintenance of normal structure. A disadvantage is the short-term viability of the tissue sections, often associated with technical issues related to tissue harvesting.

Fetal lung organ cultures have been used extensively in the study of embryonic and fetal development of the lung. Airway organ cultures have been quite useful, but adult lung organ culture has been more challenging. The advantages of organ cultures include the relatively straightforward procedures (except for adult peripheral lung culture), maintenance of normal cellular relationships within the explants, and the small amount of tissue injury during preparation of the tissue for explant. The major disadvantages include the loss of normal means of cell nutrition, gaseous diffusion, and waste excretion.

Isolated Cells and Cell Culture Systems

Isolated cells provide a powerful approach to the understanding of the biology of individual cell types. Cultures of individual cell types have been used to determine cell composition, biochemical activity, and control mechanisms. Numerous commercially available cell lines provide alternatives to harvesting and primary culture.

Lung Cancer Model Systems

Several lung cancer model systems have been developed in animals that allow the study of the histogenesis and progression of tumors in circumscribed locations of the bronchial tree. Carcinogenic agents are incorporated into an inert matrix and made into pellets that are implanted into lobar bronchi. The carcinogen diffuses out of the pellet and induces neoplastic changes in the bronchial mucosa. In a second method, tracheas are removed from rats and a carcinogen-containing pellet is introduced into the lumen. The tracheas are then grafted under the skin of syngeneic animals. Cell cultures can be established from these explants or cytological analysis performed on cells removed by flushing. In larger animals, such as dogs, bronchial explants may be implanted under the skin of the donor animal. Finally, techniques are available that allow repeated exposure of circumscribed segments of the trachea to carcinogen-containing solutions.

Pulmonary Function

Physiological measurements provide useful information in intact animals regarding adverse health effects, especially in relation to ventilatory function or gas exchange. In humans and larger laboratory animals, these tests are advantageous because they are noninvasive, may not interfere with other toxicologic tests, and can be repeated on the same subject. The disadvantage is that handling, stress, and other factors may affect the results. Therefore, sham-treated or sham-exposed animals should also be included in the test groups. In small laboratory animals, some of these tests are performed as terminal procedures. Pulmonary function tests assess the mechanical characteristics of ventilatory function in relation to pressure, air flow, and air volume within the lung; the presence and magnitude of functional impairment can be determined. They also provide an alternative means of assessing structural changes that affect function. In addition, they may detect functional changes in cases where there is no alteration in structure, for instance, in bronchoconstriction.

Bronchopulmonary Lavage

Bronchoalveolar lavage (BAL) can be used to evaluate toxicant-induced alterations in pulmonary epithelial integrity, cellular damage, and surface release/accumulation of cellular secretory products. It is also a convenient way to recover macrophages and other cells for *in vitro* studies. If the animal is large enough, BAL can be performed in the living animal, either as a single test or sequentially to monitor changes. In smaller animals, such as the rat and mouse, BAL is usually performed in the lung *in situ* or following excision after euthanasia.

The aspirated fluid can be analyzed for its cellular profile, protein content, enzymes, and lipids. Increased activity of marker enzymes, such as lactate dehydrogenase, alkaline or acid phosphatase, or angiotensin-converting enzyme, is usually an indicator of cell damage; increased serum albumin is indicative of pulmonary edema; and the presence of certain inflammatory cells and enzymes involved in collagen metabolism may predict the development of more chronic changes following exposure to harmful dusts. It has not been possible to find similar markers in the serum.

The advantages of BAL include the relative simplicity of the procedure, the rapidity with which results can be obtained, the ability to sample the whole or large portions of the lungs, and, in larger animals, the ability to perform sequential evaluations. In general, constituents of BAL fluid correlate well with morphologic changes. Disadvantages include that this is a terminal procedure in smaller experimental animals, and that only the surface of the alveoli and airways are sampled. Recent studies suggest that lavage of the nasal cavity may be useful for detection of toxicant-induced changes in this region.

Biochemical Evaluation

The biochemistry of lung cells has been extensively studied, with methods ranging from analysis of whole homogenized lung tissue to defined lung cell types *in vitro*. Data can be expressed on a whole lung or unit weight basis. In most cases, expression on a per lung or lobe basis is preferred, since lung weight may be altered by components other than those being examined. However, lung weight itself is a useful parameter for initial determination of whether or not the test agent causes a pulmonary effect. Since lung weight may be increased by edema, inflammation, fibrosis, or neoplasia, both wet and dry weight information may be useful. The metabolism of foreign chemicals by lung tissue can be examined in isolated perfused lung preparations.

Advantages of biochemical measurements are that they are quantitative and may provide mechanistic information. A major disadvantage is the difficulty of localizing or relating specific biochemical events to a defined cell population.

Morphologic Evaluation

Morphologic evaluation of the respiratory tract can be performed by a variety of methods, and the particular ones utilized by the investigator depend on factors such as the objectives of the study, species of animal used, suspected site or type of injury, other evaluations to be performed, cost, and facilities available. Animals are usually anesthetized and then exsanguinated. Evaluation begins at the macroscopic level, and can proceed through the light microscopic and ultrastructural levels. Each of these levels is important; for instance, it is possible to miss focal lesions if samples are taken for ultrastructural studies without prior localization of changes. Outline drawings of the respiratory tract may be useful to record the location of lesions.

Nasopharyngeal and Laryngeal Regions

In small laboratory animals, gross examination is usually limited to the exterior, with internal examination performed on histologic sections. In larger animals, dissection and trimming of the nasal cavity prior to fixation allows gross examination of internal structures. Nasopharyngeal structures of small laboratory animals are generally fixed *in situ* with the rest of the head, in 10% buffered formalin solution. Optimal fixation is achieved using retrograde flushing of the nasal cavity with the fixative through the nasopharyngeal orifice. In larger animals, appropriate sections are fixed by immersion. Decalcification, preferably using the slow formic acid–sodium citrate method, follows.

For light microscopic examination, standard cross-sections from decalcified tissue should be made with a razor. Because of the distribution of the different types of epithelium within the nasal cavity, it is imperative to examine sections from exactly the same location in both control and treated animals. Mapping of the location, type, and severity of lesions may be useful, especially in rodents, since the nasal passage of rodents is very complex, and lesions may occur in small but distinct regions. This method allows the susceptible site and cell type to be identified. For larger animals, sections from proximal and distal regions of the nasal cavity, pharynx, and larynx should be selected.

The larynx is also an important target site for inhaled materials in rodents, and should be routinely examined. The major target site is located on the ventral floor of the larynx near the base of the epiglottis, cranial to the ventral laryngeal diverticulum (ventral pouch).

Tracheobronchial Tree and Pulmonary Parenchyma

The macroscopic examination determines the topographic distribution of abnormalities and, especially in larger animals, provides the basis for sample selection. The lungs are examined visually and palpation is a useful adjunct in larger species; care must be taken, however, not to induce artifactual changes which interfere with morphologic and especially ultrastructural examination. The pleural cavity should be examined for the presence of fluid or abnormalities of the pleura. Determination of lesion distribution is especially important in spontaneous disease, to assist with formation of differential diagnoses.

The lungs from laboratory animals should generally be fixed by intra-airway instillation of fixative. This is also the preferred method of fixation for large animals, where detailed examination is required. However, immersion fixation is used most commonly. Intravascular fixation may be the method of choice in some studies. Buffered formalin is the usual fixative for light microscopy, while formaldehyde–glutaraldehyde fixatives are preferable for combined light and electron microscopic studies.

Fixation by immersion is best when lung tissue is no longer aerated, while airway instillation is best when lung tissue is still aerated. Airway fixation can be done simply with a syringe and blunt needle inserted into the trachea in small animals, or into a selected bronchus in larger animals, if only a portion of lung is to be fixed. The fixative is instilled at a relatively constant rate and pressure until the periphery of the lobes is uncurled. The airway should be ligated after fixative instillation to maintain inflation. This is satisfactory for routine light microscopic examination; however, fixation at a constant pressure is preferable, and essential if morphometric studies are to be performed.

The protocol for sampling lung tissue for microscopic evaluation is of critical importance. Lesions may be focal rather than diffuse, and may affect airways, parenchyma, or both. In addition, the sections examined represent a very small part of the total lung. Sampling must be standardized for each study. Minimal sites to be sampled in extrapulmonary airways are the proximal trachea and tracheobronchial bifurcation. In many cases the tracheobronchial lymph nodes should also be examined. In small animals, for simple qualitative morphologic examination, each lobe should be separated at trimming, and a longitudinal section cut parallel to the axis of the main bronchus of each lobe. This should include the bronchus and major vessels. In many studies, the lung is divided for both biochemical analyses and morphologic examination.

Quantitative Techniques

Quantitative information on changes in structure of the respiratory tract may be obtained by morphometric techniques. Light microscopy provides sufficient resolution to measure alveolar surface area, proportional volumes of tissue and air, and total number of alveoli.

Mean linear intercept (MLI), a measurement related to alveolar surface area and number of alveoli present in the lung, is frequently used to assess lung growth or the development of emphysema.

Autoradiography may be used to localize radiolabeled molecules within the respiratory tract; if the compound is not bound covalently within the tissue, frozen sections must be used. Whole-body frozen sections have been used to determine the macroscopic distribution of radiolabeled compounds in tissues such as the nasal epithelium, trachea, bronchi, and pulmonary parenchyma.

Cell turnover and cell kinetics have been studied by autoradiographic and immunohistochemical techniques. Whatever method is used, it must be noted that it is not possible to identify pulmonary cell types using standard 4–6 μm paraffin sections. Thinner, usually 1 μm sections of lung embedded in methacrylate, epon, or similar material are used. For autoradiographic studies, animals are given a single injection or a constant infusion (using a minipump) of [^{3}H]thymidine. The thymidine analog, 5-bromo-2'-deoxyuridine (BrdU), like thymidine, is incorporated into DNA, and is detected in tissue sections using a specific antibody to bromodeoxyuridine. Endogenous markers of cell proliferation, such as proliferating cell nuclear antigen (PCNA), can also be used to identify proliferating cells. This is of particular value when cell proliferation in archived tissues needs to be determined. Proliferative activity can be expressed as labeling index, that is, number of labeled cells within a defined cell population (e.g., type II alveolar cells) or within the overall cell population of the alveolar zone (e.g., number of cells labeled per total number of cells counted).

Additional Techniques

Special techniques to study various components of the respiratory tract include the preparation of whole-lung macrosections, which have been used primarily for studying emphysema in humans; corrosion casts and airway microdissection for detailed examination of airway morphology and morphometry; latex casts to study the vascular tree; elemental microanalysis; immunohistochemistry for localization of isozymes of cytochrome P450 enzymes and adducts; and energy dispersive X-ray analysis (EDXA) for detection and quantification of inorganic particles *in situ*.

Animal Models

Models of human disease are developed in laboratory animals in order to study the mechanisms involved in the initiation and progression of the disease, as well as to test potential treatments. The choice of animal species for the testing of compounds potentially toxic to the respiratory tract is made on the basis of species similarity to humans, and the type of response anticipated. Similarities include the diversity of cell types, cell size of major alveolar cell types, the allometry of lung volume and alveolar surface area to body mass, and thickness of air to blood–tissue barrier. Species differences include nasal cavity morphology, airway branching patterns, airway composition, epithelial cell distribution, Carla cell composition and metabolic function, transition from airways to alveolar duct, and alveolar number, surface area, and size. Other criteria for species selection include existence of a large or appropriate database, and cost and ease of animal handling.

CONCLUSIONS

The respiratory tract is a complex organ system both macroscopically and microscopically, with many different functions and cell types localized throughout the nasopharyngeal, tracheobronchial, and pulmonary segments. Exposure to xenobiotics occurs via inhalation and via the blood following ingestion, dermal exposure or parentral administration. Xenobiotics vary from particles of variable size, to gases, to plant toxins, thus dosimetry and site of injury are critical in interpreting the response to injury. In addition, species differences must be considered in interpretation of data to be used in risk assessment. In a diagnostic situation, since the pulmonary response to injury is often nonspecific, it is important to consider the gross distribution of pulmonary lesions, and to use detailed history and ancillary test results in conjunction with histologic evaluation to determine potential etiologic agents.

FURTHER READING

Barrow, C.S. (ed.) (1986). *Toxicology of the Nasal Passages*. Hemisphere Publishing Corp., New York, NY.

Boorman, G.A., Eustis, S.L., Elwell, M.R., Montgomery, C.A., and MacKenzie, W.F. (eds) (1990). *Pathology of the Fischer Rat*, pp. 315–367. Academic Press, New York, NY.

Cantor, J.O. (ed.) (1989). Handbook of Animal Models of Pulmonary DiseaseVols. I and II. CRC Press, Boca Raton, FL.

Dixon, D., Herbert, R.A., Kissling, G.E., Brix, A.E., Miller, R.A., and Maronpot, R.R. (2008). Summary of chemically induced pulmonary lesions in the National Toxicology Program (NTP) toxicology and carcinogenesis studies. *Toxicol. Pathol.*, 36, 428–439.

Dixon, D., Herbert, R.A., Sills, R.C., and Boorman, G.A. (1999). Lungs, pleura and mediastinum. In *Pathology of the Mouse* (Maronpot, R.R. ed.), pp. 293–332. Cache River Press, Vienna, IL.

Dungworth, D.L. (ed.) (1982). The respiratory system. *Adv. Vet. Sci. Comp. Med.*, 26. Academic Press, New York.

Gardner, D.E. (ed.) (2006). *Toxicology of the Lung*, 4th edn. CRC/Taylor & Francis, Boca Raton, FL.

Green, F.H.Y., Vallyathan, V., and Hahn, F.F. (2007). Comparative pathology of environmental lung disease: An overview. *Toxicol. Pathol.*, 35, 136–147.

Hahn, F.F., Gigliotti, A., and Hutt, J.A. (2007). Comparative oncology of lung tumors. *Toxicol. Pathol.*, 35, 130–135.

Harkema, J.R., Carey, S.A., and Wagner, J.G. (2006). The nose revisited: A brief review of the comparative structure, function, and toxicologic pathology of the nasal epithelium. *Toxicol. Pathol.*, 34, 252–269.

Haschek, W.M., Witschi, H.P., and Nikula, K. (2002). Respiratory system. In *Handbook of Toxicologic Pathology* (Haschek, W.M., Rousseaux, C.G., and Wallig, M.A. eds), 2nd edn, pp. 3–83. Academic Press, San Diego, CA.

Herbert, R.A., and Leininger, J.R. (1991). Nose, larynx and trachea. In *Pathology of the Mouse* (Maronpot, R.R. ed.), pp. 235–258. Cache River Press, Vienna, IL.

Hussain, A.N., and Kumar, V. (2006). The lung. In *Robbins and Cotran Pathologic Basis of Disease* (Kumar, V., Abbas, A.K., and Fausto, N. eds), 7th edn, pp. 711–772. Elsevier Saunders, Philadelphia, PA.

Khalil, N., Churg, A., Muller, N., and O'Connor, R. (2007). Environmental, inhaled and ingested causes of pulmonary fibrosis. *Toxicol. Pathol.*, 35, 86–96.

Lopez, A. (2007). Respiratory System. In *Pathologic Basis of Veterinary Medicine* (McGavin, M.D., and Zachary, J.F. eds), 4th edn, pp. 463–558. Mosby, Philadelphia, PA.

Renne, R.A., Gideon, K.M., Harbo, S.J., Staska, L.M., and Grumbein, S.L. (2007). Upper respiratory tract lesions in inhalation toxicology. *Toxicol. Pathol.*, 35, 163–169.

Roth, R.A. (ed.) (1997). Toxicology of the respiratory system. In *Comprehensive Toxicology* (Sipes, I., McQueen, C., Gandolfi, A.J. eds), Vol. 8, Pergamon Elsevier Science, Inc., New York, NY.

Schwartz, L.W., Hahn, F.F., Keenan, K.P., Keenan, C.M., Brown, H.R., and Mann, P.C. (1994). Proliferative lesions of the rat respiratory tract, R-1*Guides for Toxicologic Pathology*. STP/ARP/AFIP, Washington, DC.

Sells, D.M., Brix, A.E., Nyska, A., Jokinen, M.P., Orzech, D.P., and Walker, N.J. (2007). Respiratory tract lesions in noninhalation studies. *Toxicol. Pathol.*, 35, 170–177.

Van Vleet, J.F., and Ferrans, V.J. (2007). Cardiovascular system. In *Pathologic Basis of Veterinary Disease* (McGavin, M.D., and Zachary, J.F. eds), 4th edn, pp. 559–611. Mosby, Philadelphia, PA.

Wakamatsu, N., Devereux, T.R., Hong, H.L., and Sills, R.C. (2007). Overview of the molecular carcinogenesis of mouse lung tumor models of human lung cancer. *Toxicol. Pathol.*, 35, 75–80.

Witschi, R.R., Pinkerton, K.E., Van Winkle, L.S., and Last, J.A. (2008). Toxic responses of the respiratory system. In *Casarett and Doull's Toxicology* (Klaassen, C.D. ed.), 7th edn. McGraw-Hill, New York, NY.

Skin and Oral Mucosa

SECTION I SKIN

INTRODUCTION

Covering approximately 20 000 cm^2 in humans, the skin is one of the largest organs of mammals; thus it is often exposed to physical or chemical agents. This chapter provides an overview of the fundamental histopathological changes caused by toxins, points out similarities with lesions caused by other agents, and emphasizes the differences and peculiarities of the toxic reactions of skin. In addition, this chapter contains information on the pathophysiology of cutaneous toxic responses, and suggests several approaches to evaluate and test for toxic effects in the integument. Because of similar reaction patterns and the increasing importance of dental materials, relevant alterations of the oral mucosa are described in Section II of this chapter.

The information presented herein is general toxic dermatopathology, and the reader is encouraged to refer to more comprehensive treatises for detailed descriptions of the effects of specific chemical agents. To understand the fundamental histopathologic and physiopathologic cutaneous responses to toxicants, it is pivotal to first review the structure and differentiation patterns of normal skin.

STRUCTURE AND FUNCTION OF SKIN

Microscopic Anatomy

The skin consists of three main components: (1) the epidermis, a superficial lining of epithelial cells covering the body surface; (2) the dermis, a richly vascularized connective tissue situated beneath the epidermis; and (3) the cutaneous adnexa or appendages, a series of epithelial structures situated in the dermis that are connected to the epidermal surface (Figure 7.1).

The number, composition, and thickness of these three components are extremely variable, and it is impossible to describe a "normal" cutaneous structural pattern. Not only does the skin differ from species to species, but within each species there are strain variations, as well as numerous variations determined by different topographic and physiologic requirements. Additional variations can be caused by age, sex, hormonal status, and genetic constitution.

The epidermis is a stratified epithelium that is separated from the dermis by a thin basal lamina. The most superficial cells are continuously replaced by proliferation and upward migration of the deeper layers. This is accomplished by cell division of the basal cells; cuboidal or columnar cells, with proliferative capacity, can also migrate and differentiate into suprabasal cells that constitute the spinous layer. These cells are large polyhedral cells with numerous often prominent intercellular junctions known as desmosomes, and a large number of keratin bundles or tonofilaments. As these cells migrate closer to the surface they become flatter, lose many of their cytoplasmic organelles, and their nuclei become smaller and condensed. There are also irregular electron-dense keratohyalin granules in the cytoplasm; these granules contain a histidine-rich protein called filaggrin that plays an important role in aggregating and homogenizing keratin filaments. This characteristic begins to appear in the granular layer, and is clearly seen in the most superficial or horny layer. The horny layer consists of extremely flat cells that lack nuclei and have a very homogenous cytoplasm; these cells are the end stage of this migration and differentiation process (orthokeratinization).

In addition to keratinocytes, the epidermis contains several nonkeratinocytic or dendritic cells, primarily Langerhans cells (bone marrow-derived cells that act as antigen-presenting cells), Merkel cells (probably of neuroectodermal origin with neuroendocrine functions), and melanocytes (melanin-synthesizing cells of neural crest origin). As stated above, epidermal thickness can vary considerably according to species, location, age, and gender. In general, rodents and cats have a thin epidermis, only 2–3 cell layers thick, dogs and horses have a somewhat thicker epidermis, and pigs have the thickest of all. A general rule of thumb is that the more sparsely-haired a species is, the thicker its epidermis will be, in particular the horny keratin layer. Marine mammals such as whales have epidermis that is exceedingly thick, up to ten cell layers or more, with an even thicker modified keratin covering.

The dermis is a loose connective tissue compartment that is located between the epidermis and the subcutaneous adipose tissue. It contains the cutaneous adnexa and numerous nerves, as well as blood and lymphatic vessels. The superficial or papillary dermis lies immediately beneath the epidermis, and contains loose fibrous tissue within an abundant glycosaminoglycans ground substance, as well as a superficial vascular plexus. The deep or reticular dermis contains larger and more densely packed bundles of collagen intermingled with elastic fibers, which vary in number depending on species and location. In general, collagen makes up ~90%, elastin ~10%, and fine reticulin ~1% of the fibrous component of the dermis. A middle vascular plexus at the level of the sebaceous glands, and a deep vascular plexus at the dermal–subcutis junction provide blood supply to the skin. Besides fibroblasts, vascular and nerve-associated cell types, mast cells, histiocytes and lymphocytes are present in low numbers, typically near small blood vessels in the superficial vascular plexus.

The cutaneous adnexa consist of hair follicles, in addition to sweat and sebaceous glands. The hair follicles are downgrowths of the epidermis in which an ordered array of keratinized cells is gradually pushed upward in the form of hair shafts. These cells give rise to hair by a process of terminal differentiation, analogous to, but more complicated than, the process described for epidermal differentiation.

Two types of sweat glands, eccrine and apocrine, have been described in mammals. Birds lack these structures except for the uropygial gland, a modified sebaceous-type gland at the base of the tail. Eccrine glands participate in thermoregulation by secreting water and salts. Abundant throughout the skin in great apes and humans, in domestic and laboratory animals the eccrine sweat glands are limited to foot pads, nasal planum or flippers. These merocrine glands are composed of a long coiled secretory tubule

A

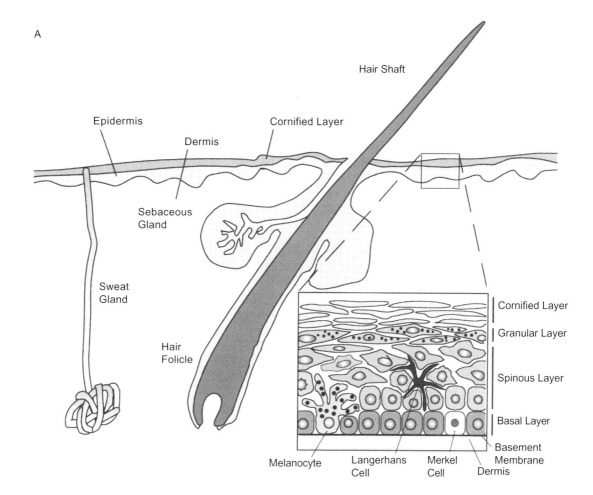

Hair Shaft

Epidermis

Cornified Layer

Dermis

Sebaceous
Gland

Sweat
Gland

Hair
Follicle

Cornified Layer

Granular Layer

Spinous Layer

Basal Layer

Basement
Membrane

Melanocyte

Langerhans
Cell

Merkel
Cell

Dermis

B

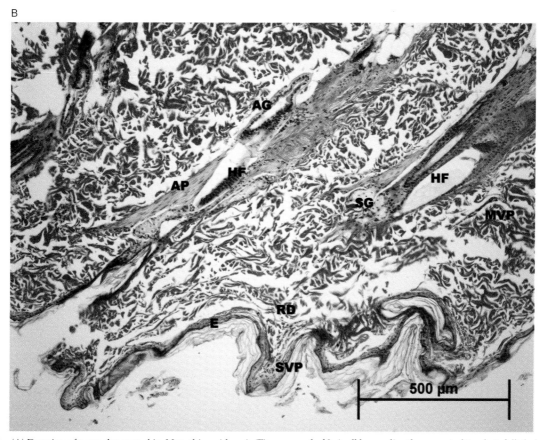

AG

HF

AP

HF

SG

MVP

RD

E

SVP

500 µm

FIGURE 7.1   (A) Drawing of normal mouse skin. Note thin epidermis (E) composed of 3–4 cell layers directly connected to a hair follicle (arrow head) that is situated in a moderately cellular dermis (D) rich in collagen fibers. (B) Normal skin from the ventrum of a beagle dog with highly folded epidermis (E), loose superficial "reticular" dermis (RD), superficial vascular plexus (SVP) immediately beneath the epidermis, hair follicles (HF), sebaceous glands (SG), and apocrine glands (AG) arising at mid-follicle level, and arrector pili (AP) muscle. The middle vascular plexus (MVP) is also evident.

and a connecting long excretory duct that ends in the epidermis separate from the hair follicle; the epithelium lining both is simple columnar. The apocrine glands, which generally empty into the hair follicle at the level of the sebaceous gland, secrete a proteinaceous material that originates from the loss of cytoplasmic pieces from the apices of the simple columnar glandular cells. Their function is not clear, but they are related to accessory scent glands that produce attractant odors during the mating season in some species. While distributed generally over the skin of most species, apocrine glands in humans are limited to armpits, groin, and nipples. Mammary glands are also modified apocrine glands, specialized to produce milk. Sebaceous glands develop from the neck or infundibulum of hair follicles, and are composed of large polyhedral lipid-laden cells that completely disintegrate after they are sloughed into the short duct to form the sebaceous secretion or sebum. Sebum is discharged into the infundibulum of the hair follicles, and spreads to the epidermal surface where it helps to keep the epidermal horny layer moist.

Skin Cell Subpopulations

Several discrete cell subpopulations have been described, especially in the epidermis. These include the group of nonepithelial cells mentioned previously, that is, Langerhans cells, Merkel cells, and melanocytes, as well as other less well-known cells that are indistinguishable from most of the basal or suprabasal keratinocytes by classical morphologic criteria. This group includes stem cells (variously characterized as slow-cycling cells, label-retaining cells, carcinogen-retaining cells, and dark keratinocytes), as well as a group of Ia-positive keratinocytes that are probably involved in immunological responses in the skin.

Langerhans cells (LCs) constitute one of the most numerous and important cell subpopulations of the epidermis. These "dendritic" cells of bone marrow origin constitute up to 2–8% of the epidermal cell population, and are usually located suprabasally. LCs have clear cytoplasm, long cytoplasmic processes, and unique paddle-shaped organelles, known as Birbeck's granules. LCs express class II molecules, as well as Fc and C3 receptors, and recognize, phagocytose and process foreign antigens to present to T-lymphocytes. They play a critical part in inducing contact hypersensitivity reactions following the epicutaneous application of antigens. In addition, LCs may play an important role in immunosurveillance against viral infection and neoplastic development in the skin.

Merkel cells constitute a small subpopulation of cells with distinctive neuroendocrine granules in the cytoplasm. Although they have been found in all layers of the epidermis and in the dermis, they do not seem to play an active role in reactive processes.

Melanocytes are DOPA-positive clear cells that appear in variable numbers and contain variable amounts of melanin depending on age, location, and race. They are most commonly found in the basal layer of the epidermis and hair follicles. Melanocytes may be involved in reactive pathologic processes, especially in the later phases of resolution or during protracted application of physical or chemical agents, resulting in areas of hyperpigmentation. Some chemicals are known for the opposite effect, hypopigmentation. This group includes compounds that are chemically related to the melanin precursors, tyrosine and dihydroxyphenylalanine (DOPA), such as hydroquinone, p-tertiary butylphenol, and p-tertiary butylcatechol. Most of these chemicals inhibit melanin production, or even destroy melanocytes.

The most important group of keratinocytes are those that reside in the basal layer, basal keratinocytes. These cells maintain the population of the epidermis by cell division, and contain the epidermal stem cells. Stem cells are the ultimate units of replacement for tissues that, like the epidermis, undergo continual renewal throughout adult life. Epidermal stem cells are a relatively small fraction of the proliferating cells. They cycle slowly to renew the stem cell population, and to produce the (amplifying) cells committed to terminal differentiation. The importance of the stem cell concept is that only a small fraction of the dividing cells may be capable of continuous renewal; the others, although able to undertake a limited number of divisions, are committed to terminal differentiation.

An interesting feature of at least one group of slow-cycling basal cells is their ability to retain electrophiles that bind to DNA; thus they have been termed carcinogen-retaining cells. These cells may play a role in the initiation phase of chemical carcinogenesis. Another group of basal keratinocytes, morphologically distinguishable by their hyperbasophilic cytoplasm and condensed nuclear chromatin, have been described in hyperplastic epithelia, and especially in phorbol-ester-treated epidermis. These cells, known as dark basal keratinocytes, or simply dark cells, seem to be associated with epidermal hyperplasia and preneoplasia.

Physiology and Biochemistry

Homeostatic Mechanisms

Of particular importance are the mechanisms that control epidermal growth and differentiation, so that a steady state in epidermal thickness is maintained. Adenyl cyclase and cyclic nucleotide phosphodiesterase are active in the epidermis, and incremental increases in the cellular levels of cyclic AMP (cAMP) inhibit proliferation of keratinocytes. In the epidermis, cAMP levels appear to be regulated by autocrine factors (chalones), produced by epidermal cells themselves, β-adrenergic receptors, prostaglandins and histamine, and cAMP may play a role in proliferative diseases like psoriasis and in tumor promotion. However, a more complex picture of epidermal regulation has evolved in the last few years. In addition to the cAMP-dependent protein kinase, it had been shown that protein kinase C (PKC) is also important in epidermal homeostasis. PKC is physiologically activated by diacylglycerol released from the cell membrane along with inositol phosphate by phospholipase C. Inositol phosphate regulates intracellular calcium, another possible signal in epidermal regulation. In tissue cultures, low levels of calcium (0–0.05 nM) in the medium maintain epidermal cells in a proliferative state, whereas higher calcium concentrations induce terminal differentiation. Calcium also is required for activation of PKC. In addition, PKC is activated by phorbol esters and is believed to play a central role in tumor promotion. Many other mechanisms have also been implicated in epidermal regulation. For example, transforming growth factor beta (TGF-β) appears to be an important negative growth factor. Growth factors, including epidermal growth factor (EGF) and related ligands for the EGF receptor, fibroblast growth factor and insulin-like growth factor appear to be responsible for the hyperproliferative response in chronic inflammatory conditions, and in other hyperproliferative diseases. Recently, there has been mounting evidence indicating a direct role for lymphokines in epidermal growth regulation.

It has become clear however, that homeostasis of the epidermis is not controlled only by regulating proliferation, but also by the rate of terminal differentiation. Research with transgenic mouse models has shown, for example, that overexpression of growth factors leads to hyperproliferation and subsequent hyperplasia of the epidermis, while overexpression of cell cycle regulatory genes produces hyperproliferation without hyperplasia, suggesting a compensatory rate of terminal differentiation as well. It would appear, then, that a delicate balance between proliferation and terminal differentiation may control epidermal thickness.

The role of apoptosis in the epidermis has only been recognized recently. Because terminal differentiation is typically the major regulatory mechanism of cell elimination, the frequency of apoptosis is relatively low in normal epidermis. More important than its potential role in regulating epidermal thickness may be the role of apoptosis in elimination of genetically-damaged cells. By eliminating cells that can no longer successfully repair their damaged DNA, apoptosis appears to

have a significant role in the prevention of cancer. An example of this role is the high rate of apoptosis in epidermal cells that have been exposed to UV radiation. In this particular case, apoptosis is a p53-mediated phenomenon that also involves the FAS/Fas-L complex.

Structural Components

The skin has a dual barrier role, the first to protect against exogenous insult, and the second to prevent water loss, both facilitated by its unique structural characteristics. The cytoskeleton of the epidermal keratinocytes has complex networks of proteins that include microtubules, actin filaments, and intermediate filaments. Keratin belongs to the family of intermediate filaments. Synthesis of keratin in any of its forms is an almost exclusive characteristic of epithelial cells. Keratin filaments in the stratum corneum have high glycine, glutamic acid, and serine concentrations, and they are cross-linked via disulfide linkages to form insoluble fibers during the process of differentiation. In a typical keratin fiber, a smaller acidic type I fiber is linked to a larger neutral or basic type II fiber.

Pathologic conditions of skin, such as psoriasis or preneoplasia, may alter the pattern of distribution of keratin filaments. In experimental models, loss of high molecular weight keratins in epidermal cells is a marker of premalignancy. Another characteristic type of protein in keratinocytes is flaggrin, a protein that facilitates aggregation of keratin filaments into large macrofibrils. Its histidine-rich, highly-phosphorylated precursor, proflaggrin, is a major component of keratohyalin granules that appear in differentiating keratinocytes. An important structural component of differentiated keratinocytes is the cell envelope, or marginal band, which develops adjacent to the cell membrane. The envelope is an alkali-resistant protective structure composed of three precursors—involucrin, keratolinin, and a sulfur-rich protein.

The epidermis is separated from the adjacent dermis by a complex structure known as the basement membrane. The basic scaffold of membrane is a mesh of type IV collagen and laminin. Associated with this core structure are several glycoproteins, such as entactin, fibline, and perlecan. Not only does the basement membrane provide anchorage to the epidermal cells, but it also regulates epidermal homeostasis, and modulates exchange of factors between the vascular dermis and the avascular epidermis.

Skin has a rich lipid content; one of the highest in the body. Not only are lipids used as sources of energy, but they also serve barrier functions, as growth regulators, and as structural components. Surface lipids are a mixture of epidermal and sebaceous components. Epidermal components include ceramide and linoleic acid, which are integral components of the water barrier, as well as cholesterol and cholesterol esters. Components derived mainly from sebum include squalene and wax esters. Triglycerides and free fatty acids appear to come from both sources. The exact roles of all these constituents in protection is controversial.

At the dermal level, the major protein is collagen, a glycine and proline-rich helical protein making up approximately 90% of dermal collagen. In contrast to the basement membrane, 80–85% of dermal collagen is type I, with the remaining being the less dense, finer, "reticular" type III collagen. Collagen is constantly undergoing renewal, being degraded and resynthesized by fibroblasts.

Percutaneous Absorption

Topically-applied substances penetrate the skin by percutaneous absorption, a passive diffusion process in which the stratum corneum plays a barrier role. This barrier is the result of the cell envelope in terminally-differentiated keratinocytes and intercellular spaces filled with lipid bilayers. The stratum corneum consists of approximately 40% protein and 40% water; the rest is mainly lipid. Therefore, lipophilic substances, such as organic solvents and organophosphorus insecticides (e.g., parathion and malathion), penetrate readily into the skin. Several other factors affect percutaneous absorption. The ionization state of the penetrant affects the rate of diffusion; electrolytes in aqueous solution have poor penetrability, and the ionization of a weak electrolyte notably reduces its permeability (e.g., salicylic acid as opposed to sodium salicylate). Ions such as Na^+, K^+, Al^{+3}, and Br^- penetrate very slowly. Simple polar substances appear to penetrate the stratum corneum at approximately the same rate as water. The addition of methylene groups on a simple polar nonelectrolyte increases the lipid solubility of the molecule. The molecular size of the penetrant, up to a certain extent, appears to influence the absorption rate. Molecules of smaller weight penetrate more rapidly, although the chemical characteristics should also be considered.

The physicochemical properties of the vehicle are also very important in influencing the rate of percutaneous absorption, since they will regulate the vehicle/stratum corneum partition coefficient. Hydration of the stratum corneum increases the permeability of both water- and lipid-soluble compounds; thus occlusive dressings of materials such as polyethylene are used in the transdermal delivery of drugs (e.g., corticosteroids). Skin occlusion raises the local temperature, which is another important factor that enhances

permeability. Other substances that increase permeability may damage the skin. These include organic solvents, such as methanol, acetone, hexane, and ether. They produce delipidization of the skin, generating interstices that transform the tissue so it behaves like a nonselective porous membrane. The stratum corneum is also damaged by anionic and cationic surfactants (soaps, detergents), even at low concentrations. Surfactants are used in cosmetics and with drugs to increase permeability; apparently they change the protein matrix of the stratum corneum.

Regional variations in permeability at different body locations will affect absorption. This is dependent on differences in the thickness of the stratum corneum; for instance, scrotal skin, which has one of the thinnest strata cornea, is very permeable. Physical integrity of the horny layer is also very important, since in most skin diseases the barrier function is notably diminished (e.g., psoriatic skin).

In some cases, the skin may serve as a storage place for toxicants. Reservoir capabilities of normal epidermis, with deposition in, and later release from, the stratum corneum, have been demonstrated (e.g., with some steroids). Certain substances, mainly ionic, may bind or form complexes with collagen in the dermis, thus remaining there for long periods of time with the potential to exert their toxicologic properties (e.g., chromium and ferric ions).

Other pathways for penetration of chemicals into the skin are the pilosebaceous appendages and the sweat glands. Although these pathways are minor in humans, in many land mammals these routes may assume greater importance, due to the greater numbers and density of pilosebaceous units.

When substances reach the living layers of the epidermis, they are exposed to the metabolic machinery of epidermal cells, which can inactivate or activate certain chemicals. Metabolic viability is a major factor affecting the *in vitro* permeation of certain chemicals (e.g., benzo[*a*]pyrene). Once chemicals have passed through the epidermis, which is an avascular tissue, they enter the dermis and are cleared by blood and lymphatic vessels. Under physiological conditions, dermal blood flow is not a rate-limiting factor for percutaneous absorption.

Frequent reference to the skin as the most effective natural barrier isolating the individual from the environment erroneously suggests a purely mechanical role played by a metabolically inert tissue. Actually, the epidermis should be viewed as a tissue in steady state growth that is very active metabolically in order to sustain itself and to regulate the body's interrelation with the environment. Extensive injury of the skin will affect the general homeostasis of the body (e.g., extensive burns). The opposite is also true, since general metabolic diseases (e.g., diabetes) will affect skin responses to injury.

Phase I and Phase II Metabolism

The presence of enzymes involved in the metabolism of steroid hormones, such as androgens, estrogens, progesterone, and glucocorticoids, has been shown in the skin. For example, testosterone is a glucocorticoid derivative that is metabolized to more potent forms in the skin via cytochrome P450-mediated 5α hydroxylation. Testosterone and its derivatives are responsible for stimulating sebum secretion and modulating hair growth. Estrogens and progesterone are also metabolized in the skin. Related to this, the skin is an important organ in the synthesis of vitamin D. In the spinous layer of the epidermis, UV light photolyzes provitamin D3 (7-dehydrocholesterol) to previtamin D3; this in turn can be isomerized to form vitamin D3 (cholecalciferol), which enters the circulation for further metabolism by liver and kidney into active Vitamin D. Epidermal cells have receptors for 1,25-dihydroxy vitamin D3, which may regulate epidermal differentiation.

The presence and induction of a variety of cytochrome P450 enzymes, as well as other oxygen and NADP(H) dependent oxidases, the mixed function oxidase (MFOs), have been demonstrated in skin. These enzymes play a fundamental role in the oxidative metabolism of endogenous substances such as steroids, prostaglandins, fatty acids, and leukotrienes, but may also play a more sinister role when they come in contact with and metabolize xenobiotics. Cutaneous cytochrome P450 enzymes play a critical role in the metabolism of certain xenobiotics; in most cases this metabolism results in detoxification. There are situations, however, where relatively innocuous, but highly lipid-soluble xenobiotics are "activated" (e.g., benzo[a]pyrene, or B[a]P), a member of the polyaromatic hydrocarbon (PAH) family of xenobiotics associated with overcooking food, or with burning of carbonaceous material in general. B[a]P, like most PAH can be metabolized by the P450-dependent aryl hydrocarbon hydroxylase (AHH) system, resulting in a variety of mostly nontoxic metabolites. There is, however, at least one "active" metabolite, a particular diol epoxide that is very reactive, and capable of binding to nucleic acids and proteins. The epoxide spontaneously forms covalent bonds with DNA bases to produce bulky adducts which ultimately produce mutations when the affected DNA segment is replicated. Adduct formation is believed to be the first step of cancer induction by this type of compound. Metabolic activation of other members of the PAH

family also occurs. For example, several oxygenated reactive metabolites of 3-methylcholanthrene and benz[a]anthracene are active carcinogens in the mouse skin bioassay. Therefore, phase I metabolism by skin may not be very efficient or may even have a counterproductive effect, transforming relatively weak carcinogens into strong carcinogens and mutagens.

Another "phase I" enzyme often expressed along with the P450s, epoxide hydrolase, is also active in animal and human skin. This enzyme converts epoxides that are often generated by P450s to dihydrodiol metabolites which, in turn, are further metabolized by AHH into the highly-reactive diol epoxides.

Phase II enzyme reactions, which involve conjugating enzyme systems, such as the glucuronosyl transferases, sulfotransferases, and glutathione S-transferases, also occur in skin and constitute an additional detoxification pathway for the reactive epoxide intermediates. Conjugation with endogenous substrates, such as glucuronic acid, sulfate, and glutathione results in the formation of water-soluble metabolites that are readily eliminated from the cells.

COMPARATIVE MECHANISMS OF CUTANEOUS TOXICITY

Because of its location, the skin acts as the main barrier against environmental toxicants. Consequently the skin, and particularly the epidermis, is frequently exposed to a wide variety of toxic agents that may act not only systemically, but also directly. There are essentially three main mechanisms of toxicity of skin: (1) direct damage produced by the toxic agent or its metabolites, for example, irritation (with or without cell death) and genotoxicity; (2) immune-mediated toxic effects; and (3) phototoxic and photoallergic effects. Table 7.1 summarizes the mechanisms of skin and oral toxicity and some of the xenobiotics that exert their effects by those mechanisms.

Direct Damage

Chemical Burns

A direct toxic action on skin can be produced by many chemical agents, environmental pollutants, occupational biohazards, and even by common cosmetic and therapeutic agents. The most extreme cases of direct toxicity are probably chemical burns produced by accidental exposure to strong acids, alkali agents, or oxidizing agents. These agents, in particular acids, coagulate cellular and intercellular proteins in the

TABLE 7.1 Mechanisms of toxicity to the skin and oral mucosa with selected examples

Mechanism	Xenobiotic
Skin	
Direct toxicity	
• Chemical "burns" (necrosis)	Strong acids, caustic (alkali) agent, or oxidizing agents
• Irritation—inflammation	Acids, alkali agents, oxidizing/reducing agents, organic solvents, keratolytic agents, *Vicia*
• Direct activation of immune effectors	Polymixin B, DMSO, aspirin, phorbol esters, biogenic amines from jellyfish and nettles
• Genotoxic agents (necrosis, hyperplasia, carcinogenesis)	UV light, ionizing radiation, inorganic arsenic, sulfur mustard, T-2 toxin, toxic organic agents or their metabolites—e.g., polyaromatic hydrocarbons, polyhalogenated hydrocarbons
Immunomediated toxicity	
• IgE-dependent reactions	Foods (urticaria), therapeutic agents (penicillin)
• Immunocomplex-mediated reactions	Penicillin, aminosalicylic acid, streptomycin
• T-lymphocyte-mediated reactions (delayed skin hypersensitivity)	Ethyl aminobenzoate, neomycin, plant toxins (poison ivy), metal (nickel and chromium), and metal derivatives (oligomercurial)
Phototoxicity/photoallergy	
• Primary phototoxicity—UV-mediated activation of compounds to produce specific photowavelengths causing skin damage (primary)	Xenobiotics—tetracyclines, sulfonamides, chlorpromazine, nalidixic acid, acridine, anthracene, phenanthrenes Plant compounds—furocoumarins (*Trifolium, Cymopterus, Ammi*), fagopyrin (*Fagopyrum*), Hypericin (*Hypericum*)
• Secondary phototoxicity due to hepatotoxicity with impairment of biliary excretion (mainly ruminants)	[Mediated by phylloerythrin] Hepatotoxic plants—e.g., *Kochia* (oxalates), *Crotalaria/Senecio/Amsinckia* (pyrolizidines), *Agave, Nolina, Panicum, Tribulus, Brassica*, alfalfa Mycotoxins—e.g., sporodesmin from *Pythium*, xenobiotics—hexachlorobenzene, lead
• Photoallergy—induce a conversion of hapten to antigen through linkage to proteins	Sulfonamides, phenothiazides, coumarin derivatives, glyceryl *p*-aminobenzoic acid, plant products (ragweed)
Adnexal damage	
• Interference with rapid growth phase of the hair follicle (anagen)	Doxorubicin, vincristine, methotrexate, cyclophosphamide, phenylglycidyl ether, dixyrazine, colchicine
• Interference with stationary phase of the hair follicle (telogen)	Mimosine (*Mimosa*), thallium, selenium, inorganic arsenic, inorganic mercury, selenium, iodine, chlorinated naphthalenes, propanolol, triparanol, anticoagulants (heparin, coumarin), oral contraceptives, selenium, phenylglycidyl ether, dixyrazine
• Acneiform lesions (hyperkeratinization and comedone formation)	Polyhalogenated hydrocarbons (e.g., dioxins)
• Anhidrosis (damage/loss of sweat glands)	Arsenic, thallium, lead, fluorine, cytarabine, bleomycin, formaldehyde
Oral mucosa	
• Interference with epithelial cell proliferation	Cytostatic drugs (e.g., methotrexate)
• Interference with immune defense mechanisms, allowing for increased secondary infections	Immunosuppressive drugs (e.g., azathioprine)
• Induce allergic reaction, including anaphylactic shock	Penicillin, sulfa drugs, antimalarial drugs, penicillamine

epidermis (and dermis if severe enough) (Figure 7.2). The coagulated necrotic tissue can form a barrier (eschar) that inhibits further penetration and damage by the acidic chemical. Alkali agents, on the other hand, saponify lipids and denature proteins, producing liquefactive necrosis, thus allowing for deeper penetration of the damaging hydroxyl ions, as well as greater extent and duration of damage. In general, the greater the degree of tissue destruction, and the greater the depth of the injury, the greater will be the secondary inflammatory reaction, in part due to the increased likelihood of bacterial or fungal colonization of the devitalized or ulcerated tissue (Figure 7.3).

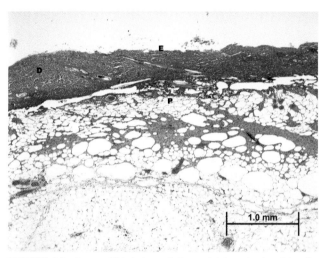

FIGURE 7.2 Severe (third degree) thermal injury in the skin of a dog, with full thickness necrosis of epidermis (E), dermis (D) and superficial panniculus (P).

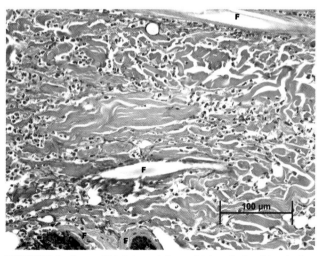

FIGURE 7.3 Severe (third degree) thermal injury in the skin of a dog illustrating the secondary suppurative inflammatory response in the dermis. Necrotic hair follicles (F) can be observed in the affected tissue.

Irritation

Skin irritation occurs more frequently than chemical burns. Among domestic animals, dermatitis due to irritation is most common in horses and dogs, generally involving glabrous skin surfaces such as the ventrum and perineal areas, where a protective hair coat that would otherwise impair contact is sparse, and the epidermis is thinner. Irritation is defined as an inflammatory process of the skin (dermatitis) that is not mediated by the immune system. Irritation can be the result of acute or chronic exposure to a large number of unrelated compounds, including acids, alkali agents, organic solvents, keratolytic agents, and oxidizing and reducing agents. Since a good correlation between chemical structure and the capacity for skin irritation has not been established, the toxicity of specific chemical compounds on skin often has to be empirically demonstrated, rather than assumed based on structure. In many cases the cellular and molecular bases of irritation remain to be determined. In most cases, however, some degree of direct damage to the epidermis is evident, which helps to distinguish contact irritant dermatitis from allergic contact dermatitis.

One possible mechanism of skin irritation is the so-called nonimmunological activation of effector pathways. This type of reaction mimics an allergic reaction to drugs or chemicals, and is produced by direct interaction of the toxic compound with immune system effectors without intervention of an antigen–antibody reaction. At least three different levels of interaction with immunoeffectors have been recognized:

1. Interaction with mast cells to release histamine, serotonin, leukotrienes, and other mediators of inflammation. This effect is produced by polymixin B, dimethyl sulfoxide, and biogenic polymers that are released by plants such as nettles, and animals such as caterpillars and jellyfish.
2. Activation of complement in the absence of antibody (i.e., via the alternate pathway). This occurs with radiocontrast media.
3. Alteration of arachidonic acid metabolism to increase prostaglandin synthesis. This occurs with aspirin, nonsteroidal anti-inflammatory agents, and phorbol esters.

Skin toxicity also results from drugs or chemicals that produce metabolic changes, such as ulceration induced by alterations in folate metabolism, or from ecological disturbance of microorganisms in the skin and mucosa, such as mycosis resulting from the use of antibiotics. Drugs which interfere with mitosis (e.g., cyclophosphamide and vincristine in humans, doxorubicin in dogs) can alter the hair development cycle, often stopping it, and leading to alopecia.

Genotoxic Agents

Since the epidermis is a tissue with high cell turnover, toxicant alteration of, or interaction with, DNA should be considered another fundamental mechanism in dermatotoxicology. The long-term or protracted effects of genotoxic agents are the induction of premalignant lesions and cancer, discussed subsequently.

The initial damage caused by genotoxic agents occurs in the basal layer of the epidermis, where the toxic agent can interact with DNA by a variety of mechanisms, such as alkylation, DNA breaks, chromosomal breaks, and adduct formation. This results in an increased rate of mutation. At lower doses, the only obvious effect may be the induction of neoplasia. At higher doses, the probability of lethal mutation increases, and a regenerative hyperplasia is observed when surviving cells attempt to replace the cells lost by death because of damage by the carcinogen/mutagen. In extreme cases, the action of the mutagen impairs the cell renewal process itself; this results in skin ulceration, since replacement of cells lost to differentiation, as well as damaged cells, is not possible. This mechanism of toxicity is thought to be the cause of the necrotizing lesions associated with sulfur mustard ("mustard gas"), which selectively targets basal cells, causing extensive alkylation of DNA to the point of cell death, leading to necrosis and vesiculation of the epidermis (Figure 7.4).

Immunomediated Cutaneous Toxicity

A common mechanism of toxic skin injury is that mediated by the immune system. In all cases in which skin reactions are mediated by immune-related mechanisms, the immune system of the individual has had previous contact with the same or a related chemical. The capacity of a chemical to elicit an immune response depends largely on the structure of the molecule, as well as factors such as route of administration, vehicle, and host factors (age, sex, individual susceptibility). Although most chemicals can activate the immune system, only macromolecules are complete antigens. Small molecules can be incomplete antigens or haptens that act as antigens after they have been bound to larger molecules (mainly proteins). In skin the proteins most frequently bound are the keratins, although intercellular proteins in some cases can also serve as binding sites for haptenic chemicals.

There are two distinct immune responses, depending on whether the reaction is mediated by humoral antibodies or by effector T-cells. The first case includes two immunotoxic mechanisms: skin anaphylactic reactions mediated by IgE antibodies (type I hypersensitivity reaction); and immunocomplex reactions mediated by IgG or IgM antibodies and complement (type III hypersensitivity reaction). These humoral reactions generally occur when antigens are introduced into the body through the gastrointestinal tract, via the respiratory tract by inhalation, or via the bloodstream by injection, but generally not by direct contact with the skin. The second type of response, mediated by effector T-cells, results in cell-mediated immunotoxic reactions, known as delayed-type sensitivity reactions (type IV hypersensitivity reaction). The cytotoxic hypersensitivity reaction (type II), the basis for some autoimmune diseases, has not been demonstrated in immunotoxicologic reactions of the skin.

IgE-dependent Reactions

The anaphylactic, also called atopic or type I, reaction is mediated by IgE antibodies, which in predisposed individuals are synthesized rather than IgM or IgG by B-lymphocytes after an antigen activates the appropriate T-cell. After re-exposure to the antigen, an interaction of the antigen and IgE, now on the surface of mast cells and basophilic leukocytes, results in degranulation of these cells, with release of histamine, leukotrienes, serotonin, and other mediators of acute inflammation. The response is primarily vascular in nature, with vasodilation (leading to erythema), increased vascular permeability, and ultimately edema. This type of reaction is generally the cutaneous expression of a systemic allergic reaction, and is most often caused by foods (especially in humans and dogs, less commonly so in cats and horses), inhaled allergens, or injected therapeutic agents (e.g., penicillin, tetracycline, Vitamin K, and vaccines).

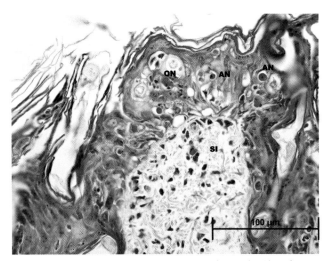

FIGURE 7.4 Direct cytotoxicity due to chemicals. Skin from a guinea pig exposed to mustard gas, illustrating the oncotic necrosis (ON) and apoptotic necrosis (AN) of the epidermal cells, as well as the secondary inflammation (SI) and edema in the underlying superficial dermis.

Immunocomplex-mediated Reactions

The type III reaction, also known as the Arthus reaction in the skin, is another member of the group of antibody-mediated hypersensitivity reactions. The immunoglobulins involved in this reaction are complement-fixing IgG or IgM. This reaction is initiated when antigen and antibodies form precipitating complexes in the bloodstream that subsequently get trapped in blood vessel walls; in some cases the immunoglobulins escape into tissues to form microprecipitates there. These antigen–antibody complexes trigger the activation of complement, with the release of chemotactic and vasoactive fragments. Since the immune complexes are usually trapped in or near small blood vessels, a vasculitis with secondary effects such as edema, purpura, thrombosis, and infarction with ulceration is the underlying mechanism of tissue damage. An Arthus reaction can be produced by a large variety of antigens, most often drugs such as penicillin, aminosalicylic acid, and streptomycin.

Delayed Skin Hypersensitivity

Type IV hypersensitivity is the main and almost exclusive mechanism of allergic contact dermatitis, the most common drug-associated immunologic condition in both humans and domestic animals, with dogs, then horses, being most often affected. The cutaneous reaction is mediated by sensitized T-lymphocytes (Figure 7.5). The antigens are small molecules (haptens) that are usually liposoluble, allowing better epidermal penetration. The haptens typically bind covalently to a "carrier" protein, which is in turn bound to the surfaces of Langerhans cells. These cells process the antigen, and present the modified antigen to the T-lymphocyte. T-lymphocytes migrate to the paracortical area of the lymph nodes, where they proliferate and form effector T-lymphocytes and memory cells.

After re-exposure (or persistence) of the antigen, effector lymphocytes become activated and secrete substances called lymphokines that mediate the inflammatory response. Typically a mixture of cytotoxic T-cells and macrophages infiltrate into the affected area, starting with the perivascular areas. The reaction is often long-standing, and chronic changes such as epidermal acanthosis and hyperkeratosis, as well as dermal fibrosis, are common.

There is an extremely long list of substances that have been documented to produce delayed hypersensitivity. The most common in domestic animals include flea collars, poison ivy/oak/sumac, rubber products, dichromates (in cement), and nickel compounds. Also implicated are therapeutic agents such as ethyl aminobenzoate and neomycin, various dyes and preservatives.

Erythema Multiforme/Toxic Epidermal Necrolysis

Erythema multiforme (EM) and toxic epidermal necrolysis (TEN) represent a spectrum of relatively rare immune-mediated diseases commonly associated with, but not limited to, adverse drug reactions. Once thought to be manifestations of type III hypersensitivity, these reactions have been linked to the inappropriate activation of cytotoxic (CD8+) T-cells against keratinocyte components in the epidermis. Haptens bound to these keratinocyte components have been demonstrated in many cases. Binding of cytotoxic T-cells to the offending keratinocytes results in apoptosis with mild erythema, superficial vesiculation (blistering) of the epidermis, and lymphocytic migration into the epidermis (exocytosis) and along the epidermal-dermal junction (interface dermatitis) in EM. In severe cases, reflective of TEN, there is full thickness necrosis of large areas of epidermis (Figure 7.6A). Unlike EM, the leukocyte response in TEN is minimal to absent (Figure 7.6B). Excessive production and release of cytokines, such as tumor necrosis factor-α and interleukin-6, have been implicated in TEN. Due to the large areas of skin affected, its fulminating nature and the full thickness necrosis of the epidermis, TEN is often life-threatening.

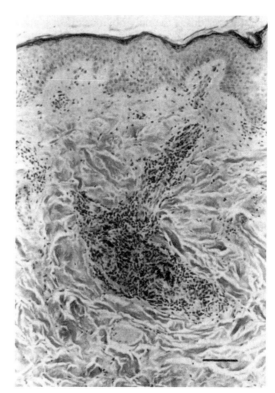

FIGURE 7.5 Delayed hypersensitivity reaction in human skin, characterized by a dense mononuclear perivascular infiltrate in the dermis. Bar = 100 μm.

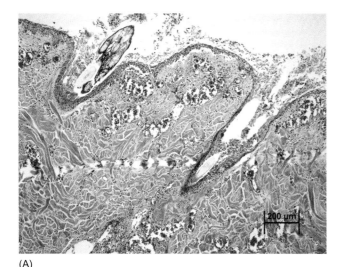

(A)

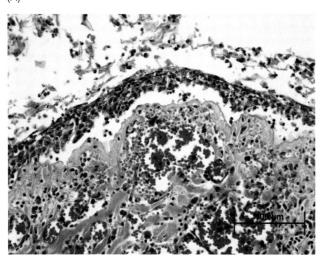

(B)

FIGURE 7.6 Toxic epidermal necrolysis in a cat secondary to flea dip. (A) Low magnification showing the extent of epidermal sloughing. (B) High magnification showing full thickness sloughing of epidermis and sparse leukocytic response despite the florid vascular response.

EM and TEN are most often reported in humans, dogs, cats, horses, and monkeys. Most often implicated are sulfonamides, penicillins, and cephalosporins, but EM after exposure to ivermectin, aurothioglucose, griseofulvin, propylthiouracil, and TEN after exposure to levamisole and D-limonene-based flea dips, have also been reported; in humans, anticonvulsive drugs and nonsteroidal anti-inflammatory drugs have also been implicated. Less frequently, dyes and preservatives have been linked to these conditions.

Phototoxicity and Photoallergy

Ingestion, injection, or contact with certain chemicals may produce hypersensitivity to light (usually UV light). Two main forms of light-associated toxicity are phototoxicity and photoallergy. Phototoxicity is a

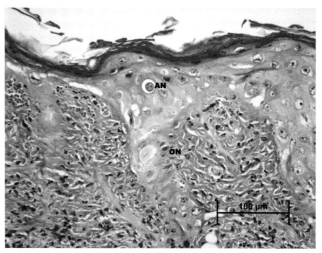

FIGURE 7.7 Primary photosensitization in the skin of a mouse exposed to the phytochemical psoralens and then exposed to UV light. Apopotic necrosis (AN) and oncotic necrosis (ON) are present in the epidermis, and there is a secondary suppurative response in the underlying superficial dermis.

direct immediate reaction involving interaction of incident light of a particular wavelength passing through the skin, resulting in either release of free electrons or an enhanced excitement state for electrons in the photosensitizing compound. As the electrons return to a less excited state, they release energy which can cleave certain molecules to produce free radicals. This release of energy, or collision with free electrons themselves, often leads to the generation of highly-reactive singlet oxygen, although other free radicals, especially from unsaturated membrane lipids, can be generated. The free radicals in turn interact with and damage proteins, membrane lipids (especially unsaturated ones), and nucleic acids via chain reactions that produce more tissue free radicals, ultimately leading to cell injury and death. The tissue damage in most cases resembles exaggerated sunburn (Figure 7.7). The molecular mechanisms of this type of reaction are complex, and not completely understood. The wavelength of the light inducing this type of reaction is variable and depends on the absorption spectra of the photosensitizer.

Many compounds have been shown to induce phototoxicity in humans—the list is very long; these include widely-used therapeutic agents such as phenothiazine, tetracyclines, sulfonamides, chlorpromazine, and nalidixic acid. Other compounds that induce phototoxicity are acridine, anthracene, phenanthrenes, and linear fluorocoumarins (also known as psoralens). The photosensitizing properties of the fluorocoumarins (mainly 8-methoxypsoralen) have been used for therapeutic purposes in the treatment of psoriasis with UV light.

Phototoxicity in domestic animals is much less common, not only because fewer photosensitizing drugs are used, but also because the heavy hair coats and generally more heavily-pigmented skin of these species limits the areas of potential damage to sparsely haired, less pigmented regions such as conjunctiva, ventrum, perineum, nares, teats, and ear tips. Grazing animals, however, can ingest photosensitizing compounds while feeding. Plants such as buckwheat (*Fagopyrum*) and St. John's wort (*Hypericum*) contain photoactive red helianthrone pigments, while spring parsley (*Cymopterus*), bishop's weed (*Ammi*) and Dutchman's breeches (*Thamnosma*) contain furocoumarins. Horses, cattle, sheep, and pigs have all suffered photosensitization after ingestion of these plants. Other plants such as rape (Brassica), alfalfa and alsike clover have been implicated in photosensitization cases.

Phototoxicity can also be caused by endogenous compounds, as in cases of porphyria. This group of disorders results from a disturbance in the metabolism of porphyrins, with accumulation of photoactive byproducts in the plasma and tissues. There are several forms of porphyria, some of which are hereditary, while others are related to hepatotoxicity or exposure to agents such as polychlorinated compounds (e.g., hexachlorobenzene), lead, or alcohol in predisposed individuals. In all cases, the skin lesions appear to be due to absorption of visible light by the porphyrin molecules, with subsequent generation of free radicals.

A third mechanism of photosensitization is associated with liver damage. In ruminants, the photoactive compound phylloerythin is formed from chlorophyll by anaerobic bacteria in the rumen. Phylloerythrin is readily absorbed into the bloodstream, but also readily excreted by the liver into the bile. Even moderate liver damage, however, especially if the biliary system is involved, leads to phylloerythrin deposition in other organs, including the skin. This triggers a photosensitization reaction with erythema, edema, exudation, and eventual necrosis of sparsely haired non-pigmented sun-exposed areas. Sporodesmin, a mycotoxin produced by *Pithomyces chartarum*, is a significant cause of photosensitization in sheep and also cattle in the southern hemisphere. As with most hepatogenous photosensitizers, sporodesmin produces damage and inflammation centered round the biliary tract, interfering with excretion of phylloerythrin. A wide variety of toxic range plants, for example, *Kochia* (fireweed), *Tribulus* (puncture vine), and *Panicum* (panic grasses), produce secondary photosensitization in grazing animals such as sheep (Figure 7.8).

Photoallergy, on the other hand, is simply a special form of delayed hypersensitivity. Although the mechanisms are not completely understood, light

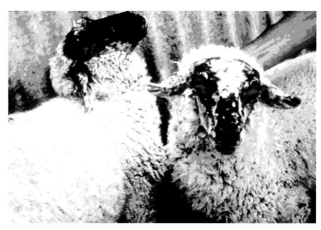

FIGURE 7.8 Secondary (hepatogenous) phototoxicity in two sheep attributed to ingestion of panic grass (*Panicum*). The sheep have encrusted ears and nasal plana with swollen red conjunctivae (image courtesy of Dr John King).

appears to modify or convert the hapten to a complete antigen, by covalently linking the hapten to cellular proteins in the epidermis. Unlike photosensitization, where the response is "immediate," the onset of photoallergy is delayed, generally taking 48 hours to become manifest. Examples of compounds inducing photoallergy are sulfonamide, phenothiazides, coumarin derivatives, glyceryl *p*-aminobenzoic acid, and plant products (e.g., ragweed).

RESPONSE OF SKIN TO INJURY

Fundamental Non-neoplastic Lesions

The cutaneous alterations induced by toxicants do not differ, in general terms, from changes caused by physical or biological agents. Since the skin is formed by various structures, the extent and degree of involvement of each component will depend on the agent itself, and on the severity of the exposure. This, in turn, depends on factors such as dose, concentration, pH, length of exposure, number of exposures, and time between exposures. Although some skin components can be spared (they rarely remain unexposed and intact), the epidermis is obviously always exposed to externally-applied toxicants. For this reason, many of the fundamental lesions are epidermal, and most studies have focused on the epidermis. For practical purposes, we will discuss fundamental cutaneous lesions according to skin component. For comparative purposes, Table 7.2 provides a partial listing of toxicants reported to cause skin lesions in common domestic animals.

TABLE 7.2   Partial listing of toxicants reported to affect the skin in common domestic animals

Lesion	Toxicant	Species affected
1. Degeneration/necrosis/apoptosis of epidermis (primary)		
	Acids and caustic (alkali) agents, oxidizing agents, ionizing radiation (e.g., UV), thermal injury, sulfur mustard	All species
	Heavy metals: inorganic mercury salts, inorganic arsenic salts	Horses
2. Degeneration/necrosis/apoptosis of epidermis (secondary)		
a. Immunologic (toxic epidermal necrolysis and erythema multiforme)	Antibiotics/antifungal agents: Trimethoprim-potentiated sulfas	Horses, dogs, cats
	Penicillin	Horses, dogs
	Amoxicillin	Cats
	Cephalosporins	Dogs
	Topical antibiotics	Horses
	Griseofulvin	Cats
	Anthelmintics/insecticides	
	Levamisole and thiabendazole	Dogs
	Ivermectin	Horses
	Organophosphates (flea dips)	Cats
	Chemotherapeutic agents	
	Aurothioglucose	Cats
	Propylthiouracil	Cats
	Plant/fungal toxins	
	D-limonene (flea dips, collars)	Dogs, cats
b. Vasoactive agents	Ergot alkaloids	Cattle
c. Phototoxic agents	Photodynamic agents (primary)	
	Hypericin (*Hypericum*)	Horses cattle, sheep, goats
	Furocoumarins (*Trifolium*, *Cymopterus*, *Ammi*, *Thamnosma*, *Cymopterus*, celery, parsley)	Cattle, sheep
	Fagopyrin (*Fagopyrum*)	Horses, cattle, sheep, pigs
	Phenothiazines	Horses, cattle, sheep, pigs
	Hepatotoxic agents (secondary)	
	Oxalates (*Kochia*)	Cattle, sheep
	Pyrrolizidine alkaloids (*Senecio*, *Crotalaria*, *Amsinckia*)	All grazing livestock
	Lantadenes A and B (*Lantana*)	Cattle
	Furanosesquiterpenoids (*Myoporum*)	Sheep
	Unknown (composite plants: *Asaemia*, *Athamasia*, *Lasiosperum*)	Cattle
	Unknown (Agave)	Sheep
	Unknown (alsike clover: *Trifolium*)	Horses
	Unknown (*Panicum*, *Tribulus*)	Horses, sheep, goats
	Sporodesmin from *Pithomyces*-contaminated ryegrass (*Lolium*) and puncture vine (*Tribulus*)	Cattle, sheep
	Microcystin (*Microcystis* algae)	All grazing livestock
3. Hyperkeratosis/parakeratosis	Chlorinated naphthalenes	Cattle

(*Continued*)

TABLE 7.2 (*Continued*)

Lesion	Toxicant	Species affected
	Iodine (kelp or supplements)	Horses, cattle
	Mercury	Horses
4. Inflammation		
a. Primary	Irritation: acids, alkali agents, organic solvents (mineral spirits, pine oils, essential oils, turpentine), phenol, oxidizing/reducing agents, keratolytic agents	All species
	Vicia villosa (hairy vetch)	Horses, cattle, sheep
b. Secondary	Strong acids, caustic agents, oxidizing agents, see 1	All species
	Immunologic agents	
	Agents inducing erythema multiforme, see 2a	Horses, dogs, cats
	Contact allergens (mainly type IV hypersensitivity)	Horses, dogs, cats
	Food allergens (mainly type I hypersensitivity)	Dogs, cats
	Photodynamic agents (primary and secondary), see 2c	Horses, cattle, sheep, goats, pigs
5. Adnexal damage		
a. Hair follicles (anagen phase)	Cancer chemotherapy drugs (e.g., doxorubicin and cyclophosphamide)	Dogs, cats
b. Hair follicles (telogen phase)	Arsenic	Horses, cattle, sheep, pigs
	Mercury	Horses
	Thallium	Cattle, sheep, dogs, cats
	Selenium	Horses, cattle
	Iodine	Horses, cattle
	Chlorinated naphthalenes	Cattle
	Mimosine	Horses, cattle
c. Sweat glands (anhidrosis)	Arsenic	Horses, cattle, cats
	Thallium	Cattle, sheep, pigs, dogs, cats
6. Disturbed growth		
a. Precancerous lesions	Arsenic	Horses, cattle, sheep, cats
	UV light (nonpigmented, hairless areas)	All species
b. Squamous cell carcinoma	UV light (nonpigmented, hairless areas)	All species

Epidermal Lesions

After exposure to any active agent, the first recognizable alterations are degenerative or involutional, and all include some degree of epidermal damage or destruction. The damage can vary from very focal keratinocyte swelling (sometimes referred to as "intracellular edema" or "ballooning degeneration") to extensive epidermal coagulative necrosis. Several degrees of epidermal damage can be found between these polar examples. The most frequent include spongiosis or intercellular edema of the spinous layer (characterized by increased space between keratinocytes), hydropic or vacuolar degeneration of the basal layer (often accompanied by spongiosis, see Figure 7.9), and individual or focal cell necrosis, also usually in the basal layer. T-2 toxin produces degeneration and necrosis in the basal layer of the epidermis (and also in the dermis), although the specific mechanism is unknown (Figure 7.10).

Epidermal necrosis can also be visualized as devitalized, sometimes hypereosinophilic and hyalinized epithelial layers with pyknotic nuclei that loosely line the dermis. Often the necrotic epithelium has already sloughed off, leaving a denuded dermal surface exposed to the environment (Figure 7.11). When the dermis is not compromised and only the epidermis is affected, the lesion is called erosion. When the epidermis is sloughed and the dermis is involved, the lesion is called an ulcer (Figure 7.12).

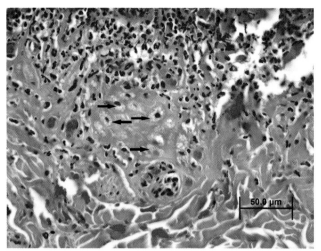

FIGURE 7.9   Ballooning degeneration (arrows) and necrosis of epidermal cells in the epidermis of a horse with a third degree thermal burn. A crust of necrotic cell debris and neutrophils overlays the affected epidermis.

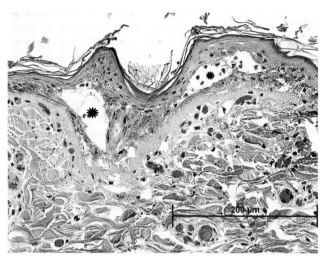

FIGURE 7.11   Necrosis of epithelium with vesiculation (*) due to lifting from the dermis in the skin of a horse with a third degree thermal injury.

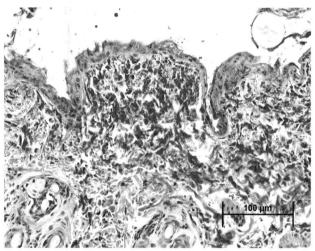

FIGURE 7.10   Epidermal and dermal necrosis due to T-2 toxicosis in the skin of rabbit.

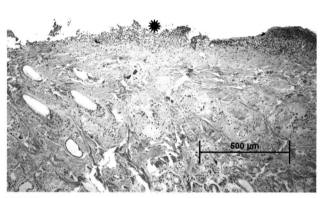

FIGURE 7.12   Ulceration (*) with adherent necrotic debris and suppurative exudate secondary to third degree thermal injury in the skin of a horse.

Inflammatory changes are frequently seen after total or partial epidermal destruction. The most intense inflammatory response typically corresponds to the depth of the injury, with injury extending into dermis producing a more vigorous inflammatory reaction (Figure 7.13). The inflammatory reaction in response to necrosis is characterized by migration of polymorphonuclear leukocytes, usually neutrophils, to the deep and lateral borders of the necrotic epidermis or ulcer. Microabscesses can sometimes be seen in the middle of the epidermis, or in the subcorneal region. The formation of intraepidermal bullae or vesicles, as well as subepidermal blisters or pustules, can be seen after exposure to caustic agents if the damage is relatively mild and limited to the upper layers of the epidermis. Frequently, especially in domestic animals, secondary bacterial or fungal contamination of the necrotic epithelium or the ulcer bed can considerably exacerbate the inflammatory response, compounding the initial damage done by the toxic agent, and often masking the inciting lesion.

After the noxious agent has ceased to act, or the tissues have adapted to a low level of injury, the epidermis responds with a series of reactive or progressive changes that usually include increased proliferation of cells (hyperplasia), and increased cell volume (hypertrophy) (Figure 7.14). These phenomena, usually associated with edema and spongiosis, can also be seen as

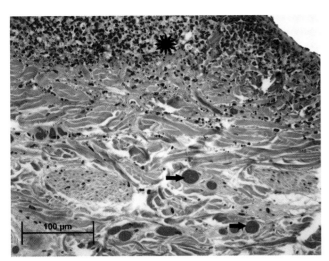

FIGURE 7.13 Inflammatory reaction in dermis in response to thermal injury of epidermis and dermis in the skin of a horse, illustrating vascuolar engorgement (arrows) and suppurative inflammation (*).

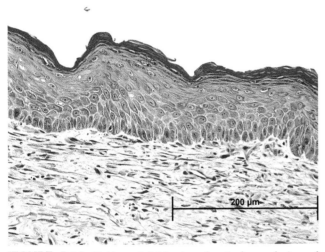

FIGURE 7.14 Epidermal thickening due to hyperplasia and hypertrophy of epidermis at the site of a recently-healed ulcer on the pinna of a dog.

an increased number of spinous keratinocytes (acanthosis). The increased proliferation of cells is reflected by an increased thickness of the epidermis, and is frequently accompanied by an increased production of superficial anucleated "squames" in the stratum corneum (hyperkeratosis). A specific increase in the number of basal keratinocytes (basal cell hyperplasia) is associated with some hyperplasiogenic agents.

Other changes in epidermal cell numbers seen after chronic exposure to carcinogens include proliferative lesions with altered growth behavior and morphology, sometimes called dysplasia or atypia. Although the just-described reactive epidermal alterations, consisting of increased number or size of layers or cells, are the usual pattern of response to chronic or protracted toxicant exposure of moderate intensity, occasionally the epidermis responds by a decrease in the size of cells or number of epidermal layers. This is usually referred to as epidermal atrophy (hypotrophy).

Dermal Lesions

The dermis can be altered by: (1) reaction to a toxicant that has injured the overlying epidermis directly; (2) diffusion through dermal capillaries of a systemically-circulating toxicant; or (3) direct penetration of the toxicant through the epidermis to cause direct damage to the dermis. As previously mentioned, during many active toxicant exposures a combination of mechanisms is likely.

Chronic dermatitis after toxicant-induced injury, either with extensive diffuse subepidermal mononuclear inflammatory cell infiltrates at the dermal–epidermal interface (lichenoid pattern), or with focal perivascular infiltrates of lymphocytes, histiocytic macrophages and mast cells, is common. These changes typically reflect an important allergic component to the lesion. Secondary infection can markedly complicate the picture, leading to a suppurative or pyogranulomatous reaction if opportunistic bacteria or fungi, respectively, colonize the area.

Two examples of skin injury induced through diffusion of toxicants from bloodstream to skin are ergotism and hairy vetch (*Vicia villosa*) toxicosis in cattle and horses. Ergot alkaloids, byproducts of metabolism produced by the fungus, *Claviceps purpurea*, a contaminant of grains, are potent vasoactive compounds that produce intense peripheral vasoconstriction, leading to ischemia and necrosis with ulceration of the skin of the distal extremities, ears, and tail of cattle ingesting the contaminated grain (Figure 7.15). Hairy vetch toxicosis, on the other hand, is postulated to have an immune-mediated mechanism, but is nevertheless an example of a systemic absorbed toxin having effects on the skin. Consumption of this range plant by cattle or horses leads to an exudative and exfoliative dermatitis with epidermal necrosis. Most striking, however, is the presence of an intense granulomatous dermal exudate containing multinucleated giant cell macrophages (Figure 7.16).

Allergic Contact Dermatitis

Acute allergic reactions which follow after local or systemic administration of toxicants are characterized by diffuse edema of both epidermis (i.e., spongiosis) and dermis, and engorgement of capillaries

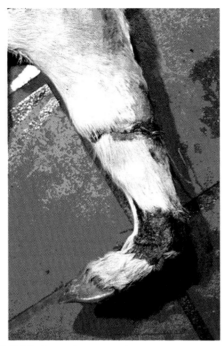

FIGURE 7.15 Dermal necrosis due to intense vasoconstriction induced by ergot alkaloids in a calf with sharp demarcation between the necrotic and non-necrotic skin (courtesy of Dr John King).

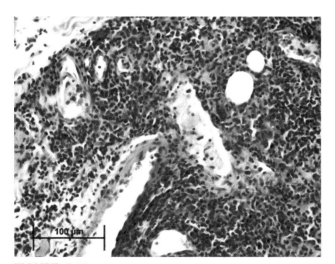

FIGURE 7.16 Intense deep dermal granulomatous inflammation in a horse induced by hairy vetch consumption.

(congestion) in the superficial dermis near the dermal–epidermal junction. As the lesion progresses, there may be eventual formation of vesicles and small blisters within the epidermis. Lymphocytes, as well as neutrophils and eosinophils (especially in horses), infiltrate into the epidermis (i.e., exocytosis) and dermis. Sometimes free red blood cells can be noted in the dermis; these are the source of hemosiderin deposits in chronic lesions.

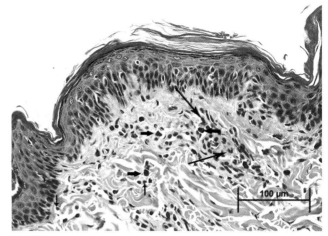

FIGURE 7.17 Chronic allergic dermatitis in a dog, with acanthosis, hyperkeratosis, perivascular infilatrates of histiocytes (long arrows), lymphocytes (short arrow), and mast cells (thick arrows) in the superficial (reticular) dermis.

The chronic phase of allergic contact dermatitis is characterized by thickening of the epidermis, with acanthosis, parakeratosis (abnormal keratinization with retention of keratinocyte nuclei), and hyperkeratosis. In the dermis there is a typical chronic superficial perivascular infiltrate that ranges from a small perivascular ring of lymphocytes to massive dermal infiltration by lymphocytes, eosinophils, and mast cells. Finally, if the injury is prolonged enough or following severe to moderate injury with significant tissue destruction, there is dermal fibroblastic proliferation together with obvious angioblastic activity. These changes, sometimes described as fibrovascular proliferation or granulation tissue, usually culminate in increased collagen content in the papillary and reticular dermis (fibrosis or scarring, Figure 7.17).

Adnexal Lesions

The cutaneous adnexa, when exposed to toxicants, undergo alterations similar to those described for the epidermis; during the alterative phase of toxicant exposure, destructive and involutional changes, such as intracellular edema, cell swelling, and focal necrosis, can be seen in these structures. After severe acute or chronic exposure, partial or total destruction of the structures or the supporting stroma may result in disappearance of the appendages from the exposed area (Figure 7.18), due to replacement by less-functional scar tissue. Although the epidermis near the affected tissue can regenerate completely by cell migration from unaffected areas, the newly-formed epidermis is unable to reconstitute the adnexal elements; less severe injury can cause adnexal atrophy or hypotrophy. Conversely, some agents are able to induce hyperplasia of sebaceous glands and hair follicles (Figure 7.19). During experimental exposure to carcinogens, epidermoid metaplasia of hair follicles has been described. Adnexotropic agents that cause selective damage to hair follicles and sebaceous glands will be considered in the next section.

Toxic Alopecia

When the hair follicle is the target of the toxic agent, alopecia is the main consequence. The agent may affect hair follicles in a specific phase of the hair cycle, such as the anagen (actively growing) or telogen (stationary) phase. In the first case, the effect of toxicity becomes evident within days or weeks of toxic exposure; telogen toxicity is slower and occurs over months of exposure. The most common mechanism of anagen toxicity is interference with the rapid mitotic activity at the base of the hair follicle (i.e., the hair bulb); this occurs with a variety of cancer chemotherapeutic agents (e.g., doxorubicin in dogs), and with the antigout agent colchicine.

Telogen toxicity is produced by different mechanisms. Heavy metals are notorious for affecting hair growth. For example, thallium (a banned, but nevertheless potent, rodenticide) produces profound skin changes, especially in dogs and cats. While acute thallium toxicosis does not produce skin lesions, chronic toxicity is typified by alopecia and ulceration affecting high friction areas (e.g., paws), as well as face, ears, ventrum, perineum, and mucocutaneous junctions. Additional changes include parakeratosis and hyperkeratosis in both epidermis and hair follicles in non-ulcerated areas (Figure 7.20). Thallium is thought to interfere with the incorporation of cysteine into keratins, and to interfere with energy metabolism of proliferating hair bulb cells, leading to premature telogen and subsequent shedding of the affected hairs. Alopecia due to chronic arsenic toxicity is suspected to have a similar mechanism, since arsenic also binds to cysteine residues in keratin and other proteins. Chronic mercury toxicosis with alopecia of long hairs in horses may also function in the same way.

The cutaneous manifestations of selenium toxicosis (Figure 7.21) is also associated with interactions with sulfur, but in this instance, it is the substitution of selenium for sulfur in sulfur-containing compounds

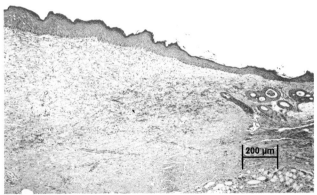

FIGURE 7.18 Dermal fibrosis and adnexal atrophy in a recently-healed wound from the pinna of a dog showing loss of hair follicles, apocrine glands, and sebaceous glands, with increased density of dermal collagen laid down in a laminar pattern.

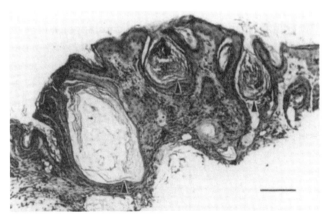

FIGURE 7.19 Chloracne. Note follicular hyperkeratosis (arrowheads), absence of sebaceous glands, and mild epidermal hyperplasia. Skin from an Skh:HR-1 mouse after 10 weeks of tetrachlorobiphenyl treatment. Bar = 120μm (from Puhvel et al., 1982, with permission).

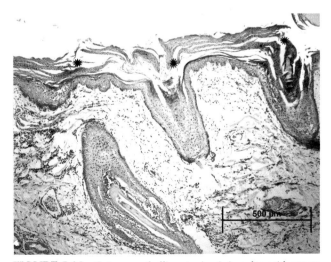

FIGURE 7.20 Cutaneous thallium toxicosis in a dog with severe parakeratotic hyperkeratosis (*) of the epidermis and superficial hair follicles.

(e.g. keratin) that is thought to produce the biochemical disruptions that result in alopecia of long hairs and hoof abnormalities in grazing animals consuming seleniferous range plants such as *Astragalus* and *Senecio*.

Mimosine, a non-protein amino acid that interferes with pyridoxine-dependent reactions, and which also chelates the essential metals iron, zinc, and copper, is present in plants such as *Leucana* (jumbey tree) and *Mimosa* (sensitive plant), grown in tropical and subtropical climates. Interference with pyridoxine metabolism presumably leads to impaired transamination, trans-sulfuration, and other basic biochemical pathways, leading to impaired amino acid metabolism. As with selenium, herbivorous mammals ingesting these plants have alopecia of long hairs (mainly horses), generalized alopecia (sheep and pigs), and hoof abnormalities (all species).

Other telogenic compounds include iodine (cranial alopecia in horses), propanolol, triparanol, and some anticoagulants, such as heparin and coumarin, and oral contraceptives. Compounds such as phenylglycidyl ether and dixyrazine have both anagen and telogen toxicity. In general, unless there is severe damage to the follicle, toxic alopecia is reversible once exposure ceases or the toxicant is metabolized and detoxified.

Chloracne

Chloracne is an occupational dermatosis of humans which occurs after exposure to a group of halogenated hydrocarbons (especially polyhalogenated naphthalenes, biphenyls, dibenzofurans, and contaminants of herbicides, such as polychlorophenol and dichloroaniline), and is characterized by an acneiform lesion, especially on the face and behind the ear (Figure 7.19). Comedones (otherwise known as "blackheads") are located in these regions, as well as on the external

genitalia, and sometimes in the axillae, shoulders, chest, back, abdomen, and buttocks; the extremities are very rarely involved. Histologically, comedones are dilations of the infundibular or suprafollicular area of the hair follicle, with accumulation of keratin and sebaceous gland secretion causing cystic dilation of the upper third of the hair follicles. Usually, there is little inflammation unless the follicle leaks or ruptures, at which point a pyogranulomatous inflammatory folliculitis generally ensues. Experimental chloracne has been induced in rabbits, monkeys, and hairless mice.

Chloracnegens have been associated with an increased incidence of soft tissue sarcomas in humans. Experimentally, 2,3,7,8-tetrachlorodibenzo-*p*-dioxin (TCDD) has been shown to be an efficient carcinogen, and a powerful inducer of the AHH system. AHH induction is used as the basis for an assay for assessing the potential chloracnegenic activity of chemicals.

Of historical interest mainly, but related to chloracne in some of its manifestations, is chlorinated naphthalene toxicosis in cattle, also known as X disease of bovine hyperkeratosis. Formerly a common additive/contaminant of petroleum-based lubricants, as well as a wood preservative, cutaneous exposure to, or ingestion of, these compounds by cattle resulted in the inhibition of Vitamin A metabolism, and signs of Vitamin A deficiency. Vitamin A is necessary for appropriate differentiation of epithelial cells, and its interference leads to impairment of normal keratinization among a series of other systemic epithelial and non-epithelial changes. Profound hyperkeratosis of epidermis and hair follicles accompanies the alopecia associated with the disease (Figure 7.22).

Sweat Gland Lesions

Several cytostatic agents such as cytarabine and bleomycin, which are used in human cancer therapy,

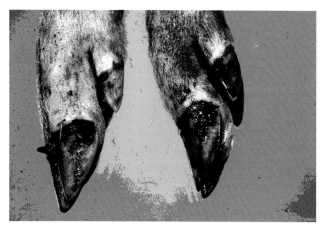

FIGURE 7.21   Selenium toxicosis in a calf, with sloughing of the hoof (courtesy of Dr John King).

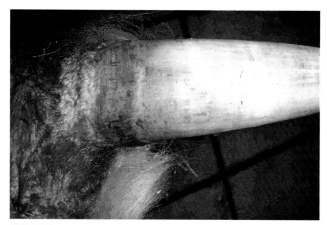

FIGURE 7.22   Hyperkeratosis ("X disease") at the base of the horn in a steer exposed to chlorinated naphthalenes (courtesy of Dr John King).

cause localized damage to the eccrine sweat ducts. This condition, called neutrophilic eccrine hidradenitis, is characterized by necrosis of the epithelial duct cells, acute inflammation, and squamous metaplasia of the remaining cells of the eccrine apparatus. The reason for the selective toxicity of these agents for eccrine glands is not clear, although high concentrations in sweat could explain this effect. Other chemicals that are toxic to sweat glands and produce generalized anhidrosis, with total or partial destruction of the eccrine system, include formaldehyde, arsenic, lead, fluorine, and thallium.

Neoplastic Lesions

Because cancer induction is one of the most important long-term effects of certain chemicals, and often constitutes the crucial endpoint of cutaneous bioassays, the most common types of skin tumors will be described.

Preneoplastic intraepithelial lesions, commonly induced in humans or domestic animals by sunlight (solar or actinic keratosis) (Figure 7.23) or by occupational or therapeutic exposure to arsenicals (Bowen's disease), are not frequently seen in experimental systems of chemical carcinogenesis. In the case of solar keratosis, there is progressive hyperplasia leading to progressive thickening of the epidermis, due to hyperplasia, parakeratosis, hyperkeratosis, and in prolonged cases, dysplasia. This is often accompanied by varying degrees of interface dermatitis and fibrosis of the underlying dermis. Some complete carcinogens, such as PAHs or nitroso compounds, will induce the types of dysplastic lesions seen in solar keratosis, but the lesions do not carry the same weight as preneoplastic alterations in other organs or tissues.

Papillomas are the most common lesion occurring in rodent skin after chemical carcinogen exposure, especially in two-stage carcinogenesis protocols of mouse skin. Papillomas are cauliflower-like structures, with either a narrow or a broad base, consisting of a series of folds united by common stalks to the underlying skin (Figure 7.24). Each of these folds consists of a central connective tissue core covered by an epidermis-like epithelium. The epithelium is usually thick, with numerous mitoses in the germinative layers, a high although variable labeling index, distinct spinous and granular layers, as well as a thick, usually fully-keratinized (orthokeratotic) horny layer. Areas of cellular atypia can be seen in many of these tumors. Papillomas in domestic animals are typically virally-induced, and generally do not progress to carcinoma, as can happen with chemically-induced papillomas in rodent models. It has been speculated, however, that papilloma virus infection can act as a cocarcinogen, especially with concomitant solar keratosis. Chemically-induced papillomas appear to arise from metaplastic or hyperplastic hair follicles, especially from the infundibular area. Papillomas may regress or continue their progression toward carcinomas.

Keratoacanthomas are morphologically very similar in all species, including humans. They often appear after exposure to UV radiation or complete carcinogens, but they are rarely seen in two-stage carcinogenesis experiments. In domestic animals, the link between carcinogen or UV exposure has not

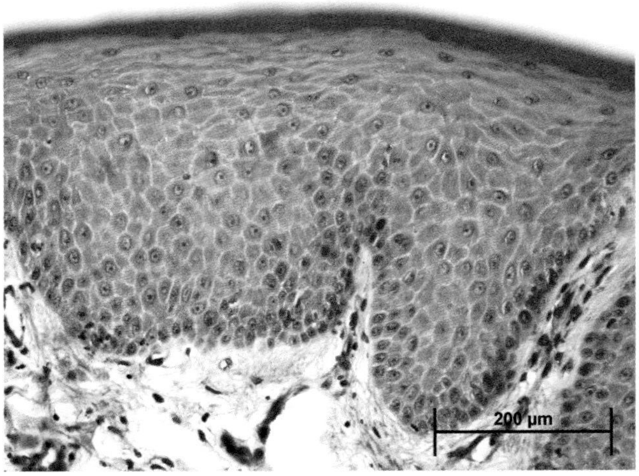

FIGURE 7.23 Actinic (solar) dermatosis on the pinna of a cat showing the extremely thickened hyperplastic/dysplastic acanthotic and parakeratotic epidermis. Nuclear atypia in both the basal and spinous layers of epidermis is evident.

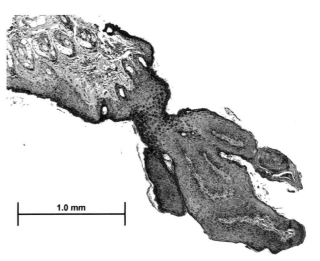

FIGURE 7.24 Cutaneous papilloma from a mouse after exposure to the carcinogen, 7,12-dimethylbenz[*a*]anthracene (DMBA) and the phorbol ester promoter, TPA.

been made. Similar to its human counterpart, murine keratoacanthoma starts as an intradermal growth of epithelial prolongations originating in the hair follicles. It usually acquires a cup-shaped architecture, with a central horny crater that has a papillomatous exophytic component and an endophytic component of deeply-penetrating epithelial cords that usually do not invade the subcutaneous tissue. Conversion to squamous carcinoma is accepted by numerous investigators. This is not the case for human keratoacanthoma, which is considered to be an abortive neoplasm that usually regresses.

Squamous cell carcinomas have been induced in many different laboratory species using UV light, ionizing radiation, or chemical carcinogens. In domestic animals UV light appears to the primary cause. In carcinogenesis models these tumors can originate from pre-existing lesions, such as papillomas, keratoacanthomas, and intraepidermal preneoplastic lesions, as well as from apparently normal or hyperplastic epidermis. Histologically, squamous cell carcinomas are usually well-differentiated, often with abundant amounts of keratin production (Figure 7.25). Less differentiated squamous cell carcinoma variants, such as spindle cell carcinoma, are less frequently seen experimentally. Metastasis to regional lymph nodes and distant sites, especially the lung, is a late occurrence. In addition to UV exposure, which is most commonly associated with squamous cell carcinoma in humans, chronic exposure to arsenic and PAHs have also been implicated in the genesis of this neoplasm.

Basal cell carcinomas, although common in dogs and cats, are generally not associated with UV exposure or chemical exposure. Basal cell carcinomas are frequent in humans, however, and usually associated with excessive exposure to UV. Basal cell carcinomas are frequently seen in rats, and occasionally seen in mice. However, since rats are not commonly used in cancer research and skin bioassays, the literature on rodent basal cell carcinomas is sparse.

Other adnexal tumors, such as sebaceous adenomas and trichoepitheliomas are relatively common in dogs, and to a lesser extent cats, but these have not been associated to date with chemical or carcinogen exposure. Adnexal tumors have been described in rats, mice, and hamsters, but also have not been linked to chemical exposure experimentally.

Melanotic tumors, a generic term that includes both benign and malignant tumors, have been produced by topical treatment of the skin with PAH in hamsters, guinea pigs, gerbils, and mice. Most chemically-induced melanotic tumors are less aggressive than the human malignant melanomas, and do not metastasize.

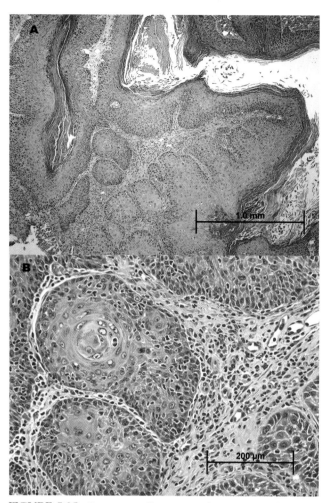

FIGURE 7.25 Squamous cell carcinoma from a mouse after exposure to the carcinogen, 7,12-dimethylbenz[a]anthracene (DMBA) and the phorbol ester promoter, TPA. (A) Low magnification image showing invasion of malignant epithelium through the basement membrane into underlying dermal stroma. (B) High magnification image showing nuclear atypia and inflammation that typically accompany this tumor.

EVALUATION OF CUTANEOUS TOXICITY

New compounds are introduced every year into the marketplace, and most of these compounds will intentionally (e.g., cosmetics) or accidentally come in contact with human skin. Therefore, reliable tests are necessary to evaluate the safety of these compounds, especially when they are intended for human use (cosmetic or therapeutic).

The animal species, and strain and the type of protocol, will depend on the objective of the toxicity bioassay. Most skin assays are used to evaluate acute irritation, chronic toxicity, and/or carcinogenesis. A few bioassays are used to evaluate specific skin reactions.

Absorption of chemicals through the skin can cause acute and chronic systemic effects, which can be monitored and assayed. The rat is the species used to evaluate systemic toxicity.

Skin Irritation Tests

Skin irritation tests have been designed to differentiate between agents that produce minor and reversible inflammatory changes (minor irritants), those that induce severe inflammation (major irritants), and those that cause massive destruction or necrosis of cutaneous structures (corrosive agents). The most frequently utilized technique is that of Draize, which has been slightly modified and adapted by the Code of Federal Regulations (1980), legislated under provisions of the Federal Hazardous Substances Act.

The technique consists of applying 0.5 g of the test substance under a gauze pad to the skin of rabbits or guinea pigs. Semifluids and liquids can be applied directly; solids should be dissolved or moistened with adequate solvents. Each animal can be used for four (guinea pig) or six (rabbit) patch tests; six animals should be used to test each substance. The Draize procedure can be modified to use abraded skin for substances that might come in direct contact with the dermis. The grossly observable skin reaction is read at 4, 24, and 72 hours after application, and scored according to Draize's scale (Table 7.3).

Although additional histopathologic examination of skin lesions would enhance the observations, this is usually not done. This procedure is valuable to screen for toxicity of household substances, such as cosmetics, soaps and detergents, but has limited value for investigating the mode of action of chemicals, or the pathogenesis of chemically-induced lesions.

Human testing has been designed to overcome some of the pitfalls of animal testing that make extrapolation to humans difficult. With adequate precautions, such as pretesting in animals and using lower concentrations, the skin test can be employed in humans using the Draize procedure; proper ethical considerations need to be addressed and fully-informed consent obtained from healthy volunteers. For humans, Draize's scale has been modified to incorporate additional skin reactions (Table 7.4).

Carcinogenesis Bioassays

Application of putative carcinogens to the skin of laboratory animals constitutes the basis of the carcinogenesis bioassay. Its objective is to determine the local and systemic carcinogenic potential of the substance, as determined by the gross and microscopic detection of neoplasms.

The general principles of chemical carcinogenesis not only apply to the skin, but were first conceived and developed from models using rodent skin. The main models are complete carcinogenesis, using one compound applied repetitively to the skin surface, and two-stage carcinogenesis, in which two different compounds are used. The first stage in the latter protocol is called initiation, and consists of a single application of a subcarcinogenic dose of a chemical that, if used in larger doses, would produce tumors. Nevertheless, the subcarcinogenic dose is sufficient to produce appropriate mutations in cellular DNA that, once perpetuated, could ultimately produce malignancy. The single application of the "initiating" compound is followed by a series of topical applications of a noncarcinogenic agent, called a promoter (usually a phorbol ester), that is able to selectively increase the

TABLE 7.3   Grading values for skin reaction following topical application of potential primary irritants[a] (Draize Scale)

Skin reaction	Value
Erythema and eschar (crust or scab) formation	
No erythema	0
Very slight erythema (barely perceptible)	1
Well-defined erythema	2
Moderate to severe erythema	3
Severe erythema to slight eschar formation	4
Edema formation	
No edema (barely perceptible)	0
Very slight edema (raised edges of area well-defined)	1
Slight edema	2
Moderate edema	3
Severe edema (raised more than 1 mm and extending beyond the area of exposure)	4

[a]Modified from National Academy of Sciences, 1977

TABLE 7.4   Scale in human skin patch test[a]

Grade	Lesion
0	No response
½	Indistinct erythema
1	Well-defined erythema
2	Erythema and edema
3	Vesicles and/or papules
4	Bulla or other severe reaction

[a]Modified from National Academy of Sciences, 1977

population of initiated cells via enhanced proliferation of the initiated cells. This eventually results in the production of skin tumors. Initially, the tumors are benign exophytic lesions (usually papillomas); some of these gradually convert into fully-invasive tumors (carcinomas). In a third model, three-stage carcinogenesis, another carcinogen in subcarcinogenic doses or a free-radical-generating compound is used as an enhancer or progressor that is applied after initiation and promotion. Enhancement is seen as an increase in conversion of papillomas to malignant tumors, and increased malignancy of the tumors (i.e., more invasion and metastasis).

The mouse is the preferred species for use in carcinogenesis bioassays, although use of a second species (rat or hamster) allows a broader interpretation of results. Several mouse strains and stocks have been used (BALB/c, B6 C3F1, SENCAR, CD-1, C3H). The test substance is applied on the shaved dorsum 2–5 times a week, in a volume of 50–200 µL, using acetone as vehicle. The dose should be close to the maximum tolerated dose (MTD). The MTD is generally determined in a pilot study, and should be the maximum dose that does not produce extensive, acute, irreversible or involutional lesions, such as necrosis or severe inflammation. Reducing the dose once the MTD is determined will facilitate dose–response studies, which usually include three dose levels in a two-year study.

Morphologic Assessment

Macroscopic evaluation of lesions is important, and should be used as an aid for the selection of tissue for histopathology. The Draize skin irritation scoring code, originally developed for rabbits, is sometimes used in rodent bioassays, but is not sufficient for precise lesion typing, and does not provide for late tumor-associated changes.

Histopathologic assessment is the most preferable and widely-used procedure for evaluating cutaneous alterations. In 1988, a panel of experts convened at the Environmental Protection Agency and made several recommendations regarding the processing of rodent skin for the histopathologic evaluation of toxicant-induced lesions. Sections of skin should be cut parallel to the longitudinal cranio–caudal axis of the animal, and should include underlying subcutis and muscular layers for complete examination of potentially affected tissues. Follicular structures are better demonstrated when skin is oriented along the longitudinal axis. Samples of skin taken at necropsy should be flattened on a piece of cardboard, gently stretched, and fixed in

10% neutral buffered formalin for several days prior to trimming. Step-sectioning every 50–75 µm allows full evaluation of all skin structures. Photographs of representative gross lesions are recommended for each treatment group. When possible, morphometric or stereologic techniques for quantification of the morphologic changes should be employed, to provide an accurate and objective evaluation.

Other Bioassays

Obviously, when tumor induction is not the objective of the investigation, an appropriate bioassay protocol should be selected. The species or strain of animals should also be carefully considered. For example, investigation of chloracnegens is best accomplished in rabbits, on the facial skin of monkeys, or more practically on the dorsal skin of hairless mice (SKh:HR-1).

For phototoxicity bioassays, the chemical is applied to a marked skin area on a mg/cm^2 or $µg/cm^2$ basis; hairless mice, rabbits, and humans have similar phototoxic reactions. Several doses of UV light above 310 nm are used. Adequate controls (chemical without UV exposure, UV exposure without chemical, and neither UV nor chemical exposure) must be used. The skin should be irradiated within 30–120 minutes of chemical application. The Draize scoring system (12–14 hours after UV exposure) is the most frequently-used system for evaluation.

Bioassays for delayed contact sensitization are designed to detect cell-mediated immune reactions (type IV hypersensitivity) that develop in previously-sensitized skin 24–48 hours after a second contact with the skin. Adult albino guinea pigs are sensitized, either by intradermal injections or by topical applications (patch test) of the test substance for three weeks. After a rest period of two weeks, the animals are rechallenged, usually with less than half the original dose of test substance. The ensuing reaction should be clearly greater than the irritation caused by the original application. A similar patch test can be used in human volunteers. A scoring scale similar to that used for irritation grading can be used.

Transgenic Animal Models

Selective breeding of mouse strains, and the advent of transgenic mice, have been developed recently and are gaining wide acceptance. The Sencar (SENsitivity to CARcinogenicity) mouse is an increasingly accepted outbred mouse strain used for testing cutaneous carcinogens and promoters. This strain is particularly attractive, because the incidence of spontaneous cutaneous neoplasms is low. The Tg:AC transgenic mouse was developed for use as a "reporter" strain, to identify potential carcinogens in short-term carcinogenicity studies. This mouse has the coding sequence of v-Ha-*ras*, linked to a ζ-globin promoter and a simian virus 40polyA signal sequence. This results in a "genetically-initiated" mouse that only requires a promoter for papilloma formation. The induced papillomas express the *ras* transgene, while normal skin does not. Use of both these strains has greatly facilitated skin carcinogenicity studies.

In Vitro Testing

As a result of opposition to the use of animals for testing purposes, and the increase in the costs of animal experimentation, attention has been directed to alternative *in vitro* methods of testing. These alternatives include the use of cell, tissue, and organ cultures. Some of the approaches under investigation include the release of mediators from cells in culture, assays of *in vitro* cell toxicity, the use of chorioallantoic membranes, and the use of lower organisms. Although many efforts are being directed toward developing reliable tests, the complexity of the actual *in vivo* response makes it very difficult to predict the response of tissues *in vivo* with a single *in vitro* test. For example, an *in vitro* test proposed for delayed skin hypersensitivity requires at least three steps: binding the test compound to Langerhans cells; activation/migration of the Langerhans cells; and the effect of these activated cells on autologous lymphocyte blastogenesis.

Some *in vitro* assays of acute toxicity using short-term rodent skin organ cultures show a good correlation between *in vivo* lesions and *in vitro* effect. Such organ cultures have been evaluated to a limited extent for histopathological and biochemical relevance, for instance for inhibition of DNA synthesis or protein synthesis, and for leakage of intracellular enzymes (e.g., lactate dehydrogenase) into the culture medium. Similar organ cultures have been used to evaluate metabolism and absorption of drugs by the skin.

For complex bioassays, the major problem is the validation of the *in vitro* tests; it will require a series of combined *in vivo* and *in vitro* efforts before new *in vitro* tests can be adopted. Therefore, it is unlikely that tests in whole animals will be replaced in the immediate future, but alternatives to replace or reduce the number of animals are being sought.

INTRODUCTION

The oral mucosa is, in many ways, similar to the skin in its architecture, function, and reaction patterns. This section only emphasizes those characteristics of the oral mucosa that influence or result in a distinct group of pathologic entities.

Because of its location at the entrance of the digestive and respiratory tracts and its proximity to the teeth, the oral mucosa is subjected to numerous natural and man-made xenobiotics. The peculiar architecture and absorption characteristics of the oral mucosa, especially in areas of extreme thinness, coupled with the rich microorganism flora of the mouth, makes the oral mucosa a peculiar site deserving separate discussion.

STRUCTURE AND FUNCTION OF THE ORAL MUCOSA

Microscopic Anatomy

The architecture of the oral mucosa is similar to that of the skin; that is, it has superficial stratified squamous epithelium covering a thin layer of connective tissue or lamina propria. In humans, the epithelium varies in thickness (50–500μm) and in morphology. Except for the mucosa covering the hard palate and some areas of the gingiva, most of the oral cavity is lined by non-keratinizing epithelium, characterized by an absence of a horny layer. Superficial epithelial cells are slightly flattened, but otherwise not very different from the underlying spinous cells. Although the oral integument has few adnexa, several hundred minor salivary glands emerge from pores in the oral mucosa. The architecture of the oral epithelium in primates and rabbits is similar to that in humans. Conversely, most rodents used as laboratory animals do not have a non-keratinizing mucosa. An orthokeratinized stratified squamous epithelium extremely similar to the epidermis covers the oral mucosa of these animals, including the mucosa of the hamster's cheek pouch, the most frequently used experimental site.

Physiology

Two main features distinguish the oral epithelium from the epidermis: a high proliferative capacity; and high absorption potential. The proliferative capacity of the oral epithelium, although variable according to the site considered (e.g., higher in the gingiva and lower in the hard palate), is approximately 2–3 times higher than that of the epidermis. This results in a tendency toward proliferative reaction patterns during chronic inflammation or irritation, as well as a very rapid normal healing process that usually takes only a few days for minor traumatic lesions.

Due to the thinness of the epithelium in certain areas (sublingual region, floor of the mouth, and gingival sulcus), and the lack of an orthokeratinized layer, the oral mucosa possesses a remarkable capacity to absorb drugs and chemicals, including those that produce systemic effects. Most chemicals penetrate the mucosa by simple diffusion, alone or in combination with a carrier molecule secreted in the saliva. The agents can be actively transported against a concentration gradient, or transported by facilitated diffusion. Penetration through the epithelial cells by pinocytosis or phagocytosis has also been described. Mucosal absorption is facilitated by organic solvents, including alcohol. Alcohol can increase the penetration of carcinogens through the oral epithelium, and thus potentiate their effects.

COMPARATIVE MECHANISMS OF MUCOSAL TOXICITY

Mechanisms of mucosal toxicity are similar to those described for skin. The reader is referred to Part I, Comparative Mechanisms of Cutaneous Toxicity, and Table 7.1.

RESPONSE OF ORAL MUCOSA TO INJURY

Fundamental Non-neoplastic Lesions

The patterns of injury and reaction are very similar to those of the skin, and will not be repeated in this section; a number of selected lesions that are peculiar to the oral mucosa will be described.

The human oral mucosa, especially the gingival, buccal, and palate mucosa, can be exposed to compounds used for restorative and therapeutic purposes. These materials can cause acute injury of the mucosa, however. Because of long-standing exposure to materials used in restorative dentistry, chronic inflammation and fibrosis are frequently the result.

Direct acute involutional changes are seen after the use of certain caustic chemicals, such as paraformaldehyde, glutaraldehyde, phosphoric acid, iodine, phenol,

and silver nitrate. Most of these materials (used mainly for pulp mummification and for improving the retention of resinous compounds to enamel) are intended to contact the dental hard tissues, but if improperly used or if cavities are inadequately sealed, they may leak and come into contact with the oral mucosa (especially within the interdental papillary area), where they can cause localized necrosis.

A chemical burn of the gingiva and buccal mucosa is commonly seen after placing aspirin tablets close to a tooth that causes pain. These regional areas of necrosis, known as aspirin burns, are painful ulcerations in the vestibular sulcus that are similar histologically to acute necrosis and ulceration described earlier for caustic agents affecting skin.

In domestic animals, consumption of plants such as Dumb cane (*Philodendron*), calla lily (Zantedeschia), Jack-in-the-pulpit (*Arisaema*), and skunk cabbage (*Symplocarpus*) can produce gingival pain and edema that, in most cases, is reversible. The cause of the reaction is disputed, but has been attributed to the physical damage by calcium oxalate crystals found in the cells of these plants.

Systemic administration of drugs can produce stomatitis with or without lesions elsewhere. Some chemicals induce vesico-bullous and ulcerative stomatitis as part of an allergic reaction that sometimes includes anaphylactic shock (e.g., penicillin, sulfa drugs, antimalarial drugs, penicillamine). Cytostatic drugs, like methrotrexate, produce lesions such as epithelial atrophy and ulceration, by interfering with normal epithelial cell proliferation. Immunosuppressive drugs, such as azathioprine, interfere with the immune defense mechanisms and with normal cell proliferation, not only causing epithelial atrophy and ulceration, but also enhancing secondary infection by pathogenic and saprophytic oral microorganisms, exacerbating the necrotizing and ulcerative processes.

Hyperplastic gingival changes and gingival fibrosis result from prolonged systemic administration of diphenylhydantoin, an anti-epileptic drug. This drug (as well as sodium valproate, another anti-epileptic agent), produces increased fibroblastic proliferation of the subepithelial connective tissue in the interdental papillae and adjacent gingiva.

Prolonged use of tobacco may produce severe lesions, such as nicotinic stomatitis (leukokeratosis of the palate of smokers), which is characterized by thickening of the hard palate epithelium, due to hyperplasia and hyperkeratosis. The mucosa has a characteristic multinodular pattern; small red dots in the center of each nodule represent the orifices of salivary ducts. This lesion is not considered preneoplastic and, thus, has to be differentiated from the precancerous leukoplakias.

Carcinogenesis

With the increased use of smokeless tobacco, moist snuff, and the persistent use of classical tobacco forms in several parts of the world, there has been an increased incidence in preneoplastic and neoplastic lesions of the oral mucosa. Leukoplakia (Figure 7.26) is the most common lesion, affecting any part of the oral cavity. It is a whitish plaque that can be homogeneously smooth or nonhomogeneous, and has three variants besides the homogeneous base lesion: (1) erythroleukoplakia or erosive leukoplakia; (2) nodular leukoplakia; and (3) verrucous leukoplakia. The three variants are considered of high preneoplastic potency, whereas the homogeneous leukoplakia has a low risk of neoplastic transformation. These lesions consist of a hyperplastic epithelium (usually in the buccal, lingual, or sublingual regions) with different degrees of cellular atypia that range from a few scattered atypical cells to a fully-developed carcinoma *in situ*. Although these lesions can be seen occasionally in non-smokers, the relationship with tobacco use is very strong. Oral cancer and its precursors have also been associated with reverse smoking and betel nut chewing.

Although the rodent oral mucosa is markedly different from the non-keratinizing mucosa that covers most of the human oral cavity, the hamster cheek pouch epithelium has been frequently used as a target organ for experimental oral carcinogenesis. Rat lip mucosa and rabbit buccal mucosa have also been used to test tobacco- or snuff-related products or fractions. A recently-developed bioassay using the rat lip mucosa surgically modeled to produce a canal or pouch has been used successfully to test the carcinogenicity of tobacco-specific nitrosamines and snuff.

EVALUATION OF ORAL TOXICITY

Most tests for toxicity of compounds that come in contact with the oral mucosa have been done using the classical cutaneous bioassays described in the section on skin. A few investigators have used the oral mucosa of rabbits or primates, but this is not a widely used approach, and there are no standard protocols or grading schemes. As pointed out earlier, the most commonly used model for oral carcinogenesis is the hamster cheek pouch. This model has been used mainly as an investigative tool for the study of oral carcinogenesis, and has not been proposed as a standard carcinogenesis bioassay system. For this purpose, the cutaneous carcinogenesis bioassay is used most frequently.

FURTHER READING

Ali, N., and Oehme, F.W. (1992). A literature review of dermatotoxicity. *Vet. Hum. Toxicol.*, 34, 428–437.

Cohen, D.E., and Rice, R.H. (2001). Toxic responses of the skin. In *Toxicology* (Klaassen, C.D. ed.), 6th edn, pp. 653–672. Macmillan, New York, NY.

Conti, C.J., Slaga, T.J., and Klein-Szanto, A.J.P. (1989). *Skin Tumors. Experimental and Clinical Aspects.* Raven Press, New York, NY.

Drill, V.A., and Lazar, P. (1984). *Cutaneous Toxicity.* Academic Press, New York, NY.

Ginn, P.E., Mansell, J.E.K.L., and Rakich, P.M. (2007). Skin and appendages. In *Pathology of Domestic Animals* (Jubb, K.V.F., Kennedy, P.C., and Palmer, N. eds), 5th edn, pp. 553–781. Elsevier Saunders, Philadelphia, PA.

Marzulli, F.N., and Maibach, H.I. (1996). *Dermatotoxicology*, 5th edn. Taylor & Francis, Washington, DC.

National Academy of Sciences (1977). *Principles and Procedures for Evaluating the Toxicity of Household Substances*, pp. 23–59. National Academy of Sciences, Washington, DC.

Nemecek, G.M., and Dayan, A.D. (1999). Safety evaluation of human living skin equivalents. *Toxicol. Pathol.*, 27, 101–103.

Pindborg, J.J. (1992). *Atlas of Diseases of the Oral Mucosa*, 5th edn. W.B. Saunders, Munksgaard, Copenhagen, Philadelphia.

Stanley, H.R. (1985). Initial tests for biological evaluation of dental materials. *Toxicity Testing of Dental Materials.* CRC Press, Boca Raton, FL, pp. 13–72.

Steinberg, M. (1984). Dermatotoxicology test techniques: An overview. In *Cutaneous Toxicity* (Drill, V.A., and Lazar, P. eds). Raven Press, New York, NY.

Wintroub, B.U., and Stern, R. (1985). Cutaneous drug reactions: Pathogenesis and clinical classification. *J. Am. Acad. Dermatol.*, 13, 167–179.

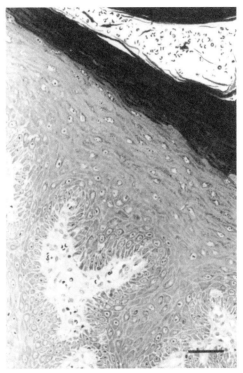

FIGURE 7.26 Leukoplakia of the buccal mucosa. Note the prominent orthokeratinized horny layer, and the thickness of the spinous layer. Human cheek mucosa. Bar = 80 μm.

Gastrointestinal Tract

INTRODUCTION

From the perspective of toxicologic pathology, the gastrointestinal (GI) tract represents one of the most fascinating organ systems to evaluate. The intrinsic ability of the GI tract to resist toxic chemicals has led to a paucity of data regarding GI toxicology. The GI tract is the entry site into the body of orally administered compounds that may be highly toxic to other internal organs, but have little or no noticeable effect on the GI tract. Nevertheless, this organ system can be readily perturbed, leading to obvious toxic responses. Some of these responses are readily identifiable, such as emesis or diarrhea. Other perturbations, such as the insufficiency of some enzymes, changes in functions (such as excess production of mucus or delayed emptying), localized inflammation or neoplastic changes, are more difficult to identify and attribute to toxicologic processes. The principal functions of the GI tract that are subject to toxic effects of chemicals include storage, propulsion, digestion, absorption, secretion, barrier

163

activity, and elimination. Due to the importance of nervous reflexes and hormones in the regulation of the GI tract, this system is relatively unique, in that toxic effects at one site (e.g., stomach) may be expressed at another site (e.g., colon).

A distinctive feature of the GI tract is the high proliferative and metabolic rate of the mucosa. The mucosa is a complex barrier that must exclude bacteria and their toxic byproducts, and yet absorb nutrients vital for homeostasis. Therefore, this organ system cannot sustain widespread toxicity without serious direct and indirect consequences to the rest of the body, if for no other reason than nutrient malabsorption.

The GI tract is also the only internal organ that contains biotransforming and toxigenic bacteria, as well as inert drug-binding materials. Consequently, when a compound is placed into the GI milieu, the ultimate toxicity to this organ system is determined by interactions of the chemical with bacterial and mammalian enzymes, as well as by the extent of detoxification or activation processes. Hence, the ability to evaluate genomic, proteomic, biochemical or morphologic changes in the GI tract can be complicated because of the matrix of interactions.

In addition, the GI tract is exquisitely sensitive to autolysis and postmortem alterations, due to its high luminal bacterial content and high metabolic activity. Many subtle toxicologic events that occur at the cellular and subcellular level may only be observed by careful and proper handling of the GI tissues at postmortem examination, or during sample collection. All of these factors, and numerous others, provide many challenges to the toxicologist or pathologist who is evaluating the GI tract as a target organ system in toxicologic pathology.

STRUCTURE AND FUNCTION OF THE GASTROINTESTINAL TRACT

A brief overview of anatomy and physiology of the GI tract with important species differences is provided, to give a foundation for the understanding of GI toxicologic physiopathology.

Macroscopic and Microscopic Structure and Function

Although many of the basic features of the GI tract are similar for various species (Figure 8.1 and

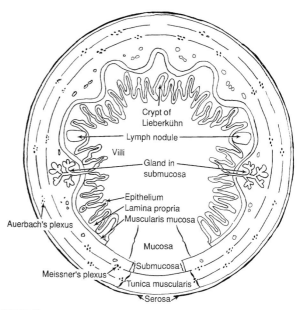

FIGURE 8.1 Schematic drawing of the intestinal tract. This basic tissue organization demonstrates the general organization of the entire GI tract. Brunner's glands are located in the submucosa of the duodenum only. Villi are present in the small intestine only.

Table 8.1), major interspecies variations are present in the fore- and hindgut (Table 8.2). Yet, within each major macroscopic variation, the cell types composing the mucosal lining of the GI tract are similar (Figure 8.2, Table 8.1).

Esophagus

The function of the esophagus in all species is to act as a conduit for material to leave the oral cavity and enter the GI tract. Interspecies esophageal variations include the presence and extent of smooth versus striated muscle, the characteristics of the gastroesophageal junction, and the presence of sacculated adaptations (e.g., forestomachs). In all species, the esophagus is lined by stratified squamous epithelium, with varying degrees of surface keratinization. The extent of keratinization of the esophageal and nonglandular gastric epithelium is dependent on the amount and type of dry foodstuff ingested in the diet. Consequently, hyperkeratosis (cornification) of the mucosa can indicate anorexia or an increase in roughage content of the feed, in both ruminants and rodents. This keratinized epithelium imparts a whitish color when the esophagus is viewed macroscopically. Keratinization is also a normal feature of the nonglandular portion of the stomach in rodents and perissodactyls (e.g., horses and tapirs).

TABLE 8.1 Cells composing the epithelial lining of the gastrointestinal tract

Cell type	Shape	Location	Product/function
Chief cell	Low columnar	Stomach (fundus)	Pepsin, rennin, lipase
Parietal cell	Pyramidal	Stomach (fundus)	HCl, intrinsic factor
Mucous cell	Cuboidal to columnar	Stomach to rectum	Mucus
Enterochromaffin cell	Pyramidal	Stomach to rectum	Hormone production
Undifferentiated cell	Low columnar	Small intestine to rectum (crypts)	Progenitor cell, secretion
Vacuolated cell	Columnar	Colon to rectum (crypts)	Progenitor cell
Paneth cell	Pyramidal	Small intestine	Lysozyme, peptidase
Absorptive cell	Tall columnar	Small intestine to colon (villi and surface)	Nutrient absorption
Goblet cell	Columnar	Small intestine to rectum (villi and surface)	Mucin
M cell	Low columnar	Dome of Peyer's patches	Antigen processing

TABLE 8.2 Variations in dietary consumption patterns in relation to gastrointestinal structure in various mammalian orders

ORDER	Dietary pattern			Gastric anatomy		Colonic anatomy	
	Carnivore	Omnivore	Herbivore	Sacculated	Stratified squamous portion	Large cecum	Sacculated or expanded colon
Carnivora	+	+		−	−	±	±
Rodentia	+	+	+	±	±	±	±
Lagomorpha			+	−	−	±	±
Primates	+	+	+	±	±	±	±
Artiodactyla		+	+	±	±	±	±
Marsupialia	+	+	+	±	±	±	±
Perissodactyla			+	−	±	±	±

[a] Modified from Stevens (2004)

The tunica muscularis of the esophagus has two muscle layers composed of striated, smooth, or a mixture of both types of muscle, depending on the species. Variations in esophageal musculature account for the ability or inability of an animal to vomit. The absence of significant amounts of striated muscle in the esophagus of rats (and horses), and the presence of a limiting ridge (margo plicatus) in the stomach, explain why these animals are unable to vomit. The ability of dogs and guinea pigs to vomit and ruminants to regurgitate is dependent on the presence of striated muscle in the esophagus. Regurgitation, not vomiting, in nonruminants indicates esophageal dysfunction or obstruction. If the esophagus is perforated by caustic compounds, repair is likely to be incomplete or defective, resulting in leakage of saliva and ingested foodstuffs into surrounding tissues. The esophagus does not heal as rapidly as other portions of the GI tract, because of a marginal blood supply and a minimal amount of adventitial and serosal connective tissue.

Stomach

Anatomical and functional variations are important considerations when designing animal studies, since compound absorption and enzyme exposure (e.g., ruminal bacteria versus acidic gastric juices) may vary from species to species, and sites of storage (e.g., nonglandular stomach) may provide prolonged contact between the host mucosa and a toxic compound.

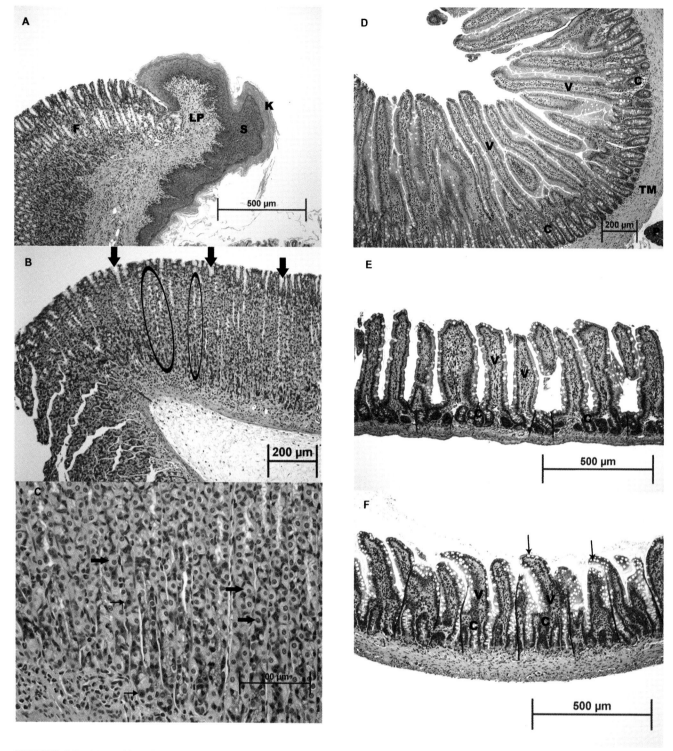

FIGURE 8.2 Normal histology of the rat GI tract. (A) Nonglandular (squamous) portion of the stomach (S) from a rat at the junction (limiting ridge) with the fundus (F) with its deep gastric glands. The stratified squamous epithelium is covered by a layer of keratin (K), and the underlying lamina propria (LP) is infiltrated by a resident population of inflammatory and immune cells. (B) Fundic (oxyntic) mucosa of the glandular stomach. Gastric pits (arrows) are lined by columnar epithelium, and are the outlet for fundic gland (ellipses) secretions. (C) In a higher magnification view of the fundus, eosinophilic pyramidal parietal cells (large arrows), as well as smaller, more basophilic chief cells (small arrows) lining the gastric glands are indicated. Identification of the enteroendocrine cells that are also present in lower numbers requires special staining techniques (e.g., Grimelius stain). (D) Duodenal portion of the small intestine, villi (V) are very long in relation to the crypts (C). Tunica muscularis (TM) and attached pancreas (P) are indicated. (E) Jejunal portion of the small intestine. Villi (V) are lined by columnar epithelial cells and have a central lacteal. Crypts (C) are composed of proliferating epithelial cells. (F) A section of ileum illustrates the shortness of the villi (V) in relation to the crypts (C). Numerous goblet cells (arrows) are also evident. (G) The cecal mucosa in the rat (as well as other species) is relatively thin, with only crypts (C) and numerous goblet cells (arrows). The submucosa (SM) is rather "loose," and the tunica muscularis (TM) is thin. (H) Colonic mucosa in the rat is highly folded, and has abundant goblet cells (arrows). Colonocytes are not as tall as enterocytes, and no villi are present, only crypts (C). (I) Peyer's patch from the ileum of a dog illustrating M cells (MC), and the mixture of lymphocytes (small arrows) and plasma cells (large arrows) in the lamina propria.

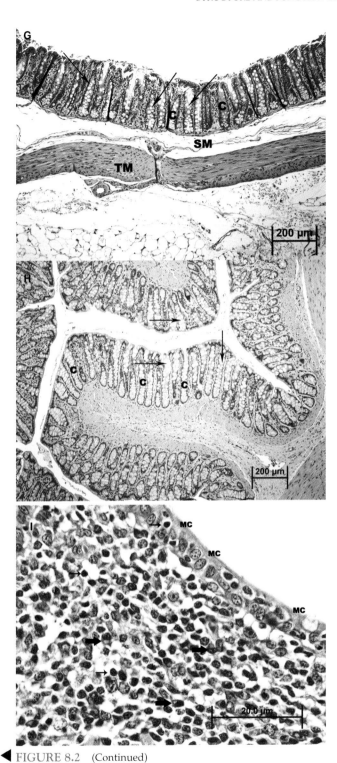

◀ FIGURE 8.2   (Continued)

Function

The stomach functions to store and macerate food, and begin early phases of food digestion. In some mammalian orders there are members that have highly sacculated forestomachs (e.g., some artiodactyls and some primates). This compartmentalization is permanent, and aids in the digestion of food. In ruminants, the "ruminal" portions of the forestomach, which are actually a modification of the esophagus, are highly permeable to volatile fatty acids released from microbial metabolism of complex carbohydrates, and are capable of active sodium and chloride absorption.

Several mammalian orders, including rodents, perissodactyls, and some artiodactyls, have a nonglandular stratified squamous portion of the stomach adjacent to the fundic or cardiac mucosa (Figure 8.2A). This squamous portion of the stomach is separated from the glandular stomach by a limiting ridge (margo plicatus), and it serves as a storage organ for ingested material. Various inflammatory cells (lymphocytes, plasma cells, and eosinophils) may be present in the lamina propria of the limiting ridge of rodents.

Structure

The topographical organization of the gastric mucosa varies widely among species. Humans, dogs, and cats are monogastric or simple-stomached mammals, in which the cardia is the first glandular portion of the stomach following the esophagus; the cardiac mucosa is macroscopically red. This portion of the stomach has foveolae (gastric pits) and tortuous mucous glands. The fundus is the next glandular region, consisting of macroscopic mucosal convolutions called rugae. The distal portion of the stomach, the pylorus, also has rugae, but they are smaller than those of the fundus and are arranged obliquely in the direction of the antrum. Unlike other portions of the stomach, the foveolae of the antrum are deeper, and make up as much as 50% of the mucosal thickness.

The fundic mucosa contains glandular epithelium composed of mucus-secreting surface neck cells, parietal (oxyntic) cells, chief (zymogen) cells, and enteroendocrine (enterochromaffin) cells (Figure 8.2B, 8.2C). Chief cells are low columnar and have a basally-located nucleus. The apical portion of the cytoplasm is filled with eosinophilic pepsinogen-filled zymogen granules. The primary function of the chief cell is to release enzymes into the gastric lumen to begin the process of gastric digestion. Parietal cells are larger, but generally less numerous than chief cells. These cells have a centrally located nucleus, and the smooth endoplasmic reticulum- and mitochondria-laden cytoplasm stains intensely eosinophilic. Parietal cells release HCl to maintain low gastric pH. They also secrete rennin in young animals, to facilitate digestion of milk. Carbonic anhydrase acting on CO_2 produces carbonic acid that provides the H^+ for excretion. Both Cl^- and H^+ are actively secreted into the lumen with water following an osmotic gradient. Food material in the gastric lumen, vagus nerve stimulation, gastric distention, and gastrin released from neuroendocrine G-cells stimulate the parietal cells to release H$^+$. Stimulation of chief cells to release pepsinogen comes from vagal nerve stimulation, high H$^+$ concentrations, gastrin, and secretin released from the duodenum. The majority of gastric glands produce acid and enzymes (e.g., pepsin), but in the antrum, mucosal glands produce mainly mucus. Cells of the gastric glands also release arachidonic acid metabolites (e.g., prostaglandins of the E series) that facilitate gastroprotection.

Intermixed with the gastric gland epithelium are enteroendocrine cells of neural crest origin. Enteroendocrine cells are usually located between the basement membrane and chief cells. The granules of enteroendocrine cells can only be visualized by silver-based stains. These cells synthesize, store, and secrete hormones in response to autonomic and intralumenal stimuli. There are at least 10 different enteroendocrine cell populations that exist in the GI tract mucosa. Enteroendocrine cells secrete serotonin, histamine, enteroglucagon (A cells), and gastrin (G cells).

Replication of mucosal epithelial cells in the stomach is somewhat different from that of the rest of the GI tract. Unlike the replication of cryptal cells in the intestines and basal cells in the esophagus, gastric mucosal cell replication occurs in the neck of the gastric glands, and differentiation proceeds both up to the surface and down into the base of the glands.

The next layer of the gastric mucosa, immediately below the epithelium, is the lamina propria. This layer is separated from the gastric epithelial cells by a basement membrane. The lamina propria of the cardia and pylorus contains high numbers of lymphocytes and plasma cells. These immune cells are abundant throughout the gastric mucosa and submucosa, and the pyloric propria may contain numerous lymphoid follicles, even in the healthy animal. This lymphoid tissue can markedly enlarge in disease states that involve antigenic stimulation.

The lamina muscularis mucosae separate the mucosa from the submucosa. The submucosa is composed of a loose reticular connective tissue matrix, supporting many blood vessels, lymphatic channels, and nerves. Peripheral to the submucosa, three smooth muscle layers constitute the tunica muscularis, which encircles the stomach. In spite of many macroscopic variations, the microscopic arrangement of the stomach is similar in all species. The mucosa rests on the submucosa, and these two layers are surrounded by a muscular coat (tunica muscularis) that is covered by the single mesothelial cell layer of the serosa.

Small Intestine

Function

This segment of the GI tract is primarily responsible for secretion and absorption of nutrients. In addition, the small intestine acts as a barrier to the passage of luminal contents (bacteria and nonabsorbed compounds) into the body, serves as a conduit for unneeded (or unwanted) ingesta to pass out of the body, and biotransforms xenobiotics. Numerous anatomical peculiarities increase the functional capacity of the small intestine, including its long length, linear plicae, circular plicae (valves of Kerkring), villi, and microvilli. These characteristics greatly enhance mucosal surface area, and can also modify the transit time of a compound through the GI tract. Relative to the stomach and large intestine, passage time through the small intestine is relatively rapid (a few hours).

Between the proximal and distal small intestine, a functional gradient of ion and water transport occurs which controls the movement of fluids and electrolytes. In the proximal small intestine, passive movement of sodium and water is from the blood to the GI tract lumen. In contrast, fluid and sodium movement is from the lumen to the blood in the distal small intestine of most species. However, net secretion occurs in the ileum and jejunum of guinea pigs, the ileum of rabbits, and the proximal portion of the jejunum in neonatal swine. The caudal small intestine for the most part absorbs sodium, chloride, and bicarbonate against an electrochemical gradient; however, this is decreased as the animal ages. Bile salts are primarily absorbed in the ileum.

Structure

The small intestine constitutes the majority of the GI tract's length. Major structural features of the small intestine vary little among different species. The general microscopic organization of the small intestine is similar to that of the stomach: three distinct layers (mucosa, submucosa, and tunica muscularis) surrounded by a thin reticular connective tissue serosa. Small intestinal mucosal morphology reflects its absorptive function, and can be artificially divided into two zones: villi for absorptive and enzyme release functions; and crypts for secretion and replacement (Figure 8.2D, F).

Crypt-depth to villus-height ratios do vary among species, however, and knowing these differences may be essential to assess the true degree of intestinal damage resulting from a toxic compound. The distance from the base of the crypt to the base of the villus is delineated by a "shoulder" at the crypt–villus junction (Figure 8.2D). This juncture can be used to demarcate the transition between the crypt and villus, and to estimate both crypt depth and villus height. The crypt-depth to villus-height ratio in the proximal small intestine ranges from a small 1:7 ratio in the pig, to a larger 1:2 ratio in the dog. This ratio varies with the extent of food material in the lumen and lumenal distention, and thus is not constant even in normal animals.

Villus height progressively decreases from proximal to distal small intestine. Villi are covered by mature and senescent epithelial cells (enterocytes) that have migrated along the basement membrane that rests on the connective tissue, the lamina propria. The center of the villus has a blind-ended lymph vessel or lacteal that is surrounded by an elaborate capillary bed subjacent to the epithelial basement membrane. These lymphatic vessels serve to carry fat-soluble compounds to the systemic circulation, thus by-passing hepatic metabolism.

The cells lining the mucosa of the small intestine are primarily composed of simple columnar enterocytes covering the villi, and a more cuboidal epithelium lining the crypts (Table 8.1). Enterocytes have extensive apical microvilli that are relatively "tall" (approximately 11 nm). Enterocytes also have multiple biotransforming and metabolizing enzymes on the luminal surface. The thickness and composition of this enzyme-rich apical membrane is maintained by cytoskeletal elements (microtubules) and the presence of tight junctions at the lateral membrane-junctional complexes.

Enterocytes originate from the small intestinal crypts which surround the base of each villus. These enterocytes progressively move along the side of the villus toward the tip. As senescent enterocytes slough from the tips of the villi, the absorptive epithelium is replaced from below by dividing epithelial cells. Most extensive replication occurs in the cells immediately above the bottom 4–6 cells in the crypt. Each crypt produces 300–400 cells per day from a relatively few stem cells that produce committed daughter cells, which in turn divide several more times in the lower and middle portions of the crypt. Negative feedback mechanisms coordinate the rate of cell proliferation in the crypts with the rate of mature cell loss at the villus tip. Epithelial cells of the small and large intestine are replaced every 2–4 days in the adult, but replacement takes longer in the neonate. Each crypt also generates terminally-differentiated goblet cells and Paneth cells as needed.

Intestinal crypt cells secrete fluids and electrolytes. These secretions are then reabsorbed by enterocytes, which absorb simple carbohydrates, amino acids, and some xenobiotics, and then actively transport the absorbed substances, with little processing, into subjacent capillaries in the lamina propria. Transport of electrolytes across enterocyte apical membranes occurs by multiple mechanisms. Uniport mechanisms move a single ion (e.g., sodium), symport systems move two ions simultaneously in the same direction (e.g., sodium and chloride), and antiports are ion exchangers which move two ions in opposite directions (e.g., sodium and hydrogen). The sodium–chloride symport system can be blocked by acetazolamide, and is sensitive to agents stimulating adenylate cyclase. These systems frequently require ATP, and are stimulated by cAMP, cGMP, or increased levels of intracellular calcium. Fluid transport is also modulated by neurotransmitters, like serotonin (increased secretion) and neuropeptide Y (increased absorption).

Toxicologic damage to membrane-bound proteins can influence the viability of mucosal epithelial cells, and the nutritional status of the animal. Within the apical membrane are proteins that consist of intimately membrane-associated calcium-magnesium-dependent ATPases and alkaline phosphatases, as well as less tightly held lactases, sucrases, maltases, and leucine aminopeptidases. The less tightly held enzymes are responsible for digestive processes, while the more tightly held ATPases control cell viability. In the thinner lateral membranes (approximately 7 nm thick) a ouabain-sensitive sodium-potassium ATPase is found in higher concentrations than in the apical surface. This enzyme is tightly linked to glucose absorption.

Other less numerous epithelial cells, such as goblet cells, are scattered among the absorptive columnar cells of the villi. The numbers of goblet cells increase in the villus mucosa from proximal to distal small intestine. The thin mucus layer which coats the surface of gastric, intestinal, and colonic mucosa is an important part of the mucosal barrier. Mucus serves as a protectant against digestive enzyme degradation, as a barrier against passage of large macromolecules, and as a lubricant to aid in the passage of ingesta through the tract.

Lysozyme- and peptidase-rich Paneth cells are found near the base of the crypts, associated with the proliferating cells. There is no known dietary or environmental factor which controls this distribution (Table 8.1). Paneth cells are found in monkeys, mice, rats, hamsters, guinea pigs, ruminants, and horses, but not in dogs, cats, swine, or raccoons. In those species which have these cells, there is an increase in Paneth cell number from duodenum to ileum. The Paneth cell secretes mercury and other heavy metals into the intestinal lumen. These cells become necrotic in chronic methylmercury intoxication of primates.

M cells are located in the surface epithelium overlying the lymphoid tissues of the intestinal tract (Figure 8.2I). These cells are recognized by the microfolds (not present in rats) on their lumenal surface, and are highly phagocytic. They are responsible for antigen sampling from the lumen contents, and for transfer of the antigen to T-lymphocytes and dendritic macrophages. Macrophages can also present antigens to T-lymphocytes in the dome region of the follicle. The M cells not only serve to shuttle antigenic material from the lumen to the mucosal immune system, but can also function as an access route for pathogenic microbes and particulate toxic agents (e.g., asbestos). Absorptive epithelial cells may also function as antigen-presenting cells, especially for soluble proteins. Enterocytes express class II major histocompatability complex (MHC) antigens, and are capable of stimulating T-cell activation and proliferation. Enterocytes may process soluble antigens, while M cells may be primarily responsible for processing particulate antigens.

Lymphocytes, plasma cells, mucosal mast cells, and eosinophils are present throughout the lamina propria, within the villi and around the crypts. The numbers of these cells increase with age. Most T-lymphocytes within the lamina propria are CD4+ helper/inducer cells, consistent with the concept that the GI tract represents a site of primary antigen exposure to the host. Although most of the cells in the lamina propria function in a similar manner as those in other regions of the body, the mucosal mast cell is functionally different from mast cells in other tissues. It does not have membrane-bound IgE, and responds to T-cell stimulation rather than to binding of antigen to surface IgE.

Large Intestine

Function

Major functions of the large intestine include storage of digesta for further breakdown or excretion, absorption of specific nutrients, and absorption/secretion of water and electrolytes. One of the main electrolyte absorbing processes is through the Na^+–K^+-dependent ATPase pathway. Herbivores secrete large volumes of salivary, pancreatic, and biliary fluids, and in horses (perissodactyls) the large intestine secretes additional fluids equivalent to 40% of the extracellular fluid volume. However, 98% of the fluid and ions secreted in the upper GI tract are reabsorbed in the cecum and colon. This reabsorptive process is critical in understanding toxicologically-induced diarrheas. The colon has very limited protein absorbing activity relative to the small intestine, but does absorb a small amount of the total body protein needs.

Although the large intestine serves as the major site of digesta retention, the duration and primary site of retention varies widely among species. Rate of passage of digesta is inversely related to the degree of colonic compartmentalization. Additionally, the normal retrograde propulsive activity of the colon may delay the passage of a toxic compound, and prolong exposure of a toxicant to various biotransforming enzymes. The high concentration of bacteria in the colon facilitates roughage digestion and compound biotransformation. Although bacterial metabolism is critical for nutrition and influences toxicologic processes, the role of bacteria in colonic physiology and toxicology has received relatively limited study.

Structure

Macroscopic morphology of the large intestine varies widely among species. A wide variety of anatomical modifications are present in relation to relative length, diameter, volume, and structural complexity of this organ. The secretory and absorptive capacity of the large intestine is also related to anatomical complexity and the need for the animal to conserve water.

Cecum

Cecal structure varies considerably among different animal species, and can be relatively quite large in some (e.g., rabbits, horses, rats). The primary function of the cecum is for microbial fermentation and storage of ingesta. Intralumenal ingesta can be passed back and forth from the cecum to the proximal large intestine, before continuing its passage down the intestinal tract. The cecal lumen contains many bacteria that are metabolically active in detoxifying or bioactivating ingested compounds and producing essential vitamins. Some aspects of antimicrobial toxicity are directly related to the modification of normal cecal microflora. The cecal mucosa (Figure 8.2G) is similar to that of the colon, and the submucosa contains lymphoid tissue that functions like Peyer's patches of the small intestine. Animals with large and functionally active ceca may have significantly different compound passage rates than species with a rudimentary cecum (e.g., rats versus dogs). Such information must be incorporated into the design of animal model studies.

Colon

The mucosa of the colon and cecum is significantly different from the mucosa of the small intestine. Goblet cells are abundant in the colonic mucosa (Figure 8.2H), and are responsible for adding mucus to the dehydrated ingesta. Villi are not present in the colon and cecum; only crypts lined by colonocytes (of mostly goblet cell morphology) are present. Inflammation of the colon can lead to epithelial metaplasia, which reduces mucus production and renders the mucosa prone to bleeding, partially due to the loss of protective mucus.

The submucosa, tunica muscularis, and serosa of the large intestine are similar to those of the small intestine, containing a mixture of lymphocytes, plasma cell, and macrophages, as well as capillaries, but lacking lacteals. The terminal end of the large intestine (rectum) is located retroperitoneally in the pelvic canal, and is not covered by a serosa.

Enteric Lymphoid System

The GI immune response is multifactorial, and involves both cellular and humoral immune mechanisms. Immunologic response of the GI tract is predominantly mediated by immunoglobulin isotype A (IgA), both with and without secretory component (sIgA) (Figure 8.3). The GI tract mucosa contains many IgA-producing plasma cells. IgA is ultimately released into the mucus layer on the luminal surface of the intestine. Additionally, cell-mediated immune mechanisms are involved in the mucosal response to toxic compounds. Cell-mediated immunity of the mucosa is distinctly different from that of nonmucosal sites. In the GI tract the columnar absorptive cells, as well as M cells of the small intestine, can function as antigen-presenting cells, Ia-antigen carriers, and activators of T-lymphocytes. Consequently, immune mechanisms in the GI tract involve multiple pathways for response to toxic compounds, which may include hypersensitivity.

Also located throughout the small intestine are lymphoid aggregates called Peyer's patches (Figure 8.2I). Peyer's patches represent the organized portion of the GI immune system, and are part of the GI-associated lymphoid tissue (GALT). The GALT composes over 25% of the body's total lymphoid mass. Peyer's patches can be composed of only a few lymphocytes, or may be well-developed lymphoid nodules with many active germinal centers (secondary follicles). They may be within the lamina propria mucosae or within the submucosa. The stronger the antigenic stimulus, the more extensive will be the response and development of the nodule. Nodules consist of follicular and parafollicular regions. Follicles are composed of B-cell-rich germinal centers. Germinal centers are surrounded by T-cells in the parafollicular area, and are capped by a dome of lymphocytes that extends up and into the specialized

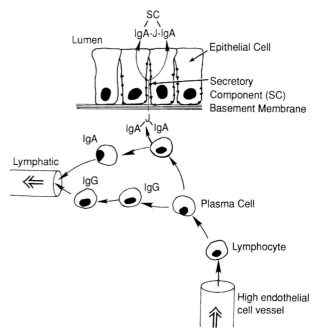

FIGURE 8.3 Schematic drawing of GI mucosal immunity the intestinal tract. The primary antibody response of the GI tract is of the IgA isotype. Monoclonal antibodies to IgA and a peroxidase-labeled secondary antibody allows the *in situ* localization of the IgA (A) present in inflamed gastric mucosal epithelial cells (E) and immunoglobulin-producing plasma cells (P). Non-immunoglobulin-A-producing plasma cells (N) are also present. Bar = 50μm. Immunoglobulin A released by plasma cells is released in a dimeric form held together by the J piece (J). Secretory component (SC) is added to the dimer on passage from the lamina propria to the lumen. This component allows the immunoglobulin to resist enzymatic degradation.

M-cell-rich epithelial covering (Figure 8.2I). GALT complexes are most extensively developed in the small intestine, but lymphoglandular complexes in the colon are also an important part of the GALT complex. Lymphoglandular complexes of the colon have germinal centers in the submucosa, but they have deep invaginations of mucosal epithelium. As in Peyer's patches, M cells partially line the surface of these complexes, and lymphocytes are closely apposed to these phagocytic cells.

When the GALT is activated, lymphocyte traffic through Peyer's patches increases. Primed and activated T- and B-lymphocytes migrate to mesenteric lymph nodes via the thoracic duct to high-endothelial-cell lined postcapillary venules (HEV), and then into intestinal lymphoid tissue. Tissue specificity of the T- and B-cells is determined by interaction with the endothelial cells of the HEV. The lamina propria not directly occupied by Peyer's patches is, nevertheless, rich in lymphoid and nonlymphoid immune cells. The ability of the immune system to respond to microbial, chemical, and dietary antigens helps prevent these agents from entering the body. GI tract mucosal hypersensitivity can be induced by circumventing the normal process in which a toxic compound is handled by the immune system. This can be done by co-administering a mucosa-damaging agent and the antigenic compound.

Lymph flows from the central lacteal to Peyer's patches, and then to many different lymph nodes, including mesenteric, pancreatic, gastric, hepatic, splenic, and colonic nodes. Lymph contains absorbed lipids, fat-soluble compounds, and recirculating lymphocytes. Some of the circulating lymphocytes have already been primed by antigen exposure, and are migrating to other mucosal sites that include the respiratory or genital tracts. This allows immune cells exposed to antigens in the GI tract to localize at other sites of the common mucosal immune system that may also be exposed to environmental toxins.

Enteric Nervous System

The nervous tissue of the GI tract is diffuse, but nevertheless highly-organized. Various motor and sensory neurons ramify throughout the wall of the GI tract, and form multiple plexuses. Nerve fibers vary in thickness and emanate from these plexuses, carrying information from one ganglion to another, and from intrinsic to extrinsic neurons.

The nervous tissue of the GI tract differs from other portions of the autonomic nervous system, because many of its neurons do not receive direct input from the central nervous system. Rather, neural information comes both from autonomic motor neurons (sympathetic and parasympathetic), and from GI sensory neurons. This results in reflex activities that act independently of the brain or spinal cord, although these basic activities can be modified by CNS input.

Neurons of the parasympathetic ganglia are in both the submucosal (Meissner's) plexus and the myenteric (Auerbach's) plexus. The myenteric plexus is responsible for the electrical rhythms of the GI tract, but is not needed for propagation of the myoelectric complex that results in peristalsis. The myenteric and submucosal plexuses are interconnected to form a single functional unit, so integration of electrical activity occurs at multiple locations in the GI tract. Parasympathetic stimulation of the GI tract leads to increased blood flow, secretions, and muscular activity. Stimulation by the sympathetic nervous system has the opposite effects. The enteric nervous tissue is also composed of integrative circuits that consist of interneurons within ganglia that process information from intramural and mucosal sensory receptors. Sensory neurons detect fluidity, volume, chemical composition, and temperature of the lumenal contents.

Specific motor neurons release neurotransmitters in the proximity of mucosal effectors, blood vessels, and muscle layers. In addition, receptors for neurotransmitters are present on and near the epithelial cells. The spatial density of myenteric neurons decreases with age.

There are three principal motility patterns of the GI tract: storage; mixing; and propulsion. Movement of a swallowed bolus of food from mouth to stomach to intestine is a propulsive event, caudally progressing in front of a contractile ring of circular smooth muscle. Gastric emptying requires coordinated propulsive contraction in the antrum, with concomitant relaxation of the upper duodenum. Contractions of smooth muscle in the GI tract occur more or less randomly, but are somewhat fixed in timing and location by the electrical slow waves or electrical control activity generated initially in interstitial cells. Propulsive contractions occur somewhat randomly, migrating clustered contraction associated with contractile rings that move caudally from 5–30 cm, thus propelling content toward the cecum. Migrating motor complexes are bands of contractile activity that move caudally from stomach to small intestine during fasting, to sweep digested food remains out of the stomach until another meal is consumed. The central nervous system exerts some degree of control over the activity of these complexes, but they are initiated in the enteric nervous system.

Biotransformation

The mucosa of the GI tract is a site of high enzymatic activity and compound conjugation (Figure 8.4). The mucosa is uniquely located so that it is exposed to the highest concentration of orally administered compounds and can modify these compounds prior to their entry into the blood. The consequences of mucosal biotransformation are compound metabolism, and activation, or deactivation (detoxification). This process can therefore lead to an increase or decrease in a compound's toxicity.

Intestinal mucosal enzymes that metabolize xenobiotics can prevent systemic absorption of many potentially toxic substances. Presystemic clearance can occur for some toxicants, either within the enterocyte or within the gut lumen itself. Gut-associated first pass effect represents the irreversible extraction and/or biotransformation of toxicants passing through enterocytes on their way into the lacteal or portal venous blood. Metabolites produced by enterocyte biotransformation can enter the intestinal lumen, the portal venous system, lacteals, or simply remain stored in the cell. Conjugated water-soluble compounds formed during transport into enterocytes tend to be excreted relatively quickly into the intestinal lumen. Xenobiotic metabolism can also be carried out by luminal microorganisms.

Several toxin-metabolizing gradients exist in the GI tract (Figure 8.4). Cytochrome P450 activity in the small intestine provides the principal initial biotransformation of most ingested xenobiotics. Most P450 isozyme activity increases in enterocytes during migration from crypt to villus. Nearly all P450 activity is attributable to villus cells. Intestinal mucosa also contains nonspecific esterases, amidases, UPD-glucuronosyl transferases, sulfotransferases, reductases, and methylases. Both glucuronidation and sulfation increase the solubility of the conjugated xenobiotics, and thus play a major role in intestinal first-pass clearance. Cytochrome P450 and UDP-glucuronosyl transferase activities are higher in the upper duodenum than in the lower small intestine. In addition, sulfation proceeds more rapidly in the proximal than in the distal small intestine.

Overall biotransformation by coloncytes is low compared to the small intestine, with most activity in the proximal 1/3 of the colon. The colon, however,

is 3–5 times more active than the small intestine in certain enzymatic processes, such as demethylation. Biotransformation in the intestine is also inducible. Several compounds, such as polychlorinated biphenyls and phenobarbital, increase P450 levels in the intestinal mucosa 2–4 days after exposure; the effect is greatest after oral administration of the compound. This augmentation of enzyme activity is similar to that which occurs in the liver. As occurs in the liver, chronic intake of ethanol will also increase the level of activity of several intestinal enzyme pathways.

Besides altering the biological activities of toxicant, biotransformation reactions in enterocytes may influence the postabsorptive fate of xenobiotics. Compounds or their metabolites entering from the blood (basal) side can be found in the GI tract lumen, independent of enterohepatic circulation. Consequently, epithelial cells of the GI tract can absorb and remove compounds both from circulating blood and from the intestinal lumen, indicating that absorption is a "two-way street" for this epithelium. Excretion of xenobiotic metabolites into the intestinal lumen permits fecal excretion, and permits escape from enterohepatic circulation (see below).

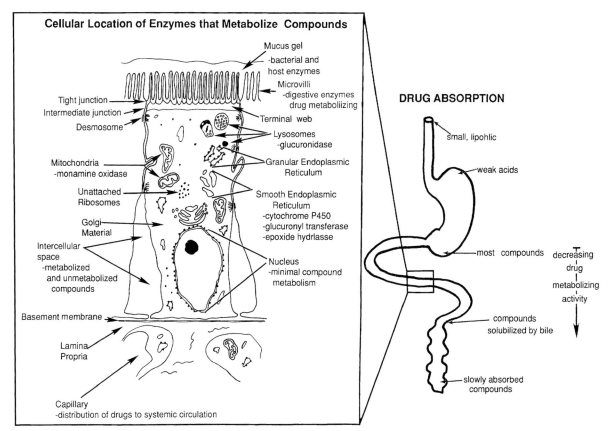

FIGURE 8.4 Biotransformation of compounds is a complex event involving absorption and metabolism gradients. Different sites of absorption will lead to different enzyme exposures. Compound solubility and transport mechanisms will result in contact with different enzymes.

Fecal excretion is a major route of elimination of many lipophilic xenobiotics, with most probably transferring by passive diffusion and a few others by excretion via non-biliary pathways. Rapid exfoliation of enterocytes also contributes to fecal excretion of some xenobiotics. In addition, excretion rates of highly-lipophilic xenobiotics can be enhanced by increasing the lipophilicity of GI contents.

Enhancement of carcinogenic activity by mucosal biotransformation may reflect incomplete metabolism of a toxic compound. In this case, the metabolized compound may form DNA-damaging intermediates, producing mutagenic molecules or superoxide anions. Dimethylhydrazine is an example of an organ-specific compound that undergoes only partial metabolism, and ultimately causes colon cancer.

Bacterial Metabolism

Ingested materials are metabolized not only by digestive and intestinal enzymes, but also by resident bacteria. GI bacteria have biotransformation enzymes that include reductases, hydrolases, demethylases, β-glucuronidases, and β-glucosidases. Since there are approximately 10^9–10^{12} bacteria per gram of feces in humans and animals, the potential enzymatic activity of this compartment of the GI tract cannot be ignored. The floral composition in mammals depends on the nutritional and health status of the host, and the host's dietary composition. Within the small intestine there is a gradual transition from sparse gram-positive microflora in the stomach, to progressively more gram-negative organisms in the ileum, to predominantly gram-negative organisms in the colon. Anaerobic bacteria outnumber aerobic species by a factor of 10^2–10^4. Anaerobic organisms include Bacteroides, Bifidobacteria, Eubacteria, gram-positive bacterial cocci and Clostridium species. Aerobic microflora includes Streptococcal and Staphylococcal bacteria, as well as yeast of the Candida group.

The influence of intestinal microbes on the host's nutritional status has been most clearly demonstrated using animals with and without gut bacteria. Consequently, overgrowth of intestinal bacteria can lead to steatorrhea, by modifying lipid absorption via hydrolysis of bile–acid conjugates and altering micelle-forming ability. Bacterial proteases also remove maltase from enterocyte brush border membranes, and cause carbohydrate malabsorption. Consequently, compounds altering microbial populations can lead to altered nutritional status.

The role of bacteria in GI toxicity is most clearly defined for carcinogen activation. Many chemical carcinogens (indirect acting) require enzymatic activation

before they can cause cellular transformation. Bacterial β-glucuronidases can deconjugate glucuronides, and lead to the release of carcinogenic aglycones. Additionally, fecal flora nitroreductases can activate procarcinogens. Bacteria also have a direct role in the detoxification process. Bacteria can deactivate carcinogens by N-dehydroxylation.

Antibiotics can not only modify bacterial populations in the GI tract, but can also directly depress neuro-effector and neuromuscular transmission. In vitro studies have demonstrated that ampicillin, lincomycin, erythromycin, and clindamycin depress contractions of the muscularis mucosa. Clindamycin and erythromycin depress the responses of the muscularis mucosa to acetylcholine. Impaired GI motility can also facilitate the proliferation of Clostridium difficile, and lead to pseudomembranous enterocolitis. These mechanisms may work in concert to induce antibiotic-associated colitis and cecal enlargement.

Various compounds from woody plants, mainly tannins and lignins, can greatly affect GI microflora. Microflora can be directly damaged by hydrolyzable tannins in oak (Quercus), for example, leading to impaired ruminal digestion, and even diarrhea.

Enterohepatic Circulation

Enterohepatic circulation allows for recycling of metabolized and nonmetabolized compounds, and is of critical importance in toxicologic processes involving the GI tract. This circulatory route is active when ingested compounds that are absorbed in the GI tract enter the portal circulation, go to the liver, and then return to the GI tract via biliary excretion. The enterohepatic circulatory pathway can also be involved with excretion and recirculation of dermally-absorbed or inhaled materials that are excreted in the bile.

A compound leaves the enterohepatic circulation if it passes out in the feces before being reabsorbed, or passes into the urine before being cleared by the liver. The ultimate destiny of a compound is dependent on the chemical composition and species of animal being studied. The importance of species differences is best illustrated by the nonsteroidal anti-inflammatory drug (NSAID) indomethacin, which undergoes enterohepatic circulation; it is excreted in the feces of dogs, but in the urine of rats. The duration of enterohepatic circulation is most extensive for this drug in dogs and rats, and least extensive in rabbits and humans.

The amount of compound that is excreted in the feces is controlled by its lipophilicity, and the extent to which it is metabolism alters its lipophilic character. Processes that increase the aqueous nature of a compound (i.e., decrease its lipophilicity) include dealkylation, glucuronidation, and sulfation, while those that increase lipophilicity (and decrease water solubility) include glucuronide hydrolysis. The rate at which a chemical is excreted in the feces is limited by the time it takes for a compound to be excreted in the bile and reabsorbed by the intestine. Factors that modify this excretion rate include motility of the intestine, distance of the site of (re)absorption from the major duodenal papilla (site of common bile duct excretion), rate of conjugate hydrolysis by GI bacteria, transport rate across the intestinal wall, and motility of the gall bladder in species which have this structure. With the exception of gall bladder motility, all factors influence intestinal transit time.

When the portal burden of a compound exceeds the liver's ability to extract it, the material will pass through the liver and enter the caudal vena cava. A compound's extractability from the blood may be altered after it has been metabolized by GI bacteria or the enteric mucosa, and then reabsorbed from the GI tract. Consequently, on reabsorption, such a metabolite may be less likely to be cleared by the liver.

Combined biotransformational processes in the liver and intestine can substantially affect the toxicity of a compound. The activation of diphenolic laxatives by microbial metabolism and conjugate hydrolysis has been clearly established. Bacteria can also modify dinitrotoluene by nitro-reduction, and give rise to elevated hepatic levels of the carcinogenic metabolite. Arylamines formed from the biliary metabolite of chloramphenicol may be responsible for the goitrogenic effect of this antibiotic in rats. Hydrolysis of polycyclic aromatic hydrocarbon (PAH) glucuronide metabolites demonstrates how enterohepatic circulation can retoxify a detoxified compound.

During enterohepatic circulation, compounds may interact with intestinal contents. This is demonstrated by the binding of bile salts to dietary fibers. Such binding will decrease the reabsorption of bile salts, and may be partially responsible for the healthful effects of soluble fibers. Alteration of bile acid circulation can influence the hepatobiliary level of several compounds which are bile soluble (cholephilic). In addition, taurocholate promotes motor activity in the colon, thereby reducing intestinal transit time. Bile acids also increase the transport of compounds across the intestinal mucosa, and may consequently enhance the toxic properties of a compound.

Enterohepatic circulation will increase xenobiotic toxicity to other organs in the enterohepatic circuit, if the compound remains active during circulation. The concentrating capacity of enterohepatic recycling may play an important role in the ulcerogenic effects of nonsteroidal anti-inflammatory drugs (NSAIDs) such as indomethacin in dogs. This same process may be important in the carcinogenic effects of colon carcinogens 3,3-dimethoxybenzidine and tris(2,3-dibromopropyl)phosphate. Biliary excretion and enterohepatic circulation have a role in colon carcinogenesis of rats induced by 2,3-dimethyl-4-aminobiphenyl (DMAB). Rats treated orally with this carcinogen excrete mutagenic agents in the bile. However, rats injected subcutaneously with DMAB do not develop colonic neoplasms.

COMPARATIVE MECHANISMS OF GASTROINTESTINAL TOXICITY

Basic functions of the GI tract include digesting and metabolizing ingested material, absorbing required nutrients (including water), and acting as a barrier. Any impairment of these basic functions will result in pathophysiological alterations to homeostasis and disease. Because the GI tract is involved in transport of nutrients, it is especially prone to injury through processes that alter absorptive functions. Additional mechanisms that can cause severe disruption of GI homeostasis include reduced blood supply or hypoxia, acid build-up and damage to the mucosal barrier, hypersensitivity reactions, and genotoxicity leading to cancer development. At a cellular level, injury to the plasma membrane and mitochondria will lead to the demise of the affected cell. At a tissue level, the difference between developing a superficial or deep mucosal lesion depends on the extent of involvement of the subepithelial capillaries and supporting stroma. In this section, general toxicologic mechanisms are discussed and summarized in Table 8.3. Several model toxicants are also discussed to illustrate these various processes.

Intestinal Barrier Function

Most ingested toxicants enter the body through the intestine, either by passing through the enterocytes or by passive paracellular diffusion. Large and polar molecules pass poorly through epithelial tight junctions, unless the epithelial barrier is disrupted (as with a high dose of ethanol). Small electroneutral molecules pass easily around the epithelial cells and into the portal circulation, but polar molecules cannot pass through the lipid barrier of the cell. Nonionized molecules can diffuse through the cell membrane into the enterocyte. Once in the enterocyte, a xenobiotic may be pumped back out of the cell by a multipurpose

TABLE 8.3   Mechanisms of toxicity to the gastrointestinal tract with selected examples

Mechanism	Xenobiotic
Altered secretion/absorption	
• Reduced nutrient absorption	Ethanol, cholestyramine, clofibrate, antimitotic agents (blunted villi), kanamycin, neomycin, polymycin, sulfosalazine, heavy metals (cadmium), plant extracts (e.g., tobacco leaf extract), NSAIDs, quinacrine, phenolphthalein, phenytoin, triparanol, phenformin, hydrolyzable tannins, proanthocyanidins
• Altered solute/water transport	*E. coli* toxins, shigatoxin, cholera toxin secretagogues; laxatives (e.g., $MgSO_4$, oil, castor oil), nonabsorbable and nonfermentable fiber (osmotic agents)
Altered blood supply	
• Blocked cyclooxygenase activity	NSAIDs (e.g., phenylbutazone, aspirin, ibuprofen, indomethacin), cadmium
• Decreased perfusion, hypoxia	Agents which induce hemorrhagic or hypovolemic shock
• Damage to endothelium	Arsenates, mercurials
Altered mucosal barrier	
• Direct epithelial damage	Bile acids, ethanol, deoxycholic acid, cadmium, hydrolyzable tannins (e.g., quercetin), *Clostridium difficile* toxin, heavy metals and metalloids, corrosive agents (i.e., caustic agents and strong acids)
• Depletion of essential sulfhydryls (e.g., cysteine, glutathione)	Ethyl acrylate, arsenates, mercurials
• Uncoupled oxidative phosphorylation	NSAIDs (i.e., aspirin), arsenates, mercurials
• Decreased synthesis of cytoprotective prostaglandins	NSAIDs, corticosteroids, cadmium
• Decreased mucus production	Corticosteroids, NSAIDs
• Altered proliferative activity of crypt cells (leading to villous atrophy)	Ionizing radiation, T-2 toxin, ricin, antimitotic agents (e.g., colchicine, 5′-fluorouracil, methotrexate), arsenates
Altered neuromuscular activity	
• Inhibition of effective peristalsis (hypomotility)	Opiates (e.g., morphine), erythromycin
• Enhanced peristalsis (hypermotility)	Organophosphate insecticides (e.g., parathion, malathion, paraoxon), nerve gases (sarin, tabu, soman), solanine (potatoes, tomatoes, and others), xanthine derivative (e.g., theobromine in chocolate)
• Induction of emesis	Cisplatin, opiates (centrally-mediated); cyclophosphamide, carnustine, dactinomycin, cisplatin (locally-mediated)
• Neurogenic atrophy	Anthraquinone
Hypersensitivity	
• Increased absorption of antigens (i.e., increased potential for hypersensitivity)	Polyvinyl chloride, metallic iron, asbestos, trinitrobenzenesulfonic acid
Increased proliferation	
• Hormonally-mediated	TCDD (dioxin), polychlorinated biphenyls, nonabsorbable, nonfermentable fiber
• Neoplastic transformation	Ptaquilosides (bracken fern), azoxymethane, hydrazine derivatives, aromatic amines, cholanthrenes, alkylnitrosamines, aflatoxin B_1, poligeenan, dextran sulfate

transporter (e.g., P-glycoprotein), biotransformed by cellular enzymes into an inactive (or reactive) metabolite, or transferred into the lymph or portal circulation.

Compounds (either nutrients or xenobiotics) that do not have specific transporters are absorbed passively around the enterocytes. Tight junctions between enterocytes are very permeable in the proximal small intestine, but become less so in the ileum. There is a net secretion of ~7 liters of fluid into the jejunum from biliary, pancreatic, and intestinal secretions in humans. Intestinal secretion is due to paracellular flow or water drawn into the lumen of the intestine by the high osmotic load in the ingesta. The fluid is then absorbed in the ileum and colon, as nutrients and electrolytes are absorbed against a concentration gradient via a variety of pumps, exchanges, and channels. As electrolytes are transported out of the gut lumen, water is also reabsorbed. When nutrients or electrolytes are not absorbed, there is an increase in luminal liquid that results in diarrhea.

Intestinal Malabsorption

A number of transport pathways exist in the GI tract that can carry materials across the mucosal epithelium. These mechanisms include active transport, facilitated diffusion or solvent drag, passive diffusion, pinocytosis, and phagocytosis. Most nutrients are absorbed by active transport mechanisms, in contrast to most toxicants which are transported by a passive diffusion process. Consequently, greater lipid solubility (lipophilicity) of a toxicant will enhance absorption. In addition, smaller molecules diffuse more rapidly, and the nonionized forms of acids and bases are absorbed more rapidly than ionized forms. A significant exception to this generalization includes the active transport of inorganic lead by calcium carrier mechanisms.

Malabsorption results from alterations in epithelial transport mechanisms, reduction in surface area (e.g., villus blunting from antimitotic agents), or binding of nutrients or compounds to unabsorbed intestinal contents (e.g., modified bile salt absorption by cholestyramine) (Table 8.3). Reduced nutrient absorption can be mediated by various toxins, including heavy metals, hydrolyzable tannins, proanthocyanins, and alkaloid-rich plant extracts. Cadmium interferes with or inhibits the absorption of calcium and alters digestion of protein and fat. Tobacco-leaf extracts reduce the activity of the loosely held intestinal brush border enzymes lactase, sucrase, maltase, and alkaline phosphatase. Proanthocyanins from wood plants can bind carbohydrates and proteins, decreasing the availability of these essential nutrients. When enzymes involved in the metabolism of complex carbohydrates are damaged, the GI epithelial cells are unable to absorb carbohydrate-derived nutrients. Malabsorption of carbohydrates and amino acids results in malnutrition, vitamin deficiencies, and osmotic diarrhea.

Toxic compounds can alter solute transport across or between mucosal epithelial cell membranes. By damaging junctional complexes between enterocytes, interfering with hydrostatic pressure gradients, or causing high lumenal osmotic pressure, a toxic compound can contribute to net water loss in the feces and lead to diarrhea. Some bacterial toxins (E. coli toxins and shigatoxin) and laxative compounds act as secretagogues and promote water loss into the lumen, eventually leading to diarrhea.

GI toxicity can also be mediated by an increased absorption of nutrients or toxic compounds. Increased toxicity of organophosphates in young mice compared with older mice is the result of an increased rate of absorption of the toxic compound.

Particulate materials may be taken up by pinocytosis (nanometer-sized particles) or phagocytosis. In mice, phagocytosis is limited to particles smaller than 6 μm in diameter. Particulate uptake plays an important role in pathological responses to polyvinyl chloride, metallic iron, and asbestos. The passage of these particles through the protective mucosal epithelium of the GI tract can lead to allergic hypersensitivity reactions, or the entry of unmetabolized compounds directly into the lymphatic and blood circulation.

Altered Blood Supply

Stomach

Hypoxia is a key factor in the pathogenesis of GI mucosal injury. This is manifested by the development of mucosal lesions in various types of shock. Thus, any toxicosis which causes shock has the potential to induce GI injury damage, whether it is directly injurious to the mucosa or not. As a general rule, the degree of mucosal damage is correlated with the extent of reduction of blood flow, even with direct toxic insults. Decreased blood flow and decreased oxygen exchange can occur locally, due to a specific toxicant, and increase the susceptibility of the mucosa to injury. For example, a local reduction in blood flow due to vascular thrombosis occurs in gastric injury induced by absolute ethanol. If the damage is confined to the epithelium only, leaving basement membrane and underlying lamina propria intact, then erosion occurs. If damage is more profound, extending into or involving underlying lamina propria, then ulceration, a more serious situation, will occur. Hemorrhagic shock in rats leads to uniform blanching of the glandular mucosa of the stomach, and a generalized reduction in blood flow. Small white ischemic foci develop on the gastric mucosa that will ulcerate and bleed after the restoration of blood pressure. Ischemia predisposes the stomach to HCl-mediated mucosal lesions, because reduced blood flow causes a build-up of H^+ in the tissue. An increase in acid back-diffusion leads to further mucosal injury. It is the combination of these two events that causes severe mucosal damage (Figure 8.5).

Arachidonic acid metabolites are inflammatory mediators that can induce gastric damage. Thromboxane A2, formed by platelets, is a potent vasoconstrictor, and causes extensive mucosal damage in the presence of the bile salt, taurocholate. Platelet aggregation is also promoted by thromboxane A2, and can lead to vascular

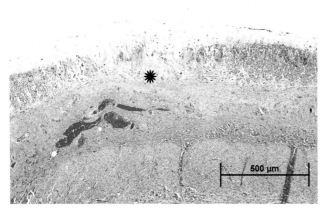

FIGURE 8.5   Gastric ulcer secondary to vascular thrombosis in a dog illustrating the loss of epithelium and lamina propria (*).

thrombosis and mucosal infarction. Both mechanisms can lead to tissue hypoxia, and are involved in the ulcerogenic effects of thromboxane. In contrast, some prostaglandins, such as PGE2 protect the mucosa from injury. Defense processes mediated through prostaglandins, such as PGE2, are thought to be a result of increased mucosal blood flow and an improved supply of oxygen.

Intestines

Ulcerative mucosal lesions can develop as a result of impaired villus microcirculation during hypotension. Hypoxia develops as a result of increased mean transit time for plasma in the villus vascular loop, which increases the efficiency of the countercurrent exchange mechanism in the villi of the GI mucosa. The time available for oxygen diffusion back into the blood is increased, resulting in reduced availability of oxygen at the villus tip. Rheological factors, such as intravascular aggregation of erythrocytes and platelets, can contribute to compromised oxygen transfer, especially when blood flow is already significantly reduced. Hypoxic injury is compounded by epithelial and intraluminal enzymes, such as trypsin, that can further damage compromised epithelial cells contributing to mucosal lesion development.

Nonsteroidal anti-inflammatory drugs (NSAIDs) have multiple mechanisms of toxicity, one of which involves altered blood flow. NSAIDs toxicosis is a two-stage sequence, the first being an early neutrophil-independent phase, and the latter being neutrophil-dependent or neutrophil-mediated. Early on, NSAIDs absorbed by the mucosal epithelium inhibit cyclooxygenase, the first enzyme in the prostaglandin synthetic pathway.

Two of the major isoforms of cyclooxygenase, COX-1 and COX-2, are inhibited to various degrees by individual NSAIDs. Inhibition of the inducible COX-2 is typically associated with the "beneficial" effects of NSAIDs, since COX-2 is the isoform associated with inflammation, being induced by a variety of inflammatory cytokines and proinflammatory mediators. Inhibition of COX-1, which is constitutively expressed in healthy tissues, is less beneficial, since this cyclooxygenase is responsible for the constitutive synthesis of prostaglandins, such as PGE2 and prostacyclin, both important in maintaining vascular tone and hence tissue perfusion. Furthermore, inhibition of cyclooxygenase shunts arachidonic acid metabolism preferentially down the lipooxygenase pathways, resulting in the increased production of proinflammatory leukotrienes, which cause vasoconstriction and promote neutrophil migration and activation, leading to enhanced potential for free radical damage and thrombosis of microvasculature.

Mucosal Barrier Damage and Cytotoxicity

Nonsteroidal Anti-inflammatory Drugs (NSAIDs)

In addition to their effects on blood flow, NSAIDs have other effects which substantially affect mucosal barrier function. NSAIDs adversely affect oxidative phosphorylation, which is uncoupled from electron transport in the mitochondria. This leads to decreased ATP production, and loss of ATP-dependent epithelial barrier function. Loss of barrier function leads to loss of protection against cytolytic bile salts, hydrogen ions, and bacterial toxins, and further mucosal damage. Neutrophil influx in response to the cellular damage and bacterial migration into the damaged tissue exacerbates the process of ongoing damage.

NSAIDs also alter acid production by the gastric parietal cells, as well as directly decreasing mucus production by goblet cells and bicarbonate secretion by pancreatic duct cells via a prostaglandin-independent mechanism. Loss of the mucus layer covering the apical surfaces of mucosal epithelium leaves both gastric and small intestinal epithelial cells prone to damage by unneutralized gastric acid. This damage is further exacerbated by activation of mucosal mast cells, which activate in response to luminal substances leaking into the mucosa past the damaged mucosal barrier, to cause edema, congestion, and exudation. All these various factors combine when toxic doses of NSAIDs are administered, either orally or parenterally, to produce typical multifocal to coalescing erythema, hemorrhage, erosion, and ulceration, along with subsequent inflammation, of the GI mucosa.

There are, however, marked species differences in sensitivity to the toxic effects of NSAIDs. Dogs are more sensitive to NSAID toxicosis than rats, which are more sensitive than monkeys. Yet, even though monkeys do not develop lesions after oral exposure to ibuprofen (300 mg/kg/day), they develop gastric ulcers when the same dose is given intravenously. Such species differences may be related in part to plasma half-life of the particular active compound. For example, the propionic acid NSAID flurbiprofen, which is toxic to dogs, has a half-life of approximately 40 hours in dogs, but only 6 hours in rats and 3 hours in monkeys, which are relatively resistant to toxicity. This demonstrates the relationship between ulcerogenic sensitivity and plasma half-life. Location of NSAIDs-induced GI lesions also shows species variation. The horse, for example, not only develops ulcers in the glandular portion of the stomach (Figure 8.6A), but also ulcerative lesions in the right dorsal colon (Figure 8.6B).

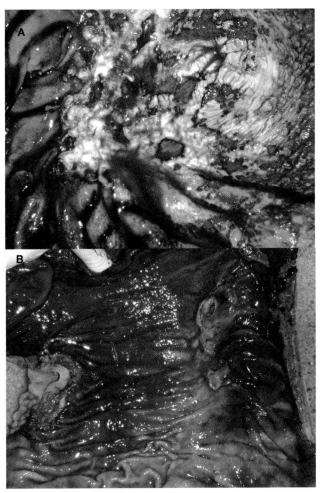

FIGURE 8.6 Gastric ulceration (A) and right dorsal colonic ulceration (B) in horses exposed to nonsteroidal anti-inflammatory drugs (NSAIDs).

Alcohol

Ethanol, like NSAIDs, causes hemorrhagic erosions in the gastric mucosa. Gastrotoxic effects of alcohols are related to their ability to increase cell membrane fluidity. Osmolality and lipid solubility are also involved, but to a lesser extent. Alcohol increases the permeability of the mucosa and causes back-diffusion of H^+, and a rise in luminal Na^+ concentrations. Depletion of the essential cellular antioxidant, glutathione, has been implicated in damage to mucosal cells, and levels of glutathione decline in proportion to the degree of alcohol injury. Treatment with glutathione depletors, such as N-ethylmaleimide, can prevent prostaglandin-mediated restoration of alcohol-induced mucosal injury.

As with NSAIDs, ethanol affects mucus and bicarbonate production. At low ethanol concentrations (10%) mucus synthesis and bicarbonate secretion are inhibited. At higher concentrations (12–15%) alcohol disperses surface mucus, depletes intracellular mucus, and promotes leakage of bicarbonate and electrolytes toward the gastric lumen.

The ultimate severity of lesion development, however, appears to be the extent of microvascular damage. At concentrations above 20% there are gastric erosions, the severity of which increases with increasing ethanol concentrations. At concentrations about 40% there is dose-dependent damage to the mucosal blood vasculature, leading to ulceration. Much of the vascular damage appears to be mediated by inflammation. Treatment with PGE2 experimentally can abolish ethanol-induced mucosal injury. As occurs with other mucosal damaging agents, injured epithelial cells are rapidly replaced if blood flow is maintained and the basement membrane remains intact.

Steroidal Compounds

Corticosteroids, like NSAIDs, also induce gastric and large intestinal mucosal alterations and damage, by altering cytoprotective mechanisms and the mucosal barrier. Long-term or high-dose steroids also induce gastric ulceration. Dogs given toxic levels of dexamethasone, a phospholipase inhibitor, develop gastric bleeding, erosions, and melena, as well as colonic ulcers that may perforate. These findings indicate that the mechanism for steroid-induced gastric lesions is partially mediated through inhibition of prostaglandin synthesis. Since the prostaglandin synthetase (cyclooxygenase) substrate arachidonic acid is reduced by inhibiting phospholipase activity, the mucosal protection provided by prostaglandins (e.g., PGE2) is lost, and gastric acid production proceeds uninhibited. In addition, production of protective gastric mucus is substantially decreased.

Bile Acids

Bile acids, and their derivatives, bile salts, are synthesized from cholesterol and function to act as emulsifiers to aid in digestion and absorption of dietary fats. However, bile salts can damage the GI tract mucosa. Bile acids are usually ionized, and occur in two forms: monomeric and micellar. Of the excreted bile acids, over 97% are reabsorbed in the ileum and returned to the liver via enterohepatic circulation. The remaining 3% undergo bacterial degradation in the colon, and are excreted in the feces or reabsorbed in the colon. GI bacteria deconjugate and desulfate bile salts, leading to the production of toxic/carcinogenic metabolites. Bile salt malabsorption during certain ileal diseases is implicated in colonic mucosal damage and diarrhea. Bile salts also stimulate colonic epithelial cell proliferation, and are capable of acting as tumor-promoters in the colon.

Bile salts induce the release of arachidonic acid, and the generation of cyclooxygenase and lipooxygenase metabolites of this fatty acid, leading to the secondary generation of active oxygen radicals. Bile salts also induce increased colonic secretion and permeability, but this occurs by mechanisms independent of endogenous arachidonic acid metabolism. Bile salts in the stomach break down gastric mucosal permeability, and solubilize the outer lipid bilayer of surface epithelium; deoxycholate inhibits active sodium transport from mucosa to submucosa. The basic mechanism of mucosal barrier damage in the stomach is similar for ethanol and deoxycholic acid.

Radiomimetic Agents

Radiomimetic compounds result in substantial cytotoxicity of mucosal epithelial cells. In this case, the mitotically active mucosal cells of the crypt are the specific targets. Ingestion of the trichothecene mycotoxin, T-2 toxin, results in widespread crypt epithelial necrosis and mucosal injury that resembles the effects of radiation exposure (Figures 8.7A, B). Necrosis of proliferating crypt cells eventually leads to loss of the remaining mucosal epithelium, as a result of continued cell senescence as enterocytes migrate up the villus and slough from the tips, with no replacement from the crypts below. Consequently, there is collapse of the mucosa, ulceration, hemorrhage, and secondary inflammation. Chemotherapeutic agents, such as colchicine and plant toxins (e.g., ricin from the castor bean), can cause similar lesions.

Dioxin

Mucosal hyperplasia has been associated with ingested chemicals, in particular 2,3,7,8-tetrachloro-dibenzo-p-dioxin (TCDD) and other related polychlorinated hydrocarbons. TCDD induces mucosal hyperplasia

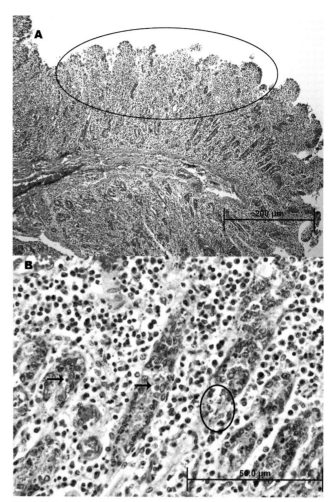

FIGURE 8.7   (A) T-2 mycotoxin-induced loss of intestinal villous epithelium (circled) secondary to crypt necrosis in a pig. Also present is engorgement of underlying capillaries and larger blood vessels in the underlying lamina propria. (B) Higher magnification image illustrating ongoing crypt cell apoptosis (arrows) and necrosis (circle).

in susceptible species, possibly by its delayed enhancement of serum gastrin levels, which then leads to a slow accumulation of gastric parietal cells.

Heavy Metals

Cellular damage to GI mucosa can occur by disrupting oxidative metabolism. Arsenates uncouple oxidative phosphorylation in the mitochondria, possibly by substituting for inorganic phosphate and forming unstable esters. Arsenic is stored in several body sites, one of which is the wall of the GI tract. Arsenicals cause GI hyperemia, and this, coupled with endothelial cell damage, leads to submucosal hemorrhage and hypoxia. Direct damage to epithelial cells, as well as suppression of epithelial cell proliferation, accentuates the damage and hemorrhagic enteritis develops. Inorganic mercurials produce a similar effect in the GI tract.

Cadmium also damages gastric mucosa, partly by damaging mucosal epithelial cells in the luminal portions of the mucosa, as well as parietal cells. This damage has been linked to lipid peroxidation, and results in decreased gastric acid and decreased mucin production, in addition to a decrease in overall epithelial cell number. Cadmium also acts partly by inhibition of PGE2 generation, hence affecting blood flow. A wide variety of heavy metals and metalloids can cause direct enterocyte damage and often necrosis in the GI tract (Table 8.4), usually by direct damage to membranes, or by several essential cellular biochemical processes.

Other Cytotoxic Compounds

Compounds that react by 1,4 addition at the β-olefinic carbon of some nucleophiles are cytotoxic. Cytotoxicity occurs because the cell is more susceptible to the reactive oxidation products that develop during normal metabolism of these types of compounds. Ethyl acrylate, for example, causes damage in the rat forestomach through depletion of sulfhydryl groups found in cysteine, glutathione, and thiol-containing peptides. Glutathione is the dominant sulfhydryl-containing constituent of epithelial cells that protects them from oxidative damage. An excessive oxidative burden, with resultant glutathione depletion, leads not only to cellular lipid and protein peroxidation, but also to genetic damage. Hydrolyzable tannins, as well as proanthocyanidins from woody plants, can be directly toxic to GI epithelial cells. This is in addition to their adverse effects on gut microflora and nutrient absorption. This cytotoxic effect, on occasion leading to hemorrhagic gastroenteritis, is especially manifest in monogastric species, but also occurs in ruminants.

A large number of plants can cause GI toxicity in herbivorous and omnivorous domestic animals (see Table 8.4 for a partial listing). The mechanisms whereby the toxic alkaloids and other compounds in these plants cause GI damage are generally unknown. The mechanisms of action appear, in many cases, to be primarily "irritative" rather than cytotoxic in nature, leading to an initial release of mucus from goblet cells, hypersecretion from crypt cells, and malabsorption, all leading to diarrhea and vomiting (in species that can vomit). At high doses, however, many of these plant compounds cause necrosis and hemorrhage (Figure 8.8), even ulceration. It should be noted that many of these plant toxins have additional and more directly life-threatening effects on other organ systems. Affected animals generally die from these effects

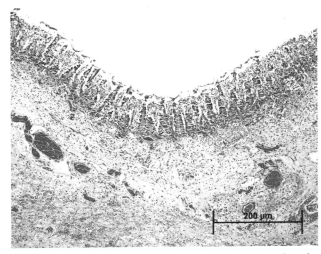

FIGURE 8.8 An "irritative" lesion caused by castor oil in the colon of a horse with pronounced vascular engorgement of both superficial and deep vasculature, edema of lamina propria and submucosa, and sloughing of superficial colonocytes.

rather than the GI effects, suggesting that the GI toxicosis may be secondary and associated with the high concentration of an irritating substance, rather than a GI specific toxic effect.

Hypersensitivity

Immunomediated hypersensitivity mechanisms of toxicity require some form of damage to the mucosal barrier, so that there is inadequate clearance of the offending antigenic or haptenic compound by the mucosal immune system. Although multiple examples of immunomediated toxicity exist, specific antigen models provide the clearest evidence of the interaction between the mucosal barrier and GI tract-associated immune responses.

The pathogenesis of hypersensitivity in the GI tract is best exemplified by an experimental model using ethanol to break down the mucosal barrier to increase permeability to trinitrobenzenesulfonic acid which acts as the hapten. Severe transmural granulomatous inflammation develops in the distal colon as a result of this treatment. The inflammatory response is characterized by mucosal and submucosal infiltrations of neutrophils, macrophages, Langhan's-type giant cell macrophages, lymphocytes, and mast cells. Immunomediated inflammatory responses such as this one ultimately lead to severe colonic ulceration. Once the animal is sensitized to an antigenic compound, an immune reaction can be generated without first causing damage to the mucosal barrier. Such "intact barrier" reactions are likely the result of hapten

TABLE 8.4   Partial list of plants which cause gastrointestinal toxicity when ingested

Plant	Toxic principle	Species affected	GI lesions/syndrome	Other systems affected
Castor bean (Ricinus communis)	Ricinine (seed)	All species	Necrotizing enteritis due to cryptal necrosis	–
	C-18 hydroxy fatty acid (in oil)	Horses mainly (all animals can be affected)	Erosive to hemorrhagic enterocolitis	–
Rosary pea (Abrus precatorius)	Abric acid (bean)	All species	Necrotizing enteritis due to cryptal necrosis	–
Common cocklebur (Xanthium strumarium)	Sesquiterpene lactones, carboxyatractyloside	Cattle, pigs, sheep and poultry (all species can be affected)	Vomiting (in species that can vomit)	Endocrine (profound hypoglycemia), liver damage
Easter Lily (Lilium longiflorum)	Unknown	Cats	Vomiting	Urinary (renal tubular necrosis)
Bulbs: Lily of the valley (Convalaria), amaryllis (Hippeastrum), hyacinth (Hyacinthus), iris (Iris), daffodils and related plants (Narcissus)	Unknown	Cattle, pets	Vomiting, diarrhea, self-limiting irritant gastroenteritis	Cardiovascular (cardiotoxic glycosides in lily of the valley)
Nightshades (Solanum spp.), including tomato, potato, black nightshade, and others	Solanine alkaloids	Cattle, horses, pets	Hypersalivation, vomiting (in species that can vomit), irritant gastroenteritis that may become hemorrhagic	Central nervous system (convulsions)
Mustards (certain Brassica spp.), pennycress (Thlaspi) and peppergrasses (Lepidum)	Allyl isothiocyanate and related compounds, irritant oils	Cattle, sheep, horses	Hypersalivation, vomiting (in species that can vomit), colic, diarrhea, irritant gastroenteritis vesicles in oral cavity, esophagus, upper GI tract	Endocrine (goiter), reproductive (abortion), hematopoietic (anemia), skin (photosensitization)
Tobacco (Nicotiana spp.)	Nicotine	Pigs mainly, pets (via tobacco products like cigarettes)	Vomiting (in species that can vomit), diarrhea, irritant gastroenteritis	Central nervous system (shaking, trembling, convulsions), respiratory (dyspnea), reproductive (abortion, teratogenesis)
Azalea (Rhododendron spp.)	Grayanotoxins (andromedotoxins)	Cattle, sheep, horses, pigs, pets (rarely)	Hypersalivation, vomiting (in species that can vomit), diarrhea, gastroenteritis	Cardiovascular (cardiotoxic glycosides)
Black walnut (Juglans nigra)	Juglone	Horses, dogs (rarely)	Colic, diarrhea, gastroenteritis	Musculoskeletal (laminitis in horses)
Chestnuts (Aesculus glabra, A. hippocastanum)	Aesculin	All grazing animals	Vomiting (in species that can vomit), colic, diarrhea, irritant gastroenteritis	Central nervous system (paralysis, coma)
Oak (Quercus spp.)	Tannins (including tannic acid, gallic acid, pyrogallol)	Cattle mainly, pets (rarely)	Diarrhea or constipation, irritant gastroenteritis	Urinary (renal tubular necrosis)
Black locust (Robinia pseudo-acacia)	Robin, robinine	Horses	Colic, diarrhea, irritant enterocolitis leading to hemorrhagic enterocolitis	Central nervous system (paralysis), cardiovascular cardiac arrhythmias
Yews (Taxus cuspidate, T. baccata)	Taxines	Grazing animals (all species can be affected)	Vomiting (in species that can vomit), diarrhea, irritant gastroenteritis (death usually intervenes before GI signs occur)	Cardiovascular (cardiac bradyarrythmia)
Soapwort (Saponaria officinalis)	Saponins	Grazing animals	Vomiting (in species that can vomit), colic, diarrhea, self-limiting irritant gastroenteritis, occasionally hemorrhagic	–
Oleander (Nerium oleander)	Oleandrin and nerioside	Grazing animals	Vomiting (in species that can vomit), diarrhea, hemorrhagic gastroenteritis (death usually intervenes before GI signs)	Cardiovascular (digitalis-like cardiotoxicity)

transport through the barrier by mucosal epithelial cells or leukocytes.

Neurotransmitter Effects

Acetyl cholinesterase is the enzyme responsible for inactivating acetylcholine at cholinergic neuromotor and neurosecretory synapses in the enteric nervous system. Inhibition of acetyl cholinesterase leads to accumulation of acetylcholine at smooth muscle M3 muscarinic receptors and M1/M3 muscarinic receptors in salivary glands, stomach, exocrine pancreas, and intestine to produce hypermotility and hypersecretion, respectively. The large volumes of secreted fluid, combined with the hypermotility, results in profuse, watery diarrhea. Acetyl cholinesterase inhibitors, such as neostigmine, edrophonium and pyridostigmine, as well as organophosphate insecticides, such as parathion, malathion, and paraoxon, are all capable of causing diarrhea by irreversible blockage of acetyl cholinesterase activity. Nerve gas agents, including tabu, sarin, and soman, also function by the same mechanism as the solanine alkaloids common in potatoes, tomatoes, and nightshade plants sometimes consumed by herbivorous (or omnivorous) domestic animals. Theobromine, a xanthine present in chocolate, may alter GI motility leading to vomiting and diarrhea. This is a centrally-mediated effect (see next section). Other toxic substances, such as anthraquinone, injure the nerve fibers and may alter the number of neurons. Thus, the loss of neuron mass may reflect an adaptational atrophy associated with the aging process, or exposure to toxic substances.

Premature migrating motor complexes can be induced by opiates and erythromycin, which results in hypercontraction with hypomotility, often resulting in constipation rather than diarrhea, a common finding in individuals addicted to opiate compounds.

Perturbation of Microflora

Administration of antibiotics has a profound effect on colonic and fecal flora, depending on the specific antimicrobial activity of the agent, route of administration, and local luminal concentration of the drug. The effect of reducing bacterial concentrations, sometimes tremendously so depending on the route, leaves a void in the microbial ecosystem that can be readily filled by pathogenic or opportunistic bacteria. Toxigenic strains of one such bacterium, *Clostridium difficile*, a normal inhabitant of the GI tract, can proliferate tremendously when other competing bacteria are eliminated by antibiotics, such as clindamycin or ampicillin. The toxigenic strains elaborate a pore-forming protein toxin which can cause apoptosis or necrosis, followed by pseudomembrane formation on the denuded colonic surface. Other opportunistic bacteria can produce similar effects when conditions are favorable for massive proliferation of the opportunistic pathogen.

Carcinogenicity

Compounds that are carcinogenic to the GI tract of laboratory animals may act by direct or indirect actions. Direct-acting (genotoxic) carcinogens cause genetic damage and "initiate" cells, with subsequent progression to morphologically-verifiable neoplasms. Indirect-acting (nongenotoxic) compounds act mainly by causing persistent proliferation that leads to a substantial increase in the number of dividing cells; consequently, the tissue is more vulnerable to background errors in DNA replication and initiating stimuli. The exact relationships between the genetic alterations and the phenotypic expression of cancer for nongenotoxic carcinogens are incompletely understood. Regardless of mechanism, all organs of the GI tract are vulnerable to carcinogenic compounds.

Stomach

Naturally-occurring tumors of the forestomach are rare in rats and mice (1%); however, hamsters can have an incidence as high as 12%. Tumors of the forestomach in common domestic animals are even rarer, except in certain localities where poor grazing conditions lead to consumption of high quantities of bracken fern (*Pteridium aquilinum*). In addition to urinary bladder lesion and hematological abnormalities, esophageal and ruminal squamous cell carcinomas are common. Ptaquilosides in the plant have been implicated experimentally in the pathogenesis of these tumors. Many agents are capable of inducing or modulating forestomach neoplasia in laboratory animals. Nongenotoxic carcinogens, in contrast to genotoxic carcinogens, must be in contact with the epithelium of the forestomach for extended periods of time (e.g., butylated hydroxyanisole—BHA). Morphologically, both genotoxic and nongenotoxic agents lead to dysplastic areas of the forestomach. However, in general, early lesions induced by nongenotoxic carcinogens are reversible, whereas those induced by genotoxic agents are irreversible.

Epithelial dysplasia and metaplasia with glandular distortion is a consistent feature of chemically-induced precancerous lesions in the glandular portion of the stomach in rodents. The metaplastic process is also associated with changes in epithelial cell enzymes (alkaline phosphatase, β-glucuronidase) and mucin glycoprotein (neutral and acid mucopolysaccharides) content. In humans, "intestinalization," that is, metaplastic replacement of normal gastric epithelium by goblet cells and tall columnar enterocyte epithelium, is considered a precancerous condition; it is not an established criterion for preneoplasia, however, in laboratory animals. Carcinomas of the glandular stomach can be induced by a variety of chemical carcinogens (e.g., N-methyl-N-nitro-N-nitrosoguanidine) in mice, rats, hamsters, and dogs; however, adenocarcinomas directly linked to carcinogen exposure under natural conditions in common domestic animals are virtually non-existent.

Intestines

Spontaneous small and large intestinal tumors in laboratory rodents and common domestic animals are rare; however, the high incidence of colon cancer in humans has led to the development of animal models which utilize chemical carcinogens to initiate colon tumors. Chemically-induced tumors of the colon are polypoid or sessile. Sessile tumors are usually mucinous, and can progress to malignancy that is characterized by local invasion, metastasis to mesenteric lymph nodes, lung, or liver, and intussusception.

Several aromatic amines induce intestinal cancers in laboratory animals through genotoxic processes. However, extensive metabolism is generally required before many chemicals become carcinogenic. Target specificity is affected by chemical structure, and is often also species-specific. For example, many nitrosamines induce tumors of small and large intestine in rats, hamsters, or guinea pigs. For many nitrosamines organ specificity appears to relate to the affinity of these compounds for enterocyte versus nonenterocyte receptors, or to site-specific cellular biotransformation that results in the formation of the ultimate carcinogenic metabolite. Another example is azoxymethane, an alkylating agent that only methylates DNA in colonic epithelium of rats and hamsters. This alkylation partially accounts for the site-specific carcinogenic activity of these compounds.

Organ specificity in response to carcinogen exposure also relates to the sites of specific carcinogen-induced genetic mutations. An example is the dominant mutation that occurs in the germline of mice APC min/+, which predisposes the animal to multiple intestinal tumors. The propensity for tumor development is dependent on a single allele, and tumors develop in the duodenum, ileum, and colon. Since all cells of these mice carry the mutation, and tumors occur only in the intestinal tract, somatic events are needed for neoplasia to develop in addition to the predisposing mutation.

Genotoxic-carcinogen-induced changes in rat colonic epithelium are similar to those observed in spontaneously developing colorectal cancer in humans. In rats, sulfomucins are the primary glycoprotein of the normal colonic epithelium. Shortly after treatment with azoxymethane and N-methyl-N-nitro-N-nitrosoguanidine, cryptal epithelium mucus changes to express primarily sialomucins. These features support the *de novo* histogenesis of colon carcinoma.

RESPONSE OF THE GASTROINTESTINAL TRACT TO INJURY

Most responses that occur as results of GI intoxication are ulcerative, proliferative, or inflammatory (Table 8.5). Because of variation in structure and function, each segment of the GI tract is affected by toxic compounds in a slightly different manner. In addition, each segment has a different range of pathophysiological responses to a toxic compound. Clinically, most alterations of the GI tract are manifested as abnormal functions, such as vomiting (if the animal is capable of such activity), diarrhea, constipation, or nutrient malabsorption. Additionally, occult or large amounts of blood may be present in the stools. Of these possible manifestations, diarrhea is perhaps the most commonly observed and most life-threatening.

One process that almost inevitably results from injury, the inflammatory response, is discussed in detail below, because many of the disease processes resulting from chemical injury ultimately involve this host reaction. Finally, the response of the enteric nervous tissue to toxic GI injury is discussed. Although the GI tract has a large amount of nervous tissue, most neural responses are manifested on a functional basis.

Pathophysiological Responses

Diarrhea

Identification of mechanisms responsible for diarrhea should focus on the small and large intestine, both separately and collectively. Small-intestinal diarrheas are generally associated with increased mucosal permeability, hypersecretion, or malabsorption. Small-intestinal malabsorption, in particular, has effects on the colon by allowing fermentable nutrients to enter the colon, where resident bacteria generate fermentation products that lead to subsequent osmotic overload. Major mechanisms of large-intestinal diarrhea include hypersecretion, large-bowel malabsorption, or colonic mucosal

TABLE 8.5 Classification of alterations to the gastrointestinal tract with selected examples

Alteration/lesion	Xenobiotic
Mucosal necrosis/ulceration/ hemorrhage	
• Esophagus and stomach	Corrosive agents: mineral acids, iodine, sodium fluoride, strong bases, phenol, ethyl acrylate
• Stomach	Inhibitors of prostaglandin synthesis/production: NSAIDs, corticosteroids
	Volatile organic agents: ethanol, methanol, chloroform, gasoline, and kerosene
• Stomach and small intestine	Inhibitors of prostaglandin synthesis/production: NSAIDs,
	Antimitotic agents: colchicine, methrotrexate, cyclophosphamide, 5'-fluoruracil
	Bile acids
	Ionizing radiation
	Vasoactive drugs: catecholamines, antihypertensive agents (e.g., reserpine), sympatholytic agents (e.g., priscoline), antihistamines
	Metal and metaloids: Arsenic, bismuth, copper salts, gold salts, iron salts, lead, manganese, mercury, nickel, thallium, vanadium, zinc salts
	Nonmetallic compounds: Phosphorus, short chain aliphatic nitriles (e.g., propionitrile)
• Large intestine	NSAIDs, metals and metalloids (see above), *Clostridium difficile* toxin, hydrolyzable tannins, *Clostridium difficile* toxin
Irritation/inflammation	
• Stomach	Volatile organic agents (see above), xanthines, dimethylhydrazines, nitrosamines, nitrosoguanines
• Small intestine and large intestine	Arsenates, mercurials, plant alkaloids, condensed tannins
• Esophageal, stomach, and intestinal cancer, and/or acute gastritis	Nonvolatile organic agents (dimethylhydrazines, nitrosoguanidines, nitrosamines)
Neoplastic proliferation	
• Forestomach and stomach neoplasia	Nitroso compounds, aliphatic/aromatic hydrocarbon, nitro, polycyclic/aromatic hydrocarbon, halogenated hydrocarbon, sodium saccharin
• Intestinal tumors	Pyrrolysis products of amino acids and proteins, 1,2-dimethylhydrazine, azomethane, azoxymethane, methylazoxymethanol acetate, nitrosomethylurea, nitrosomethylnitroguanidine, and metabolites
• Colon tumors	Nitroso-*n*-butyl-hexylurea, *n*-amyl-hexylurea, *n*-hexylurea, azoxymethane, *N*-methyl-*N*-nitro-*N*-nitrosguanine

injury. In both organs, mucosal damage and subsequent inflammation lead to release of PGE2, which stimulates electrolyte secretion and activation of mast cells, with subsequent release of histamine to further enhance fluid loss. Inflammatory cells can also release mediators that stimulate nerve activity that may lead to localized GI tract hypermotility. Given these factors, the pathogenesis of diarrhea after toxic insult can be generally divided into four major categories: (1) increased mucosal permeability and exudation; (2) hypersecretion; (3) malabsorption; and (4) abnormal GI motility.

Although the pathogeneses of diarrhea can vary, some of the most injurious involve toxins that affect the GI tract's ability to transport fluid. Since a major function of the GI tract is to absorb and secrete large amounts of fluid, such toxins are life-threatening,

even though little overt morphologic damage may be present. This process, and the extent of the resulting diarrhea, is best demonstrated with cholera toxin. Cholera toxin activates adenylate cyclase, resulting in the secretion of large amounts of fluid into the small-intestinal lumen, overloading the large intestine's ability to absorb lumenal water. This process leads to severe diarrhea and death, with little morphologic evidence of mucosal damage.

The consequences of diarrhea are systemic in nature, and include dehydration, acidosis, and electrolyte alterations. Direct loss of bicarbonate in the feces causes acidosis, and intracellular hydrogen ion concentrations increase as potassium concentrations decrease. Consequently, there is inadequate maintenance of electrochemical gradients, which leads to increased extracellular potassium and mass excretion of this electrolyte in the urine and feces, leading to lethal systemic effects.

Malabsorptive diarrheas associated with loss of enterocytes, crypt cells or both, often accompanied by hemorrhage and inflammation, are commonly associated with GI toxicosis. This type of diarrhea is more often accompanied by morphologic changes, although they are relatively nonspecific. These lesions may be site-specific, however, providing a clue to the type of toxicant involved. For example, corrosive agents are far more likely to cause necrosis and inflammation in the pharynx and esophagus than lower down in the GI tract.

Coordinated peristalsis can be altered by bulking agents such as fiber. By causing distension, these compounds elicit contractions that occur in either direction along the bowel. In a few cases, for example in organophosphate insecticide toxicosis, diarrhea is via prolonged stimulation of muscarinic receptors, due to inhibition of acetylcholinesterase at the synapse. The greatly enhanced peristaltic activity, combined with stimulation of secretion, leads to decreased transit time through the GI tracts and diarrhea.

Vomiting (Emesis)

Vomiting is a clinical response to toxicity that occurs in some animal species. Vomiting requires the presence of skeletal muscle in the wall of the esophagus. Vomiting may be stimulated by direct mucosal irritation/damage, or by stimulation of the vomiting center in the central nervous system. Toxicants can act directly on the mucosa to induce vomiting via activation of sensory nerves traveling via sympathetic or vagal pathways to the center in the medulla of the brain controlling emesis. Most plant toxins that induce vomiting probably do so via this mechanism. A major neurotransmitter involved in the vagal sensory pathway is 5-hydroxytryptamine (5-HT), which binds to 5-HT3 receptors on the endings of sensory nerves in the mucosa. Compounds such as cyclophosphamide, carmustine, dactinomycin, and cisplatin induce enterochromaffin cells in the mucosa to release 5-HT, triggering vomiting by this peripheral mechanism.

Other compounds, however, including cisplatin, act "centrally:" that is by directly stimulating centers in the brain that trigger or regulate vomiting. The area postrema of the medulla, where the chemoreceptor trigger zone and emesis center are located, as well as the solitary nucleus in the brain stem, are two regions that can stimulate vomiting if appropriately stimulated. Apomorphine, L-dopa, bromocryptine, and emetine (from the ipecac plant), all produce vomiting via their effects on various components of the central vomiting pathways. Compounds which act centrally may not induce GI lesions directly, and thus may not produce visible morphologic changes.

Constipation

Constipation is both a structural and functional phenomenon. Compounds which add bulk to feces (e.g., fiber) may cause constipation if there is a concomitant reduction in water intake. Polyps and neoplastic masses induced by carcinogenic agents may result in physical obstruction. The constipating effects of certain analgesic compounds (e.g., morphine) have a neurological component to their pathogenesis. By neurogenically decreasing motility, these increase transit time, allowing for more water absorption, leading to firming of fecal material.

GI toxicity modulated by changes in nervous tissue responses is generally identified by functional abnormalities first detected clinically. Normal intestinal motility is typified by peristaltic activity that moves intralumenal contents down the GI tract via coordinated contraction of both longitudinal and circular muscle layers. Neuronal networks involved in peristalsis are complex and incompletely understood, but it is known that cholinergic excitation plays a major role. Opiate (e.g., morphine) toxicity is manifested clinically as a nonpropulsive, and hence constipating, pattern of segmental motility. Normal segmentation movements mix intraluminal contents. This activity involves reciprocal neural inhibition, and concomitant disinhibition of adjacent muscle segments. Endogenous opioid peptides may be involved in normal segmentation motility, since morphine locks the intestine into a continuous segmentation pattern of motility that actually prohibits normal propulsion of ingesta through the tract. In morphine-dependent rats, diarrhea, which is opposite the acute effects of morphine, is a primary withdrawal event.

Inflammatory Response

Because of the high number of bacteria, and the compositional characteristics of the luminal contents, inflammation is frequently involved in many lesions of the GI tract regardless of the underlying mechanism of injury. However, the inflammatory response is generally less severe in primary toxicologic lesions than in primary bacterial diseases. Even so, inflammation will be greater if the toxicant damages not just mucosal epithelium, but also underlying lamina propria. Ulcerative lesion will generate a far greater inflammatory response than erosive lesion, and healing is more likely to be complicated by fibrosis with loss of function.

Inflammation of the stomach (gastritis) is essentially a process that is restricted to the mucosa. Gastritis is usually catarrhal (i.e., involving large amounts of mucus) with irritants, but there may be ulceration, hemorrhage, and lymphoid hyperplasia with both cytotoxic agents and irritants (at high doses). Gastritis glandularis, a disease of primates, has additional features of mucosal hyperplasia, and mucus-filled cysts in the mucosa and submucosa. This lesion may be induced by ingestion of polychlorinated biphenyls.

Inflammation of any part of the intestinal tract can be called enteritis. However, this term is frequently used to designate only small-intestinal inflammation; in contrast, the term colitis is used to designate large-intestinal inflammation. Direct-acting toxic compounds usually cause more severe inflammation in the proximal GI tract (duodenum) than in the distal tract (ileum and large intestine). Mercury can cause lesions of the large-intestinal mucosa, as a result of transport of this agent from the blood into the colonic lumen.

Chronic inflammatory reactions can be a primary or secondary effect in toxicologically-mediated lesions. Immunomediated responses are characterized by accumulations of chronic inflammatory cells (lymphocytes, plasma cells, and macrophages), although there may be a superimposed active cellular component consisting of neutrophils and eosinophils.

Diseases which cause chronic inflammation or injury to the lamina propria or lymphatic vessels may lead to malabsorption of fatty acids and weight loss. Fatty acids and monoglycerides are packaged into chylomicrons by the enterocytes, before being exported to the central lacteal and into the lymphatic circulation. Consequently, damage to the lymphatic circulation that is long-standing can result in significant malabsorption-related disorders. Systemic complications, such as septicemia and bacteremia, may develop as a result of chronic inflammation and ulceration of the GI tract. Secondary lesions may be present in the liver (e.g., abscesses), skin (e.g., perianal ulcers developing secondary to chronic diarrhea), or urinary tract (e.g., females can develop an ascending infection of the urethra via fecal contamination associated with malabsorption-induced diarrhea).

Mucosal Response

General

The exposure of GI mucosal epithelial cells to ingested toxins would suggest that the GI tract should be a frequent site of toxicologic injury. The actual frequency of toxicity, however, is lower than one would expect. Factors that account for the GI tract's ability to escape damage include its capacity for compound biotransformation, and the large surface area that permits extensive contact between the toxic compound and multiple toxin-metabolizing enzymes. Additionally, mixing of the injurious compound with lumenal contents dilutes it, and thus decreases its undesirable effects. Finally, mucosal barrier components, such as mucus, protect cells while the short half-life of GI epithelial cells results in relatively rapid removal of those that have had both structural and molecular damage, for example damage to DNA.

Since the epithelium of the GI tract is the first layer of host cells to contact ingested compounds, these cells can respond to toxic compounds before they enter the circulation. Epithelial cells can also undergo biochemical changes which allow them to functionally reconstitute mucosal integrity and function after an insult. The presence of inducible detoxification enzymes in GI epithelial cells—including the cytochrome P450, alcohol dehydrogenase, monoamine oxidase, epoxide hydrolases, esterases, amidases, glucuronidases, sulfatases, and glutathione S-transferases—allows the epithelial cells to adapt to toxicant exposure and maintain a barrier function.

In addition, unique forms of adaptive mucosal protection occur after exposure of the mucosa to irritants. When there is mucosal irritation, increased levels of PGE2 are elaborated to protect the mucosa from strong irritant damage by increasing blood flow and stimulating bicarbonate secretion in the small intestine. Rapid and profound release of mucus from goblet cells is another response that has been observed in response to irritating toxicants, the mucus providing a barrier to further penetration of the offending substances. Sublethally injured GI epithelial cells are able to reseal damaged membranes. Mucosal epithelial cells can also participate in covering discontinuities in the epithelial barrier by "flattening out" to cover denuded portions of lamina propria. Viable epithelial cells at the margins of ulcers and erosions become active participants in GI barrier restitution, by migrating over denuded basal lamina. Furthermore, GI epithelial cells are protected from injury by a microvillus-rich apical membrane that can be sloughed off if damaged, and underlying cytoskeleton then can be utilized to seal the remaining viable cell body. Membrane resealing is a key process in maintaining an intact epithelial layer, if the injury does not cause widespread and severe loss of epithelial cells.

Rapid replacement of lost epithelial cells is one of the GI mucosa's primary defense mechanisms against more severe injuries that result in necrosis of epithelium. Each segment of the GI tract has a basal rate of mucosal proliferation that varies with species, age, diet, and disease state. Under normal dietary conditions and health, the range of proliferation rates for the most actively dividing mucosal cells (stomach to colon) is 3–6 days. When the intestine encounters a noxious agent, enterocyte half-life is reduced. If the damage is transient, mucosal replacement and normal microarchitecture can recover within three days under ideal conditions.

Stomach

Several mechanisms are responsible for preventing gastric mucosal damage by both normal digestive processes and injurious compounds. These include increasing the amounts of, or modifying, the mucus gel covering the mucosal surface, increased secretion of bicarbonate to neutralize the acidic environment of the gastric lumen, increasing resistance to acid back-diffusion, and increasing blood flow. Several of these processes are mediated by prostaglandin synthesis in mucosal and submucosal tissues. Additionally, mucosal protection is mediated in part by lipids (neutral lipids and phospholipids) within the mucus gel layer. These lipids increase the hydrophobicity of the mucus gel, leading to repulsion of water-soluble compounds. Mucus, nevertheless, can be lost when the stomach is exposed to mucolytic agents like bile acids or ethanol, or when subjected to mechanical trauma.

Mucosal damage can occur, however, without mucus-layer disruption. For example, the adherent mucus gel is not extensively disrupted by gastrotoxic agents, such as indomethacin. These agents readily permeate the mucus barrier and directly damage the underlying epithelium. Yet, since the mucus layer remains intact, epithelial repair is facilitated and the damage can be self-limiting. With persistent mucosal damage, however, mucus gel secretion will be reduced, due to the net loss of functional epithelial cells. Collapse of the mucus barrier results in further loss of surface epithelial cells, further reducing mucus release, vascular occlusion, and ultimately ulceration and scar formation.

Cellular proliferation is a key epithelial cell mechanism in maintaining/restoring mucosal barrier function. Repair of chemically or mechanically induced gastric epithelial cell discontinuities can be complete within 30–90 minutes of injury; however, the rapidity of repair is dependent to a large extent on the amount of damage the compound inflicts on the proliferating cell population. Minor damage to the proliferative compartment leads to mild gastritis, and any loss of nonproliferating surface epithelial cells is compensated for by increased proliferation of the undamaged proliferative epithelial cells. However, severe mucosal damage does occur when the proliferating population

is destroyed. One of the mechanisms by which PGE2 enhances healing of the gastric mucosa is by protecting the cells in the isthmus of the gastric pits, and allowing these replicative cells to reconstitute the surface epithelium rapidly.

In cases of mild injury, changes in the proliferative epithelial cell population may be the only morphologic indication of mucosal injury. Low doses of indomethacin and aspirin increase epithelial proliferation in rat gastric mucosa, but have no visible effect in the antrum and duodenum, and do not cause inflammation. In contrast, corticosteroids depress epithelial cell proliferation in fundic, antral, and duodenal mucosa of rats, and predispose them to gastric ulcers.

Small and Large Intestines

Damage to small intestinal mucosa by toxicants results in a variety of changes, depending on the degree and extent of injury. Damage to enterocytes, without damage to underlying lamina propria or to the proliferative epithelial cell population lining the crypts, will result in a temporary shortening of villi and a decrease in height of remaining enterocytes as they flatten out to cover the denuded mucosal surface (Figure 8.9). Restitution of the lost enterocytes can happen within a matter of a few days. As the proliferative rate of crypt cells increases, and the cell cycle time decreases, crypts will elongate as the number of newly-formed epithelial cells increases. Complete differentiation and restoration of function generally takes longer than replacement, since newly-formed epithelial cells must leave the proliferative compartment and develop the specialized biochemical and morphologic features associated with absorptive cells.

Damage to the crypt cells by toxicants is a more serious matter, leading to "mucosal collapse" (Figure 8.10). The mechanisms of restitution after proliferative unit ablation are not well understood. Death of crypt cells without underlying damage to lamina propria, in particular the vasculature, will eventually result in complete restitution of cryptal and villous epithelium, provided complicating factors associated with loss of the mucosal barrier are minimized. Secondary events, such as fluid loss from the denuded mucosal surface, leakage of ingesta into the lamina propria, colonization of the lamina propria by resident gut bacteria (Figure 8.11), and the inevitable inflammatory response are minimized. Any one of these complicating factors, if unchecked, can lead to severe systemic consequences, and defective restitution of the mucosal barrier. Damage to underlying vasculature, especially if thrombosis occurs, can exacerbate injury even further and also lead to ulceration and hemorrhage. It is

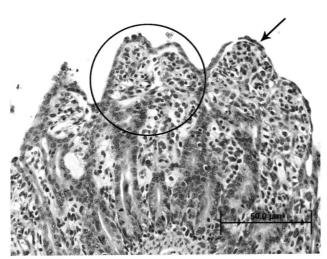

FIGURE 8.9 Villous atrophy and cryptal atrophy in the small intestine of a pig secondary to loss of enterocytes. An atrophied villous is circled. The arrow points to flattened, regenerating enterocytes migrating to cover the denuded villus.

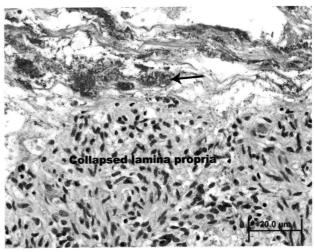

FIGURE 8.11 Secondary bacterial colonization of denuded and collapsed small intestinal mucosa in a dog, secondary to loss of villous and cryptal epithelium. The arrow points to one of many bacterial colonies on the surface.

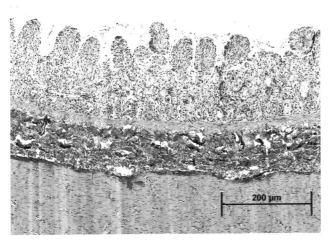

FIGURE 8.10 "Mucosal collapse" due to necrosis of cryptal enterocytes, leading to loss of enterocytes covering the villi in the small intestine of a cat.

thought that maintenance of regional blood flow in areas of damage is essential for the minimization of ongoing damage, and enhancement of repair and restitution in all sections of gut.

Restitution of the colonic mucosal barrier is slow compared to the stomach and small intestine. Migration of surviving colonocytes to cover the denuded mucosa surface is more than twice as slow as in the stomach. The proliferative response on the part of colonic crypt cells, however, is similar to that of the small intestine once replication begins. As with the small intestine, complete restitution of the mucosal barrier is possible if mitigating factors, such as secondary bacterial colonization, inflammation, and thrombosis are not present.

PGE2, which helps maintain perfusion and enhances mucus production, as well as fermentable fibers (e.g., guar), which stimulate the release of endogenous growth factors, are examples of inducers of mucosal proliferation and healing in the intestinal tract. Growth factors such as TGFα, TGFβ, and gastrin also enhance cell proliferation by influencing stem cell kinetics.

Organ-specific Responses

Esophagus

Various species have unique anatomical adaptations of the esophagus (e.g., forestomach of ruminants), but the lining mucosa and its response to injury are similar among species. The esophagus in general has a poor vascular supply. Therefore, substantial injury to the mucosa, particularly if blood supply is compromised, is liable to result in permanent loss of function. Highly-caustic agents fed to animals often lead to severe mucosal damage, followed by ulceration, inflammation, fibroplasia, and scar formation with stricture (Table 8.5).

Spontaneous esophageal cancer is rare in animals and humans living in countries with a "Western" style of civilization. However, esophageal cancers are commonly found in humans living in certain regions of China, Iran, South Asia, and Africa. The exact reasons for this are not clearly defined, but environmental factors, including N-nitroso compounds contaminating foods, spicy foods, and fungal toxins have been implicated at various times. When rats are exposed to chemical carcinogens in model systems, for example to *N*-methyl-*N*-nitrosoaniline, the mucosa of the esophagus progresses through a sequence of hyperkeratosis/hyperplasia, dysplasia, papilloma, and finally carcinoma. Esophageal cancer can also be induced in rats with dihydrosafrole, and in mice with γ-irradiation. Additionally, zinc-deficient rats treated with carcinogens may develop multiple neoplasms of the esophageal mucosa.

Stomach

Ulceration and Inflammation

Gastric ulceration, with associated inflammation and mucus loss, are responses not only to toxicant exposure, but also to stress, as well as various mucolytic agents that are not necessarily inherently toxic themselves. Active ulcerogens include NSAIDs, ethanol, taurocholate (bile acids), aliphatic nitriles, certain thiols, and amines (Table 8.5). In addition to these direct-acting compounds, antimitotic and antineoplastic agents (e.g., colchicine and 5′-fluorouracil) which inhibit mitosis, and hence interfere with replacement of senescent, sloughed surface epithelial cells, cause ulceration not only in the stomach, but in other parts of the GI tract as well.

Proliferative Response

Hyperplasia of gastric mucosa can be induced by duodeno-gastric reflux, by impairment of outflow, or by abnormal hormonal stimulation (Figure 8.12). The hyperplastic epithelial cells maintain normal anatomical boundaries (i.e., they do not infiltrate into the subepithelial tissues), but there are significant changes in mucosal maturation and differentiation. Animals with gastric hyperplasia have decreased chief cells containing cytoplasmic zymogen granules, decreased mature surface cells, glandular atrophy, loss of regular parietal cell distribution, and decreased mucus production. Although not considered preneoplastic *per se*, hyperplasia of sufficient duration may increase the risk of neoplastic development. The onset of progression toward carcinoma is demonstrated by loss of cellular differentiation, abnormal gland structure, invasion of mucosa into surrounding tissue, abnormal glycoprotein expression, and displacement of normal tissue. When cellular changes include tissue invasion or areas of severe epithelial atypia, metaplasia, or dysplasia, with or without extensive proliferative activity, the lesion should be considered a carcinoma.

A hormone-mediated proliferative response of the stomach can occur when there is prolonged gastrin release, resulting in hyperplasia of enterochromaffin-like (ECL) cells, or even neuroendocrine-cell tumors ("carcinoids"). Hyperplasia of enteroendocrine cells

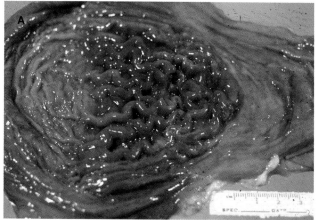

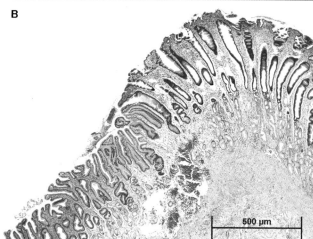

FIGURE 8.12 Hyperplastic gastric mucosa from a dog under prolonged hormonal stimulation from a gastrin secreting tumor. (A) Gross image of hyperplastic mucosa. (B) Microscopic image of affected mucosa showing loss of differentiation of glandular epithelium.

has been demonstrated after exposure to ranitidine and substituted benzimidazoles like omeprazole, both of which produce hypergastrinemia.

Small Intestine

Damage to the small intestinal mucosa frequently results in villus atrophy and crypt cell hyperplasia. Villous atrophy and concomitant crypt hyperplasia may resolve if the damage is mild or superficial; however, atrophy may be permanent if there is damage to and inflammation in, the underlying lamina propria (see discussion above). If ulceration occurs, an associated inflammatory reaction ensues. Duodenal sites are more frequently found to have ulcers than other small intestinal segments. The same ulcerogens which affect the stomach frequently damage the duodenum as well. On the other hand, the distal small intestine is a frequent site of functional abnormalities, such as diarrhea, rather than a location for morphologic damage. The small intestine is an infrequent site of neoplasm development. However, lymphosarcomas may originate in the lymphoid nodules of the lamina propria and submucosa. Adenocarcinomas induced by a carcinogenic agent or natural causes generally originate from the mucosal epithelium, and invade the submucosa and tunica muscularis mucosa.

Large Intestine

Ulceration and Inflammation

Responses of the large intestine to toxic injury can be studied using models that induce either acute or chronic lesions. Acute erosive injury to the colonic mucosa can be induced using the bile salt, deoxycholate (15 mM, 30 minutes). Damage to the surface cells is mediated by reactive oxygen metabolites and complete ablation of the surface epithelium occurs within eight minutes. Mucosal permeability is regained after 40 minutes, and recovery of absorptive activities occurs when the epithelium is restored to a columnar phenotype (two hours). The reparative process of the mucosa occurs by active cell migration from the proliferative zone in the crypts to the surface. This process will be delayed or not take place if damage to the mucosa is severe enough to eliminate stem cells in the crypts; ulceration, inflammation, fibrosis, and permanent loss of function at the affected site will occur in such situations.

Proliferative Response

One common response seen in the colon with prolonged toxic injury is mucosal hyperplasia and polyp formation. Hyperplastic polyps of the colon may be either inflammatory or regenerative in nature. Benign lymphoid polyps occur in the colon or rectum as a result of lymphoid tissue hyperplasia, and can protrude into the intestinal lumen. Inflammation of the lymphoid polyps is a frequent concomitant event.

Proliferative polyps of the mucosal epithelium can be classified as adenomatous polyps or adenomas. Adenomatous polyps are composed of elongated glandular tubules of neoplastic non-malignant epithelium with little stroma. In contrast, villous adenomas have multiple projections of epithelial-lined lamina propria supporting the benign neoplastic epithelial cells. Regardless of classification, the mucus content of neoplastic epithelial cells is reduced, and mitotic figures are common in these polyps. The presence of multiple polyps should be regarded as an early cancerous event in rodents, since there is an adenoma–carcinoma sequence in the colon in most rodent models.

Cecal Enlargement

Cecal enlargement is a response to various compounds and food additives observed in several rodent species. These materials include antibiotics, modified starches, polyols (e.g., sorbitol and mannitol), some fibers, and lactose. Many of these compounds share the feature of being poorly absorbed and osmotically active. The mechanism for the distention has not been clearly defined. Other features include mucosal hypertrophy and hyperplasia. The morphologic response is associated with functional changes leading to soft stools or diarrhea, and increased large bowel mucosal permeability. These functional alterations are likely to be mediated by the increased osmotic activity of the cecal contents. The morphologic and functional changes probably represent an adaptational process, since the changes are reversible when the diets are returned to normal.

Generalized large intestinal enlargement is a common change observed with incompletely digested and poorly-absorbed substances that are subjected to microbial metabolism in both cecum and colon. Increased microbial metabolism of the offending substances leads to the generation of osmotically active byproducts that cause soft stools and cecal distention.

EVALUATION OF GASTROINTESTINAL TOXICITY

The ability of the GI tract to adapt to various diets and nontoxic compounds is well-established. Both adaptational and toxicologic processes can be manifested by altered structure or function, or both together. Evaluation of these processes requires a basic understanding of the mechanism of action of the toxic compound, or at least a suspected pathogenesis for the toxic injury observed. Routine approaches involve *in vitro* and *in vivo* methods. Because alterations in numerous other organ systems can occur as a result of GI toxicity, whole animal studies are generally required in order to properly interpret GI toxicity. As a result of this complex interrelationship between organ systems and the inherent complexity of the GI tract, numerous animal models have been developed to study various GI diseases and toxicities.

In Vitro Strategies

In vitro studies can be used to detect alterations of the mucosal lining as a whole, or within individual cellular components. Mucosal lining studies conducted with Ussing chambers can be used to evaluate solute transport by large regions of isolated mucosa from various isolated segments of the GI tract. Long-term organ or explant cultures of GI tract can also be used to conduct carcinogen metabolism studies. Advances in cell culture techniques for GI epithelial cells, isolation of membrane vesicles, and molecular biological methods have been very useful in providing information about binding of agents to epithelial cells, location of enzyme systems, mechanisms of molecular transport, and genetic damage.

Cellular and organelle markers have been established to identify cells from various portions of the GI tract. Keratin can be used as a general marker of epithelial cells and the extent of differentiation. Identification of colonic epithelial cells can be verified using antibodies to colon specific antigen (CSAp), colon antigen 3, or 5E-113. Disaccharidases of small intestinal epithelium can be identified using antibody or enzyme assays. Chromogranin immunohistochemistry, neuron-specific enolase histochemistry, argyrophilic stains, and classic morphology studies can be used to identify neuroendocrine cells. Goblet cells can be identified morphologically using Schiff reagent for mucins.

A biochemical anatomy of cells in the GI tract can be obtained through *in vitro* assays of enzymatic activities in biopsied mucosa. Enzyme markers can be used to detect alterations of brush border (disaccharidases), lysosomes, peroxisomes, mitochondria, and endoplasmic reticulum.

Evaluation of lumenal contents is also part of the search for GI tract toxicity. Lumenal fluid can be used to determine if altered bacterial populations and abnormal enzyme secretions are present. Occult blood can be detected in stool samples, and represents a noninvasive means of evaluating the integrity of the mucosa.

Because the GI tract is the first organ system exposed to ingested xenobiotics, highly sensitive assessments of genotoxic potential, such as single cell electrophoresis to measure DNA breakage in isolated GI epithelial cells, can be utilized. The comet-like appearance of DNA bands on an agarose gel, derived from a single epithelial cell immobilized in an agarose matrix, can be correlated to DNA strand breaks caused by the test chemical, giving the investigator an idea of its genotoxic potential.

In Vivo Strategies

Whole animal studies must include proper structural and functional evaluation of the entire animal, as well as more focused assessment of the GI tract. Attention to other organs, such as liver and pancreas, may provide essential clues to GI tract disorders of uncertain origin. Altered lipid absorption (a primary intestinal disorder) and abnormal bile acid release (a primary liver disorder) may lead to similar clinical abnormalities, but clearly have different causes. Consequently, proper in-life and postmortem evaluations are needed to establish a cause and effect relationship properly.

Since the major function of the GI tract is nutrient absorption, the extent and rate of absorption should be quantitatively assessed by administering a test agent and determining the concentration of this agent in blood, tissues, and feces. Passive permeability of markers (e.g., ^{51}Cr-labeled EDTA) from the intestinal lumen into the blood may be used to detect small intestinal diseases. Additionally, various agents that are nonabsorbed (e.g., polyethylene glycol 4000) or absorbed (e.g., radiolabeled amino acids) can be used to answer different questions about nutrient absorption.

Propulsive activity of the GI tract can also serve as an indicator of toxicity. Tracking unabsorbable markers can serve as a net indicator of motility. Specific aspects of motility, such as muscle contractility or electrical activity, can also be quantified. The extent of the evaluation and the exact approach used will be dictated by the goals of the study.

Organ weights and volumes and their ratios to body weight are sensitive allometric measurements of GI tract response and toxicity. The ability of the stomach and intestine to adapt to various diets and compounds can be established using such methods. Since both adaptational and toxic response can be manifested by changes in tissue volumes or weights, more refined structural and functional methods may be required for this screening approach.

Molecular Pathology

The newly-developed methodologies in the areas of genomics and proteomics have and will continue to provide useful mechanistic insights into toxicologic processes and resultant morphologic alterations. The rapid development of microarray analysis techniques allows a quantitative assessment of gene expression in tissues, and even within lesions. Real-time polymerase chain reaction (RT-PCR) and two-dimensional polyacrylamide gel electrophoresis methodologies allow further evaluation of gene expression and protein profiles, respectively. Coupled with *in situ* hybridization and immunohistochemical analysis to localize mediators and the cells producing them, these procedures provide the essential tools for integration of molecular and morphologic data to establish definitive mechanistic information for toxicologic pathologists.

Application of molecular methods has been particularly important in defining the role of inflammatory cytokines and growth factors in the morphogenesis of tissue damage and repair. Microarray analysis, coupled with other more standard evaluative methodologies, can provide vast amounts of information regarding induction and suppression of not only the cytokines and growth factors themselves, but also the pathways involved in their regulation and expression. The number of genes typically up- or down-regulated in a particular lesion, or during a particular pathologic process, as well as their potential interactions, is typically vast and highly complex, at times almost defying logical analysis. The diversity of genes changing during a process illustrates the need to integrate genomic and proteomic findings with standard physiologic and morphologic observations, to ensure proper interpretation and attribution of the role of a gene or protein in a toxicologic process.

Morphologic Methods

Evaluation of the GI tract for toxicity should be conducted using macroscopic, microscopic, and ultrastructural methods. Macroscopic evaluation includes identification of ulcers, enlarged lymphoid tissues (e.g., Peyer's patches), neoplasms, and foreign bodies. Microscopic studies should be conducted on all lesions observed macroscopically, and at preselected tissue sites. In an attempt to standardize communications, specialty organizations are adopting standardized nomenclature for the description of microscopic lesions in certain portions of the GI tract. For structural studies of the GI tract, attention to detail is required for proper tissue fixation.

Assessment of morphologic alterations of the GI tract should consist of close evaluation of the mucosa and its specializations. The mucosa consists of surface epithelium, crypts/glands, lamina propria, and a thin layer of muscle separating the mucosa and submucosa. Specializations of the mucosa include glands of the esophagus, foveolae of the stomach, villi of the small intestine, and glands of the large intestine. The submucosa and the tunica muscularis (outer smooth muscle layers) should also be examined for changes in thickness and cellularity.

Villi should be evaluated critically when assessing small intestinal toxicity. Since villi bend in various directions, and have shapes that vary with species (e.g., tongue-like in rats and finger-like in humans), and location (longer in the duodenum than in the ileum), close comparisons with control animals is required to prevent misinterpretation.

Changes in the lamina propria at all levels of the GI tract can be detected by carefully assessing alterations in the make-up of the normal resident cell population. Neutrophil, eosinophil, lymphocyte, and plasma cell populations may change in response to a toxicologic insult. Increases in any of these populations, or a change in the relative proportions of each cell type, are indications of a potential underlying toxicologic or disease process. It must also be kept in mind that inflammatory infiltrates frequently occur secondary to epithelial cell toxicity. Lymphoid follicles may develop and be associated with an extensive increase in lymphocytes and plasma cells. These follicles may occur in the lamina propria or submucosa. Additionally, lymphomas may be associated with a substantial number of abnormal lymphocytes in the lamina propria. Changes in the submucosa generally involve blood vessels and lymphatics, and may involve nerves as well. Alterations in this region are frequently characterized by edema, lymphangectasia, and inflammatory or neoplastic cell infiltrates.

Different fixatives are used for evaluation of GI toxicity, depending on the purpose of the study and the technique being used. The most routinely used multipurpose fixative is 10% neutral buffered formalin. Because of rapid postmortem autolysis, GI tract tissues must be placed into any fixative within 1–2 minutes of death for optimum evaluation.

Ultrastructural studies can be conducted using scanning or transmission electron microscopy. Scanning electron microscopy (SEM) provides information on surface alterations. This technique is particularly useful for examining altered villus structure in the small intestine. Morphometric and stereological analyses are additional powerful morphologic methods that can be used to correlate biochemical and morphologic data.

Cellular proliferation, differentiation, and senescence are processes that have distinctive phenotypic and genotypic characteristics. Phenotypic alterations reflecting these processes can be examined by using plant lectins (e.g., wheat germ agglutinin) in combination with histochemical stains (e.g., periodic acid—Schiff or Alcian blue) to identify specific markers associated with each process. Specific lectins bind to specific membrane glycoproteins that serve as useful biomarkers to detect epithelial cell differentiation occurring in the GI tract. Additional understanding of the genetic control of these processes can be obtained using techniques such as *in situ* hybridization. Although not as sensitive as *in vitro* blotting technology, *in situ* hybridization allows localization of genes active in organ and tissue alterations to specific cell and tissue locations.

Animal Models

General Considerations

Variations in mammalian GI tract morphology show closer correlation with diet composition, body weight, and the need for water consumption, than with taxonomical classification. The capacity of the GI tract to hold digesta decreases with decreasing body weight in herbivorous animals; however, the rate of metabolism increases with decreasing body weight. Smaller animals have various strategies to compensate for this phenomenon. These adaptive mechanisms include an increase in cecal volume, and the practice of coprophagy (e.g., lagomorphs and rodents). Because of these modifications, the GI tract in these species may render them unsuitable in some situations as animal models for humans.

Nutritional issues must be considered when extrapolating results from GI studies performed in healthy animals to humans. Generally, compounds of therapeutic importance are administered to human patients that are ill and consequently undernourished. Toxicologic effects of therapeutic or other beneficial compounds are tested in healthy animals. These animals are fed nutritionally balanced commercial diets for their lifespan, and are allowed to grow and develop under ideal conditions of lighting, temperature, and humidity. Since macronutrients in the diet markedly affect the drug-metabolizing enzyme systems associated with the GI tract, such conditions might result in estimation of a maximally-tolerated dose that does not reflect what the dose would be in the disease state.

Evaluation of the GI tract for toxicity must also take into consideration dietary effects on the mucosa. For example, all rodent diets support normal growth and healthy condition, yet the mucosal absorption sites in animals fed a semipurified diet are significantly different from those in animals fed plant-based rodent chow, thereby affecting absorption kinetics and metabolism of a potential toxicants. Yet, since many mammalian systems have similar mechanisms of response to toxic compounds, animals serve as ideal test systems for the evaluation of toxic potential, pathophysiological responses, and systemic complications of an ingested or injected compound.

Specific Models

Ulcerative Lesions of the Stomach and Small Intestine

Propionitrile, cysteamine, 3,4-toluenediamine, and 1-methyl-4-phenyl-1,2,3,6-tetrahydropyridine (MPTP) produce acute and chronic gastric and duodenal ulcers in rodents. The morphologic appearance of duodenal ulcers produced by these alkyl compounds in rats is similar to that seen in humans.

Colitis and Typhlitis

Experimental models of colitis have been created in a number of laboratory animals (e.g., rats and guinea pigs) with ricinoleic acid, bile acids, poligeenan, melphalan, formaldehyde, alcohol, dextran sulfate, and acetic acid. Some of the lesions observed in these models may be mediated by mechanisms involving hypersensitivity or alterations in prostaglandin synthesis pathways, and are frequently associated with colon cancer if the compound induces an inflammatory process that is long-standing (e.g., poligeenan). Intracolonic administration of the hapten trinitrobenzene sulfonic acid will also lead to an immunologically-based colitis.

Colon Cancer

Colon cancer represents a leading cause of cancer-related death in Western civilization, but is relatively rare in laboratory animals. Consequently, a number of experimental models have been generated to evaluate this process. In addition, various animal species and dosing regimens have been used to produce colon cancer in animals. Both genotoxic and nongenotoxic models of colon cancer are used, but the chemically-induced genotoxic models are most consistent.

The rat is most widely used as a rodent model of colon carcinogenesis, with the mouse used somewhat less frequently. The F344 rat strain has a colon with many of the same structural and histochemical features of the human colon. This animal model may be better than the mouse, since the mouse colon structure and epithelial cell histochemical composition differ from that of the human.

Of the various chemical models available, the hydrazine derivatives have several properties that make them useful for evaluating the two-step mechanisms of colon carcinogenesis. Unlike the skin, colon carcinomas can be induced in 1,2-dimethylhydrazine-treated rats without a preliminary benign tumor stage. The incidence rate is constant, and directly proportional to total dose, with an average of one carcinoma/colon/year. This hydrazine derivative produces the promutagenic DNA lesion of O^6-methylguanine. Hydrazine models demonstrate that dysplastic or adenomatous changes are not obligatory stages before cancer; however, these lesions do indicate an increased risk of cancer development. The models may also be used to determine if the major factors in determining malignancy are ones that cause benign lesions to become larger, or ones that initiate specific cancerous changes in the DNA.

Azoxymethane is another carcinogen used frequently to study colon carcinogenesis, with the rat as the model animal. Besides inducing malignant tumors without progression through benign papillomatous lesions first, azoxymethane induces putative preneoplastic lesions—aberrant crypt foci (ACF)—which can be readily identified and quantified as biomarkers of carcinogenesis. ACF can be readily identified in whole mounts of colon, because they stain with methylene blue due to their altered morphology. This includes altered surface mucus, increased epithelial height, branching of the crypt, dilated cryptal opening, and increased pericryptal connective tissue. ACF also exhibit genotypic and proliferative atypia, as well as dysplasia, and show heterogeneity between individual crypts and among individual cells. Quantification of ACF is being used more and more as a biomarker of cancer induction. In F344 rats, azoxymethane produces colon cancer within three months, and the neoplasms readily metastasize to regional lymph nodes and the liver. This biological behavior is similar to that of certain human colorectal carcinomas.

Enterohepatic Circulation

Species differences in enterohepatic circulation are primarily determined by variations in biliary excretion. Since the rat is a very efficient biliary excretor of xenobiotic metabolites, extrapolation of toxicity data on drugs undergoing enterohepatic circulation from rats to other species may result in overestimation of a compound's safety or toxicity.

Species differences in the metabolism and toxicity of drugs and undergoing enterohepatic circulation exist between species such as rats, deer, and horses, which lack a gall bladder, and species which do have a gall bladder. Because of the concentrating capacity of the gall bladder, compounds may be concentrated to levels 10 times greater than in hepatic bile. Such concentrating activity, coupled with prolonged biliary retention, may favor passive reabsorption through the gall bladder mucosa. Additionally, reabsorption would be markedly enhanced by concomitant mucosal injury to the gall bladder epithelium.

Knockout/Transgenic Models

Transgenic mice and mice with targeted gene recombinations are now being widely used to study the basic biology and toxicology of the gut. These genetically-modified animals have been used to study cell growth and regulation, metabolism, mutagenesis, and carcinogenesis. A few examples will be briefly discussed below.

Cell Growth and Regulation

In both the small and large intestines there is regional variation in the expression of the growth factors EGF and TGFβ. Transgenic mice with a metallothionein-inducible promoter in the regulatory region of the TGFβ gene have a phenotype similar to human Menetrier's disease, including hypertrophic gastritis, mucosal hyperplasia, reduced gastric acid production, and altered mucin production. Mice overexpressing TGFβ in the duodenum have a pronounced increase in crypt cell proliferation, and increased crypt-villus dimensions.

An important component of the Wnt signaling pathway and an important effector of cell–cell adhesion, β-catenin, is associated with human colon cancer, due to its regulation by the APC gene product. Chimeric mice with a truncated β-catenin gene have marked increases in cell proliferation and apoptosis in small intestinal crypts, and altered cellular migration along the crypt-villus axis, resulting in abnormal architecture.

Carcinogenesis

A variety of transgenic mouse models, such as BigBlue and Mutamouse, have been used to investigate mutagenesis on exposure to various dietary factors (e.g., high fat content), and potentially-carcinogenic food contaminants. Although there is a general correlation between mutation rate and carcinogenicity, a high frequency of mutations in an organ did not always correlate with carcinogenicity, indicating other factors at play, such as cell turnover, apoptosis, and cell proliferation rates.

Transgenic and knockout models for a wide range of cancer genes, such as p53, APC and *ras* have also been created and used to investigate both spontaneous and environmentally-induced tumorigenesis in the intestine. Although these models allow for understanding of specific gene changes within the content of a genomic environment of the model species, it is clear from the complexity of gene regulation in different species that extrapolation from one species to another requires information that is currently beyond the state of the art.

Metabolism

Transgenic knockout mice of various cytochrome P450 genes (e.g., CYP1A2, CYP2E1) and the Ah receptor have been constructed to investigate the role of these proteins in phase I metabolism of various tissues, including intestine.

FURTHER READING

Bertram, T.A. (2002). Gastrointestinal Tract. In *Handbook of Toxicologic Pathology* (Haschek, W.M., Rousseaux, C.G., and Wallig, M.A. eds), 2nd edn, Volume II, Chapter 30, pp. 121–185. Academic Press, San Diego, CA.

Bertram, T.A., Markovitz, J.I., and Juliana, M.M. (1996). Nonproliferative lesions of the alimentary canal in rats, G1-1. In *Guides for Toxicologic Pathology*. STP/ARP/AFIP, Washington, DC.

Boorman, G., Eustis, S.C., Elwell, M.R., Montgomery, C.A., and Mckenzie, W.F. (eds) (1990). *Pathology of the Fischer Rat*, pp. 9–29. Academic Press, San Diego, CA.

Dixon, D., Heider, K., and Elwell, M.R. (1985). Incidence of non-neoplastic lesions in historical control male and female-344 rats from 90-day toxicity studies. *Toxicol. Pathol.*, 23, 338–348.

Gad, S.C. (2007). *Toxicology of the Gastrointestinal Tract*. CRC Press, Boca Raton, FL.

Jones, T.C., Mohr, U., and Popp, J.A. (1997). *Digestive System. Monographs on Pathology of Laboratory Animals.* Springer-Verlag, Berlin, Germany.

Pasual, D.W., Kiyono, H., and McGhee, J.R. (1994). The enteric nervous and immune systems: Interactions for mucosal immunity and inflammation. *Immunomethods*, 5, 56–72.

Rozman, K., and Hanninen, O. (1986). *Gastrointestinal Toxicology*. Elsevier, Amsterdam, The Netherlands.

Smith, M.W. (1986). New ways to measure intestinal injury at the cellular level. *Br. J. Cancer*, 53(S), 23–25.

Stevens, E.C., and Hume, I.D. (2004). The mammalian gastrointestinal tract. In *Comparative Physiology of the Vertebrate Digestive System*, 2nd edn., Chapter 4, pp. 64–93. Cambridge University Press, Cambridge, UK.

Walsh, C.T. (2007). Methods in Gastrointestinal Toxicology. In *Principles and Methods of Toxicology* (Hayes, A.W. ed.), 5th edn. Boca Raton, FL, Taylor & Francis.

Whiteley, L.O., Anver, M.R., Botts, S., and Jokinen, M.P. (1996). Proliferative lesions of the intestines, salivary gland, oral cavity and esophagus of rats, GI-1/2/4. In *Guides for Toxicologic Pathology*. STP/ARP/AFIP, Washington, DC.

The Liver

INTRODUCTION

Toxic responses occur relatively frequently in the liver compared with other organs. The reasons for this are numerous, but important factors include the high metabolic capability and the portal blood supply of the liver. The liver is a major site of metabolism resulting in the activation of exogenous chemicals or xenobiotics to toxic metabolites. Organs that lack such metabolic capabilities, or have lower metabolic capabilities, are less susceptible to toxicants requiring metabolic activation. The liver is also the first major organ to be exposed to ingested toxicants, due to its portal blood supply. Therefore, toxicants may be at least partially removed from the circulation during this "first pass," providing protection to other organs while increasing the likelihood of hepatic injury.

STRUCTURE AND FUNCTION

The liver has two blood supplies, the hepatic artery and the portal vein. The hepatic artery provides oxygen and nutrition, while the portal vein delivers substances absorbed by the gastrointestinal tract for metabolic conversion and/or removal. The gross appearance of the liver is similar in all species, although the lobes vary in shape and size. Histologically, the liver has a lobular architecture that is similar in all species. While hepatocytes are the major cell type in the liver, all of the cell types are important for normal hepatic function and participate in toxicologic responses.

Gross and Microscopic Anatomy

The liver is located in the cranial abdomen and accounts for 1–4% of body weight in adults of most species, with a greater percentage for neonatal liver. In rats and mice it accounts for approximately 4% of the body weight, in adult omnivores about 2%, in herbivores about 1%, and in humans about 2.5%. The liver is divided into lobes that vary according to species. In mice and rats, it consists of four lobes: left, median, right, and caudate. The gall bladder, when present, stores and concentrates bile; in mice, it is located in a cleft between the two sublobes of the median lobe. It collects bile from the hepatic duct via the cystic duct, which then continues on to the duodenum as the common bile duct. Rats, horses, and elephants lack a gall bladder, and thus continuously secrete unconcentrated bile.

The blood supply to the liver arrives at the hilum from two sources: the portal vein, which drains the gastrointestinal tract, providing 60–70% of the afferent hepatic blood flow; and the hepatic artery, providing the remainder. Blood flow from the liver is via the hepatic vein, which enters the caudal vena cava. The hepatic lobule is the classical subunit of the liver (Figure 9.1A). At the center of this hexagonal structure is a central vein, a tributary of the hepatic vein. At the angles of the hexagon are portal tracts that contain bile ducts, the hepatic artery, branches of the portal vein, as well as nerves and lymphatics. The sinusoids provide a conduit for blood flow from the portal tract (hepatic artery and portal vein) toward the central vein. The sinusoids (Figure 9.1B), lined by endothelial cells, separate the hepatic plates which consist of cords of hepatocytes. Bile canaliculi are specialized structures formed by the lateral aspects of adjacent hepatocytes. Hepatocyte microvilli protrude from the apical surface into the space of Dissé, which lies between the endothelial cells and the hepatocyte. Stellate cells (previously termed Ito cells) are also present within the space of Dissé. Küpffer cells or fixed hepatic macrophages are attached to the endothelium.

Cell Components

The Hepatocyte

The parenchymal cell of the liver is the hepatocyte, which represents approximately 60% of the hepatic cells and 80% of the hepatic volume. Hepatocytes are polyhedral cells with round central nuclei and abundant cytoplasm. The cell membrane has three domains: perisinusoidal; intercellular; and pericanalicular. The canaliculi are located at the pole opposite the sinusoid. Bile secreted into canaliculi flows toward the portal bile ducts. Hepatocytes are oriented in cords composed of a single row of cells separated from vascular sinusoids by endothelial cells (Figure 9.1B). Blood flows through the sinusoids from portal to central venous regions. This directional blood flow results in the metabolic zonation of hepatocytes across the sinusoid, reflecting the physiological variations among hepatocytes, depending on their location along the sinusoid. These physiological variations are considered to represent the adaptation of hepatocytes to gradients in concentrations of nutrients, oxygen tension, and other substances along the sinusoid. Distribution of hepatocytes along sinusoids has thus been described in both anatomic and functional terms (Figure 9.1C).

Anatomically, hepatocytes are distributed in three indistinctly separate areas of a lobule: periportal; midzonal; and central lobular. Functionally, hepatocytes are considered to reside in acini composed of three metabolic zones, the first (Zone 1) reflecting greatest proximity to vascular supply of substrates and oxygen; this roughly approximates the periportal area. Zones 2 and 3 reflect decreasing proximity to vascular supply, and approximate the midzonal and central lobular areas respectively. Differences in anatomic distribution and metabolic function result in subtle morphologic variations in hepatocytes. For example, central lobular hepatocytes tend to be larger than periportal hepatocytes, and contain more smooth endoplasmic reticulum and less cytoplasmic lipid.

The lifespan of the hepatocytes is estimated to be 200 days in rats. Although highly differentiated, hepatocytes undergo cell division to support liver growth or replace those which are lost, either through normal attrition or due to injury. While hepatocytes may divide to produce additional hepatocytes, stem cells and oval cells (see subsequent text) have also been proposed as hepatocyte progenitor cells, at least in rodents.

The importance of the liver in numerous homeostatic activities is attributed to the extreme diversity of hepatocyte function. Many of these functions are related to the intermediary role of hepatocyte metabolism between dietary sources of energy and extrahepatic tissue demands for energy. Most of these

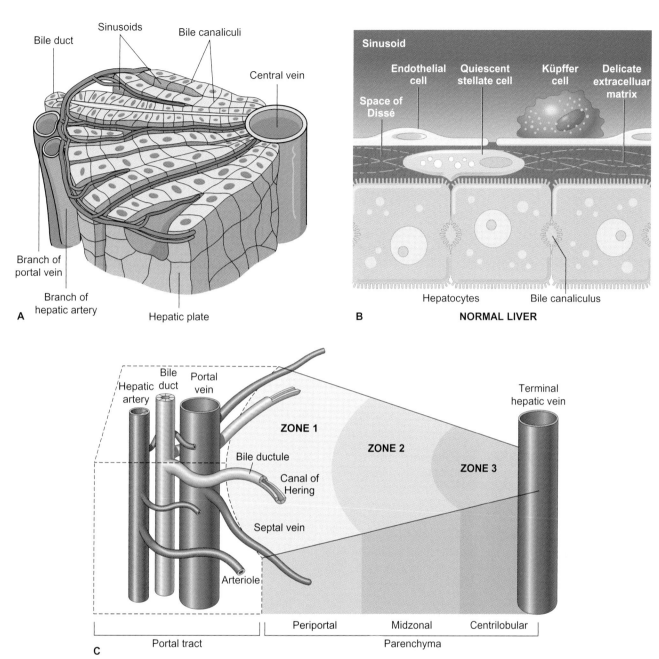

FIGURE 9.1   Schematic representation of the microscopic and functional organization of the liver. (A) Microscopic organization of the liver. A central vein is present in the center of the lobule with radially arranged plates of hepatocytes. Branches of the portal vein and hepatic artery are located in the periphery of the lobule, and blood from both the artery and vein enter the sinusoids. Peripherally-located bile ducts drain the bile canaliculi that are formed by and lie between the hepatocytes. (From McCance, K.L., and Huether, S.E. (2002). *Pathophysiology: The Biologic Basis for Diseases in Adults and Children*, 4th edn. Mosby, St. Louis.) (B) Schematic representation of the hepatic sinusoid. The sinusoid is a vascular lumen lined by discontinuous endothelium. Küpffer cells are attached to the endothelial cells and project into the sinusoid. The space of Dissé lies between the endothelial cells and the hepatocytes, whose microvilli extend into this space. Stellate (Ito) cells are present within the space of Dissé and extend between hepatocytes. (From Crawford, J.M. (2005). Liver and biliary tract. In *Robbins and Cotran Pathologic Basis of Disease*, Kumar, V., Abbas, A.K., and Fuasto, N. eds, 7th edn, pp. 877–938. Elsevier Saunders, New York. Figure 18-3, p. 884.) (C) Functional organization of the liver. Both the classical lobule and the functional acinus are represented. The lobule is a hexagonal unit with portal areas at the margin and a terminal hepatic vein (central vein) at the center. The lobule is divided into the periportal, midzonal, and centrilobular areas. The acinus is a diamond-shaped structure with the distributing branches of the vessels from the portal areas at the center of the structure. Zone 1 of the acinus is closest to the afferent blood supply, and zone 3 is at the tip of the diamond-shaped structure, close to the terminal hepatic vein. Zone 2 is between zones 1 and 3. (From Crawford, J.M. (2005). Liver and biliary tract. In *Robbins and Cotran Pathologic Basis of Disease*, Kumar, V., Abbas, A.K., and Fuasto, N. eds, 7th edn. Elsevier Saunders, New York. Figure 18-1, p. 879.)

hepatocyte functions represent variation in magnitude of activity relative to other cells in the body. However, some functions are qualitatively specific for hepatocytes, including urea cycle metabolism (nitrogenous waste handling) and bile formation.

Nonparenchymal Cells

Nonparenchymal cells consist of sinusoidal, peri-sinusoidal, and biliary cells. Biliary epithelial cells form a system of ducts that move bile out of the liver. Bile ducts, along with hepatic arterioles and portal venules, are found in portal areas which are normally separated from the sinusoidal hepatocytes by a so-called "limiting plate" of hepatocytes. Bile ducts are lined by cuboidal to columnar epithelial cells, and are surrounded by connective tissue of the portal area. These epithelial cells have fewer mitochondria than hepatocytes. The ducts are connected with the canaliculi by short intermediate canals (canals of Hering) or ductules lined by low cuboidal epithelial cells with scant cytoplasmic organelles and small dark nuclei.

The sinusoids are separated from the perisinusoidal space of Dissé by fenestrated flat endothelial cells that are devoid of basement membrane, permitting the rapid exchange of cell-free constituents between the blood and the perisinusoidal space.

The Küpffer cells, which differentiate from mononuclear phagocytic cells derived from bone marrow, are stellate and sit on the sinusoidal surface of the endothelial cell, projecting into the vascular space (Figure 9.1B). They are the major phagocytic cell of the liver, and also a major source of cytokines following hepatic injury. Most blood-borne particulate material is cleared by Küpffer cells, except in certain species such as pigs, goats, and cattle (family Artiodactyla) in which the pulmonary intravascular macrophage is primarily responsible for this function. Two other intrasinusoidal cell populations are the dendritic cell and the pit cell. Pit cells contain cytoplasmic granules, are defined morphologically as large granular lymphocytes, and function as liver-specific natural killer (NK) cells. They adhere to the endothelium and to Küpffer cells.

The perisinusoidal space contains stellate cells which contain cytoplasmic lipid droplets and store vitamin A. Although stellate cells only constitute approximately 5% of hepatic cells, they play an important role in hepatic injury, because once activated they can be stimulated to produce collagen which is important in hepatic fibrosis.

Cells of the hematopoietic system are present in fetal liver, and may be present but considerably decreased in number in the postnatal period in rodents. These cells may appear in adult liver in response to anemia or inflammation, especially in rodents. In rare instances, foci of hematopoiesis have been described in association with chemical carcinogenesis.

In summary, several general concepts are crucial for understanding hepatic function and disease. Exocrine, endocrine, and metabolic functions of the hepatic parenchyma occur in the hepatocytes. The liver receives a double blood supply, consisting of arterial circulation and portal circulation from the splanchnic venous drainage. Circulation and biliary secretion are compartmentalized, and exchange between blood and hepatocytes is greatly facilitated.

Xenobiotic Metabolism

The role of the liver in activation and detoxification of xenobiotics is of central importance. Metabolic reactions of xenobiotics in liver occur primarily in hepatocytes, and are grouped into two major categories: Phase I and Phase II. Phase I reactions consist of oxidations and reductions, which usually result in a more polar metabolite. Phase II reactions consist of conjugations with glucuronide, sulfate, glutathione, acetyl, amino acid, or methyl groups.

Detoxification and increasing water solubility (hence aiding elimination) may be considered the optimal goal of these reactions, in which a potentially toxic xenobiotic is rendered inactive and/or excreted. However, sometimes the same enzymatic machinery for detoxification may result in a metabolite that is more toxic than the parent xenobiotic, thereby resulting in bioactivation. Metabolism by the enzyme alcohol dehydrogenase is also important in the liver. Metabolism in the liver by both enzyme systems is responsible for most of ethanol's toxic effects.

MECHANISMS OF TOXICITY

Factors important in hepatic injury include those related to the xenobiotic, as well as the target organ. Hepatocytes have high metabolic activity and high capacity for biotransformation. Blood flow is important in exposing the liver to toxicants, especially those absorbed from the gastrointestinal tract, and in the lobular pattern of injury due to intrahepatic delivery of toxicants. The enterohepatic circulation is important in many species where hepatotoxicants excreted in bile are recirculated from the intestinal tract back to the liver. This can result in prolonged hepatic exposure to the xenobiotic. Pre-existing injury or disease can alter metabolism and excretion of xenobiotics. Interaction of xenobiotics can be additive or synergistic, as with alcohol potentiation of acetaminophen toxicity.

The mechanism of action of hepatotoxicants can be direct or indirect, where reactive metabolites are responsible for toxicity. Reactive metabolites are generally formed through cytochrome P450-mediated reactions in the liver, which occasionally may be preceded by deconjugation of the xenobiotic by intestinal bacteria.

Species, race, strain, breed, and individual differences can affect susceptibility to hepatotoxicants. A classic example is the marked susceptibility of rats, as compared to mice, to aflatoxin-induced hepatotoxicity, because of differences in cytochrome P450s. In companion animals, cats are relatively deficient in hepatic glucuronly transferase, and thus more susceptible to many hepatotoxicants, such as acetaminophen, than dogs where conjugation of Phase I metabolites with glucuronide in Phase II reactions is limited. While dogs occasionally develop hepatic necrosis as an idiosyncratic response to the anti-inflammatory agent carprofen (Rimadyl), Labrador retrievers are more susceptible than other breeds of dog, indicating genetic polymorphism within species of animals. Ethnic genetic polymorphisms in aldehyde dehydrogenase affect ethanol metabolism in humans. Individual genetic differences in hepatic metabolism of xenobiotics play a major role in individual susceptibility to hepatotoxicants.

Classification of Hepatoxicants

Classification Based on Type of Response

Hepatotoxicants can be classified based on the type of response they induce, predictable (intrinsic) or unpredictable (idiosyncratic). Predictable hepatotoxicants induce a dose-dependent effect which occurs in the majority of those exposed. However, as discussed above, a variety of factors influence the severity of injury manifested in an individual. Most hepatotoxicants recognized in domestic animals fall into the category of predictable hepatotoxicants.

Unpredictable or idiosyncratic responses depend on a specific individual reacting in a manner different to the population at large, and therefore affect only a small proportion of those exposed. Idiosyncratic drug reactions account for 6–10% of all adverse drug reactions and the majority of hepatic adverse reactions to marketed drugs in humans. Predictable hepatotoxicants are usually identified early during drug development, and either eliminated from further development or approved under stringent regulations.

Potential mechanisms for idiosyncratic reactions include the rate at which the host metabolizes the xenobiotic, e.g., chlorpromazine, atypical metabolism, or the host's propensity to mount an immune response to an antigenic stimulus, e.g., halothane. The hapten hypothesis provides an explanation for an immune mechanism. Chemically-reactive drugs, or more likely their metabolites, act as haptens and bind to endogenous proteins. These drug–protein adducts are seen as foreign, and induce an immune response. It has been suggested that immunological tolerance against these drug–protein adducts develops as a default in most patients, and it is only when there is interference with this tolerance in a susceptible individual that an idiosyncratic response occurs. The Küpffer cell is believed to play a central role in induction of tolerance to hapten–protein adducts. Other drugs that cause idiosyncratic reactions in humans include sulfonamides, α-methyldopa, and allopurinol. The potential for induction of an idiosyncratic reaction cannot be identified during current safety evaluation studies, due to species differences and infrequency of the finding. In domestic animals, acute idiosyncratic reactions have been identified in cats, due to diazepam (valium), and in dogs, due to mebendazole and carprofen, and chronic reactions have been identified in dogs due to anticonvulsants, such as primadone, phenobarbital, and phenytoin.

Classification Based on Functional Characteristics

Classes of hepatotoxicants include drugs, natural toxicants, metals (e.g., copper and iron), vitamins (e.g., vitamin A), and chemicals. Hepatotoxic drugs include acetaminophen, nonsteroidal anti-inflammatory drugs (NSAIDs), glucocorticosteroids, antibiotics and antifungals, anesthetic agents, and anticonvulsants. Drug-induced liver injury (DILI) accounts for about 10% of acute hepatitis in humans. Herbal and botanical products are also an important cause of hepatic injury. Natural toxicants include mycotoxins such as aflatoxin B_1, fumonisins, sporodesmin, phomopsins, amatoxins, and phalloidin from *Amanita* sp of mushrooms; plant toxins such as pyrrolizidine alkaloids, lantedene from *Lantana camara*, and the glycoside carboxyatractyloside in cocklebur (*Xanthium* spp); and algal toxins such as microcystin-LR from *Microcystis aueroginosa*, and cylindrospermopsin from *Cylindrospermopsis raciborskii*. Hepatotoxic chemicals include those used for industrial (e.g. alcohol, carbon tetrachloride) or agricultural purposes (white phophorus used as rodenticide), as food additives (xylitol toxic to dogs), or from environmental contamination.

Cellular Mechanisms of Toxicity

While many potential mechanisms of hepatic cell injury have been characterized, it is often not clear which mechanism is of primary importance in the pathogenesis of cell injury for any particular toxin. Some of these mechanisms are listed in Table 9.1, and discussed elsewhere in this chapter.

NON-NEOPLASTIC RESPONSES TO INJURY

Each of the different cell types in the liver may respond to a toxic insult (Table 9.2). The lesion produced depends on which cells are injured, and the different responses of each cell type. Injury may result in apoptopsis, necrosis, or both. Less severe injury or other forms of injury may result in adaptation, or the accumulation of various cytoplasmic infiltrations and pigments. It is important to remember that exposure to a xenobiotic may not necessarily result in degenerative or necrotic responses. Cells, particularly hepatocytes, have a remarkable capability to adapt to various exogenous agents. While adaptive responses are not toxic manifestations of exposure to xenobiotics, they are important indicators of exposure, and potentially of altered hepatic function. Hepatocellular necrosis is usually followed by regeneration. Inflammation may also occur. Chronic hepatic injury can result in fibrosis or cirrhosis which is irreversible. Potential consequences of hepatic failure include hepatic encephalopathy, metabolic disturbances such as hemorrhagic diathesis and hypoalbuminemia, and vascular and hemodynamic alterations.

In domestic animals, acute, severe exposure to a hepatotoxicant will often result in a readily classifiable type of alteration (Tables 9.3 and 9.4); however, chronic exposure often results in complex changes that can lead to fibrosis and cirrhosis. In addition, it is not uncommon to have exposure to multiple hepatotoxins. For example, plant toxins such as pyrrolizidine alkaloids may cause minor morphologic alterations, but these may prevent excretion of copper, thus increasing susceptibility to copper toxicosis. In addition, pyrrolizidine alkaloids can prevent normal cell division which is important in the normal reparative responses, and thus predispose to fibrosis. Impairment of liver function can lead to extrahepatic effects, including hepatic encephalopathy and cutaneous effects, such as epidermal necrosis in dogs (hepatocutaneous syndrome), and photosensitization (secondary [hepatogenous] photosensitization) in herbivores, when phylloerythrin enters the circulation and reaches the skin instead of being excreted in bile (see Chapter 7, Skin and Oral Mucosa).

TABLE 9.1 Potential mechanisms of hepatic injury with selected examples

Mechanisms	Xenobiotic	Lesion
Metabolic activation		
Cytochrome P450 enzymes	Acetaminophen, carbon tetrachloride, thioacetamide, bromobenzene, aflatoxin B_1	Centrilobular necrosis (acute)
Alcohol dehydrogenase	Allyl alcohol, ethanol, ethylene glycol	Periportal necrosis
Disruption of calcium homeostasis and cell membrane injury		
Cytoskeletal effects	Microcystin-LR	Centrilobular hepatocyte disassociation and necrosis
ATP production	D-galactosamine	Steatosis
Mitochondrial injury		
β-oxidation	Aspirin, antiviral nucleosides, valproic acid, tetracyclines, aflatoxin B_1	Steatosis
Oxidative phosphorylation	Bile acids, amiodarone, cyanide	Cholestasis
DNA synthesis	Some antiviral nucleosides	Necrosis
Apoptotic pathways	Hydrophobic bile acids, fumonisins	Apoptosis
Autoimmunity	Tienilic acid, dihydralazine	Hepatitis
Canalicular injury	Estrogen, erythromycin, lantadene	Cholestasis
Bile salt transporter	High fat diet	Steatosis
Canalicular cytoskeleton	Phalloidin	Actin filament changes, necrosis
Idiosyncratic	Humans: halothane, phenytoin. Cats: diazepam (valium) Dogs: carprofen, sulfonamides	Severe hepatocellular necrosis

TABLE 9.2 Classification of non-neoplastic liver lesions with selected examples

Lesion	Toxicant		
	Chemicals/other	Drugs	Toxins (plant, fungal, algal)
Parenchymal cell (hepatocyte)			
Cell death			
Central lobular necrosis	Carbon tetrachloride, bromobenzene, dimethylnitrosamine, chlorinated hydrocarbons	Acetaminophen, hypoxia in conjunction with many drugs	Microcystin-LR, aflatoxin, gossypol, pyrrolizidine alkaloids, wild coffee, red maple, Russian knapweed, sporidesmin
Midzonal necrosis	Furan (mice), hexachlorophene (cats)	Concanavalin A, cisplatin	Aflatoxin (rabbit), *Myoporaceous* furanosesquiterpinoid essential oil, nutmeg
Periportal necrosis	Allyl alcohol, N-hydroxy-acetylaminofluorene, phosphorus	Cocaine, rifampicin, some anesthetics	Aflatoxin (poultry), cyclochlorotine
Massive necrosis	Dichloropropanol	Cisplatin, diazepam (cats)	Microcystin LR, cycads, *Amanita phalloides*
Focal necrosis and granulomas formation	D-galactosamine	Isoniazid, phenothiazine, α-methyldopa, allopurinol, quinine, phenytoin	*Eupatorium adenophorum*, *Penicillium* sp
Apoptosis	Cyproterone acetate, lead nitrate, ethanol, dioxin, 2-acetylaminofluorene, hexavalent chromium	Tacrine, zerumbone, rezulin; chemotherapeutic drugs, tunicamycin, prostaglandins	Fumonisins, sesquiterpene lactones, citrinin, ochratoxin, clivorine, lipopolysaccharide, monocrotaline, gliotoxin,
Accumulations and pigments			
Triglyceride accumulation	Carbon tetrachloride, phosphorous, orotic acid, 4-aminopyrazolpyrimidine, ethanol, carbon tetrachloride, L-carnitine trans-fats, ethanol, diethylnitrosamine	Tetracycline, methotrexate, amiodarone, valproic acid, antiviral nucleosides, estrogens, cholestyramine, β-blockers, steroids, prostaglandin E$_2$, valproate	Aflatoxin, canola oil, plant sterols, omega-6-fatty acids, plant stanols, retinoids, nutmeg
Phospholipidosis	2-methylnaphthalene, lead, pentamidine	Chlorphenterimine, azithomycin, amiodarone, ketoconazole, fluoxetine, cationic amphiphilic drugs	*Oxytropis* sp
Other accumulations and pigments	Iron, copper, antimony	Glucocorticosteroids (dogs), β3 adrenergic receptor agonists	Fagopyrin, hypericin, polyphenolic pigments
Nucleolar lesions	Nitrosamines, 1-nitro-9-aminoacridine, ethidium bromide	Daunomycin, proflavin	α-amanitin, aflatoxins
Other hepatocellular changes			
Megalocytosis, megalokaryosis	Nitrosamines, 1-(4-dimethylamino-benzyldene)-indene, methylazoxymethanol, N-hydroxyacetylaminofluorene, xanthine 3N-oxide	Vidarabine, hydroxyurea	Pyrrolizidine alkaloids, aflatoxins, lasiocarpine, protoberberine alkaloids, *Urtica dioica*
Cholestasis	Methionine, methyl isobutyl ketone, manganese, α-naphthylisocyanate	Griseofulvin, estrogen, erythromycin, chlorpromazine, rifamycin, novobiocin, carbamazepine, anabolic steroids, chemotherapeutic agents, tolbutamide, tricyclic antidepressants	Lantadene A and B, phalloidin, sporidesmin, *Larrea tridentate*, Ackee fruit, sesquiterpenes

(Continued)

TABLE 9.2　(*Continued*)

Lesion	Toxicant		
	Chemicals/other	Drugs	Toxins (plant, fungal, algal)
Hypertrophy			
Smooth endoplasmic reticulum increase	Cyproterone acetate, PCBs	Phenobarbital	Aflatoxins
Peroxisome proliferation	Diethylhexyl phthalate, dichloroacetic acid, haloacetates	Clofibrate, fenofibrate, troglitazone	
Mitochondrial hypertrophy	Cuprizone, ethionine, orotic acid	Reverse transcriptase inhibitors	Aflatoxins, *Acremonium exuviarum*
Bile duct epithelium			
Acute bile duct necrosis	Alpha-napthylisothiocyanate, phenylisocyanate, 2-acetylaminofluorene	Trimethoprim sulfa (dogs)	Sporodesmin
Bile duct hyperplasia	Allyl alcohol, coumarin, piperonyl butoxide, alpha-naphthylisothiocyanate, diethylnitrosamine	Methapyrilene, praziquante	Aflatoxin, pyrrolizidine alkaloids, sporidesmin, methyleugenol
Oval cell hyperplasia (rodents)	2-Acetylaminofluorene, PCBs,TCDD, o-nitrotoluene, furans, cobalt sufate	Asparaginase, 2-amino-3-methylimidazo-[4,5-f]quinoline (IQ), methapyriline	Aflatoxin, citrinin, methyl eugenol, estragole
Nonparenchymal cells			
Endothelial cell necrosis	Nitrosamines, beryllium, arsenicals, diquat, carbon teterachloride, bromobenzene	Anti-VEGF, acetaminophen, chemotherapeutic drugs, cyclosporine A, antiviral drugs, HIV-AIDS drugs, antifibrotic drugs, TNF-α, dimethylnitrosamine	Pyrrolizidine alkaloids, microcystin-LR, lipopolysaccharide, ergot, aflatoxin
Stellate (Ito) cell toxicity	Vitamin A, carbon tetrachloride, iron toxicity	Retinoic acid, methotrexate	
Küpffer cell necrosis	Beryllium, gadolinium chloride, carbon tetrachloride	Pentoxifylline, antifibrotic drugs	Ricin, *Penicillium cyclopium*
Hepatitis	β-naphthylisothiocyanate, ethanol, carbon tetrachloride, trinitrotoluene (TNT)	Halothane, sulfonamides, methyldopa, NSAIDS, phenytoin, diclofenac, augmentin, nitrofurantoin, halothane, methamphetamine, methotrexate	*Chelidonium majus, Cassia siamea*, dandelion (*Taraxacum officinale*), *Teucrium pol, Chelidonium majus*, Kava kava, aloe vera
Liver as a whole			
Fibrosis/cirrhosis	Carbon tetrachloride, ethanol, dithethylnitrosamine, iron	α-methyldopa, acetaminophen metabolites, arsenic, deferiprone, celecoxib, methotrexate, oxyphenisatin, iproniazid, methyldopa, sulphonamides, propylthiouracil	Pyrrolizidine alkaloids, aflatoxins, *Capillaria hepatica, Pueraria lobata*

TABLE 9.3 Selected toxicants causing hepatic disease in domestic animals

Category	Type of toxicant	Toxicant	Source of toxicant	Source of contamination	Species affected	Acute toxicity/disease	Chronic toxicity/disease	Other organ systems affected/disease	Classification of mechanism
Natural toxins	Mycotoxins	Aflatoxins, especially B_1	*Aspergillus* spp., e.g., *A. flavus*	Corn and other cereal crops, peanuts, cottonseed, contaminated pet food	Cattle, pigs, dogs, horses, poultry, humans; all susceptible	Necrosis (mainly centrilobular), lipidosis, biliary hyperplasia / Acute aflatoxicosis	Megalocytosis, biliary fibrosis, cirrhosis, neoplasia / Chronic aflatoxicosis	Immune and other systems	Electrophile, cytochrome P450 bioactivation
		Fumonisins, especially B_1	*Fusarium verticillioides*	Corn	Horses, pigs, all (humans?) susceptible	Apoptosis, necrosis possible	Fibrosis (pigs, horses)	CNS (horses, equine leukoencephalomalacia), lung edema (pigs), kidney (rats, ruminants)	Alteration of sphingolipid metabolism
		Sporidesmin	*Pithomyces chartarum*	*Lolium perenne* (rye grass)	Sheep, cattle	Biliary duct necrosis, cholestasis	Chronic cholangitis, biliary hyperplasia, fibrosis	Skin: secondary photosensitization ("facial eczema")	Biliary obstruction
		Phomopsins	*Phomopsis leptostromiformis*	*Lupinus* sp (lupines)	Sheep, cattle, horses	Scattered necrosis, mitotic arrest / Lupinosis	Fibrosis, biliary hyperplasia Hepatic atrophy	Photosensitization, skeletal myopathy	Cytoskeletal disruption (binds tubulin)
		Amatoxins	*Amanita* and other spp.	Mushroom	All	Centrilobular to massive disassociation/necrosis, nucleolar fragmentation, hemorrhage, lipidosis			Cytoskeletal disruption (inhibits nuclear RNA polymerase II)
	Cyanobacterial toxins	Microcystin-LR	*Microcystis aeruginosa* and other algal species	Freshwater blue green algal blooms	All	Centrilobular to massive disassociation/apoptosis/necrosis, hemorrhage	Fibrosis		Cytoskeletal dysruption (inhibits cytoplasmic protein phosphatases 1 and 2A)
		Nodularins	*Nodularia Spumigena*	Brackish water algae	All	Centrilobular necrosis			
		Cylindrospermopsin	*Cylindrospermopsis raciborskii*	Freshwater algal blooms	All	Centrilobular necrosis, lipidosis		Kidney	Protein synthesis inhibitor

(Continued)

TABLE 9.3 (Continued)

Category	Type of toxicant	Toxicant	Source of toxicant	Source of contamination	Species affected	Acute toxicity/disease	Chronic toxicity/disease	Other organ systems affected/disease	Classification of mechanism
Plants and plant toxins		Carboxyatractyloside	*Xanthium* spp (cocklebur)	Plants or grains contaminated by seed	Pigs, cattle, horses, sheep	Centrilobular to massive necrosis		Cardiac hemorrhage	Inhibit oxidative phosphorylation
		Pyrrolizidine alkaloids	*Senecio, Crotalaria, Heliotropium, Echium, Amsinckia, Cynoglossum* spp	Plants or grains contaminated by seed	Horses, cattle, pigs All susceptible	Centrilobular necrosis, hemorrhage	Megalocytosis, fibrosis (centrilobular, periportal, sinusoidal), biliary hyperplasia Veno-occlusive disease (humans)	Lung, kidney possible Secondary: hepatoencephalopathy, photosensitization	Electrophile, cytochrome P450 bioactivation
		Triterpenes, lantadenes A and B	*Lantana camara*	Plants	Ruminants	Necrosis, cholestasis	Megalocytosis, biliary hyperplasia, cholestasis	Kidney, heart; secondary photosensitization	
		Saponins	Some *Panicum* spp. e.g., *P. coloratum* (kleingrass), *P. virgatum* (switchgrass)	Grasses	Horses, ruminants	Crystal-associated cholangiopathy	Fibrosis and biliary hyperplasia	Secondary: hepatoencephalopathy, photosensitization	Biliary obstruction
			Trifolium hybridum (alsike clover) Also red clover	Pasture	Horses	Cholangiohepatitis	Biliary hyperplasia, fibrosis "Big liver" disease	Skin: photosensitization Oral: stomatitis ("slobbers")	
		Methylazoxymethanol	*Zamiaceae* and *Cycadaceae* spp	Cycads (Sago palm nuts)	Ruminants, dogs, pigs, horses	Centrilobular necrosis	Megalocytosis, cholestasis, biliary hyperplasia, fibrosis (ruminants)	CNS (ruminants, "Zamia staggers")	Alkylation of DNA and RNA
		Gossypol	*Gossypium* sp (cotton)	Cotton seed meal	Pigs, cattle	Centrilobular necrosis		Heart: cardiomyopathy; male reproductive system	Oxidative stress
		Furanosesquiterpenoid oils (ngaione)	*Myoporum* spp	Leaves and branches	Ruminants horses, pigs	Centrilobular or variable necrosis	Bile duct hyperplasia	Lung (sheep); secondary photosensitization	
		Steroidal sapogens	*Tribulus terrestris*	Forage	Sheep	Crystalline material in bile ducts	Bile duct hyperplasia and fibrosis		Biliary obstruction
		Phorbol esters	*Pimlea* spp	Forage	Cattle	Angiectasis (*peliosis hepatis*)		Lung	

Metals		Copper	Anthelmintics, pesticides, foot baths, feed additives	Dietary, supplements, environmental	Ruminants (especially sheep), pigs, dogs (metabolic defect in susceptible breeds)	Centrilobular necrosis	Ruminants: centrilobular and multifocal necrosis with Cu release; Cu pigment Dogs: cirrhosis	Ruminants: intravascular hemolytic anemia; nephrosis secondary to methemoglobinuria Nonruminants: gastric ulcers	Free radical formation
		Iron		Injectables, supplements	All	Periportal to massive necrosis	Hemachromatosis (dogs and cats); periportal fibrosis, biliary hyperplasia, bile stasis (foals)	Acute gastroenteritis	Free radical formation
Chemicals	Food additives	Xylitol	Sweetener	Baked good, desserts, toothpaste, candy	Dogs	Centrilobular necrosis		Coagulopathy	Insulin release
		Vitamin A		Diet, liver	Cats	Stellate cell and hepatocellular toxicity	Centrilobular fibrosis (veno-occlusion, captive cheetahs) Veno-occlusive disease	Skeletal system, teratogenesis	
	Other	Polycyclic aromatic hydrocarbons (PAHs)	Phenolics and coal tar derivatives	Clay pigeons, asphalt shingles, creosote, disinfectants	All (especially cats, pigs)	Centrilobular to massive necrosis			
		Carbon tetrachloride	Anthelmintic, cleaning agents	Household products	All	Centrilobular necrosis		Kidney, bone marrow (aplastic anemia)	Free radical fomation, cytochrome P450 bioactivation
		Phosphorus	Rodenticide (white), fireworks (yellow)		All	Periportal necrosis, fatty change		Heart, kidney	Free radical formation, cytochrome p450 bioactivation

TABLE 9.4   Selected drugs causing hepatic disease in domestic animals

Category	Drug	Species affected	Acute toxicity/ disease	Chronic toxicity/ disease	Mechanism of toxicity
Anthelmintics	Mebendazole	Dogs (breed susceptibility)	Centrilobular to massive necrosis		Idiosyncratic
	Thiacetarsamide	Dogs			
Anticonvulsants	Phenobarbital, primidone, phenytoin	Dogs	Multifocal apoptosis/necrosis, inflammation	Cirrhosis	Idiosyncratic
Anti-inflammatory	Carprofen	Dogs (Labrador)	Centrilobular necrosis		Idiosyncratic
	Ibuprofen	Dogs	Centrilobular necrosis		
	Acetaminophen	All; dogs mainly	Centrilobular necrosis		Electrophile, cytochrome P450 bioactivation
	Glucocorticoids	Dogs only	Glycogen accumulation		
			Steroid hepatopathy		
Sedative	Diazepam	Cats only	Massive necrosis		Idiosyncratic
Anesthetic	Halothane		Centrilobular necrosis, lipidosis		Idiosyncratic
	Methoxyflurane				
Antimicrobial	Trimethoprim-sulfa	Dogs	Periportal to massive necrosis	Necrotizing cholangitis	Idiosyncratic
	Tetracycline	Dogs, cats	Lipidosis, massive necrosis		β-oxidation of mitrochondrial fatty acids
Antifungals	Ketaconazole	Cats mainly	Necrosis		

Histologic Types of Hepatic Necrosis

Cell death or necrosis is a frequent sequel to liver injury. While necrosis may affect any cell type in the liver, necrosis of hepatocytes is most frequent and most completely studied. Xenobiotic-induced necrosis of hepatocytes may occur in several different histologic patterns, based on its relationship to the lobular architecture of the normal liver. The specific pattern of necrosis seen after the administration of a hepatotoxin is reproducible within a given species, and most often between species, although species differences may be seen (see Table 9.2). For aflatoxins, central lobular necrosis is the most common pattern; however, periportal necrosis has been described in poultry, cats and rats, and midzonal necrosis in rabbits. Patterns of hepatocellular necrosis have been widely studied in experimental animals, and similar patterns of necrosis have been observed in humans exposed to chemicals and drugs.

While xenobiotics are generally believed to be specific for a single area of the lobule, at least within a given species, it is interesting to note that the lobular effect may shift with a change in dose, duration of exposure, or coexposure to another agent.

Central Lobular (Centrilobular) Necrosis

Central lobular necrosis is by far the most frequent form of hepatocellular necrosis following acute exposure to a variety of hepatotoxic agents, including carbon tetrachloride, acetaminophen, thioacetamide, and bromobenzene (see Tables 9.2, 9.3, and 9.4, Figures 9.2 and 9.3). As the term implies, central lobular necrosis occurs in the central lobular area, with the necrotic hepatocytes completely encircling the central vein (terminal hepatic venule). Based on this morphologic distribution, central lobular necrosis has also been referred to as centrilobular, centrolobular, and pericentral, indicating the relationship to the classic hepatic lobule, or periacinar, and the relationship to metabolic zonation. In some literature, this pattern of necrosis has been referred to as perivenous, based on the distribution around the terminal hepatic venule. The lesion is generally found uniformly throughout the

A

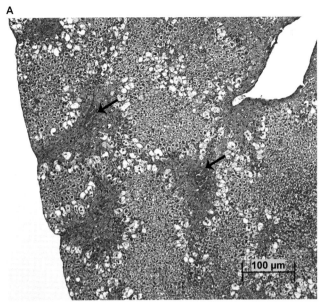

B

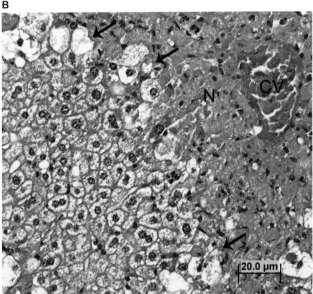

FIGURE 9.2 Central lobular necrosis; carbon tetrachloride, single dose, rat. H&E stain. (A) A zone of coagulation necrosis around central veins (arrows) is separated from viable periportal hepatocytes by a zone of hepatocytes undergoing hydropic degeneration. (B) Higher magnification of (A). Necrotic hepatocytes (N) surround the central vein (CV) with adjacent hepatocytes undergoing hydropic degeneration (arrows).

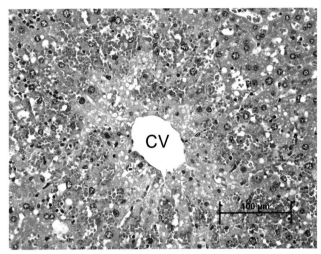

FIGURE 9.3 Central lobular necrosis with hemorrhage; acetaminophen, single intraperitoneal dose, rat. Hemorrhage is present amid a zone of necrosis that surrounds a central vein (CV). H&E stain.

liver, with the central areas of most, if not all, lobules affected. Within each lobule, the percentage of cells involved depends on the inciting agent and the dose.

Necrosis generally appears as coagulative necrosis, and may be limited to a single row of hepatocytes surrounding the central vein, or may extend up to half the width of the lobule. While an increase in the dose of the toxic agent will expand the lesion, to involve a greater portion of the lobule extending toward the portal triad,

even maximum doses of some hepatotoxicants, such as carbon tetrachloride, may fail to expand the lesion past the midzonal area. The demarcation between necrotic hepatocytes is frequently abrupt when examined by light microscopy. However, in some cases a thin zone of swollen, lipid- or fluid-filled hepatocytes may separate the obviously necrotic hepatocytes from the more peripheral hepatocytes that appear normal by light microscopy. Despite the rather extensive destruction of tissue in more severe instances of central lobular necrosis, inflammatory cell infiltration is generally limited, especially during acute toxicity.

Cellular injury induced by central lobular hepatotoxicants is frequently restricted to the hepatocytes, as occurs after the administration of carbon tetrachloride. With this toxicant, endothelial cells and Küpffer cells appear to be normal, while the adjacent hepatocytes are uniformly destroyed. The swollen and necrotic hepatocytes appear to compress the vascular spaces, so that little blood is observed in the sinusoids in the necrotic central lobular areas. With other toxicants, such as various nitrosamines, the endothelial cells lining the sinusoids adjacent to the necrotic hepatocytes are also destroyed. The destruction of multiple cell types results in the destruction of normal architecture, having profound ramifications for the histologic appearance of the lesions, as well as the subsequent reparative process. Hepatocellular necrosis, when accompanied by destruction of the endothelial cells, results in central lobular hemorrhage into the zone of necrotic hepatocytes (Figure 9.3). Because central lobular necrosis may also be associated with hemorrhage, the gross appearance may be variable.

Central lobular necrosis of hepatocytes is generally repaired rapidly following a single or short toxicant exposure; the liver can return to near normal light microscopic appearance within a week of the toxic insult. However, if sinusoidal cells and the normal scaffolding are destroyed, replacement of the necrotic hepatocytes through regeneration is accompanied by fibrosis, which may be minimal, in the previously necrotic zone around the central vein.

Central lobular necrosis provides an interesting biological phenomenon, since the central lobular hepatocytes are the last cells to receive the blood constituents as the blood percolates in a normal portal to central lobular route. This is consistent with the observation that central lobular necrosis occurs as a sequel of heart failure, as oxygen is depleted by passage of blood through the periportal areas. Based on the blood flow, the periportal hepatocytes might be expected to be more sensitive to toxic injury, because they are first to receive the blood-borne toxicant, and presumably in the highest concentration.

In most, if not all, instances a metabolic basis accounts for the distribution of central lobular necrosis. Many toxic agents are not inherently toxic, but only become so after being metabolized by the target organ or cell (see above). Compared with periportal hepatocytes, the central lobular hepatocytes have a much higher concentration of cytochrome P450 and associated enzymes that metabolize and thereby activate xenobiotics. It is the distribution of the metabolizing system, resulting in a higher concentration of the ultimate toxicant in the central lobular region, which accounts for the occurrence, as well as the frequency, of central lobular toxicity in the liver. In addition, oxygen tension is lower as one approaches the central vein, due to consumption of oxygen from the blood which enters via the portal vein in the portal triad.

Other mechanisms of central lobular necrosis include acute hypoxia/anoxia and uptake of toxin, such as microcystin-LR (MCLR), via the bile acid uptake pathway, which is located primarily in centrilobular hepatocytes. MCLR results in severe disassociation of hepatocytes in the central lobular regions (Figure 9.4). Severe acute anemia often causes paracentral necrosis, characterized by an incomplete rim of necrotic hepatocytes around the central vein.

Information on potential hepatotoxicant exposure, and presence and character of lesions in other organs, assist the diagnostic pathologist in narrowing the differential list (see Table 9.3). However, a specific cause for central lobular necrosis is often not identified.

Midzonal Necrosis

Midzonal necrosis is the least common histologic pattern of lobular hepatocellular necrosis following

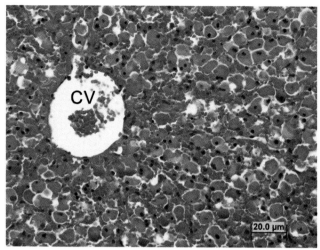

FIGURE 9.4 Severe disassociation of central lobular hepatocytes with hemorrhage, microcystin-LR, single intraperitoneal dose, rat. Hepatocytes surrounding a central vein (CV) are disassociated and undergoing apoptosis, as evidenced by peripheralization of the nucleus and condensation of the cytoplasm. H&E stain.

exposure to hepatotoxicants. It has been described following furan treatment of mice, aflatoxin treatment of rabbits, and hexachlorophene exposure of cats. As the name implies, this pattern of necrosis is found as a band of necrosis equidistant between the portal triad and the central vein (Figure 9.5). The zone is generally very thin, affecting only two to three cells in the middle of the lobule. Therefore, midzonal necrosis is generally not noted grossly. Because hepatocytes are extremely variable in their metabolic capacity and oxygen tension, midzonal necrosis of hepatocytes is presumably dictated by a unique susceptibility of these hepatocytes, based on their location in the lobule.

Periportal Necrosis

Although not rare, periportal necrosis of hepatocytes is a much less frequently observed pattern of hepatocellular injury than central lobular necrosis. In periportal necrosis, necrotic hepatocytes surround the portal area; this has also been referred to as peripheral lobular necrosis. Periportal necrosis may be evident grossly by its distinctive lobular pattern. However, it is extremely difficult to discern, from the gross appearance, whether the necrotic area is central lobular or periportal.

Several different reasons have been proposed for the periportal distribution of injury. First, the periportal area is the first area of the hepatic lobule to be exposed to a toxin being delivered through the bloodstream via the portal vein. This suggests that the periportal hepatocytes may receive the largest

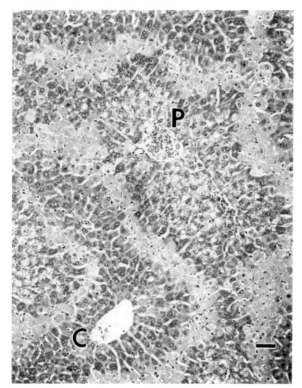

FIGURE 9.5 Midzonal necrosis; furan, single dose, mouse. Central (C), portal (P). H&E stain. Bar = 48μm.

dose of the toxin, as cells further down the sinusoid may be partly protected by removal of the toxicant in the periportal area. Toxicants affecting the periportal hepatocytes are usually primary toxicants, without a requirement for biotansformation for induction of their toxic effects. Although this rationale may be correct in some instances, and is attractive because of its simplicity, in some instances the periportal distribution of hepatotoxicity is apparently due to metabolic zonation, including the greater oxygen tension in the portal than in the central lobular area of the lobule. Küpffer cells, which are greater in number in periportal regions, have also been implicated in susceptibility of the periportal region to necrosis.

The most widely studied toxicant inducing periportal necrosis is allyl alcohol, although N-hydroxy-2-acetylaminofluorene and, in some species, especially poultry, aflatoxin B_1, will also induce a similar lesion. Phosphorus will also cause periportal necrosis, via its conversion to the toxicant phosgene in the stomach, and absorption via the portal vein. Necrotic hepatocytes completely surround most portal triads (Figure 9.6). Hemorrhage is infrequently, if ever, observed in periportal necrotic areas. As with central lobular necrosis, inflammatory response to the necrotic tissue is very limited, and sometimes not evident, especially during acute toxicity.

Following periportal necrosis, repair begins rapidly. Regeneration of hepatocytes results in repopulation of the area with hepatocytes. Minimal fibrosis may also extend from the portal area in the reparative process. In addition, bile ductule proliferation (biliary hyperplasia) may be associated with repair. Proliferated bile ductules, composed of cuboidal bile duct epithelial cells, may be limited to the portal area, or may extend into the area of necrosis during the first week following periportal necrosis of hepatocytes. In the latter instance, the periportal area may be repopulated by a mixture of hepatocytes and normal-appearing bile ductules complete with a central lumen. With additional time after the toxic insult, the bile ductules usually regress, so the portal area is once again composed of normal-appearing hepatocytes. In rodents, numerous oval cells may also be found in the periportal area within one week of the acute necrosis. Oval cells are characterized light microscopically by small, oval, uniformly-stained nuclei surrounded by a minimal amount of indistinct cytoplasm (see below). Oval cells appear to be most numerous when hepatocyte regeneration is completely, or at least partially, blocked.

Massive (Diffuse) Necrosis

Massive necrosis in the liver is characterized by necrosis involving the entire liver lobule (Figure 9.7). Although not every lobule may be equally affected, the necrosis extends from the central vein to the portal area in at least some portion of the lobule (bridging necrosis), and frequently affects the entire lobular structure of multiple lobules (multilobular necrosis). Necrotic hepatocytes lyse, and residual stroma becomes condensed, resulting in blood-filled spaces within a connective tissue stroma. Due to the massive reserve in liver function, destruction of a large portion of the liver may in some cases be compatible with life.

Hepatocytes remaining as small islands of unaffected cells or entire lobules in an unaffected area of the liver will effectively repair the damaged liver by regeneration. However, the complete destruction of hepatocytes and their associated scaffolding in a lobule renders that lobule incapable of participating in the reparative process, so the lobule is permanently lost from the liver. Lobules with only a few hepatocytes remaining will mount a regenerative attempt. However, severe destruction of the lobular support structure will result in an aborted regenerative effort, and variably sized regenerative nodules without normal lobular structure. Therefore, lobules in less-affected areas will be the main source of the regenerative response, resulting in the enlargement of those lobules, but retention of normal structure. Where complete

A

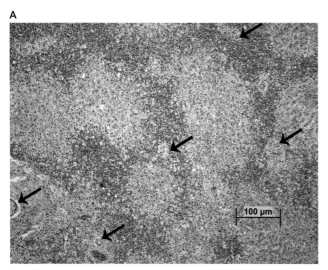

B

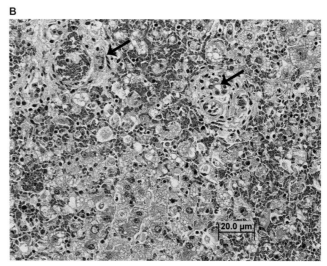

FIGURE 9.6   Periportal necrosis with hemorrhage; tribrissen (trimethoprim-sulfadiazine combination) treatment, dog. H&E stain. (A) Hemorrhage is present periportally (portal tract, arrows). (B) At higher magnification, necrotic hepatocytes and hemorrhage surround the portal tract (arrows).

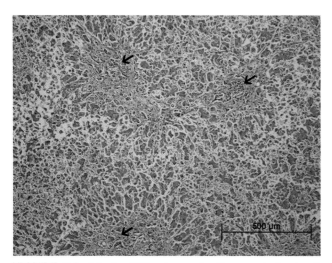

FIGURE 9.7   Massive (diffuse) necrosis, diazapem (valium), cat. Hepatic lobules contain disassociated hepatocytes undergoing necrosis; only the portal regions (arrows) are clearly defined. H&E stain.

or substantial destruction of the lobule occurs, fibrosis will constitute the major reparative effort. With time, dense vascular channels will appear, with a few interspersed regenerative nodules from residual hepatocytes.

Massive necrosis is clearly evident on gross observation. In the early phase, the affected liver areas are abnormal in color (frequently pale) and appear slightly swollen. After several days, the affected area is depressed below the surface of the adjacent tissue. If the whole liver is affected, the liver may be smaller than normal and flaccid. As the repair process progresses to fibrosis, the affected areas become firm.

At all phases of injury and repair, the affected areas are irregular in both size and shape.

Massive necrosis of the liver generally occurs when exposure is to extremely high doses of a hepatotoxicant, or as an idiosyncratic response. The early lesion may be found in either the central or portal lobular areas; progressive extension of the lesion across the lobule occurs over time. Massive necrosis may also be noted when toxicants are delivered directly into the vascular system, particularly into the portal vein or a major tributary. Massive necrosis in this instance may be limited to certain areas or lobes of the liver, as a result of incomplete mixing of the toxic agent in the portal vascular supply, resulting in massive doses to small portions of the liver.

In humans, approximately one third of cases of massive hepatic necrosis in the USA are due to acetaminophen toxicity. Other causes include halothane, antituberculosis drugs (rifampin, isoniazid), antidepressant monoamine oxidase inhibitors, industrial chemicals such as carbon tetrachloride, and mushroom poisoning (*Amanita phalloides*). Examples of massive necrosis in domestic animals include dogs that ingested *Amanita* spp. and cats treated with diazepam (valium) (Figure 9.7).

Focal (Non-zonal) Necrosis

Focal necrosis of hepatocytes may be observed following exposure of an animal to a hepatotoxicant. Although this pattern of necrosis has been described following the exposure of humans to a variety of pharmaceuticals (e.g., isoniazid and phenothiazine), it is infrequently observed in toxicological studies in

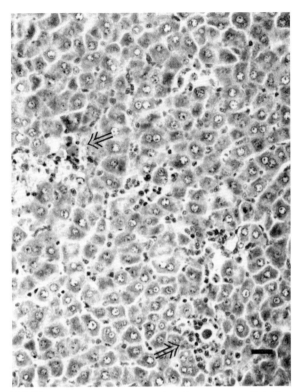

FIGURE 9.8 Focal necrosis with inflammatory cell infiltrates (arrows); galactosamine, single dose, rat. H&E stain. Bar = 24 48 μm.

animals. Despite the rarity of this pattern, focal necrosis has been described in detail following the acute treatment of rats with *d*-galactosamine. Focal necrosis consists of discrete areas of hepatocytic necrosis that can be found at any location within the hepatic lobule (Figure 9.8). The necrotic areas are frequently small, involving only three to four cells. In addition to the necrotic hepatocytes, a small number of mononuclear inflammatory cells are frequently found in the lesion.

Focal necrosis may be observed grossly as small pale foci, usually less than 1 mm in diameter. The lesions are particularly evident when they include inflammatory cells. Because the lesions are randomly located throughout the liver tissue, they do not form a recognizable pattern when observed grossly, and are noted on both capsular and cut surface of the liver.

Focal necrosis may be repaired by removal of the dead hepatocytes and replacement by adjacent hepatocytes. Complete regression may be delayed by the presence of inflammatory cells. No fibrosis is observed. When macrophages predominate, these cell aggregates are sometimes called granulomas or granulomata. The basis for the focal pattern of necrosis is poorly understood, but probably due to microvascular dynamics. The focal pattern is reminiscent of necrosis caused by bacteremia and viral hepatitis (which are differentials for this lesion), in which the

immune response and localized release of inflammatory cytokines have been implicated.

Apoptosis

Apoptosis is a special form of individual hepatocellular death, with specific histologic features (see Chapter 2 and Figure 2.5) and generally a non-zonal distribution. Unlike necrosis, there is no release of cellular contents from dying cells since the cell membrane is intact; thus, inflammatory cells are not recruited. Apoptotic cells in the liver are characterized by rounding of dying hepatocytes with hyper-eosinophilic cytoplasm and surrounding clear halo resulting from contraction of the dying cell. As individual hepatocytes undergo programmed shrinkage, apoptotic bodies are histologically characterized as small, densely-eosinophilic structures that may have dense, sometimes fragmented, chromatin (Figure 9.9). Apoptotic bodies may be free, or within Küpffer cells or normal adjacent hepatocytes.

In the liver, very low rates of apoptosis are found, primarily representing the physiologic loss of senescent hepatocytes. Apoptotic bodies are increased in livers that are regressing in size after cessation of treatment with a chemical or agent that causes dramatic hepatocyte hyperplasia, such as phenobarbital, cyproterone acetate, or lead nitrate. This enhancement of apoptosis during liver regression suggests that apoptosis is important in the readjustment of the tissue to a normal size. Enhancement of apoptosis has also been observed during the chronic administration of chemicals that induce both hepatic hyperplasia and peroxisome proliferation in rodents. With long-term high doses of peroxisome-proliferating chemicals, and perhaps of other inducers of hepatic hyperplasia, apoptosis is associated with an enhanced rate of hepatocellular replication. In contrast, short-term treatment may be associated with decreased rates of apoptosis. Apoptosis is also elevated in developing hepatic neoplasms that have an enhanced replicative rate. The cause and effect relationship of enhanced cell replication and enhanced apoptosis in the livers of animals treated with chemicals that induce hepatic hyperplasia is unclear. However, chemicals acting as promoters are known to shift cell signaling pathways away from apoptosis and toward proliferation. For discussion of the biochemical basis of apoptosis, see Chapter 2.

Apoptosis is a characteristic feature of some hepatotoxicants, such as the fumonisin mycotoxins. In the past, apoptosis was described morphologically as "individual" or "single cell" necrosis. Apoptosis can be induced by triggering proapoptotic pathways, or via immune-mediated events that lead to the release of TNF-α, or activate FAS pathways. The relationship

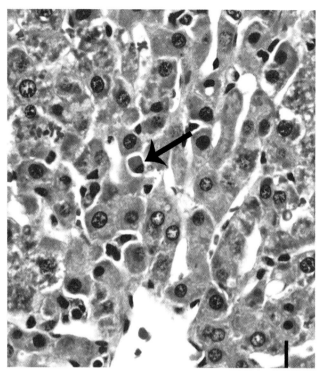

FIGURE 9.9   Hepatocellular apoptosis, fumonisin B₁, rat. Early changes (arrow) characterized by individualization and cytoplasmic condensation of cell, with margination of chromatin in eccentrically-located nucleus. Apoptotic bodies are phagocytized by adjacent hepatocytes or Küpffer cells (not shown). H&E stain.

between apoptosis and necrosis can be confusing. By altering the study design, particularly the dose, a toxic agent can sometimes induce either or both lesions, as observed with fumonisin B₁. The mechanism of fumonisin toxicity is believed to be due to its alteration of sphingolipid metabolism. Mitochondrial injury can trigger apoptosis, by cytochrome c release, and necrosis, if more severe injury is present.

Intracellular Accumulations

Hepatic Lipidosis

To understand the potential mechanisms of hepatic lipidosis, the central role of the liver in normal lipid metabolism must be appreciated. Fatty acids are constantly cycled between liver and adipose tissue. Accumulation of triglyceride in liver results from an imbalance between uptake of fatty acids and their secretion as very low density lipoprotein (VLDL). Different toxins may cause this imbalance by different means. For example, carbon tetrachloride and phosphorus impair protein synthesis, thereby reducing apoprotein available for VLDL formation. The central lobular location of carbon tetrachloride lipidosis and periportal location of phosphorus lipidosis may

reflect differences in metabolic activation of the toxicant. However, hepatocytes from both sites are involved in VLDL apoprotein production. Orotic acid causes lipidosis by interfering with VLDL formation in the Golgi apparatus. In contrast to the examples just given, 4-aminopyrazolopyrimidine interferes with the secretion of VLDL from the Golgi body to the perisinusoidal space. Antiviral nucleosides and intravenous tetracyclines damage mitochondria, interfering with β-oxidation of lipids, which leads to accumulation of free fatty acids and triglycerides.

Hepatic or hepatocellular lipidosis (fatty change, fatty degeneration, steatosis) refers to the accumulation of triglycerides within hepatocytes. Membrane-bound lipid inclusions which develop near, and possibly from, endoplasmic reticulum may coalesce until they are visible as clear vacuoles by routine light microscopy. Unambiguous determination of vacuolar lipid content depends on avoiding embedment procedures that extract lipid such as paraffin embedment. Thus frozen sections (formalin fixed tissue can be used) are needed for lipid special stains (oil red O, osmium).

In some cases, hepatocytes contain a central large clear vacuole which displaces the nucleus to the periphery of the cell (macrovesicular lipidosis, Figure 9.10). In humans, macrovesicular lipidosis has been described in methotraxate and amiodarone toxicity. In other cases, hepatocytes contain several smaller vacuoles which do not displace the nucleus (microvesicular lipidosis). In humans, microvesicular lipidosis is described as a feature of tetracycline, salicylate, and yellow phosphorus toxicities. These morphologic variants of lipidosis may be somewhat specific with respect to cause, but the difference in pathogenesis is not understood. In humans, both micro- and macrovesicular lipidosis occur as a feature of ethanol toxicity. Microvesicular steatosis has recently been described as a characteristic feature of mitochondrial injury, e.g., due to valproic acid, in which there is interference with beta-oxidation of lipid. Grossly, severe hepatic lipidosis is characterized by an enlarged liver with soft yellow hepatic parenchyma (Figure 9.11A). Although lipidosis may be associated with hepatic necrosis, it has been generally (but not universally) held that lipidosis, unless severe or possibly microvesicular in nature, does not impair hepatic function or, of itself, cause hepatic injury.

In domestic animals, centrilobular lipidosis is a prominent lesion of aflatoxicosis in several species, including dogs (Figure 9.11B). Canine diets containing aflatoxin B₁-contaminated corn have caused hepatotoxicity resulting in death. Other changes consistent with aflatoxicosis, such as bile duct proliferation, were also found. Centrilobular lipidosis has also been observed in halothane toxicity in ponies.

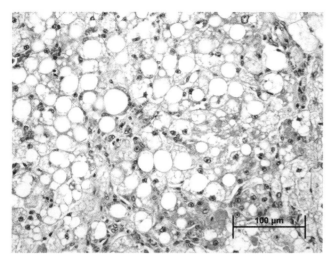

FIGURE 9.10 Hepatic lipidosis, macrovesicular, dog. Severe hepatic lipidosis is characterized by large intracytoplasmic vacuoles that peripheralize the nucleus and remaining cytoplasm within hepatocytes. To confirm that vacuoles represent accumulated fat, a special stain such as oil-red-O or osmium can be performed on frozen sections (not shown). H&E stain.

Toxic chemicals are only one cause of lipidosis. Diabetes mellitus and acute starvation cause lipidosis, by increasing delivery of fatty acids from adipose tissue to liver. Lipidosis is a manifestation of pregnancy toxemia in the rabbit and ewe, and can also be due to diet and anoxia. Species-specific disorders include bovine and feline fatty liver syndromes, and hepatic lipidosis of ponies, miniature horses, and donkeys.

Phospholipidosis

Phospholipidosis is a distinct form of lipidosis caused by amphiphilic drugs, such as chlorphentermine. These toxicants bind to phospholipids and inhibit their catabolism. Hepatocytes, Küpffer cells, and extrahepatic cells are enlarged and have foamy cytoplasm, resembling hereditary metabolic lipidosis. Crystalloid and lamellated inclusions are found within distended lysosomes of affected cells by electron microscopy.

Hydropic Change

Hydropic change is an accumulation of water within the cytosolic matrix or rough endoplasmic reticulum of hepatocytes. Hydropic change of the latter type occurs in the liver of rats given either carbon tetrachloride or carbon disulfide (CS_2), and in mice given cylindrospermopsin. Hydropic change is characterized by enlarged pale-staining cytoplasm, with narrowing of the sinusoids and the perisinusoidal

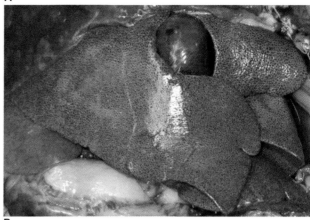

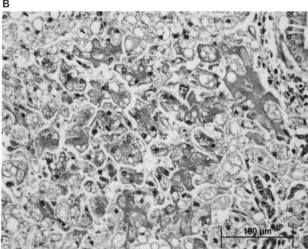

FIGURE 9.11 Hepatic lipidosis, aflatoxin contaminated pet food, dog. (Courtesy of Dr. B. Summers, Cornell University.) (A) The liver is swollen and yellow because of hepatocellular lipidosis. The gall bladder is distended. (B) Hepatocytes contain variably sized cytoplasmic vacuoles which often displace the nucleus peripherally. Brown canalicular bile plugs may also be seen. H&E stain.

space of Dissé (Figure 9.12). This form of injury is reversible, and can be attributed to a failure to maintain intracellular sodium ion balance. Glycogen is usually depleted. In its mildest form, hydropic change may be difficult to observe by light microscopy. When routine histologic stains are used, hydropic change may not be easily distinguished from mild lipidosis or glycogen accumulation.

Glycogen Accumulation

Although glycogen content of the liver is variable, depending on the physiologic state of the animal, glycogen accumulation may be observed in hepatocytes as a manifestation of toxicity, and also with diabetes mellitus. Glycogen accumulation results in a clear

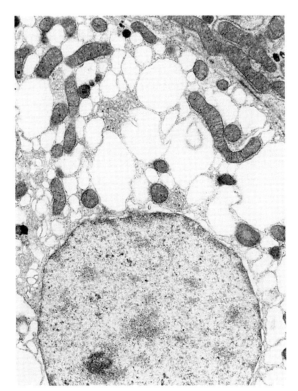

FIGURE 9.12   Hydropic degeneration characterized by dilated endoplasmic reticulum, rat.

cytoplasm with indistinct vacuoles which do not displace the nucleus; this is apparently due to impairment of enzymatic activity for glycogen catabolism, or an increase in glycogen synthesis. Diffuse periportal glycogen accumulation was observed following acetaminophen treatment in rats. Glycogen storage can also occur in foci of cellular alteration (see below). Alternatively, glycogen depletion can occur either as a primary toxic effect, or due to fasting or cachexia. Periodic acid-Schiff (PAS) stain with and without diastase is used to confirm glycogen within tissues.

Glucocorticosteroid-induced hepatocellular degeneration due to exogenous or endogenous sources is a specific disorder resulting from severe glycogen accumulation in dogs, often called "steroid hepatopathy." Histologically, a poorly-defined lobular pattern, often including midzonal regions, is evident, with markedly swollen hepatocytes (up to 10 times normal volume, Figure 9.13). A characteristic feature of this disease is increased activity of serum ALP, due to the corticosteroid-induced isoenzyme.

Lipofuscin Accumulation

Small amounts of lipofuscin pigment accumulate in hepatocytes with aging and following sublethal injury. In sublethal injury, such as hydropic degeneration, steatosis, or atrophy, damaged organelles are often

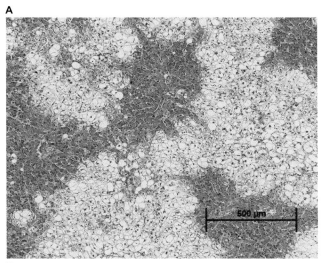

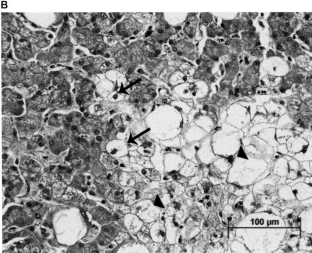

FIGURE 9.13   Glucocorticoid hepatopathy; glucocorticosteroid treatment, dog. H&E stain. (A) Hepatocytes are pale and swollen in a central lobular to midzonal pattern. (B) Glycogen accumulation results in hepatocellular swelling and clearing of the cytoplasm (arrows). Peripheralization of the nucleus (arrowheads) may be observed.

removed by forming autophagosomes, with undigested residual material retained as lipofuscin. Several chemicals, most notably the peroxisome proliferators, result in dramatic lipofuscin accumulation. The pigment is granular and brown in unstained or routinely stained sections, and located adjacent to bile canaliculi. Lipofuscin can be distinguished from other liver pigments by staining positively by Schmorl's technique, or by autofluorescing under ultraviolet light. Lipofuscin is believed to represent lysosomal accumulation of poorly-digested lipid.

Iron Accumulation and Toxicity

Abnormally increased storage of iron in hepatocytes (hemochromatosis) may occur as a consequence of excessive dietary intake or treatment with hepatotoxiants, and results in hepatic dysfunction. Iron is stored in hepatocytes in the form of ferritin, ferric iron bound to the protein apoferritin. Excess ferritin aggregates form hemosiderin, which is observed as gold-brown granules and can be confirmed with the Prussian blue reaction. Ultrastructural studies demonstrate that these membrane-bound granules, siderosomes, may derive from secondary lysosomes, and are often pericanalicular. Biliary excretion of iron from lysosomes may represent an important route for excretion of excess iron. While most hemosiderin in hepatocytes is derived from iron present in transferrin and, to a lesser extent, hemoglobin, that in Küpffer cells and other macrophages in the body is derived from breakdown of red blood cells.

Acute iron toxicosis, e.g., iron dextran injection in piglets, can cause periportal necrosis, as well as gastroenteritis. Of historical interest, equine neonatal hepatic failure syndrome followed administration of a supplement, primapaste, to pregnant mares. This dietary supplement contained ferrous fumerate, which caused severe hepatic necrosis in the unborn foal. Foals were born with severe periportal fibrosis, bile duct hyperplasia, and bile stasis.

Copper Accumulation and Toxicity

Excess storage of hepatic copper may occur as a consequence of increased copper intake or prior liver damage. Normally, serum copper is bound to ceruloplasmin, and hepatic copper to metallothionen. It is excreted from the liver in bile. Excess copper is initially distributed within the cytoplasm but later concentrates in lysosomes, leading to formation of reactive oxygen species that can initiate lipid peroxidation. Copper accumulation may be demonstrated in histologic sections by either rubeanic acid or rhodamine staining. In rats fed a high copper diet, copper is localized in the periportal and sometimes midzonal hepatocytes. Sufficient copper accumulation is associated with enlarged hyperchromatic hepatocytes and necrosis, with accumulation of neutrophils and mononuclear inflammatory cells. In mice, copper intoxication has been associated with Mallory body formation.

In domestic animals, species-sensitivity to copper toxicosis is greatest in sheep, followed by dogs, with cattle and pigs being much less sensitive. Acute toxicity is characterized by central lobular necrosis, together with intravascular hemolysis and gastroenteritis (Figure 9.14). Chronic toxicity, with progressive accumulation of copper, occurs in ruminants, especially sheep which are exquisitively sensitive.

Dietary sources of copper include mineral blocks (formulated for cattle), copper sulphate supplementation, and pastures with normal copper but low molybdenum. Hepatotoxic plants, such as those that

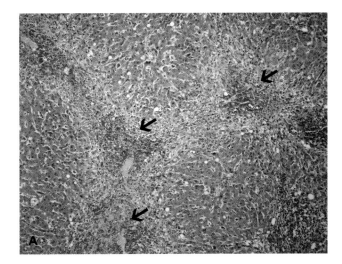

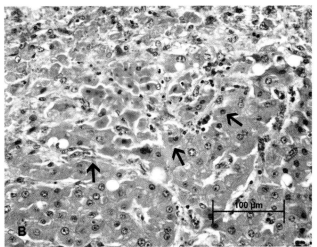

FIGURE 9.14 Chronic copper hepatotoxicity, sheep. H & E stain. (A) Patchy hepatocellular necrosis is present within the lobule, with biliary proliferation and congestion within portal regions (arrows). (B) Focal hepatocellular necrosis with cell loss and small aggregates of inflammatory cells are present (affected area delineated by arrows).

contain pyrrolizidine alkaloids, result in cholestasis and prevent biliary excretion, thus exacerbating copper accumulation. Cell death, characterized by multifocal hepatocellular necrosis, results in release of copper which is phagacytosed by remaining hepatocytes and Küpffer cells, and is followed by regenerative hepatocyte proliferation. Toxicity induced by the pyrrolizidine alkaloids, found in many different plants, not only decreases biliary excretion, but also inhibits cell proliferation, resulting in markedly increased copper concentration in remaining hepatocytes.

Once a threshold for storage is reached, some event triggers a massive release of copper from the liver into the circulation, leading to an acute, often fatal, hemolytic crisis, and severe hepatocellular necrosis. Acute intravascular hemolysis results in anemia, jaundice, hemoglobinemia, and hemoglobinuria. The characteristic gross lesions are icterus, a soft, swollen and often pale liver, black "gun metal" kidneys, and an engorged dark spleen. In addition to the lesions of copper toxicosis, paracentral to central lobular necrosis due to acute anemia/hypoxia, and evidence of plant toxicity are often present. Chronic liver disease due to copper toxicity can be found in pigs and cattle, and from a hereditary disorder of copper metabolism in dogs.

Pathology of Transcription and Translation

Alterations in transcription and translation may result in subtle morphologic changes. Although massive and prolonged inhibition of these events is incompatible with the life of the cell, minor or more acute alterations of these events may be recognized as minimal morphologic changes.

Nucleolar Lesions

The nucleolus is the first organelle of the hepatocyte to develop morphologic changes when the rate of RNA synthesis is altered. A wide variety of hepatotoxins, such as α-amanitin (the toxic agent in the mushroom *Amanita phalloides*), and various hepatocarcinogens, including aflatoxin B_1 and nitrosamines, interfere with RNA synthesis by direct interaction with the DNA, or by inhibiting the nuclear RNA polymerase involved in transcription. Intracellular ATPase deficiency, induced experimentally by the ATPase trapping agent ethionine, results in similar nucleolar lesions, which are apparently mediated through reduced RNA synthesis. As a result of this inhibition, the nucleolus is reduced in size, as noted in histologic sections routinely processed for light microscopy. A lobular distribution may be noted for this lesion; abnormal hepatocytes are recognized in either central or periportal areas of the lobule, depending on the area of the lobule primarily affected by that particular toxin.

Transmission electron microscopy provides a better definition of the nucleolar lesion. In addition to being reduced in size, the nucleolus is frequently fragmented or segregated (Figure 9.15). In contrast to the normal mixture of granular and fibrillar components forming the nucleolonema of the nucleolus (see Figure 9.12), segregated nucleoli have the granular and fibrillar components separated into distinct homogeneous zones, and the altered nucleolus maintains a normal location near the center of the nucleus. Fragmented nucleoli have separated granular and fibrillar portions of the nucleolus and portions of altered nucleolus are scattered across the nucleus, rather than present in a single segregated structure. Some hepatotoxins primarily

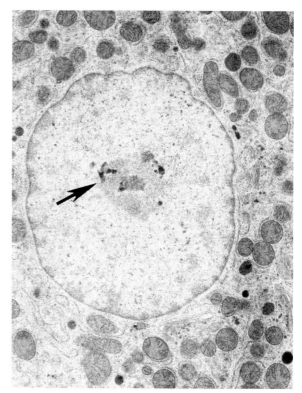

FIGURE 9.15 Nucleolar segregation (arrow); dinitrotoluene treatment, single dose, rat.

cause fragmentation, while others primarily cause segregation of the nucleolus.

Reduction of nucleolar size is an acute lesion. It can be recognized within several hours of administration of a single dose of specific hepatotoxins, and may persist up to several days after treatment if the cells remain viable. Although the lesion is subtle when viewed by light microscopy, it is identifiable at a time when other evidence of hepatocytic injury is not yet morphologically detectable.

Nucleolar enlargement in hepatocytes may also occur in response to exposure to hepatotoxins. Nucleolar enlargement is identified routinely and used as an aid in the diagnosis of neoplasms, but it is less frequently used in the evaluation of non-neoplastic tissue. The occurrence of this lesion indicates an enhancement of protein synthesis, and is identified most frequently in hepatocytes that are undergoing rapid cell proliferation. In livers undergoing chemically-induced cell proliferation or cell proliferation in response to pre-existing hepatocellular necrosis, nucleolar enlargement may be the most sensitive morphologic index.

Polysome Breakdown

In normal protein synthesis, ribosomes are evenly spaced along single strands of messenger RNA, forming polysomes that can be observed by transmission electron microscopy. If RNA synthesis is blocked by a toxin, e.g., T-2 toxin, the lack of messenger RNA results in the disappearance of polysomes. By light microscopy, polysome breakdown results in loss of basophilic granules in hepatocytic cytoplasm. However, polysomes are extremely fragile, and require appropriate and rapid fixation to be observed.

Cholestasis

Cholestasis can be defined in one of three ways: biochemically; physiologically; and morphologically. Defined biochemically, cholestasis consists of altered serum constituents, i.e., hyperbilirubinemia, bile acidemia, and elevated enzymes, such as alkaline phosphatase (ALP) and γ-glutamyl transpeptidase (GGT). Defined physiologically, cholestasis consists of reduced bile flow, which can only be assessed by experimental preparations in which the bile duct has been cannulated.

Morphologically, cholestasis consists of accumulation of bile pigment in canaliculi. This change is often accompanied by deformation and loss of canalicular microvilli. Bile pigment accumulation may be observed by light microscopy and confirmed by Hall's stain, but alterations of microvilli can only be observed by electron microscopy. Initially, cholestasis is usually observed in centrilobular areas. With progression, other lobular areas are involved, and irregular vacuolation of hepatocytes may develop. With severe cholestasis, the liver appears greenish brown. Following cholestatic insult, morphologic evidence of cholestasis is observed rarely in routine toxicology studies using rats or mice, although bile accumulation is observed following chronic administration of griseofulvin to mice.

Several mechanisms lead to cholestasis and model systems have been developed to characterize these mechanisms. Cholestasis can be divided into extrahepatic and intrahepatic. Extrahepatic cholestasis is related to obstruction of bile flow outside the liver, and results from backing up of bile in the biliary tree. Intrahepatic cholestasis is a primary hepatocellular disorder, related to alterations in bile acid load, bile salt transport, membrane fluidity, and cytoskeletal function, so that the hepatocyte is unable to metabolize and excrete bile. Examples of cholestatic agents include chlorpromazine, contraceptives, lantadene from *Lantana camara*, and phalloidin. Lantadene A and B have a direct effect on canalicular transport. Estrogen and erythromycin bind to and disrupt the molecular pumps that secrete bile constituents into the canaliculi. Intrahepatic cholestasis can also result from hemolysis or inherited abnormalities.

Hepatocellular Adaptive Responses

Exposure of the liver to xenobiotic agents may result in responses in the liver that generally are not considered toxic effects. The responses simply may reflect the attempts of the liver to adjust to the new environment or conditions, as muscle enlargement represents a response to increased workload. Although a number of the adaptive responses of the hepatocyte are of a metabolic nature, morphologic changes frequently may be noted microscopically and, on some occasions, grossly.

Endoplasmic Reticulum

Since cytochrome P450 mono oxygenase enzyme (CYP) activity is localized in the smooth endoplasmic reticulum (SER), many compounds that cause an increase in CYP isozymes also result in increased SER. Induction of CYP may lead to altered metabolism, with resulting imbalance of detoxification and bioactivation pathways. Phenobarbital and 3-methylcholanthrene are considered model compounds for enzyme induction. Other enzyme inducers include synthetic steroids, ethanol, DDT, and PCBs. Phenobarbital causes an increase in a wide variety of monooxygenase activities, and may be associated with a two to five-fold increase in SER. This leads to the appearance of centrilobular hypertrophy with amorphous eosinophilic hepatocytic cytoplasm (Figure 9.16, also see Figure 2.2). Although the increase is mainly due to additional production of SER, part of the SER increase may be related to impaired membrane catabolism. Compounds such as 3-methylcholanthrene cause increases in only a few specific mono-oxygenase activities, and may not show morphologic evidence of SER increase. *Trans*-stilbene oxide has an intermediate effect: it induces several of the enzymes that phenobarbital does, with less extensive increases in SER. SER changes and associated enzyme induction are reversible following withdrawal of chemical exposure.

Peroxisomes

A variety of xenobiotics (including certain hypolipidemic drugs, herbicides, plasticizers, and solvents) and some dietary modifications cause an increase, sometimes dramatic, in hepatocytic peroxisomes and peroxisome-associated enzymes. Hyperplasia and induction of microsomal CYP 4A family members invariably accompany peroxisome proliferation. Treatment of rodents with peroxisome proliferators results in centrilobular hypertrophy characterized by granular eosinophilic cytoplasm (Figure 9.16C). By ultrastructural analysis, increases in peroxisome number, and sometimes alteration of peroxisomal size,

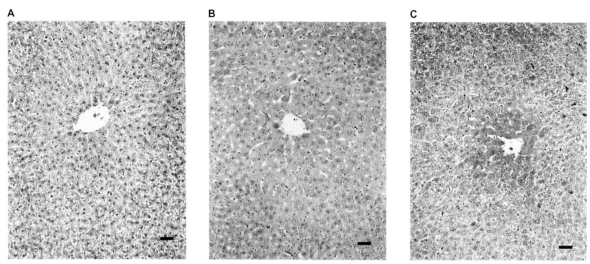

FIGURE 9.16   Hepatocellular adaptive responses, rat. (A) Control, central lobular region. (B) Phenobarbital treatment associated central lobular hepatocellular hypertrophy. (C) WY-14,643 treatment-associated central lobular hepatocellular hypertrophy with granular cytoplasm. Central veins (center) in each micrograph. H&E stain. Bar = 48 μm.

are observed. Associated increases in pericanalicular lipofuscin may also be observed after prolonged treatment. The prolonged treatment of rodents with chemicals that cause peroxisome induction often results in development of hepatocellular neoplasia.

Increases in peroxisomes, enzyme induction, and hyperplasia have been linked to a receptor known as PPAR-α (peroxisome proliferator-activated receptor). This member of the steroid/thyroid receptor superfamily activates the transcription of responsive genes following xenobiotic ligand binding and heterodimerization with one or more subtypes of RXR-alpha (retinoid X receptor), another nuclear receptor.

Mitochondria

Hypertrophy or enlargement of mitochondria, termed megamitochondria, may be induced by a variety of processes. Large mitochondria result from fusion of pre-existing ones, as occurs with cuprizone and isonicotinic acid derivatives. In the case of mitochondrial fusion, mitochondrial hypertrophy is not discernible by light microscopy. By electron microscopy, hypertrophic mitochondria have normal cristae and normal matrix density. This should be distinguished from swollen mitochondria, which have swollen cristae and irregular densities in the matrix. Mitochondrial hypertrophy and swelling have also been distinguished biochemically and ultrastructurally. Mitochondrial swelling is associated with uncoupling of oxidative phosphorylation, whereas mitochondrial hypertrophy is associated with normal oxidative phosphorylation. Agents that uncouple oxidative phosphorylation, such as NSAIDs, tolcapone, and dintrophenol, greatly reduce ATP synthesis.

Mild to severe enlargement of mitochondria is seen with dysruption of mitochondrial β-oxidation, an important mechanism of drug-induced hepatic injury. Ultrastructurally, the amount of mitochondrial matrix increases, and becomes increasingly electron lucent. By light microscopy these changes may be visualized as cytoplasmic vacuolation. Microvesicular steatosis, inflammation, and necrosis occur in humans and rats as a feature of chronic or severe interference with mitochondrial free fatty acid β-oxidation. The antidiabetic drugs phenformin (withdrawn from the market) and troglitazone can cause this change.

Hepatocellular Proliferation

Normally, hepatocytes are long-lived, and proliferation occurs at a very low rate following juvenile growth. However, proliferation of hepatocytes as a manifestation of toxicity may occur in two ways. The first is regeneration, which serves to restore liver mass lost by chemically-induced necrosis (e.g., carbon tetrachloride toxicity). This response is comparable to that induced in residual liver lobes following partial hepatectomy. Regenerating hepatocytes, prior to division, can be recognized by loss of cytoplasmic basophilia (dispersion of ribosomes from rough endoplasmic reticulum) and glycogen depletion. Occasional mitotic figures are observed, and an increase in mitotic rate may be quantified.

The second form of hepatocellular proliferation is chemically-induced hyperplasia, which is caused by compounds such as phenobarbital, cyproterone acetate, hexachlorocylohexane, and peroxisome proliferators in rats and mice. It is usually accompanied by induction of cytochrome P450 enzyme activity and liver enlargement, caused by both hyperplasia and hypertrophy of hepatocytes. It is not associated with necrosis detectable by microscopy or serum enzyme alterations. Hyperplasia may be recognized by increased mitosis and cytoplasmic changes that indicate enzyme induction. This form of proliferation never continues beyond a few days, even though animals may be subjected to continued exposure. That is, the hepatocellular proliferation ceases and the new increased liver weight is maintained. However, on withdrawal of the chemical exposure, liver weights return to pretreatment levels. Reversion to normal liver weight involves the loss of hepatocytes through apoptosis (see previous text). A persistent increase in liver weight caused by prolonged treatment of animals with chemicals that cause hyperplasia may be associated with subsequent hepatocellular carcinogenesis. It should be noted that hepatocyte multinucleation can occur in response to some hepatotoxicants.

Hepatocellular Ploidy

From birth to two weeks of age, most rat hepatocytes are mononuclear and diploid. With increasing age, the ploidy state shifts so that by adulthood 50% to 70% of hepatocytes are mononuclear tetraploid. A transient increase in binuclear diploid hepatocytes occurs during this shift. Increase in ploidy may be recognized by light microscopy as larger diameter nuclei (karyomegaly, cytomegaly). This change is more prominent in mice, however it is not observed as an age related change in humans or domestic animals. Shifts in ploidy may be stimulated as a consequence of chemical toxicity, especially where regeneration or carcinogenesis occur. Severe karyomegaly and cytomegaly can be as observed following chronic chlordane or fumonisin B$_1$ exposure (Figure 9.17). Most cancers are associated with the development of diploid hepatocytes.

Hepatocellular Megalocytosis

Megalocytosis is characterized by a markedly-enlarged hepatocyte (cytomegaly), with an enlarged and hyperchromatic nucleus (karyomegaly) and increased cytoplasmic volume (Figure 9.18). It occurs when hepatocytes are stimulated to divide, usually following a regenerative stimulus, when there is inhibition of mitosis but not DNA synthesis. In domestic animals, megalocytosis is commonly observed following pyrrolizidine alkaloid toxicity, and has also been reported following ingestion of aflatoxins, cycad (sago) palms (*Zamiaceae* sp), *Lantana camara*, and nitrosamines.

Bile Ductular Lesions

Of the numerous natural and man-made hepatotoxins, most agents cause preferential injury to the

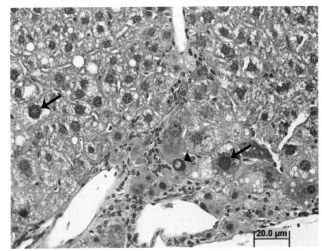

FIGURE 9.17 Chronic fumonisin B$_1$ treatment, mouse. Many hepatocytes (arrow) have enlarged and hyperchromatic nuclei (karyomegaly). Karyomegaly and cytomegaly (arrowhead) with nuclear membrane invagination (pseudo inclusion) and oval cell proliferation are also present. (Slide courtesy of Dr D. Caldwell, Health Canada.) H&E stain.

hepatocytes compared to the several other cell types in the liver. Injury to hepatocytes also may result in secondary responses in other hepatic cells, such as the epithelium lining the bile ductules that are found in each portal triad. Injury to bile ductular epithelium and hepatocytes can, of course, coexist. However, a select group of hepatotoxins preferentially injure bile ductular epithelium, resulting in lesions that take one of three morphologic forms: acute necrosis; bile ductular hyperplasia; and oval cell proliferation.

Acute Necrosis of Bile Ducts

Acute necrosis of bile duct epithelium is observed infrequently, although it has been extensively characterized following experimental treatment with the toxicant α-naphthylisothiocyanate (ANIT), (Figure 9.19) in both mice and rats. By 12 hours, there is cytoplasmic swelling of the epithelium of both intrahepatic bile ducts and bile ductules. By 24 hours, epithelial cells are necrotic and slough into the dilated ducts which are surrounded by edematous connective tissue containing inflammatory cells. Focal hepatocellular necrosis may be observed adjacent to the portal triads, presumably caused by the leakage of bile.

Following acute necrosis, bile duct epithelium is regenerated rapidly, most probably from the few residual ductular epithelial cells, or from proliferation of the small epithelial cells in the adjacent canal of Hering. Regeneration tends to result in a slight overproliferation of duct epithelium, so each portal triad contains several fully-formed bile ductules by one week after initial insult.

A

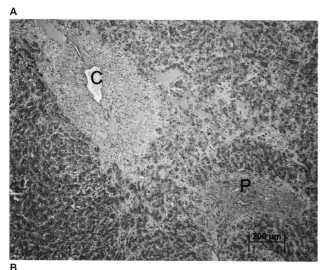

B

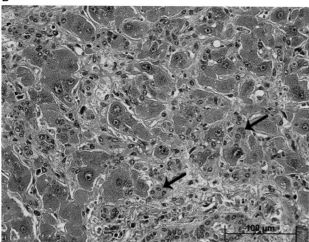

FIGURE 9.18   Chronic pyrrolizidine hepatotoxicity, cow. H&E stain. (A) Severe fibrosis is present around the central vein (C), portal tract (P), and within sinusoids. Multiple bile ducts (reduplication) are present in the portal region, and sinusoidal fibrosis (arrows). (B) Greatly enlarged hepatocytes (megalocytosis), sinusoidal fibrosis and biliary proliferation.

Chemically-induced acute necrosis of bile duct epithelium may be relatively specific for different levels of the biliary tract, depending on either species or chemical. ANIT causes extensive epithelial necrosis in the extrahepatic ducts in the mouse, but not in the rat. Phenylisothiocyanate causes acute necrosis of epithelium in the interlobar ducts, but not in the epithelium of the bile ductules found in the portal triad. In domestic animals, acute biliary epithelial necrosis occurs in sheep and, to a lesser extent, cattle ingesting the mycotoxin sporidesmin, from spores of *Pithomyces chartarum*, which grows well on dead rye grass (*Lolium perenne*). The resulting cholestasis often leads to secondary photosensitization (facial eczema), due to inability to excrete phylloerythrin via the bile.

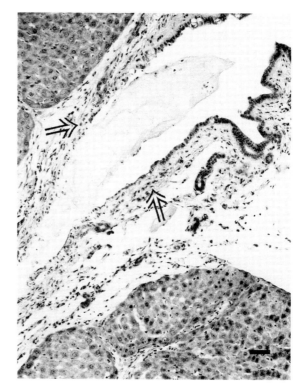

FIGURE 9.19   Bile duct necrosis (arrows); α-naphthylisothiocyanate, rat. H&E stain. Bar = 48 μm.

Biliary necrosis has also been reported in dogs following treatment with trimethoprim sulfa.

Bile Duct Hyperplasia

Bile duct hyperplasia is a common finding in both rodents and domestic animals. Hyperplastic ducts may be restricted to the immediate periportal area, or may extend from the immediate periportal area and form foci of proliferated ducts. To assess bile duct hyperplasia, a clear appreciation of normal bile duct numbers is needed. In the young rodent, one or two bile ductules are found in each portal triad. However, with increasing age, a typical portal triad will have several bile ductules that will continue to be restricted to the triad. In addition, small foci of cholangiofibrosis can be found in the liver of the aged rat. This lesion typically contains several histologically normal bile ductules that are each surrounded by a thin zone of mature collagenous connective tissue. Inflammatory cells in the lesion are rare. Foci of cholangiofibrosis are found throughout the liver, and do not always have an apparent association with portal triads, although this may be a false impression due to the plane of sectioning.

Bile duct hyperplasia induced by chemicals may take several forms. Simple hyperplasia is characterized by several histologically normal bile ductules restricted to each portal triad that would normally have only one

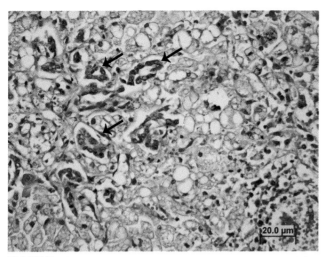

FIGURE 9.20 Bile duct hyperplasia; aflatoxin contaminated dog food, dog. Multiple bile ducts (arrows) are present within a portal area. Adjacent hepatocytes contain variably sized vacuoles (see also Figure 9.11). H&E stain.

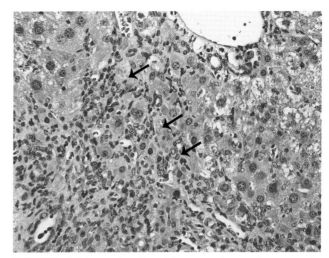

FIGURE 9.21 Oval cell proliferation; chronic fumonisin B_1, mouse. Large numbers of oval cells, small basophilic cells (arrows), extend out from the periportal region separating hepatocytes. H&E stain. (Slide courtesy of Dr D. Caldwell, Health Canada.)

or at most two ductules (Figure 9.20). Inflammation in or surrounding the proliferated ducts may be present. Simple bile duct hyperplasia is found within days or a few weeks after treatment with a bile ductular toxin. Simple bile duct proliferation may remain static for some time, regress, or progress to a more extensive form, including the appearance of cholangiofibrosis.

Cholangiofibrosis is most common in the rat, and is characterized by proliferated ducts surrounded by collagenous connective tissue. However, the morphologic pattern of cholangiofibrosis may be extremely variable, depending on the inciting chemical, the duration of chemical treatment, or the time since a single exposure to the chemical. The epithelium may be squamous or columnar, may undergo mucous metaplasia, or may resemble intestinal epithelium. Cysts and inflammatory cell infiltrates may be present. Cholangiofibrosis may partially regress over time if the original inciting agent is removed. Cysts and collagenous material may remain without obvious biliary epithelium. The ultimate lesion following regression may be a focus of scar tissue, although progression to cholangiocarcinoma has been demonstrated with some studies.

Oval Cell Hyperplasia

The oval cell is characterized by a nucleus that has an oval shape and is uniformly basophilic. The surrounding cytoplasm is extremely scant, without distinct cytoplasmic borders. Ultrastructurally, oval cells closely resemble normal bile duct epithelium and appear to arise from the small epithelial cells that line the terminal biliary ductules, also referred to as the Hering canals.

Oval cell proliferation is readily noted by light microscopy. The characteristic cells may be restricted to the periportal area in mild to moderate cases of proliferation. In more extensive proliferation, oval cells extend from the portal triads, and are found interspersed with histologically normal hepatocytes (Figure 9.21). Extensive oval cell hyperplasia has a diffuse distribution, and the cells rarely form packets or nodules.

Oval cell hyperplasia occurs after the treatment of rodents with a variety of hepatocarcinogens, including 2-acetylaminofluorene, aflatoxin B_1, and various azo dyes. Oval cell proliferation is also prominent following the treatment of rodents with ethionine or a choline-deficient diet. Extensive oval cell proliferation may be a relatively unique response of the rodent liver. Similar morphologic responses have been reported only rarely in humans or domestic animals, such as rabbits, guinea pigs, and dogs. However, a marker of rat oval cells, OV-6, has been identified in small hepatocytes and biliary epithelial cells in livers of non-rodent species, including humans.

Oval cell proliferation can occur independently, or can be associated with conventional bile duct proliferation. Proliferated oval cells may regress if the inciting agent is removed, so that the liver resumes a normal histologic pattern without remnant effects. In some instances, areas of cholangiofibrosis may develop from, or at least in conjunction with, oval cell proliferation.

Although the origin of oval cells is still partly obscure, the identification of phenotypic markers for oval cells in hepatocytes and biliary epithelial cells in livers following injury has led to the concept that oval cells are facultative stem cells in the liver. The oval cell has been proposed as a precursor to hepatic tumors in rodents, because of its response following the treatment of rodents with hepatocarcinogens and its pleuripotential characteristic when transformed *in vitro*.

Cholelithiasis

Cholelithiasis is a rare spontaneous disease in laboratory animals, characterized by the appearance of choleliths or gallstones. However, in an attempt to develop a model for human cholelithiasis, this disease has been induced experimentally in several laboratory animal species, including the mouse, rabbit, ground squirrel, prairie dog, and guinea pig. In most instances, cholelithiasis is induced by feeding a diet high in cholesterol and/or a specific bile acid. In the guinea pig, choleliths also may be induced by the parental administration of the antibiotic lincomycin.

Experimentally, while epithelial hyperplasia with resultant pseudostratification and mucous secretion of the surface epithelium occurs within several days, the appearance of choleliths takes at least several weeks. Morphologic changes in gall bladders containing choleliths may include a thickened gall bladder wall composed of excess smooth muscle and connective tissue, hyperplastic epithelium forming outpocketings, and vacuolated epithelium due to mucosubstance accumulation.

Nonparenchymal Cell Toxicity

Although the nonparenchymal cells are less conspicuous and probably affected less frequently by hepatotoxins, they are nevertheless occasionally involved in toxic responses. When nonparenchymal injury is noted, it is most frequently associated with hepatocellular injury.

Endothelial Lesions

Endothelial necrosis has been specifically described following the treatment of rats with single large intraperitoneal doses of dimethylnitrosamine. The endothelial injury accounts for the hemorrhagic nature of the lesion, noted both grossly and microscopically. However, it is uncertain whether the endothelial injury occurs due to a primary response of the endothelial cell to the nitrosamine, or to activated nitrosamine crossing from the adjacent hepatocyte. When the endothelial cells are destroyed, as happens with dimethylnitrosamine, the repair process includes fibrosis, in addition to the expected regenerative process. Pyrrolizidine alkaloids also appear to damage endothelial cells. The fibrosis resulting from pyrrolizidine alkaloid toxicity is

more severe around central veins, and has been characterized as veno-occlusive disease.

Very rapid destruction of hepatic endothelial cells follows the administration of microcystin-LR, a toxin produced by the cyanobacterium, *Microcystis aeruginosa*. Destruction of the endothelium can result in the embolization of hepatocytes to the lung. Hepatocyte dissociation, probably related to the aggregation of actin filaments, precedes endothelial cell injury. Arsenicals and beryllium can also cause necrosis of sinusoidal endothelium.

Although necrosis of the endothelial cells is an extreme manifestation of endothelial injury, some toxins have more subtle effects on this cell type. Enlargement of the fenestrations in the sinusoidal endothelial cells of the liver is observed after ethanol treatment. This may seem to be a relatively minor alteration, but enlargement of these pores in the endothelium may have important effects on the material that comes in direct contact with the apical region of the hepatocyte. The similarity in the response of rat liver endothelial cells to diverse insults such as hypoxia, irradiation, and endotoxin suggests that this cell has a very limited response to injury. In each case, the appearance of intracellular holes and intercellular gaps, similar to those induced by ethanol, are accompanied by blebs on the surface of the endothelial cell.

Angiectasis (*peliosis hepatis*, telangiectasia) is characterized by clusters of greatly dilated sinusoids, usually occurring randomly throughout the liver parenchyma. The resultant lacunae are filled by blood, and may be either lined by or devoid of endothelium. Angiectasis may be an incidental finding, especially in aged mice. Angiectasis is rarely reported, but may be associated with toxins that induce endothelial injury. Localized endothelial injury may result in a weakened vascular wall in the sinusoid that subsequently leads to angiectasis. In humans, angiectasis can occur following use of anabolic steroids and, rarely, oral contraceptives. In cattle, it can occur following ingestion of *Pimlea* sp.

Stellate Cell Lesions

The stellate cell is also known as the Ito cell, fat-storing cell, lipocyte, and perisinusoidal cell. Although it is a minor cell in the liver, constituting only 5% of the total hepatic cell numbers, it plays a central role in several toxin-induced hepatic lesions. Because the stellate cell is the vitamin A storage site in the liver, its response is central in the development of hepatic lesions associated with hypervitaminosis A. On administration of excessive doses of vitamin A, stellate cells enlarge due to the development of large cytoplasmic lipid deposits. With continued treatment, collagen is formed by activated stellate cells, whose phenotype is now similar to myofibroblasts. Prolonged hyper-vitaminosis A will result in severe hepatic fibrosis in the rat and several other species. Vitamin A toxicity is believed to be the cause of veno-occlusive disease of captive exotic cats, especially cheetahs.

Stellate cells are responsive to hepatic injury induced by a variety of hepatic necrogenic agents. When carbon tetrachloride induces central lobular necrosis, or when ethionine causes periportal necrosis, stellate cells accumulate in the local area of injury, apparently because of a proliferation of the local population of stellate cells. These cells participate in the reparative process by producing collagen. It is now well-established that hepatic fibrosis occurring within the lobule is due to collagen production by the stellate cell. This process depends on activation, proliferation, and stimulation of collagen production in stellate cells by TGF-β. In contrast, fibrosis in the portal area that occurs with chemically-induced bile duct injury is the result of collagen production by the resident fibroblasts in the portal area.

Cystic degeneration, also known as *spongiosis hepatis*, is a unique microscopic lesion of rodents believed to represent a degenerative change of stellate cells. It is characterized by multilocular cyst-like structures containing finely granular or flocculent eosinophilic material. Each cystlike structure may range in size from the diameter of a hepatocyte to many times the diameter of a hepatocyte. It may be seen in normal hepatic parenchyma, as well as in proliferative hepatocellular lesions such as foci and neoplasms.

Küpffer Cells

Küpffer cells, hepatic macrophages, are the major phagocytic cell of the liver, as well as antigen-presenting cells. Therefore, any particulate material that is injected intravascularly and often intramuscularly into an animal may be found in this cell type, e.g., iron following intramuscular injection in piglets. The specific response of Küpffer cells to foreign particulate material is well known, and several toxins, as well as physiological substances, also have primary effects on this cell. More recently, Küpffer cells have been implicated in idiosyncratic hepatotoxicity.

Endotoxin normally released by the intestine is routinely removed and detoxified by the Küpffer cells. Therefore, any chemically-induced alteration in the Küpffer cells to perform this vital function may result in injury to the underlying hepatocytes, as well as other tissues in the body. Several of the model hepatotoxic chemicals, such as carbon tetrachloride and galactosamine, decrease the endotoxin-removing activity of the Küpffer cell. The resultant endotoxemia probably plays some role in the subsequent hepatotoxic response. While some chemicals may injure or decrease the activity of Küpffer cells, other agents may enhance Küpffer cell activity. For example, exogenous estrogen will cause the enlargement and proliferation of Küpffer cells (hyperplasia), as well as enhance their phagocytic activity. Küpffer cell hyperplasia (histiocytosis) generally manifests as small aggregates of Küpffer cells that may contain pigment. Küpffer cells can be activated to produce a variety of cytokines, eicosanoids, nitric oxide, and oxygen radicals, and thus interact with hepatocytes, endothelial cells, and stellate cells. As a result, Küpffer cells can participate in the pathogenesis of toxic hepatic injury and repair.

Although the major emphasis in chemically-induced hepatotoxicity is frequently placed on the hepatocyte, hepatotoxic agents may affect the Küpffer cells, either preferentially or prior to induction of hepatocytic injury. Ricin, a potent protein synthesis inhibitor produced by the castor bean plant, *Ricinus communis*, initially injures the Küpffer cells of the liver. Beryllium can also cause Küpffer cell death via necrosis or apoptosis.

Hepatitis

In humans, hepatitis (inflammation of the liver) with or without cholestasis, is a common manifestation of drug induced liver injury (DILI). It is associated with many therapeutic drugs, including oxyphenisatin, methyldopa, nitrofurantoin, isoniazid, and dantrolene. The occurrence of hepatitis as a manifestation of hepatotoxicity of these agents in experimental animals has not been reported and injury is believed to be an idiosyncratic response. Granulomatous hepatitis, characterized by multifocal accumulation of macrophages and giant cells without necrosis, was observed in rats following α-naphthylisothiocyanate administration, and with a small number of other chemicals. In humans, granuloma (granulomata) formation has been reported in response to a number of drugs, including sulfonamides, methyldopa, quinidine, and allopurinol.

Spontaneous multifocal inflammation is commonly observed in rodent livers as a background lesion. It appears as randomly scattered inflammatory cell accumulations that usually include macrophages, and may also include neutrophils and lymphocytes. Necrotic hepatocytes may also be present, although usually limited in number. Multifocal inflammation may also be induced by viral agents, such as the newly-recognized norovirus. A more severe and progressive form of hepatitis in mice has been recognized to result from *Helicobacter hepaticus* infection. Other infectious causes of hepatic inflammation should also be considered.

Hepatic Fibrosis and Cirrhosis

Hepatic Fibrosis

Hepatic fibrosis is defined as an overall increase in extracellular matrix; there are changes in collagen types and their site of deposition (see Figure 9.18A). Phenotypically-altered stellate cells and myofibroblasts (located within connective tissues of portal and central areas) are responsible for this collagen deposition. Collagen deposition may be related to lobular structure (perisinusoidal, periductular and portal), or the site of injury. The excess collagen accentuates normal features, while architecture is not disrupted. This is accompanied by minimal regeneration, and there may be collapse of lobules. This type of fibrosis generally occurs following chronic low-level toxicant exposure.

Cirrhosis

Cirrhosis can be defined as hepatic fibrosis with nodular regeneration (Figure 9.22). It is the final, irreversible result of many disease processes, and is often called "end-stage liver." For example, it occurs following exposure to aflatoxin B_1 in many species, as a result of repeated carbon tetrachloride administration in rats and mice, and alcohol abuse in humans. The regeneration and fibrosis apparently result from repeated hepatocellular necrosis (Figure 9.23). Grossly, cirrhotic livers are nodular, and tan or yellow in color (Figure 9.24). Early cirrhosis may result in liver enlargement, although progression of the disease may result in a reduction in liver size. When advanced, cirrhosis may lead to hepatic failure.

Microscopically, nodules of regenerating hepatocytes are characterized by cell plates greater than two cells thick, and are separated by connective tissue. In humans, cirrhosis is among the top ten causes of death in the Western world, with alcohol abuse the major contributor. Drug-induced cirrhosis can occur with α-methyldopa, acetaminophen, arsenic, deferiprone, celecoxib, methotrexate oxyphenisatin, isoniazid, sulfonamides, and propylthiouracil. Regenerative nodules associated with fibrosis are a feature of the response of some dogs to anticonvulsant drugs.

Specific Etiologic Examples

In most cases of chronic hepatic injury it is not possible to determine the cause of initial injury. The presence of megalocytosis (see Figure 9.18B), induced by exposure to pyrrolizidine alkaloids, aflatoxins, cycads, or nitrosamines may help in reaching an etiologic diagnosis. Pyrrolizidine alkaloids, present in many plant families (e.g. *Senecio*, *Crotalaria*, and *Echium* sp; comfrey

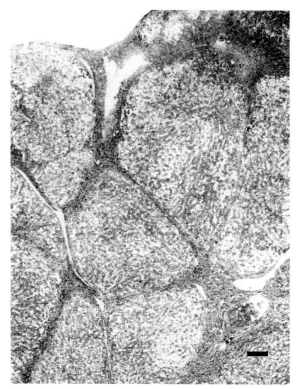

FIGURE 9.22 Cirrhosis in a rat, characterized by collagenous septa and nodular regeneration. H&E stain. Bar = 120 μm.

(*Symphytum officinale*), used as an herbal tea) are converted via the cytochrome P450 enzymes to pyrrolic esters, which are alkylating agents. Among domestic animals, pigs are most susceptible to toxicity, followed by cattle and horses, with sheep and goats least susceptible. While the liver is the major target organ, the lung and kidneys may be affected, depending on the species and the specific alkaloid. Experimentally, acute toxicity results in central lobular hepatocyte necrosis and damage to the sinusoidal endothelium.

In domestic animals, the typical manifestation is chronic disease with hepatic fibrosis (see Figure 9.18A), megalocytosis and biliary proliferation; nodular regeneration may also be present (cirrhosis), especially in cattle. Extrahepatic changes include ascites, diarrhea, icterus, and photosensitization. In humans, pyrrolizidine alkaloid toxicity is termed veno-occlusive disease (VOD), due to the extensive fibrosis of the central vein or sinusoidal obstruction syndrome based on the pathogenesis of sinusoidal endothelial destruction.

Aflatoxins, mycotoxins produced primarily by *Aspergillus flavus*, frequently contaminate corn, peanuts, and cottonseed used in human and animal food. Aflatoxin B_1 is the most common and potent mycotoxin. Metabolism to the reactive species is via cytochrome P450 enzymes with severity of toxicity being both species- and age-dependent. Mice are relatively

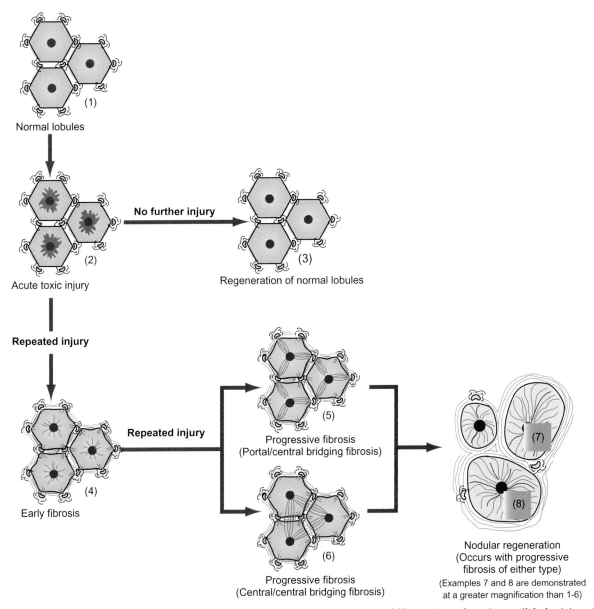

FIGURE 9.23 Schematic diagram of the effects of hepatic injury on the development of fibrosis. Acute hepatic centrilobular injury (2) that occurs only once usually resolves, and normal liver architecture returns (1, 3). Repeated bouts of injury or severe injury can initiate hepatic fibrosis (4). In the earliest stages, fibrosis may be reversible, but as fibrosis progresses it reaches a point at which repair is unlikely. Fibrosis starts as fine branches of collagen deposition between portal areas or central areas, or dissecting into the hepatic parenchyma (5, 6). Over time, greater amounts of collagen and other extracellular matrix are deposited, and the lobular architecture becomes progressively distorted. In the end-stage liver, nodular regeneration (7, 8) and extensive, circumferential fibrosis are typical. The regenerative nodules shown here (7, 8) are at an early stage of regeneration. As shown in Figure 9.24, they will regenerate to form nodules that will commonly exceed the size of normal hepatic lobules. These nodules will often compress (7) the central vein(s) of hepatic lobules within and adjacent to those from which they arose. (From Cullen, J. (2007). In *Pathologic Basis of Veterinary Disease*, McGavin, M., and Zachary, J.F., eds, 4th edn. Mosby Elsevier, St. Louis. Figure 8-22, p. 410.)

resistant to toxicity. In acute toxicity, central lobular necrosis occurs in most species, although midzonal necrosis has been described in rabbits, and periportal necrosis in poultry, cats, and rats. In addition to necrosis, hemorrhage, lipidosis, and biliary proliferation are common features (see Figures 9.11 and 9.20). Recent outbreaks of acute aflatoxicoses have been reported in humans in Africa, and dogs in the USA and Israel. Chronic toxicity is manifested as fibrosis, with or without nodular regeneration, as well as biliary proliferation and megalocytosis. In humans, aflatoxins are a cause of hepatocellular neoplasia; coexposure to hepatitis B virus and other mycotoxins may also play a role.

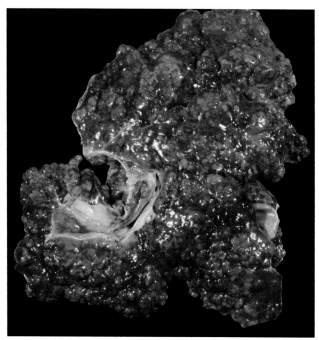

FIGURE 9.24 Cirrhosis; liver, dog. The liver is small, firm and irregular, with multiple regenerative nodules separated by tracts of fibrous connective tissue (end-stage liver).

Alcoholic liver disease accounts for about 65% of cirrhosis in humans in the Western world. Ethanol and its metabolites cause hepatocellular injury through glutathione depletion, mitochondrial injury, altered metabolism of methionine, and cytokine release from Küpffer cells. Acute toxicity is characterized by lipidosis, Mallory bodies, and necrosis with neutrophil accumulation. Lipidosis results in enlargement of the liver, but is reversible in the early stages. Alcoholic hepatitis follows with continuing injury. In 10–15% of alcoholics, with continued alcohol abuse, hepatitis progresses to cirrhosis, which is irreversible.

HEPATIC NEOPLASIA

Like most neoplasms, hepatic neoplasia may occur spontaneously, most often associated with increasing age. In humans, primary hepatic carcinomas are relatively uncommon in the USA and Western Europe, but represent up to 40% of cancers in some countries where viral hepatitis is common. Aflatoxicosis has also been linked to human hepatic carcinomas. In domestic animals, hepatic neoplasms have not been linked to chemical exposure. However, the induction of hepatic neoplasms is the most common neoplastic response found in rodents exposed to exogenous chemicals. Over 50% of all chemicals that induce neoplasms in rodents cause neoplasms in the liver, although these chemicals may also cause neoplasms in other organs. Partly due to their frequent occurrence, liver neoplasms in rodents have been the basis of controversy for many years.

The controversy has several different facets. Most importantly, the relevance of the rodent liver neoplasm as an indicator of risk in humans who may be exposed to the chemical has been challenged. Those who question the relevance of the rodent liver tumor frequently note that human liver tumors are a relatively rare form of human cancer in industrial societies, where the exposure to man-made chemicals would be expected to be greatest. The resolution of the controversy awaits a better understanding of the mechanism of liver tumor induction by chemicals.

A second controversy concerning rodent liver tumors is the issue of diagnostic classification. As in other areas of diagnostic pathology, the active biological potential of a neoplasm is interpreted from tissue taken at a single point in time. Whereas most malignant neoplasms generate little discussion, the distinction between hyperplastic and benign neoplastic lesions has proven very difficult. The morphologic distinction between benign and malignant hepatic neoplasms is also not always obvious. Despite these difficulties, there are diagnostic criteria for the various types of benign and malignant liver tumors. For rats and mice, the Society of Toxicologic Pathology's website (https://www.toxpath.org, standardized nomenclature, position papers) and GoRENI (http://www.goRENI.org) can be accessed for nomenclature and diagnostic criteria of proliferative and neoplastic lesions in toxicologic pathology. GoRENI is the internet discussion platform for the global initiative "INHAND"—the *In*ternational *Ha*rmonization of *N*omenclature and *D*iagnostic criteria—which will provide a unified nomenclature for use in toxicologic pathology. In addition, valuable organ sampling guides are provided on the GoRENI website (http://reni.item.fraunhofer.de/reni/trimming/index.php).

Hepatocellular Neoplasia

Hepatocellular neoplasia is a frequent consequence of carcinogen exposure in a variety of laboratory animal species. Spontaneous hepatocellular neoplasia is observed with a variable incidence in different strains of mice and rats. In mice, a relatively high incidence (30–50% in males) of hepatocellular carcinoma occurs in the C3H strain, and a relatively low incidence (~5% in males) occurs in the C57B1/6 strain mice. In the F_1 hybrid of these two strains, an intermediate incidence is observed. Much of the high background incidence and heightened sensitivity to carcinogens in the C3H strain comes from a gene at the Hcs locus. The resulting phenotype is attributed to higher rates of proliferation and growth in preneoplastic lesions in hepatocytes. Most rat strains, such as F344, have a relatively low incidence of hepatocellular neoplasia. Spontaneous incidence rates vary with age at examination (two years as opposed to lifespan), gender and laboratory conditions. In humans, hepatocellular carcinoma has been linked to both chronic aflatoxin and alcohol exposures.

Malignant hepatocellular neoplasms are referred to as hepatocellular carcinomas. These lesions are grossly visible nodules which are frequently firm, have a smooth or multinodular surface, and are grayish white. However, in other instances the lesion may be soft, with variable dark red areas due to hemorrhage (Figure 9.25). Microscopically, hepatocellular carcinomas consist of cells which usually resemble hepatocytes. In rats, trabecular, acinar, and solid patterns are recognized, sometimes within the same neoplasm (Figure 9.26). In mice, carcinomas are similarly composed of cells resembling hepatocytes, usually in a trabecular pattern. Differentiation between acinar hepatocellular carcinoma and cholangiocarcinoma, which arise from bile duct epithelium, without mucus production may be difficult. Hepatocholangiocellular carcinomas have the features of both hepatocellular carcinomas and cholangiocarcinomas.

Benign proliferative lesions of hepatocytes are referred to as hepatocellular adenomas. In rats, previously used terms included nodular hyperplasia and neoplastic nodules, reflecting an inability to clearly distinguish hyperplasia from neoplasia in the rodent liver. It is known that some of these lesions may regress, while others may progress to hepatocellular carcinoma.

Adenomas must be differentiated from foci of cellular alteration and hepatocellular regenerative hyperplasia. In rats, adenoma can be distinguished from carcinoma by preservation of the hepatic cords, composed of fairly uniform hepatocytes which are separated by sinusoids. In mice, hepatocellular adenomas are usually solid nodules of closely-packed hepatocytes, surrounded by apparent sinusoids. The cells are usually basophilic, and may also be vacuolated. Hepatocellular adenomas should be differentiated from hepatocholangiocellular adenomas which have the features of both hepatocellular adenomas and cholangiomas.

Foci of cellular alteration may represent progenitor lesions from which hepatocellular neoplasia may arise. These foci are composed of hepatocytes which have cytological or histochemical alteration, but merge imperceptibly with surrounding hepatocytes (Figure 9.27). Their boundaries have little or no compression

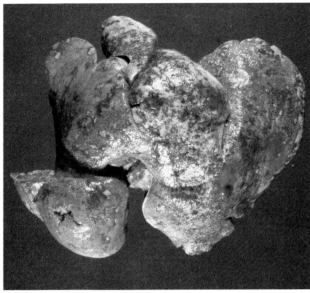

FIGURE 9.25 Hepatocellular carcinoma; liver, dog. A multinodular hemorrhagic mass protrudes from the surface of the liver and affects multiple lobes.

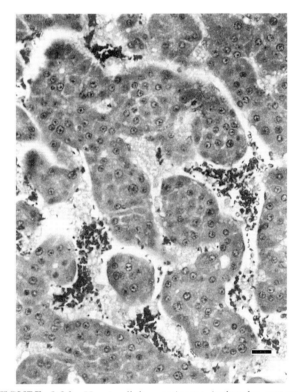

FIGURE 9.26 Hepatocellular carcinoma (trabecular pattern), rat. H&E stain. Bar = 24 μm.

of adjacent parenchyma. Foci occur spontaneously in rats and mice, and are generally found in much greater numbers following treatment with carcinogens. As mentioned earlier, hepatocellular foci and

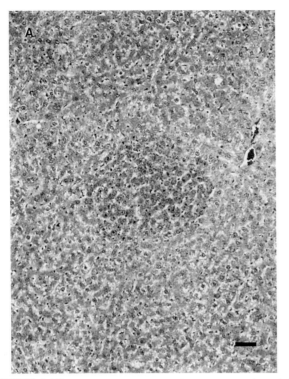

FIGURE 9.27   Foci of hepatocellular alteration, rat. A basophilic focus (center) is present. H&E stain. Bar = 48 μm.

neoplasms have been characterized using a variety of histochemical markers.

The regression of early hepatocellular proliferative lesions following chemical removal is seen in some, but not all, experimental protocols for induction of hepatocellular neoplasia. This variability in progression or regression makes it difficult to predict future events for any single lesion, or group of lesions, observed at one distinct point in time.

The hepatoblastoma has been reported in mice and in humans during young childhood. This neoplasm is a spontaneous lesion in the B6C3F$_1$ and BALB/c strains. Hepatoblastomas have also been increased in B6C3F$_1$ mice fed 2-acetylaminofluorene. In these tumors a variable cell population includes islands or sheets of poorly-defined cells with oval nuclei and elongated cells, arranged in rosettes and ribbons. At low magnification, the lesion is basophilic, due to the numerous small nuclei surrounded by scant cytoplasm. Cystic and large vascular spaces are often present. The histogenesis is unknown with liver blastema cells, neoplastic hepatocytes, oval cells, and biliary epithelial cells proposed.

In domestic animals, hepatocellular nodular hyperplasia is common in the dog. This is a proliferative, but non-neoplastic and non-regenerative, hepatocellular lesion. Multiple hyperplastic nodules are typically present, and may be several centimeters in diameter.

Histologically, they are characterized by a normal but distorted lobular pattern. Hepatocellular adenomas and carcinomas are uncommon, but have been described most commonly in ruminants and dogs.

Bile Duct Neoplasms

Neoplasms of bile duct epithelium are extremely rare as spontaneous lesions in the rodent, even though bile duct proliferation is relatively common. Bile duct neoplasms may be induced on administration of several chemical carcinogens, including azo dyes, furans, and some nitrosamines such as N-nitrosomorpholine. Although early bile duct proliferation, including oval cell proliferation and cholangiofibrosis, is associated with the development of bile duct neoplasms, bile duct carcinogenesis should not be predicted based on bile duct proliferation. Indeed, many chemicals that induce substantial bile duct proliferation fail to cause the formation of bile duct neoplasms.

Neoplasms of the bile ducts may be noted grossly in laboratory animals. They are generally present as multiple white nodules of varying consistency, depending on the degree of fibrosis. The characteristic light color and the frequent firm consistency make bile duct neoplasms easily distinguishable from other primary hepatic neoplasms when observed grossly. However, it may be relatively difficult to distinguish a primary bile duct neoplasm from metastatic epithelial neoplasms derived from other sites.

Histologic types of bile duct neoplasms recognized in the livers of rodents include cholangiocarcinoma and cholangioma. The cholangiocarcinoma is generally characterized by a moderate collagenous connective tissue stroma surrounding neoplastic cells that form nests, irregular cords, or gland-like structures (Figure 9.28). The gland-like structures of cholangiocarcinomas have very little to no mucous material. The neoplastic cells are irregular in shape and size, varying from a flattened, almost squamous, to a low columnar appearance. Mitotic figures may be relatively numerous. Cholangiocarcinomas clearly invade into vessels, lymphatics, and connective tissue surrounding the liver.

Cholangioma is a benign lesion of bile duct epithelium that is characterized by a distinct border, and composed of numerous irregular bile ducts. Simple cholangiomas have scant connective tissue stroma, and may have a thin connective tissue capsule. Although the individual bile ducts may be slightly irregular in shape, the epithelium lining these ducts is usually homogeneous in cell size and shape. The cells are cuboidal, similar to normal intrahepatic bile duct epithelium. Mitotic figures are rare. Cystic cholangiomas are characterized by irregular cystic cavities,

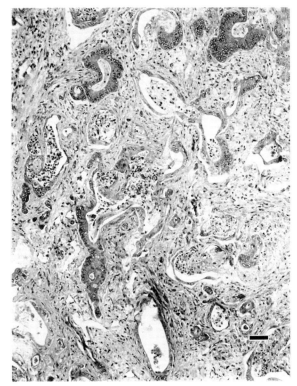

FIGURE 9.28 Cholangiocarcinoma, rat. Ducts are lined by neoplastic cells and surrounded by extensive collagenous stroma. H&E stain. Bar = 48 μm.

usually lined by a uniformly low cuboidal to squamous epithelium. These must be differentiated from bile duct cyst(s), which do not have expansive growth and are lined by flattened epithelium that does not form acini or papillary structures, as well as bile duct hyperplasia and cholangiofibrosis. Both the simple cholangioma and the cystic cholangioma are clearly benign structures.

In humans, cholangiocarcinomas are relatively uncommon, except in geographic regions where the liver fluke, *Opisthorchis sinensis*, is found. A risk condition for this tumor was the use of Thorostat. In domestic animals, bile duct neoplasms are termed cholangiocellular (bile duct) adenoma (consistent with cholangioma of rodents), and carcinoma (consistent with cholangiocarcinoma). These tumors are uncommon, except for adenomas in the cat which may be the most common primary hepatic neoplasm in that species. Cystic variants, usually referred to as cystadenomas, are most common.

Endothelial Neoplasms

Spontaneous primary hepatic endothelial neoplasms are uncommon in all laboratory animals. When they are chemically-induced, primary endothelial neoplasms can occur concurrently with, or independent of, hepatocellular carcinomas. In humans, the primary liver form of hemangiosarcomas (angiosarcomas) has been associated with exposure to vinyl chloride, arsenic, and Thorostat. When noted grossly, endothelial cell neoplasms have a characteristic dark red, or mottled dark red and white, appearance. Primary endothelial neoplasms are variable in size and may be multicentric. When found on the capsular surface, endothelial cell neoplasms may rupture, causing hemorrhage into the abdominal cavity, complete exsanguination, and death.

Hemangiomas are characterized histologically by a single layer of densely-packed endothelial cells along disrupted hepatic cords. The more common hemangiosarcoma is characterized by numerous pleomorphic neoplastic endothelial cells that densely line the remnant and disorganized hepatic cords. As the lesions progress in size, the remaining hepatocytes are slowly replaced as the neoplasm becomes composed predominantly of neoplastic endothelial cells.

Küpffer Cell Neoplasms

The Küpffer cell sarcoma is a rare neoplasm in rodents induced by only a very few chemicals that are given intravascularly, most notably trypan blue and thorium dioxide. Küpffer cell sarcomas form multiple gray macroscopic nodules that occur randomly through the liver. Histologically, they are composed of macrophage-like cells characterized by a pale, oval, indented nucleus surrounded by abundant vacuolated cytoplasm. The differential diagnosis of Küpffer cell sarcoma is extremely difficult and includes malignant fibrous histiocytoma, histiocytoma, and histiocytic sarcoma.

EVALUATION OF TOXICITY

Toxic responses in the liver can be evaluated by several different technical approaches. The liver can be evaluated as part of the entire animal, or as an isolated perfused organ. The response of the individual cells in the liver may be studied in primary cultures.

The initial identification and evaluation of hepatic toxic responses is generally done in a laboratory animal. The administration of the toxic agent to the whole animal most clearly mimics exposure of humans and domestic animals. Experimental animals may be exposed by a variety of routes, although the oral route is most common. The evaluation of hepatotoxicity in whole animals has several distinct advantages. Because the whole animal has all normal physiologic functions intact, chemical uptake and delivery to the target organ are intact. The metabolic function of the animal is intact, within the liver and other body sites. This is particularly important if a toxic response is dependent on metabolism at a distant site, such as the intestine, where the normal bacterial flora may be essential for activation of the chemical.

The whole animal is the only system in which a chronic response can be evaluated over its entire course. For example, the induction of liver neoplasms requires at least several months, a time period that cannot be achieved by liver perfusion or cultured hepatocyte techniques. Likewise, the development of cirrhosis requires many months, and cannot be duplicated using other approaches. Liver perfusion and cultured hepatocyte techniques may be used to understand processes at a single point in time, but cannot reproduce the entire pathogenesis of the response. The major disadvantage of whole animal studies is the complexity of the system, which hinders the evaluation of the response and the possible mechanisms by which that response occurred. Nonetheless, the whole animal is the relevant system by which responses in the perfused liver and cultured hepatocyte must be judged.

Morphologic Evaluation

General Evaluation

Morphologic evaluation of the liver can use simple or complicated approaches. Macroscopic evaluation is best achieved by removing the liver from the animal. All lobes should be identified, to ensure a complete specimen. The liver may be rinsed with physiologic saline to remove blood and other materials, blotted, and weighed. After weighing, the capsular surfaces (diaphragmatic and abdominal) are examined. Cut surfaces can be examined following sectioning of each lobe at uniform predetermined intervals.

Evaluation of the liver for toxicity generally includes a measurement of liver weight. Since liver weight is obviously dependent on animal size, liver weight is generally best expressed in relation to the body weight. In most animals the relative liver weight (liver weight divided by body weight) is 3–4%. The relative liver weight will be slightly higher in young growing animals and slightly lower in obese animals. Hepatic toxicity may result in a reduced or increased liver size. Reduced size may be due to either acute or chronic hepatic injury resulting in cell loss. Interpretation of increased liver weight is more difficult. An enlarged

liver can be due to proliferation of hepatocytes resulting in a hyperplastic liver, or simply due to enlargement of the individual hepatocytes.

Routine microscopic evaluation utilizes immersion fixation with 10% buffered formalin, paraffin embedment, and hematoxylin and eosin staining of 4–6μm sections. Examination of liver sections should include evaluation of lobule size and distribution of lesions, often best done at low magnification. Each structure within the lobule should be evaluated, as well as each cell type. Hematoxylin- and eosin-stained sections demonstrate many alterations of hepatocytes and bile duct epithelial cells, but do provide less information on nonparenchymal cells.

In addition to focal gross lesions, representative samples which include capsule and underlying parenchyma should be prepared. These samples should be taken in a uniform fashion with respect to lobe, site, and orientation, and more than one lobe should be sampled. In this way, intralobar and interlobar variation may be accounted for. Interlobular variation in response has been reported and may be due to portal streamlining of toxic agents absorbed via segments of the gastrointestinal tract, as well as transperitoneal migration of volatile toxicants out of the stomach. In addition, if intraperitoneal exposure is used, one may see localized capsular or subcapsular lesions. A liver organ sampling guide is provided for the mouse on the GoRENI website (http://reni.item.fraunhofer.de/reni/trimming/index.php).

Specialized Evaluation

Exsanguination of the animal prior to removing the liver is adequate for routine examination. However, perfusion of the liver with buffered saline to remove blood constituents is done in some laboratories. Perfusion of the liver with fixative, generally via the portal vein, is often chosen for ultrastructural examination, but immersion fixation may be adequate for some studies. Numerous fixatives have been used to prepare liver specimens for electron microscopy. Although aldehydes, particularly glutaraldehyde, are easy to use, primary fixation in osmium tetroxide is preferable for some evaluations, such as nucleolar structure evaluation.

Immunostaining techniques have been described for numerous proteins, including enzymes, present in the liver. Sample preparation, especially fixation, must be optimized for each antigen of interest and for each staining technique. Often, stains for enzymatic activity are utilized in studies of hepatotoxicity. Many of these techniques require preparation of frozen sections. Frozen sections of fixed tissue are used for lipid stains, such as oil red or osmium. Liver tissue may be frozen with embedding media to a microtomy chuck at the time of dissection, and stored frozen until sections are cut.

Morphometric analysis has had several uses in evaluation of hepatotoxicity. Changes in organelle number or size may be quantitated from electron micrographs. For ultrastructural morphometry, intralobular variation may be minimized by sampling strategy. Morphometry may also be used to quantitate changes at the light microscopic level. Volume density is easily determined, since it is equivalent to an area ratio that can be easily determined on light or electron microscopic sections. This approach can be applied to a variety of tissue responses, providing information that may not be apparent by nonquantitative techniques. In the case of foci of hepatocellular alteration, additional information can be derived regarding size and number of lesions using stereologic estimations.

In recent years, the toxicologic significance of chemically-induced hepatocellular proliferation has been studied. Increased rates of hepatocellular turnover may indicate cytotoxicity or adaptive hyperplasia, and may be mechanistically related to neoplastic development. Quantitation of cell replication has usually been approached by determining the fraction of cells in mitosis or replicative DNA synthesis (S phase). In addition to cell proliferation, DNA replication may also reflect changes in hepatocellular ploidy or nuclearity. To determine S phase, the incorporation of a nucleoside into DNA over a specified time period can be used. Isotopically-labeled thymidine can be detected by liquid scintillation counting, or by quantitative autoradiography. Bromodeoxyuridine, a thymidine analog, can be detected by monoclonal antibody, making it applicable for quantitative immunohistochemistry or cell-sorter analysis of suspensions of individual hepatocytes. The administration of either nucleoside may be by pulse or continuous dosing regimens. The latter uses a constant rate delivery system over several days. This technique is much more reliable for detecting small differences in levels of DNA replication, since circadian and day-to-day variation in rate of cells entering S phase is averaged over the period of nucleoside administration for each animal. The determination of increased DNA replication, coupled with constant liver weight, may detect minimal hepatocellular loss through necrosis or apoptosis that is not detectable by routine light microscopy or clinical chemistry.

Immunohistochemical detection of proliferating cell nuclear antigen (PCNA) has been used as a surrogate for detection of S phase nuclei by labeling techniques. PCNA is a protein associated with DNA polymerase δ, and its expression begins in late G_1 cells, and continues through S phase and beyond. The chief advantage of PCNA detection over other techniques is that the administration of labeled nucleoside or nucleoside analog is not necessary, so that it can be performed on archival materials where a need to estimate hepatocellular proliferation was not forseen. However, it is a less precise methodology, partly due to a lack of precise phase-dependent cut-off in expression level, and partly due to its sensitivity to variations in tissue fixation and processing. Other antibodies, such as Ki67 may also prove useful for determination of cell proliferation in the liver.

Clinical Chemistry Evaluation

Alterations in clinical chemistry parameters may be associated with hepatocellular injury, decreased functional mass, cholestasis, altered hepatic blood flow, metabolic adaptation (e.g., enzyme induction), or altered Küpffer cell activity. The pattern of findings in a selected battery of tests may indicate the type and severity of liver lesions. Because the liver has large functional reserves, it is possible that significant loss of functional tissue may occur with minimal or no detectable change in routine laboratory tests.

Hepatotoxicity can be monitored by measuring the activity of more-or-less liver-specific enzymes in serum. These enzymes are indicators of cellular degeneration or necrosis, and increase membrane permeability. Alanine aminotransferase (ALT) is an excellent enzyme for evaluation of hepatocyte injury in most species, however half-life varies according to species. Aspartate aminotransferase (AST) tends to parallel serum ALT activity following liver injury, but is not specific for liver as muscle also has high activity. Serum ALT and AST activities increase within hours of significant liver injury. Other enzymes that may be elevated due to hepatocellular injury, but less frequently measured, include lactate dehydrogenase (LDH, not specific for liver), sorbitol dehydrogenase (SDH), glutamate dehydrogenase (GDH), isocitrate dehydrogenase and arginase. Increased serum γ-glutamyl transferase (GGT) activity is indicative of bile duct cell injury and cholestasis in the rat. Other indicators of cholestasis include increased serum and urine bilirubin, and increased serum bile acids and alkaline phosphatase (ALP) activity. Alkaline phophatase is not specific for liver since isoenzymes for bone (high in young growing animals), intestine (especially in the rat), and steroid-induced (in the dog only) can contribute significantly to serum activity.

Another approach is an assay of liver function by administration of a dye that is taken up, conjugated, and excreted, usually into the bile. One such dye is sulfobromopthalein (BSP), which can be measured in plasma following pulse administration. Persistence of

BSP in plasma (prolonged BSP retention) may indicate impaired hepatic function.

Noninvasive Imaging

Another whole animal approach to characterizing liver lesions is noninvasive imaging. Changing technologies in this area have led to magnetic resonance imaging (MRI) as one current major imaging advance. As resolution improves with development, MRI may eventually be valuable in monitoring progression or regression of focal hepatic lesions that are submacroscopic to microscopic in size. Therefore, MRI may prove useful in characterization of neoplastic development following chemical administration. In addition to MRI, the development of new probes for utilization with positron emission tomography (PET) scanning may make the functional characterization of molecular changes in the live animal an available option in the future.

In Vitro Approaches

Perfused Liver Preparations

The use of perfused liver preparations may uniquely address certain issues in hepatotoxicity. This preparation involves perfusion of livers with physiological buffer solutions of appropriate pH, temperature, and O_2 concentration. Viability can be assessed by monitoring LDH release, oxygen consumption, and trypan blue uptake. The advantages of the perfused liver preparation over isolated hepatocytes include the maintenance of normal hepatic architecture, which allows continuous monitoring of liver uptake of chemicals and biliary excretion of hepatic metabolites. In addition, the role of oxygen tension in hepatotoxicity can be evaluated by comparing anterograde (portal vein) and retrograde (hepatic vein) perfusion. Liver perfusion has the unique advantage of allowing instantaneous delivery, or cessation of delivery of a toxin or physiological substance, while monitoring the integrated metabolic response of the liver. These preparations are limited by time, that is, maintenance beyond a few hours is not practical.

Cultured Hepatocytes

Many investigations of hepatocellular toxicity have utilized cultured hepatocytes. These investigations have studied metabolism, cytotoxicity, genotoxicity, and carcinogenicity. Advantages of cultured hepatocytes include the ability to prepare multiple cultures from a single animal, thereby increasing replicates and

decreasing animal usage. The need for large amounts of chemicals and response modifiers is reduced when compared with whole animal studies. Extrahepatic responses in whole animals can be eliminated as potential contributors to hepatic responses. Finally, human hepatocytes can be used in comparative animal hepatocyte studies for increasing reliability in risk estimation using animal data.

In routine cultures, many xenobiotic metabolic functions decrease within four days, but modifying culture media and attachment matrix, or co-culturing with other cells can prolong maintenance of these functions. In routine cultures of hepatocytes, there is very little DNA replication or cell division. Conditions can be altered to stimulate or inhibit hepatocyte proliferation in culture.

Liver Slices

The use of precision-cut liver slices to evaluate the effect of potential and actual toxicants in liver represent another technical approach for hepatic pharmacology and toxicology. In this technique, viable liver is cut to slices of specified thickness which are maintained in roller vials containing liquid media for several hours. Advantages of this system are that it maintains the normal hepatocyte and matrix contacts that are disrupted in the preparation of primary cultures.

Use of Animals as Models

Studies in laboratory species have served a very useful purpose in the identification of hepatobiliary toxins and carcinogens, and in providing an in-depth understanding of the mechanism of action of many chemicals. The use of genetically-engineered mouse models and molecular biology techniques has greatly facilitated this process. The combination of identification, of and elucidation of the mechanism of action of hepatobiliary toxins, is essential in determining the relative importance of toxins for potentially exposed humans.

Despite the importance of animal models for identifying and providing a basic understanding of the mechanism of action of hepatobiliary toxins, the limitations of these models must be considered. Different species may have different, or at least unequal, responses when exposed to a given toxin. For example, aflatoxin B_1 is a potent hepatotoxin and hepatocarcinogen in the rat, but produces minimal effects in the mouse. When such differences occur, it must be determined which animal is most predictive of a response in potentially exposed humans. The resolution of this dilemma resides in developing a basic understanding of the response in the two species, and then determining which factors in the response also may be relevant to humans.

SUMMARY AND CONCLUSIONS

Toxic injury to the hepatobiliary system is a relatively frequent response when experimental animals are exposed to xenobiotics. However, the diversity of responses is extensive. The different cell types provide an opportunity for the toxin to preferentially affect a single cell type, while producing little effect on other cell types. Even when a single cell type is affected, most frequently the hepatocyte, the response may vary greatly in terms of either the distribution within the liver or the severity. Toxic responses in the liver may be manifest in relatively short periods of time; for example, hepatocyte necrosis can occur within 24 hours of exposure. In contrast, the induction of cirrhosis and neoplasia require a relatively long period of toxin exposure. The type of response is a key indication of the action of the toxin.

FURTHER READING

Abboud, G., and Kaplowitz, N. (2007). Drug-induced liver injury. *Drug Saf.*, 30, 277–294.

Arias, I.M., and Boyer, J.L. (2001). *The Liver: Biology and Pathobiology.* Lippincott Williams & Wilkins, Philadelphia, PA.

Bischoff, K., and Ramaiah, S. (2007). Liver toxicity. In *Veterinary Toxicology Basic and Clinical Principles* (Gupta, R.C. ed.), pp. 145–160. Elsevier Academic Press, New York, NY.

Boone, L., Meyer, D., Cusick, P., Ennulat, D., Bolliger, A.P., Everds, N., Meador, V., Elliott, G., Honor, D., Bounous, D., and Jordan, H. (2005). Selection and interpretation of clinical pathology indicators of hepatic injury in preclinical studies. *Vet. Clin. Pathol.*, 34(3), 182–188.

Burt, A.D., Portmann, B.C., and Ferrell, L.D. (eds) (2006). *MacSween's Pathology of the Liver*, 5th edn. Churchill-Livingstone, New York, NY.

Cattley, R.C., Popp, J.A., Haschek, W.M., Rousseaux, C.G., and Wallig, M.A. (eds) (2002). Handbook of Toxicologic Pathology, 2nd edn. Vol. 2. Academic Press, San Diego, CA, pp. 187–225.

Crawford, J.M. (2005). Liver and biliary tract. In *Robbins and Cotran Pathologic Basis of Disease* (Kumar, V., Abbas, A.K., and Fausto, N. eds), 7th edn, pp. 877–938. Elsevier Saunders, New York, NY.

Cullen, J.M. (2007). Liver, biliary system, and exocrine pancreas. In *Pathologic Basis of Veterinary Disease* (McGavin, M., and Zachary, J.F. eds), 4th edn, pp. 393–461. Mosby Elsevier, St. Louis, MO.

Cullen, J.M., and Miller, R.T. (2006). The role of pathology in the identification of drug-induced hepatic toxicity. *Expert Opin. Drug Metab. Toxicol.*, 2, 241–247.

Dambach, D.M., Andrews, B.A., and Moulin, F. (2005). New technologies and screening strategies for hepatotoxicity: Use of *in vitro* models. *Toxicol. Pathol.*, 33, 17–26.

Deleve, L.D., and Kaplowitz, N. (2007). *Drug-Induced Liver Disease*, 2nd edn. USC Medical Center, Los Angeles, CA.

Eustis, S.L., Boorman, G.A., Harada, T., and Popp, J.A. (1990). Liver. In *Pathology of the Fischer Rat* (Boorman, G.A., Eustis, S.L., Elwell, M.R., Montgomery, C.A. Jr., and MacKenzie, W.F. eds), pp. 71–94. Academic Press, San Diego, CA.

Foster, J.R. (2005). Spontaneous and drug-induced hepatic pathology of the laboratory beagle dog, the cynomolgus macaque and the marmoset. *Toxicol. Pathol.*, 33, 63–74.

Gunawan, B.K., and Kaplowitz, N. (2007). Mechanisms of drug-induced liver disease. *Clin. Liver Dis.*, 11, 459–475.

Harada, T., Enomoto, A., Boorman, G.A., and Maronpot, R.R. (1999). Liver and gallbladder. In *Pathology of the Mouse* (Maronpot, R.R. ed.), pp. 119–183. Cache River Press, St Louis, MO.

Hardisty, J.F., and Brix, A.E. (2005). Comparative hepatic toxicity: prechronic/chronic liver toxicity in rodents. *Toxicol. Pathol.*, 33, 35–40.

Hussaini, S.H., and Farrington, E.A. (2007). Idiosyncratic drug-induced liver injury: an overview. *Expert Opin. Drug Saf.*, 6, 673–684.

Jaeschke, H. (2008). Toxic responses of the liver. In *Casarett and Doull's Toxicology. The Basic Science of Poisons* (Klaasen, C.D. ed.), 7th edn, pp. 557–582. McGraw-Hill, New York, NY.

Lee, W. (2003). Drug-induced hepatotoxicity. *N. Engl. J. Med.*, 349, 474–485.

Lee, W.M. (2008). Etiologies of acute liver failure. *Semin. Liver Dis.*, 28, 142–152.

Lee, W.M., and Senior, J.R. (2005). Recognizing drug-induced liver injury: current problems, possible solutions. *Toxicol. Pathol.*, 33, 155–164.

Parker, G.A., and Picut, C.A. (2005). Liver immunobiology. *Toxicol. Pathol.*, 33, 52–62.

Peters, T.S. (2005). Do preclinical testing strategies help predict human hepatotoxic potentials? *Toxicol. Pathol.*, 33, 146–154.

Ramachandran, R., and Kakar, S. (2009). Histological patterns in drug-induced liver disease. *J. Clin. Pathol.*, 62, 481–492.

Schiff, E.R., and Sorrell, M.F. (eds) (2007). *Schiff's Disease of the Liver.* Lippincott Williams & Wilkins, Philadelphia, PA.

Solter, P.F. (2005). Clinical pathology approaches to hepatic injury. *Toxicol. Pathol.*, 33, 9–16.

Stalker, M.J., and Hayes, M.A. (2007). Liver and biliary system. In *Jubb, Kennedy, and Palmer's Pathology of Domestic Animals* (Maxie, M.R. ed.), 5th edn, pp. 297–388. Elsevier, New York, NY.

Watkins, P.B. (2005). Idiosyncratic liver injury: Challenges and approaches. *Toxicol. Pathol.*, 33, 1–5.

Pancreas

SECTION I EXOCRINE PANCREAS

INTRODUCTION

The pancreas is usually a "silent" internal organ that is not often directly involved in the absorption of ingested xenobiotics, or involved directly in their detoxification. The recognized frequency of xenobiotic toxicity for the pancreas is low, but when toxicity occurs there can be a major impact on health. Even though direct xenobiotic toxicity of the pancreas is infrequently reported, a large number of acute and chronic pancreatitis cases are of unknown etiology and often linked indirectly to toxin exposure, in particular in economically underdeveloped areas of the

237

world, where exposure to environmental pollutants and contaminants is high.

The pancreas constitutes about 0.1% of adult body weight in humans, and is of similar relative size in many domestic animals. Both the exocrine and endocrine portions are highly specialized to synthesize and secrete a wide variety of specific proteins. More than 80% of the gland consists of exocrine pancreatic acinar cells. These cells secrete digestive enzymes into the intestine through the pancreatic duct system, a system which composes 2–4% of the mass of the pancreas.

NORMAL STRUCTURE OF EXOCRINE PANCREAS

Gross Anatomy

The normal pancreas is pale relative to the liver and spleen, and less translucent than retroperitoneal and mesenteric fat. Lobules of acinar tissue and major ducts are grossly visible, but islets and intralobular ducts cannot be perceived grossly.

The pancreas extends from the duodenum to the hilum of the spleen. Its configuration varies with species and, to a lesser extent, within individuals of a species. The organ is compact and elongate in the dog and human, triangular to quadrilateral and exceedingly compact in ruminants and horses, whereas it is less compact in several rodent species. In the rat and mouse, for example, the tail (splenic portion) is relatively compact, whereas the head is dispersed within the mesentery of the duodenal loop. The central portion of the gland, between head and tail, is designated as the body. These general topographical regions (head, body, tail) are useful for descriptive reference; however, the body and tail are not divided by distinct anatomical landmarks. In the human, the pancreas is narrow along the axis of the superior mesenteric vessels. This segment is designated as the neck, and marks the boundary between the body and head; these vessels also provide a landmark in the rodent. The rodent pancreas also includes a gastric lobe which has no counterpart in other larger species. Five lobes have been described in the hamster pancreas. In ruminants and horses the pancreas is quite compact, and dorsally located just beneath the caudal thoracic or cranial lumbar vertebrae and cranial to the right kidney. In dogs, cats, and pigs, pancreatic anatomy is similar to that of humans. The pancreatic duct system extends from its entry into the duodenum to all portions of the pancreatic lobules. Successively smaller branches of the pancreatic duct end as ductules connected to acinar tubules. The main pancreatic duct (duct of Wirsung) is

easily identified in most species. In humans, an accessory duct, named for Santorini, may open separately into the duodenum. By contrast, multiple small ducts enter the rodent duodenum directly from adjacent pancreatic tissue, thereby bypassing the main duct. Whatever the species, pancreatic ducts are classified according to size and location as main duct, interlobular ducts, and intralobular ductules.

Microscopic Anatomy and Ultrastructure

The exocrine pancreas is composed of two basic parenchymal cell types: acinar cells and ductal cells. Cells of the terminal ductules which contact or are interspersed among acinar cells are commonly designated as centroacinar cells. In Figure 10.1, a section of normal rat pancreas, the typical morphology and arrangement of acinar cells, ducts and pancreatic islets is illustrated.

Acinar cells are pyramid-shaped cells arranged to form a convoluted, often interconnecting, tubuloacinar network within the lobules. The tubules and acini are surrounded by a basement membrane (basal lamina), and have a small central lumen. Acinar cells make and secrete digestive enzymes. Histologically, this function is reflected by the presence of basophilic staining in the paranuclear basal portion of the cell, which corresponds ultrastructurally to stack-like accumulations of rough endoplasmic reticulum (RER). The apical granular eosinophilia (near the acinar lumen) reflects the presence of zymogen granules, the secretory granules which actually contain the digestive enzymes. In adult rats, 60% or more of acinar cells have two nuclei.

Ultrastructural characteristics of acinar cells (Figure 10.2) reflect the histologic features just described (abundant RER and zymogen granules). In addition, junctional complexes between the lateral cell membranes

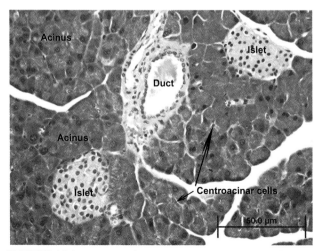

FIGURE 10.1   Pancreas from a rat showing zymogen-rich acinar cells, centroacinar cells, ducts and islets.

of adjacent cells, elongate mitochondria, and well-developed Golgi complexes at the interface between the RER and zymogen granules can be visualized using electron microscopy. The intercellular occluding junctions are in the apical region near the acinar lumen; the lumenal cell membrane forms microvilli. Some of the cells give rise to kinocilia. Gap junctions between adjacent acinar cells are an important feature, allowing for rapid communication of biochemical signals.

Ductal cells, smaller than acinar cells, have a single nucleus. Normal main and interlobular ducts are lined by a single layer of cuboidal or low columnar cells. The main pancreatic duct has a thick collagenous layer, two to three times the thickness of the epithelium. This layer is penetrated by numerous small ductular branches. Interlobular ducts have a collagenous layer, approximately as thick as the epithelial cell layer. In the smallest branches of the duct system, the intralobular ductules have cells that are cuboidal or slightly flattened, and are surrounded by a basement membrane of extracellular matrix; they lack a fibrous wall. Histologically, the cytoplasm of ductal cells is pale and eosinophilic. Ultrastructurally, the cytoplasm contains relatively small amounts of RER, smooth endoplasmic reticulum (SER), and prominent mitochondria. Mucoprotein secretory granules may be present. Lateral cell membranes are linked by occluding junctions, and the lumenal surface forms microvilli. The basal cell membrane abuts the basal laminae.

The delicate fibrous stroma which surrounds acinar cells and ductules also supports vessels and nerves. Blood supply to each lobule is via an interlobular artery which enters the lobule to produce separate capillary beds for acini, ductules, and islets. Capillaries from at least some of the islets form a portal system that empties into the periacinar capillaries. Small sympathetic ganglia are present within the pancreas. Fat cells are normally interspersed within pancreatic lobules, and increase in number with age or obesity.

Acinar and ductal cells can divide in experimental animals, so regeneration of the exocrine pancreas can occur following toxic injury. When the injury is mild or moderate, the pancreas may be restored to normal size and structure; however, when injury is more severe, regeneration may be incomplete, with replacement of a portion of the lobular tissue by fat, or more commonly by fibrous scar tissue that can progressively constrict and "squeeze out" remaining functional parenchyma (Figure 10.3).

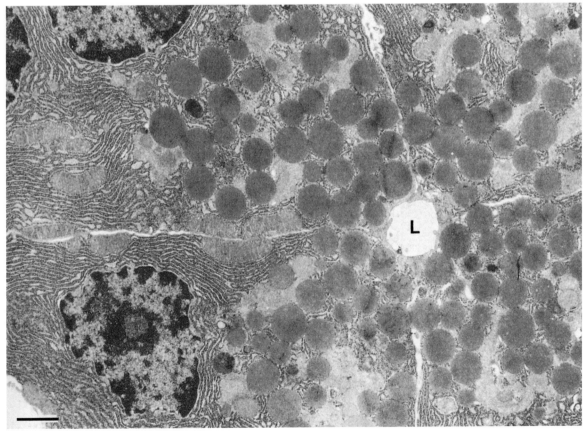

FIGURE 10.2 Normal acinar cells from a control animal (rat). Nuclei, rough endoplasmic reticulum, and mitochondria occupy the basilar portion of the cells, left, while zymogen granules surround an acinar lumen (L), right of center. Electron micrograph. Bar = 1 μm.

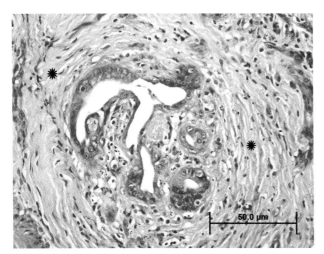

FIGURE 10.3   Fibrotic pancreas from a dog with severe chronic pancreatitis. Note the concentric layers of dense collagenous scar tissue (*) trapping residually inflamed ductules and acini.

The ability of pancreatic cells to divide implies that hyperplasia can be induced by appropriate stimuli. Peptide hormones which stimulate pancreatic secretion (see below) also serve as growth factors for the pancreas. In excessive concentrations, they have caused pancreatic hypertrophy and hyperplasia.

PHYSIOLOGY OF EXOCRINE PANCREAS

Acinar cells secrete zymogen by exocytosis of zymogen granules into the acinar lumen. They do this in response to cholinergic vagal nerve stimulation, or to specific circulating peptide hormones for which the cells have receptors. Cholecystokinin (CCK) and bombesin are two peptides that stimulate pancreatic secretion. CCK is the major humoral mediator of enzyme secretion, and is secreted by the proximal small intestine and controlled by a negative feedback loop. An increase in the level of trypsin activity in the intestinal lumen results in decreased secretion. A peptide (monitor peptide) is secreted in the pancreatic juice as a stimulus for CCK secretion by the intestinal mucosa (Figure 10.4A). When there is no competing substrate, or there is no trypsin inhibitor in the intestinal lumen, the monitor peptide is destroyed, and CCK secretion decreases. Excess CCK secretion can be induced by the presence of trypsin inhibitors in the diet, such as those in raw soy meal. Feeding of such diets has been associated with hyperplasia of the pancreas in some species, such as the rat (Figure 10.4B).

Several of the exocrine digestive enzymes are synthesized as inactive proenzymes, which are activated

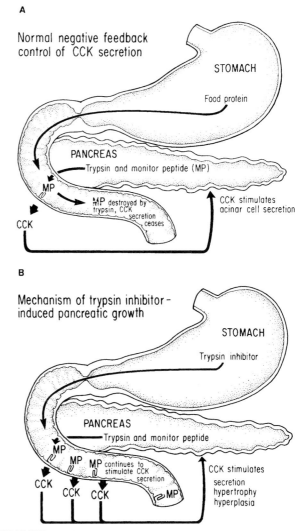

FIGURE 10.4   Diagram of the monitor peptide (MP) mechanism for feedback regulation of cholecystokinin (CCK) secretion by the small intestine. (A) MP stimulates CCK secretion during the digestive phase after a meal, but is destroyed by trypsin and chymotrypsin in the postdigestive phase when these enzymes are no longer occupied by food proteins. Pancreatic secretion is also stimulated by cholinergic vagal nerves following a meal. (B) Destruction of MP is prevented by a trypsin inhibitor, prolonging CCK secretion and leading to pancreatic growth. (Illustration by Joan Thomson.)

by cleavage in the intestinal lumen. Trypsin is normally activated by enterokinase, a protease secreted by the intestinal mucosa, but it can also be activated by active trypsin or certain lysosomal enzymes. Trypsin activates the other proenzymes secreted by the pancreas.

Duct cells secrete water and bicarbonate, which buffer the pancreatic juice at about pH 8.3, which favors stability of the proenzymes. Duct secretion is stimulated by the vagal nerves and by secretin, which reaches the cells through the circulation. Ductal secretion is required to carry enzyme proteins into the duodenum.

Pancreatic enzymes are required for normal digestion and absorption of food in the gastrointestinal tract, especially for the hydrolysis of lipids. The exocrine pancreas appears to possess great functional reserves. In humans with chronic pancreatitis, it appears that atrophy and scarring must progress to the point that enzyme secretion is reduced below 10% of normal levels before malabsorption occurs, causing fat and nitrogenous compounds to increase in the feces.

COMPARATIVE MECHANISMS OF EXOCRINE PANCREATIC TOXICITY

For the most part, xenobiotics reach the pancreas through the bloodstream after absorption and systemic distribution. Thus, exposure may occur by several routes, such as skin contact, inhalation, injection, or ingestion. Exposure *per os* poses an additional threat to the pancreas, since ingested xenobiotics in the duodenum may reflux into the pancreatic duct and reach the ductal cells. Such reflux has been documented in experimental animals when duodenal lumenal pressure is increased, but this is not regarded as a regular or predictable occurrence unless an additional predisposing factor is present.

The pancreas contains both phase I and phase II drug-metabolizing enzymes, although the levels of cytochrome P450-related enzymes is perhaps 1% of that in hepatocytes. Most P450 enzyme activity appears to be localized in the acinar cell, making that cell more prone to bioactivation of xenobiotics, and hence more likely to be injured by reactive intermediates. Induction of such enzymes by xenobiotics, for example, β-naphthaflavone, has been demonstrated. Both acinar and ductal cells contain phase II enzymes, such as the glutathione S-transferases, and abundant antioxidant enzymes, such as the quinone reductases. The activation of indirectly-acting toxicants and procarcinogens by the pancreas has been documented. For example the β-oxidized di-*n*-propylnitrosamines are activated to form mutagens by pancreatic microsomal cell fractions. There are significant species differences in the effect of xenobiotics, notably the response to pancreatic carcinogens.

A frequently studied rat (and canine) model of pancreatitis is based on hyperstimulation of the pancreas by caerulein, a CCK analog with high affinity for CCK receptors. Hyperstimulation causes loss of secretory polarity, and subsequent sequestration of zymogens in lysosomes, or alternatively release of zymogens across the basolateral portions of the acinar cell into the interstitial space. Lysosomal enzymes activate the zymogens. This mechanism of hypersecretion is hypothesized to be key in the pathogenesis of pancreatitis in this model. These, and additional studies with xenobiotics such as cyclosporin A, ethanol, and organophosphates (e.g., diazinon in dogs and cats) suggest that CCK-induced hypersecretion has a significant role in the often multifactorial etiology of pancreatitis. Typically, another inciting agent that is cytotoxic for acinar cells, combined with hypersecretion, is needed to induce pancreatitis experimentally.

Persistent stimulation by caerulein has also been used to develop a model of chronic pancreatitis, a severe problem in humans. Persistent stimulation of the pancreas by CCK (or its analogs) also induces hyperplasia, which can promote carcinogenesis. Therefore, chronic pancreatitis enhances the risk of carcinogenesis in the injured organ.

The role of free radical damage in the pathogenesis, or at least the progression, of pancreatitis is becoming apparent in experimental and clinical studies. There is a great deal of flux between oxidized and reduced glutathione during the synthesis of zymogens, and particularly during the process of excitation–secretion, putting the pancreas at risk of oxidant stress, especially during its secretory phase. Furthermore, the presence of inducible P450 enzymes in acinar cells increases the possibility that reactive intermediates, or even free radicals, may be generated on exposure to the appropriate xenobiotics. The use of antioxidants of various types (e.g., N-acetylcysteine, Vitamin E) to dampen the severity or diminish the progression of pancreatitis clinically and experimentally is evidence that oxidant stress also has a key role in the pathogenesis of pancreatitis.

Numerous chemical agents are known or suspected to induce acinar cell damage or necrosis, to alter acinar cell or duct cell function, or to induce neoplastic change in the pancreas. Although there is a wealth of anecdotal and clinical evidence linking numerous xenobiotics to pancreatic injury in humans, experimentally these linkages have been difficult to prove. Ethanol, the toxicant most commonly associated with pancreatitis in humans, appears to have a direct cytotoxic effect on the pancreas, and to alter pancreatic acinar cell function in a way that promotes protein precipitation in the duct system. Impairment of ductal outflow is a major predisposing factor for pancreatitis, both in humans and experimentally in rodent models. Excessive intake of alcoholic beverages is regarded as a major cause of both acute and chronic pancreatitis in humans, although it is not generally a problem in domestic animal species.

TABLE 10.1 Agents and drugs reported to cause pancreatitis in humans

Association with Pancreatitis	Agent
Strong causative association with pancreatitis	Alcohol (ethanol)
	Azathioprine
	l-Asparaginase
	Corticosteroids
	Cytarabine
	Didanosine
	Estrogens
	Furosemide
	Mercaptopurine
	Mesalamine
	Opiates
	Pentamidine
	Pentavalent antimonials
	Sulfasalazine
	Sulindac
	Trimethoprim-associated sulfonamides
	Valproic acid
Probable causative association with pancreatitis	Acetaminophen
	Carbamazeprine
	Cisplatin
	Cyclopenthiazide
	Enalapril
	Erythromycin
	Hydrochlorothiazide
	Interferon α-2β
	Lamuvidine
	Methyldopa
	Octreotide
	Phenformin
	Procainamide
	Rifampin
Other agents associated with pancreatitis	Clozapine
	Cyclosporine
	2′,3′-Dideoxyinosine
	Lisinopril
	Metronidazole
	Salicylates
	Zalcitabine

TABLE 10.2 Selected agents reported to cause toxic effects in exocrine pancreas experimentally in rodents

Agent	Species
2-Acetaminofluorene and 4-acetaminofluorene	Rat
Aflatoxin	Rat
β-3-thienyl-dl-alanine	Rat
Arginine	Rat
Azaserine	Rat
Carbon Tetrachloride	Rat
Chloraquine	Rat
Crambene	Rat
Dibutyl tin	Rat
Diethanolamine	Rat
Ethanol	Rat
5-Fluorouracil	Rat
Lysine	Rat
Manganese	Rat
N-nitrosomethyl(2-oxopropyl)amine	Rat
Puromycin	Rat
Triparanol	Rat
Actinomycin D	Mouse
Chlorothiazide	Mouse
Neutral red	Mouse
Vinblastine	Mouse
Cobalt chloride	Guinea pig
Diazinon	Guinea pig
N-nitrososbis(2-oxopropyl)amine	Hamster
Cortisone	Rabbit
Ethionine	Rat, mouse, guinea pig, hamster
4-Hydroxyaminoquinoline-1-oxide	Guinea pig, rat
Methionine	Hamster, rat
N_6-(N-methyl-N-nitrosocarbamoyl)-L-ornithine	Rat, hamster
N-nitroso(2-hydoxypropyl)(2-oxypropyl)amine	Hamster, rat

Medical literature also contains numerous reports of acute pancreatitis in association with specific therapeutic products (Table 10.1). The risk of pancreatitis, although low, seems well-established for some of these agents, for example, asparaginase and azathioprine, but for others only rare sporadic cases have been reported. For the latter agents, the proof that the agent was the cause of pancreatitis is often weak and circumstantial. This list continues to expand.

Experimentally, rodents are susceptible to pancreatic damage by an overlapping, but somewhat different, spectrum of xenobiotics (Table 10.2). By contrast, however, relatively few xenobiotics are clearly linked to pancreatic injury in common domestic animals (Table 10.3), even though there are sporadic anecdotal reports in the veterinary literature.

TABLE 10.3 Selected agents associated with exocrine pancreatic toxicity in common domestic animals[a]

Agent	Species
Chocolate[b]	Dog
Corticosteroids	Dog
Deoxyvalinol (DON)	Pig
Dichloroacetate	Dog
Ethanol	Dog
dl-Ethionine	Dog
Fumonisin B_1	Pig
Organophosphates (especially diazinon)	Dog
T-2 toxin (vomitoxin)	Pig
Trimethoprim-enhanced sulfonamides	Dog
Zinc	Dog, cow, sheep, pig, chicken

[a] Experimental and "naturally-occurring" reports, idiosyncratic occurrences not listed
[b] Associated with the high fat content of chocolate rather than toxicosis

RESPONSE OF EXOCRINE PANCREAS TO INJURY

Most xenobiotics effect pancreatic injury by appearing to damage the acinar cell in some manner. Although the exact mechanism of damage in most cases is not known or only poorly understood, the acinar cells undergo a variety of changes. In the few cases where ducts may be affected initially, evidence suggests that alterations in duct function ultimately affect acinar cell function, resulting in initiation of pancreatitis. Table 10.4 summarizes the basic alterations that result from pancreatic injury.

Cytotoxic Effects on Acinar Cells

Sublethal Injury

Acinar cells undergo swelling or accumulate fat in the cytoplasm, as a result of toxic injury. They also frequently degranulate prior to swelling or vacuolation, particularly if hypersecretion is part of the pathogenesis of the injury. At the ultrastructural level, cell swelling is accompanied by vesiculation of the rough endoplasmic reticulum and dilatation of ER cisternae, giving the acinar cell a pale, "feathery" appearance histologically. Dense inclusions in the endoplasmic reticulum (intracisternal granules) have been noted in rats following exposure to puromycin (Figure 10.5)

and 1-cyano-2-hydroxy-3-butene (crambene), agents which also induce acinar cell death.

One hallmark of sublethal injury to acinar cells is the presence of autophagic vacuoles (AV). These are best appreciated at the ultrastructural level (Figure 10.5), but can be identified in histologic sections when they are large (Figure 10.6A). In electron micrographs, autophagy manifests as segregation of cytoplasmic organelles within a membrane probably derived from the endoplasmic reticulum. Mitochondria, zymogen granules, and even nuclei may be recognizable in the vacuoles. Degradation of the contents of an AV ensues promptly after its formation, so that only lipid, membranous or granular debris may remain. In histologic sections, AVs appear as dense acidophilic or basophilic cytoplasmic inclusions.

Cell Death

Apoptosis

Apoptosis may be identified as dense cell-sized bodies, almost always surrounded by a clear, well-defined halo. The cells frequently contain round, membrane-bound nuclear fragments, with extremely condensed chromatin clumped into a "cap" or "crescent" at one pole of the nuclear fragment. An entire acinus is seldom affected; rather, only one or two cells show the apoptotic morphology at any one point in time, and the number of apoptotic cells will vary widely from lobule to lobule. Fragments of apoptotic acinar cells may be engulfed by resident tissue macrophages, or by adjacent parenchymal cells. This process does not elicit an acute inflammatory response, although macrophages engorged with newly-formed apoptotic cells or digested apoptotic bodies (residual bodies) become more obvious as apoptosis progresses and the acinar cell population diminishes. When there is diffuse mild injury, the presence of scattered apoptotic cells, expanded interstitial space (in part due to loss of acinar cells), and more prominent tissue macrophages may be the primary histologic evidence of injury (Figure 10.6B). Loss of characteristic morphologic features of remaining acinar cells may occur if cell loss is severe, as the remaining ductal cells condense and attempt to regenerate the lost parenchyma. Even with large-scale apoptosis, inflammation and fibrosis are minimal, although numerical atrophy may be quite marked. Complete recovery and regeneration generally occur after a bout of apoptosis, provided the inciting stimulus is removed.

There is accumulating experimental evidence that apoptosis is a frequent occurrence in the exocrine pancreas, especially in cases of mild or persistent low-grade injury. In pigs, for example, the mycotoxins

TABLE 10.4   Classification of pancreatic alterations with selected examples

Alteration	Xenobiotic
Exocrine	
• Vacuolation and autophagy (degeneration)	Crambene, ethanol, fumonisin B$_1$, organophosphates, puromycin, T-2 toxin
• Acinar cell apoptosis	Arginine, crambene, organophosphates, T-2 toxin
• Acinar cell necrosis followed by inflammation	Actinomycin D, arginine, azaserine, crambene, ethioinine, 4-hydroxyaminoquinoline-1-oxide (4-HAQO), lysine, organophosphates, puromycin, zinc
• Acute inflammation with variable acinar cell necrosis	alcohol, azathioprine, l-asparaginase, chlorthalidone, chlorothiazide, furosemide, 6-mercaptopurine, methyldopa, oral contraceptives, pentamidine, riftampicin, sulindac, tetracycline, thiazide diuretics, valproic acid
• Chronic interstitial inflammation	Alcohol
• Duct cell degeneration/necrosis	Dibutyl tin, Zinc
• Neoplasia (experimental animals) well-characterized	Azaserine, 7,12-dimethylbenz[α]anthracene, 4-hydroxyaminoquinoline-1-oxide (rat); N-nitroso (2-hydroxypropyl) (2-oxypropyl) amine, N-nitrosobis (2-hydroxypropyl) amine (rat and hamster); N-nitrosobis (2-oxypropyl) amine (hamster)
• Weak or sporadic association	Aflatoxin B1 (monkey); colfibrate, nafenopin, nitrofen, N-nitrosodimethylamine (rat); N$_δ$-(N-methyl-N-nitrosocarbamoyl)-L-ornithine (rat, hamster); N-nitroso-2,6-dimethylmorpholine, N-nitrosomethyl (2-oxopropyl) amine (hamster); N-methyl-N-nitrosourea (guinea pig, mouse), N-ethyl-N'-nitro-N-nitrosoguanidine (dog)
Endocrine	
• Increased secretory granules	Benzothiodiazines (chlorothiazide, diazoxide, furosemide, trichlorothiazide, and hydrochlorothiazide)
• Degeneration, vacuolation and degranulation in β-cells	Cyclosporin, cyproheptadine
• Apoptosis	Streptozotocin
• Necrosis	Alloxan, α-amanitin, streptozotocin
• Insulitis (inflammation of islets)	Streptozotocin
• Neoplasia	Alloxan and streptozotocin (rat), azinophosmethyl, 6-diethylaminomethyl-4-hydroxyaminoquinoline-1-oxide, heliotrine

fumonisin B1 and T-2 toxin (vomitoxin) frequently induce vacuolation and "single cell necrosis," consistent with what is now interpreted to be apoptosis in acinar cells (Figure 10.7), resulting in degeneration of the pancreas without substantial inflammation. Apoptosis may actually be the "preferred" response to injury, since inflammation is generally minimal and cells are eliminated before they can burst and release their intensely pro-inflammatory contents, which are highly attractive to neutrophils. Acinar cells express high levels of the pro-apoptotic protein, Bax, in their mitochondria, but express very little bcl-2, the prime anti-apoptotic protein. Acinar cells also express death receptors for apoptosis, including the TNFα receptor, and CD95. The milder form of acute pancreatitis, known as "edematous pancreatitis," appears to have an apoptotic component as well, especially at the milder end of the spectrum. This is speculated to be the reason for its typically self-limiting nature. Experimentally, mild pancreatitis is typically associated with acinar cell apoptosis, while severe pancreatitis is associated with a large degree of necrosis and relatively little apoptosis. It should be noted, however, that there is evidence for species differences in response to an insult to acinar cells. In rats, for example, caspases, the effector enzymes of the apoptotic process, are rapidly activated during acinar cell injury, whereas in the mouse caspases typically are not activated as readily, and necrosis occurs preferentially after injury.

Necrosis

When necrosis of acinar cells occurs, groups of lethally injured acinar cells—usually entire acini or even groups of acini—are only briefly identifiable. The dead cells quickly pass through the stage of coagulation necrosis to liquefaction, because of the high content of hydrolytic enzymes. The release of lipase and phospholipase into the interstitium results in destruction of adjacent fat cells; fat necrosis commonly accompanies the liquefactive necrosis of acinar tissue. Release of enzymes and necrotic debris incites

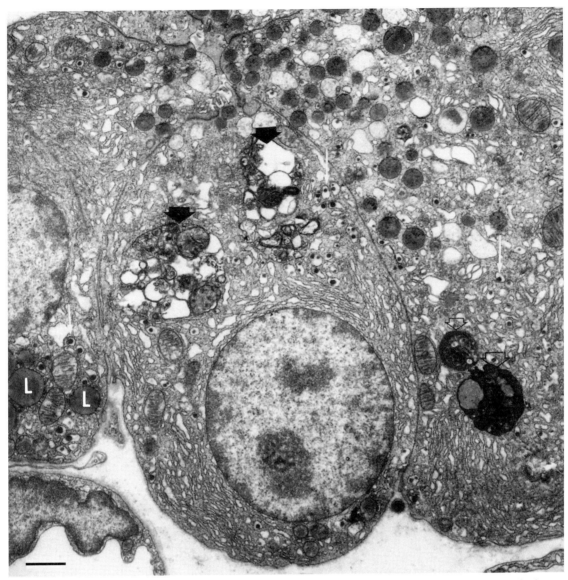

FIGURE 10.5   Acinar cells from a puromycin-treated rat. Intracisternal granules are present in vesiculated rough endoplasmic reticulum (small arrows). Autophagic vacuoles (wide arrows) are present in the cytoplasm. Lipid vacuoles (L) are present in the cytoplasm of one cell, lower left. Electron micrograph. Bar = 1 μm.

acute inflammation, and the classic histologic picture of acute necrotizing pancreatitis (Figure 10.8). At this stage of injury, significant degrees of necrosis are detectable by biochemical evaluation of serum for pancreatic exocrine enzymes such as amylase or lipase. Necrosis of acinar tissue is usually explosive, and is best recognized 12–48 hours after the initial toxic injury. Gross changes at this time include edema and marked congestion, especially around the margins of the lobules. This is typically followed by an intense neutrophil response, and often necrosis of surrounding mesenteric fat. At later times, the pancreas may appear atrophic or fibrotic, and chronic inflammation may be seen histologically if the injury is persistent

or very severe (Figure 10.3). During regeneration, the pancreas shows an increased rate of mitosis in both acinar and ductal cells. In the early stages of the regenerative phase after severe injury, newly-regenerated acinar cells arise from surviving ductal cells, and then produce additional acinar cells as regeneration progresses. The regenerated acinar cells generally do not produce zymogen granules until regeneration is complete. Thus, during the healing phase regenerating acinar cells are not functional as digestive cells.

Some xenobiotic-induced pancreatic necroses mimic the most severe forms of acute hemorrhagic pancreatitis, for example, after ethionine administration in female mice fed a choline-deficient diet. Intermediate

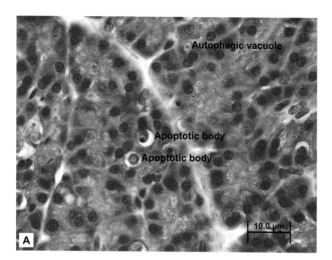

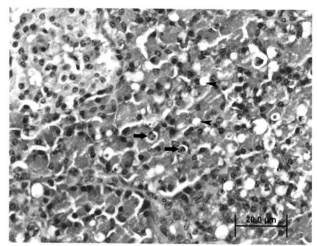

FIGURE 10.7   Acinar cell apoptosis (arrows) and vacuolation (arrowheads) in a porcine pancreas after exposure to T-2 toxin.

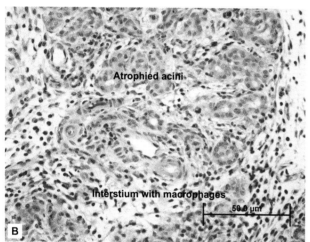

FIGURE 10.6   (A) Pancreas from a rat treated with crambene, showing autophagic vacuoles and apoptotic bodies. (B) Pancreas from a rat after repeated crambene exposure, with persistent acinar cell apoptosis leading to atrophy, increased interstitial space and prominence of tissue macrophages.

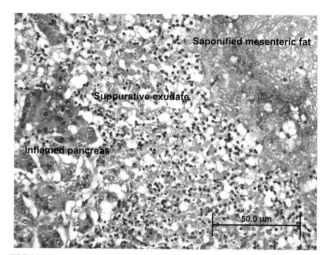

FIGURE 10.8   Acute necrotizing pancreatitis in a dog, with an intense suppurative exudate and necrosis of mesenteric fat with saponification.

degrees of pancreatic necrosis simulating nonfatal degrees of pancreatitis have been induced by puromycin, azaserine, and hydroxyaminoquinoline 1-oxide in rodents, organophosphates in dogs and cats, or zinc in sheep. Lower doses of these and other agents, or treatment with less cytotoxic agents, may induce milder degrees of damage, typified by apoptosis or a mixture of apoptosis and necrosis typical of edematous pancreatitis or human interstitial pancreatitis. Amino acid analogs, and even certain amino acids themselves (e.g., lysine and arginine), have a specific propensity to affect the acinar cells experimentally in rodents, probably because of the cells' high affinity for uptake of α-amino acids. The pancreas has been shown to concentrate both normal and several amino acid derivatives to a greater degree than most other tissues.

Absorbed products of tissue breakdown in acute pancreatitis appear to have a variety of effects systemically, such as pulmonary and renal dysfunction. Depression of cellular respiration has been described in such cases, and may contribute to the development of shock.

Mutation

Nonlethal mutations appear to occur in acinar and ductal cells exposed to mutagens or carcinogens. The induction of DNA damage in both acinar and ductal cells by carcinogens has been documented in hamsters and rats. Focal phenotypic changes appear to be clonal, and are the basis of short-term assays for pancreatic carcinogens. At present, it is not possible to determine which focal lesion has the potential to progress to a neoplasm except by observation in long-term studies, since it has been estimated that less than 1% of such foci actually complete the progression to neoplasia.

Metaplasia

Acinar cells may show reduced zymogen and RER content, and take on a ductal appearance in areas of chronic pancreatitis. This has been referred to as ductular metaplasia.

Cytotoxic Effects in Ductal and Centroacinar Cells

Changes in ductal and centroacinar cells are less distinct than those described in acinar cells. These cells may show swelling, hypertrophy, or undergo necrosis. Ductal changes often appear to be secondary to inflammation or necrosis in adjacent acinar tissue. Their lumens may contain eosinophilic condensates of the proteinaceous pancreatic secretions, and squamous or mucous cell metaplasia of ductal epithelium has been described. Hyperplastic and dysplastic changes have been described in carcinogen-treated rodents, as has transdifferentiation of ductal cells (or differentiation of stem cells) to form hepatocytes in response to toxic injury in the pancreas of hamsters and rats. This is a focal phenomenon, perhaps clonal, which does not clearly result from mutation, since it can be induced in rats by a period of copper deficiency to induce extreme atrophy followed by recovery that allows for regeneration. It should be noted that any damage to duct cells which results in impairment of outflow to produce actual or relative obstruction to outflow can trigger acinar cell injury and acute pancreatitis. Therefore, xenobiotics which may not be inherently toxic to ductal, centroacinar, or acinar cells, but which impair outflow, for example, by altering the viscosity of secretion, can trigger pancreatitis, especially if additional predisposing factors are present. Zinc pancreatotoxicity in sheep has been postulated to induce pancreatitis in this way.

Carcinogenesis

Chemical carcinogens of diverse structure have been shown to affect the pancreas (Table 10.5), although it should be noted that nitrosamines dominate the list. Several long-term models for chemical induction of carcinomas in the pancreas of experimental animals have been developed. Two of these have been extensively characterized and studied: (1) azaserine used as a pancreatic carcinogen in rats; and (2) N-nitrosobis (2-oxopropyl)amine (BOP) used in the Syrian golden hamster. Several carcinogens induce microscopically-detectable focal hyperplasia and dysplasia of acinar cells in the exocrine pancreas of rats (Figure 10.9). Some of these lesions grow to become grossly visible nodules 1mm or larger in diameter. These foci and

TABLE 10.5 Summary of chemicals that cause carcinoma in the pancreas of experimental animals[a]

Agent	Species
Group A (well-characterized model carcinogens)	
Azaserine	Rat
7, 12-Dimethylbenz[a]anthracene	Rat
4-Hydroxyaminoquinoline-1-oxide	Rat
N-Nitroso(2-hydroxopropyl)(2-oxopropyl)amine	Hamster, rat
N-Nitrosobis(2-oxopropyl)amine	Hamster
N-Nitrosobis(2-hydroxypropyl)amine	Hamster, rat
Group B (reported as carcinogens once or in a limited number of papers)	
Aflatoxin B1	Monkey
Clofibrate	Rat
Nd-(N-methyl-N-nitrosocarbamoyl)-L-ornithine	Rat, hamster
N-Methyl-N-nitrosourea	Guinea pig, mouse
Nafenopin	Rat
Nitrofen	Rat
N-Ethyl-N'-nitro-N-nitrosoguanidine	Dog
N-Nitrosodimethylamine	Rat
N-Nitroso-2,6-dimethylmorpholine	Hamster
N-Nitrosomethyl(2-oxopropyl)amine	Hamster
Group C (reported to cause islet cell tumors)	
Alloxan	Rat
Azinophosmethyl	Rat
6-Diethylaminomethyl-4-hydroxyaminoquinoline-1-oxide	Rat
Heliotrine	Rat
Streptozotocin (plus nicotinamide)	Rat

[a]Groups A and B list carcinogens for the exocrine pancreas

nodules have collectively been termed atypical acinar cell nodules (AACN); however, some observers prefer other designations, such as focal cellular change, and focal hyperplasia. Aged dogs and cats not infrequently develop hyperplastic nodules within the exocrine pancreas composed entirely of acinar cells, which are often somewhat larger and more intensely staining than surrounding normal acinar cells (Figure 10.10). The nodules are irregularly distributed, and seldom if ever develop into true neoplasms. The pathophysiologic significance appears negligible, and a connection to toxin exposure has not been established.

Benign pancreatic tumors in domestic animals are rare, although pancreatic adenocarcinomas in dogs and cats do occur. These tumors can be acinar, ductular, or a combination of morphologies, many also elicit a dense fibrotic (scirrhous) stromal response. Morphology does not necessarily correlate with aggressiveness, and a link to toxin exposure has not been made.

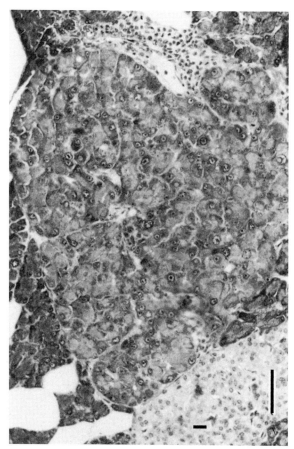

FIGURE 10.9   Focus of atypical acinar cells (center) from the pancreas of a rat treated with azaserine. The acinar cells of the focus are paler, and most have larger nuclei than the surrounding normal acinar cells. An islet (I) borders the focus at the lower right. Hematoxylin and eosin stain. Bar = 100 μm.

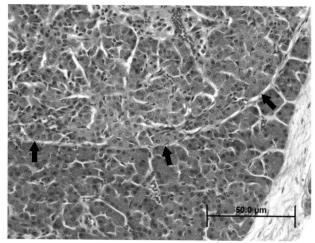

FIGURE 10.10   Nodular acinar cell hyperplasia in a dog. The arrows define the border between the paler hyperplastic cells and normal pancreas.

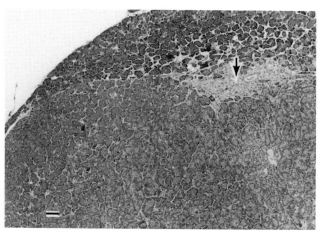

FIGURE 10.11   Acinar cell adenoma in the pancreas of an aza-serine-treated rat. The cells of the adenoma (lower two-thirds of the field) stain more lightly than the normal acinar cells. A small islet is compressed at the junction of the adenoma and normal pancreas (arrow). Hematoxylin and eosin stain. Bar = 100 μm.

Rats and mice characteristically develop acinar cell neoplasms that exhibit several histologic variants, while hamsters characteristically develop neoplasms with a ductal phenotype, also containing several sub-types. In addition, aged rats spontaneously develop a low incidence of well-differentiated, apparently benign, acinar cell neoplasms (adenomas). The incidence and number of acinar cell adenomas is often dramatically increased among rats after treatment with carcinogens, such as azaserine and 4-hydroxyaminoquinoline 1-oxide (Figure 10.11). Acinar cell carcinomas in rats have been classified as well-differentiated, poorly differenti-ated, and undifferentiated (Figure 10.12). Duct-like, cystic, and microcystic areas have been encountered in tumors, in which the dominant phenotype is acinar, but mucin secretion is rare in rat pancreatic carcinomas. In contrast, duct-like carcinomas in hamsters often show some evidence of mucin secretion (Figure 10.13). Cystic and mucinous variants have been described.

Adenosquamous carcinomas have been described in both rats and hamsters, but are rare.

EVALUATION OF EXOCRINE PANCREATIC TOXICITY

Evaluation of the toxicity of agents to the exocrine pancreas must be done almost entirely *in vivo*, for practical reasons. To culture acinar cells is difficult because they self-destruct, but they can be isolated and examined immediately *in vitro*. Freshly-isolated acinar cells have been used to detect DNA damage by *in vitro* exposure to carcinogens, and to evaluate

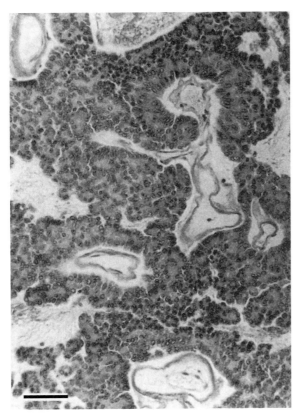

FIGURE 10.12 Acinar cell carcinoma from the pancreas of a rat that was treated with *N*-nitroso(2-hydroxypropyl)(2-oxopropyl)amine (HPOP) one year earlier. Vascular channels and connective tissue divide the tumor cells into irregular masses. Hematoxylin and eosin stain. Bar = 100 μm.

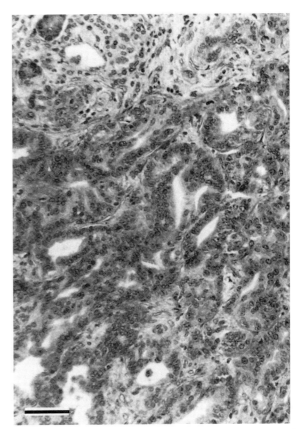

FIGURE 10.13 Duct-like carcinoma from the pancreas of a hamster treated with multiple injections of *N*δ-(*N*-methyl-*N*-nitroso-carbamoyl)-ornithine, beginning eight months earlier. Hematoxylin and eosin stain. Bar = 100 μm.

the activity of drug-metabolizing enzymes. Ductal cells can be cultured for longer periods, but isolation is demanding and laborious. Such primary cultures have also been used for studies of DNA damage.

Methods of Testing

Gross and microscopic postmortem examinations of the pancreata of experimental animals, such as rodents, offer the most direct approach for toxicity testing. Blood can be collected for amylase or lipase assays, since these enzymes are released interstitially and enter the blood with pancreatitis or duct obstruction.

Determination of urine or serum amylase can be applied *in vivo*, and this offers the most practical initial screen for detection of acute exocrine pancreatic injury. This technique lacks specificity for pancreatic damage, unless additional isoenzyme studies are done to allow separation of amylase from the pancreas (P-amylase) from amylase originating from the salivary glands and intestine. The relative amount of salivary amylase in serum varies from species to species, being quite

high in the rodent and pigs, but virtually absent in the dog. High levels of salivary amylase in many species, its production by other tissues under certain circumstance, and its unpredictability in species such as the cat, limit its usefulness as a sole marker for pancreatic injury. Serum lipase, on the other hand, is specific for pancreatic cell injury in most species except the cat. Serum lipase activity is as reliable as serum amylase, but somewhat more difficult, time-consuming, and expensive to perform. Other tests for pancreatitis, such as trypsin-like immunoreactivity (TLI) show promise, especially in species such as the cat, where serum amylase and serum lipase activities may not be elevated even with substantial pancreatic damage.

Several biochemical methods have been used to detect DNA damage in the pancreas, including determination of unscheduled DNA synthesis, and alkaline elution analysis to detect DNA strand breaks.

Short-term studies to detect chronic toxicity or the induction of focal preneoplastic lesions have been conducted in the azaserine-rat model using protocols of 2–6 months duration. The number of preneoplastic lesions is regarded as an indicator of initiation, and the rate of growth of such lesions is used to assess promotion in the short-term studies. Recently, a similar approach has been utilized in the BOP-hamster model in experiments lasting four months.

Carcinogenicity studies in rats are done by giving the potential carcinogen, and performing a postmortem examination in which the size and number of preneoplastic lesions in the pancreas are measured. Typically, counts and measurements of size in hematoxylin- and eosin-stained, paraffin-embedded sections are used for assessment of AACN size and number. The raw data are expressed as number per cm^2 of tissue, and then formulae for quantitative stereology are applied to calculate the focus number per cm^3, the true focus size (diameter or volume), and the fraction of the pancreatic tissue that is replaced by foci and nodules (volume %). It has been shown that at least some carcinogens induce a large number of foci if they are given when acinar cells are dividing actively, for example, when the animals are 2–3 weeks old.

BOP and several related metabolites and derivatives of dipropylnitrosamine are effective pancreatic carcinogens in the pancreas of Syrian golden hamsters. The spectrum of lesions in the hamster includes cystic ductal complexes, intermediate ductal complexes, tubular ductal complexes, intraductal hyperplasia, carcinoma *in situ*, and microcarcinoma.

Morphologic Evaluation of Toxicity

Acute toxic injury to the pancreas usually causes diffuse change which may be reflected as a change in pancreatic weight, or as grossly visible edema. The gland should be dissected free of fat and lymph nodes, and then weighed. Representative sections from the head, including major ducts, and the tail should be taken for histologic study. There is no need to fix the entire gland for recognition of acute or subacute toxic injury, since these are diffuse processes. Fixation may be in 10% neutral buffered formalin or in Bouin's solution, which is preferred for preservation of secretory granules. Staining with hematoxylin and eosin is typically sufficient for morphologic assessment.

In rodent carcinogenesis bioassays, or in studies of four months' duration undertaken for the detection of focal carcinogen-induced lesions, it is preferable to fix the whole pancreas. It is possible to fix the pancreas of rodents in a flat configuration, for example, in a cassette, so that a broad surface of tissue is present in the section. Although a normal-sized rat pancreas can be preserved in two paraffin blocks, in larger species multiple samples should be taken to represent head, body, and tail. Extensive sampling is required to

detect small and localized carcinomas, adenomas, and preneoplastic lesions which may escape gross detection. This is especially true in intermediate-term studies, in which the number and size of the lesions is to be evaluated quantitatively. In carcinogenesis studies of 1–2 years' duration, large tumors (sometimes multiple) may be encountered, so that it is impossible to embed the entire pancreas. Representative sections of all grossly-identified lesions and remaining normal pancreas (if present) should be taken.

Animal Models

Studies of normal pancreatic physiology and models of experimental pancreatitis have primarily used rats and dogs. Classic studies of acinar cell biology have employed guinea pig and rat pancreas, whereas mice have been used as a source of acinar cells for *in vitro* studies. *In vivo*, mice provide a useful model of acute pancreatitis, and a model for pancreatic cancer in transgenic lines. Because hamsters have been used extensively in pancreatic carcinogenesis studies, the anatomy, physiology, and cell biology of their pancreas is well-characterized. The dominance of acinar cell tumors in the rat versus ductal tumors in the hamster is striking. It apparently represents a fundamental difference in the response of the two species to initiating agents. The spectrum of tumors induced in animals is similar to that found in humans, although human carcinomas are predominantly duct-like in phenotype. Thus, the phenotypes of the pancreatic cancers induced in hamsters by nitrosamines are closer to those found in humans than those found in rats and mice.

SUMMARY AND CONCLUSIONS

The preceding sections suggest several approaches to detecting toxic injury to the exocrine pancreas. Toxicologic evaluation of new chemicals that might be used in ways that will result in significant human exposures should include acute and chronic tests focused on: (1) acinar cell cytotoxicity; (2) effects on the duct system or pancreatic secretions which will lead to duct obstruction; and (3) carcinogenicity. Evaluation should include acute and chronic toxicologic studies for all compounds, and carcinogenesis bioassay for potential carcinogens. Since so many α-amino acid analogs have been shown to affect the exocrine pancreas, such compounds should be especially suspect in regard to their effects on acinar cells. Because a significant fraction of pancreatic disease is of unknown etiology, the recognition and control of pancreatotoxic agents may reduce the incidence of pancreatitis and pancreatic carcinoma.

SECTION II ENDOCRINE PANCREAS

STRUCTURE OF ENDOCRINE PANCREAS

Gross Anatomy

In the adult pancreas of most animal species, the endocrine portion comprises only 1–2% of cells. The endocrine cells are contained in small ovoid clusters (100–200 μm diameter) called the islets of Langerhans, and are distributed throughout the pancreas; however, the population density of islets is higher in the tail than in the head of the pancreas. The number of islets in a normal pancreas varies, depending on the size of the organ. A normal pancreas from a mouse will contain between 500 and 800 islets, while a human pancreas contains approximately 500 000 islets.

Microscopic Anatomy and Ultrastructure

Pancreatic islets are typically arranged in tight variably sized clumps of pale-staining polyhedral cells having clear cytoplasm, variably distinct cell borders, and a centrally-located round nucleus (Figure 10.14). The cells are surrounded and supported by a delicate reticular stroma. Fenestrated capillaries permeate each islet, entering at the periphery and exiting centrally, to further perfuse surrounding exocrine pancreatic lobules. Islets are most often found near the center of the lobule, although they can also be present near intralobular ducts.

Despite their virtually identical histomorphology, three major cell types were originally identified in the islets, using differential histochemical staining. These cells have been termed alpha (α), beta (β), and delta (δ) cells. The α-cells contain the hormone glucagon; the β-cells, insulin; and the δ-cells, somatostatin. It is now possible to identify these three cell types easily, using immunocytochemical staining directed at the hormonal products of these cells. More recent studies have identified other hormone-containing cells in the islets, the most numerous of which contain a 36-amino-acid linear polypeptide. These cells have been termed pancreatic polypeptide (PP) cells.

The β-cells are the most abundant cells found in the endocrine pancreas. Although the numbers of these cells vary from islet to islet, approximately 80% of endocrine cells are of this cell type. By comparison,

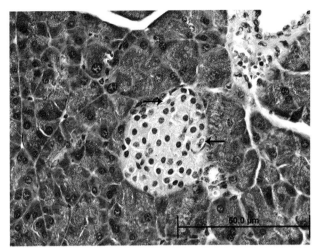

FIGURE 10.14   Normal pancreatic islet from a mouse. The islet is composed of a cluster of pale cells that are smaller and paler than surrounding acinar cells. Note the finely-granulated cytoplasm, and the centrally-located small round hyperchromatic nucleus at the center of each cell. Arrows point to two small fenestrated capillaries entering the islet.

the α-cells comprise approximately 15% of the endocrine cells; and the δ-cells, nearly 4%. The remaining 1% consists mainly of the PP cells. In humans and rodents, the β-cells occupy the core of the islets, while the other cell types form the periphery. Penetrating the β-cell core of human islets are large vascular channels lined with α- and δ-cells.

Regional variations in the cellular composition of islets from different areas exist. Islets in the body or the tail of the human pancreas contain β-, α-, and δ-cells in a normal proportion of 80:15:4; however, in the posterior half of the head there are fewer β- and δ-cells, and almost no α-cells. PP cells replace α-cells in this region.

In addition to hormone-containing cells, the islets also contain small numbers of fibroblasts and pericytes for the support of the capillary network surrounding the islet cells. Autonomic nerve fibers enter the islets and innervate the hormone-containing cells and the vasculature. Ultrastructurally, the various endocrine cells in the pancreas are readily-identified by the unique characteristics of their granules.

β-cells

The β-cells contain secretory granules which are about 300 nm in diameter (Figure 10.15). These granules feature a moderately electron-dense core which is variably shaped, depending on the species. This core possesses a periodic substructure which appears crystalloid in nature; this structure contains insulin. The space between the core and the limiting membrane is filled with fine granular material, but some paler

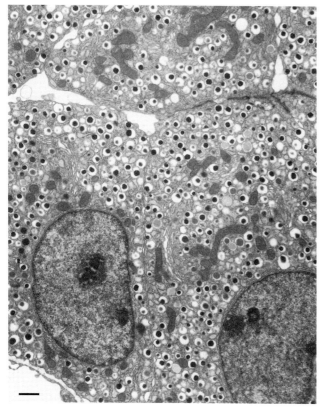

FIGURE 10.15   Pancreatic β-cells from a mouse showing insulin-containing secretory granules. These granules are characterized by a space between the dense core and the limiting membrane. Bar = 1 μm. (Courtesy of Dr Michael Appel, University of Massachusetts, Worcester, Massachusetts.)

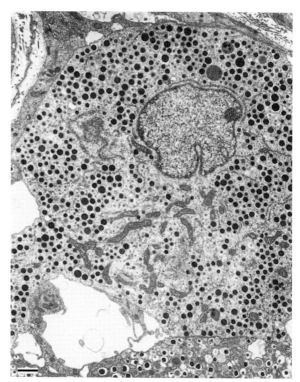

FIGURE 10.16   Pancreatic α-cell from a mouse showing gluca-gon-containing secretory granules. The nucleus of this cell is charac-teristically indented, and the granules have an eccentrically-located core of high density. Bar = 1μm. (Courtesy of Dr Michael Appel, University of Massachusetts, Worcester, Massachusetts.)

granules can be seen that do not contain a crystalline core. The Golgi apparatus is large and extensive in the β-cell, and the mitochondria are rounder and more numerous than in the other endocrine cells.

α-cells

An indented or lobulated nucleus, filamentous mitochondria, and a small Golgi apparatus are prominent features of α-cells (Figure 10.16). Their secretory granules are densely packed and are uniform in size, with a diameter of approximately 250 nm. These vesicles are characterized by an eccentrically-located core of high electron density, embedded in a matrix of less dense material. The core is closely surrounded by the limiting vesicle membrane.

δ-cells

The δ-cells, which are slightly larger than the α-cells and usually abut them, contain secretory vesicles which vary in size, but are usually larger than those seen in α- or β-cells (Figure 10.17). These vesicles contain a fine granular matrix of low or moderate electron density, which is relatively homogeneous and extends almost to the vesicle membrane. There is a subpopulation of δ-cells, referred to as δ1-cells. The secretory vesicles in these cells are relatively small (150–200 nm) and contain a homogeneous granular interior and peripheral narrow electron lucent space.

PHYSIOLOGY OF ENDOCRINE PANCREAS

The islets can be viewed as a microorgan whose major function is to manage fuel distribution and storage for the whole organism. Glucose is the primary fuel used to provide energy for life and, therefore, is the chief substance to be regulated.

Two biologically-antagonistic hormones provide this important regulatory function. Insulin, the secretory product of the β-cells, is the fuel storage hormone; its antagonist is glucagon, the secretory product of the α-cells, responsible for fuel mobilization. These two hormones are intimately coupled in such a way that in times of circulating fuel excess, as is the case after

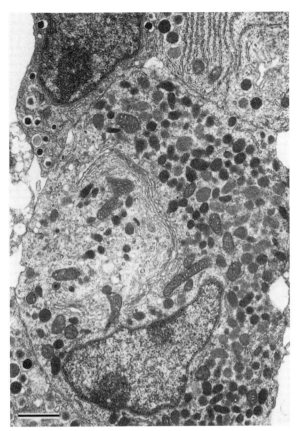

FIGURE 10.17 Pancreatic δ-cell from a mouse showing somatostatin-containing secretory granules. Granules from δ-cells are irregular in shape and of moderate density. Usually they are larger than either α- or β-cell granules. Bar = 1 μm. (Courtesy of Dr Michael Appel, University of Massachusetts, Worcester, Massachusetts.)

a meal, the amount of insulin secreted by the islets is proportionally greater than the amount of glucagon. Insulin favors nutrient uptake and synthesis of glycogen, fat, and protein in peripheral tissues. Conversely, at times when the circulating concentration of nutrients drops, and when endogenous nutrients are needed to sustain the organism, the secreted hormone mixture contains more glucagon than insulin. This mixture favors the production of glucose from the breakdown of hepatic glycogen stores, as well as from other gluconeogenic precursors. In addition, this hormone ratio promotes the production of free fatty acids, glycerol, and ketones, all substances which can be used as alternative energy substrates. Somatostatin, the secretory product of the δ-cells, inhibits the secretion of both insulin and glucagon, and hence damps excessive secretion and helps fine-tune the delicate balance between these hormones. Any factor which alters the function of α- or β-cells can disrupt the critical balance between insulin and glucagon, with subsequent loss of control of fuel management, and dire consequences for the organism.

MECHANISMS OF ENDOCRINE PANCREATIC TOXICITY

By far the most common lesion seen in the endocrine pancreas involves the β-cells. Decreased insulin secretion results in the collection of diseases termed diabetes mellitus. Idiopathic diabetes mellitus is a collection of diseases in which defective carbohydrate metabolism results in inappropriate hyperglycemia. Most individuals with diabetes mellitus can be categorized into two groups: individuals who require insulin therapy to maintain life, a syndrome termed insulin-dependent diabetes mellitus (IDDM); and individuals who would survive without insulin replacement therapy, a syndrome termed non-insulin-dependent diabetes mellitus (NIDDM). Although the etiologies and clinical manifestations of the two syndromes differ, the initial lesion in both syndromes involves the β-cell.

Insulin-dependent Diabetes Mellitus

Islet cells are substantially reduced numerically in IDDM. Although the factors responsible have yet to be fully defined, genetic influences and immunological phenomena are involved. However, a role for environmental factors in the etiology of IDDM has recently been suggested by epidemiological studies that demonstrate a marked increase in newly-diagnosed cases of IDDM associated with changes in environmental influences. An example of the potential threat of ingested xenobiotics has been provided by epidemiologic studies in Iceland. These studies suggest that IDDM may occur in some male offspring of mothers who have ingested smoked mutton. Analysis of this meat has revealed that it contained significant amounts of various N-nitroso compounds. However, to date, experimental studies linking these compounds to IDDM have been inconclusive.

Direct evidence that xenobiotics can cause IDDM in humans has been provided by case reports of individuals who ingested the rat poison Vacor, N-(4-nitrophenyl)-N9-(3-pyridinylmethyl) urea; many developed severe IDDM. In toxicity studies in animals, Vacor was either nontoxic (dogs, cats) or so lethal that the islet toxicity was not detected (rats). Thus, species differences precluded detection of β-cell toxicity in animals.

Other xenobiotics have induced some forms of IDDM studies in laboratory animals (Table 10.6), implying further that environmental toxins may have a role in IDDM. N-nitroso compounds (streptozotocin, chlorozotocin) and other complex amines (alloxan)

TABLE 10.6   Agents reported to cause cytotoxic effects in the endocrine pancreas

Cytotoxic effect	Agent	Species
Permanent β-cell damage	Alloxan	Rat, mouse, rabbit, dog, cat, sheep, monkey, pigeon, turtle
	Chlorothiazide	Human
	Dithizone	Rabbit
	Oxine	Rabbit
	Streptozotocin	Rat, mouse, dog, lamb, human
	Vacor	Human
Permanent hyperglycemia	Azoxyglycosides	Rat, human
	Chlorozotocin	Rat, mouse, hamster
	Methylnitrosourea	Hamster, mouse
	Streptozotocin	Neonatal rat
	Vacor	Human
Transient hyperglycemia	Cyproheptadine	Rat, mouse, fetal mouse, human
	Cyclosporin	Rat, mouse
	Diazoxide	Rat, mouse, dog, human
	Furosemide	Rat, mouse, dog, human
	Hydrochlorothiazide	Rat, mouse, human
	l-asparaginase	Human
	Styrylquinoline 90	Rat, rabbit
	Trichlormethiazide	Rat, mouse, dog, human
	Xylazine	Cat, cow

can cause disease very similar to that seen in humans. These, and other structurally similar compounds, pose a potential threat to all mammals, either through contamination of the environment and inadvertent exposure, or by formation of these agents in the body through biotransformation reactions.

Until recently, the abrupt onset of clinical symptoms of IDDM was considered to be strong evidence for an environmental agent as a cause of massive β-cell destruction. However, the finding that some forms of IDDM are slowly progressive has led to a conceptual change with regard to how environmental influences may impact upon this disease. Rather than precipitating IDDM abruptly by massive β-cell destruction, environmental xenobiotics may trigger the development of autoimmune processes directed against β-cells in genetically-susceptible individuals. Alternatively, β-cell tropic agents may possibly augment ongoing immunological processes, thereby hastening the onset of clinical manifestations of IDDM. The naturally-occurring antibiotic streptozotocin (SZ) apparently does trigger an autoimmune response against β-cells in mice. Repeated subdiabetogenic doses of SZ administered to certain strains of mice can cause diabetes associated with islet inflammation and β-cell destruction. Diabetes can only be prevented by combined

treatment with nicotinamide, to block the direct toxicity of SZ, and antilymphocyte serum to negate cell-mediated immunity directed against β-cells.

SZ also augments the diabetogenic activity of some viruses. Subdiabetogenic doses of SZ, in combination with Coxsackie B3 or B5 virus, or the B variant of encephalomyocarditis virus, can cause clinical diabetes in mice. In the absence of SZ, none of these viruses precipitate diabetes. In humans, where some forms of IDDM are strongly associated with autoimmunity, it is possible that xenobiotics that interact with or exacerbate ongoing immunological phenomena will be identified in the future. This interaction, like those described earlier, would hasten the destruction of β-cells and produce IDDM.

Non-insulin-dependent Diabetes Mellitus

In NIDDM, the β-cell lesion is a functional defect in the glucose-stimulated secretory mechanism for insulin. Comparison of insulin-dependent versus non-insulin-dependent diabetic patients receiving intravenous glucose stimulation has revealed that only the second phase of normal biphasic insulin secretion is preserved; the rapid first phase is generally absent. The absence of a rapid first-phase insulin release forces the individual with NIDDM to secrete greater concentrations of insulin to control a glucose challenge. In contrast, the insulin response to nonglucose substrates, such as certain amino acids and neural and hormonal secretagogues, in NIDDM is often normal. However, the ability of glucose to potentiate the response of these secretagogues is markedly impaired. A second insulin secretory defect in NIDDM appears to be at the level of basal-insulin release. As NIDDM progresses, basal-insulin levels tend to decrease as β-cell function declines. This fall in plasma insulin results in abnormal glucose production, and a rise in plasma glucose levels. Therefore, functional defects are manifested in the β-cells from patients with NIDDM, in both the stimulated and unstimulated state. Based on studies with identical twins, it has generally been believed that genetic factors were solely responsible for the pathogenesis of NIDDM. However, with the discovery that a disease very similar to NIDDM can be produced in adult rats by treating them as neonates with a large bolus of SZ, it is plausible to assume that environmental factors can play a role in the etiology of this disease. Animals treated with an SZ bolus exhibit almost no elevation in fasting plasma glucose concentrations compared to controls, and have only slightly elevated non-fasting glucose levels. However, SZ-treated animals are markedly glucose intolerant when challenged with a bolus of glucose (2 g/kg). Like their human counterparts with NIDDM, rats with chemically-induced NIDDM have a defective first phase insulin release. Although the insulin response to glucose is defective, these animals exhibit normal responses to arginine, glyceraldehyde, sulfonylureas, isoproterenol, and glucagon. As rats with this chemically-induced diabetes age, they eventually develop a resistance to the actions of insulin in peripheral tissues such as adipocytes and the heart. In the heart, the insulin resistance leads to a cardiomyopathy that is similar to that seen in human NIDDM, and significantly different from cardiac effects seen in IDDM. From these experiments with SZ, it is apparent that an environmental insult to the β-cells early in life can have dire consequences much later. Therefore, if identical twins develop NIDDM it is still possible that this disease is toxin-induced, since both would be exposed to the same environment. There is a subgroup of NIDDM characterized by familial hyperinsulinemia that has abnormal circulating insulin. The structurally abnormal insulin is the result of a point mutation at a position in the insulin gene that codes for an essential amino acid. Since many environmental toxins also are mutagenic, one can speculate that mutagenic chemicals could be one factor responsible for initiating this syndrome of hyperinsulinemic NIDDM.

Glucose Intolerance

A variety of chemicals have been identified as causing mild hyperglycemia and glucose intolerance. For the most part these effects are temporary; when the chemical is removed the hyperglycemia resolves. A description of the better-characterized chemicals follows.

Benzothiodiazines

The benzothiodiazines are a group of diuretic and antihypertensive drugs. The diuretic chlorothiazide is a good model for this class, since hyperglycemia occurs in some individuals treated with this drug. Chlorothiazide also exacerbates glucose intolerance in pre-existing diabetics. Other members of this class (e.g., diazoxide, furosemide, trichlorothiazide, and hydrochlorothiazide) have similar hyperglycemic effects.

The benzothiodiazines cause hyperglycemia by two specific mechanisms: through inhibition of insulin release by hyperpolarizing the plasma membrane and preventing the opening of voltage-gated Ca^{2+} channels needed for insulin release. They also have extra-islet effect(s), since they increase hyperglycemia in insulin-deficient severely diabetic animals, presumably by causing release of catecholamines. β-cells from animals treated with benzothiodiazines have increased numbers of secretory granules. When the drugs are withdrawn, diabetogenic effects are reversed, and the β-cells appear normally granulated.

Cyproheptadine

Cyproheptadine is an antiserotonin, antihistaminic compound used in adults and children to stimulate weight gain. When given to adult rats in repeated high doses, this chemical produces an inhibition of proinsulin synthesis, a reduction in pancreatic insulin, and glucose intolerance. Morphologically, extensive vacuolation can be seen in β-cells by light microscopy, and a progressive degranulation of β-cells, dilation of endoplasmic reticulum, and loss of ribosomes from the surface of the RER can be observed ultrastructurally. All these effects are reversed when treatment ceases; however, permanent changes in β-cells can be induced in the offspring of pregnant rats given repeated low doses of cyproheptadine during the last eight days of gestation. This treatment initially causes a 50% reduction in fetal pancreatic and serum insulin concentrations, but mothers exhibit no changes in insulin levels. By 50 days after birth, the progeny of the drug-treated dams are glucose intolerant, have two-fold increased levels of pancreatic insulin, and have an accentuated response to the insulin-lowering action of cyproheptadine. These results demonstrate that a permanent postnatal defect in β-cell function can be produced by prenatal exposure to xenobiotics.

l-Asparaginase

l-Asparaginase causes a temporary nonketogenic hyperglycemia. The pathogenesis of this effect has yet to be elucidated; however, the antineoplastic activity of this compound is mediated by decreasing the availability of l-asparagine to neoplastic cells which require exogenous l-asparagine because of a deficiency in the l-asparagine synthetase. In a similar manner, β-cells may also be deficient in this enzyme, and require an exogenous supply of l-asparagine in order to maintain insulin synthesis.

Cyclosporin

The polypeptide cyclosporin blocks the onset of spontaneous autoimmune diabetes in the BB rat, and is currently undergoing clinical trials in humans with recently-diagnosed cases of IDDM, to suppress autoimmune attack directed at the β-cells. This chemical inhibits insulin secretion in mice, rats, and humans *in vivo* and *in vitro*. β-cells in cyclosporin-treated animals exhibit severe degranulation, cytoplasmic vacuolization, and dilation of the endoplasmic reticulum. When cyclosporin is removed, both the functional and morphologic abnormalities disappear. The mechanism of cyclosporin-induced effects on β-cells is not yet known; however, the drug may be selectively taken up by β-cells and cause destabilization of mRNA.

RESPONSE OF ENDOCRINE PANCREAS TO INJURY

Apoptosis

Apoptosis is a common pathological feature seen in both NIDDM and IDDM (Figure 10.18, Table 10.4). In mice that develop IDDM following treatment with multiple subdiabetogenic doses of SZ, two phases of β-cell destruction by apoptosis were found. The first is before insulitis has developed, and is likely due to the direct toxic effects of SZ. The second phase is subsequent to insulin, and is likely triggered by reactive oxygen

or nitrogen species resulting from the inflammation. Studies using cultured β-cells have confirmed that they will undergo apoptosis when given lower concentrations of SZ. However, when treated with higher doses, the cells die via necrosis.

Evidence that the inflammation can cause a slowly progressive apoptosis of β-cells is provided by the observation of β-cell death seen in the NOD mouse model of spontaneous autoimmune IDDM. Because apoptosis of β-cells is observed before T-cells are present, it is likely that it is initiated by either macrophages or cytokines. Both of these components are associated with the production of reactive oxygen and nitrogen species, and have been found to induce apoptosis in cultured β-cells.

In the case of NIDDM, apoptosis has been associated with islet amyloid polypeptide (IAPP), which is co-secreted with insulin. An increased secretion of IAPP causes islet amyloid to accumulate during the progression of NIDDM. It seems reasonable to expect that xenobiotics that enhance the production of IAPP would augment the ongoing pathogenesis of NIDDM. This may be how the ingestion of betel nuts or flour made from the cycad plant augments NIDDM in humans.

Necrosis

Xenobiotic induced β-cell damage, with subsequent abrupt diabetes, has been seen in a variety of animals including the rat, mouse, Chinese hamster,

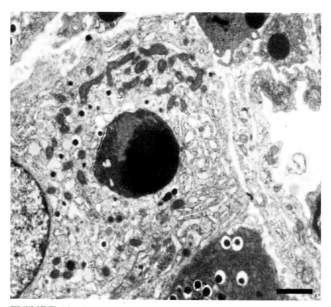

FIGURE 10.18   An apoptotic β-cell. The nucleus with condensed chromatin in a cell with intact organelles is characteristic of apoptosis. Bar 1 μm. (Courtesy of Dr Susan Bonnar-Weir, Harvard Medical School, Boston, MA.)

dog, sheep, rabbit, and monkey (Table 10.4). Damaged β-cells initially exhibit vacuolated cytoplasm (Figure 10.19), followed by pyknosis of the nuclei as the cells detach from one another. Generally, β-cell disintegration is complete within 24 hours. Following significant β-cell loss, islets in these diabetic animals are small and inconspicuous. Cells within the islet are arranged in small cords surrounded by connective tissue. It has

been demonstrated, using immunocytochemical techniques, that these cords are composed of two-thirds glucagon-containing α-cells and one-third somatostatin-containing δ-cells (Figure 10.20A–D). Insulin-containing β-cells are almost totally absent in these islets. Inflammation tends to be fairly inconspicuous in response to the dying islet cells. This regeneration, arising from remnant islet cells or via budding from ductules, is termed nesidioblastosis. Even so, regeneration is not functionally complete, because recovered animals are glucose-intolerant as adults.

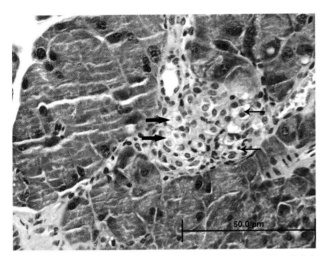

FIGURE 10.19   Islet cell vacuolation (large arrows), shrinkage and pyknosis (small arrows), and in a mouse after exposure to streptozotocin.

Insulitis

Inflammation of the islets, termed insulitis, is observed in some animal models of diabetes (Table 10.4). This condition is characterized by an infiltration into the islets of leukocytes, predominantly lymphocytes; however, a few macrophages are often also present. Only rarely are eosinophils, plasma cells, or polymorphonuclear cells observed in the infiltrate. Insulitis has also been found in the islets of humans with IDDM of short duration. The exact pathogenic consequences of insulitis in chemically-induced models of diabetes are not yet fully defined. Nevertheless, this inflammation is an integral part of an autoimmune response directed against β-cells in some animal models of spontaneous diabetes.

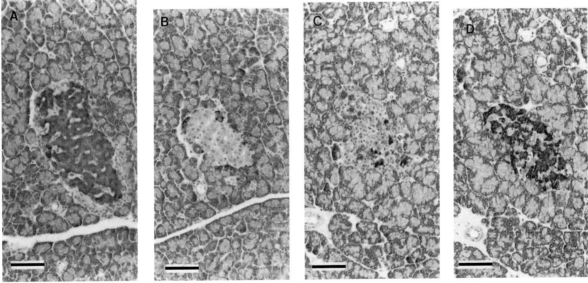

FIGURE 10.20   (A) Normal pancreatic islet from a rat stained by immunoperoxidase techniques to reveal insulin-containing pancreatic β-cells. Approximately 80% of the cells within the islet stain positively for insulin. Bar = 100 μm. (B) The same pancreatic islet stained by immunoperoxidase techniques, to reveal glucagon-containing α-cells and somatostatin-containing δ-cells. These cells are confined to the periphery of the islet. Bar = 100 μm. (C) Pancreatic islet from a rat, treated with streptozotocin (70 mg/kg), stained by immunoperoxidase techniques to reveal insulin-containing β-cells. Only a few cells stain positively for insulin, many necrotic cells are visible, and the normal architecture of the islet is disrupted. Bar = 100 μm. (D) The same islet stained by immunoperoxidase techniques, to reveal glucagon-containing α-cells and somatostatin-containing δ-cells. These cells are the predominant cell types found in this islet, and can be seen penetrating as cords into the center of the islet. Bar = 100.

Regeneration

No effective regeneration of lost β-cells occurs in the islets of adult animals treated with chemical diabetogens. Marked regeneration, however, can be seen in neonates following a toxic insult. Replication of surviving β-cells, and the budding of new islets from ducts, is termed nesidioblastosis. This regenerative process, however, is not functionally complete because these animals are glucose-intolerant in adult life.

Carcinogenesis

Tumors in the endocrine pancreas have been reported after exposure to xenobiotics. The known diabetogens alloxan and SZ cause islet cell tumors in rats, usually detectable seven months after exposure. The incidence of animals with tumors can be increased by treatment with nicotinamide and the toxin concomitantly. Other chemicals that have been reported to induce islet cell neoplasia are 6-diethylaminomethyl-4-hydroxyaminoquinoline 1-oxide, heliotrine, and azinophosmethyl. All these chemicals cause tumors in rats; mice appear resistant to these carcinogenic effects. Most neoplasms are adenomas, although a small proportion of carcinomas have been reported. β-cells are the predominant type of cell found in islet cell tumors. The number of secretory granules within the cytoplasm of these cells is variable, as is the amount of insulin secretion and associated hypoglycemia. Neoplasms may contain scattered α- or δ-cells, which can be identified either immunohistochemically or ultrastructurally.

EVALUATION OF ENDOCRINE PANCREATIC TOXICITY

In Vivo Testing

Tests of β-cell function *in vivo* include determination of serum glucose and serum insulin concentrations. Glucose tolerance tests can be performed in animals by measuring blood glucose concentrations in serial samples taken over a 2-hour period following administration of a bolus of glucose by stomach tube or intraperitoneal injection.

Elevated fasting blood glucose or glucose intolerance, and deficient serum insulin levels in response to glucose are the most sensitive parameters for evaluation of β-cell function. Reversibility of β-cell injury can be assessed by re-evaluating these parameters following removal and elimination of the xenobiotic. α- and δ-cell function are usually not tested *in vivo*, although

levels of both glucagon and somatostatin can be determined by radioimmunoassay.

The morphologic integrity of all islet cell types can be evaluated histologically and ultrastructurally postmortem. The subtle, and often slowly progressive, nature of many islet lesions, and the relative lack of tissue response to injury, degeneration and death, can make qualitative assessment difficult. Immunohistochemical stains using antibodies raised against islet hormones are now standard for identification of specific cell types at the histologic level. These stains may be applied to fixed tissues using immunoperoxidase staining.

In Vitro Testing

In vitro techniques may be more suitable for establishing the pathogenesis of toxin-induced β-cell injury, because *in vivo* biotransformation and other whole animal effects may hinder mechanistic investigations. Several cell lines which secrete insulin are available for investigating potentially diabetogenic chemicals. Primary cultures of islets obtained via enzymatic digestion of the pancreas are the best *in vitro* tools.

In vitro toxicity testing has the major drawback of uneven distribution of either nutrients or toxins throughout the 100–200 μm islets in static culture. To overcome this problem, methods have been developed to culture β-cells in monolayers, utilizing pancreata from neonatal animals. Cultured β-cells are selectively-sensitive to the toxic effects of the known diabetogens SZ and alloxan. Although these cells must be prepared from fresh pancreata for every experiment, they closely approximate the functions of β-cells *in vivo*. Therefore, these cells are ideally suited for screening and elucidating the mechanisms of action for specific β-cell toxins.

Animal Models

SZ and alloxan are the toxins most often used to induce experimental diabetes. These agents are effective in most rodent species, and in some higher species including dog, sheep, and monkey. The types of diabetes which can be modeled have been discussed in previous sections.

SUMMARY AND CONCLUSIONS

Toxicologic studies of new chemicals, to which humans might be significantly exposed, should include evaluation of cytotoxicity for islet cells.

Structural analogs of glucose are particularly suspect for potential endocrine effects, because they may enter or bind to β-cells via glucose receptor pathways. Since a significant fraction of diabetes is of unknown etiology, the recognition and control of toxic agents that affect islets may reduce the incidence of diabetes. Since IDDM is a heterogeneous collection of diseases with more than one distinct etiologic pathway, environmental influences can operate in an individual by several scenarios, including direct destruction of a critical mass of β-cells, triggering of autoimmune processes against β-cells, or augmentation of separate ongoing diabetogenic factors (e.g., autoimmune processes and viruses) to hasten the onset of disease. Experimental evidence also suggests that xenobiotics can predispose to the development of NIDDM.

FURTHER READING

Clark, A., de Koning, E.J., Hattersley, A.T., Hansen, B.C., Yajniek, C.S., and Poultous, J. (1995). Pancreatic pathology in non-insulin dependent diabetes (NIDDM). *Diabetes Res. Clin. Pract.*, 28, 539–547.

Go, V.L.W., DiMagno, E.P., Gardner, J.D., Lebenthal, E., Reber, H. A., and Scheele, G.A. (eds) (1993). *The Exocrine Pancreas: Biology, Pathobiology, and Diseases.* Raven Press, New York, NY.

Kore, M. (1998). Role of growth factors in pancreatic cancer. *Surg. Oncol. Clin. N. Am.*, 7, 25–41.

Longnecker, D.S. (1994). Preoplastic and neoplastic lesions of the pancreas in hamster, mouse and rat. In *EULEP Pathology Atlas* (Bannasch, B., and Gossner, W. eds), pp. 64–81. Schattauer, Stuttgart, Germany.

Longnecker, D.S., and Wilson, G.L. (2002). Pancreas, Chapter 32. In *Handbook of Toxicological Pathology* (Haschek, W.M., Rousseaux, C.G., and Wallig, M.A. eds), 2nd edn, Vol. II, pp. 227–254. Academic Press, San Diego, CA.

Wiebkine, P., Schaeffer, B.K., Longnecker, D.S., and Curphey, T.J. (1984). Oxidative and conjugative metabolisms of xenobiotics by isolated rat and hamster acinar cells. *Drug Metab. Dispos.*, 12, 427–431.

Wilson, B.L., and Longenecker, D.S. (1999). Pancreatic Toxicology. In *Endocrine and Hormonal Toxicology* (Harvey, P.W., Rush, K.C., and Cockburn, A. eds), pp. 125–153. Wiley, London, UK.

Kidney and Lower Urinary Tract

INTRODUCTION

The kidney is particularly susceptible to the toxic effects of drugs and environmental chemicals, due to its high blood flow-to-mass ratio, and its unique function of concentrating urine and urine constituents (including xenobiotics) through a countercurrent mechanism. As such, the kidney is often exposed to a higher concentration of xenobiotics than other tissues. Since most xenobiotics or their metabolites are excreted in the urine, the urothelium, particularly that lining the urinary bladder, is frequently a target for toxicity.

Xenobiotic-induced kidney effects are manifested clinically either as the nephrotic syndrome, or as acute and chronic renal failure. In one survey of human hospital patients, 18.3% of all acute renal failure cases were drug-related. An estimated 500 000 new patients on a worldwide basis develop drug-related end stage renal failure each year.

This chapter emphasizes xenobiotic-induced structural and biochemical changes that occur in the kidney and lower urinary tract, and the potential mechanisms involved. The rat is the species of focus, since it is the most important model in renal safety assessment, due to the excellent concordance in response to xenobiotics between rats and humans. In addition, common xenobiotic-induced renal diseases in domestic animals are briefly reviewed. The gross, microscopic, and ultrastructural anatomy is presented, followed by a discussion of relevant physiologic mechanisms. Mechanisms of renal injury, and the methods used to recognize and characterize these mechanisms, are reviewed on a subtopographical basis using specific xenobiotics as examples.

RENAL STRUCTURE AND FUNCTION

Site localization of injury forms the basis for understanding and predicting the functional consequences of a lesion. Additionally, cellular and subcellular localization of the primary xenobiotic effect (site of earliest and most sensitive alteration) is a prerequisite step for establishing a subcellular organelle target in mechanistic studies.

Gross, Microscopic, and Ultrastructural Anatomy

Since the rat is the most frequently used model in renal toxicology, the following review of the anatomy of the kidney and lower urinary tract will focus on the rat, with brief mention of species differences.

Gross and Subgross Anatomy

Embryologically, the functional unit of the kidney, the nephron, arises from the nephrogenic mesodermal mass, whereas the collecting tubes and urothelium of the urinary tract originate from the Wolffian (mesonephric) duct. The renal pelvis represents a dilatation of the ureter.

The kidney of the mature rat is bean-shaped, and weighs approximately 0.51% to 1.08% (with a mean of 0.65%) of the body weight, varying with age and sex. The kidneys are located retroperitoneally, ventrolateral to the vertebral column. The right kidney is located cranially to the left, and is within the protective

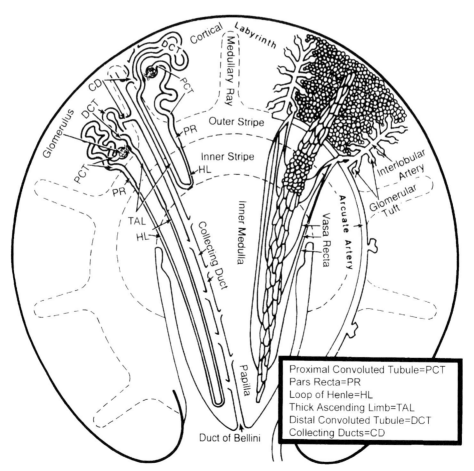

FIGURE 11.1   Schematic drawing of the nephron and vasculature, denoting subtopographical anatomic relationships.

province of the rib cage. It has a basic unipapillary architecture, the simplest type of mammalian kidney. Other types can generally be regarded as adaptations to larger body sizes. In transverse section, the cortex and outer stripe of the outer medulla can be differentiated from the inner stripe of the outer medulla and the inner medulla with the papilla extending into the renal pelvis. A subgross photograph of a 5 μm thick periodic acid-Schiff (PAS)-stained transverse section enables differentiation of the outer stripe of the outer medulla from cortex, and the inner stripe from inner medulla. Furthermore, the arcuate vessels are readily visualized (Figures 11.1 and 11.2). Nephrotoxins typically have predilection sites in specific zones of the kidney, dependent on the mechanisms of injury (Table 11.1 and Figure 11.2).

The lower urinary tract extends from the kidney pelvis bilaterally through the ureters, into the urinary bladder, and ultimately out the urethra. It functions primarily to transport urine formed in the kidneys to the urinary bladder for storage until ultimate excretion. The structure and function of the lower urinary tract is similar in all mammals, including the structure of a unique lining epithelium, the urothelium (also referred to as transitional cell epithelium).

The urinary bladder, a highly-distendable organ, is located in the posterior abdominal cavity. The most anterior portion of the bladder in rodents is referred to as the dome, and the more posterior portion, formed by a triangle-like area where the ureters enter and the urethra exits the bladder, is referred to as the trigone. The urethra of the female is short, slightly flattened dorsoventrally, and extends from the urinary bladder to the clitoral fossa just anterior to the vaginal orifice. The urethra of the male is considerably longer, extending from the bladder through the pelvic girdle (membranous urethra), and continuing through the penis as the penile urethra, opening at the tip of the penis.

Vasculature and Innervation of the Kidney

The kidney receives 25% of the cardiac output, with the cortex receiving 850% of renal blood flow. The outer medulla receives 14% and the inner medulla 1%. In the adult kidney, the renal artery branches in the pelvis into 6 to 10 interlobar arteries, giving rise in turn to arcuate arteries coursing parallel to the capsule along the corticomedullary junction. Interlobular arteries arise from the arcuates, coursing perpendicular to the capsule, each supplying a cortical labyrinth.

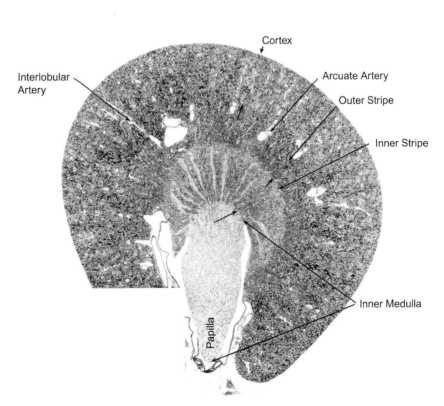

FIGURE 11.2   Subgross topographical anatomy of the rat kidney, illustrating the zones of the kidney with correlative sites of functional activity, and nephrotoxin examples targeting the zone or function in Table 11.1.

TABLE 11.1   Site of target functional activity and associated nephrotoxicants

Target functional activity	Associated nephrotoxicants
Glomerulus	
Direct effect on epithelial cells	Puromycin
Oxidative activation	Adriamycin
Increased GFR	Hypertension, aldosterone, high protein diet
Decreased GFR (efferent arteriole constriction)	Cyclosporin, tacrolimus, amphotericin B, radio-contrast agents, antiprostaglandins
Decreased GFR (via systemic effects)	ACE inhibitors, inotropic and vasodilator cardiotonics
Mesangiolysis	Mitomycin C, croton oil, snake venom
Nephron lumen precipitation	Folic acid, ethylene glycol, glycine, glycolic acid, oxalic acid, methotrexate, peptide mimetics (e.g., integrin receptor antagonists), sulfanomides
Proximal convoluted tubule	
Sodium pump-linked transport	Phosphate, lithium
Endocytosis, pinocytosis, protein-linked uptake	Aminoglycosides, α_{2u}globulin, Bence-Jones protein, hemoglobin, myoglobin, lead, cadmium, bismuth, sucrose, manitol, nitrilotriacetic acid
Pars recta	
Oxidative activation	Chloroform, acetaminophen, acetamide, paracetamol, p-aminophenol, 1,1-dichloroethylene, bromobenzene, epichlorohydrin, 1,2-dichloropropane, n-succinimide
Activation by glutathione conjugation	1,2-Dibromomethane, trisphosphate, 1,2-dibromo-3-chloropropane, 1,2-dichloroethane
β-lyase-mediated bioactivation	Trichloroethylene, hexachlorobutadiene, trichloroethene, tetrachloroethane, chlorinated and fluorinated olfins
Organic acid transport (with metabolism to reactive intermediate)	Carbapenems, cephalosporin, citrinin, procainamide, methotrexate
Organic base transport (with oxidative activation)	Cisplatinum
Cell respiration	Mercury salts, ischemic/hypoxic reperfusion injury
Distal nephron	Fluoride, methoxyflurane, 5-azacytidine, furosemide (thick ascending tubule), thiazide-like diuretics (distal convoluted tubule), amiloride (cortical collecting ducts)
Papilla	
Interstitial concentration via counter current exchanger and oxidative activation via endoperoxide synthetase	NSAIDs, phenacetin, 2-bromoethylamine, 5-nitrofurans

Each interlobular artery gives rise to 6 to 11 afferent arterioles. All renal artery branches are end arteries without significant collateral supply. The renal circulation is a portal system as capillary beds (glomerular) reunite into an efferent arteriole, running for a varying distance before again forming a capillary bed surrounding portions of the nephron. All circulation to the medulla is of postglomerular capillary derivation. Veins run parallel to the main arterial and arcuate system. Lymphatics run parallel only to the cortical vasculature, being absent in the medulla. The interstitium of cortex and medulla are not functionally contiguous.

Efferent arterioles of subcapsular nephrons are long, breaking into capillary beds that supply the same nephron, then subsequently coalescing to form an interlobular vein. Efferent arterioles of midcortical and juxtamedullary nephrons, in contrast, give rise to descending vasa recta which break up into capillary plexuses, forming the exclusive blood supply to the medulla. Capillary plexuses reunite, forming ascending vasa recta. Capillary plexuses are dense in the inner stripe, but sparse in the outer stripe and inner medulla. Ascending vasa recta join the arcuate veins at the corticomedullary junction.

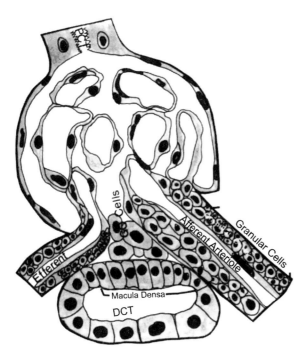

FIGURE 11.3 Drawing of juxtaglomerular apparatus. Proximal convoluted tubule (PCT); distal convoluted tubule (DCT) and Goormaghtigh cell (GO).

Nerves that are associated with intrarenal arterioles have been noted to have ramifications in the afferent and efferent arterioles, as well as in the juxtaglomerular apparatus. These nerve fibers are monoaminergic with norepinephrine and dopamine activity.

Microscopic and Ultrastructural Functional Anatomy

Histologic and ultrastructural cytologic characteristics of the following nephron subunits are important in toxicologic pathology: glomerulus; proximal convoluted tubule; pars recta; loop of Henle; thick ascending limb; juxtaglomerular apparatus (Figure 11.3); distal convoluted tubule; collecting ducts; and interstitium.

Glomerulus

The glomerulus is composed of a capillary network lined by a thin layer of endothelial cells, a central region of mesangium, and epithelial cells (podocytes). The glomerulus represents the filtering unit for blood through which the plasma filtrate is derived in the first part of the uriniferous space. The filtering membrane of the glomerulus consists of fenestrated capillary endothelial cells, a glomerular basement membrane, and the visceral epithelial cells or podocytes (Figure 11.4). The glomerular basement membrane principally consists of

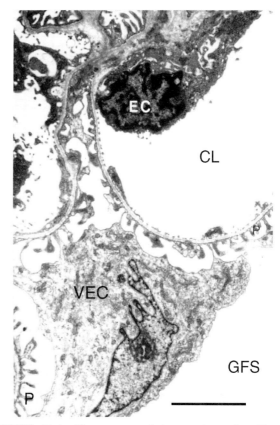

FIGURE 11.4 Ultrastructure of the rat glomerulus, illustrating a visceral epithelial cell (VEC), foot processes (P) of the VEC, and an endothelial cell (EC) of a capillary loop (CL). Lower right, Glomerular filtration space (GFS). Bar = 10 μm.

Type IV collagen and polyanionic proteoglycans, particularly heparan sulfate.

The mesangium is an extremely important component of the glomerulus, forming the supporting framework in which the glomerular tuft capillaries ramify. The mesangium includes an extracellular matrix comprising Type IV collagen, proteoglycans, and other proteins, and two cell types. The mesangial stellate cell is contractile, responding to vasoactive hormones such as angiotensin II. This stellate cell synthesizes and secretes the mesangial matrix. The second mesangial cell is phagocytic, has a clearing role, and participates in local immune reactions. Mesangial uptake lags behind the systemic reticuloendothelial system, in the appearance as well as the disappearance of antigen. The lymphatic system receives the end products of mesangial phagocytic cell processing.

Bowman's capsule surrounding the glomerulus has two layers, the visceral, mentioned earlier, and the parietal. The parietal layer and its basement membrane are continuous with the proximal convoluted tubule. Frequently, in the normal mature male mouse, and occasionally, in the mature male rat, the proximal convoluted tubular epithelial cells extend into Bowman's capsule, practically surrounding the glomerulus. These cells retain their cuboidal shape, and suffer the same toxicologic fate as those in the proximal convoluted tubule.

Proximal Convoluted Tubule

The proximal tubule begins at the urinary pole of the glomerulus and consists of an initial convoluted portion, the proximal convoluted tubule (PCT), which is a direct continuation of the parietal epithelium of Bowman's capsule, and a straight portion, the pars recta, which is located in the outer stripe and/or medullary ray. In the rabbit, a well-defined neck segment is shown to be present between the parietal epithelium of Bowman's capsule and the PCT. This segment is not present in the rat or human.

The vast majority of structural subunits in the cortex represent proximal convoluted tubules (PCTs). The PCTs, as well as the pars recta, are qualitatively differentiated from the remainder of the nephron and collecting duct by their lumenal brush border, recognized in routine hematoxylin and eosin (H&E) sections, in electron micrographs (microvilli), and by using special stains such as periodic acid-Schiff or alkaline phosphatase. These cells are cuboidal, with eosinophilic cytoplasm and a central large round nucleus. Ultrastructurally, endocytotic vesicles, lysosomes, phagolysosomes, endoplasmic reticulum (predominantly smooth), Golgi apparatus, and mitochondria are prominent. Peroxisomes and lipid vacuoles also occur in PCTs. Because of the convolutions of the PCT tubules, these are consistently recognized as transverse sections in histologic sections.

The proximal tubule is divided into three segments (P_1, P_2, and P_3) in several animal species including rat, rabbit, mouse, and the rhesus monkey. Only the PCT and pars recta have been positively identified in the normal human kidney. The P_1 segment is short, connecting with the glomerular filtration space. Cells of this segment have the highest rate of oxidative metabolism in the kidney. The P_2 segment represents the vast majority of the PCT, and extends a short distance into the pars recta. The vast majority of the pars recta consist of the P_3 segment.

Pars Recta

The pars recta, or straight portion of the proximal tubule of the juxtamedullary nephron, are located in the outer stripe of the medulla (Figure 11.5A). Pars recta of short-looped (subcapsular) nephrons are found within the medullary rays, or within the outer stripe. The ratio of long-to-short-looped nephrons is approximately 1:2. Histologically and ultrastructurally, the cells of the pars recta are similar to those of the PCTs, with two exceptions: phagolysosomal proteinic reabsorption droplets are much less prominent in the pars recta and the brush border in the rat is highest and most developed in the pars recta. Pars recta tubules histologically may be seen as both transverse, as well as longitudinal, profiles. Differentiation between PCT and pars recta has significant functional and toxicological relevance.

Thin Limbs of the Loop of Henle

The transition from the proximal tubule to the thin descending limb of the loop of Henle is abrupt, and it marks the boundary between the outer and inner stripes of the outer medulla. Four epithelial cell types are described in the thin descending and the thin ascending limbs of the loop of Henle; each, however, is histologically flattened and has amphophilic cytoplasm.

Ultrastructurally, cell types vary from non-specialized cells without interdigitation to cells with interdigitation and specialization. Specialization is evidenced by a variation (increase) in cytoplasmic numbers of mitochondria and intra-membranous particles, and the surface number of microvilli (always sparse). No toxicologic significance has been determined for the differentiation of cell types.

The length of Henle's loop varies, with subcapsular nephrons having a very short loop (thus short-looped nephrons) extending only into the outer stripe. Nephrons arising in midcortex have loops extending midway through the inner medulla. Juxtamedullary nephrons (or long-looped nephrons) extend deep into the papilla (see Figure 11.1). However, only about 250 nephrons reach the last millimeter of the tip of the papilla.

The transition from the pars recta to the descending loop of Henle results in reduction in outside diameter, with only a slight change in lumenal diameter. The inner stripe of the outer zone of the medulla consists of Henle's loops, thick ascending tubules (the thick ascending segment or straight portion of the distal tubule), and collecting ducts (Figure 11.5B). The inner zone of the medulla consists of Henle's loops and collecting ducts.

Thick Ascending Limb

The distal tubule is comprised of three structurally-distinct segments: the thick ascending limb of the loop of Henle (TAL); the macula densa; and the distal convoluted tubule (DCT). The TAL is found in

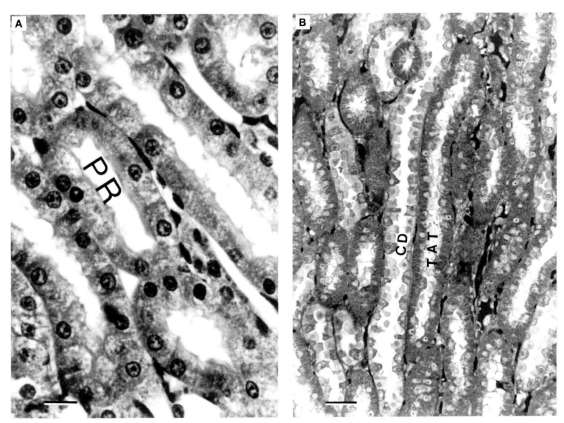

FIGURE 11.5   Rat kidney. (A) Outer stripe illustrating normal pars recta (PR) or straight portion of the proximal tubule. Bar = 20 μm. (B) Inner stripe illustrating normal thick ascending tubule (TAT) and collecting ducts (CD). Plastic-embedded section (2 μm) stained with Lee's hematoxylin. Bar = 50 μm.

the outer zone of the medulla and in the cortex, ending near its own glomerulus, just past the macula densa. In the rat and rabbit, the cortical TAL extends beyond the vicinity of the macula densa, and forms an abrupt transition with the DCT. Cells lining the TAL are cuboidal, with eosinophilic cytoplasm and round central nucleus. TAL cells are smaller than PCT and pars recta cells. Thus, in the tubule cross-section, several more cells are found in the thick ascending tubule than in the PCT or pars recta tubule. Ultrastructurally, cells of the TAL have prominent mitochondria and rough endoplasmic reticulum. Glycogen or lipid droplets and phagolysosomes may also be found in the cytoplasm. Although significant ultrastructural heterogeneity occurs at various levels of the thick ascending tubule, no relevant toxicologic correlate has been described. Tamm–Horsfall protein covers the lumenal membrane surface of the cells lining the TAL.

Juxtaglomerular Apparatus

The juxtaglomerular apparatus (JGA) is located at the vascular pole of the glomerulus, where a portion of the distal nephron comes into contact with its parent glomerulus. The main components of JGA are the macula densa of the thick ascending limb, the renin-producing granular cells of the afferent arteriole, and the extraglomerular mesangial cell (Goormaghtigh or GO cell, lacis cell; see Figure 11.3). The macula densa is a specialized region of the TAL adjacent to the hilum of the glomerulus. The cells of macula densa are low columnar, and exhibit an apically-placed nucleus. With electron microscopy the macula densa cell base is seen to interdigitate with the adjacent lacis cells to form a complex relationship.

Distal Convoluted Tubule

The DCT is approximately 1 mm in length, begins at a variable distance beyond the macula densa, and extends to the connecting tubule that connects the nephron with the collecting duct. The connecting tubule is well-defined in the rabbit, but not in the rat, mouse, or human kidney. Cytologically the DCT cells are taller, but otherwise similar to those of the thick ascending limb of the loop of Henle. However, the Tamm–Horsfall protein is not found covering the luminal cell membrane.

Collecting Ducts

The collecting ducts extend from the connecting segment in the cortex through the outer and inner medulla to the tip of the papilla. Cells lining the collecting duct are low cuboidal in the cortex, increasing in height to low columnar in the papilla. Two cell types occur: the intercalated cell (a dark cell); and the principal cell with amphophilic or clear cytoplasm. In the inner medulla the intercalated cell disappears. Collecting ducts progressively anastomose from cortex to papilla. In the papilla, collecting ducts form the ducts of Bellini, which empty into the pelvis.

Renal Interstitium

The renal cortex in the rat consists of 7% interstitium by volume, of which only 3% represents the interstitial cells. In contrast, in the medulla the amount of interstitium continuously increases toward the tip of the papilla, reaching up to 29% by volume. The interstitium of the papilla consists of mucopolysaccharides and three cell types: stellate; monocyte; and pericyte. The stellate cell synthesizes prostaglandins. The stellate cells are interconnected and subcompartmentalize the interstitium, forming a barrier to axial diffusion of solutes. The corticomedullary junction connective tissue and outer stripe apparently serve to isolate the increasingly-hypertonic medullary interstitium from the cortex. The proportion of interstitium in the inner medulla increases with age and ischemia.

Lower Urinary Tract

The urothelium is a unique, highly-specialized epithelium lining the lower urinary tract. The basal cell layer is composed of cuboidal cells with larger intermediate cells superimposed. The superficial cell layer is composed of extremely large, flat, polygonal cells ($>100\,\mu m$ in diameter), with a scalloped surface which is lined by a unique asymmetric unit membrane containing distinctive proteins, the uroplakins.

Comparative Considerations

Among domestic animals, the kidney of carnivores and horses is unipapillary (unipyramidal). In the dog kidney, the renal pyramids are fused into a crest-like papilla with pyramidal vestiges, recognized as recesses or invaginations of the renal pelvis. These renal recesses are separated by interlobar artery branches of the renal artery, which form the arcuate arteries at the corticomedullary junction. Both the dog and cat have venous drainage (without parallel arteries) of subcapsular parenchyma, with veins grossly visible on the surface. The cat kidney has veins in the capsule, while those of the dog are subcapsular. The cat kidney contains sufficient fat to cause a yellow color, visible grossly. Lipid vacuoles are present within the epithelium of the PCT. This fat deposition is hormonally-dependent; yellow coloration is absent in the anestrus female. Collecting duct epithelial cell cytoplasm in the dog frequently contains sufficient fat to create yellow streaks in the cortex that are visible grossly.

The bovine kidney is multipapillary and externally lobulated. The human kidney is multipapillary, but not externally lobulated. The cynomolgus monkey kidneys are unipapillary with fusion of renal pyramids into a relatively short crest-like papilla. The equine kidney has glomeruli of sufficient size to be grossly visible on the cortical surface. The capsule strips easily from the surface in common mammalian species, except for the horse.

The rat has the most prominent outer stripe (of outer medulla) visible subgrossly, constituting one-third of the medulla by volume. The outer stripe in cat and human is thin. In the dog, the outer stripe is virtually absent. This forms the basis of the frequent misrecognition in the rat of the junction of the inner and outer stripe as corticomedullary junction. The dog has only long-looped nephrons, in contrast to rat and human. In the dog, the pars recta joins Henle's loop near the corticomedullary junction; thus all Henle's loops turn in inner medulla. In the dog, the pars recta occur only in medullary rays. Development of the inner medulla varies proportionately with urine-concentrating capacity of the species.

While species differences are found at the gross level, the organization of renal parenchyma at the cellular level is basically comparable among the commonly-studied mammalian species. One exception of defined toxicologic impact occurs in the proximal convoluted tubule of the male rat. It is characterized by unique large crystalloid alpha$_{2u}$globulin cytoplasmic phagolysosomal inclusions, recognized as hyaline droplets by light microscopy (Figure 11.6A).

Intraglomerular reflux occurs in the dog in hyperthermia, or as a postmortem artifact, and in humans as an ischemic or toxicologic change in early renal failure. This detachment and upward displacement of the proximal convoluted tubular epithelium into Bowman's filtration space contrasts with the occasional normal appearance of PCT cells lining the parietal layer of Bowman's capsule in the mouse and rat.

Tamm–Horsfall, a protein of relevance in cast formation in humans, lines the lumenal membrane of cells of the distal convoluted tubule in humans, but not in rats. Tamm–Horsfall protein lines the lumenal surface of cells in the thick ascending limb in both species.

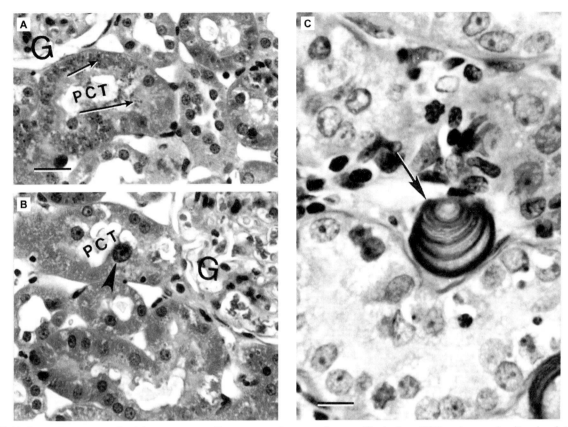

FIGURE 11.6   Light micrograph of the young sexually-mature male rat renal cortex, illustrating: (A) Spontaneous hyaline droplets (arrows) (Bar = 40 μm); (B) Spontaneous karyomegaly (arrowhead) glomerulus (G), and proximal convoluted tubule (PCT) (Bar = 15 μm); (C) Interstitial mineralization reflecting mineralized dedundant basement membrane (arrow). Bar = 15 μm.

Physiology

The primary functions of the kidneys can be separated into four major categories: control of the body's water and electrolytes; excretion of the waste products of metabolism; elaboration of hormones; and selected metabolic activities.

Control of Body Water and Electrolytes

Water and Sodium Balance

The kidneys play a major role in the control of fluid and electrolyte composition of the body. The size of the body fluid compartment and total body water are kept remarkably constant by control of fluid osmolality, through control of thirst centers and renal sodium and water excretion. Sodium and its attendant anions contribute 90–95% of the osmotic activity of the body fluid osmolality. Renal activity in electrolyte and fluid balance is mediated by modulation of glomerular filtration rate (GFR), adrenergic nerve activity, antidiuretic hormone (ADH), aldosterone, and natriuretic hormones. Reabsorption of NaC1 accounts for most of the energy expenditure in the kidney.

Normal renal function is predicated on adequate perfusion (pressure and volume). The kidneys typically receive 25% of the cardiac output. However, only about 10% of oxygen consumption occurs in the kidneys. Approximately 85% of renal flow can be associated with the cortex, 14% with the outer medulla, and 1% with the inner medulla, reflecting heterogeneity in intrarenal distribution.

Glomerulus

Filtration is the basic determinant in urine formation, and a key measurement of kidney function. Discrimination in glomerular filtration for larger molecules occurs based on molecular size, configuration, and charge. Transport of cationic molecules is facilitated, whereas that of anionic molecules is restricted more than that of neutral ones. Quantitation of the filtration process or glomerular filtration rate (GFR) is readily accomplished by the standard formula:

$$\text{GFR (ml/min)} = [\text{urinary creatinine (mg/ml)} \\ \times \text{urine volume (ml/min)}]/\text{serum} \\ \text{creatinine (mg/ml)}$$

Vascular resistance varies within the kidney, so renal blood flow remains constant (autoregulation) over a wide range of systolic pressures, from 90 to 220 mm Hg. Neural regulation of renal blood flow is minimal in the normal steady-state.

Proximal Tubule

The proximal tubule represents the site of reabsorption of the most sodium, without regard to body needs at this level. Obligatory water reabsorption occurs, also regardless of body needs. This water reabsorption is passive, accompanying active reabsorption of solutes.

Active transport of sodium is mediated by Na^+–K^+-ATPase in the basolateral cell surface membranes. A widespread correlative ultrastructural feature of salt-transporting epithelia across species is basolateral cell-process interdigitation and tight junctions.

Henle's Loop

An osmotic gradient is established and maintained by selective permeability in the loops of Henle (countercurrent multipliers) and passive diffusion in the vasa recta (countercurrent exchangers). This forms the basis for a countercurrent system, in which inflow runs parallel to, in intimate proximity with, and opposite to, outflow. The ability of the kidneys to concentrate urine is dependent on the gradient of increasing interstitial osmolality running from the outer medulla to the tip of the papilla created by the countercurrent system.

All sodium and water transport in Henle's loop is passive. Permeability is high to water, but low to salt, in the descending limb. In contrast, in the ascending limb, sodium permeability is high, but water permeability is low. As filtrate passes down Henle's loop, osmolality increases, due to osmosis of water into the hypertonic interstitium. The interstitium is rich in osmotically-active urea, because of reabsorption by the collecting ducts.

Distal Nephron

The distal nephron includes the thick ascending limb (TAL), distal convoluted tubule, and collecting ducts. Sodium is transported passively in the TAL, but actively elsewhere in the distal nephron, and is dependent on body needs with responsiveness to aldosterone. In contrast, chloride is actively transported in the TAL. Facultative reabsorption of water occurs, regulated according to body needs by ADH. Permeability to water is low in the absence of ADH in the distal nephron.

Potassium Transport

The potassium ion is the principal intracellular electrolyte. The kidney is responsible for controlling the concentration of potassium in the body. A marked decrease in urinary potassium clearance does not occur until body potassium stores are depleted 20% to 40%. An increase in potassium load, however, results in a prompt rise in urinary potassium clearance. There is a connection between sodium reabsorption and potassium excretion, reflecting passive K^+ transport. A connection also exists between urinary potassium and hydrogen ion excretion. Potassium excretion is also influenced by aldosterone. The proximal tubule is the site of 70% of potassium reabsorption. The hormonal control (aldosterone) of secretion, however, occurs in the distal nephron. Alkalosis results from increased excretion of potassium in urine, while acidosis results in diminished renal potassium excretion.

Calcium and Phosphate

Calcium and phosphate (PO_4) balance is profoundly influenced by active transport in the proximal tubule. The glomerular filtrate concentration of calcium is 50% to 75% of the plasma level. Calcium is 99% reabsorbed, 60% in the PCT, two-thirds of which is passive in exchange for sodium. The phosphate glomerular filtrate concentration is 90% of the plasma level. Two-thirds of the phosphate is reabsorbed in the proximal tubule, whereas 20% typically is cleared in the urine.

Magnesium

Of plasma magnesium, 75% is filterable. Over 80% of filtrate magnesium is reabsorbed, predominantly in Henle's loop, but also in the proximal tubule.

Excretion of Waste Products

Nitrogenous waste products consisting of urea, creatinine, and ammonia ion are excreted in the urine.

Elaboration of Hormones and Regulatory Peptides

The kidney may be regarded as a primary or secondary organ for the generation of various hormones and growth factors. Erythropoietin, renin, prostaglandins, and various growth factors are produced by the kidney, which have important local or systemic effects. In addition, the kidney is a site of degradation (metabolism) of hormones, such as insulin and aldosterone. The kidneys are also involved in the metabolism of vitamin D, with the active metabolite of vitamin D_3 produced under the influence of parathyroid hormone.

Erythropoietin

Erythropoietin is largely produced by renal peritubular interstitial cells. Plasma levels of erythropoietin are controlled by a recruitment of additional peritubular cells, rather than increased production by individual cells. Renal hypoxia and androgens cause increased erythropoietin secretion.

Renin

Renin is produced within JG cells after processing and cleavage of prorenin, which is produced in the liver. The primary stimuli for renin release from JG cells include reduction of renal perfusion pressure and hyponatremia. Renin release is also influenced by the sympathetic nervous system, and by endocrine influences including angiotensin II (AII), ADH, endothelin, and prostaglandins. Renin activates AII, which causes secretion of aldosterone by the adrenal cortical zona glomerulosa. The net effect is systemic vasoconstriction, intrarenal vasoconstriction, and increased aldosterone release. The effect of aldosterone is predominantly on the distal tubular network, affecting an increase in sodium reabsorption in exchange for potassium.

Prostaglandins and Cyclooxygenases

The kidney is a major site of prostaglandin (PG) synthesis; it synthetizes prostaglandins (PG) and thromboxanes from arachidonic acid by the cyclooxygenase enzyme system. This enzyme system is present in various cell types, including vascular, glomerular, tubular, and interstitial cells (Figure 11.7). Cyclooxygenase (prostaglandin endoperoxide synthase) catalyzes the committed step in PG biosynthesis. Mammalian cells contain two related, but unique, isozymes, cyclooxygenase-1 (COX-1) and cyclooxygenase-2 (COX-2). COX-1 is primarily expressed constitutively, and is involved in the production of PGs which modulate normal physiologic functions in several organ systems, including the kidneys. COX-2 expression is inducible, and is involved in the production

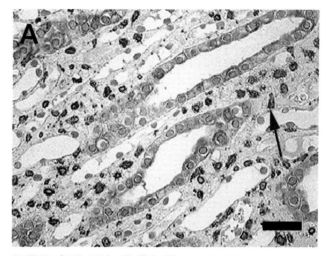
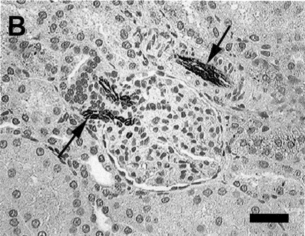
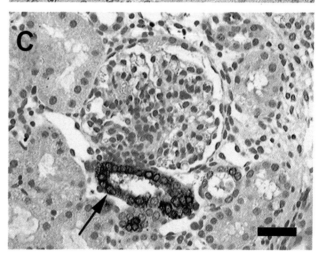

FIGURE 11.7 Immunohistochemical staining showing COX-1 immunoreactive protein in: (A) the collecting ducts, and the papillary interstitial cells (arrow); (B) the efferent and afferent arterioles and a small artery (arrow); and (C) COX-2 immunoreactivity in the macula densa (arrow) in the dog kidney. Bar = 30 μm.

of PGs which modulate physiological events in development, ovulation, cell growth, and inflammation. The predominant cyclooxygenase enzyme activity metabolites are prostacyclin (PGI_2) and prostaglandin E_2 (PGE_2), which play important roles in regulating the physiological action of other hormones on renal vascular tone, mesangial contractility, and tubular processing of salt and water.

Renal Metabolism

Secondary Active Transport

The glucose transporter in the brush border has characteristics typical of carrier-mediated transport, exhibiting saturation kinetics, competitive inhibition, accelerated exchange diffusion, and active transport via Na^+, K^+-ATPase.

Protein and Amino Acid Transport

Of the amino acids in the glomerular filtrate, 99% are actively reabsorbed. This occurs within the first millimeter past the glomerulus in the dog and human; different transport systems are responsible for transport of neutral, acidic, and glycine-shared amino acids.

Proteins of a size up to that of albumin, or slightly larger, enter urine in the glomerular filtrate. Hemoglobin, though of similar size to albumin, enters urine more readily, because of its shape. The absence of hemoglobin in normal urine is predicated on hemoglobin binding to the large protein, haptoglobin.

Protein reabsorption is thought of as a low-affinity, high-capacity, and low-specificity process. Filtered proteins bind to the brush border, and then are taken up by endocytosis. Endocytotic vacuoles then fuse with lysosomes, forming proteinic phagolysosomes, where catabolism occurs. Transport of proteins is affected by size, charge, and configuration. For example, cationic albumin is reabsorbed in a five-fold greater amount than anionic albumin.

Sex differences in protein handling do occur. For example, the female rat reabsorbs more labeled protein, and then degrades the reabsorbed protein more rapidly, than the male in the same unit of time. Proximal tubular cell endopeptidase and exopeptidase activity is greater in the female than in the male rat.

Organic Acid Transport

There are a wide variety of organic acids existing as anions, both endogenous products of catabolism and exogenous substrates, which are transported by the proximal convoluted tubule. Probenecid blocks organic acid transport.

Control of Acid–Base Balance

The kidneys play a very important role in regulation of acid–base balance. Endogenous acid production comes from incomplete metabolism of fats and carbohydrates, from oxidation of sulfur-containing amino acids, and from oxidation and hydrolysis of phosphoprotein residues. The kidneys regulate hydrogen ion concentration by three mechanisms: reabsorption of filtered bicarbonate, secretion of titratable acid, and secretion of ammonia. In the dog, 85% of bicarbonate reabsorption takes place in the proximal tubule. In tubular cells, hydrogen ions are produced by hydration of carbon dioxide. This hydrogen ion is secreted into the tubular lumen in exchange for a sodium ion, leaving sodium and bicarbonate ions behind within the cell. Buffers in the tubular lumen (predominantly monohydrogen phosphate) accept the hydrogen ion, passing down the nephron as a titratable acid.

Renal tubular cells synthesize ammonia by enzymatic deamination of amino acids. Ammonia diffuses down its concentration gradient into the tubular fluid, where it acts as an acceptor of hydrogen ions, forming ammonium ions. The ammonium ion is lipid-insoluble; thus it is trapped in the tubule lumen and excreted in the urine.

Insulin

Plasma insulin concentration is controlled to a great extent by the kidney. After nephrectomy, the removal rate of insulin from the circulation is reduced by approximately 65%. Insulin is reported to directly influence calcium conservation by the kidney.

Fatty Acid Utilization

The kidney extracts and utilizes glucose, lactate, palmitate, citrate, glutamine, and other fatty acids from plasma. Besides the liver, the kidney is the only organ to metabolize glycerol to a major extent. Proximal tubules utilize a variety of substrates for energy metabolism, but fatty acids are preferred. The rate of respiration in the kidney parallels the rate of active transport. The proximal tubule accounts for 70% of all reabsorptive activity in the kidney. Lactate is one of the main metabolic substrates oxidized by the proximal tubules.

Cholesterol Control

Hepatic cholesterologenesis is controlled by negative feedback of the cholesterol precursor mevalonic acid. The kidney plays the dominant role in metabolizing mevalonate by a nonsterol shunt pathway. Thus, renal disease may cause hypercholesterolemia. The female rat metabolizes mevalonate at twice the male rate, thus the male converts more mevalonate to cholesterol than the female.

Xenobiotic Metabolism

Xenobiotic-metabolizing enzymes, including cytochrome P450-dependent mixed-function oxidases, are present in the kidney. Mixed-function oxidase activity occurs in the proximal tubule, primarily in the pars recta or P_3 segment in the rat. Cytochrome P450 content of the kidney is only 10% to 20% of liver content. However, at the cell level, the cells of the pars recta are comparable to hepatocytes in concentration of P450s. Rat renal mixed-function oxidases are not induced by phenobarbital, as in the liver. Polycyclic aromatic hydrocarbons are inducers of rat renal P450 microsomal enzymes. In the rabbit, both phenobarbital and polycyclic aromatic hydrocarbons induce renal mixed-function oxidase activity. Microsomal P450 activity in the rabbit is highest in the P_2 segment of the proximal tubule.

In contrast, fatty acid hydroxylation enzyme activities are greater in the kidney than the liver. During the biosynthesis of prostaglandin, structurally unrelated chemicals may be cooxygenated, as an alternative to the mixed-function oxidase system, as an important mechanism in the metabolic activation of xenobiotics. Induction of metabolizing enzymes in the kidney can lead to elevations in absolute kidney weights.

Xenobiotic Clearance

The liver and kidney are largely responsible for inactivation and excretion of drugs and other chemicals. Clinically, in instances of renal impairment, the clearance of a drug can be compromised, resulting in increased systemic levels with continuing administration, subsequently achieving toxic levels. In drug discovery, physiochemical properties of the drug are recognized to correlate with effective renal clearance. Compounds with low molecular weights, low lipophilicity, and preferentially ionic at pH 7.4 are eliminated effectively. Substances with high molecular weight, protein binding, and lipophilicity, while almost completely nonionic, will be ineffectively cleared, if at all, in the urine.

Adaptation to Demands for Altered Function

The kidney adapts to altered demands by functional and structural changes. Several stimuli are recognized as causes of renal hypertrophy, including administration of increased protein, amino acids, urea, or NaCl. Testosterone treatment, ACTH-mediated hyperadrenocorticism, and diabetes mellitus also cause renal hypertrophy. Xenobiotics metabolized by the kidney can cause renal enlargement, presumably through adaptive increase in metabolizing-enzyme synthesis activity. Biochemically, compensatory hypertrophy leads to an increase in the RNA:DNA ratio. In contrast, this change in RNA:DNA ratio apparently does not occur in renal parenchyma undergoing tissue repair.

MECHANISMS OF TOXICITY

Overview and Classification

General Considerations

Xenobiotic-associated kidney injury typically depends on selective concentration of the toxic moiety at the target cell or subcellular organelle. This concentration is favored by normal function of the kidney. The magnitude of blood flow per gram of renal parenchyma is higher than for any other tissue. Glomerular filtration with tubular reabsorption serves to further concentrate potentially toxic moieties. Tubular transport occurs via protein-binding with endocytosis, via active or passive link with ATP hydrolysis-dependent transport such as the sodium pump, or via organic anion or cation transport. Concomitantly, selective membrane permeability may serve to maintain critical concentrations of molecules concentrated via transport.

The kidney has the capacity to dissociate protein-bound toxicants, such binding serving to protect other tissues from the injurious agent. The kidney also has the capability to alter the pH of tubular fluid, which can serve to transform solutes to a reactive form. Finally, the kidney participates in metabolism of xenobiotics. Renal metabolism with derivation of reactive electrophilic intermediates causes injury following covalent reaction or peroxidatic reaction with the target cell macromolecules.

Classification of Nephrotoxins

Classification According to Functional and Structural Characteristics of the Xenobiotic

Nephrotoxicants can be categorized according to intrinsic structural or functional characteristics of the xenobiotic into one (or more) of the following classes: functional/structural characteristics of the xenobiotic; mechanism of injury; and subtopographical target. This classification has relevance, since members of the class often act through similar mechanisms. Furthermore, this classification serves to help categorize and organize thinking concerning the otherwise exhaustive numbers of individual nephrotoxins. The listing of nephrotoxins by functional class in Table 11.2

TABLE 11.2   Listing and classification of selected nephrotoxicants according to functional characteristics
of the inducing agent

Hemodynamic and prerenal factors
Angiotensin-converting enzyme inhibitors
Hypertension
Cardiotonics
Ischemia
Shock

Proteins and amino acids
Albumin
Alpha$_{2u}$ globulin
Bence–Jones
D-serine
Dietary protein
Hemoglobin
Lysinoalanine
Lysozyme
Maleic acid
Myoglobin

Naturally occurring toxins
Aflatoxin
Ochratoxin A
Citrinin
Aristolochic acid
Bacterial toxins
Monocrotaline
Furan derivatives
Lantana camara
Halogeton
Rhubarb
Isoniazid
Methyldopa
Propanolol
ACTH
Bilirubin
Calcium
Fluoride
Glucose
Iron
Magnesium
Phosphate
Potassium
Sodium
Serotonin
Vitamin D$_2$
Zinc

Physical agents
Electrical shock

Heat stroke
Radiation

Metals
Aluminum
Antimony
Arsenic (organic)
Beryllium
Bismuth
Cadmium
Copper
Gold
Lead
Lithium
Mercuric chloride
Nickel
Rubidium
Trimethyltin
Uranium

Antibiotics/antifungals/ antimalarials
Amikacin
Amoxicillin
Amphotericin B
Bacitracin
Beta-lactam compounds
Cefalexin
Cephaloridine
Ciprofloxacin
Colistin
Erythromycin
Gentamycin
Kanamycin
Netilmicin
Neomycin
Polymixins
Quinadones
Rifampin
Sulfonamides
Streptomycin
Tobramycin
Vancomycin

Osmotic agents and diuretics
Carbonic anhydrase inhibitors
Dextran
Ethacrynic acid
Furosamide
Mannitol

Sucrose
Thiazides
Torasemide

Organic solvents
Carbon tetrachloride
Chloroform
Halogenated aliphatics
Toluene
Trihalomethanes
Trichloroethylene

Synthetic biological toxicants
Fumigants/nematocides
1,2-dibromomethane
1,2-dibromethane-3-chloropropane

Germicides
O-Benzyl-p-chlorophenol

Herbicides
Bipyridium compounds, e.g., paraquat

Insecticides
Chlorinated hydrocarbons
Hexachlorocyclohexane
Organophosphorus compounds
Toxaphene

Gasoline additive
1,2-dichloroethane

Miscellaneous therapeutics
Interferon
IV gamma-globulin
Acyclovir
Aziothioprine
Cimetidine
Foscarnet
Probenicid
Captopril
Clofibrate

Glycols
Diethylene glycol
Diethylene glycol monoethyl
Ethylene dichloride
Ethylene glycol
Ethylene glycol dinitrite
Hexachloro-1,3-butadiene
Organonitriles
Propylene glycol
Acrylonitrile

(*Continued*)

TABLE 11.2 (Continued)

Industrial chemicals
Styrene
Chelators
Diphosphonates (Cl$_2$ MDP, EHDP)
Ethylenediamine tetraacetic acid (EDTA)
Nitrilotriacetic acid (NTA)

Analgesics/anesthetics/ anticonvulsants
Halothane
Methoxyflurane
Carbamazepine
Hydantoin
Heroin
Procacainamide

Cancer therapeutics/ immunosuppressors
Adriamycin

5-azacytidin
Carboplatin
Cisplatin
Cyclophosphamid
Cyclosporin A
Doxorubicin
Gallium nitrate
Ifosfamide
Methotraxate
Mitomycin
Nitosourea
Puromycin
Streptozotocin
Tacrolimus
Vincristine

Diagnostic agents, radiocontrast
Diatrizoate
Iodide

Hyperuricacidemia therapeutics
Allopurinol

Male antifertility agents
α-chlorohydrin

Nonsteroidal anti-inflammatories
Acetaminophen/paracetamol
Ibuprofen
Indomethacin
Naproxen
Meloxican
Phenacetin
Salicylates
Sulindac
Rofecoxib
Fenoprofen
Piroxicam
Tolmeitin

is not considered inclusive. Obscure chemicals or chemicals that cause functional perturbation without overt evidence of morphologic alteration are excluded. This listing emphasizes laboratory and domestic animal nephrotoxicants, although most agents induce comparable injury in all laboratory and higher species. Notable exceptions are addressed in subsequent sections. This listing further primarily considers xenobiotics or agents for which kidney injury occurs as a major toxic host response. More detailed information regarding toxicants causing renal and lower urinary tract injury in domestic animals is shown in Tables 11.3 and 11.4.

Classification According to Mechanism of Injury

Xenobiotics causing kidney injury can also be classified by mechanism in one of the following five categories: xenobiotics directly perturbing cellular or subcellular organelle function; xenobiotics causing injury via reactive intermediates or peroxidative stress; xenobiotics perturbing levels of cellular, interstitial or lumenal substrate; xenobiotics perturbing renal hemodynamics; and xenobiotics eliciting immune-mediated injury.

Classification According to Subtopographical Target

Further subclassification of nephrotoxins occurs by subtopographical, as well as subcellular, organelle target site. Localization of subtopographical and subcellular organelle predilection requires time-course sequence studies with light and electron microscopic evaluation. Target site identification is an integral step in pathogenesis studies. However, simply identifying the target site for a xenobiotic does not identify the mechanism of injury. The following section discusses well-characterized nephrotoxicants based on defined subtopographical and subcellular organelle target site to exemplify specific mechanisms of injury.

Glomerular Injury

Glomerular disease is a major disorder in humans, and the most common cause of chronic renal failure. The glomerulus is a target for nephrotoxicity, because it is the first to see the xenobiotic, because filtration is its major role, and because of hemodynamics. Xenobiotics can directly affect any of the components

TABLE 11.3　Selected toxicants causing renal and lower urinary tract toxicity in domestic animals

Category	Type of toxicant	Toxic agent	Source of toxicant	Source of contamination	Species affected	Lesions	Other organ systems affected/disease	Mechanism
Natural toxins	Mycotoxins	Ochratoxin	*Penicillium ochraceus* and *Aspergillus verrucosum*	Contaminated grain, grapes, coffee, pork products	All species susceptible, pigs most commonly exposed	Tubular degeneration/necrosis, proximal tubules; interstitial fibrosis (porcine nephropathy); carcinogenesis experimentally	Immune suppression	Electrophile, cytochrome P450 bioactivation; proapoptotic
		Citrinin	*Penicillium* and *Aspergillus* spp.	Contaminated grain	All species susceptible, pigs most commonly exposed	Tubular degeneration/necrosis		Mitochondrial effects and inhibition of respiration
	Plants and plant toxins	Oxalic acid, sodium and potassium oxalates	Halogeton (*Halogeton glomeratus*), greasewood (*Sarcobatus vermiculatus*), rhubarb (*Rheum rhaponticum*), sorrel, dock (*Rumex* sp.), lamb quarters (*Chenopodium* spp.)	Weeds	Ruminants mostly, pigs	Tubular degeneration/necrosis, oxalate crystals	Rumenitis in sheep	Oxalates complex with calcium and precipitate causes physical damage
		Pigweed (*Amaranthus retroflexus*)		Weed	Pigs, calves	Tubular degeneration/necrosis; perirenal edema		
		Red maple (*Acer rubrum*)			Horses	Tubular degeneration/necrosis; hemoglobin casts	Hematopoietic	Intravascular hemolysis causes ischemic tubular necrosis augmented by hemoglobin casts
		Vetch (*Vicia* spp.)		Pasture legume	Cattle mainly, horses rarely	Esinophilic granulomatous nephritis	Any organ	

Category	Toxic principle	Source	Type	Species affected	Lesion	Target organ	Mechanism
	1,25-dihydroxy-vitamin D glycoside	Cestrum diurnum, Solanum spp., Trisetum spp.	Weed	All susceptible, ruminants and horses most common	Tubular degeneration/necrosis, mineralization	Stomach, lung, bone	Renal ischemia from vasoconstriction and mitochondrial calcification
		Lilium spp. e.g., Easter lily	Ornamentals, cut flowers	Cats only	Tubular degeneration/necrosis; proximal tubules	Pancreas	
	Ptaquiloside	Brackern fern (Pteridium aquilinum/esculentum)	Weed, native fern	Cattle (enzootic hematuria)	Necrosis and hemorrhage, urinary bladder; neoplasia	Bone marrow, GI	
		Sorghum spp.	Forage crops and escapes	Horses (equine cystitis ataxia syndrome), uncommon	Necrosis and hemorrhage, urinary bladder	CNS	Hydrocyanic acid and nitrates present but mechanism unknown
	Pyrrolizidine alkaloids	Senecio, Crotalaria, Heliotropium, Echium, Amsinckia, Cynoglossum spp.	Pasture or grain contaminated by seed	Horses, cattle, pigs. All susceptible	Tubular degeneration/necrosis, megalocytosis of tubular and glomerular cells	Liver mainly, lung possible Secondary: hepatoencephalopathy, photosensitization	Electrophile, cytochrome P450 bioactivation
	Triterpenes, lantadenes A and B	Lantana camara	Weed, ornamentals	All grazing animals except horses	Proximal tubular degeneration/necrosis	Liver mainly, heart; secondary photosensitization	
	Gallotannins, polyhydroxyphenolic compounds and metabolites	Oaks (Quercus spp.)	Leaves, buds, or acorns	All grazing animals, cattle most common	Tubular degeneration/necrosis; perirenal edema	GI tract, developmental	
Insects	Cantharidin	Blister beetle (Epicauta spp.)	Alfalfa hay	All susceptible; horses mainly exposed, also cattle	Necrosis, urinary bladder	GI tract, heart	
Snake venom		Crotalid snakes (rattlesnakes, water moccasins, copperheads)		All susceptible	Mesangiolysis (glomeruli); tubular necrosis	Local tissue necrosis, hematologic and CNS effects in some cases	

(Continued)

TABLE 11.3   (Continued)

Category	Type of toxicant	Toxic agent	Source of toxicant	Source of contamination	Species affected	Lesions	Other organ systems affected/disease	Mechanism
Metals		Mercury, inorganic salts	Environmental	Industrial	All susceptible	Proximal tubular degeneration/necrosis	CNS with organic mercury	Inhibits mitochondrial enzymes, thus uncoupling of oxidative phosphorylation; binds to free sulfhydryl groups depleting glutathione
		Lead	Batteries, paint, gasoline	Industrial	All susceptible	Proximal tubular degeneration/necrosis, intranuclear inclusion bodies, karyomegaly	CNS, hematopoietic, reproductive	Binds to free sulfhydryl groups depleting glutathione; also other mechanisms
		Arsenic	Environmental, pesticide, feed additive	Industrial, pest control	All susceptible	Tubular degeneration/necrosis; medullary necrosis (dogs)	GI tract, vascular; CNS with some organic arsenicals	Interacts with sulfhydryl enzymes, resulting in disruption of cellular metabolism; arsenate can uncouple oxidation and phosphorylation
		Copper	Anthelmintics, pesticides, foot baths, feed additives	Dietary supplements, environmental	Ruminants (especially sheep), all susceptible	Tubular degeneration/necrosis; hemoglobinuric and bile nephrosis (gunmetal kidney)	All species: liver necrosis Ruminants: intravascular hemolysis. Non-ruminants: gastric ulcers	Free radical
		Cadmium	Environmental	Industrial	All susceptible	Proximal tubular degeneration/necrosis	Bone, testes	Free radical injury by cadmium released from metallothionein in lysosomes of renal tubular cells

Food	Food additives/supplements	Vitamin D₃		Oversupplementation, improper mixing	All species; horses, pigs mostly	Tubular degeneration/necrosis, mineralization	Vascular system, bone	Renal ischemia from vasoconstriction and mitochondrial calcification
	Fruit	Grapes, raisins			Dogs only	Tubular degeneration/necrosis		
		Melamine and cyanuric acid	Plastics/resin industry	Contaminated pet food	Dogs, cats	Distal tubular degeneration/necrosis, melamine-cyanuric acid crystals		Crystal precipitates from melamine-cyanuric acid complexes which damage renal tubules
Chemicals	Other	Ethylene glycol	Antifreeze	Automotive use, contaminated products	All species, dogs, cats most common	Proximal tubular degeneration/necrosis, oxalate crystals		Metabolized by alcohol dehydrogenase to metabolites including oxalate, which complexes with calcium and precipitates as crystals that damage tubules
		Pine oil	Cleaners and disinfectants	Household products	Cats	Tubular degeneration/necrosis	Liver	
		Carbon tetrachloride	Anthelmintic, cleaning agents	Household products	All susceptible	Tubular degeneration/necrosis	Liver	Free radical, cytochrome P450 bioactivation
		Paraquat	Herbicide	Agricultural, household	All susceptible	Tubular degeneration/necrosis	Lung	
		Vitamin D	Calciferol in rodenticide (quintox)	Pest control	All susceptible, dogs, cats most common	Tubular degeneration/necrosis, mineralization	Lung, stomach, vasculature	Renal ischemia from vasoconstriction and mitochondrial calcification

TABLE 11.4   Selected drugs causing renal and lower urinary tract toxicity in domestic animals

Category	Drug	Species affected	Toxicity	Mechanism of toxicity	Other organs affected
Anti-inflammatory, analgesics	Phenyl butazone, flunixin meglumine	Horses, cattle	Papillary necrosis	Inhibition of prostaglandin synthesis and vasoconstriction	Gastrointestinal (GI) tract
	Some NSAIDS, analgesics (e.g., aspirin, carprofen, ibuprofen, naproxen, diclofenac)	Dogs, cats, vultures	Tubular degeneration/ necrosis, papillary necrosis occasionally in dogs	Electrophile, bioactivation in some cases	Liver, GI tract in some cases
Antineoplastics	Cisplatin	Dog	Tubular degeneration/ necrosis	Metabolic activation, affects cell respiration; proapoptotic	Intestinal tract, bone marrow
	Cyclophosphamide	Dog	Urinary bladder hemorrhage and necrosis	Cytochrome P450 bioactivation, acrolein is active metabolite; proapoptotic	
Antimicrobials	Aminoglycosides: gentamycin, neomycin, kanamycin, streptomycin, tobramycin	All species including snakes	Proximal tubular necrosis	Lysosomal injury; oxidative stress	
	Tetracyclines	All species	Tubular degeneration		Teeth and bone (in young), liver occasionally
	Cyclosporine (immunosuppressive agent)	Dogs, cats	Acute tubular necrosis Vasculopathy Glomerulopathy Chronic nephropathy with interstitial fibrosis		Immune system
	Sulfonamides	Ruminants	Tubular degeneration, crystals on gross examination	Crystal formation	
Antifungals	Amphotericin B	Dogs, cats	Tubular necrosis	Vasoconstriction	

of the glomerulus, including visceral epithelial cells (podocytes), endothelial cells (e.g., cyclosporine A), mesangial cells, and the basement membrane. They can also alter blood flow, and induce immune-mediated reactions which can indirectly affect the glomerulus.

Direct Xenobiotic Perturbation of Cell or Subcellular Organelle Function

Changes in Polyanionic Binding Sites in the Glomerular Filtration Barrier

Protamine (a heparin antagonist) induces charge reduction in the glomerular filtration barrier, followed by functional evidence of injury, manifested as proteinuria. Fixed polyanionic-binding sites in the filtration barrier serve to retain anionic plasma proteins such as albumin in the circulation. Otherwise, nontoxic doses of circulating polycationic agents such as protamine cause protein leakage, which secondarily induces morphologic lesions. Podocyte injury in this model is a consequence of albuminuric or protein overload.

Interference in Formation of Cross-links in Glomerular Basement Membrane Collagen

D-penicillamine affects glomerular basement membrane directly in rats, possibly by interfering with collagen cross-link formation. D-penicillamine is used in the treatment of rheumatoid arthritis. Adverse effects of the drug include development of membranous glomerulonephritis as an apparent consequence of defective basement membrane synthesis.

Glomerular Podocyte (Visceral Epithelial) Injury

The target site for puromycin aminonucleoside (a cancer chemotherapeutic) nephrosis has been critically examined, with detailed sequential ultrastructural evaluation of glomeruli in a daily low-dose rat model. The earliest change occurs as effacement of podocytic foot processes by broad expanses of epithelial cytoplasm, followed by proteinuria. With persistent proteinuria, puromycin induces focal segmental glomerulosclerosis. Adriamycin (following metabolism) and histamine receptor antagonists also damage the epithelial cells and induce proteinuria.

Mesangiolysis

Mesangiolysis, capillary endothelial cell loss, and glomerular capillary cysts (aneurysms) occur as acute phase responses to snake venom, croton oil, glomerular ischemia, hypertension, hemolytic–uremia syndrome, thrombotic thrombocytopenic purpura, transplant rejection, radiation, and immune-mediated glomerulonephritis (Figure 11.8). Hemolytic–uremia syndrome represents a serious complication of bacterial endotoxemia. Hemolytic–uremia is characterized by leukocyte-mediated intravascular fibrin deposition in, and occlusion of, glomerular capillaries, with resultant renal cortical necrosis (generalized Schwartzman reaction model). Drugs such as cyclosporin, mitomycin-C, and estrogen-containing contraceptives have been identified as risk factors for hemolytic–uremia in humans.

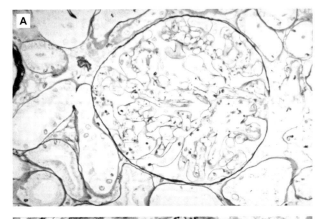

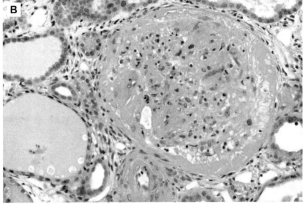

FIGURE 11.8 Mesangiolysis. (A) Early stage of thrombotic microangiopathy in a dog. Silver stain. (Courtesy of Drs B. Harmon and C. Brown, University of Georgia.) (B) Florid lesions of malignant hypertension in a SHR rat treated with DOCA. Salt-loading lesions are characterized by fibrinoid necrosis of the arterioles and glomerular tuft, caused by sustained diastolic pressure exceeding 110 mm Hg.

Reactive Intermediates and Oxidative Stress

The current hypothesis for reactive oxygen intermediate (ROI)-induced damage is that these compounds are formed at rates that far exceed the capacity of the cellular antioxidant defense mechanisms. ROI have been implicated in the pathogenesis of inflammatory, immune, and toxic insults in glomerular injury.

With continuous treatment, cytotoxic properties of adriamycin may arise from metabolism to a quinone, by prostaglandin endoperoxide synthetase present in the glomerular tuft endothelial cells. An electron reduction, catalyzed by flavoenzymes such as NADPH- cytochrome and P450 reductase, produces semiquinone electrophilic intermediates, with covalent binding and injury, or production of superoxide anions, with transformation into the more deleterious oxygen species, the hydroxyl radical and singlet oxygen.

Perturbation of Levels of Cellular, Interstitial, or Luminal Substrate

Diabetic hyperglycemia is associated with glomerular and mesangial basement membrane thickening, characteristics of diabetic glomerulopathy. Glycosylation of basement membrane protein proportional to the level of glucose in the local environment has been hypothesized as a mechanism of the basement membrane injury. Xenobiotics perturbing glucose levels could thus potentially act through such a mechanism.

Perturbation of Renal Hemodynamics

Increased Glomerular Filtration Rate

Persistent elevation of glomerular capillary flow causes glomerular injury, characterized by mesangial expansion and proteinuria, progressing to focal glomerular sclerosis. Two interrelated, but potentially independently-acting, hemodynamic functional alterations causing injury include increase in single nephron glomerular filtration rate (SNGFR), and increase in glomerular capillary hydraulic pressure (GCHP). Increased SNGFR and GCHP can be induced by deoxycorticosterone injection, and by saline as the drinking water source, which is a model for inducing hypertension.

Increased transglomerular traffic of plasma protein would be expected to occur in the hyperfiltering nephron with increased SNGFR or GCHP. Protein overload of the glomerular filtration barrier is considered a mediator of the glomerular injury in hypertension. Concomitantly, increased capillary network hydraulic pressure may mechanically injure the glomerular capillary structure. A low protein diet prevents the increase in SNGFR and GCHP, and thus protects the hypertensive rat from developing injury (proteinuria and glomerular morphologic alteration, Figure 11.8B). Decrease in dietary protein in the normal rat leads to decreased SNGFR and GCHP. Dietary protein plays an important role in the development and progression of kidney injury. An increase in dietary protein can cause an increase in kidney size and GFR, with subsequent glomerular injury, accumulation of mesangial deposits, and, eventually, glomerulosclerosis.

Associated at least in part with protein overnutrition, chronic progressive nephropathy (CPN) occurs in nearly all two-year-old male laboratory rats (see below), with female rats less affected. These lesions are substantially reduced by limiting either protein or total diet consumption. Humans also have glomerular sclerosis of 10% to 30% of nephrons between the fourth and eighth decades of life.

Reduction in renal mass also results in increases in SNGFR and GCHP in the parenchyma, as a compensatory response to maintain renal function. Reduction in renal mass results in nephron injury morphologically similar to that associated with hypertension and protein overnutrition. Reduction of dietary protein significantly reduces the severity and rate of progression of disease in the remnant parenchyma.

Reduced renal mass with individual nephron hyperfiltration, subsequent mesangial expansion, and sclerosis with further nephron loss thus represents the final common pathway to progressive renal failure, regardless of the primary injury mechanism (Figure 11.9). Restriction of dietary protein is correspondingly universally beneficial in ameliorating chronic progressive kidney disease, regardless of instigating factors.

Decreased Glomerular Filtration Rate

Cyclosporin may cause renal toxicity via signal transduction. Transmembrane signal transduction refers to the process whereby a ligand binds to the external surface of the cell and, without necessarily penetrating the cell membrane, elicits a physiological response specific for that hormone and cell type. Cyclosporine, used in transplant patients to prevent rejection, causes two forms of toxicity. The first is an acute decrement in the glomerular filtration rate which is reversible on cessation of treatment, possibly mediated by endothelin receptor binding. Cyclosporin markedly augments the glomerular vasoconstrictor response to vasoactive hormones. Thus, cyclosporin induces an unfavorable perturbation in transmembrane signaling response, serving as a prototype for a transmembrane signaling disorder. The second form of toxicity is a chronic and reversible attrition of nephron function following chronic exposure. It is believed that episodes of acute vascular effect, when sustained, eventuate in a chronic form of tubulointerstitial disease in humans. The chronic disease is characterized by striped areas of tubulointerstitial fibrosis, tubular atrophy, and efferent arteriolopathy, beginning in the outer medulla, with extension to the medullary rays.

Immune-mediated Injury

A plethora of therapeutics has been associated with immune-mediated renal injury in humans (Table 11.5). Immune-mediated kidney injury accounts for most forms of primary glomerular disease, and many secondary glomerular disorders. There are two major

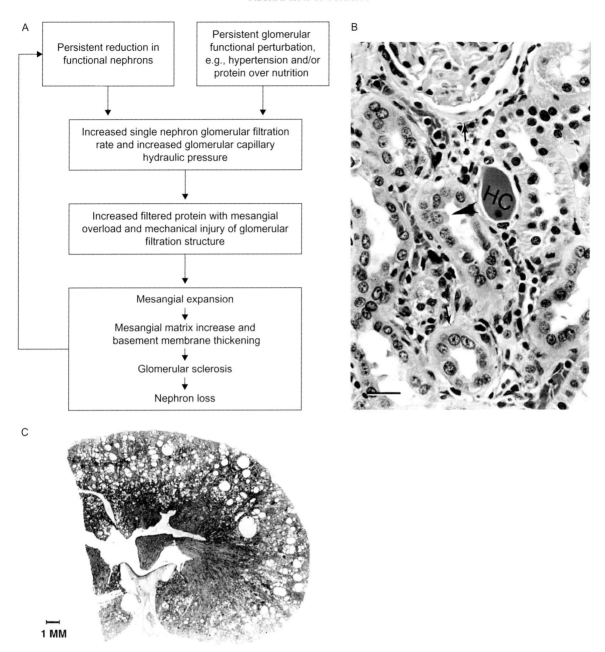

FIGURE 11.9   (A) Pathogenesis of chronic progressive nephropathy. (B) Kidney of a 2-year-old Sprague–Dawley rat, illustrating the hallmarks of chronic progressive nephropathy, including hyaline casts (HC), thickened basement membrane (arrows), and regenerative proximal tubular epithelium (arrowhead). Interstitial inflammatory cells are also present (Bar = 32 μm). (C) Subgross photomicrograph of kidney of a 2-year-old Sprague–Dawley rat illustrating cystic changes in severe chronic progressive nephropathy. Bar = 1 mm.

forms of immune-mediated glomerular disease. The first consists of injury by antibody reacting *in situ* within the glomerulus, either with insoluble fixed (intrinsic) glomerular antigen, or with molecules planted within the glomerulus (either exogenous, such as drugs, or endogenous). The second form involves

injury from deposition of circulating antigen antibody complexes in the glomeruli.

Drug-associated immune-mediated kidney injury represents an important differential etiologic diagnosis for all renal diseases in humans. Xenobiotic-associated immune-mediated renal disease in humans typically

TABLE 11.5 Xenobiotic-induced immunologically mediated renal injury in humans

Membranous glomerulonephritis

Gold salts, mercurials, D-penicillamine, captopril

Nephrotic syndrome with minimal glomerular change

Lithium, NSAIDs, rifamcin

Immunologically mediated glomerulonephritis

Hydantoin, mephenytoin, heroin, hydralazine (lupus), interferon

Immunologically mediated acute interstitial nephritis without the nephrotic syndrome

Antibiotics, including penicillin derivatives, most notably methicillin and cyprofloxacin, cephalosporins, tetracyclines, rifamcin, eythromycin, and vancomycin

Sulfonamides, including sulfasalazine

Diuretics, including chlorothiazide, chlorthalidone, cyclothiazide, furosemide, hydrochlorothiazide, tienilic acid, and triamterene

Analgesics, most prominently clometacin, but also including antipyrine, aminopyrine, antrafeine, flactafenine, glaphenine, noramidopyrine, paracetamol, and sulphinpyrazone

Other therapeutics, most prominently cimetidine, but also including allopurinol, carbamazepine, clofibrate, captopril, and diphenylhydantoin

is expressed in a relatively small percentage of exposed individuals. Additionally, a substantial number of drugs associated with immune-mediated kidney injury in humans depend on host factor variability for expression, as well as interaction with pre-existing disease. A few industrial and environmental chemicals have also been implicated, by association, in development of immune-mediated kidney disease, such as Goodpasture's syndrome. Mercurials and drugs with a sulfhydryl group, such as gold salts, penicillamine and captopril, are associated with membranous glomerulopathy. Immune-mediated renal disease is not recognized as a significant xenobiotic-induced spontaneous disease in domestic animals.

Proximal Tubular Injury

The propensity of the proximal tubule to injury is due to its reliance on oxidative metabolism, high concentration of cytochrome P450 enzymes and beta-lyases, and reabsorption and active secretion function. The proximal tubule is a major site for xenobiotic injury, and is the most common target of nephrotoxicants in domestic animals. Proximal tubular toxicants frequently affect both convoluted and straight segments, although these segments may be differentially affected.

A xenobiotic may be metabolized in the kidney to a reactive intermediate. Cells of the pars recta contain a much greater proportion of smooth endoplasmic reticulum than any other portion of the nephron. Phase I reactions involve oxidation, reduction, or hydrolysis to produce more water-soluble metabolites facilitating excretion. In Phase II metabolism, conjugation occurs, e.g., with glutathione. The same family of enzymes responsible for metabolism, detoxification, and excretion may catalyze the metabolic activation. Thus, the outer stripe (pars recta) is typically the primary site of injury for xenobiotics acting via metabolic activation; the PCT is often also affected.

Reactive intermediates at sufficiently high levels may react with critical cellular targets, leading to toxicity. Electrophiles may bind covalently, and cause irreversible inactivation of protein, DNA, RNA, and lipid macromolecules. To protect against covalent binding, cells possess high concentrations of thiols, primarily glutathione for the conjugation of reactive intermediates. However, these thiols can become depleted, leading to reactive metabolite covalent binding to critical biomacromolecules. In addition, certain xenobiotics that are metabolized to sulfur containing metabolites conjugated with glutathione can be further metabolized to cysteine S-conjugates, and then further metabolized by cysteine conjugate β-lyases to reactive thiols. Xenobiotic injury via this β-lyase pathway is also preferentially expressed in the outer stripe. The metabolism to cysteine conjugates may occur in the liver with transport, uptake, and injury in the pars recta, the site of the highest concentration of the beta-lyase activity.

In addition to cell metabolism, in considering proximal tubule toxicity, the organic acid–base transporters must be considered. Several xenobiotics require transport as an organic ion to initiate cell injury, including cephalosporin antibiotics, critinin, mercuric anion, and cysteine conjugates. The organic anion transporter has been the most characterized, and may be the most important, relevant to renal toxicity. This transporter is localized in the basolateral and apical margin of cells at all levels of the proximal tubule, but in higher levels in P3 in the rabbit. Organic anion transport is presumed to be involved in the transport of important proximal tubule nutrient substrates such as succinate. p-Aminohippuric acid (PAH) represents a model organic anion in the study of this transporter. Transport of PAH is inhibited by organic anions such as probenecid and penicillin. PAH and probenecid reduce toxicity of drugs requiring transport as an organic anion in mechanistic studies. Mepiperphenidol, quinine, and quinidine have been used as inhibitors of organic base transport. Organic ion transporters in the kidney and liver are now recognized as linked to the multidrug resistant gene plaguing the efficacy of chemotherapeutics through a role in drug efflux, evidenced by the overexpression of p-glycoproteins. Numerous interactions of clinical importance occur through interference in clearance dependent on organic ion transporters, such as cimetadine reducing zidovudine elimination. Furthermore, creatine clearance can be reduced by organic anions, simulating nephrotoxicity in the absence of renal injury.

Finally, relevant to expression of injury in the proximal tubule, the unique portal system must be considered. There is a marked cortical medullary gradient in oxygen tension, with relative hypoxia in the outer medulla. This is related to the lower medullary blood flow, the countercurrent exchange of oxygen, and the high metabolic requirements of the thick ascending limb and pars recta. Blood flow to the outer stripe is postglomerular. The number of mitochondria is significantly lower in the P3 segment compared to the P1 and P2 segments. The outer stripe is the most sensitive in the rat kidney to hypoxia, and is a site for synergism between toxicity and hypoperfusion. Synergism between compromised perfusion and toxicity occurs clinically because the majority of cases of human drug-induced nephrotoxicity occur in the presence of compromised renal perfusion.

The following discussion regarding the five basic mechanistic categories across the proximal tubule will draw on selected xenobiotic injury for which substantial knowledge of pathogenesis exists. Through this approach, understanding of potential mechanisms, as well as morphologic findings correlating with different mechanisms, should be expanded. The proximal convoluted tubule contains a very active endocytosis/lysosomal apparatus, thus representing the site of injury related to the lysosomal overload, as well as protein-bound toxic moieties. It must also be noted that tubular epithelial cells are also very sensitive to ischemia which may accompany direct xenobiotic induced tubular injury.

Direct Perturbation of Cell or Subcellular Organelle Function

Aminoglycoside Antibiotic Lysosomal Overload

Renal toxicity of the aminoglycoside antimicrobials such as gentamycin, neomycin, kanamycin, tobramycin, amikacin, and streptomycin, correlates with the concentration of the compound in the renal cortex, with neomycin being the most toxic. Gentamycin, a prototypical aminoglycoside antibiotic, has a low molecular weight, binds only weakly to plasma proteins, and is freely cleared into the glomerular filtrate as the primary route of excretion. Serum half-life is inversely correlated with GFR. Serum half-life is 30 minutes with normal GFR. Within minutes after administration, intense binding of drug to brush border can be demonstrated. This binding is specific, and receptor-mediated. A charge interaction exists between cationic sites on the gentamycin molecule and anionic sites on the brush border. Propensity for binding phospholipids, charge, and toxic potential are strongly correlated when comparing different aminoglycoside antibiotics. After binding, gentamycin is taken into the cell by endocytosis, followed by fusion of the endocytic vesicles with phagosomes. Within the phagolysosome, gentamycin inhibits phospholipases and sphingomyelinase responsible for degradation of phospholipid-rich cell membranes. Thus, the drug and phospholipid membranes are sequestered and accumulate in the phagolysosome. This phenomenon is reflected ultrastructurally by the appearance of myeloid bodies. This process occurs at all levels of the proximal tubule, with predilection for the PCT. Since calcium competes with gentamicin for binding sites, calcium loading ameliorates gentamycin toxicity.

Lysosomal overload of gentamicin and phospholipid membranes results in compromised lysosomal membrane integrity, and lysosomal enzyme leakage occurs. This may explain cell necrosis as the overt manifestation of toxicity. There is also evidence for oxidative stress in gentamycin-induced tubular injury.

Heavy Metals

Heavy metals typically injure the proximal tubule, while some can also affect the glomerulus and the vascular system. They typically accumulate in the kidney, liver, bone, and brain. The spectrum of heavy metal renal effects, as well as pathogenesis, can be appreciated by considering the effect of cadmium, inorganic mercury, and lead. Other heavy metals, such as thallium and arsenic, are less studied, but share features of injury with one or more of these three.

Cadmium

Cadmium is a widespread environmental and occupational contaminant. Upon uptake from digestive or respiratory portals of entry, cadmium binds to albumin and other high molecular weight proteins. It is taken up by the liver, binds to the low molecular weight metal transport protein, metallothionein, and is then released into the bloodstream.

Plasma levels of cadmium bound to metallothionein (6500 Da) remain low, since this complex passes freely into the glomerular filtrate. The complex is reabsorbed, as are many low molecular weight proteins, in the proximal tubules by endocytosis. Metallothionein is hydrolyzed in the phagolysosome, releasing cadmium, which stimulates metallothionein synthesis *de novo*. Cadmium (Cd^{2+}) rapidly binds newly-synthesized or reabsorbed metallothionein. The renal toxicity of cadmium occurs on the intralysosomal release of free ligand, which may also interact with proteins other than metallothionein. Cadmium accumulates in the kidney, bound to metallothionein, in a time- and dose-responsive manner. A biological half-life in the human is approximately 10 years.

Threshold levels of cadmium must accumulate prior to induction of overt tubular injury. The threshold varies widely in experimental animals, from 10–200 μg Cd/g wet weight, because of variations in dose rate, route, and form of cadmium administered. Impaired reabsorption of beta$_2$-microglobulin is a sensitive marker of cadmium injury to the proximal tubule. The earliest ultrastructural alteration of cadmium toxicity occurs as phagolysosomal change. Tubular necrosis, or an increase in the incidence or severity of lesions of CPN, characterizes the light microscopic changes in cadmium injury in the rat. The mechanism of Cd^{2+}-effect on the proximal tubular cell involves free radical damage. Cadmium induced chronic renal failure in humans can result in osteoporosis with spontaneous fractures (Itai–Itai disease). Multiparous women are most susceptible.

Mercury

As with cadmium, the toxic potential of mercury depends on dose rate, form, and route of administration. Toxicity of the inorganic salts is quantitatively different than organic mercurials, because of differential solubility. Mercury salts are most nephrotoxic. Organic mercury intoxication can lead to central nervous system injury. Environmental contamination of Minamata Bay in Japan with industrial waste containing mercury led to the name Minamata disease. Chronic mercurial nephrotoxicity in humans today is almost always a consequence of chronic occupational exposure. Acute mercury poisoning represents a classical cause of proximal tubular cell necrosis. This response preferentially occurs in the pars recta, but with increased time and dose, affects all segments.

Mercuric ions enter the proximal tubular cells from both the luminal and peritubular sides, and initially concentrate in the endoplasmic reticulum. The mechanism of proximal tubular cell injury traditionally has centered on uncoupling of oxidative phosphorylation in mitochondria, and mercury does inhibit mitochondrial enzymes. Furthermore, this mechanism is consistent with subtopographical localization in pars recta, the site of predilection for hypoxic injury.

As with other heavy metals, mercury also reacts with free sulfhydryl groups, and thus leads to depletion of glutathione. As with cadmium, peroxidative processes also can be considered a cause underlying tubular cell injury. Male rats are significantly more sensitive to mercury-induced tubular cell injury; this is associated with correlative sex differences in renal levels of sulfhydryl groups. Mercuric chloride-induced nephrotoxicity has been used as a model to suggest that toxicologic evaluations conducted only at the end of a subchronic study may significantly underestimate nephrotoxic potential. In the acute phase of treatment, overt tubular necrosis and functional evidence of renal failure occur. In subchronic exposures (20 to 90 days) functional indices may return to normal. However, histopathologic evidence of regeneration and repair persist, so the antecedent injury must be recognized.

Chronic exposure of the rat to mercury results in increased incidence and severity of lesions of CPN. Chronic mercury poisoning has been reported to occur because of immune-mediated mechanisms of injury resulting in glomerulonephritis. These reports of immune-mediated renal injury in chronic mercury poisoning fail to differentiate chronic cytotoxicity with an expected secondary immune-mediated component in the spectrum of injury from a primary immune complex disease, independent of cytotoxicity.

Lead

Rapid and selective accumulation of lead occurs in the kidney, initially isolated to the cytosolic fraction of proximal tubular epithelium. Lead is highly reactive with the sulfhydryl group of two cytosolic proteins having molecular weights of 11 500 and 63 000 Da; this accounts for the accumulation. These high-affinity lead-binding proteins regulate the bioavailability of lead, as well as transport into the nucleus. These two proteins are also shown to be present in the brain. Lead pretreatment results in a 30–40% decrease in binding of lead to renal mitochondria. Renal toxicity is reduced through this specific cytosolic protein binding.

Acute or subchronic lead nephrotoxicity is characterized by the presence of intranuclear inclusions in proximal tubular epithelial cells in most species. In the kidney, 80% to 90% lead is concentrated in nuclei, suggesting that the intranuclear inclusions represent a storage site. Extrusion of the nuclear inclusion into the cytoplasm, and increasing tubular lysosomal activity, may represent a sequence of lead metabolism by the proximal tubule. Cytoplasmic lead can bind to mitochondria, inhibiting mitochondrial respiration, with resultant mitochondrial swelling as a potential mechanism of injury. Acute lead exposure is also characterized by increased apoptotic necrosis and proximal tubular cell replication. This stimulated replication may be related to the carcinogenic potential of lead in the rat. Karyomegaly is a sensitive morphologic indication of lead toxicity in the rat, and has been noted in other species. Chronic lead exposure may lead to increased incidence and severity of lesions of CPN in rats, or induction of CPN in humans. Chronic exposure at dosages which show cytomegaly and karyomegaly is associated with eventual tubular tumor formation in the rat. Lead exposure in humans does not appear to represent a risk for renal tumorigenesis.

In domestic animals, spontaneous lead toxicosis is associated with exposures to batteries and other vehicle components (mainly calves), as well as lead-based paints (calves, dogs, zoo animals). Acute exposure may be associated with nephrotoxicity, with typical intranuclear inclusion bodies within tubular epithelial cells. These stain with a modified acid-fast stain (Figure 11.10). Polioencephalomalacia may be a more common manifestation of lead toxicosis in calves. Hematopoietic and reproductive toxicity may occur with lead toxicity.

Xenobiotics Which Cause Injury via Metabolic Activation

Organohalides

The kidney is the primary target organ for toxic organohalides. Organohalides form a class bridging three functional categories: synthetic biologic toxicants; organic solvents; and chemicals involved in plastics and resin manufacturing. A significant portion of the American population is chronically exposed to small amounts of these chemicals in water. The acute necrotizing effects (Figure 11.11), as well as teratogenic and carcinogenic effects at high doses in the laboratory animal, are dependent on conversion of the parent compound to toxic metabolites. Species, sex, and tissue differences in susceptibility to injury are

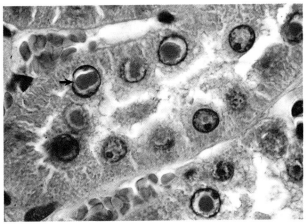

FIGURE 11.10 Nephrosis, lead toxicosis, kidney, cortex, rat. Acid-fast intranuclear inclusion bodies (arrow) present in the proximal convoluted tubular epithelium are diagnostic of lead poisoning. Acid-fast stain with H&E counterstain. (Courtesy of Dr J. King, College of Veterinary Medicine, Cornell University; From Newman, S.J., Confer, A.W., and Panciera, R.J. (2007). Urinary System. In *Pathologic Basis of Veterinary Disease* (McGavin, M., and Zachary, J.F., eds), 4th edn, Fig 11-41, p. 654. Mosby Elsevier, St. Louis, MO.)

expected, related to differences in pharmacokinetic behavior of the specific chemical.

Chlorine disinfection of drinking water results in the formation of trihalomethanes, primarily chloroform. Chloroform is considered a prototypical organohalide; its mechanism of injury has been extensively studied. Renal metabolism of chloroform results in derivation of phosgene as the potential reactive intermediate.

Covalent adduct formation with DNA may be causally associated with the hepatic and renal carcinogenic potential of chloroform in the rat. Phosgene depletes renal glutathione, subsequently initiating an autocatalytic peroxidative degradation of membranes. Glutathione conjugation with the injurious chloroform metabolite reduces or prevents covalent binding with tissue macromolecules.

Cephalosporins

Cephalosporins and other β-lactam antibiotics cause proximal tubular necrosis in humans and laboratory animals. Selective toxicity to the PCT occurs because of high intracellular concentrations achieved by active transport by the organic anion transporter. PCTs represent the segment of the nephron with greatest organic anion transport activity. Cephaloridine, as a model cephalosporin, is metabolized in the proximal convoluted tubular cell and, at sufficiently high concentrations, induces lipid-peroxidation-type injury to membranes via oxidative stress.

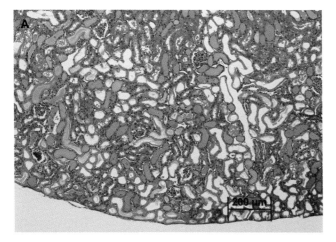

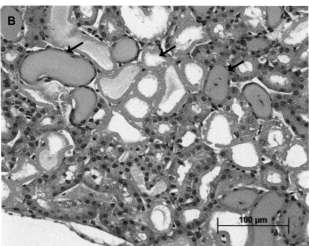

FIGURE 11.11   Tubular epithelial necrosis primarily affecting the pars recta in a male mouse kidney 24 hours after treatment with a single dose of carbon tetrachloride (0.25 ml/kg). (A) Dilated tubules often contain hyaline casts. (B) Tubular epithelium is absent or markedly attenuated (arrows) and hyaline casts often fill the lumen.

Mycotoxins

Mycotoxins represent an important class of xenobiotics which cause renal injury in humans and food animals. Ochratoxin A, an organic anion, causes proximal tubular injury which first appears as cytoplasmic vacuolation with phagolysosomal hydropic swelling and myelin figure formation, followed by tubular necrosis. Ochratoxin A is an important cause of chronic renal disease in swine, often in combination with citrinin. Ochratoxin A is actively transported via the organic anion transporter, resulting in tubular accumulation. Ochratoxin A is metabolized to a reactive intermediate, and is a renal carcinogen in laboratory rodents.

Plant Toxins

Endemic (Balkan) nephropathy (EN) is an important human disease in Eastern Europe, characterized by chronic tubulointerstitial disease with increased incidence of upper urinary tract transitional cell (urothelial) carcinoma. Although ochratoxin A was believed to play a central role in this disease, recent studies suggest that dietary exposure to aristolochic acid (AA) is responsible. Aristolochic acid is present in the seeds of *Aristolochia* spp., with *A. clematitis*, which often grows in cultivated wheat fields in regions where EN is prevalent, being of most interest. The major components of the plant extract AA are nitrophenanthrene carboxylic acids, which, after metabolic activation, are genotoxic mutagens. Studies using human microsomes have shown that cytochrome P450 (CYP) 1A2 and CYP1A1, as well as prostaglandin H synthase (cyclooxygenase, COX), have a role in the metabolic activation of AA to species forming DNA adducts. These DNA adducts have been found both in renal tissue and in transitional cell carcinomas of affected humans. Renal failure was reported in horses fed hay contaminated with *A. clematitis* in the Balkan region in the 1950s, and similar nephrotoxic changes, as well as carcinogenesis, have been induced experimentally in rats and rabbits.

A. clematitis was used as a medicinal plant by the ancient Egyptians, Greeks, and Romans, and is used to a minor extent in traditional Chinese medicine. Chinese herbs nephropathy, now called aristolochic acid nephropathy or AAN, has been reported following consumption of herbal compounds containing *Aristolochia* spp. *Aristolochia* containing herbal compounds are classified as a Group 1 carcinogen by the International Agency for Research on Cancer.

Halogenated Alkenes

Conjugation in Phase II metabolism, for example with glutathione (GSH), typically decreases the reactivity of the metabolic intermediate, correspondingly reducing toxicity potential. However, stable GSH conjugates which are degraded to cysteine conjugates may be subsequently bioactivated to a toxic metabolite by a renal cysteine conjugate β-lyase (β-lyase pathway). β-lyase cleaves S-cysteine conjugates to putative reactive thiols. β-lyase enzyme activity is mainly localized in the pars recta. Hexachloro-1,3-butadiene, tetrafluoroethylene, chlorotrifluoroethylene, trichloroethylene, and dichlorovinyl cysteine may produce nephrotoxic effect via such a mechanism. These agents correspondingly produce selective necrosis in the pars recta.

Cisplatin

The clinical use of cisplatin, a platinum-containing cancer chemotherapeutic agent, is limited by nephrotoxicity, because it accumulates in the pars recta. Injury is mediated by metabolic activation with reactive intermediates affecting cell respiration.

Xenobiotics Perturbing Cellular, Interstitial, or Lumenal Substrate

Phosphate Toxicity

Administration of phosphates causes proximal tubular necrosis. Histologically, there is consistent mineralization of the necrotic cells in contrast to only occasional cellular mineralization associated with most other causes of tubular necrosis.

Iron Toxicity

Bisphosphonates chelate cations, and are used therapeutically in the treatment of Paget's disease and hypercalcemia of malignancy. A limiting factor in the parenteral use of these chelators is their nephrotoxic potential. A prototype, chloromethane diphosphonate (Cl_2MDP), preferentially sequesters iron. Cl_2MDP perturbation of iron at the subcellular level may be associated with the nephrotoxic response, specifically through peroxidative processes. Cl_2MDP causes proximal tubular necrosis, with quantitative predilection for pars recta. Cl_2MDP is not metabolized, but does accumulate in renal cortex and outer stripe (as well as in bone).

Zinc Toxicity

Induction of zinc toxicity through dietary manipulation is very difficult. In contrast, dietary administration of high levels of the chelator trisodium nitrilotriacetate monohydrate (NTA) results in zinc nephrotoxicity. When plasma glomerular ultrafiltrate levels of NTA exceed $20\,\mu M$, an increase in plasma and, thus, glomerular ultrafiltrate zinc occurs. In the proximal tubules, zinc is reabsorbed, but NTA is not. NTA is not metabolized, and is excreted unchanged in the urine. The increased tubular zinc uptake rapidly leads to persistent changes of osmotic nephrosis, possibly through zinc stabilization of lysosomal membranes. Osmotically-altered proximal convoluted tubules become hypertrophic, and then hyperplastic. Doses sufficient to cause the osmotic type of nephrosis also cause an increase in incidence or severity of lesions of chronic progressive nephropathy in the rat.

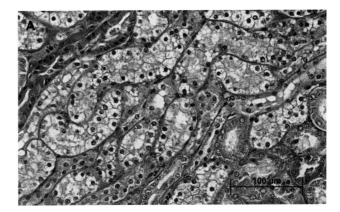

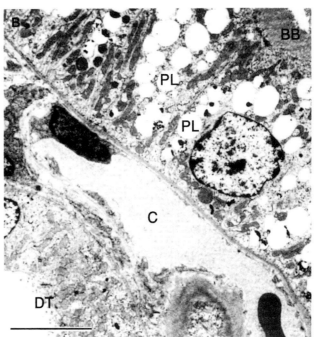

FIGURE 11.12 Osmotic nephrosis, kidney. (A) Tubular epithelial cells show marked cytoplasmic vacuolation following ethylene glycol intoxication (H&E stain). (B) Ultrastructure of proximal convoluted tubule; rabbit; polyethylene glycol treatment. Hydropic swelling of the phagolysosomes (PL) is present. Peritubular capillary (C); distal tubule (DT); brush border (BB). Bar = $5\,\mu m$. (Courtesy of Dr B. Sturgill, University of Virginia.)

With lifetime exposure, proliferative sequelae associated with the toxic response are associated with development of rodent renal tubular tumors.

Osmotic Nephrosis

Glucose and sucrose are reabsorbed by pinocytosis, leading to vacuolization of PCTs (Figure 11.12). This vacuolization represents hydropic swelling of the phagolysosome, and has been designated osmotic nephrosis. Mannitol and dextran induce the same change. The functional impact of this change is minimal, and the vacuolization actually may be a transient adaptive response. Lifetime rodent studies of mannitol have not revealed toxic or tumorigenic consequences of the osmotic change.

Oxalate Nephrosis

Ethylene glycol is a prototype for chemicals causing oxalate nephrosis. It is found in antifreeze, and is an important cause of spontaneous nephrotoxicity in dogs and cats. It has also been found as a contaminant in other products, such as toothpaste. Non-metabolized ethylene glycol has similar toxicity to ethanol. Ethylene glycol or its metabolites can be associated with osmotic nephrosis which is unassociated with oxalate deposition (Figure 11.12A). Reduced renal function may occur in acute exposure, without oxalate deposition.

Ethylene glycol is absorbed from the gastrointestinal tract, and a small percentage is oxidized by hepatic alcohol dehydrogenase to the toxic metabolites glycolaldehyde, glycolic acid, glyoxylate, and oxalate. These metabolites act directly on the tubular epithelium to cause necrosis. Oxalic acid in the renal tubular lumen sequesters calcium, and precipitates as calcium oxalate crystals which obstruct the nephron and lead to additional damage. Marked deposition of calcium oxalate crystals is the consistent finding in fatal cases of acute ethylene glycol poisoning (Figure 11.13).

Oxalate nephrosis in domestic animals, especially pigs and cattle, can also be caused by oxalate-containing plants, genera such as *Halogeton*, *Sarcobatus* (greasewood), *Rheum* (rhubarb leaves), and *Rumex* (sorrel and dock) (see Table 11.3). Oxalates from these plants are absorbed from the intestine, and form deposits with calcium in the renal tubules where they cause obstruction and necrosis. Other causes include methoxyflurane, ascorbic acid (vitamin C), rust-removing chemicals, and *Aspergillus niger* present on grains. It should be noted that small numbers of calcium oxalate crystals may be present in some species unassociated with disease, or secondary to nonspecific renal injury.

Inducible Alpha$_{2\mu}$ Globulin Nephropathy Syndrome

Normal mature male rats spontaneously develop hyaline droplets in PCT epithelial cell cytoplasm (see Figure 11.6A). Ultrastructurally, these represent large crystalloid phagolysosomal proteinic reabsorption droplets. Biochemically these hyaline bodies consist of alpha$_{2\mu}$ globulin. Hyaline droplets reflect the normal

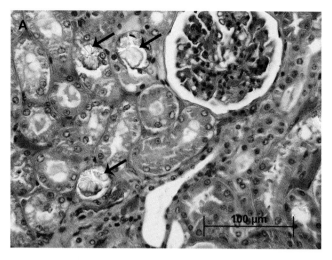

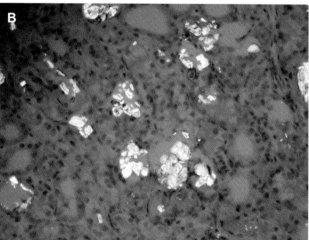

FIGURE 11.13   Ethylene glycol (antifreeze) toxicity; kidney. (A) Cat. Prominent refractile oxalate crystals (arrows) are present in the lumen of proximal tubules which show variable loss and attenuation of epithelium (H&E stain). (B) Dog. Multiple tubules contain birefringent radiating sheaves of calcium oxalate crystals (H&E stain under polarized light). (From Sebastian, M.M., Baskin, S.I., and Czerwinski, S.E. (2007). Renal Toxicity. In *Veterinary Toxicology: Basic and Clinical Principles*, (Gupta, R.C. ed.), Figure 4. Elsevier Academic Press, New York, NY.)

glomerular filtration with PCT uptake and accumulation of this poorly-hydrolyzable low molecular weight protein. The mature male rat liver synthesizes and secretes approximately 50 mg of alpha$_{2\mu}$ globulin per day, which is rapidly cleared in the glomerular filtrate and serves as a pheromone. Approximately 15 to 20 mg of alpha$_{2\mu}$ globulin is lost in the urine each day in the normal mature male rat, creating a physiologic proteinuria. Normal female rats, and higher species of either sex, including humans, do not develop this change, and do not normally excrete a large quantity of poorly-hydrolyzable protein in their glomerular ultrafiltrate for PCT cell reabsorption. Furthermore, neither normal humans nor humans with perturbed urinary protein profiles excrete significant levels of alpha$_{2\mu}$ globulin proteins. The male mouse also is a physiologic proteinuric, because of a mouse urinary protein (MUP) which has similar electrophoretic characteristics, but does not accumulate in the proximal tubule.

Several chemicals of societal importance affect the male rat through perturbation of alpha$_{2\mu}$ globulin. These include *d*-limonene and unleaded gasoline; *d*-limonene is widespread in natural foods, with average daily adult consumption estimated at over 2.5 mg/kg body weight. In the male rat, 10 mg/kg body weight per day is injurious to the kidney. *d*-limonene and unleaded gasoline induce a specific triad of subchronic renal lesions in the male rat. The primary response in the male rat kidney is exacerbated hyaline droplet formation, again consisting specifically of alpha$_{2\mu}$ globulin, which causes PCT cell injury, evidenced by increased apoptotic necrosis. This leads to the additional lesions in the triad, specifically, granular cast formation in the outer medulla and increased incidence or severity of CPN. This specific triad of pathologic alterations persists through 91 days of exposure.

These chemicals also cause renal tubular tumors in male rats, but not in female rats or mice of either sex. A specific spectrum (quadrad) of chronic injury includes linear medulla mineralization, urothelial hyperplasia, increased incidence and severity of CPN, and tubular tumorigenesis (Figure 11.14; Tables 11.6 and 11.7). *d*-Limonene and unleaded gasoline do not exert their effect through a direct genotoxic mechanism. A direct and specific interaction occurs between alpha$_{2\mu}$ globulin and the inducing xenobiotics (or metabolites). This reversibly-bound conjugate resists hydrolysis to a greater extent than alpha$_{2\mu}$ globulin alone, thus accumulating to a pathologic degree. Finally, the alpha$_{2\mu}$ globulin PCT cell-overload results in accelerated apoptosis, with replicative response persisting through the first year of treatment of the male rat. This replicative response has been demonstrated to be linked with the subsequent tubular tumor response.

Because of the PCT cell peculiarities described, this specific male rat response is not considered predictive for female rats or other common mammalian species such as mice, dogs, monkeys, and humans.

Light Chain Nephropathy

In the normal human, 5 mg/kg/day of κ light chain is filtered; 0.04 mg/kg/day is excreted in the urine, with much larger amounts in patients with multiple myeloma, primary amyloidosis, or monoclonal gammopathies. These light chains are approximately 22 000 Da, and designated as Bence–Jones protein. Light chain proteinuria is seen in 40% to 80% of myeloma patients, because of overproduction by neoplastic cells. The capacity of the proximal tubular epithelium to reabsorb and catabolize the protein may be exceeded. The Bence–Jones protein in these cases resists normal lysosomal proteolytic degradation, and thus accumulates in the phagolysosome. Spontaneous, as well as experimentally-induced, cases of Bence–Jones nephrosis are characterized by phagolysosomal protein overload, with propensity for crystalloid change in proximal tubular epithelium, cast formation, and nephron atrophy or regeneration. This nephropathy is important because it illustrates the nephrotoxic potential of endogenous proteins, and presents similarities to the renal changes in the inducible alpha$_{2\mu}$globulin nephropathy syndrome.

Inhibition of Sphingolipid Metabolism

The mycotoxin fumonisin B$_{1,}$ is produced by *Fusarium verticillioidies* and other *Fusarium* spp. which grow on corn. It alters sphingolipid metabolism and causes renal injury in the rat, rabbit, and some ruminants such as sheep and young cattle. The most sensitive target tissue, the pars recta, develops accelerated apoptosis (Figure 11.15) and, in male rats, tubular neoplasms. The mechanism of carcinogenicity is thought to be mediated through increased cell proliferation.

Myoglobin and Hemoglobin

Myoglobin can induce acute renal failure. Myoglobinuria occurs secondary to rhabdomyolysis. Causes of rhabdomyolysis include trauma, ischemia, hyperpyrexia, electrolyte disturbance, and toxicants. Myoglobin nephropathy is of interest because it causes a pigmented cast nephropathy. Hemoglobin can also induce a morphologically-comparable pigmented cast nephropathy (Figure 11.16). Hemoglobinemia can follow severe intravascular hemolysis and, once the normal carrier molecule is depleted, hemoglobin can pass into the glomerular filtrate. Causes of intravascular hemolysis include exogenous chemicals, such as phenothiazine. Hemoglobinuria with accompanying nephrosis occurs in sheep with chronic copper toxicity and in horses with red maple toxicity. While hemoglobin and myoglobin are not themselves nephrotoxic, they can increase the severity of the necrosis, due to renal ischemia that may occur secondary to severe anemia or hypovolemic shock. The concentration of hemoglobin sufficient to injure the kidney typically is associated with red discoloration of plasma. In contrast, in myoglobinuria, because of the smaller

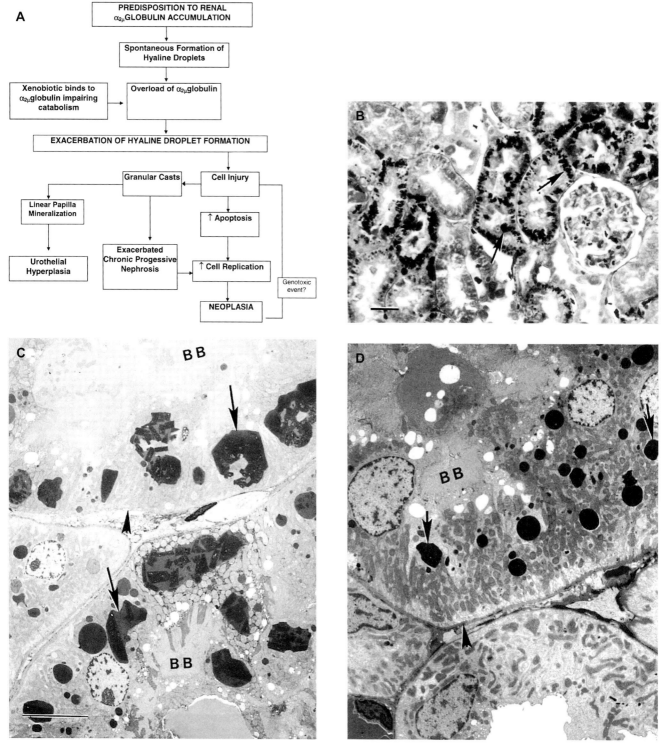

FIGURE 11.14 Inducible male rat alpha$_{2u}$ globulin nephropathy syndrome. (A) Schematic pathogenesis of the specific lesions occurring in this syndrome. (B) Exacerbated hyaline droplet formation in the cytoplasm of the proximal convoluted tubular cells (arrows) as a consequence of decalin treatment (Mallory's Heidenhain stain. Bar = 30 μm). (C) Decalin-treated and (D) control animals. Ultrastructural correlate of the hyaline droplets observed by light microscopy. Note the increased size and propensity for crystalloid change of phagolysosomes (arrows) with decalin treatment. Basement membrane of the PCT (arrowhead); brush border (BB). Bar = 10 μm.

TABLE 11.6   Criteria for including xenobiotics as inducers of the alpha$_{2\mu}$ globulin nephropathy syndrome

1. The xenobiotic or its metabolites bind reversibly and specifically with alpha$_{2\mu}$ globulin in the kidney
2. The xenobiotic or its metabolite and the bound alpha$_{2u}$ globulin accumulate in the mature male rat kidney in hyaline droplets (other proteins do not accumulate)
3. Subchronic treatment results in injury to the male rat kidney, characterized consistently by a specific spectrum of lesions, including exacerbated hyaline droplet formation, granular casts in the outer medulla, and exacerbated changes undifferentiable from those of chronic progressive nephropathy
4. Chronic treatment ($\geq$1 year with sacrifice after 2 years) consistently results in a specific triad of injury, including linear papilla mineralization, urothelial hyperplasia, and exacerbated chronic progressive nephropathy plus renal tubular tumors in male rats
5. Renal injury, including tumor formation, cannot be forced in the female rat or mice of either sex in short-term or in long-term testing; furthermore, the xenobiotics or their metabolites do not accumulate, nor does protein accumulate in the exposed female rat or mouse kidney
6. The xenobiotics or their metabolites are not considered genotoxic

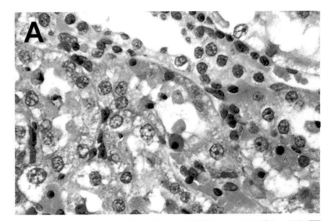

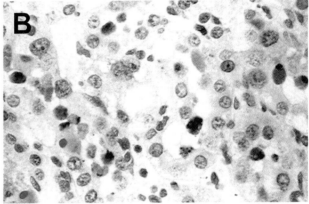

FIGURE 11.15   Rat kidney following subchronic treatment with fumonisin B$_1$, outer stripe apoptosis. Immunohistochemical stains for apoptotic cells, although not specific, facilitate quantitative evaluation ((A) H&E stain; (B) Tunel stain). (Courtesy of Drs Tom Bucci and Paul Howard, NCTR.)

TABLE 11.7   Xenobiotics that produce the alpha$_{2\mu}$ globulin nephropathy syndrome including tumors in male rats[a]

Jet fuels: JP-4, JP-TS, JP-7, RJ-5, JP-10

Dimethyl methylphosphonate

Hexachlorobenzene

Nitrotoluene

Cl-986 (COX and 5 lipooxygenase inhibitor)

Hexachloroethane

Isophorone

d-Limonene

Lindane

Paradichlorobenzene

Pentachloroethane

Unleaded gasoline

[a]Test system specific response

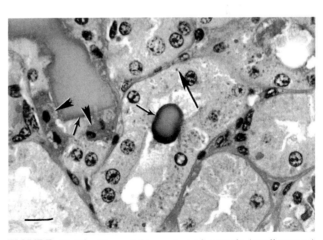

FIGURE 11.16   Hemoglobin casts and crystals (small arrows) in the proximal tubular lumen of horses in red maple poisoning. Hyaline droplets (large arrows) and proximal tubular cell degeneration and necrosis (arrowheads) are evident. Bar = 17 μm. (Courtesy of Dr W. Crowell, University of Georgia.)

molecular weight, renal clearance is sufficiently high to maintain normal colored plasma.

Amino Acid Toxicity

Lysinoalanine, an amino acid formed during alkali treatment of protein, may be found in processed foods for human consumption. Lysinoalanine is of interest since it induces cytomegaly or karyomegaly in the rat and mouse kidney. This effect has not been observed in hamsters, monkeys, or rabbits. This change seems largely reversible. Furthermore, long-term studies have not led to renal tumor formation or any other adverse change. This karyomegaly develops in the pars recta. Karyomegaly also develops spontaneously in the rat PCT (see Figure 11.6B).

Lysine, a component of some parenteral nutrition therapies, and D-serine injection in the rat, induce necrosis of the proximal tubule. D-Serine is of interest since it induces necrosis restricted to the pars recta. Serine is also normally synthesized *in vivo* in the rat, as well as in the human kidney.

Synthetic Diet-induced Nephrocalcinosis

Within a few weeks of feeding certain commercially-available semi-purified diets to rats (e.g., AIN 76), intratubular mineral deposits consisting of calcium and phosphate salts become marked in the pars recta (Figure 11.17). The alteration primarily affects the female. Changing dietary calcium-to-phosphorus ratios by increasing calcium, or by adding magnesium to the diet decreases or prevents this mineral precipitation. Altering water load and intratubular pH also affects mineral deposition in the kidney.

Vitamins D and K

Vitamin D_3 toxicity causes widespread mineralization within the body with kidney, lung, and stomach the most severely affected. Mineralization occurs along basement membranes, and often affects the vasculature. The source of excess vitamin D is usually dietary such as over-supplementation, improper mixing of diet, and ingestion of plants that contain calcinogenic glycosides (e.g., *Cestrum diurnum*, *Solanum malacoxylum*, *Trisetum flavescens*). In addition, calciferol is the active component of the rodenticide, Quintox, which is frequently ingested by dogs. Excessive vitamin D activity results in hypercalcemia. Renal ischemia from vasoconstriction and mitochondrial calcification results in tubular necrosis, with epithelial and basement membrane mineralization. Intratubular mineralized deposits may be present. If renal changes are severe, uremia may be present.

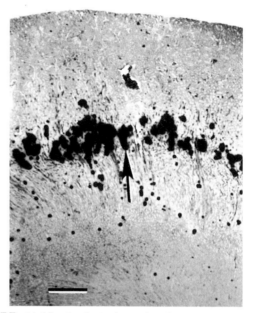

FIGURE 11.17 Synthetic-diet-induced nephrocalcinosis in a female rat. Notice the extensive mineralization in the outer stripe (arrow) (Alizarin Red S Stain; Bar = 0.6 mm).

Vitamin K_3 (menadione sodium sulfate) can cause acute tubular degeneration and necrosis in horses. Chronic changes consist of tubular dilation with casts and chronic interstitial fibrosis.

Xenobiotics Causing Crystal Nephropathy

Intratubular precipitation of xenobiotics or endogenous crystals (induced by xenobiotics) can cause or promote acute and chronic kidney injury. A number of xenobiotics, including drugs, are known to precipitate within renal tubules, due to their insolubility within urine. Risk factors for xenobiotic or endogenous crystal precipitation within the kidney tubules include true or effective intravascular volume depletion, underlying kidney disease, and certain metabolic disturbances that promote changes in urinary pH favoring crystal precipitation (see below under Lower Urinary Tract). In human medicine, the major causes of crystal nephropathy are drugs such as methotrexate, acyclovir, and rarely sulfonamides. In veterinary medicine, the most common cause is oxalate nephrosis (see above), which is most frequently induced by ethylene glycol (antifreeze) ingestion in dogs and cats, and by oxalate-containing plants in large animals.

More recently, the focus has been on melamine adulteration of food products. Melamine, 1,3,5-triazine-2,4,6-triamine, is used primarily for manufacturing melamine resins and melamine-based resins that are used in production of a wide variety of products including laminates, adhesives, molding compounds, textiles, and flame retardants. The addition of melamine, which is high in non-protein nitrogen, to food constituents in order to boost the apparent protein content has been a widespread practice in China.

Melamine-cyanuric Acid: Pet Food Nephropathy

In 2007, an outbreak of renal failure in domestic cats and dogs associated with renal tubule crystalluria resulted in a major recall of pet food in North America. The outbreak was traced to wheat gluten imported from China. Analysis of the pet food and gluten demonstrated the presence of simple triazine compounds, primarily melamine and cyanuric acid. Experimentally, a mixture of melamine and cyanuric acid produced melamine cyanurate crystalluria and acute renal toxicity in cats, fish, and rodents. Cyanuric acid complexing with melamine was critical for the precipitation of crystals in the kidney. A similar outbreak in Asia in 2004 resulted in the deaths of 6000 dogs and fewer cats, due to renal failure. This outbreak was the result of pet food contamination which was incorrectly attributed to mycotoxins at the time. Retrospective analysis for melamine and cyanuric acid in paraffin sections from affected animals was positive.

Clinically, animals ingesting pet food contaminated with melamine and cyanuric acid were azotemic with hyperphosphatemia, and urinalysis revealed isostenuria and crystalluria. In acute cases, the kidneys were pale and swollen, with congested vasculature. Crystals could be identified on impression smear. Histologically, distal nephron injury was characterized by tubular dilation, epithelial tubular degeneration and necrosis, and intratubular crystal deposition. Unique striated crystals were present in distal tubules and collecting ducts (Figure 11.18). These dissolved over time in neutral buffered formalin, so timely processing is important. Tubular rupture with inflammation can occur. In more chronic cases, intratubular crystals may be found in the medulla. Inflammation, fibrosis, and sometimes granulomatous lesions may be present.

The major differential for melamine cyanurate nephrotoxicity in dogs and cats is oxalate nephrosis. Hypocalcemia is prominent in oxalate nephrosis, but absent with melamine/cyanurate toxicity. Crystal morphology and location within the nephron differs. Oxalate crystals are pale yellow, occur as sheaves and rosettes, are stable and prominent on polarization, and are located primarily in proximal tubules (see Figure 11.13). Melamine/cyanurate crystals are gold to brown, occur as pinwheels or granules, and are

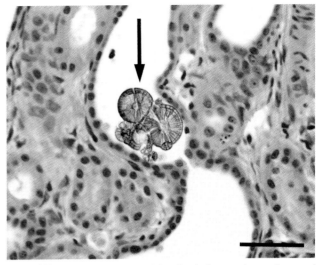

FIGURE 11.18 Cat. Dilated distal tubule contains a cluster of round green melamine/cyanuric acid crystals with radiating spokes and concentric striations (arrow). Surrounding proximal tubules appear unaffected (H&E stain; Bar = 45μm). (With permission from Brown, C.A., Jeong, K.S., Poppenga, R.H., Puschner, B., Miller, D.M., Ellis, A.E., Kang, K.I., Sum, S., Cistola, A.M., and Brown, S.A. (2007). Outbreaks of renal failure associated with melamine and cyanuric acid in dogs and cats in 2004 and 2007. *J. Vet. Diagn. Invest.*, 19, 528. Fig 1(A).)

located in the distal nephron. Sulfonamides have also caused crystal nephropathy, affecting the distal nephron in domestic animals and humans. Crystals may be observed grossly, but have poor stability in formalin and during processing. Currently used sulfonamides have good solubility, and do not form crystals unless predisposing factors are severe.

Melamine-associated Retrograde Nephropathy

Retrograde or reflux nephropathy, characterized by tubular dilation extending from the papilla to the cortex, has been reported in rats treated with melamine. This is thought to be due to melamine precipitation in the lower urinary tract creating pressure effects through transient obstruction. These renal changes are similar to human reflux nephropathy of early childhood, when urinary tract infection is superimposed on congenital vesiculouretral reflux. Microscopic changes of human reflux nephropathy primarily involve the tubules and interstitium, and are characterized by tubular atrophy and dilation, and corticomedullary scarring. The epidemic of infant kidney disease in China linked to melamine adulteration of milk products may have a similar etiology. Affected infants developed urinary tract calculi; premature birth and melamine-contaminated formula were the precipitating factors.

Xenobiotics Perturbing Renal Hemodynamics

Ischemia and Hypoxia

When the rat kidney is subjected to ischemia via clamping the renal artery and then reperfused, necrosis occurs in the proximal tubule (invariably accompanied by medullary congestion), which is most marked in the outer stripe. This tubular injury appears in periods of ischemia as short as 15 minutes. The shorter the period of ischemia, the longer the reperfusion interval required before necrotic cells can be visualized in this model. With slightly longer periods of ischemia (45 to 60 minutes) and reperfusion (up to 24 hours), necrosis appears in PCTs; but the pars recta is most prominently affected. Distribution of proximal tubule necrosis in ischemia–reflow injury has features in common with a pattern produced by hypoxia, as well as by mitochondrial toxicants such as mercury.

Three interrelated mechanistic explanations for the irreversible cell injury are impaired mitochondrial oxygen uptake, with anaerobic ATP depletion then oxidative stress on reperfusion; precipitous calcium influx from the extracellular to intracellular compartment, with activation of calcium-dependent catabolic processes; and release of cytotoxic lysosomal enzymes into the cytosol. Interestingly, ischemic proximal tubule damage is more severe in old rats than in young rats, possibly associated with corresponding age-associated reduction in basal renal adenine nucleotide content and nephron number in the old rat.

Prolonged ischemia (over two hours) results in infarction. Prolonged ischemia induced by temporary clamping of the renal artery results in cortical infarction, whereas occlusion of venous return results in medullary infarction. Obstruction of an interlobular artery results in a wedge-shaped area of cortical necrosis (Figure 11.19).

Other Sites of Renal Injury

Distal Nephron

The importance of primary xenobiotic injury of the loops of Henle, the thick ascending tubule, or the distal convoluted tubule is not well established. Tilorone, an interferon inducer, causes phospholipidosis in the DCT as a limited example of a primary toxic response for the distal nephron. Crystal formation by precipitation of melamine and cyanuric acid occurs in the distal nephron, due to the low pH in that region (see above). Other reports of distal nephron perturbation are often based on functional tests, without concomitant demonstration of the site of specific structural change. These reports fail to differentiate functional from toxic alterations, or primary from secondary changes in the nephrotoxic response.

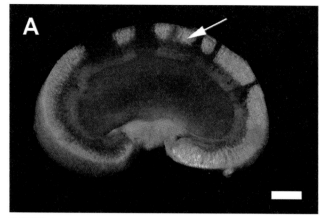

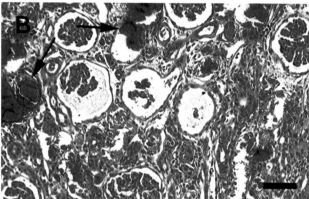

FIGURE 11.19   Effect of reduced renal perfusion due to interlobular artery obstruction with outer cortical necrosis in a beagle dog. (A) Diffuse necrosis in the outer cortex (arrow) with sparing of the inner cortex, medulla, and papilla (Bar = 5 mm). (B) Same kidney showing tubular epithelial necrosis, tubular mineralization (arrows) and glomerular tuft atrophy (Bar = 50 μm).

Collecting Duct

2-Amino-4,5-diphenyl Thiazole HCl

2-Amino-4,5-diphenyl thiazole HCl can be used to induce renal polycystic disease. Of interest are factors considered prerequisite to cyst development in the absence of tubular obstruction and in the presence of normal transtubular pressure gradient. Specifically, this model chemical causes a structural defect of the basement membrane as an integral step in the pathogenesis. The primary site of basement membrane injury is in the collecting duct of the outer medulla. Tubular basement membrane is principally responsible for limiting distensibility of the renal tubule. Altered basement membrane also represents an early change in chronic progressive nephropathy. This basement membrane change, in addition to concomitant increased transtubular pressure, may represent the underlying explanation for prominent cystic dilatation with hyaline cast formation, frequently occurring as an early change in chronic progressive nephropathy of the rat. The site of basement membrane injury and cyst formation in CPN involves proximal nephron rather than collecting duct.

Renal Papilla and NSAIDs Toxicity

The renal papilla is a target of nephrotoxicants, primarily due to its low and poorly-oxygenated blood supply. Renal papillary injury can occur under various conditions that affect medullary blood flow or solute concentration, e.g., amyloidosis, diabetic nephropathy, and various xenobiotics including arsenic and NSAIDs. Dehydration is a predisposing factor in papillary injury. Papillotoxins include NSAIDs, acetaminophen, and arsenic.

Drug-induced renal papillary injury is widely-recognized following treatment with NSAIDs in domestic animals, but is rare in humans (Figure 11.20). Multifocal RPN occurring in the clinical setting in large animals, especially horses and calves, is associated with phenylbutazone (butazolidin) and flunixin meglumine (banamine). Phenylbutazone is a nonselective inhibitor of COX-1 and COX-2. In small animals, especially dogs, phenylbutazone, ibuprofen, aspirin, carprofen, flunixin meglumine, and naproxen

treatment have been associated with acute renal failure; concurrent dehydration often presdisposes dogs, and other species, to papillary necrosis.

In addition to renal papillary injury, other renal effects of NSAIDs include acute renal failure, interstitial nephritis, and fluid and electrolyte disturbances in humans, monkeys, rats, dogs, and vultures; nephrotic syndrome, interference with hypertensive and diuretic therapy, and allergic-type interstitial nephritis with peripheral eosinophilia, and eosinophiluria in humans; and outer cortical atrophy with interstitial fibrosis in dogs and infants of monkeys and humans. With the exception of renal papillary injury, these NSAID-related renal effects are reported most commonly in humans. Phenacetin abuse, often associated with NSAID abuse, also results in capillary sclerosis in humans. The following is a brief description of the mechanisms and pathophysiology of the NSAID-related renal effects described in different species.

Inhibition of Cyclooxygenases

In general, nonsteroidal anti-inflammatory drugs (NSAIDs) are nonselective inhibitors of both the cyclooxygenase (COX) isoforms; cyclooxygenase-1 (COX-1) and cyclooxygenase-2 (COX-2). Long-term

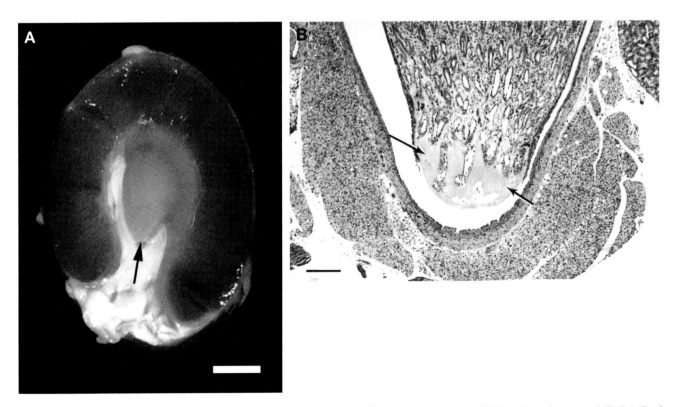

FIGURE 11.20 Nonsteroidal anti-inflammatory drug-induced renal papillary necrosis (arrows). (A) Dog (Bar = 5 mm); and (B) Rat, Grade II (Bar = 0.6 mm). (Courtesy of Dr G. Clark, Upjohn.)

use of NSAIDs is associated with toxic effects in multiple organ systems, specifically the GI tract and the kidneys. COX-1 inhibition by NSAIDs is considered responsible for these toxicities.

The isoform and species variations in the renal distribution of COX may, in part, explain the renal effects of NSAIDs in humans and laboratory animals. The renal medulla and papilla predominantly express COX-1, and are the major sites of PG production in the kidney (see Figure 11.7A and B). The constitutive expression of COX-2 in rats, dogs (see Figure 11.7C), mice, and pigs indicate that this isoform is involved in regulation of normal renal functions in these species. Much more limited distribution of COX-2 in the human and monkey kidneys suggests that COX-2-mediated PGs may have little role in regulating normal renal function in primates. Thus, if NSAID-induced effects on renal functions and toxicity (e.g., RPN) in laboratory animals are linked to COX-2 inhibition, it is probably of little relevance to humans. Rats, and to a lesser degree dogs, are especially sensitive to developing RPN, as are horses and calves.

The increased susceptibility of laboratory animals to RPN could also be complicated by species-related differences in renal anatomy and physiology compared with humans, in addition to the differences in COX-2 expression. Selective COX-2 inhibitors do not result in RPN in rats or dogs, confirming that selective COX-2 inhibition is not the cause of RPN. The rat commonly develops RPN at exposures to NSAIDs that are comparable to human recommended-use guidelines, while RPN in humans is rare. This indicates greatly increased sensitivity of the rat to RPN compared to the human.

The cause of RPN remains unknown, and its linkage to NSAIDs is generally circumstantial. Ischemic injury, by inhibiting the vasodilatory effects of PGs by NSAIDs, has been suggested as one possible mechanism. The distribution of COX isoforms suggests that inhibition of COX-1-mediated PGs may play some role in the development of RPN in humans.

Acute Renal Failure (ARF)

This is the most common form of NSAID-related renal toxicity in humans, and is caused by a hemodynamic effect due to loss of counter-regulatory PGs. Conditions that may reduce actual or effective circulation volume, e.g., plasma volume contraction (hemorrhage, salt loss, hypoalbuminemia), congestive heart failure or cirrhosis, and ascites, cause a homeostatic increase in vasoconstrictors, including norepinephrine and AII. Vasodilatory effects of PGs at the afferent arteriole counterbalance this vasoconstrictor effect to maintain GFR and renal perfusion. Loss of PGs by

NSAID-inhibition of COX (especially at the afferent arteriole) results in pronounced vasoconstriction and a decrease in glomerular capillary pressure, resulting in a decline of GFR.

The clinical laboratory changes in subjects developing ARF in response to conventional NSAIDs include oliguria, decreased fractional excretion of sodium, decreased GFR, and increase in BUN and creatinine. Withdrawal of NSAIDs results in a complete reversal of ARF; however, if not recognized early in the course of therapy, prolonged renal ischemia may cause acute tubular necrosis and permanent renal damage.

NSAIDS can also induce acute renal failure in dogs. Of interest is the recently-documented vulture die-off in India, due to diclofenac-induced acute renal failure. Diclofenac was used widely in cattle in India. When carcasses from treated cattle were ingested, vultures died in large numbers.

Acute Interstitial Nephritis (AIN) With or Without Nephrotic Syndrome (NS)

This toxicity occurs following months-to-years of NSAID treatment. AIN alone is more common than AIN with NS and NS alone. The mechanism of this toxicity is not known. One possibility is a reaction to non-COX reactive arachidonic acid metabolites. Clinical laboratory changes in this syndrome include elevated BUN, creatinine (often exceeding >6 mg/dL), oliguria, proteinuria (>3.5 g/24 hr with NS), microscopic hematuria, and pyuria. Histopathologic evaluations reveal severe interstitial edema and multifocal infiltrates of lymphocytes and plasma cells surrounding proximal and distal tubules. Lymphocytes are predominantly $CD8^+$ T-cells, with small numbers of B-cells. Eosinophiluria, eosinophilia, rash, and fever are absent. Ultrastructurally, patients with NS show minimal change glomerulopathy, with marked epithelial foot process-fusion.

Fluid and Electrolyte Disturbances

Prostaglandins exert modulatory influences on many ion transport sites along the nephrons, and are important in sodium and water homeostasis in the kidney. Thus, NSAID-inhibition of renal PGs interferes with PG-mediated sodium chloride transport, antidiuretic hormone, and distribution of blood flow from cortical to juxtamedullary nephrons. Sodium and water retention manifests clinically as edema. The clinical laboratory changes may include oliguria, decreased urinary sodium and chloride excretion, and an increase in serum chloride levels.

PGs also regulate renin release, and thus indirectly affect aldosterone production. NSAID treatment may result in hyporeninemic hypoaldosteronism. Aldosterone is important in potassium excretion from the distal convoluted tubules and collecting ducts. However, it is rare to see hyperkalemia with NSAIDs in the absence of other defects in potassium homeostasis. Elevated serum potassium and decreased urinary potassium excretion are observed in the clinical laboratory profile.

Chronic Renal Failure or Analgesic Nephropathy

The loss of vasodilatory PGs, accumulation of drug in papilla at higher concentrations, and production of reactive metabolites are considered responsible for renal papillary necrosis (RPN) as the primary manifestation. RPN occurs with structurally-dissimilar compounds that share the ability to inhibit PG synthesis, suggesting that redistribution of PG-dependent medullary blood flow may contribute to the development of RPN, due to prolonged papillary and medullary ischemia. No remarkable changes in renal function occur if lesions are localized to the tip of the papilla. RPN lesions may progress, causing chronic inflammation of medulla and cortex.

Experimentally, chemically-induced RPN has also been associated with other agents including cyclophosphamide, dapsone, radiocontrast media, 2-bromoethanamine hydrobromide (2-BEA), ethyleneimine, and jet fuel petroleum. The least severe and earliest morphologic change observed following treatment with most papillotoxic agents is decreased alcian blue staining of the interstitial matrix, due to loss of glycosaminoglycans, followed by degeneration and necrosis of the interstitial cells. With progression, vascular congestion and degeneration of capillary endothelia become apparent, followed by degeneration and necrosis of the epithelial cells of the loops of Henle, collecting ducts, and urothelium. These changes start at the tip of the papilla and involve increasing proportions of the papilla, reflecting increasing severity (Figure 11.20B).

Blood flow and drug concentration in the papilla are inexorably influenced by factors influencing body fluid and solute concentrations. Specifically, a reduced urine flow and increased interstitial medullary solute concentration are associated with increased drug concentration and decreased blood flow in the papilla. Correspondingly, depletion of effective plasma volume or increased solute load increase propensity for RPN occurrence. The decreased flow may be mediated by renin release. The homozygous Brattleboro rat, devoid of endogenous ADH, is resistant to RPN, but becomes susceptible with ADH injection, supporting the interactive influence of urine flow and papilla solute concentration on RPN development.

The pig is similar to the human with regard to renal anatomy and physiology, as well as salicylate pharmacokinetics and renal concentration. RPN only develops in humans after prolonged high-level use, and in the presence of chronic renal disease, the pig is similarly refractive to RPN. RPN has been produced experimentally mainly in rats, occasionally in rabbits and dogs, and rarely in monkeys. The laboratory rodent, as a chronic consequence of RPN, develops urothelial neoplasia. Several interrelated differences in rats compared to humans and other species influencing the integrity of inner medullary blood flow include well-developed inner medulla, unipapillary kidney, high urine concentrating capacity, exclusive postglomerular tuft blood supply to the papilla, and increased NSAID or metabolite papilla concentration on a mg drug/kg body weight basis. These factors, along with interspecies differences in COX isoform distribution, may explain the enhanced susceptibility of rats to develop RPN.

Lower Urinary Tract

Urinary Chemistry

Alterations in urinary chemistry can be a cause of toxicity to the urothelium, and can greatly influence the toxicity of administered chemicals. Major differences in the composition of urine between species, particularly between rodents and humans, have led to significant insights into the extrapolation of potential hazards to humans based on observations in rodents. This is especially true for nongenotoxic chemicals.

A major influence on urinary toxicity is pH. The pH of rodent urine generally lies between 5.0 and 8.0, and is greatly influenced by diet. Urinary pH can influence the formation of solids, and the ionization of numerous chemicals and their metabolites, greatly influencing the reactivity of these chemicals, their interaction with the urothelium, and their ability to be absorbed by the urothelium.

A major difference between rodent and human urine is the overall osmolality. Rodent urine is usually highly-concentrated, the osmolality ranging from 1200 to 2000 mosmol/L, with male urine having higher protein concentrations than female urine. In rats, this is due to the production and excretion of alpha$_{2u}$ globulin, and in mice, mouse urinary protein (MUP). These can influence not only toxicity in the kidney, but also in the bladder, but by different mechanisms.

Differences in concentration of calcium and phosphate can influence the toxic and carcinogenic response to a variety of chemicals, but this is largely due to their involvement in the formation of various urinary solids. Similarly, urinary silicate levels can reach sufficiently high levels, depending on dietary sources, to lead to the formation of various urinary solids and the production of toxicity. This is particularly true in sheep and other domesticated animals. Monovalent ions such as sodium and potassium are also thought to influence the toxicity of some chemicals.

Urinary Solids

Small quantities of solids are normally present in urine, including cells, cellular debris, casts, and crystals (normally magnesium ammonium phosphate). Collectively, this material is referred to as urinary sediment, and is not toxic to the lining urothelium. In contrast, solids can form and collect in the urine, ranging from small (precipitate), to microscopic (crystals), to macroscopic (calculi) material. The extent of the toxicity produced by these solids is related to the quantity of the foreign matter produced, and to the coarseness of its surface. Precipitate generally causes relatively minor degrees of toxicity, whereas calculi can produce gross toxicity, including ulceration. In addition, calculi can be large enough to obstruct the urinary stream, usually of the ureters or urethra, leading to formation of hydronephrosis and hydroureter.

Solids can be produced by excessive concentrations of normal constituents of the urine, leading to precipitation, or can form secondary to high concentrations of the administered chemical or its metabolites. Numerous factors of normal urine contribute to the formation of these solids, including urinary pH, citrate (acting as a chelating substance for calcium), calcium, magnesium, and phosphate concentrations as related to solids formed from these substances, the overall osmolality of the urine, and the concentrations and types of proteins and mucopolysaccharides. In general, rodents are considerably more susceptible than are primates, including humans. Table 11.8 lists the substances which have been identified in the formation of calculi in rodents and/or humans.

The formation of solids from normal urinary constituents occurs as a consequence of marked alterations in normal urinary physiology. For example, any treatment resulting in excess excretion of calcium and phosphate in the urine will lead to calcium phosphate lithiasis.

When urinary precipitates and microcrystalluria lead to superficial damage to the urothelium without full thickness injury or ulceration, there is no inflammation. In contrast, if there is massive accumulation of certain types of crystals, such as silicates, or

TABLE 11.8 Substances producing urinary calculi when administered to rodents and/or humans

Uracil	Diethylene glycol	Glycine
Thymine	4-Ethylsulfonylnaphthalene-	Triamterene
Fosetyl-al	1-sulfonamide	Sulfonamides
Melamine	Oxamide	Ampicillin
Urate	Acetazolamide	Amoxicillin
Homocysteine	Terephthalic acid	Indinavir
Cysteine	Dimethylterephthalate	Glafenic acid
oxalates	Nitrolotriacetate	Orotic acid
Calcium	Polyoxyethylene-8-stearate	Biphenyl
phosphate		

the presence of calculi, there is severe trauma to the urothelium, leading to ulceration, consequent hemorrhage, and an inflammatory reaction. Of critical importance in risk assessment is the fact that urinary solid formation is a threshold phenomenon, based predominantly on the attainment of sufficiently high concentrations of the offending substance in the urine to produce precipitation. Second, solids, including precipitate, microcrystals, and calculi, are in a state of dynamic flux, and can increase or decrease in size, depending on the composition of the urine. It is not unusual, even for calculi, to be present transiently and then to be excreted. In contrast to primates, including humans, in which calculi frequently produce obstruction and consequently severe pain, calculi can accumulate in the bladder in quadrapeds since they are horizontal. These animals can potentially live a normal lifespan with urinary calculi present without complete obstruction. This has considerable implication for inter-species extrapolation with respect to the chronic effects of the presence of calculi.

Renal Carcinogenesis

Comparative Aspects

Approximately 2% of all noncutaneous malignancies in humans arise in the kidney. Of these, 80% to 90% arise in the proximal convoluted tubule, and are designated tubular cell adenocarcinomas. These renal carcinomas arise after 40 years of age, with peak incidence in the sixth and seventh decades of life. Males are affected approximately 2–3 times as frequently as females. Renal cancer is the cause of 12 000 deaths annually in the United States. Renal adenomas are much more frequent, with incidence as high as 20% of randomly-autopsied patients. Over 85% of these adenomas occurred in kidneys with glomerulosclerosis.

Despite vigorous epidemiologic attempts to associate renal cancer with environmental and nutritional agents, only two factors emerge in the United States: cigarette smoking and obesity. Association with other factors such as caffeine, soda pop, hydrocarbon solvents, and gasoline has not been substantiated. Three medical conditions associated with an increased risk for renal carcinoma in humans are end-stage renal disease with dialysis, transplanted kidneys, and membranous glomerulonephritis.

Genotoxic Xenobiotics

Many chemicals require metabolic conversion to exert their genotoxic and consequent carcinogenic potential. Resultant electrophilic intermediates covalently bind renal macromolecules, including nucleic acids. Aflatoxin B_1, aristolochic acid, dimethylnitrosamine, trisphosphate, daunomycin, and 2-aminofluorene exemplify this concept. Genotoxic renal carcinogens share the propensity to exert their biological effect in multiple species, strains, sexes, and tissues. Tissue site, strain, sex, and species differences in response to exposure parallel the capability of the target site to accumulate and metabolize the xenobiotic. Nitridazole and dimethylnitrosamine studies illustrate this association. Furthermore, genotoxic renal carcinogens typically induce tumors rapidly, in high incidence, and with minimal duration of exposure. Rodent experiments with bleomycin sulfate, 1,2-dimethylhydrazine, azoxymethane, and dimethylnitrosamine demonstrate this potential.

The mammalian nephron and renal interstitial connective tissue are of mesodermal origin. The metanephrogenic blastema is endowed with capacity for bipotential differentiation into the epithelium of the nephron or the tissue comprising the interstitium. Some genotoxic renal carcinogens (e.g., ENU), when administered *in utero*, induce nephroblastoma which is a counterpart of Wilm's tumor in juvenile humans. Genotoxic chemicals (dimethylnitrosamine, DMN) administered postnatally (during renal immaturity) typically induce renal mesenchymal tumors (RMT) in the rat. In contrast, after onset of sexual maturity, agents such as DMN primarily, if not exclusively, induce tubular neoplasms.

Xenobiotics inducing renal tumors in multiple species and both sexes suggest the presence of human renal carcinogenic potential (e.g., ochratoxin A). Variations in tumor response can be quantitative, based on varying levels of metabolic conversion and adduct formation at the target cell level. Species and sex variability frequently exists in metabolism of xenobiotics. Correlative differences in sensitivity to

the toxic and carcinogenic effect of xenobiotics causing injury following derivation of reactive metabolites can be observed. Genotoxic renal carcinogens are nephrotoxic; however, the cytotoxic event and associated repair processes are not considered essential factors in eventual tumor development. Cytotoxic responses typically include proximal tubular cell necrosis, as well as cytomegaly or karyomegaly of proximal tubular epithelium. These genotoxic xenobiotics can also cause increased relative kidney weight in animals on repetitive exposure. This is presumably associated with stimulated renal mixed-function oxidase activity.

Heavy Metal Carcinogens

Several heavy metals share structural and functional renal effects in the rodent species. Metals that have been carefully scrutinized, including chromium, mercury, nickel, and lead, induce genetic injury, and may interact or bind directly with DNA, for example, nickel. Several metals are carcinogenic in rodent kidneys, for example, lead, nickel, gold, chromium, and mercury (organic). The carcinogenic response typically is not species-, or strain-specific. The accumulation of the metal at the tissue target site is prerequisite to the carcinogenic response. The solubility of the metal complex, the vehicle for the metal, and the dose level and duration of treatment all influence the carcinogenic potential in the rodent. These latter factors presumably each influence the critical target tissue level. Similarly, the chemical form of the metal influences its carcinogenic potential.

The carcinogenic heavy metals each have nephrotoxic potential, characterized by acute tubular necrosis if administered at sufficiently high levels. Increased tubular replicative rate occurs, even at doses failing to induce oncotic cell necrosis, presumably associated with increased apoptotic necrosis. In subchronic and chronic studies at carcinogenic levels, these metals induce karyomegaly and cytomegaly in proximal tubular epithelium. The karyomegalic cell has not been demonstrated as a precursor lesion (preneoplastic change) in the cancer response. Nonetheless, karyomegaly may represent a useful short-term marker of renal events occurring relevant to the carcinogenic process. Heavy metals that induce nephrotoxicity, interact with DNA, or accumulate in the nucleus, and that are nephrotoxic (with karyomegaly) in subchronic studies, can be predicted to be rodent renal carcinogens if tested in lifetime studies at doses inducing these short-term effects. The relevance of this rodent response for higher species, including humans, has not been demonstrated. In part, this may be because the high levels required to induce precursor lesions are unlikely to be encountered outside the laboratory setting.

Nongenotoxic Rodent Renal Carcinogens

Several chemicals exert a nephrotoxic response which apparently forms a prerequisite event in the tumorigenic process. The toxic injury is typically accompanied by increased apoptosis, replicative rate increase, and hyperplastic response in tubular epithelium (Table 11.9). Exposure must occur over the majority of the rodent's lifespan and tumors appear late, usually well after one year of treatment.

Tumor incidence is often low, and toxic tubular tumorigens typically do not interact directly with DNA and are not considered genotoxic, as evaluated in short-term assays. Renal toxicity *per se* is a weak risk factor for rodent tubular tumor development. Sufficiently weak tumor responses with incidence less

than 8.5% in a group size of 50 at a 99% confidence level may not be recognized in cancer bioassays. Kidney tumor response, however, is easier to detect than tumor response in several other rodent tissues, because of the typically low spontaneous incidence (<3%) in the rat at 24 months.

All rat nongenotoxic renal carcinogens (for which sufficient data has been published for comparison) are injurious to the kidney at carcinogenic doses in subchronic studies. Chronic toxicity can be presumed to be associated with persistent replicative increase and perturbed apoptotic rate. Examples include beta-cyclodextrin, folic acid, agents inducing the $alpha_{2\mu}$ globulin syndrome (see Table 11.7), and fumonisin B_1.

However, several chemicals tested in rodent cancer bioassays have not been demonstrated to cause tumors, despite the presence of chronic toxic injury, possibly because of the limitations of the bioassay in detecting weak tumorigens. Aminoglycoside antibiotics induce replicative rate increase and toxicity at

TABLE 11.9   Classification of tubular proliferative lesions

Designation	Subclass	Criteria
Tubular regeneration	—	Tubule lined by cells with basophilic cytoplasm and often increased numbers, but without increase in size of the tubule[a]
Simple tubular hyperplasia	Predominantly basophilic, eosinophilic, clear, oncocytic	Definite increase in cross-sectional diameter of the tubule and number of cells lining the tubule; single layer of cells lining the tubule; marked cellular atypia may occur[a]
Atypical tubular hyperplasia	Predominant basophilic, eosinophilic, clear, oncocytic; Cystic or solid	Tubules increase in size because of increase in cell number, with multiple layers and orderly growth in relation to nephron basement membrane; marked cellular atypia may occur[a]
Adenoma	Cell type is basophilic, eosinophilic, clear, oncocytic; Predominant growth pattern is tubular, lobular, solid	Unequivocal loss of continuity with original nephron unit; often with compression of adjacent parenchyma; synthesis of new basement membrane; frequent cellular atypia; typically greater in cross-sectional diagram than twice a normal glomerular tuft
Adenocarcinoma/carcinoma	Cell type is basophilic, eosinophilic, clear; Predominant growth is tubular (more or less distinct formation of tubules), lobular (nests of cells separated by scanty connective tissue), solid (continuous sheets of cells); Scirrhous response (prominent dense fibrous connective tissue proliferation)	Disorderly basement membrane synthesis and invasiveness, or growth without regard to limiting basement membranes; frequently necrosis; neovascularization; size typically greater than 3 mm in diameter; usually marked cellular atypia (non-neoplastic lesions may also exhibit cellular atypia)

[a]Regenerative, simple, and complex hyperplasias occur on a nephron basis, so several adjacent affected tubules typically are noted in cross-section with perpendicular orientation to the medulla

doses used in cancer bioassays without carcinogenic response. Cancer bioassays, however, apparently have not included groups treated over the majority of the rodent's lifespan. Thus, the tumor potential of nephrotoxic antibiotics, such as netilmycin and gentamycin, has not been assessed with the duration criterion for chemicals in this mechanistic class.

Lower Urinary Tract Carcinogenesis

Urothelial tumors most frequently occur in the urinary bladder. The two basic mechanisms of xenobiotic-induced urothelial carcinogenesis are via direct damage to DNA (genotoxicity), or an increase in cell proliferation. Rodents have been excellent models for evaluation of a variety of classes of genotoxic chemicals, several of which are relevant to known human carcinogenesis, in particular, the aromatic amines and the phosphoramide mustards. Although most aromatic amines produce tumors of other tissues in addition to the bladder, several urothelial-specific carcinogens have been identified, including N-butyl-N-(4-hydroxybutyl)nitrosamine (BBN), nitrofurans and other nitroaromatics, nitrosoureas, or phosphoramide mustards such as cyclophosphamide. Recently, DNA adducts of aristolochic acid (AA) have been identified in human urothelial carcinomas (see above).

These genotoxic chemicals are metabolically-activated to reactive electrophiles which covalently bind to DNA, leading to mutations and ultimately to the formation of cancer. However, in general, these chemicals induce detectable incidences of urothelial tumors in animal bioassays only when administered at doses sufficient to also produce hyperplasia as a consequence of cytotoxicity and regenerative hyperplasia. In contrast to these chemicals are numerous others which produce cancer without being genotoxic. Most of these chemicals produce cancer of the urothelium by increasing cell proliferation due to cytotoxicity with consequent regenerative hyperplasia. The toxicity can be produced either by formation of urinary solids, reaction of the chemical and/or its metabolites with the urothelium, or alteration of normal urinary constituents leading to toxicity.

RESPONSE TO INJURY

Introduction

Cell Death

Apoptosis plays an important role in nephron development in fetal kidney, and in tubular repair following renal insult. Numerous toxicants have been implicated to trigger or block the intracellular processes resulting in abnormal regulation of apoptosis mediating a wide range of pathologic consequences ranging from renal agenesis to neoplasia.

Apoptosis is increased in atrophy, after reversal of organ hypertrophy, after radiomimetic cancer chemotherapeutics and ionizing radiation, as well as after administration of numerous tubular toxicants. The agents affecting renal apoptosis are comprised of heavy metals, pharmacological agents, and naturally-occurring toxins. Many tubular toxicants, such as lead and aminoglycosides, which induce oncotic necrosis at high exposures, induce apoptotic necrosis at lower exposures. Accelerated apoptosis has been defined as a pivotal feature in renal toxicity, such as the alpha$_{2\mu}$ globulin nephropathy syndrome and fumonsin nephrotoxicity. Increased apoptosis can be recognized by an increased tissue replicative rate in the absence of hyperplasia, or by demonstration of increased apoptotic cells in urine, tissue, and/or uriniferous spaces (see Figure 11.15).

Nephron Unit Response

A major concept in toxicologic pathology of the kidney is the propensity for the nephron to respond to injury as a unit, rather than to respond only at the subtopographical site of injury. The nonspecific hallmark of the nephron response to injury (cell death) is the alteration of the tinctorial characteristics of the proximal tubular cell cytoplasm from the normal functional eosinophilia to the basophilia of a regenerating cell. This occurs concomitantly with basement membrane thickening (see Figure 11.9B). These changes are present in continuous segments of a single nephron, and are observed histologically in several tubules in cross-section with adjacent tubules often oriented perpendicular to the inner medulla. This change initially appears in a subacute time frame (three to seven days). However, individual xenobiotics or classes of xenobiotics may, in addition, also induce morphologically-specific primary injury, based on the cellular or subcellular organelle target site. Responses to injury are thus usefully considered on a subtopographical basis.

Glomerulus

Any process that interferes with the structural integrity of the glomerulus can result in abnormal loss of protein in the urine, predominantly albumin. Glomerular injury may be non-inflammatory (glomerulopathy) or inflammatory (glomerulonephritis). Affected glomeruli may be observed grossly in some cases. Histologic changes are characterized by one or more of the following: hypercellularity due to cellular proliferation or leukocytic infiltration; basement membrane thickening; and hyalinization and sclerosis.

Non-inflammatory Glomerular Injury

A non-inflammatory glomerular injury of potential importance in toxicologic pathology is designated "focal segmental glomerulosclerosis" by medical pathologists.

Focal Segmental Glomerulosclerosis

"Focal" denotes absence of involvement of all nephrons, in contrast to diffuse involvement. The term "segmental" denotes involvement of only part of an individual glomerulus, in contrast to global involvement. Aminonucleosides and heroin exemplify agents with this effect. Light microscopically, increased PAS-positive staining occurs in the affected tuft, with increased silver staining in the thickened basement membrane. Ultimately the tuft becomes sclerotic or scarred (>3 weeks), and may stain positively with Masson's trichrome for collagen. Occasionally, immune-complex trapping can be demonstrated, but is considered secondary. The medical pathologist examining the kidneys of old rats with chronic progressive nephropathy would designate this spontaneous lesion in early stages as focal segmental glomerulosclerosis.

Membranous Nephropathy

Membranous nephropathy is thought to be caused by immune-complex deposition in the glomerular tuft, and is the most common cause of nephrotic syndrome in adults. Repeated (chronic) injection of soluble antigens produces this lesion, characterized by subepithelial immune-complex (IgG and C3) deposition, recognized light microscopically with silver stains as spikes of argyrophilic material on the epithelial surface of the basement membrane. In routine histologic sections, the capillary wall of the affected glomerulus is diffusely slightly thickened. Membranous nephropathy is sometimes classified as membranous glomerulonephritis, especially in veterinary medicine.

Mesangiolysis

Capillary endothelial cell loss and glomerular capillary cysts, as well as leukocyte-mediated intravascular fibrin deposition, occur in the hemolytic uremia syndrome, with subsequent cortical necrosis. Some snake venoms produced by the Crotalidae family can cause mesangiolysis with mesangioproliferative glomerulonephritis in survivors (see Figure 11.8).

Inflammatory Glomerular Injury

Inflammation of the glomerulus is termed glomerulonephritis. It is frequently due to immune-mediated disease during which antigen, antibody, or immune complexes are deposited within the glomerulus. Localization within the glomerulus is partially due to molecular charge and size of the molecule, as well as by glomerular factors. Fluorescence and electron microscopy are used to define the type and location of the deposits, which help to identify the specific type or origin of the glomerular disease.

Hypercellularity due to leukocyte infiltration and/or cell proliferation are the hallmarks of an inflamed glomerulus. If the proliferating cell is mesangial, the process is designated mesangioproliferative glomerulonephritis. If neutrophils are increased in the tuft, the process is designated exudative glomerulonephritis. Severe tuft inflammation may lead to proliferation of parietal epithelial cells which, together with leukocytes, form crescents, thus, crescentic glomerulonephritis.

Membranoproliferative glomerulonephritis denotes a combination of mesangial cell proliferation and basement membrane thickening, with ultrastructurally-evident subendothelial deposits. Glomerulonephritis typically has a primary immunologic etiology. Because of the rare occurrence of glomerulonephritis as a primary injury mechanism in the practice of toxicologic pathology, it will not be further discussed.

Proximal Tubule and Interstitium

Tubule-interstitial Disease

In humans and dogs, injury to the tubules and interstitium are typically lumped together under the heading tubule-interstitial disease. Disorders that affect the tubules cause immediate reaction in the interstitium and vice versa. Also, in humans and dogs in advanced stages, tubule-interstitial diseases tend to resemble each other, and are given the common morphologic designation of chronic interstitial nephritis. In contrast, in rats, primary interstitial disease is poorly-documented, other than in purposeful attempts to induce immunologic disease models. Furthermore, the consistent minimal expression of renal toxicity in the rat is designated as exacerbated CPN, rather than chronic interstitial nephritis. This species-difference in interstitial response is exemplified by direct comparison of the chronic renal effects of a diphosphonate drug at high dosages (used in the treatment of Paget's EHDP) in the dog and the rat. The dog response is that of chronic interstitial nephritis, whereas the rat response is characterized as increased incidence and severity of CPN.

Chronic interstitial nephritis is characterized by interstitial fibrosis, interstitial inflammatory infiltrates, tubular atrophy, and glomerular sclerosis. Numerous additional examples exist in which common agents including gentamycin, mercury, and cadmium, induce tubular disease or exacerbated CPN in rats, and tubule-interstitial disease or chronic interstitial disease in humans. Data strongly support the concept that common mechanisms exist for these comparative nephrotoxins, with the expression of injury varying between rat and human. The concept that the exacerbation of CPN is not of relevance in risk assessment lacks merit, based on the plethora of published data on comparative nephrotoxicants.

If interstitial inflammation occurs without evidence of tubular injury, is severe, and appears early in the process, contains eosinophils or polymononuclear leukocytes, or occurs with peritubular immune-complex antibody deposition, the process should be regarded as a primary interstitial nephritis. If focal areas of tubular necrosis accompany the interstitial reaction, it is called tubulo-interstitial nephritis. The process most commonly producing this pattern of renal injury is hypersensitivity to synthetic penicillins, especially methicillin, as well as other synthetic antibiotics, diuretics, and NSAIDs. The response typically has a delayed onset (approximately 15 days after initiation of exposure), and is not dose-responsive.

Acute Tubular Nephrosis

Acute tubular nephrosis (ATN) is a clinicopathologic entity, characterized morphologically by destruction of tubular epithelial cells and clinically by acute diminution and loss of renal function. It is the most common cause of acute renal failure. The two most common causes of ATN are ischemia and direct toxic injury to the tubular cells by agents such as drugs, heavy metals, radiocontrast dyes, and radiation. Acutely affected kidneys may be pale and swollen, with bulging of the cortex on cut section. The medulla may be pale or congested.

In spontaneous renal injury, it may be difficult to differentiate ischemic and toxic tubular injury, and a combination may be present. Ischemic ATN is characterized by focal tubular epithelial necrosis at multiple points along the nephron, with unaffected segments in between. The pars recta and the ascending thick limb of the medulla are most affected in humans. Degenerative changes, rather than necrosis, are often

present. If necrosis is present, it is often accompanied by rupture of basement membrane (tubulorrhexis). Interstitial edema, leukocytes within dilated vasa recta, and evidence of epithelial regeneration are often present. In contrast, in toxic ATN, the pars recta and the proximal convoluted tubule are affected diffusely, and basement membrane remains intact. In both types, protein casts are often present in the distal tubules. Tubules often appear dilated, due to loss or flattening of the epithelium.

Xenobiotic-induced acute alteration of proximal tubular epithelium, degeneration with or without necrosis, should be designated acute tubular nephrosis in the laboratory rodent and other animals. Several patterns of specific alterations occur, depending on the inciting agent and thus on the mechanism. The type of cell death, necrosis or apoptosis, should be differentiated. Most tubular toxicants, if given at sufficiently high concentrations, can induce tubular cell death. The responsibility of the toxicologic pathologist is to report the site of tubular cell death. Cell death can readily be identified as primarily occurring in the PCT, or in the pars recta. Although a few agents induce specific alterations, such as lead-induced intranuclear inclusions, which stain with the modified acid-fast stain, most toxicants induce very nonspecific injury.

Regeneration following ATN is largely dependent on the basement membrane being intact, the xenobiotic being removed, and adequate epithelium remaining. Initially, remaining epithelium flattens out to cover the basement membrane. Regeneration may be seen three days after injury, and is characterized by cuboidal epithelium with basophilic cytoplasm, hypertrophic nuclei, and occasional mitotic figures. Normal-appearing tubular epithelium may be seen after 7 to 14 days, and a return to normal structure after 21 days. If regeneration does not take place, tubular atrophy and interstitial fibrosis result. If basement membrane damage is severe, there is loss of regenerative capacity, and interstitial inflammation takes place.

Agents that induce proximal tubular necrosis at higher doses typically induce accelerated apoptosis at lower doses. For example, gentamycin and mercury, at high doses (but below the dose sufficient for inducing light microscopic lesions), causes replicative and apoptotic rate increases in PCT. Increases in proximal tubular cell replicative rate and urine apoptotic cell count may reflect a more sensitive indication of cell injury than light microscopic examination in short-term studies.

Osmotic Nephrosis

Osmotically-active agents such as mannitol and sucrose can induce osmotic nephrosis. Microscopically, the change in proximal convoluted tubules is diffuse and characterized by cytoplasmic vacuolation; hydropic change is limited to the phagolysosome (see Figure 11.12). Osmotic nephrosis or hydropic change occurs in ethylene glycol toxicity, but here the vacuolation may also occur between the proximal tubular cell and basement membrane.

Hyaline Droplet Nephrosis

This represents phagolysosomal protein overload. Increased glomerular filtrate protein, derived via glomerular disease, primarily represents albumin, and typically stains PAS positive. In contrast, the protein overload associated with the inducible alpha$_{2\mu}$ globulin nephropathy syndrome results in hyaline droplets that are PAS negative, but Mallory's Heidenhain positive (see Figure 11.14). Mallory's stain is not specific to alpha$_{2\mu}$ globulin, but rather it is specific to the biochemical attributes of this protein. Purity of the protein within the phagolysosome may result in crystalloid change, such as is associated with alpha$_{2\mu}$ globulin, Bence–Jones protein, myoglobin, and hemoglobin nephropathies.

Lipidosis

Lipidosis of proximal tubular epithelium occurs spontaneously, but is not severe in the rat and the mouse (Figure 11.21). These cytoplasmic fat droplets can be confirmed by the oil red-O staining of frozen sections. Increased fat or lipid nephrosis is not a common toxicologic response, but can be observed, for example, as a transient acute change when corn oil is

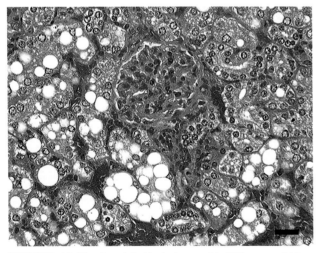

FIGURE 11.21   Renal lipidosis in an old CD1 mouse kidney. Bar = 20 μm.

used as a vehicle for xenobiotics. Subtle light microscopic differences exist between osmotic nephrosis and fatty degeneration so that, with experience, differentiation is possible in routine sections.

Phospholipidosis

Phospholipidosis in the kidney is most typically induced by aminoglycoside antibiotic therapy. On light microscopy, the proximal tubular epithelial cells may have subtly increased cytoplasmic lucency. Special stains for phospholipids, such as Baker's, have not proved useful in light microscopic confirmation of this process. In toluidine blue-stained plastic sections, however, cytoplasmic bodies are readily apparent by light microscopy. Ultrastructurally, the hallmark of phospholipidosis is the presence of concentric multilaminated phospholipid membrane whorls in the phagolysosome, designated myelin figures. Toluidine blue staining is useful for presumptive diagnosis of tubular phospholipidosis.

Necrosis

Oncotic necrosis of tubular cells can be induced by ischemia, heavy metals, and xenobiotics requiring metabolic transformation to exert their toxic potential (see Figure 11.11). Ischemia, certain metals that affect cell respiration (such as mercury), and xenobiotics requiring metabolic transformation preferentially effect the pars recta. This propensity may require time–dose studies for demonstration since, with increased severity, all segments of the proximal tubule may be injured. Other heavy metals, such as lead, and xenobiotics bound to proteins preferentially injure the PCT. Because protein reabsorption activity predominates at this level, xenobiotics requiring transport, such as organic acids or bases, also preferentially affect the PCT.

In domestic animals, causes of tubular degeneration and necrosis include antibiotics such as oxytetracycline, amphotericin B, and sulfonamides; heavy metals, mycotoxins, and plant toxins (see Tables 11.3 and 11.4). Many of these have been described under mechanisms of toxicity. Ochratoxin A and citrinin induce tubular epithelial degeneration and necrosis in swine. This can progress to renal fibrosis in chronic toxicity.

Many plants cause tubular necrosis in domestic animals. Several species of pigweed, especially *Amaranthus retroflexus*, a plant high in oxalate and nitrate, causes tubular injury in swine, cattle, and uncommonly in horses. Leaves, buds, or acorns from oak trees or shrubs (*Quercus* spp.) cause tubular necrosis in cattle and sheep, thought to be due to tannins and their metabolites such as gallic acid. Following ingestion of either plant, there is severe perirenal edema and the kidneys are pale.

In cats, lily toxicity has been recently recognized, with many different members of *Lilium* sp. being nephrotoxic. Leaves and, to a lesser extent, the flowers are responsible. Acute proximal tubular necrosis occurs (Figure 11.22). Easter lilies are a common source of the toxic plant. Lily toxicity has not been reported in other species. Raisins and grapes can cause proximal tubular necrosis in dogs, characterized by scattered mineralized casts and brown intracellular and intralumenal pigment in many cases (Figure 11.23). Hypercalcemia also occurs in many cases. Raisin/grape toxicity has not been reported in other species.

Apoptotic necrosis of tubular epithelium is a feature of experimental fumonisin toxicity in rats, rabbits, and young ruminants (see Figure 11.15). Apoptosis has also been described in cadmium toxicity experimentally.

Necrosis with Crystal Formation

Poorly-soluble sulfonamides can crystallize in the tubules and cause direct toxicity to the tubular epithelium via mechanical means. Crystals are usually detected on gross, but not histologic, examination, since they dissolve with tissue processing. Proximal tubular degeneration and nephrosis occur in oxalate nephrosis, which can be induced by ingestion of ethylene glycol (see under Mechanisms of Toxicity) or some plants. The specific findings are pale yellow, birefringent, calcium oxalate crystals in the tubular

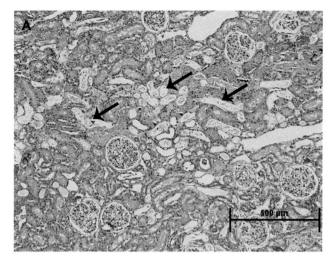

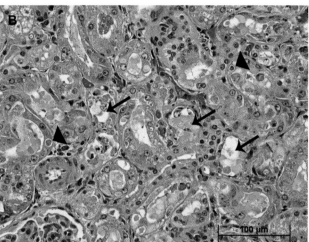

FIGURE 11.23   Tubular necrosis due to ingestion of raisins, dog, kidney. (A) Within the cortex, tubules appear dilated (arrows) and often contain granular material. (B) Tubular epithelium has undergone degeneration with necrotic cells sloughing into the lumen (arrows). Intracytoplasmic hyaline bodies are present within some remaining epithelial cells (arrowheads). Intralumenal and intracellular pigment may occasionally be observed (not shown) (H&E stain).

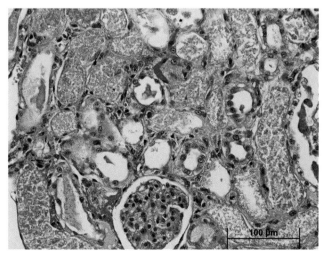

FIGURE 11.22   Tubular necrosis due to ingestion of Easter lily, cat, kidney. Tubular epithelium is largely absent and granular casts fill the lumens (H&E stain).

lumens, and sometimes also in the tubular epithelium and interstitium. These crystals are arranged in rosettes or sheaves, and can be readily identified with polarized light (see Figure 11.13). Distal tubular necrosis was reported in cats and dogs following ingestion of pet food contaminated by melamine and cyanuric acid (see under Mechanisms of Toxicity). Crystals are pinwheel shape, granular, and readily-visualized without the need for polarized light (see Figure 11.18).

Necrosis with Hemoglobin Casts

Hemoglobin casts may be seen with some toxicants, such as copper toxicity in sheep and red maple

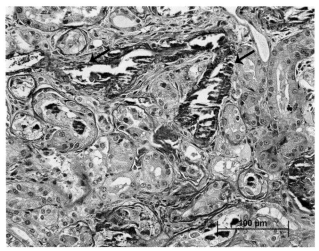

FIGURE 11.24   Tubular necrosis and mineralization due to chole-calciferol toxicity following ingestion of quintox rodenticide, dog, kidney. Linear areas of mineralization outline tubules with necrotic tubular epithelium (arrows). Mineral deposits are also present within the tubular lumens and on tubular basement membranes (H&E stain).

(*Acer rubrum*) toxicity in horses, where hemoglobinuria occurs secondarily to severe intravascular hemolysis (see Figure 11.16). Pigmented casts accompany ischemic tubular necrosis. Grossly, with copper toxicity, the kidneys are blue-black, so-called "gunmetal" kidneys, and the medulla is also darkly-stained. There is severe proximal tubular epithelial degeneration and necrosis, and tubular lumens are filled with orange-red heme casts.

Mineralization

Excess Vitamin D and xenobiotics exerting vitamin D-like biologic activity, at sufficiently high doses, cause mineralization of renal basement membranes, both vascular and tubular (Figure 11.24). A commercially-available rodenticide contains cholecalciferol and has this potential for rodents, as well as domestic animals, mainly dogs, consuming the agent. Ingestion of plant-derived calcinogenic glycosides by cattle and horses can also induce mineralization (see discussion under Mechanisms).

Perturbation of calcium phosphorus ratios, for example, through the use of certain commercially-available synthetic rodent diets (AIN 76), results in severe tubular lumenal mineralization, predominantly restricted to the pars recta (see Figure 11.17). Special stains, such as Alizarin Red S or Von Kossa's, are recommended for demonstration of mineralization. Calcium salt precipitation in tissue can go undetected in routinely stained sections.

Inner medullary and pelvic mineralization occurs spontaneously, but can be exacerbated by certain test agents, such as sucralose, kaolin, sorbitol, and magnesium sulfate. These agents cause cecal enlargement and increased calcium absorption, evidenced by increased urinary calcium with urothelial hyperplasia as a sequela to the mineral deposits.

Chronic Progressive Nephropathy

Chronic progressive nephropathy is the term for a common spontaneous disease of rats (see Figure 11.9). The cause of the spontaneous disease, at least in part, is protein and caloric overnutrition. The association of protein overnutrition has been discussed under glomerular hemodynamic perturbation. Exacerbation of lesions of CPN represents the most commonly-reported minimal expression of nephrotoxicity in the rat. Most nephrotoxicants, at doses below those that induce overt evidence of nephron or tubular injury, cause or exacerbate injury morphologically the same as the lesions of CPN. Gentamycin represents a prototypical compound exemplifying this concept. Many nephrotoxicants that exacerbate CPN at lower doses induce specific toxicological injury at higher doses, such as proximal convoluted tubular necrosis and intranuclear inclusions, with lead as the example. Many nephrotoxicants that induce specific injury simultaneously exacerbate the lesions of CPN. Agents inducing the unique alpha$_{2\mu}$ globulin nephropathy syndrome exemplify this concept. Recognizing the cause of CPN as single nephron hyperfusion enables understanding as to why the CPN change is nonspecific, as any cause of nephron injury can indirectly cause the hyperfiltration of uninjured nephrons as a compensatory change. Looking across a multitude of tubular toxicants in the rat, exacerbation of the lesions of CPN represents the unifying designation for chronic injury.

In chronic progressive nephropathy of rats, three predominate changes occur in extracellular matrix over time. The first change is a generalized thickening of basement membranes that is characterized immunohistochemically by increase in laminins. Second, an increase in extracellular matrix occurs in the interstitium, characterized by increased fibronectin and thrombospondin. The third change observed with aging is interstitial scarring in areas of tubular atrophy. The most predictive clinical laboratory pathology correlate with CPN is urinary albumin increase. An age-related spontaneous occurrence of chronic progressive nephropathy becomes apparent by 20 weeks of age, utilizing urinary albumin as the biomarker.

Kidney disease processes that have sufficient injury to be recognizable as irreversible and progressive, even in the absence of the initiating event, have progressed sufficiently in the vicious cycle of nephron loss, with responsive increased perfusion in residual nephrons so that insufficient nephrons remain to accomplish urinary function without hyperfiltration on an individual nephron basis. Chronic progressive nephropathy in this context represents the final common pathway of renal failure, regardless of the instigating mechanism.

Nephrotoxicants, after a single or acute exposure period, can also induce or exacerbate CPN. The pivotal feature seems to be whether the integrity of the basement membrane is compromised in this acute injury process. Acute tubular necrosis of a moderately severe extent can be completely reversible if basement membrane integrity is maintained.

Renal Papillary Necrosis

Renal papillary necrosis (RPN) develops microscopically, and can be graded in terms of severity. Each of these grades may represent an endpoint in the lesions for the individual animal. In an animal with the most severe grade of lesion, the papilla still presumably goes through these antecedent, less-severe stages. Grade one is characterized by the loss of microvasculature, loops of Henle, and interstitial cells, with replacement by eosinophilic homogenous substrate. This occurs with complete preservation of collecting ducts. Epithelium covering the papilla may be intact or focally disrupted. In grade two, focal necrosis of all structures occurs, but is limited to the apex of the papilla (see Figure 11.20B). In grade three, confluent necrosis extends to mid-papilla. In grade four, confluent necrosis extends to the base of the papilla. In grade five, confluent necrosis extends to outer medulla. The necrotic papilla may mineralize, or the mineralization may be restricted to a transverse band at the junction, with viable medulla. Abscission of the necrotic papilla may occur, followed by re-epithelization of remaining viable medulla.

Secondary cortical changes develop as a consequence of nephron obstruction in RPN, reported as glomerulosclerosis. Re-epithelialized medulla or urothelium in proximity to nonviable tissue may become hyperplastic. Neoplasia may ultimately develop from this hyperplastic urothelium, if the rat is carried through its normal lifespan. Neoplasia occurring secondary to RPN is of limited relevance in risk assessment, since RPN is uncommon in humans and linked with analgesic abuse when associated with toxic xenobiotic exposure.

In domestic animals, horses, calves, and dogs, gross lesions of papillary necrosis are often multifocal, sharply-delineated, with a greenish yellow appearance (see Figure 11.20A). The necrotic papilla may slough, leaving an attenuated inner medulla. Small pieces of sloughed tissue may be passed through the ureter; however, larger pieces may obstruct the ureter resulting in hydronephrosis, or serve as a nidus for mineralization and develop into concretions. However, functional effects are rare.

Renal Tubular Hyperplasia and Neoplasia

Carefully-studied models of renal tumor development in the rat, regardless of mechanism, demonstrate a dose-responsive increase in hyperplastic tubules, morphologically representing a continuum of change up to and including neoplasm development. Furthermore, in toxic tubular tumorigenesis, the increased incidence and severity of CPN has been demonstrated to parallel an increase in regenerative and hyperplastic tubules, again up to and including neoplasm formation (Figures 11.25 and 11.26A; Table 11.10).

The distinctive criterion differentiating hyperplasia from neoplasia in the proximal tubule is growth, which is constrained within the boundaries of the tubule of origin in hyperplasia. In neoplasia, tubular epithelial growth disrupts and compromises the integrity of the otherwise constraining basement membrane. The reversibility or progression of the lesion, with discontinuation of dosing, forms the definitive criterion for differentiation of borderline lesions. If definitive neoplasms are increased ($\geq$10% difference) and all types of hyperplasias are increased, including borderline lesions in a group, then a tumorigenic process has probably occurred. The universal criterion of malignancy, metastasis, is an uncommon feature of renal tubular carcinomas. The primary criteria for differentiating between benign and malignant, in the absence of metastasis, include cellular and invasive growth, cellular anaplasia, and basement membrane reduplication.

Several additional kinds of renal neoplasms that are associated with xenobiotic exposure may occur. These neoplasms uncommonly occur spontaneously. The renal mesenchymal tumor occurs in young rats, associated with genotoxic insult at an immature age. The predominant cell type is a fibroblastic spindle cell, with predisposition to encircle sequestered pre-existing tubules. Smooth muscle fibers, vascular structures, and occasionally striated muscle and cartilage can be found in these tumors. This tumor is often very malignant. The nephroblastoma is a tumor of the young rat, rarely occurring spontaneously, but inducible with specific *in utero* genotoxic insult. This tumor consists of islands of densely-packed blastema-like basophilic

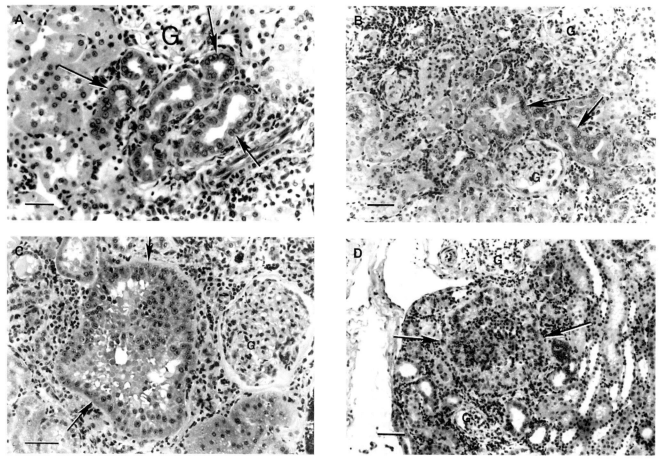

FIGURE 11.25   Proximal tubule proliferation and neoplasia (arrows). Glomerulus (G). (A) Tubular regeneration (Bar = 25 µm). (B) Simple hyperplasia, basophilic cell type (Bar = 50 µm). (C) Complex (or nodular) hyperplasia with atypia, basophilic cell type (Bar = 50 µm). (D) Complex hyperplasia with atypia, basophilic cell type. This particular lesion represents the most extreme degree of hyperplasia. Interstitial constituents, small size, preservation, and thickness of section contribute to the uncertainty about the integrity of, and continuity with, the nephron of origin of this proliferative process. This is a prerequisite to definitive differentiation of neoplasia from hyperplasia (Bar = 100 µm). (Courtesy of Dr R. Bruner, Pathology Associates, Inc., Cincinnati, Ohio.)

cells, with scant cytoplasm and ill-defined cytoplasmic margins, often with a tubular structure at their center (Figure 11.26B). Glomeruloid formation is typically found.

Of 230 chemicals tested by the National Toxicology Program (NTP), only 4% were associated with renal tumorigenesis, while 25% were nephrotoxic. Two classes of agents identified with high potential for nephrotoxicity were organohalides and aromatic amines. The majority of chemicals inducing tumors were organohalides. The organohalides are generally considered as genotoxic, as well as cytotoxic in the proximal tubule.

Lower Urinary Tract: Non-neoplastic Lesions

Cytotoxicity and Necrosis

Acute toxicity of the urothelium can be produced either by reaction of the chemical and/or its metabolites with the urothelium, by production of urinary solids, or by significant alterations of normal urinary constituents. The resulting acute injury can be of two major types, either superficial, involving the superficial cell layer and possibly the intermediate cell layer, or the injury can be more profound, leading to damage of the full thickness of the epithelium with ulceration.

If the injury is superficial, histologic changes by light microscopy can be minimal, with necrosis only detected by electron microscopy. The necrosis is usually followed by a mild degree of simple hyperplasia. The epithelium quickly returns to normal, unless the inciting stimulus is prolonged, in which case papillary and/or nodular hyperplasia can ensue.

Toxicity which results in ulceration follows a rather typical course. Vacuolization of the epithelium is rapidly followed by necrosis and denudation of the epithelium. The basement membrane is usually breached, and there is acute hemorrhage, edema, and

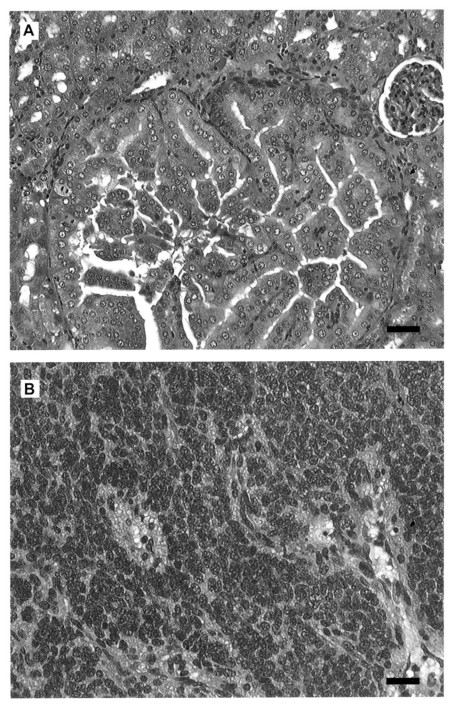

FIGURE 11.26   Renal tumors in CD1 mouse kidneys. (A) Tubular adenoma (Bar = 40 μm). (B) Nephrobastoma (Bar = 20 μm).

inflammation (cystitis). If the inciting toxic agent is administered briefly, the ulcer is repaired within 3–6 weeks, with the epithelium and bladder wall returning to normal. However, fibrosis in the submucosa and even in the underlying muscle wall, as well as lymphocytes and macrophages can remain for a long time after the ulcer heals. Ulceration, in contrast to superficial erosion, is usually accompanied by a much

more prominent, regenerative process with not only simple hyperplasia, but also papillary and/or nodular formation and even papilloma formation. These epithelial changes are completely reversible if the inciting agent is removed before the formation of malignancy.

Necrosis, inflammation, and hemorrhage due to xenobiotic exposure occurs in domestic animals. In cattle, ingestion of bracken fern (*Pteridium aquilinum*)

TABLE 11.10   Suggested descriptive nomenclature for reporting common nonproliferative alterations[a]

Congenital lesions	Cell death
Renal agenesis	Apoptosis (single cell death)
Renal hypoplasia	Oncosis (necrosis)
Polycystic kidney	
Adrenal rest	
Hydronephrosis	
Disturbances of cell growth/differentiation	**Degenerative changes**
Glomerular atrophy	Tubular epithelial vacuolation
Tubule atrophy	Hyaline droplets
Cell/tubule hypertrophy	Intracellular inclusion bodies
Tubule regeneration	Cytoplasmic pigmentation
Karyomegaly/karyocytomegaly/multinucleation	Tubular dilatation
Bowman's capsule metaplasia/hyperplasia	Tubular casts (hyaline or grannular)
Squamous cell metaplasia of pelvic epithelium	Crystal formation
Osseous metaplasia	Mineralization (tubular, vascular, interstitial, or renal pelvic)
	Renal calculi
	Amyloidosis
	Glomerulosclerosis
Inflammatory changes	**Vascular changes**
Glomerulonephritis (membraneous, mesangioproliferative, or crescentic)	Vascular thrombosis
	Infarction (acute or chronic)
Pyelonephritis	Periarteritis
Interstitial nephritis	
Interstitial fibrosis	
Microabscesses	
Miscellaneous changes	**Special disease processes**
Extramedullary hematopoiesis	Chronic progressive nephropathy (CPN)
Cortical necrosis	Alpha$_{2\mu}$ globulin nephropathy
Papillary necrosis	Obstructive nephropathy

Severity modifiers: minimal (<1%); mild (1–10%); moderate (10–25%); moderately severe (25–75%); severe (75%)

Duration modifiers: acute, subacute, or chronic

Distribution modifiers: focal, multifocal/segmental, or diffuse/global

[a]Modified from Hard et al., 1999

causes chronic hemorrhagic cystitis (enzootic hematuria) which is accompanied by proliferative urothelial lesions and neoplasia (see below). Hematoxicity resulting in anemia is also present. In horses, cystitis and ataxia have been associated with ingestion of hybrid strains of *Sorghum* spp. Ingestion of blister beetles (*Epicauta* spp.) found in alfalfa hay causes ulceration and necrosis of the urinary bladder and gastrointestinal tract of horses, as well as myocardial necrosis. The toxic agent is cantharadin, a bicyclic terpenoid. In dogs and cats, cyclophosphamide treatment can cause hemorrhagic cystitis, due to the effect of acrolein, a metabolite of cyclophosphamide.

Hyperplasia

Hyperplasia can be either focal or diffuse. Simple hyperplasia is defined as an increase in the number of cell layers greater than normally present, and is frequently associated with an increase in mitosis and is sometimes accompanied by inflammation. Nodular hyperplasia (Figure 11.27) represents an endophytic growth, with epithelial cells accumulating in what appears to be the subepithelial connective tissue, similar to von Brunn's nests in human pathology. Although these frequently do not appear to be connected to the overlaying epithelium, serial sections can usually demonstrate the connection. Such lesions should not be mistaken for invasive carcinoma. Papillary hyperplasia is an exophytic growth, consisting of fronds of well-differentiated epithelial cells layered around a central fibrovascular core (Figure 11.28). Distinguishing between papillary hyperplasia and papillomas can be difficult.

Squamous Metaplasia

Squamous metaplasia of the urothelium can be produced by chronic inflammation, administration of bladder toxicants or carcinogens, or vitamin A deficiency. It can be reversible if the inciting stimulus is removed. The metaplasia is usually non-keratinizing, but keratinization can occur. Squamous metaplasia is frequently accompanied by chronic inflammation. Squamous cell carcinoma can arise from areas of squamous metaplasia.

Mineralization

Calcification of the lower urinary tract is commonly seen at the fornix of the kidney pelvis, and is usually accompanied by chronic inflammation and epithelial hyperplasia. In other portions of the lower urinary tract, calcification is frequently associated with the presence of calculi. In fact, the presence of mineralization in the urothelium, in association with proliferative and neoplastic lesions, can be taken as evidence of the former presence of urinary calculi or crystals. Remnants of calcification can also be seen in the lumen associated with neoplastic lesions, even if calculi are not obvious. Calculi composed of substances other than calcium, especially those composed of organic chemicals, may not be detectable by histologic analysis, since they may be lost during fixation, embedding, or staining.

Intracytoplasmic Granules

Intracytoplasmic, eosinophilic-to-clear inclusions are occasionally seen in urothelial cells as a response to toxicity, but are considered normal in rhesus monkeys.

Lower Urinary Tract Epithelial Neoplasms

Most malignancies of the lower urinary tract arise from the epithelium, and show urothelial differentiation. In humans, bladder cancer appears to represent two distinct diseases. The more common disorder consists of low-grade, papillary neoplasms which do not

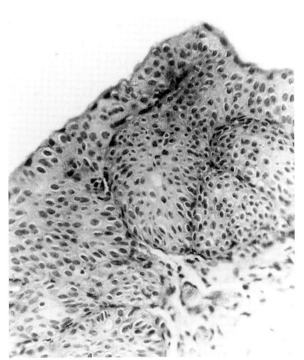

FIGURE 11.27 Nodular hyperplasia of the rat urinary bladder induced by FANFT (H&E stain). (From Cohen, S.M. (1983). *The Pathology of Bladder Cancer*, II:9. With permission.)

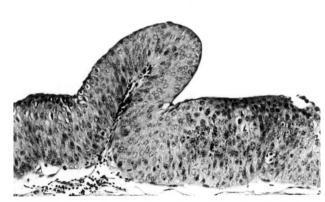

FIGURE 11.28 Papillary hyperplasia of the rat bladder induced by FANFT, with adjacent severe simple hyperplasia (H&E stain).

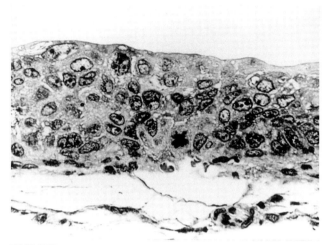

FIGURE 11.29   Urothelial carcinoma *in situ* in a male mouse treated with BBN for 12 weeks.

invade or metastasize, but have a strong propensity to recur. The second disease is non-papillary, high grade, and frequently presents as an invasive lesion which commonly metastasizes. This type of disease begins as a flat, dysplastic abnormality of the epithelium, progressing to carcinoma *in situ* (CIS, Figure 11.29), and eventually to invasive carcinoma. These two diseases are mimicked to a great degree in rodents. In the rat, papillary neoplasms occur most commonly, but in contrast to humans, they can further evolve to high-grade and invasive lesions. In mice, non-papillary neoplasms are most common. Papillomas are benign epithelial lesions of the bladder which project into the lumen as polypoid formations. In rodents, these frequently have the appearance of inverted papillomas. There is no cellular or nuclear pleomorphism or anaplasia, and they can have a narrow or broad base. Mitoses are uncommon, and the epithelial lining of the papillary fronds and nodules is generally limited to three to five cell layers in thickness. Focal areas of atypia, mitotic activity, increased basophilia, or invasiveness of the underlying connective tissue are indicators of a transition to carcinoma.

The classic example of xenobiotic-induced urothelial carcinoma in domestic animals is in cattle, due to ingestion of bracken fern (*Pteridium aquilinum*). Chronic hemorrhagic cystitis (enzootic hematuria) is accompanied by hyperplasia of the urothelium in the urinary bladder, ureter, and renal pelvis. Adenomas, papillomas, fibroma, hemangiomas, adenocarcinomas, and transitional cell and squamous carcinomas have been reported, with papillomas most common. The carcinogen is believed to be ptaquiloside which forms adducts with DNA. Humans are potentially at risk if they consume rhizomes or croziers of bracken fern, since young growing portions of the fern contain the highest levels of ptaquiloside. In addition, this toxin may be present in milk from cows grazing bracken fern.

EVALUATION OF TOXICITY

Diagnostic Evaluation of Renal Disease

Kidney weight can easily be obtained, and both absolute and organ to body weight ratio may be useful. The kidney can be evaluated *in situ* for location, size, presence of perirenal edema, and any capsular alterations. In larger animals, the capsule should always be removed, so that the surface can be evaluated for changes in color and contour. On cut section, the cut surface should be evaluated for swelling (bulging), the ratio of cortex to medulla, and the presence, distribution, and character of any lesions. In acute disease, often little is seen with death due to potassium-induced cardiotoxicity, metabolic acidosis and pulmonary edema. In chronic renal disease, readily observable changes may be present in the kidneys, as well as in other organs. In uremia there may be mineralization of the lung, kidney, stomach, and to a lesser extent other tissues. In the nephrotic syndrome, edema, ascites, and pleural effusions may be present. Impression smears can identify the presence of crystals. Urinalysis on urine collected from the bladder may provide useful insights (see below).

In larger animals, midsagittal and transverse sections of the kidney, including the papilla, are immersion-fixed in 10% neutral buffered formalin, embedded in paraffin, and sectioned at 3 to 4 um. Rodent kidney are often fixed whole (see below). Histologically, all components of the kidney need to be examined including glomerulus, tubules, interstitium, vasculature, and papillae for changes, as described in Table 11.10.

Routine Screening for Nephrotoxicity

Rats are typically used in the safety assessment of new molecular entities, as the concordance in response to xenobiotics between rats and humans is excellent. Exceptions include immune-mediated xenobiotic injury in humans, xenobiotic-induced alpha$_{2\mu}$ globulin nephropathy in male rats, and indirect injury due to extremely high xenobiotic doses. Safety assessment based on rat data is complicated by age-associated changes in human renal structure and function, and factors affecting glomerular filtration rate (GFR), including hydration status, hypertension, heart failure, and cirrhosis.

In acute toxicity studies, the recognition that death from renal toxicity with renal failure typically takes three days in the rat is important. Death within 24 to 48 hours of initial treatment probably cannot be attributed to nephrotoxicity with renal failure as the primary mechanism. Familiarity with spontaneous disease is essential for the establishment of the nature and cause of morbidity or mortality in an individual animal.

The most minimal expression of nephrotoxicity may occur simply as a slight exacerbation of the severity of a spontaneous type of lesion. Spontaneous disease may also mask or mimic a toxicologic response. Spontaneous renal lesions include chronic progressive nephropathy and parenchymal mineralization in the rat; amyloidosis in the CD1 mouse and Syrian hamster; granulomatous nephritis due to *Encephalitozoan cuniculi* and mineralization in New Zealand White rabbits; early chronic interstitial nephritis or mineralization in the laboratory beagle under three years of age; eosinophilic crystalline intranuclear inclusions in tubular epithelial cells of old dogs; mineralization and interstitial infiltrates in nonhuman primates, as well as tubulointerstitial nephritis due to *Klossiella equi* in horses. Multifocal segmental to global glomerulosclerosis is often noted in older marmosets and cynomolgus monkeys. Eosinophilic intracytoplasmic inclusions affect the urothelium of approximately 10% of rhesus monkeys, and should not be confused with viral inclusions.

In evaluating new test agents for their nephrotoxic potential in laboratory animals, routine methodologies are appropriately sensitive. At the end of the exposure period, these include clinical chemistry screens with blood urea nitrogen (BUN), creatinine, and electrolytes, urinary excretion of protein and electrolytes, routine urinalysis (with volume, specific gravity, and microscopic sediment evaluations), relative kidney weight determination, and gross and microscopic examination of kidney tissue.

The assessment of nephrotoxicity by the measurement of BUN and creatinine only is less sensitive and nonspecific. For robust assessments of urinary biomarkers, it is essential to collect urine specimens of good quality over a 16 to 24 hour period, and to consider the age of animals being evaluated. In rats, the urinalysis results may become more variable due to the development of spontaneous age-related renal diseases (see Table 11.10). The main age-related changes in these parameters include increases in kidney weights; increased urinary excretion of protein and calcium; decreased urinary excretion of sodium, chloride and *N*-acetyl-β-D glucosaminidase (NAG);

decreased creatinine clearance; increased serum levels of urea, creatinine, sodium, and chloride; and decreased serum levels of albumin.

For routine microscopic examination, immersion fixation in 10% neutral buffered formalin of a single midsagittal section of left and transverse section of the right kidney represents a practical approach. Histopathology is generally recognized as the single most appropriate screen for evidence of renal injury. Evaluations of BUN and creatinine can represent prerenal or postrenal mechanisms, rather than kidney injury. Some reports suggest that urine analyses are more sensitive than histopathology for demonstration of injury. While this may be true on an individual chemical or chemical class basis, convincing evidence on a broader scale remains to be developed. A complicating factor for confirmation is differentiating overt toxicity from physiologic adaptive change in the presence of perturbation of a urine constituent property.

Classification of renal disease should use unambiguous descriptive terminology, including subtopographical anatomy, description of the basic pathologic process, modifiers, and quantitative measure of lesion distribution and extent (see Table 11.10).

Special Techniques

In the event a nephrotoxic potential is recognized, special techniques may be utilized to refine the risk assessment, to explore structure–activity relationships, and to search for sensitive predictors of nephrotoxic events. Thorough characterization of the nephrotoxic event can begin retrospectively with existing wet tissues. Special stains for protein, fat, amyloid, and mineral can be applied to the routine or frozen fixed sections. Reprocessing with plastic embedding, sectioning at 1 μm, and staining with Lee's hematoxylin readily enables the subtopographical identification of lesion site.

To optimally prepare the kidney for examination of lumenal surfaces, for immunohistochemistry, or for electron microscopy evaluation, perfusion fixation should be prospectively employed.

For further understanding of the injury process, morphogenesis and pathogenesis studies are indicated. These are designed to establish or confirm subtopographical, as well as subcellular, organelle targets, to establish interrelationships of renal lesions and biochemical or functional perturbations, to differentiate prerenal and postrenal injury from primary renal insult, and to search for early biomarkers of the injury process. The next step is to conduct time- and dose–response studies using doses sufficiently high to manifest acute injury. One must be aware that, by substantially increasing the dosage to develop an acute model, new or different types of injury may occur. However, models requiring weeks to months of exposure simply are impractical for making rapid progress in the understanding of disease mechanisms.

Several parameters become routine in time- and dose–response studies. The determination of urinary para-aminohippurate (PAH) and inulin clearances for determination of GFR and renal plasma flow (RPF), respectively, are performed. GFR changes developing before onset of renal injury indicate probability of pre-renal (hemodynamic) factors in the cause of the renal injury. Onset of GFR changes after onset of overt renal injury indicates the GFR change to be a consequence of the primary renal injury.

Because increased apoptosis can occur as a more sensitive indicator of injury than routine light microscopy, renal epithelial cell counts in urine or apoptotic cells in tissue sections should be included as an important parameter. This should be combined with replicative rate determinations on day 7. Typically, after examination of the sections by light microscopy, the earliest time points of observed effect and the lowest dose exerting this effect are identified, establishing the subtopographical target.

Specimens for ultrastructural evaluation to determine organellar target should be selected to include one or two affected animals from this earliest time point and lowest affected dose group, and one or two animals from the antecedent period time point, in addition to appropriate controls. Time intervals for sacrifice in the acute injury model to establish the time response could include 1, 3, 5, and 7 days after initiation of treatment. Interrelationship of acute and subacute lesions with subchronic and chronic lesions, of course, might require subchronic studies with sequential interim evaluation. Additional parameters should be included in time–course studies, based on specific knowledge of the test agent and results of previous testing.

After the acute model has been designed, characterized, explored ultrastructurally, and evaluated in the clinical laboratory, a mechanistic hypothesis and proposed early specific biomarkers of injury should be emerging. At this time, the knowledge should exist to design studies to demonstrate early molecular and biochemical premonitors prerequisite in the injury process. The concept that the earliest and most sensitive indicators of perturbation lead to discovery of the primary mechanism of injury in contrast to the consequence of the injury must be continuously considered. With confirmation of a sensitive specific biomarker, a series of studies can be accomplished more efficiently.

The biomarker, of course, may be morphologic or biochemical. At this stage, the pathologist can begin to test the mechanistic hypothesis by experimental manipulation designed to modify the toxic response. Objective quantitation of the biomarker by automated image analysis provides an important tool for improving the sensitivity, reliability, and efficiency of the evaluation. Examples of application include quantitation of mitotic figures in specially-stained sections, identification of the segment of the nephron unit undergoing hypertrophy, and quantitation of hyaline droplet response in specially-stained sections.

Further exploration of the mechanism of toxicity typically requires additional techniques, and must be tailored to each situation. Techniques of value include analytical electron microscopy, analytical chemistry, *in situ* hybridization, proton-nuclear magnetic resonance imaging spectroscopy (PNMR), identification of specific antigenic markers in the tissues and urine via two-dimensional protein electrophoretic separation, and *in vitro* systems for studying nephrotoxic mechanisms.

Evaluation of the Lower Urinary Tract

Evaluation of Urine

Examination of urine has become a critical part of the assessment of mechanisms involved with chemical toxicity and carcinogenicity of the lower urinary tract. Centrifugation and examination of urinary sediment for the presence of increased numbers of crystals or abnormal crystals, formation of urinary precipitate, or presence of calculi is an essential evaluation step. Any variation in diet and water intake may affect urinary composition. pH, osmolality, and urinary chemistries should be assessed. Analysis of urine for the presence of the administered chemical and its metabolites may be useful. Fresh voided urine may be examined cytologically, although typically too few cells are present for this to be done routinely.

Morphologic Evaluation

Urinary bladder is best evaluated microscopically if it is inflated to its normal size with the fixative while the animal is under anesthesia and still alive, because of rapid autolysis. Inflation of the bladder can be done either by injection of fixative through the dome of the bladder, or better, by insertion into the urethra. Ten percent buffered formalin, pH 7.4, is routinely used, but Bouin's fixative provides better fixation if lesions are minimal or absent. This also provides excellent fixation for histochemical, immunohistochemical, and electron microscopic observations. If transmission electron microscopy is to be performed, phosphate-buffered glutaraldehyde remains the fixative of choice. Examination under the dissecting microscope is also a useful adjunct for evaluation.

The presence of calculi or other solids in the lumen should be noted at necropsy. This is particularly important since some calculi may dissolve during fixation, processing for embedding, or during staining procedures. Some calculi, especially those containing calcium, can be observed microscopically. Retrograde seminal ejaculation into the urinary bladder lumen frequently occurs during sacrifice and the concretions of seminal fluid are observed microscopically, usually as homogenous eosinophilic material. This can be mistaken as calculi. Sperm may be present in this coagulum or free in the urine.

For routine processing, the bladder is sliced longitudinally for embedding. Additional examination is required for more detailed studies. Light microscopic evaluation is usually performed on hematoxylin and eosin-stained sections. Von Kossa staining for calcium can be useful under some circumstances. Numerous immunohistochemical and molecular techniques have been developed to further investigate mechanisms involved in the various toxicologic and pathologic changes that develop in the lower urinary tract.

CONCLUSION

The primary method for identification of renal and lower urinary tract toxicity is light microscopic examination of the kidney and urothelium-lined tissues, supplemented with selected serum and urine analyses. In diagnostic pathology, it is often not possible to identify the causative agent from the morphologic changes. Exposure to possible toxicants must be explored, and ancillary information considered.

In development of products with nephrotoxic potential, time–course studies utilizing ultrastructural pathology also play a pivotal role. To refine the risk assessment process through research, determination of the cellular and subcellular organelle target of xenobiotic injury forms the cornerstone in understanding the mechanism of injury. Through identification of cellular or subcellular organelle target sites, the most sensitive biomarkers can be identified to noninvasively monitor for the presence of a specific xenobiotic insult.

Demonstration of the pathogenesis of the full spectrum of toxic lesions enables the definition of primary or secondary changes and reversible, irreversible, or progressive processes. Understanding of the prerequisite molecular and biochemical events and test substance pharmacokinetics that lead to the primary organellar perturbation facilitates precision in hazard identification. Subsequently, comparative test substance metabolism, and pharmacokinetic, as well as anatomic and functional similarities in humans, must be assessed for the equivalent precision in extrapolation for human risk assessment.

By understanding basic tissue responses to diverse etiologic agents, potential mechanisms of injury may be examined in the refinement of risk assessment. Based on this understanding it may be possible to predict the potential functional and long-term consequences after short-term toxic responses. These predictions are important for guidance in long-term product development planning.

FURTHER READING

Alpers, C.E. (2005). The kidney. In *Robbins and Cotran's Pathologic Basis of Disease* (Kumar, V., Abbas, A.K., and Fausto, N. eds), 7th edn, pp. 955–1021. Elsevier Saunders, New York, NY.

Arend, L.J., and Nadasdy, T. (2009). Emerging therapy-related kidney disease. *Arch. Pathol. Lab. Med.*, 133, 268–278.

Barbier, O., Jacquillet, G., Tauc, M., Cougnon, M., and Poujeol, P. (2005). Effect of heavy metals on, and handling by, the kidney. *Nephron Physiol.*, 99, 105–110.

Brenner, B.M. (ed.) (2008). *Brenner & Rector's The Kidney*, 8th edn. Saunders Elsevier, Philadelphia, PA.

Brown, C.A., Jeong, K.S., Poppenga, R.H., Puschner, B., Miller, D.M., Ellis, A.E., Kang, K.I., Sum, S., Cistola, A.M., and Brown, S.A. (2007). Outbreaks of renal failure associated with melamine and cyanuric acid in dogs and cats in 2004 and 2007. *J. Vet. Diagn. Invest.*, 19, 525–531.

Choudhury, D., and Ahmed, Z. (2006). Drug-associated renal dysfunction and injury. *Nat. Clin. Pract. Nephrol.*, 2, 80–91.

Cohen, S.M., Wanibuchi, H., and Fukushima, S. (2002). Lower urinary tract. In *Handbook of Toxicologic Pathology* (Haschek, W. M., Rousseaux, C.G., and Wallig, M.A. eds), 2nd edn, Vol. 2, pp. 337–362. Academic Press, San Diego, CA.

Cristofori, P., Zanetti, E., Fregona, D., Piaia, A., and Trevisan, A. (2007). Renal proximal tubule segment-specific nephrotoxicity: An overview on biomarkers and histopathology. *Toxicologic Pathology*, 35, 270–275.

Dobson, R.L., Motlagh, S., Quijano, M., Cambron, R.T., Baker, T.R., Pullen, A.M., Regg, B.T., Bigalow-Kern, A.S., Vennard, T., Fix, A., Reimschuessel, R., Overmann, G., Shan, Y., and Daston, G.P. (2008). Identification and characterization of toxicity of contaminants in pet food leading to an outbreak of renal toxicity in cats and dogs. *Toxicol. Sci.*, 106, 251–262.

Fogo, A.B., Bruijn, J.A., Cohen, A.H., Colvin, R.B., and Jennette, J.C. (eds) (2007). *Fundamentals of Renal Pathology*. Springer, Berlin, Germany.

Ghanta, N.R. (2002). Diet and kidney diseases in rats. *Toxicol. Pathol.*, 30, 651–656.

Gwaltney-Brandt, S.M. (2002). Heavy metals. In *Handbook of Toxicologic Pathology* (Haschek, W.M., Rousseaux, C.G., and Wallig, M.A. eds), 2nd edn, Vol. 1, pp. 701–733. Academic Press, San Diego, CA.

Hard, G.C., Alden, C.L., Bruner, R.H., Frith, C.H., Lewis, R.M., Owen, R.A., Kreig, K., and Durchfeld-Meyer, B. (1999). Nonproliferative lesions of the kidney and lower urinary tract in rats. *Guides Tox. Path.*, 1–31.

Hard, G., Flake, G., and Sills, R. (2009). Re-evaluation of kidney histopathology from 13-week toxicity and 2-year carcinogenicity studies of melamine in the f344 rat: morphological evidence of retrograde nephropathy. *Vet Pathol.*, Jul 15. [Epub ahead of print].

Haschek, W.M., Voss, K.A., and Beasley, V.R. (2002). Selected mycotoxins affecting animal and human health. In *Handbook of Toxicologic Pathology* (Haschek, W.M., Rousseaux, C.G., and Wallig, M.A. eds), 2nd edn, Vol. 1, pp. 645–699. Academic Press, San Diego, CA.

Hau, A.K., Kwan, T.H., and Li, P.K. (2009). Melamine toxicity and the kidney. *J. Am. Soc. Nephrol.*, 20, 245–250.

Heyman, S.N., Lieberthal, W., Rogiers, P., and Bonventre, J.V. (2002). Animal models of acute tubular necrosis. *Curr. Opin. Crit. Care*, 8, 526–534.

Hook., J.B., Tarloff, J.B., and Lash, L.H. (eds) (2004). *Toxicology of the Kidney*, 3rd edn. CRC Press, Boca Raton, FL.

Keenan, K.P., Coleman, J.B., Mccoy, C.L., Hoe, C.M., Soper, K.A., and Laroque, P. (2000). Chronic nephropathy in *ad libitum* overfed Sprague-Dawley rats and its early attenuation by increasing degrees of dietary (caloric) restriction to control growth. *Toxicol. Pathol.*, 28, 788–798.

Khan, K.N.M., and Alden, C.L. (2002). Kidney. In *Handbook of Toxicologic Pathology* (Haschek, W.M., Rousseaux, C.G., and Wallig, M.A. eds), 2nd edn, Vol. 2, pp. 255–336. Academic Press, San Diego, CA.

Maxie, M.G., and Newman, S.J. (2007). Urinary system. In *Jubb, Kennedy, and Palmer's Pathology of Domestic Animals* (Maxie, M.E. ed.), 5th edn, pp. 425–522. Elsevier, New York, NY.

Newman, S.J., Confer, A.W., and Panciera, R.J. (2007). Urinary system. In *Pathologic Basis of Veterinary Disease* (McGavin, M., and Zachary, J.F. eds), 4th edn, pp. 613–691. Mosby Elsevier, St. Louis, MO.

Perazella, M.A. (2005). Drug-induced nephropathy: an update. *Expert Opin. Drug Saf.*, 4, 689–706.

Puschner, B., Poppenga, R.H., Lowenstine, L.J., Filigenzi, M.S., and Pesavento, P.A. (2007). Assessment of melamine and cyanuric acid toxicity in cats. *J. Vet. Diagn. Invest.*, 19, 616–624.

Rosen, S., and Stillman, I.E. (2008). Acute tubular necrosis is a syndrome of physiologic and pathologic dissociation. *J. Am. Soc. Nephrol.*, 19, 871–875.

Schnellmann, R.G. (2008). Toxic responses of the kidney. In *Casarett and Doull's Toxicology. The Basic Science of Poisons* (Klaassen, C.D. ed.), 7th edn, pp. 583–608. McGraw-Hill, New York, NY.

Sebastian, M.M., Baskin, S.I., and Czerwinski, S.E. (2007). Renal toxicity. In *Veterinary Toxicology: Basic and Clinical Principles* (Gupta, R.C. ed.), pp. 161–176. Elsevier Academic Press, New York, NY.

Seely, J.C. (1999). Kidney. In *Pathology of the Mouse* (Maronpot, R.R. ed.), pp. 207–234. Cache River Press, Vienna, IL.

Silva, F.G. (2004). Chemical-induced nephropathy: a review of the renal tubulointerstitial lesions in humans. *Toxicol. Pathol.*, 32(Suppl 2), 71–84.

Swenberg, J.A., Short, B., Borghok, S., Strasser, J., and Charbonneau, M. (1989). The comparative pathobiology of alpha$_{2U}$ globulin nephropathy. *Toxicol. Appl. Pharmacol.*, 97, 35–46.

Thukral, S.K., Nordone, P.J., Rong Hu, L.S. et al (2005). Prediction of nephrotoxicant action and identification of candidate toxicity-related biomarkers. *Toxicol. Pathol.*, 33, 343–355.

Van Vleet, T.R., and Schnellmann, R.G. (2003). Toxic nephropathy: environmental chemicals. *Semin. Nephrol.*, 23, 500–508.

Verlander, J.W. (1998). Normal ultrastructure of the kidney and lower urinary tract. *Toxicol. Pathol.*, 26, 1–17.

CHAPTER

12

Cardiovascular and Skeletal Muscle Systems

OUTLINE

SECTION I HEART

INTRODUCTION

Many agents are capable of altering cardiovascular function and causing an adverse effect. The major causes of cardiovascular toxicity in humans include smoking, alcohol, and adverse drug reactions. Major causes of cardiovascular toxicity in animals include ionophores (used as growth promoters) and toxic plants in horses and ruminants, gossypol (found in cottonseed meal) in pigs, and anthracyclines (antineoplastic drugs) in dogs. Altered cardiac function may result from abnormalities in ion movement, membrane function, contractile function, and energy producing systems. Cardiac responses to xenobiotic exposure range from developmental abnormalities to alterations in the myocardium, conduction system, valves and endocardium/pericardium. Morphologic alterations following xenobiotic exposure include hypertrophy, degeneration, apoptosis and necrosis, and cardiomyopathy. However, many xenobiotics that induce arrhythmias or interfere with metabolic function can cause death without accompanying morphologic alterations.

A wide spectrum of toxicity testing procedures are utilized to detect cardiotoxicoses. These procedures include monitoring contractile function, electrical activity, and blood pressure, and assessment of morphologic alterations. During drug development, the majority of cardiotoxic agents are identified using *in vitro* and *in vivo* safety evaluation methods. However, adverse drug reactions are sometimes identified after drugs have been approved for use (post-marketing). A recent example is that of the cyclo-oxygenase-2 (COX-2) inhibitors, Vioxx and Bextra, which were found to cause prolongation of the QT interval in some patients and thus serve as a potential trigger for generation of arrhythmias.

STRUCTURE AND FUNCTION

Gross and Microscopic Anatomy

The heart is a four-chambered muscular pump that lies within the pericardium. The heart is interposed as a pump into the vascular system; the right side supplies the pulmonary circulation and the left side the systemic circulation. The chambers of the atria and ventricles are separated from each other by atrioventricular valves (tricuspid on the right and mitral on the left) and from the outflow tracts by the semilunar valves, pulmonary valve on the right that opens into the pulmonary artery, and the aortic valve on the left that opens into the aorta. The right atrium receives systemic venous blood from the cranial vena cava, caudal vena cava, azygos vein, and the coronary sinus. Blood from the lungs enters the left atrium from the pulmonary veins.

The heart is composed of three layers: the epicardium, the myocardium, and the endocardium. The epicardium or outer layer of the heart is the visceral layer of the serous pericardium. The entire surface of the pericardial cavity is covered by mesothelium. The subepicardial layer contains a thin layer of fibrous connective tissue, adipose tissue, as well as numerous blood vessels, lymphatic vessels, and nerves.

The myocardium, the muscular portion of the heart, is composed of cardiac muscle cells or myocytes arranged in overlapping spiral patterns. The myocardial thickness is related to the pressures present in each chamber; the atria are thin and the ventricles are thick. The thickness of the left ventricular free wall is approximately three-fold greater than that of the right ventricle when measured in a transverse section across the middle of the chambers.

The endocardium is the inner layer of the heart that lines the chambers. The inner surface of the endocardium is lined by endothelium lying on a thin layer of connective tissue with the subendocardial layer containing blood vessels, nerves, and connective tissue with Purkinje fibers throughout the ventricles.

The valves consist of a fibrosa (dense collagenous layer), a spongiosa (loose connective tissue layer) and a ventricularis (elastic fiber rich layer).

The arterial supply to the heart is met by the left and right coronary arteries, which arise from the aorta. Extensive anastomoses occur between the capillaries that run parallel to the cardiac muscle cells. On cross-section, the ratio of capillaries to muscle cells is approximately 1:1. The coronary veins tend to follow the course of the arteries (except in birds) and open into the left atrium by the coronary sinus. The lymphatic vessels course in the epicardium and converge into trunks that lie adjacent to the coronary arteries in the coronary groove and eventually enter the tracheobronchial lymph nodes.

The cardiac conduction system includes the sinoatrial node at the junction of the anterior vena cava and the right atrium; the atrioventricular node and bundle located beneath the septal leaflet of the tricuspid valve and traversing the lower atrial septum onto the upper portion of the muscular ventricular septum; and the right and left bundle branches that descend on each side of the muscular ventricular septum and eventually ramify over the ventricles as the Purkinje fiber network.

Normal features in animal hearts may occasionally be misinterpreted as lesions. The epicardial lymphatics, especially in cattle, may appear as prominent white streaks that might be interpreted as necrosis. The septal cusp of the tricuspid valve is normally rather tightly attached to the ventricular septum. In young ruminants, the ductus arteriosus and foramen ovale may be patent. The overall shape of normal hearts vary from the elongated somewhat flattened conical profile in the horse, cow, and chicken to the somewhat shortened and rounded shape of the pig and dog. Cardiac weight (as % body weight) vary greatly among species; pigs and rats have small hearts (approximately 0.3% of body weight), cows, mice and guinea pigs have intermediate-sized hearts (approximately 0.5% of body weight), and dogs, cats and horses have large hearts (from 0.75% of body weight in nonathletic dog breeds to 1.25% in athletic breeds).

Cellular and Extracellular Elements of the Heart: Biology and Clinical Relevance

Atrial and ventricular myocardium are composed of a variety of cells, of which the myocytes are the force-generating cells. Myocytes are elongated and joined to one another by intercellular junctions. The latter mediate electrical coupling of the myocytes and render them able to act as a functional syncytium. The myocytes are surrounded by a rich network of blood vessels and capillaries and are embedded in a matrix of connective tissue. Also present in this matrix are nerves and lymphatics, as well as mast cells, histiocytes, fibroblasts, pericytes, and poorly differentiated mesenchymal cells. Valvular interstitial cells (VICs) are the most prevalent cells in the valves with characteristics of fibroblasts, smooth muscle cells and myofibroblasts.

Ventricular Myocytes

Ventricular myocytes are approximately cylindrical, but branch freely, and are 80–100 μm in length and 10–20 μm in width (Figures 12.1 and 12.2). The ends of myocytes have a step-like appearance, which corresponds to the intercalated discs. Myocytes are limited by the sarcolemma, a structure formed by the plasma membrane (plasmalemma) and the external lamina (laminar coat, basement membrane, basal lamina, glycocalyx). The plasmalemma has the usual trilaminar

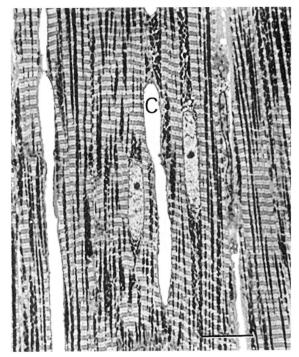

FIGURE 12.1 Longitudinal section of perfused rat myocardium with open capillaries (C) and prominent banding patterns. Plastic-embedded, toluidine blue stain. Bar = 10 μm.

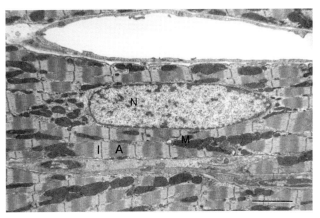

FIGURE 12.2 Electron micrograph of section in Figure 12.1. Several myocytes lie adjacent to an open capillary (top). Sarcomeres are relaxed and have prominent A (dark) and I (light) bands. N, nucleus; M, mitochondria. Bar = 5 μm.

structure and is 99 nm wide. The external lamina contains basement membrane collagens (types IV and V) and noncollagen glycoproteins.

The T system is a network of tubular invaginations of the sarcolemma. Their lumina are continuous with the extracellular space. The T system allows close direct contact between the extracellular environment and the deeper regions of the cells, and functions in facilitating the inward spread of electrical events at the cell surface, in ionic exchange with the interstitium and in the excitation-contraction coupling in the ventricular myocardium. Neighboring myocytes are connected end-to-end and, to a lesser extent, side-to-side by intercellular junctions. These mediate intercellular adhesions and transmission of the electrical impulse. The end-to-end junctions are known as intercalated discs, the side-to-side junctions as lateral junctions.

Myocytes contain one or two nuclei that are centrally located and oblong. Myofibrils course around the nucleus, leaving at the nuclear poles a conical area free of contractile elements but densely packed with other cellular organelles. The contractile elements occupy about 50% of the cytoplasm of myocytes and form a continuous mass which is separated into myofibrils of varying size by the interfibrillar matrix. This matrix contains mitochondria, sarcoplasmic reticulum and T tubules, glycogen particles, and other organelles. Myofibrils are highly ordered arrays of contractile elements. They exhibit a periodicity that is clearly evident by light microscopy in the form of dark anisotropic A bands and light less anisotropic I bands. The I bands are bisected by a thick dark Z band. The array of contractile elements between two adjacent Z bands is known as a sarcomere and constitutes the contractile unit of cardiac muscle.

The ultrastructural differentiation of the sarcoplasmic reticulum (SR) is closely related to that of the myofibrils and the T system. An important function of the SR is to actively take up and release calcium ions, by mechanisms that involve calsequestrin, during the contraction-relaxation cycle of the myocyte. The SR also functions in the metabolism of glycogen and lipids.

Ventricular myocytes are rich in mitochondria, which constitute 35% of the cell volume. Mitochondria are situated between the myofibrils, in subsarcolemmal and perinuclear areas. Mitochondria are the sites of oxidative phosphorylation and of synthesis of high-energy phosphates and thus provide the energy needed for muscular contraction. Cardiac mitochondria are very sensitive to noxious influences; at the ultrastructural level they can be drastically changed even by short periods of ischemia.

Lysosomes, phagosomes, and multivesicular bodies are commonly observed in myocytes, as are residual bodies of lysosomal origin (lipofuscin granules); all of these structures are usually located in the perinuclear region. The Golgi apparatus in ventricular myocytes is usually found in the form of multiple stacks of cisterns and associated vesicles in the perinuclear areas. Ventricular myocytes contain moderate amounts of glycogen. Small numbers of free ribosomes are found throughout the cell, whereas rough endoplasmic reticulum (RER) is mostly confined to the perinuclear region.

Atrial Myocytes

The architecture of atrial myocytes basically resembles that of ventricular myocytes; however, the two cell types differ in a number of fine structural features, including the intercellular junctions, the T system, the SR, the mitochondria, and the specific "atrial" granules. Atrial myocardium contains not only working atrial myocytes but also less well-defined types of myocytes which resemble Purkinje fibers and transitional cells. The arrangement of atrial myocytes is less regular than that of ventricular myocytes.

Atrial myocytes contain a population of cytoplasmic granules that are the source of important regulatory hormones, the atrial natriuretic peptides (ANP). The prohormone atriopeptigen is released in response to elevated vascular volume. Natriuresis and diuresis are produced by atriopeptin acting to increase glomerular filtration rate, renal blood flow, urine volume, and urinary sodium excretion and to decrease plasma renin activity.

Conduction System

The conduction system of the heart consists of the sinoatrial node, the atrioventricular node, and the bundle of His. The morphology of the specialized conducting cells shows great variation, not only among different species but also in different components of the conductive system in a given species.

Components of Myocardial Interstitium

The myocardial interstitium contains small numbers of fibroblasts, spindle-shaped connective tissue cells, myofibroblasts and a small number of undifferentiated connective tissue cells (primitive mesenchymal cells), which probably function as reserve cells. Macrophages (histiocytes) and mast cells are normally present in small numbers in the myocardial interstitium. Anitschkow cells are small and spindle-shaped and have oblong nuclei that contain a centrally located bar of chromatin. Anitschkow cells are probably activated myocardial fibroblasts or fibroblast-like mesenchymal cells. Small bundles of collagen fibrils ("collagen struts") constitute a fibrous skeleton that mechanically interconnects adjacent myocytes and also connects myocytes to neighboring capillaries. Elastic fibers in normal myocardial interstitium are small, inconspicuous, and few in number.

Cellular Components of the Myocardial Vasculature

The detailed structure of the various types of vascular cells is presented subsequently with the discussion of the vessels.

Myocardial Innervation

Unmyelinated nerve fibers are commonly found in cardiac muscle, where they course in the proximity of blood vessels.

Physiology and Functional Considerations

The heart propels blood through the lungs and peripheral circulatory system, providing oxygen and nutrients to all tissues. The efficiency of the heart and its ability to perform its task depend on the coordinated conduction of the cardiac impulse and rapid coordinated activation of the contractile apparatus. The functional unit of the myocardium is made of cylindrically shaped striated muscle fibers as described earlier.

Resting and Action Potential

The electrical activity of the heart is generated at the level of the individual muscle cells. The principal diffusible ions responsible for the electrical activity of the myocardial cells are sodium, potassium, calcium, and chloride. Electrical currents and chemical mediators act on the cardiac cell to change its membrane potential. When the membrane potential attains a threshold value, a characteristic sequence of self-propagated de- and repolarization occurs (action potential). During depolarization the potential difference between the inside and outside of the cardiac cell reverses as the inside of the cell becomes positive with respect to the outside. The time course of de- and repolarization essentially falls into two basic patterns: slow response and fast response. Disease processes and certain drugs and other chemicals which alter membrane properties can convert a fast-response cell to a cell with properties similar to those of a slow-response cell.

Slow-response fibers normally are found in only a few specific locations in the heart, for example, the sinoatrial (SA) and atrioventricular (AV) nodes. Conduction velocity is slow in fibers from these areas.

The resting potential in slow-response cells is near $-60\,mV$. At this level, fast sodium channels are virtually inactive and thus only slow sodium and calcium channels are functional. The slow channels are activated when the transmembrane potential reaches $-40\,mV$.

Initiation and Conduction of Cardiac Impulse

The coordinated pumping action of the heart is initiated and controlled by pacemaker cells in the SA node and conducting tissue. Both slow- and fast-response fibers are involved in this impulse initiation and conduction system. The impulse originating in the SA node travels rapidly to all parts of the atria and AV node. Conduction of the impulse through the AV node is slow and limits the frequency with which impulses can enter the ventricles. Once past the AV node, the impulse is again conducted rapidly through the specialized conducting fibers of the bundle of His. This bundle subdivides into the many branches forming the subendocardial Purkinje system which ultimately delivers the impulse to the ventricular muscle cells. The propagation of excitation initiates the contractile process in both ventricles.

Excitation-Contraction Coupling

Myofibrillar contraction involves the sliding of the thick myosin filaments of the sarcomere past the thin actin filaments. This process is modulated by changes in the cytosolic concentration of calcium, which binds to the regulatory proteins tropomyosin and troponin in the thin filament. Myosin ATPase is activated. ATP is hydrolyzed and the energy is used to form cross-bridges between actin and myosin. The force and velocity of contraction depend on the amount of calcium that reaches the contractile sites. Calcium and sodium entering the cell as a result of the membrane action potential may cause depolarization of the sarcoplasmic reticulum and release large quantities of bound intracellular calcium. The intracellular concentration of calcium is decreased by reuptake into the sarcoplasmic reticulum. When the level decreases sufficiently, the actin-myosin interaction is inhibited and relaxation occurs.

Myocardial Metabolism

Heart muscle utilizes chemical energy to initiate and sustain the work of contraction. The majority of the energy liberated from fuel substances occurs as a result of the production of ATP. Energy sources such as lactate, glucose, triglycerides, and fatty acids ultimately enter the tricarboxylic acid (TCA) cycle to generate ATP. Within the TCA cycle, the carbons from pyruvate are oxidized through intermediate steps to carbon dioxide, and oxidative phosphorylation is initiated in the mitochondria. The energy produced by the reactions is stored in the heart as ATP or creatine phosphate. The process of energy utilization also involves calcium ions. The action potential allows both externally and internally sequestered calcium to move into the cytosol of the myofibrils. The released calcium then activates the myofilaments by binding ATP into reactive sites between the myosin and the actin filaments. An ATPase enzyme splits ATP in the presence of magnesium and the myofibril contracts.

Innervation of the Heart

Nervous control of the heart is mediated by the parasympathetic and sympathetic divisions of the autonomic nervous system. The vagal nerve fibers (parasympathetic) supply the SA node, atrial muscle fibers, AV node, and, to a limited degree, the ventricles. The main effects of acetylcholine, released from the vagal nerve, are a decrease in the force of atrial and ventricular contraction, a decrease in conduction velocity through the AV node, and a decrease in heart rate.

The release of norepinephrine by sympathetic nerve stimulation increases the slope of diastolic depolarization so the threshold potential is reached more quickly and the rate of SA nodal discharge is increased (positive chronotropic response). This effect is attributed to an augmentation of slow inward calcium currents. The effects on the AV node and other conducting fibers are similar to those of the SA node. Sympathetic stimulation of myocardial contractile fibers leads to an increase in force of contraction (positive inotropic response). This action is mediated by cyclic adenosine monophosphate (cAMP). cAMP is thought to activate a kinase enzyme that ultimately makes more calcium available for the contractile proteins.

Xenobiotic Exposure

It is known that the heart and blood vessels are susceptible to a variety of chemicals and drugs. Some chemical agents exert myocardial effects selectively while many may produce cardiovascular alterations through nonspecific actions. As with other organs, the blood provides the vehicle by which exposure can occur. A substance in the blood may cause only a functional alteration which lasts during the exposure period. However, because of its unique function, the heart will be exposed to maximal concentrations of substances or metabolites for prolonged periods of time. As a consequence, additional problems can

arise since the risk of irreversible myocardial effect increases with the duration of exposure. Substances producing myocardial effects may enter the vascular compartment from any exposure route. For example, sufficient amounts of inhaled carbon monoxide (CO) can lead to decreased O_2 availability and thereby produce tachycardia and other electrocardiographic changes suggestive of hypoxia. Likewise, inhaled low molecular weight halogenated alkanes used for industrial purposes, as well as volatile anesthetics, can cause arrhythmias and sensitize the heart to sympathoadrenal discharge or to exogenous catecholamines.

A substance in the blood capable of producing myocardial toxicity need not have a direct effect on cardiovascular function. Chemically induced alterations in other organs such as the kidney could lead to acid-base balance and electrolyte concentration changes of sufficient magnitude to cause significant alterations in cardiovascular function.

MECHANISMS OF TOXICITY

Cardiotoxic reactions are potentially serious events; for this reason their detection in non-clinical safety studies of drug candidates or in premarketing safety studies of other chemicals is of great importance. The detectability of cardiotoxic reactions in these studies depends greatly on the mechanism of action of the chemical on the heart. Although reactions due to exaggerated pharmacological effects (termed "on target" effects) are readily elicited in laboratory animals, those due to unrelated mechanisms (termed "off target" effects) may or may not develop under the conditions of safety studies. The latter, and particularly those reactions that require preconditioning factors for their occurrence, are often detected only in clinical trials or with extensive use of the product. Nevertheless, many of these reactions can be reproduced in laboratory animals; the identification of appropriate animal models is instrumental in the development of new drugs that are devoid of cardiotoxic effects. Table 12.1 lists selected agents from the major use or exposure classes with known cardiotoxic effects while Table 12.2 lists the major mechanisms of cardiotoxicity and provides selected examples.

Physiological Mechanisms of Functional Alterations

The intrinsic properties of myocardial tissue such as automaticity, excitability, and conductivity endow the heart with a variety of chemically sensitive pathophysiologic mechanisms. The most important disruptions

TABLE 12.1   Selected agents with cardiotoxic potential by class or use category

Agents (chemical class or use category, exposure)	Examples (exposure)	Comment
Industrial and environmental chemicals		
Solvents (industrial)	Chloroform, benzene	Highly lipophilic; disrupt cardiac function directly and via neuro-hormonal effects; sensitize heart to arrhythmogenic effects of endogenous catecholamines
Halogenated alkanes (mainly industrial)		CNS depressants (highly lipophilic crossing blood–brain barrier readily); depress heart rate, contractility, and conduction
	Fluorocarbons (freons) (also environmental)	Sensitize heart to arrhythmogenic effects of endogenous catecholamines; reduce cardiac output and coronary flow
	Haloanesthetics (medical use): halothane, methoxyflurane	Myocardial depression. Negative chronotropic, inotropic, and dromotropic effects
Alcohols and aldehydes (mainly industrial)		Acute cardiodepressant effects
	Ethanol (mainly dietary)	Alcoholic cardiomyopathy following long-term ingestion. Decreased cardiac contraction, arrhythmias and ventricular fibrillation
	Other alcohols (industrial): methanol, isopropanol	
	Acetaldehyde (also ethanol metabolite)	At high dose release catecholamines with sympathomimetic effects
Particulate matter in air pollution (environmental)	Combustive byproducts and crystalline materials	ECG changes
Heavy metals (industrial, environmental, or food/water contaminant)		Negative inotropic and dromotropic effects. Form complexes with intracellular macromolecules and antagonize endogenous Ca_2
	Cadmium, cobalt	Cardiomyopathy
	Lead	Sensitize heart to arrhythmogenic effects of endogenous catecholamines
Other metals	Manganese, nickel, lanthanum (environmental, industrial)	Block Ca^{2+} channels
Metalloids	Arsenic (environmental, therapeutic)	Affinity for sulfhydryl proteins. Tachycardia, cardiomyocyte apoptosis
Pharmaceutical chemicals		
Cardioactive drugs		
Antiarrhythmic agents		Decrease conductivity and automaticity of the myocardium
	Class I: quinidine, procainamide, phenytoin	Na^+ channel blockers
	Class II: propananol	β adrenergic receptor blocking
	Class III: amiodarone	K^+ channel blockers
	Class IV: verapamil	Ca^+ channel blockers
Inotropic drugs		Adrenergic receptor agonists.
	Catecholamines, epinephrine, and isoproterenol	Myocardial hypoxia; cellular Ca^{2+} overload; subendocardial necrosis
	Sympathomimetics (nasal decongestants): ephedrine, phenylephrine	α-adrenergic receptor agonists
	Cardiac glycosides (also plant toxins): digoxin, digitoxin	Can result in Ca^{2+} overload.

(Continued)

TABLE 12.1   (*Continued*)

Agents (chemical class or use category, exposure)	Examples (exposure)	Comment
CNS active drugs	Tricyclic antidepressants: imipramine, amitryptyline	Postural hypotension, prolongation of the PR, QRS, and QT interval; supraventricular and ventricular arrhythmias (including TdP)
	General anesthetics: halothane, propofol, methoxyflurane	Insert in membrane lipid bilayer; stabilize membranes. Depress myocardial contractility
Local anesthetics	Cocaine	Ventricular fibrillation, myocyte death, myocardial infarction
	Procainamide, lidocaine	Na^+ channel blockers
Anti-inflammatory agents	COX-2 inhibitors: rofecoxib (Vioxx), celecoxib (Celebrex)	Thrombotic effects. For Vioxx—QT prolongation, risk of TdP
Antihistamines	Terfenadine, astemizole	Histamine H1 receptor antagonists. Ventricular arrhythmias, risk of TdP
Antineoplastic agents	Anthracyclines: doxorubicin or adriamycin, daunorubicin	Acute: anaphylactoid-type reaction. Chronic: dilated cardiomyopathy
	Fluorouracil	Myocardial ischemia; cardiac arrest
	Cyclophosphamide	Hemorrhagic necrosis; pericarditis
Antimicrobial/antiviral agents	Aminoglycosides: gentamycin	Cardiodepression. Blockade of sarcolemmal Ca^{2+} channels
	Macrolides: erythromycin	QT prolongation, risk of TdP
	Fluoroquinolones: grepafloxacin, moxifloxacin	QT prolongation, risk of TdP
	Tetracycline, chloramphenicol	Depress contractility
	Penicillin, sulfonamide	Hypersensitivity myocarditis
	Furazolidone	Biventricular cardiac failure in turkeys, ducklings, and chicks
	Antifungal: amphotericin B	Depress contractility
	Antiviral agent: zidovudine (AZT)	Affects Ca^{2+} homeostasis, mitochondrial toxicity Main risk when multiple drugs used.
Anorexigens	Fenfluramine, dexfenfluramine	Valvulopathy
Growth-promoting agents	Clenbuterol	Myocardial hypertrophy
	Monensin, lasalocid, narasin, salinomycin, maduramicin	Positive inotropic effect. Increase excitation–contraction coupling; enhance metabolism of cardiac cells; increase sarcolemmal cationic trap for Na^+/K^+ (lasalocid)
Natural/endogenous products		
Catecholamines	See Inotropic drugs above	
Steroids and related hormones	Anabolic–androgenic steroids	Dilated cardiomyopathy
	Glucocorticoids, aldosterone	Stimulate cardiac fibrosis. Cardiac hypertrophy with dexamethasone use in infants
	Thyroid hormones	Hypothyroid: decreased heart rate, contractility and output
		Hyperthyroid: increased heart rate, contractility, output, ejection fraction and mass
Cytokines	Proinflammatory:IL-2, TNF-α	
	Anti-inflammatory: IL-4	
	Interferon	Dilated cardiomyopathy, arrhythmias, ischemia

(*Continued*)

TABLE 12.1 (*Continued*)

Agents (chemical class or use category, exposure)	Examples (exposure)	Comment
Toxins		
Animal toxins	Snake venom cardiotoxins (Cobra, rattlesnake)	Cobra cardiotoxin: systolic arrest; disruption of myocardial cell membranes and myofibrils Ultimate Ca^{2+} overload
	Bratrachotoxin (steroidal alkaloid, poison dart frog)	Opens Na^+ channels in nerves and myocytes resulting in depolarization and paralysis
	Tetrodotoxin (TTX, puffer fish), saxitoxin (STX, dinoflagellates)	Conduction defects. Binds to Na^+ channels. STX accumulates in shellfish, and is the cause of paralytic shellfish poisoning (PSP) in humans
	Canthadrin (from the blister beetle, *Epicauta* sp)	Myocarditis, with horse most sensitive Mitochondrial damage
Bacterial toxin	Endotoxin	Reduces coronary perfusion; depresses contractility; negative inotropic and chronotropic responses to NE and histamine. Depresses Ca^{2+} ATPase activity
Plant toxins	Toxic alkaloids: water hemlock (*Cicuta douglasii*)	Toxic alkaloids induce arrhythmia, myocardial necrosis
	Cardiac glycosides: avocado (*Persea americana*)	Cardiac glycoside interferes with Na^+/K^+-ATPase enzyme. Myocardial necrosis
	Gossypol (*Gossypium* sp, cotton)	Cardiomyocyte atrophy, dilated cardiomyopathy
Fungal toxins		Negative inotropic and chronotropic effect
	Moniliformin	Myocardial necrosis/fibrosis and sudden death syndrome in chicks and turkey poults
	Fumonisin	Sphingolipid alterations; decrease in contractility lead to left sided heart failure and pulmonary edema in swine

TdP: Torsades des Pointe

TABLE 12.2 Mechanisms of cardiotoxicity with selected examples

General mechanism	Specific mechanism	Xenobiotic
Pharmacologic action/side-effects	Beta-adrenergic agonists	Isoproterenol, catecholamines
	Vasodilating antihypertensive agents	Minoxidil, hydralazine
Direct effect	Free radical injury	Anthracyclines
	Imbalance of ionic movement	Monensin and other ionophores
	Calcium overload	Vitamin D, calcinogenic plants
	Interference with energy production	Emetine, carbon monoxide
	Damage to proteins	Furazolidone, metallic salts
	Formation of reactive metabolites	Allylamine
	Specific metabolic blocks	Cobalt, fluoroacetate
	Injury by activated lymphocytes	IL-2, other cytokines
	Apoptosis	Antineoplastic agents, oxygen free radicals
	Altered lysosomal function	Amiodarone, choloroquine
	Induction of arrhythmias	Amitryptyline, lithium carbonate
Allergic/hypersensitivity reactions		Penicillin, sulfonamides, methyldopa

in normal cardiac functions arise from alterations in membrane function, particularly in ion transport and in the contractile or energy producing systems.

Arrhythmias are among the most serious immediate functional cardiac abnormalities. Abnormalities in impulse formation and in impulse conduction, individually or in combination, are the primary causes of arrhythmias. Substances can directly influence the initiation or propagation of the cardiac electrical impulse by altering the ionic gradients and fluxes that are involved in these processes.

The two types of electrical activity (fast and slow responses) that have been detected in cardiac tissue and in chemically altered cells have a major role in the precipitation of arrhythmias. Fast-response cells are located in the working atria and ventricles and in most portions of the conducting system except the SA and AV nodes. Exposure to certain agents or ischemic conditions can reduce the resting membrane potential of the cardiac cell. The reduction in membrane potential causes a decrease in the speed of impulse conduction and enhances the chance for a block in conduction of electrical activity. The fast-response fibers possess a second slow inward current carried by Ca^{2+} ions which develops only when the fast Na^+ depolarizing current has decreased the membrane potential. Sustained partial depolarization of the membrane to about -60 mV, by abnormal conditions such as increased extracellular potassium concentration or hypoxia, inactivate the fast sodium channel while leaving the slow calcium component functional. The initiation and conduction of the slow-response action potential in fibers that are partially depolarized by damage or hypoxia may provoke abnormalities of cardiac rhythm. Paradoxically, the effect of antiarrhythmic agents such as quinidine on the heart may be to initiate rhythm disturbance. Such a proarrhythmic action can occur when fast sodium channel activity is decreased without interference with the development of slow calcium channel responses.

Certain specific functional properties of myocardial tissues appear to increase the susceptibility of the heart to structural perturbations. One predilectional site for necrosis is the left ventricular subendocardium. The susceptibility of the subendocardium, especially the left ventricular papillary muscles, is related to a high oxygen requirement and a low capillary supply per mass of tissue. Subendocardial necrosis, particularly of the left ventricular papillary muscles, has been found following treatment with isoproterenol and vasodilating antihypertensive agents such as minoxidil or diazoxide. The subendocardial necrosis is thought to be of ischemic origin due to the hemodynamic effects of these agents. Vasodilation-induced

hypotension leads to a reflex increase in heart rate. Myocardial energy requirements increase without a corresponding augmentation of energy supply because the diastolic period when blood perfusion occurs is shortened. Thus, the pharmacological effects of vasodilators lead to ischemic myocyte death due to the combination of increased energy utilization and underperfusion in the susceptible subendocardium.

Biochemical Mechanisms of Cardiotoxicosis

Xenobiotics can cause myocardial alterations by reacting with functional or structural molecules of vital significance. The high-energy requirement of the heart predisposes the myocardium to the adverse effects of metabolic poisons. Toxic reactions may involve suppression of an enzyme system. Cobalt-induced cardiotoxicity is due to inhibition of certain mitochondrial energy-generating systems.

Adverse myocardial effects may be elicited when a compound or a reactive metabolite of a compound interacts with structural macromolecules in the myocyte. Since myocardial enzymes that metabolize endogeneous substances may also utilize xenobiotics as substrates, the biotransformation of the latter could occur in the heart. The role of metabolically derived chemically reactive substances in the initiation of certain myocardial toxicities has been described. After acute exposure to the industrial chemical allylamine, rats develop focal degenerative and necrotic myocardial changes, whereas prolonged dosing leads to myocardial and vascular fibrosis. An amine oxidase enzyme found in the heart and blood vessels metabolizes allylamine to acrolein. This reactive metabolite is responsible for the observed myocardial alteration. Acrolein is conjugated by glutathione and is excreted as a mercapturic acid conjugate. It is likely that the extent of injury is a function of the role of acrolein formation and the availability of glutathione at the site of biotransformation.

The role of reactive chemical species in myocardial toxicity is of considerable consequence in other ways. Two factors of significance regarding the development of reactive radical-induced injury include the rate of formation of the reactive products and the availability of sufficient amounts of protective substances. Some agents can stimulate the formation of reactive oxygen radicals in the heart and produce myocyte alterations. Anthracycline antineoplastic agents such as doxorubicin produce a distinctive type of chronic congestive cardiomyopathy in humans and experimental animals. Two major morphologic lesions are found in the myocyte: dilatation of the sacroplasmic reticulum and loss of myofibrils. The pathogenesis of these lesions is linked to the generation of toxic oxygen free radicals. A key factor in this concept was the finding that doxorubicin can form a complex with iron that is capable of mediating production of reactive oxygen radicals. This complex can bind to cell membranes and, by reacting with endogenous thiols, is capable of oxidative destruction of structural macromolecules such as those found in the cell membrane. The unique sensitivity of the heart to the cardiotoxic effects of doxorubicin may be secondary to the low cellular concentrations of enzymes such as catalase that are capable of preventing accumulation of damaging reactive oxygen radicals. In addition, doxorubicin suppresses the activity of glutathione peroxidase, another enzyme capable of protecting against injury by oxygen free radicals. Thus the low levels of potential protective enzymatic activity make the myocardium quite vulnerable to the effects of certain reactive substances.

Cardiotoxicoses Due to Direct Cellular Injury

Direct cardiotoxic effects are the result of a selective or random interaction of the chemical with molecules of vital importance in the myocytes. Direct cardiotoxicosis is of great significance in the commercial or medicinal utility of a chemical. Since effects occurring by a direct mechanism are dose and time related, they are usually detectable in laboratory animals. However, species differences in drug metabolism should be considered and, therefore, carefully designed studies, involving doses from the therapeutic dose to a sublethal dose in both acute and subacute treatment regimens, should be conducted in at least two species of laboratory animals.

Cardiotoxicoses Due to Indirect Acting Injury

Cardiotoxicoses Due to Pharmacological Mechanisms

The most frequent adverse cardiac reactions are caused by cardiovascular drugs, for example, digitalis glycoside, antiarrhythmics, and antihypertensives. These reactions are the result of exaggerated pharmacological effects following an overdose or occurring because of an unusual sensitivity to the patient brought about by old age, a specific disease, or drug interactions. The heart can also be a target of pharmacologic side effects, for example, when the drug acts on an organ other than the desired one. Examples of cardiac effects of drugs that act on the central nervous system are the neuroleptic and antidepressant-induced arrhythmias.

If the desired pharmacological effect occurs in a laboratory animal species, it is likely that the exaggerated effect can also be elicited. Effects of this nature are dose related and may appear only at doses that are nearly sublethal in laboratory animals. However, they could occur at therapeutic doses in humans, since several conditions may predispose to their development. Of particular significance are those conditions that are frequently encountered in the greatest users of drugs, the elderly. Altered physiological functions that may be associated with adverse effects are decreased glomerular filtration rate or pre-existing heart disease, for example, congestive heart failure. For example, the toxicity of digoxin is increased with a decreased glomerular filtration rate, and β-adrenergic blocking agents cause potentially fatal effects in patients with congestive heart failure. Life-threatening cardiovascular effects may develop following a therapeutic dose of β-blockers in patients whose cardiac function depends upon the maintenance of sympathetic drive.

Arrhythmias and QT-interval prolongation have occurred in patients receiving overdoses or even therapeutic doses of tricyclic antidepressants or neuroleptics. However, several conditions sensitize to these effects. Sudden cardiac deaths associated with ventricular fibrillation have occurred in patients who had pre-existing heart disease and were taking therapeutic doses of these drugs.

Thioridazine is one of the most cardiotoxic phenothiazine neuroleptic drugs. One of its metabolites, a ring sulfoxide, appears to be responsible for cardiotoxicity. Patients at risk are those who rapidly metabolize thioridazine to this cardiotoxic metabolite. Neuroleptic- induced electrocardiographic changes may be enhanced by a glucose load that increases the intracellular to extracellular ratio of potassium in response to an increase in insulin.

Hypersensitivity Reactions

The heart is also a target of immune mediated effects of xenobiotics. Allergic skin reactions are occasionally accompanied by subtle electrocardiographic changes and, in rare instances, by hypersensitivity myocarditis. Diagnostic testing for suspected allergens in humans carries some risk of cardiac reaction. In systemic anaphylaxis, mediators such as histamine and leukotrienes cause constriction of coronary arteries and decrease the force of contraction of the heart muscle; thus, a primary cardiac event occurs and can include arrhythmia or even heart failure. Penicillin has now replaced horse serum as the most frequent cause (1–10%) of anaphylaxis in humans. Fatal reactions, however, are less than one per one million injections.

Detection of a sensitizer can be facilitated by use of the isolated perfused guinea pig heart, pretreated and challenged with the test compound.

In addition to anaphylaxis, antibody-mediated cytotoxic immune- complex-elicited injuries can affect the heart. Methyldopa-induced myocarditis fits into this category. Numerous drugs can cause immune-complex-mediated reactions in the coronary vessels (e.g., sulfonamides, penicillin, procainamide, quinidine), and autoimmune mechanisms have been implicated with some of these drugs. Development of the reactions in humans has been associated in some instances with a specific haplotype (a set of alleles) of the major histocompatibility complex (MHC). The great polymorphism of the gene product is responsible for variability in the sensitivity to antigens. The predictability of cardiotoxic effects due to hypersensitivity reactions from laboratory animals to humans is uncertain.

Organellar Localization of Injury

It is obvious that many highly specific biochemical and pharmacological mechanisms can mediate the cardiac cellular damage produced by certain toxic drugs and chemical agents. It is of interest to try to establish structural-functional correlations with respect to such lesions; however, the time course of these changes presents a complex variable. Even highly specific, localized disturbances of the delicate equilibria of cell functions can lead rapidly to a picture of generalized cell damage or cell necrosis. Various subcellular organelles of cardiac muscle cells subject to specific damage by toxic agents include:

1. Mitochondria: Compounds which interfere with mitochondrial enzymes (cyanide, thyroid hormone), uncouple oxidative phosphorylation (dinitrophenol, cobalt, lead, mercury), bind to mitochondrial DNA (acriflavin), produce mitochondrial mineralization (dehydrotachysterol, sodium phosphate), or produce selective mitochondrial damage by undetermined mechanisms (ionophores such as monensin, *Cassia occidentalis*).
   Mitochondrial control of cell death is through modification of mitochondrial permeability transition (MPT) which behaves like a membrane pore that allows diffusion of solutes < 1500 DA in size. Modification of MPT can be temporary or become irreversible, with loss of mitochondrial homeostasis and high amplitude swelling that can result in rupture of the outer membrane and release of cytochrome c into the cytosol. Release

of cytochrome c can also be due to the effect of Bax, a pro-apoptotic protein of the Bcl-2 family that increases following oxidative stress, or occur in the early phase of defective mitochondrial oxidative phosphorylation. Cytochrome c, when present in the cytosol, activates caspase 9, followed by caspase 3, leading to apoptosis. Defective mitochondrial oxidative phosphorylation also leads to depletion of cellular ATP levels, resulting in necrosis. Abnormal mitochondrial protein biosynthesis can follow damage to nuclear or mitochondrial DNA. Mitochondrial DNA is subject to far more oxidative damage than nuclear DNA and repair processes are less efficient. Cumulative mitochondrial DNA damage, under oxidative stress conditions such as with Adriamycin, leads to irreversible mitochondrial dysfunction in the heart. AZT appears to be cardiotoxic due to inhibition of replication of mitochondrial DNA.

2. Sarcoplasmic reticulum: Compounds that cause selective dilatation of SR elements (anthracyclines) and other SR alterations (guanidine, volvatoxin A)
3. Contractile material: Compounds which primarily cause myofibrillar lesions (sympathomimetic amines, plasmocid, diuretics, or other conditions leading to potassium deficiency), furazolidone in birds, halothane, corticosteroids
4. Sarcolemma: Compounds which selectively affect the sarcolemma (tetrodotoxin, verapamil, cardiac glycosides)
5. Nucleus/nucleolus: Compounds which selectively affect the nucleus/nucleolus (anthracyclines)
6. Lysosomes/residual bodies: Compounds which cause accumulations of electron-dense lamellae (chloroquine)

Although these changes seldom are specific (some changes can resemble the degenerative lesions seen in the late stages of hypertrophy), they can provide valuable clues about the mode of action of a given agent. Many of the changes in the contractile apparatus, nucleus, or membrane system (plasma membrane, T tubules, and sarcoplasmic reticulum) are associated with complex alterations in the concentrations of Ca^{2+}, Mg^{2+}, Na^+, and K^+, as well as with changes in the intracellular compartmentalization of these ions. In addition, these changes and changes in intracellular pH can be associated with activation and release of lysosomal hydrolytic enzymes, including cathepsin D and other proteases, and phospholipases. These variously interrelated changes, coupled with alterations in the permeability of plasma membranes, act as determinants of whether or not cellular injury progresses to the point of irreversibility, that is, cellular necrosis.

Xenobiotic Interactions

Drug interactions play a significant role in the development of serious cardiotoxic reactions. The myocardial sensitivity to the arrhythmogenic actions of cardiac glycosides is increased by diuretic agents which deplete potassium and magnesium. Digitalis glycosides and extracellular potassium have competitive affinities for the membrane Na^+-K^+-ATPase enzyme. Exposure to potassium may simultaneously increase Na^+-K^+-ATPase activity and decrease the binding of glycosides to this enzyme. A decrease in extracellular K^+ would intensify the inhibitory effect of glycosides on the Na^+-K^+-ATPase system, resulting in an increase in intracellular sodium concentration. As a result the magnitude of the membrane potential may approach the threshold for initiation of diastolic depolarization and thus initiate serious arrhythmias. Concurrent exposure to cardiovascular agents that have similar effects, but which act by different mechanisms, can cause potentiation of specific adverse effects. For example, the simultaneous administration of propranolol, a β-adrenergic receptor blocker, and verapamil, a calcium channel antagonist, has caused profound AV block and marked hypotension.

Normally, catecholamine administration causes a predictable series of dose-related myocardial effects. Initially sinus tachycardia occurs, but a variety of arrhythmias are induced as the dose is increased (ventricular bigemeny, multifocal premature ventricular contractions, ventricular tachycardia) and finally, at high concentrations, ventricular fibrillation ensues. Exposure to certain halogenated hydrocarbon chemicals reduces the amount of catecholamines necessary to cause these arrhythmias.

The role of sensitizing factors has also been demonstrated in laboratory animals. For example, age- or weight-dependent susceptibility to the cardiotoxicity of β-adrenergic agonist and vasodilating antihypertensive agents occurs in the rat and to some extent in other laboratory animal species.

RESPONSE TO INJURY

Any of the tissue components of the heart may be specifically targeted by toxic agents and may respond individually, or the heart may respond as an organ. The morphologic reactions of the heart to toxic injury include cardiac hypertrophy, cardiomyopathies, cardiac cellular damage, myocardial necrosis and apoptosis, inflammation, and vascular changes (Tables 12.3 and 12.4). Of the tissue components, cardiac muscle cells are the most commonly affected. Cardiac muscle cells have a limited morphologic response to injury. Reversible alterations include cellular growth disturbances that lead to atrophy or hypertrophy. Distinctive myocyte alterations can result from sublethal injury or degeneration, such as fatty degeneration, lipofuscinosis, vacuolar degeneration or myocytolysis (Figure 12.3). Lethal injury to myocytes results in cell death, either necrosis or apoptosis, or both (Figure 12.4). Apoptosis is increasingly recognized for its role in the development of cardiotoxicity.

Unlike many other organs, regeneration in the heart is limited with necrosis frequently followed by fibrosis. While some information has recently been generated on myocardial regeneration and remodeling, little information is available on this response following toxic injury. Cell death is usually followed by an increase in size (hypertrophy) of remaining cardiomyocytes and fibrosis from excess accumulation of extracellular matrix (ECM), especially collagen (types I and III). Degradation of ECM is dependent on activation of matrix metalloproteins (MMPs) that may lead to reversibility of fibrosis. Cardiac stem cells that are self renewing, clonogenic and multipotent have been described. These can differentiate into cardiomyocyes and form vascular structures.

Drug-induced myocardial lesions usually consist of multifocal areas of myocardial degeneration, necrosis, inflammation, or fibrosis. However, large confluent areas of necrosis and fibrosis resembling myocardial infarcts have been produced by agents such as isoproterenol or by various combinations of drugs, sometimes in association with other factors, as in the electrolyte-steroid stress models of Selye. The human cardiomyopathies produced by most experimentally documented cardiotoxic drugs have the features of either an acute toxic or an acute allergic reaction. These features develop either shortly after administration of a single dose of a particular drug or during the course of treatment, requiring administration of multiple doses. These cardiomyopathies demonstrate an unequivocal cause and effect relationship, whether they result from an overdose, a side effect, or a hypersensitivity reaction. The clinical features of these reactions usually are those of acute toxic phenomena, with ischemic changes detected in the electrocardiogram, arrhythmias, acute cardiac failure, and sudden death. Myocardial lesions in acute drug-induced cardiotoxicity vary from multifocal damage to absence of anatomic changes. The latter is the case with certain agents such as digitalis and quinidine, which cause considerable functional changes without accompanying morphologic alterations. Cardiomegaly noted in these circumstances is attributable to pre-existing heart disease. Less frequently, drugs or chemicals

TABLE 12.3   Cardiotoxic agents that can produce myocardial necrosisa

Catecholamines	arsenic	*Dichapetalum cymosum*	Vitamin D and calcinogenic plants
isoproterenol	cadmium	Other plants	*Cestrum diurnum*
epinephrine	selenium	*Ateleia glazioviana*	*Solanum malacoxylon*
norepinephrine	nickel	*Brassica napus*	*Solanum torvum*
salbutamol	lead	*Cicuta* sp (water hemlock, cicutoxin)	*Trisetum flavescens*
terbutaline	Gossypol (*Gossypium* spp, cottonseed)	*Eupatorium rugosum* (white snakeroot, tremetone)	cholecalciferol (some rodenticides)
ephedrine	Cantharidin (*Epicauta* spp, blister beetle)	*Pachystigma pygmaeum*	Fungal toxins
Vasodilating anti-hypertensive agents	Histamine	*Pachystigma thamnus*	moniliformin
minoxidil	Methylxanthines	*Pavetta harborii*	T-2 toxin
hydralazine	theobromine	*Pavetta schumaniana*	Chloroquine
Beta adrenergic bronchodilators	theophylline	*Fodogia monticola*	Plasmocid
salbutamol	caffeine	*Cassia occidentalis* (coffee senna)	Brown FK
terbutaline	Ionophores	*Cassia obtusifolia*	Insulin
Cytokines	monensin	*Karwinskia humboldtiana* (coyotillo)	Phenylenediamine
IL-2	lasalocid	*Vicia villosa* (hairy vetch)	Brominated vegetable oils
IL-4	salinomycin	*Trigonella foenum-graecum*	Rancid fat
interferon	narasin	*Palicourea marcgravii*	High erucic-acid rapeseed oil
tumor necrosis factor-alpha (TNF-alpha)	A204	*Persea americana* (avocado)	Carbon monoxide and cigarette smoke
Isoproterenol	maduramicin	*Cicuta douglasii* (water hemlock)	Papain
Metaproterenol	Fluoroacetate containing plants	*Baileya multiradiata*	Allylamine
Digoxin	*Acacia georginae*	*Nerium oleander* (cardiac glycosides)	Hyperoxia
Corticosteroids	*Gastrolobium* spp.		Emetine
Metals	*Oxylobium* spp.		
cobalt			

TABLE 12.4   Cardiac responses to toxic injury with selected examples

Tissue component	Response	Xenobiotic
Heart as an organ	Defects: septal, valvular, vascular	Trypan blue, salicylates, griseofulvin, thalidomide, cortisone, dexamethasone, retinoic acid
Myocardium	Functional alteration, no morphologic alterations	Myocardial depressants (e.g., inhalation anesthetics), cardiotonic agents (e.g., some ionophores, cardiac glycosides) (see Table 12.5)
	Hypertrophy	Thyroid hormone, growth hormone, catecholamines, carbon monoxide
	Dilated cardiomyopathy	Ethanol, anthracylines, furazolidone, cocaine, interferon, some cytokines (e.g., IL-2), tumor necrosis factor (TNF), gossypol
	Degeneration	
	A. Vacuolar degeneration	Anthracyclines (e.g., adriamycin), antivirals (e.g., AZT)
	B. Fatty degeneration	Erucic acid
	C. Myocytolysis	Furazolidone
	Necrosis/fibrosis	Catecholamines, some ionophores, methylxanthines (see Tables 12.3 and 12.6)
	Apoptosis	Adriamycin

(Continued)

TABLE 12.4 (*Continued*)

Tissue component	Response	Xenobiotic
	Inflammation (myocarditis)	See Table 12.7
	Neoplasia	1,3-butadiene, nitrosamines
Conduction system/cardiac nerves	Cardioneuropathy, fibrosis of sinus node	Spanish toxic oil syndrome (oleoanilide contamination of rapeseed oil), eosinophilia-myalgia syndrome (contaminated typtophan)
Endocardium	Fibrosis	Methylsergide, ergotamine, serotonin
	Neoplasia	N-methyl-N-nitrosourea, dimethylnitrosoamide, triazine compounds
Valves	Valvulopathy	Fenfluramine
Pericardium	Hemorrhage	Minoxidil, theobromine, anticoagulants
	Inflammation (pericarditis)	Hydralazine, procainamide

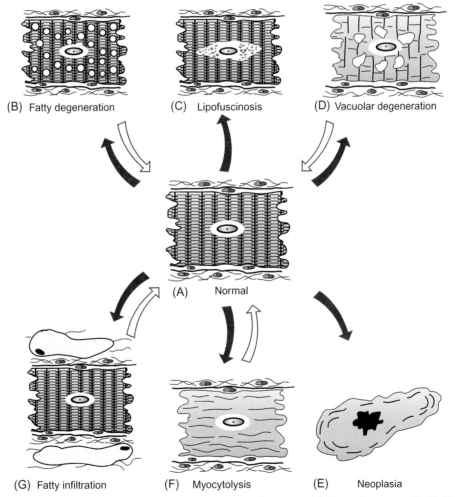

FIGURE 12.3 Schematic diagram of various sublethal cardiac muscle cell injuries. (A) Normal muscle cell. (B) Fatty degeneration. (C) Lipofuscinosis. (D) Vacuolar degeneration. (F) Myocytolysis. Also illustrated is fatty infiltration of interstitium (G) and neoplastic transformation of myocytes (E). (A–G, redrawn with permission from School of Veterinary Medicine, Purdue University.) From Van Vleet, J. F. and Ferrans, V.J. (2007). Cardiovascular System. In *Pathologic Basis of Veterinary Disease*, 4th ed. (McGavin, M., and Zachary, J.F., eds), Mosby Elsevier, St. Louis, Figure 10-6, p. 563.

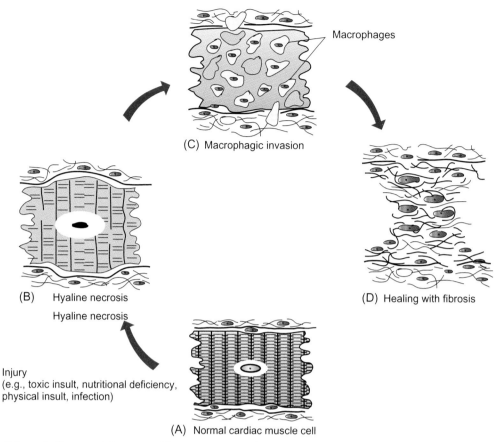

FIGURE 12.4   Schematic diagram of the sequential events in myocardial necrosis. (A) Various injuries lead to (B) hyaline necrosis or apoptosis of myocyte. (C) Healing with phagocytosis of cellular debris by macrophages, and (D) subsequent healing with fibrosis, rather than by regeneration. (A–D, Redrawn with permission from School of Veterinary Medicine, Purdue University.) From Van Vleet, J. F. and Ferrans, V.J. (2007). Cardiovascular System. In *Pathologic Basis of Veterinary Disease*, 4th ed. (McGavin, M., and Zachary, J.F., eds), Mosby Elsevier, St. Louis, Figure 10-7, p. 564.

may produce long-term cardiac alterations which may show clinical and morphologic manifestations of a chronic cardiomyopathy. In domestic animals, cardiotoxicity most commonly occurs without morphologic changes or manifests as myocardial necrosis. Cardiotoxicity may be acute or chronic depending on manner of exposure. In livestock, exposure is usually through ingestion of contaminated feed or exposure to toxic plants in pasture. Companion animals may be exposed to cardiotoxic drugs during chemotherapy or inadvertently by ingestion of human drugs. Myocardial necrosis due to toxins and chemicals (Table 12.3) must be distinguished from nutritional deficiencies (e.g., vitamin E/selenium deficiency), physical injuries and shock.

Developmental Cardiotoxicities

Abnormal cardiac function in the newborn is usually a consequence of a malformation. Ventricular and atrial septal defects are the most common structural changes. These have been associated with prenatal treatments with diphenylhydantoin and thalidomide in human infants, with phenobarbital and caffeine in rats, and with acetylsalicylic acid and cortisone in dogs.

Chemicals can also influence the functional development of the heart. Central control of cardiovascular reflexes is established prenatally, but the peripheral sympathetic system develops over the first postnatal weeks. Administration of reserpine to pregnant rats caused a permanent elevation of sympathetic tone in their offspring. Neonatal treatment with reserpine or with glucocorticoids slowed development of the sympathetic nervous system. Perinatal exposure to ethanol, opiates, or thyroid hormone accelerated development of the sympathetic nervous system in rats, but a deficit in the number of nerve terminals and neurotransmitter receptors occurred, resulting in subsensitivity to sympathetic stimulation that persisted in adulthood.

Treatment with cardiovascular drugs during pregnancy can cause adverse effects on the fetus or the newborn. For example, a β-agonist given as a tocolytic

TABLE 12.5 Cardiotoxic agents that can cause death without morphologic alterations

Cardiotonic agents increase force of myocardial contraction

1. Agents that inhibit Na^1/K^1-ATPase

Cardiac glycosides and aglycones—digitalis (*Digitalis purpurea*), digoxin, digitoxin, ouabain, Asclepin (*Asclepias* sp), oleandrin and neriine (*Nerium oleander*), bufodienolides (*Bufo marinus*)

2. Agents that increase Na^1 influx

Interact with electrogenic Na^+ channel; alkaloids (aconitine, veratrum), polypeptides (scorpion venom, anthopleurin-A)

Increase resting membrane permeability to Na^+; grayanotoxin (*Kalmia* sp, *Rhododendron* sp, *Pieris japonica*) batrachotoxin, ciguatoxin

Create artificial Na^+ channels in sarcolemma; carboxylic acid ionophores (monensin, salinomycin)

3. Agents that increase Ca^{21} influx

Calcium ionophores (X-537A, A23187), catecholamines, fluoride, digitalis, histamine

Myocardial depressants

1. Agents that decrease Na^1 permeability

Tetrodotoxin, saxitoxin, local anesthetics, antiarrhythmic drugs (quinine), higher alcohols, polyethylene glycol

2. Agents that replace sarcolemmal Ca^{21} and increase Ca^{21} influx

Metals (Cd, Mn, Ba)

3. Agents that alter contractility

Inhalation anesthetics (enflurane, halothane, isoflurane, methoxyflurane)

Halogenated hydrocarbons used in fire extinguisher compounds, propellants, solvents, refrigerants (chlorinated or fluorinated methane or ethane derivatives)

Cardiodepressant peptides produced during circulatory shock (myocardial depressant factor)

Fungal toxin (fumonisin B_1)

Other agents with cardiac action

Taxine (*Taxus cuspidata*), aconite (*Aconitum columbianum*), hyoscyamine and atropine (*Datura stramonium*), *Zygadenus* sp, selenium

---

(antilabor) agent can cause arrhythmia and a β-blocker given as an antihypertensive may cause cardiac depression in the newborn child. Delayed or long-lasting effects have also been demonstrated in animal experiments. Exposure of neonatal rats to low concentrations of lead caused an enhanced response to the arrhythmia- inducing effect of norepinephrine later. These findings indicate the need for evaluation of effects of this nature in preclinical studies, particularly when the drug is destined for use during pregnancy or in neonates.

Myocardium

Agents which Alter Cardiac Functions without Causing Morphologic Alterations

The heart's intrinsic properties of automaticity, excitability, conductivity, and contractility endow it with a variety of drug- sensitive mechanisms. Consequently, exposure of the heart to certain agents could lead to effects such as functional changes in rhythm and the force of contraction leading to death without morphologic alterations (Table 12.5).

Arrhythmias

Arrhythmias are among the most serious immediate functional cardiac abnormalities. As discussed previously, disturbances of impulse formation and of impulse conduction, either singly or in combination, are the main causes of cardiac arrhythmias. Arrhythmias are most commonly manifested as tachycardia (increased heart rate) that includes sinus tachycardia, atrial tachycardia, ventricular tachycardia and Torsade des Pointes (TdP), a ventricular tachycardia with distinct ECG characteristics that is potentially life threatening. The trigger for TdP is the long QT syndrome (LQTS), which may be congenital or acquired, and which involves abnormal repolarization of the heart. The abnormal repolarization causes differences in the "refractoriness" of the myocytes. After-depolarizations (which are more common in LQTS) can be propagated to neighboring cells due to the differences in the refractory periods, leading to re-entrant ventricular arrhythmias. Since many drugs such as haloperidol, erythromycin and methadone can prolong the QT interval, prolongation of the QT interval is of major concern in drug discovery and development, and special testing is mandated by the USFDA.

Environmental exposure to particulate matter pollutants as well as cardiomyopathies have also been shown to be risk factors.

Changes in Contractility

As a consequence of the ionic events responsible for the action potential there is an increase in the intracellular free calcium concentration. Myocardial contractility increases when more calcium is available inside the cell. Catecholamines activate the adenyl cyclase system by stimulating membrane β-receptors. The resulting increase in cAMP affects the sarcoplasmic reticulum that provides calcium ions to the contractile proteins. This action leads to a positive inotropic effect. By interfering with the actions of norepinephrine, β-adrenergic blocking agents such as propranolol exert negative inotropic and chronotropic effects. Vagal impulses or cholinergic substances can also produce negative inotropic and chronotropic effects. Fumonisin B_1 decreases myocardial contractility in pigs. This is thought to be mediated by increased sphingosine inhibiting the L-type calcium channels in the myocardium. Left sided heart failure results in pulmonary edema.

Impaired contractility may be the result of a decrease in cardiac energetics (availability of fuel substrate, oxygen extraction, metabolic process for energy production, or utilization of energy) or impairment of the process of excitation-contraction coupling. Toxic agents can interfere with the process of energy liberation, storage, or use. For example, ergot derivatives and vasopressin all can produce coronary vasoconstriction and decrease the myocardial oxygen supply. Some substances may affect oxyhemoglobin association or dissociation, thereby interfering with oxygen delivery. When coronary blood flow or oxygen extraction is reduced, the metabolism and function of the heart can be disrupted at all levels. Agents can alter the energy liberation and supply process by interfering with the rate-limiting steps in the tricarboxylic acid cycle. For example, some anesthetics and several cytotoxins (rotenone, cyanide) interfere with electron transport systems or uncouple phosphorylation.

Cardiac Hypertrophy

Cardiac hypertrophy is defined as an increase in the mass of the heart muscle beyond the normal limits for age, sex, and body weight. This increase usually develops as a compensatory response to an increase in work load and may result from congenital lesions, acquired valvular dysfunction, pulmonary disease (cor pulmonale), systemic hypertension, variously mediated drug effects (thyroid hormone, growth hormone,

catecholamines), or from unknown causes. Changes in structure and function of the ventricular myocardium are referred to as myocardial adaptation or remodeling. Hypertrophy may be adaptive, as with increased exercise, or maladaptive or pathological as with xenobiotic injury. Cell death, if extensive, is followed by compensatory hypertrophy of remaining myocytes but is frequently accompanied by fibrosis and often manifests as dilated cardiomyopathy. It is a risk factor for arrhythmias, heart failure and sudden cardiac death. Cardiac hypertrophy due to hyperthyroidism is the result of enhanced protein anabolism and regresses after restoration of normal thyroid functional status.

Cardiac hypertrophy may be concentric, as seen in adaptive hypertrophy, or eccentric as seen in dilated cardiomyopathy. In concentric hypertrophy there is an increase in width of individual myocytes due to new contractile protein units assembled in parallel, while in eccentric hypertrophy there is a relatively greater increase in length than width.

Dilated Cardiomyopathies

Dilated cardiomyopathy (DCM) is characterized by progressive cardiomegaly, dilation of both ventricular chambers and contractile (systolic) dysfunction. The terms congestive or ventricular-dilated cardiomyopathy have also been used. Dilated cardiomyopathy describes a heterogeneous group of heart muscle diseases including the cardiomyopathy associated with chronic alcoholism (alcoholic cardiomyopathy), sequelae of viral infection, or administration of toxic agents including cytokines. The etiology of the disorder remains unknown in many human patients (idiopathic dilated cardiomyopathy). Environmental exposure to particulate matter in the air has recently been recognized as a cause of cardiomyopathy.

Causes of dilated cardiomyopathies in domestic animals include exposure to furazolidine, anthracyclines and gossypol. Gossypol is the toxic principle in cottonseed which is often used as a source of protein in swine and cattle feed in areas where cotton (*Gossypium sp*) is grown. It is a yellow polyphenolic pigment that makes the cotton plant more insect resistant. Gossypol is cardiotoxic and causes infertility. Within the heart, it interferes with the conduction system by affecting the movement of K^+ across cell membranes. Adult ruminants are relatively insensitive since free gossypol is largely bound to protein in the rumen; however, calves can develop toxicosis. If gossypol is present at toxic doses in feed, large numbers of animals are often affected. At necropsy, dilated cardiomyopathy with secondary pulmonary edema and centrilobular hepatic necrosis are observed (Figure

12.5A). The characteristic histologic feature of gossypol toxicity in swine is myocyte atrophy with perinuclear clearing (Figure 12.5B). Myocardial toxicity also occurs in pre-ruminal ruminants.

Alcoholic Cardiomyopathy (ACM)

Ethyl alcohol has detrimental effects on myocardial metabolism; nevertheless, the pathogenetic mechanisms of alcoholic cardiomyopathy remain uncertain.

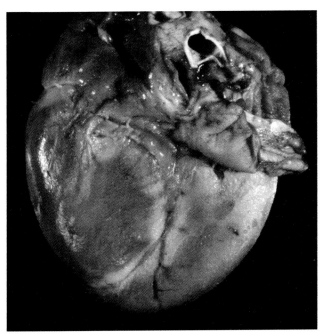

(A)

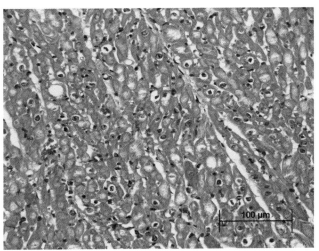

(B)

FIGURE 12.5 Cardiomyopathy in a pig, due to gossypol toxicosis. (A) Both ventricles are dilated resulting in a rounded apex. The pericardium is roughened from long-standing hydropericardium. (B) Cardiomyocyte atrophy. Myocytes are small, with perinuclear sarcoplasmic clearing. Paraffin-embedded, hematoxylin and eosin stain.

Reactive oxidative metabolites generated from the biotransformation of ethanol are thought to lead to lipid peroxidation of myocytes and oxidation of protein thiols. Acetaldehyde produced in the liver from metabolism via alcohol dehydrogenase may also reach the heart and produce adverse effects. Cardiomyopathy develops only in a small percentage of alcoholic patients. It is a dilated cardiomyopathy with hypertrophy and fibrosis. It has been difficult to reproduce experimentally, except for the pig, until recent studies using a liquid alcohol-containing diet in a metallothionen (MT) knockout mouse. MT is a zinc regulatory protein with release of zinc under oxidative stress. The addition of zinc to the diet prevented the occurrence of cardiac fibrosis but not hypertrophy. It appears likely that the toxic effect of ethanol on myocardium is modified by other factors and that the "alcoholic" cardiomyopathy observed clinically in human patients is a multifactorial disease that may include malnutrition, cigarette smoking, systemic hypertension and additives used in production of alcoholic beverages.

Anthracycline Cardiomyopathy

Although anthracycline antibiotics also can produce acute (ventricular arrhythmias and depression of contractility) and subacute (pericarditis and myocarditis) cardiac toxicity, these antineoplastic agents are well known for the distinctive type of chronic congestive cardiomyopathy that they produce in humans, dogs and experimental animals. The pathogenesis of this cardiotoxicity, which generally is dose dependent (usually at least 400 mg/m² total cumulative dose) remains uncertain; however, a number of possible mechanisms have been proposed, including drug binding by intercalation into the DNA of cardiac muscle cells; inhibition of several enzyme systems; and promotion of peroxidative damage, mediated by free radicals, to cell membranes, mitochondrial membranes, DNA, enzymes, and membranes of sarcoplasmic reticulum. Cumulative DNA damage due to oxidative stress leading to irreversible dysfunction may explain the late onset of cardiomyopathy. The drug toxicity leads to two major lesions; ventricular dilatation and myocardial cellular degeneration characterized by myofibrillar loss and cytoplasmic vacuolization (Figures 12.6 and 12.7). The latter is caused by massive dilatation of tubules of sarcoplasmic reticulum. These changes also can involve the conduction system of the heart.

Considerable efforts have been made to diminish the cardiotoxicity of anthracyclines without compromising their therapeutic effectiveness. The most successful results in this regard have been obtained with

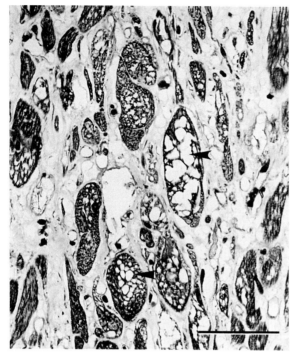

FIGURE 12.6   Severe vacuolar degeneration (arrowheads), and atrophy of myocytes with surrounding edema and fibrosis in a doxorubicin-treated rabbit (15 mg/kg total cumulative dose over 16 weeks). Plastic-embedded, toluidine blue stain. Bar = 50 μm.

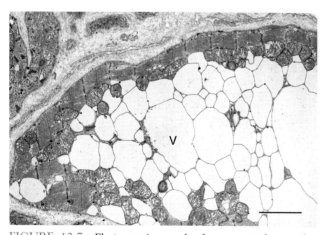

FIGURE 12.7   Electron micrograph of a myocyte from a dog given 16 mg/kg (total cumulative dose) of doxorubicin over four months. The myocyte has severe vacuolar (V) degeneration, due to distention of the sarcoplasmic reticulum. Bar = 2 μm.

ICRF-187, a compound which probably chelates iron (needed to mediate the peroxidative reactions promoted by anthracyclines). When given concomitantly with doxorubicin (adriamycin), ICRF-187 markedly reduces the severity of cardiomyopathy Compounds that act as free radical scavengers (vitamin E, *N*-acetylcysteine) have been much less successful in blocking the cardiotoxic effects of doxorubicin.

Antineoplastic agents other than the anthracyclines are also capable of producing cardiac damage, but only rarely. Among these are cyclophosphamide, busulfan, mitomycin C, cisplatinum, 5-fluorouracil, and vincristine.

Cytokine Cardiovascular Toxicity

The cardiovascular effects of cytokines can be classified as pro-inflammatory (TNF-α, IL-1β, IL-2, IL-6, IL-8, Fas ligand and chemokines), anti-inflammatory (IL-4, IL-10, IL-13, and TGF-β) and cardioprotective (cardiotrophin-1 and leukemia inhibiting factor). Cardiotoxicity has been observed from various cytokines utilized for cancer immunotherapy including interleukin-2 (IL-2), IL-1, IL-4 and interferon. The most frequently recognized cardiovascular complication of cancer immunotherapy provoked by IL-2 is the vascular leak syndrome which is thought to result, at least in part, from the interaction between IL-2-activated lymphocytes (lymphokine activated killer cells or LAK cells) and endothelial cells. The vascular leak syndrome is characterized by an increase in vascular permeability, with fluid retention, peripheral edema, ascites, pleural effusion and pulmonary edema. IL-2 may also decrease the mechanical performance and metabolic efficiency of the heart through changes in NO synthesis and Na^+/H^+ exchange. Interferon can cause cardiac arrhythmias, dilated cardiomyopathy and signs of myocardial ischemia. TNF-α has been shown to induce cardiomyocyte apoptosis and has a negative inotropic effect potentially through increased sphingosine. However, TNF-α is also protective to stresses such as ischemic injury.

Furazolidone Cardiomyopathy

When administered to young ducks, chickens, and turkeys, furazolidone causes congestive cardiomyopathy, severe ventricular dilatation, and diffuse myofibrillar lysis (Figure 12.8). Supplementation with selenium, vitamin E, and taurine does not protect against furazolidone-induced cardiomyopathy; however, propranolol has been reported to be protective. The biochemical mechanisms mediating this cardiomyopathy remain unknown.

Degeneration Due to Sublethal Cardiac Muscle Cell Injury (See Figure 12.3)

The common types of sublethal inury consist of hydropic degeneration, myofibrillar degeneration, fatty degeneration and lipofuscinosis. Myocyte atrophy occurs in gossypol toxicosis and perinuclear clearing is prominent (see Figure 12.5B).

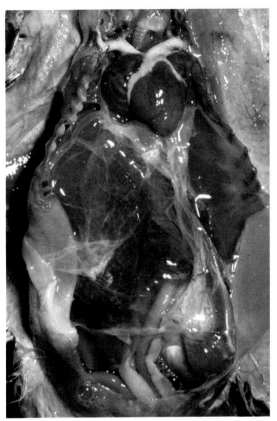

FIGURE 12.8 Cardiac dilatation and congestive heart failure in a duckling with furazolidone toxicosis. Serous fluid accumulation is present in the body cavities, and fibrin deposits are present over the liver. From Van Vleet, J. F. and Ferrans, V.J. (2007). Cardiovascular System. In Pathologic Basis of Veterinary Disease, 4th ed. (McGavin, M., and Zachary, J.F., eds), Mosby Elsevier, St. Louis, Figure 10-13, p. 566.

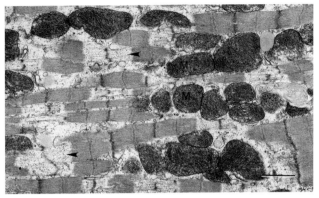

FIGURE 12.9 Selective disruption and lysis of I bands (arrowheads) in left ventricular myocardium of a rat with acute plasmocid toxicosis. M, mitochondria. Bar = 1 μm.

Hydropic Degeneration

Hydropic degeneration is a distinctive microscopic alteration in cardiac muscle cells associated with chronic administration of anthracyclines (see Figure 12.6). Gross lesions of doxorubicin cardiotoxicity in pigs, rabbits, and dogs were hydropericardium, hydrothorax, and ascites. In some animals the myocardium was pale and the hearts were dilated; however, many animals did not have gross evidence of cardiotoxicity. The microscopic and ultrastructural alterations in the myocardium were similar across all species including humans. The three major lesions observed in myocytes were sarcoplasmic vacuolization, myocytolysis, and hyaline necrosis. The distinctive vacuolar lesions resulted from distention of elements of the sarcoplasmic reticulum and the T tubules (see Figure 12.7). Vacuolar degeneration and myocytolysis also were present in Purkinje fibers.

Vacuolar lesions have also been reported in rat cardiomyocytes following treatment with antiviral drugs such as FIAC (1-(2-deoxy-2-flouro-β-d arabinofuranosyl)-5-iodocytosine) and Zidovudine (azidothymidine, AZT) which are used for AIDS therapy. With FIAC, early lesions consisted of dilatation of the sarcoplasmic reticulum while with AZT the vacuolar lesions were due to marked and widespread mitochondrial swelling with disruption of cristae. Chronic AZT use in AIDS patients can result in cardiomyopathy.

Myofibrillar Degeneration or Myocytolysis

Myofibrillar degeneration represents a distinctive sublethal injury of cardiac muscle cells. Affected fibers have pale eosinophilic sarcoplasm and lack cross striations. Ultrastructurally, myofibrils have variable extent of dissolution (myofibrillar lysis). This lesion has been described in furazolidone cardiotoxicity in birds, potassium deficiency in rats, anthracycline toxicosis (see above), and plasmocid toxicosis in rats (Figure 12.9).

Fatty Degeneration

Fatty degeneration (fatty change) is the accumulation of abundant sarcoplasmic lipid droplets in myocytes. Grossly, in severe cases the myocardium will be pale and flabby. Microscopically, affected myocytes have numerous variably sized spherical droplets that appear as empty vacuoles in paraffin sections but stain positively for lipids with lipid-soluble stains in frozen sections. This lesion may occur with systemic disorders such as severe anemia, toxemia, and copper deficiency but is less often seen in the heart than in the liver and kidney. It has also occurred in rats, rabbits, monkeys, gerbils, turkeys, chickens, ducklings, and pigs fed diets containing long-chain monoenoic fatty acids such as erucic acid, which is found in rapeseed oil. New varieties of rape plants produce rapeseed oil that contains only small amounts of erucic acid.

Lipofuscinosis

Lipofuscinosis or brown atrophy of the myocardium occurs in healthy aged animals and in animals with severe cachexia, as well as a hereditary lesion in healthy Ayrshire cattle. Affected hearts appear brown and microscopically have clusters of yellowish-brown granules at the nuclear poles of myocytes. These granules represent intralysosomal accumulation of membranous and amorphous debris (residual bodies).

Similar microscopic and ultrastructural lesions with accumulations of concentric lamellar bodies in myocytes were produced in rats by Brown FK, a food-coloring agent and in rats and mice given chloroquine.

Necrosis, Myocarditis, and Postnecrotic Resolution (see Figure 12.4)

Myocardial necrosis is a nonspecific response with many different etiologies, including toxicants, nutritional deficiencies, ischemia, metabolic disorders, and trauma. Necrosis can be focal, multifocal or diffuse with functional effects dependent on location with the heart. Necrosis of cardiac muscle cells is generally followed by leukocytic invasion and phagocytosis of sarcoplasmic debris. The end result is persistence of sarcolemmal "tubes" of basal lamina surrounded by condensed interstitial stroma and vessels. In some lesions with severe disruption of the myocardium, the residual effects will be fibroblastic proliferation and collagen deposition to form scar tissue. Regeneration of cardiac muscle cells is generally not observed. Rarely, in very young animals and especially in avian hearts, a limited amount of myocyte regeneration will occur. Hyperplasia of myocytes is a normal component of cardiac growth in the first several months of life but then ceases; the remainder of growth is the result of hypertrophy of myocytes until normal cell sizes are reached.

On the basis of the pathogenesis and morphology of the resulting lesions, toxic cardiac damage can be classified into the following categories: myocardial necrosis or toxic myocarditis, myocardial infarcts and infarct-like lesions, and hypersensitivity myocarditis.

Myocardial Necrosis or Toxic Myocarditis

Chemicals can cause myocardial injury by direct toxic effects which result in cell damage and cell death, either via apoptosis or necrosis (Table 12.3). In humans this type of injury is most frequently drug induced, while in domestic animals it can be caused by many different types of agents, some of which also cause skeletal muscle injury (Table 12.6). This type of toxicity is dose related; depending upon its rate of progression, it can cause either acute toxic myocarditis or

a more chronic cardiomyopathy. Acute toxic myocarditis is characterized by interstitial edema, multifocal areas of cardiac muscle cell necrosis with contraction bands, and an inflammatory cell infiltrate consisting of lymphocytes, plasma cells, and polymorphonuclear leukocytes. Eosinophils may be present, but seldom are prominent. The paucity of eosinophils and the presence of various stages of cell death and healing by fibrosis serve to differentiate toxic myocarditis from hypersensitivity myocarditis. A true vasculitis is not present. Microthrombi have been reported in toxicity due to ADP, cyclophosphamide, catecholamines, and thromboxane A. Selected chemicals known to produce myocarditis by direct toxic mechanisms are presented in Table 12.2. It should be remembered that a cellular inflammatory reaction may be poorly developed or totally absent in toxic myocarditis due to antineoplastic or immunosuppressive agents.

Chronic inflammatory myocarditis has been observed in atrial myocardium of dogs and pigs treated with minoxidil, a vasodilating antihypertensive agent that also can produce foci of left ventricular papillary muscle necrosis. The atrial lesions in dogs are localized mainly in the right atrium, whereas those in pigs are found in the left atrium. The papillary muscle necroses are thought to be consequences of the tachycardia, hypotension, and hypoperfusion which occur when large doses of minoxidil are given. Similar right atrial lesions are produced in dogs by the administration of large doses of theobromine.

Some of the more commonly observed toxic causes of myocardial necrosis in domestic animals include ionophore toxicity in horses and ruminants, anthracyline toxicity in dogs, white snakeroot toxicity in horses and gossypol toxicity in pigs. Deaths in ruminants have resulted from consumption of plants such as *Acacia georginae* and *Dichapetalum cymosum* that occur in localized areas of the world.

Ionophores, polyether acid ionophore antibiotics such as monensin, lasalocid, and narasin, are often added to ruminant feed as growth promotants and coccidiostats. Toxicity occurs when target species (species in which use is approved by FDA) are exposed at high doses or when nontarget species (species in which use is not approved) such as horses are exposed. Toxicosis has been reported in most species, including avian. Ionophores are extensively metabolized via the P450 cytochrome pathway. Ionophores form lipid soluble dipolar reversible complexes with cations, allowing movement of cations across cell membranes causing a disruption of ionic equilibrium. Mitochondrial damage affects oxidative metabolism. Necrosis of cardiac (Figure 12.10) and skeletal muscle is due to ionophore induced calcium overload. Horses

TABLE 12.6 Common agents inducing cardiac and/or skeletal muscle degeneration/necrosis in domestic animals

Agent	Myocardial necrosis	Skeletal muscle degeneration/necrosis	Other organs affected	Primary species affected
Drugs and feed additives/contaminants				
Ionophores—monensin, lasalocid, narasin, A-204, maduramicin, salinomycin	±	+		All, mostly livestock, horse most susceptible
High erucic acid rapeseed oil, brominated vegetable oils, rancid fat	+			
Antineoplastic drugs—anthracyclines (e.g., doxorubicin, daunorubicin)	+	+		Dog, cat
Corticosteroids—cortisone, triamcinolone, fluorocortisone	+	+	Liver	Dog
Anesthetics—halothane and others (via malignant hyperthermia)	±	+		Pig
Methylxanthines (theobromine, theophylline, caffeine)	+			Pets exposed
Catecholamines	+			All
Vasodilator antihypertensives	+			Pets exposed
Vitamin D (supplements, rodenticide, calcinogenic plants, analog in psoriasis medication)	+		Kidney, lung, stomach, other	All, soft tissue mineralization
Iron dextran (injected)	+	+	Hemosiderosis of lymph nodes	Pig
Thallium	+		Gastrointestinal tract, skin	Dog
Selenium (acute)	+	+	Variable: liver, lung, pancreas, kidney, CNS	Pigs, ruminants
Biological agents				
A. Plants (toxins)				
Cassia occidentalis, C. obtusifolia (*coffee senna*)	+	+		Ruminants, horse, pig
Karwinskia humboltiana (coyotillo)	+	+		Ruminants, horse, pig
Eupatorium rugosum (white snakeroot, tremetone)	+	+		Horse, cow, man
Gossypium spp (gossypol in cottonseed products)	+	+	Liver, lung secondarily	Pig, pre-ruminal ruminant, dog
Neruim oleander (cardiac glycosides)	±			Livestock, dog
Trigonella foenumgraecum	+	+		Cattle
Petiveria alliacea	+	+		Cattle
Diaporthe toxica (lupinosis)	−	+		Sheep
Persia americana (avocado)	+	−	Lung secondarily; mastitis in some species	Goats, caged birds, ostriches, horses
Cicuta spp (water hemlock, cicutoxin)	+	+	CNS stimulant	All
Vicia villosa (hairy vetch)	+		Granulomatous lesions in skin, other organs	Horse, cattle
Fluoroacetate containing plants	+	−		All

(Continued)

TABLE 12.6   (*Continued*)

Agent	Myocardial necrosis	Skeletal muscle degeneration/necrosis	Other organs affected	Primary species affected
Calcinogenic plants (e.g., *Solanum* sp)	+	+		Livestock
Thermopsis montana	−	+		Calves
B. Animal and insect toxins				
Epicauta sp (cantharidin in blister beetle)	+	−	Urinary bladder, gastrointestinal tract	Horse
C. Bacterial and fungal toxins				
Clostridium chauvoei, *C. septicum*, *C. novyi*, *C. perfringens* toxins	±	+	Gastrointestinal tract, liver, muscle	Cattle, sheep, horse, pig
Moniliformin	+	−		Poultry

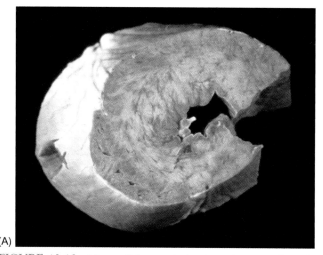

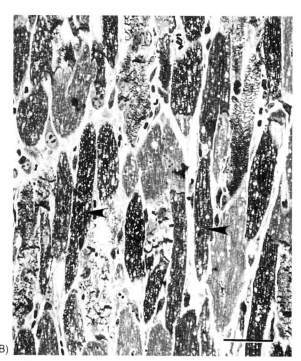

FIGURE 12.10   Myocardial necrosis due to acute monensin toxicosis in a calf. (A) Cross-section of the left ventricular myocardium with pale, mottled areas (arrows) due to necrosis. (B) Numerous dense necrotic fibers (arrowheads) in ventricular myocardium. Note intrasarcoplasmic lipid vacuoles. Paraffin-embedded, hematoxylin and eosin stain. Bar = 50 μm. From Van Vleet, J. F. and Ferrans, V.J. (2007). Cardiovascular System. In *Pathologic Basis of Veterinary Disease*, 4th ed. (McGavin, M., and Zachary, J.F., eds), Mosby Elsevier, St. Louis, Figure 10-55, p. 586.

are exquisitively sensitive to ionophore toxicity with cardiotoxic effects predominating (LD$_{50}$ 2–3 mg monensin/kg). Cardiac muscle necrosis can be observed if the horse survives for 3 to 4 days after exposure. Skeletal muscle toxicity predominates in ruminants exposed to ionophores at excessive doses (goats and sheep LD$_{50}$ 12–24 mg monensin/kg; cattle LD$_{50}$ 50–80 mg monensin/kg).

White snakeroot (*Eupatorium rugosum*) is a perennial that grows in moist shaded areas of timber stands in the eastern half of the USA and Canada. The primary toxic component is a ketone, called trematone, which requires bioactivation by the cytochrome P450 system. Toxicoses have been observed in many species but occur most commonly in horses, and also in cattle. Toxicity generally occurs after ingestion of 0.5% to 1.5% of the body weight of the plant over 1–3 weeks. The toxin is excreted in the milk and has induced toxicity in humans ("milk fever"), calves and cats. Abraham Lincoln's mother is said to have died from drinking milk from cows that ingested white snakeroot. Clinically, muscle tremors (especially cattle),

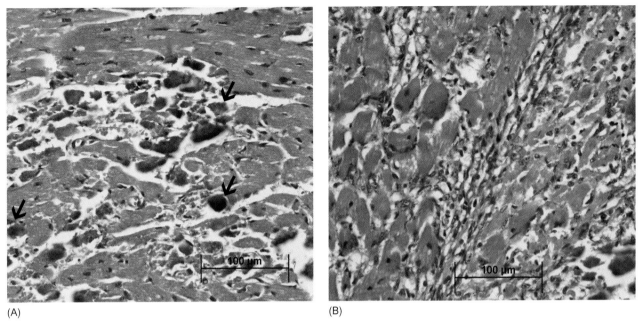

(A)   (B)

FIGURE 12.11   Myocardial necrosis with mineralization and fibrosis in a horse, due to white snakeroot (*Eupatorium rugosum*) toxicosis. Paraffin-embedded, hematoxylin and eosin stain. (A) Acute myocardial necrosis. Necrotic myocytes are fragmented and heavily mineralized (arrows). (B) Myocardial fibrosis. Fibroblasts replace and separate degenerating and necrotic myocytes.

sweating and cardiovascular effects (especially horses) occur. Myocardial and skeletal muscle necrosis with prominent mineralization is the primary lesion (Figure 12.11). Mineralization is also a prominent feature of vitamin D toxicity including that due to ingestion of calcinogenic plants.

Myocardial Infarction Associated with Toxic Reactions

Grossly evident myocardial infarction may occur in drug-induced coronary arteritis (as from amphetamines), fibromuscular intimal proliferation (estrogen- and/or progesterone-containing oral contraceptives), embolization from infective endocarditis (associated with intravenous drug abuse), or, in patients with normal coronary arteries, following exposure to toxic levels of carbon monoxide, nitrates, thyroid preparations, methylsergide or ergot derivatives, and certain antineoplastic agents. Large infarct-like areas of necrosis, not related to obstruction of large extramural coronary arteries, have been produced in experimentally with toxic doses of isoproterenol. Isoproterenol increases cardiac rate, contractility, and oxidative metabolism as well as increasing calcium uptake, stimulating the adenyl cyclase system, causing aggregation of platelets and formation of free radicals capable of causing peroxidative damage. Other sympathomimetic amines (norepinephrine, epinephrine) are capable of inducing lesions of myocardial necrosis, which are small, multifocal, and usually localized in left ventricular subendocardium.

Catecholamine-induced cardiac lesions occur in conjunction with pheochromocytomas, tetanus, subarachnoid hemorrhage, and other central nervous system (CNS) lesions which result in increased intracranial pressure. Ischemic cardiac damage can be aggravated by high circulating levels of catecholamines in patients with acute myocardial infarction. Similar changes occur in domestic animals that have neurologic lesions ("brain-heart" syndrome) and are most commonly observed in the dog. Cocaine induced myocardial damage also occurs via catecholamine mediated mechanisms.

Hypersensitivity Myocarditis

Hypersensitivity myocarditis represents the most common form of drug-induced heart disease in humans. The clinical criteria for the diagnosis of this disorder are previous use of the drug without incident; the hypersensitivity reaction bears no relationship to the magnitude of the dose of the drug; the reaction is characterized by clinical signs consistent with classic allergy, serum sickness, or infectious disease; immunologic confirmation; and persistence of symptoms until the drug is discontinued.

Hypersensitivity myocarditis associated with drug therapy is characterized by infiltration of the heart muscle with numerous eosinophils admixed with mononuclear cells, predominantly lymphocytes and plasma cells. The cellular infiltrate may be focal or diffuse and is associated with foci of myocytolysis.

Fibrotic changes are absent and all lesions are similar in age and appearance. Vascular involvement is frequent and consists of vasculitis affecting small arteries, arterioles, and venules. The inflammatory reaction may also involve the pericardium but characteristically spares the cardiac valves. The absence of extensive myocardial necrosis or fibrosis distinguishes drug-related hypersensitivity myocarditis from other forms of myocarditis in which eosinophils are prominent. Endocardial fibrosis is not a feature of hypersensitivity myocarditis. Selected drugs associated with hypersensitivity myocarditis are listed in Table 12.7. Some of these drugs have also been associated with hypersensitivity vasculitis. The pathogenesis of drug-induced hypersensitivity myocarditis remains unclear. The condition appears to be immunologically mediated, perhaps as a reaction in which the drug or one of its metabolites acts as a hapten and combines with an endogenous macromolecule; it is this combination that is antigenic. Hypersensitivity myocarditis also has developed after injection of horse serum, tetanus toxoid, and smallpox vaccine.

In domestic animals, hypersensitivity myocarditis is not recognized except possibly for the granuloma-tous lesions induced by ingestion of vetch (*Vicia villosa*) in horses and cattle. Granulomatous dermatitis is usually the presenting clinical syndrome, but lesions can be present in many organs.

Cell Death

Cell death can occur via necrosis or apoptosis and both can occur simultaneously in response to injury. Apoptosis has only recently been described in the heart leading to extensive research in this area. It has been shown to be an important form of cell death in adriamycin induced cardiotoxicity. Both mitochondrial and non-mitochondrial pathways can lead to apoptosis and necrosis. Release of mitochondrial cytochrome c into the cytosol is a critical factor in cardiomyocyte apopotosis. Cytochrome c leads to activation of caspase 9 which is followed by caspase 3 activation and apoptosis. Necrosis is initiated by a decrease in ATP production due to decreased electron transport. Both release of cytochrome c and collapse of electron transport can occur if mitochondrial permeability is altered, as with defective mitochondrial oxidative phosphorylation, providing one explanation how both apoptosis and necrosis may be induced at the same time.

Two basic forms of cardiac muscle cell necrosis are distinguishable: coagulation necrosis and necrosis with contraction bands (myofibrillar damage leading to myocytolysis).

Coagulation Necrosis

Ischemia of less than 20 min duration produces damage characterized by glycogen depletion, mitochondrial swelling, mild intracellular edema, and relaxation of sarcomeres (reflecting loss of contractility). These changes are reversible upon reflow. However, when the period of ischemia exceeds 20 min, irreversible injury develops with the features of coagulation necrosis. By 60 min, most of the cells in the ischemic area become irreversibly injured. Coagulation necrosis is characterized by intramitochondrial flocculent precipitates, thought to be derived from mitochondrial lipids; margination of nuclear chromatin, indicating irreversible nuclear damage; small holes or defects in the plasma membrane, signifying loss of its permeability barrier function; relaxed myofibrils with indistinct myofilaments; and various degrees of dissociation of the intercellular junctions. Coagulation necrosis is limited to central areas of infarcts, in which reflow does not occur following ischemic damage.

Necrosis with Contraction Bands

In contrast to coagulation necrosis, peripheral areas of infarcts show a different type of necrosis, known as necrosis with contraction bands, which is characterized

TABLE 12.7   Drugs associated with hypersensitivity myocarditis in human patients

Acetazolamide	*p*-Aminosalicyclic acid[+]
Allopurinol[*]	Penicillin[*]
Aminophylline	Phenindione
Amitriptyline	Phenylbutazone[*,+]
Ampicillin	Phenytoin
Carbamazepine[*,+]	Procainamide[*,+]
Cephalothin	Pyribenazamine
Chloramphenicol[*]	Quinidine[*]
Chlorpropamide[*]	Reserpine[+]
Chlorthalidone[*]	Spironolactone[*]
Colchicine[*]	Streptomycin
Diclofenac	Sulfonamides[1]
Digitalis/digoxin	Sulfadiazine
Diphenylhydantoin[*,+]	Sulfamethoxazole
Furosemide[*]	Sulfisoxazole
Hydrochlorothiazide	Sulfonylureas
Indomethacin	Tetracycline[*]
Isoniazid[*,+]	Theophylline
Lidocaine	Triamterine
Methyldopa[+]	Trimethoprim
Oxyphenbutazone[*]	

[*]Also associated with hypersensitivity non-necrotizing vasculitis
[+]Also associated with lupus-like syndrome
[1]Sulfonamides have been associated with toxic necrotizing vasculitis

by hypercontraction of myofibrils, intramitochondrial electron-dense calcific deposits, and progression to myocytolysis (Figures 12.12 and 12.13). The distinctive features of this type of necrosis are related to the entry of large amounts of calcium ions, which originate from partial perfusion of peripheral areas of ischemic lesions, into cells which are damaged by ischemia. The passage of calcium through damaged abnormally permeable plasma membranes is responsible for the hypercontraction. This passage occurs either when severely but temporarily ischemic tissue is reperfused with arterial blood or when necrosis develops because of factors not related to a reduction in coronary blood flow. For these reasons, necrosis with contraction bands is seen in many forms of cardiac toxic injury, including the lesions caused by catecholamines, vasodilating antihypertensive agents, and other cardiotoxic compounds.

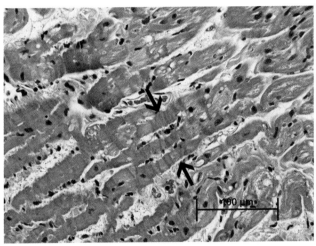

FIGURE 12.12 Myocardium with contraction bands in a rat. Transverse bands (arrows) of densely eosinophilic material are separated by pale, sometimes granular or vacuolated sarcoplasm. Paraffin-embedded, hematoxylin and eosin stain.

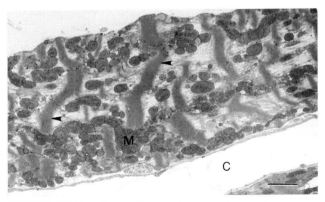

FIGURE 12.13 Contraction band necrosis in ventricular myocyte of a rat with acute plasmocid toxicosis. Dense transverse masses of contractile material are prominent (arrowheads). M, mitochondria; C, capillary. Bar = 2 μm.

Progression of necrosis with contraction bands to myocytolysis is mediated through lysis of the myofilaments, a change that results in an empty appearance of the cells. The time course of this progression is highly variable.

Progression of Morphologic Alterations Following Myocardial Necrosis

Grossly, affected areas appear pale initially and may progress to prominent yellow to white dry gritty areas with dystrophic mineralization (see Figure 12.10A). The lesions may be focal, multifocal, or diffuse. The most frequent sites of focal lesions are the left ventricular papillary muscles and the subendocardial myocardium, especially when such lesions are related to disturbances of vascular perfusion. These lesions may be overlooked at necropsy unless multiple incisions are made in the ventricular myocardium. In diseases with diffuse necrosis, such as so-called "white muscle disease" of calves and lambs with selenium-vitamin E deficiency and in white snakeroot toxicosis, the pale lesions may be readily observed on the epicardial and endocardial surfaces.

Microscopically, fibers in areas of recent necrosis often appear swollen and hypereosinophilic (hyaline necrosis). Striations are indistinct and nuclei are pyknotic. Necrotic fibers often have scattered basophilic granules that represent mitochondrial accumulation of calcium salts as confirmed by electron microscopy (see Figure 12.11A).

Another pattern of necrosis may also be observed when affected myocytes have a "shredded" appearance from hypercontraction and formation of multiple transversely oriented bars of disrupted contractile material (often termed contraction band necrosis) (see Figure 12.12). A third type of appearance is seen in necrotic myocytes within large areas of ischemic necrosis (infarcts). Affected fibers have features of coagulation necrosis but have relaxed rather than hypercontracted contractile elements.

Areas of necrosis will have infiltration of inflammatory cells 24 to 48 hr after injury. These cells are mainly macrophages, with occasional neutrophils, that phagocytose and lyse the necrotic cellular debris. In early stages of resolution of necrosis it may be difficult to distinguish the lesions from those produced by some types of myocarditis (see previous text). Later lesions of resolving necrosis will have persistent stromal tissues (interstitial fibroblasts and collagen, capillaries) and empty "tubes" of basal laminae from necrotic myocytes (see Figures 12.6 and 12.11B). The healing phase is further characterized by proliferation of connective tissue cells (fibroblasts, capillary endothelial cells) and by deposition of connective tissue (collagen, elastic tissue, acid mucopolysaccharides). Grossly, these areas will appear as white scars.

The outcome of cases with myocardial necrosis will vary depending on the extent of the damage. Many animals will die acutely from cardiac failure if the extent of myocardial damage is extensive. Early deaths from necrosis-related arrhythmias may also occur. Some cases may eventually develop cardiac decompensation and die with cardiac dilatation and scarring and lesions typical of chronic congestive failure. Finally, with minimal damage, lesions may resolve completely or only microscopically detectable residual myocardial lesions may be found when death eventually occurs from other causes.

Endocardium

Endocardial morphologic alterations are infrequently associated with cardiotoxic agents. Examples include drug-induced endocardial fibrosis and neoplasia.

Fibrosis

Endocardial mural fibrosis can occur in association with toxic or ischemic myocardial necrosis. Mural endocardial thickening also occurs in the late stages of allylamine cardiotoxicity and in radiation-induced myocardial fibrosis.

Neoplasia

Chemically induced cardiac neoplasms are infrequent but have been described in rats, mice, and hamsters. The compounds involved included carbamates (1,1-diphenyl-2-butynyl-N-cyclohexyl carbamate), fluorenylacetamide, urethan, ethylnitrosourea, methylnitrosourea, dimethylnitrosamine, methylnitrosamine, ethyl methanesulfonate, ethylnitrosobiuret, hydrazine, triazene, diethylnitrosamine, and 1,3- butadiene. Most of the induced neoplasms were of endocardial origin (endocardial mesenchymal tumors, mostly Schwannomas) but a few arose from the vasculature of the myocardium or pericardium (hemangiosarcoma).

Pericardium

Pericardial lesions induced by toxic agents are infrequent. Examples include drug-induced epicardial hemorrhage and pericarditis.

Hemorrhage

Minoxidil, a vasodilating antihypertensive drug, produced hemorrhagic right atrial lesions in dogs.

Minoxidil can also produce left ventricular papillary muscle necroses and superficial endocardial and epicardial hemorrhages in various regions of the heart. Pericardial hemorrhage can occur as a result of cyclophosphamide toxicity and of therapy with anticoagulants, as in some patients with uremia who are given heparin during the course of hemodialysis.

Pericarditis

Pericarditis with or without effusion has been reported to occur in patients with drug-induced systemic lupus erythematosus. The syndromes have been most clearly documented in the case of hydralazine and procainamide. Drugs that cause toxic myocarditis, hypersensitivity myocarditis, or large areas of myocardial necrosis often also cause pericarditis by extension of the inflammation to the pericardium, particularly the visceral pericardium. Pericarditis is commonly seen as a response to effusion within the pericardial sac, irrespective of the cause of the effusion.

Valves

Valvulopathy, characterized by nodular or segmental thickening of heart valves due to fibromyxoid proliferation, can be induced by methylsergide and ergotamine tartrate, and may occur with the carcinoid syndrome. Similar alterations of cardiac valves occurred in humans chronically treated with the appetite-suppressant drugs (anorexigens) such as fenfluramine and dexfenfluramine. The lesions consisted of thick white fibrous plaque of leaflets and chordae. Mitral valve involvement was most common but aortic and tricuspid regurgitation was also observed. The pathogenesis of anorexigen-induced valvulopathy appears to be mediated via activation of the 5HT 2B receptor (5HT2BR). The antiparkinsonian drugs, pergolide and cabergoline, are potent 5HT2BR agonists and have also been reported to cause valvulopathy in humans.

EVALUATION OF CARDIOTOXICITY

The ability to detect cardiovascular toxicities in animals is subject to a number of complicating factors. The exaggerated pharmacological effects of an agent might be recognized in one species but be absent or entirely different in another species. A pre-existing cardiovascular disease, old age, or poor nutritional status could predispose to cardiovascular toxicity. Since toxicological evaluations of chemicals are usually carried out in normal animals, those toxicities that occur as a result of a predisposing condition may not become apparent. The consequences of myocardial drug interactions could increase the potential for adverse cardiovascular effects; two agents when given separately may be relatively nontoxic, but when given together could elicit severe cardiovascular toxicity, for example, propranolol and verapamil. A toxic effect is less likely to be detected when the mechanism is unrelated to the primary pharmacologic activity, for example, when a reactive metabolite is responsible for the injury. The biotransformation of the substance, as well as the degree to which a given reactive metabolite is formed, commonly varies among species. Substances intended for the treatment of cardiovascular diseases are generally examined in much greater detail for specific effects on the heart or arterial blood pressure than are agents intended for noncardiovascular use. The ratio between therapeutic and toxic doses is generally higher for those agents with a secondary rather than a primary cardiovascular action. The physiologic and biochemical methods used to characterize the desired properties of a new substance are often nearly identical to those employed in identification of toxic effects. Adverse cardiovascular reactions usually involve the heart (myocardium and specialized tissue), the arterial resistance vessels in various vascular beds, or blood pressure regulation in general. An assessment of cardiovascular toxicity should, therefore, include monitoring of basic functions such as contractility, rhythmogenicity, and arterial blood pressure. Myocardial damage may also be assessed by determination of activities of muscle-origin serum enzymes and isoenzymes, as well as troponins (see Skeletal Muscle) and natriuretic peptides.

Serum biomarkers used in myocardial infarction in humans include the MB isoenzyme of creatine kinase and myoglobin. Neither is specific to the myocardium. BNP is used as a biomarker for chronic heart failure since it appears directly correlated with the degree of ventricular wall tension. However its control is not well understood. Cardiac troponins T (cTnT) and I (cTnI) are constituents of myofilaments and exclusive to cardiomyocytes, therefore this assay has absolute specificity. Any measurable concentration of serum cTn reflects myocardial injury.

Physiologic Evaluation of Toxicity

Monitoring Myocardial Contractile Function

Mechanical energy in cardiac muscle is reflected in two measurable contractile properties of the muscle; the ability to shorten and the ability to develop force. All indices of the contractile state are based on these two characteristics of muscle contraction or some derivative of them, such as velocity of shortening or force development. A positive inotropic agent will increase both the extent and velocity of muscle shortening and the extent and rate of force development. In the intact animal, an increased force can be accompanied by changes in ventricular loading conditions as a result of effects on arterial blood pressure and ventricular chamber size. The change in ventricular load can influence the degree of muscle shortening and force development. In order to accurately quantitate a change in myocardial contractility, the influence of changes in muscle loading conditions must either be eliminated or taken into account. The influence of loading conditions on myocardial contractility, whether the experimental model is an isolated cardiac muscle or an intact ventricle, is determined by the preload and afterload. The preload sets the initial resting muscle length and, as a result, the level at which the muscle functions along its length-tension curve. The extent of muscle shortening and the velocity of muscle shortening both decrease as afterload increases.

Isolated Muscle Preparations

There are a variety of isolated muscle preparations that have been developed for evaluating myocardial contractility. Because there is a complex relationship between inotropism and chronotropism, force of contraction measurements are best made in test systems where the cardiac tissue is electrically stimulated at a constant rate. The papillary muscle, the left atrium, and atrial or ventricular strips from the cat, guinea pig, or rabbit are the most frequently used areas of the heart for this purpose. In these types of preparations, contractile force is best determined as isometric tension development and the isotonic force-velocity relation. Isometric tension development can be evaluated from the rate of tension development (dp/dt), the peak development tension (p), and the time to peak tension (TPP). The force-velocity relationship can be obtained by monitoring the velocity of isotonic shortening as the afterload is increased.

Isolated Perfused Heart

The isolated heart allows a definitive evaluation of chemical effects directly on the heart without interference or interactions with other tissues and organs present in the body. In addition, it is possible to maintain control over variables, such as perfusion pressure and blood flow, that are likely to change during the course of an experiment in an intact animal. The structural composition of the heart is retained in such an isolated system. The principle limitation to use of isolated organ preparations is that adequate physiological and biochemical integrity can be retained for only limited periods of time (up to 4 hr). The isolated heart can be a useful tool in the identification and exploration of cardiotoxic actions on ventricular contraction, heart rate and rhythm, and coronary vasculature.

In Vivo *Invasive Preparations*

A major advantage of *in vitro* studies is that the determinants of cardiac performance such as heart rate, preload, and afterload may be fixed. For intact animal studies the analysis of drug effects on myocardial contractibility is more difficult unless these three functions are carefully controlled. However, studies with intact animals will provide information concerning adaptive responses to xenobiotics. In a closed-chest anesthetized dog, cat, or pig, indirect assessment of contractility is possible if certain variables such as heart rate, arterial blood pressure, and cardiac output are recorded simultaneously. A strain gauge arch will give the most direct assessment of myocardial contractility.

Noninvasive Methods

Noninvasive techniques are available for evaluating myocardial contractility. Echocardiography allows examination of cardiac function by reflected ultrasound. Echocardiography can detect alterations in contractility resulting from a variety of pathologic conditions that affect the myocardium, pericardium, and cardiac valves. Echocardiography has been successfully used in detecting drug-induced myocardial alterations in dogs.

Left ventricular function may be assessed by the measurement of systolic time intervals. Changes in systolic time intervals diverge from normal at the same time and in the same direction as hemodynamic parameters monitored by invasive techniques. However, correlations between these two methodologies are not perfect because they reflect different functions, that is, time periods rather than pressure or volume changes. Concurrent use of the systolic time intervals with echocardiology can be advantageous because the two methods are complementary by providing information on the isometric and ejection phases of left ventricular contraction.

Monitoring Myocardial Electrical Activity

Cardiac arrhythmias are the most common and generally the easiest drug- or chemical-induced adverse cardiovascular response to detect. Xenobiotics can interfere with the formation and conduction of cardiac impulses and thereby initiate supraventricular and ventricular premature contractions, disturbance of conduction, bradycardia, or tachycardia. Disturbances of impulse formation may be due to changes in normal automaticity of the specialized conduction tissues or to abnormal autonomic activity generated in any area of the heart. A typically fast or slow propagation of impulses may occur anywhere in the myocardium. The most important arrhythmogenic actions of xenobiotics can be reproduced and monitored in heart muscle preparations, isolated heart preparations, and intact animals.

Heart Muscle Preparation

The use of isolated Purkinje fibers to evaluate possible toxic effects of substances can provide significant preliminary information. Purkinje fibers from dogs and sheep are the most frequently used. The number of usable fibers varies with each heart, and in the dog, ranges from three to eight. Long-term continuous recording from cardiac Purkinje fibers is possible because they contract less vigorously than atrial or ventricular muscle.

In contrast to Purkinje fibers, many contractile myocytes suitable for isolated tissue studies can be obtained from each heart. Normally these muscle cells are not spontaneously active and must be electrically stimulated to evoke action potentials. The electrical activity of contractile muscle fibers is often studied concurrently with Purkinje fibers. Alterations in membrane potentials can be used to evaluate arrhythmic activity. Membrane action potentials are a reflection of and result from changes in membrane ionic permeability.

Cultured Heart Cells

Cultured cells in monolayer networks and sheets regress to the embryonic state. These reverted cells are helpful for examining certain myocyte properties such as changes in type of cation channels, K^+ permeability, and the electrogenesis of pacemaker potentials. Reaggregated cultured heart cells can be prepared that retain highly differentiated electrical properties and their normal pharmacological receptors. Simultaneous monitoring of transmembrane potentials and contractions can be made on single cells by using appropriate microelectrode and photoelectric techniques. Since the cells are denervated, the direct effect of various chemicals and pharmacological agents on the myocyte can be evaluated without involvement of neural and systemic influences.

Intact Animals

All data regarding the effects of xenobiotics on myocardial electrical action potentials obtained from studies using isolated tissues should ultimately be correlated with whole animal studies. The information from whole animal studies is most often obtained from electrocardiographic or His-bundle recordings.

Significant changes in the electrocardiogram following exposure to xenobiotics may result from functional alterations to the myocyte cell membrane or structural damage to the myocyte.

A major problem with studies examining potential arrhythmogenesis is the extrapolation of results obtained from animal studies to humans. In an effort to minimize this problem, dogs have been used as the standard animal model for electrocardiogram (ECG) analysis. Mouse and rat arrhythmogenesis screens are being developed.

Common ECG alterations detected after exposure to cardioactive substances include QRS interval prolongation, lengthening or shortening of QTs, characteristic changes in the shape of the ST-T complex, various degrees of AV block, right bundle branch block, left bundle branch block, intraventricular block, increases in P-wave amplitude and duration, and ectopic arrhythmias.

Monitoring Arterial Blood Pressure

The recording of arterial blood pressure in toxicity studies complements electrocardiography by adding a hemodynamic variable to routinely monitored cardiovascular functions. A majority of the toxicity studies in which blood pressure is recorded are carried out in the dog and rat. Single and multiple blood pressure measurements have been reported in these and other species using both direct and indirect methods.

Direct blood pressure measurements entail either direct percutaneous puncture or exposure and catheterization of a major artery. A widely used indirect method to measure systemic arterial blood pressure in the rat is tail cuff sphygmomanometry. However, this method in rats measures only systolic pressure A major disadvantage to all tail cuff techniques is that it is not possible to record blood pressures continuously. A variety of noninvasive techniques for indirect blood pressure measurements in conscious dogs and pigs have been evaluated. More recently, many noninvasive techniques have been modified for use in mice.

Morphologic Evaluation of Toxicity

Toxic injuries to the heart that result in expression of morphologic alterations must be detected by careful gross and microscopic evaluation (Figure 12.14). In specific instances, further study may be desirable, including ultrastructural evaluation, histochemical procedures, and morphometric analysis. Special attention must be given to problems that accompany morphologic evaluations. These include possible sampling errors, presence of postmortem alterations, misinterpretation of tissue artifacts, and failure to recognize normal variations in structure, incidental lesions, and lesions of spontaneous diseases.

Gross Examination

Many thorough descriptions have been published on the methods of gross dissection and examination of the exterior and interior features of the heart at necropsy. Any one of these methods can be used successfully and will result in a systematic and thorough evaluation of the heart for gross lesions. However, variations in the standard necropsy method may be desirable to best expose certain lesions and to optimize the display of the heart for photography. All gross lesions detected including alterations in size, shape, color, consistency, and weight should be recorded and, in many cases, also photographed. A special search for congenital anomalies should be done. Care must be taken to avoid misinterpretation of postmortem alterations including rigor mortis, prerigor and postrigor muscular relaxation, imbibition of blood, alterations from terminal intracardiac injection, postmortem blanching of the myocardium, and intracardiac blood clots. Hearts should be weighed following removal of blood clots from the chambers and the data recorded as absolute weight and relative weight in terms of body weight. Other necropsy procedures that may be utilized in special instances include measurements of ventricular wall thicknesses and valve ring circumferences but these determinations vary greatly depending on the state of contraction of the heart. Other optional procedures include determinations of weights of walls of individual chambers and the septum, use of a macroscopic enzyme histochemical technique to detect and quantitate myocardial ischemic injury, and gross or radiographic evaluation of the coronary arterial tree following infusion of radiopaque or pigmented material. Color photography may be improved if the heart is fixed for a few hours or overnight in Jore's or Klott's solution, since this will subdue highlights while retaining color.

The conduction system may be evaluated microscopically by collection of a series of blocks of tissue that include the SA node, AV node, His bundle and specialized conduction fibers.

Microscopic Examination

Tissue specimens for microscopic study may be obtained at the time of necropsy or by endomyocardial

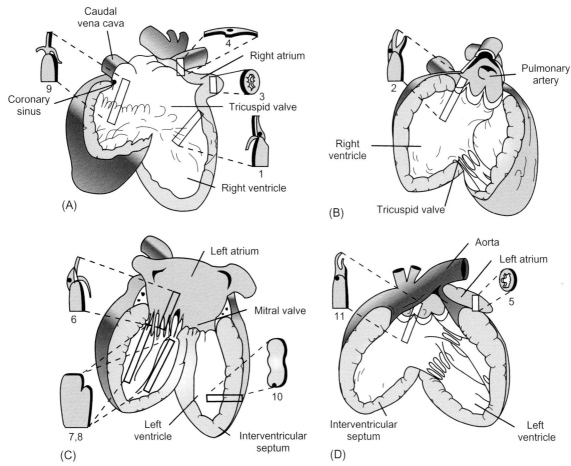

FIGURE 12.14   Schematic diagram of the gross and microscopic examination of the heart. Diagrams A to D illustrate the heart opened. The numbers indicate the area and the shape of the blocks of tissue removed for histopathology. (A) Right ventricle and right atrium. (B) Right ventricular cavity and pulmonary outflow tract. (C) Left ventricle and left atrium. (D) Left ventricle and aortic outflow tract. 1. Right ventricular free wall, atrioventricular valve, and atrium. 2. Pulmonic valve, right ventricular outflow tract, and pulmonary artery. 3. Right auricular appendage. 4. Sinoatrial node. 5. Left auricular appendage. 6. Left atrioventricular valve, ventricle, and atrium. 7 and 8. Left ventricular free wall and papillary muscles. 9. Atrioventricular node, right atriocentricular valve, and atrium. 10. Interventricular septum. 11. Aortic valve, left aortic outflow tract and aorta. (A–D, from Bishop, S.P. (1999). Necropsy techniques for the heart and great vessels. In *Textbook of Canine and Feline Cardiology*, Fox, P., Sission, D., and Moise, N. eds, 2nd edn. Saunders, Philadelphia, PA.)

biopsy from living patients. Endomyocardial biopsies, although used extensively now in human medicine, have had limited application in animal studies except for occasional use in dogs and nonhuman primates. Samples from hearts at necropsy should be multiple to detect lesions that are not diffusely distributed and lesions that are not grossly apparent. Tissue blocks should include samples of any gross lesion and routine collection of specimens from both atria, both ventricular free walls, ventricular septum, left ventricular papillary muscle, and the coronary arterial tree. Sampling should be increased in regions where lesions are predicted to be produced by a specific agent. In small laboratory animals, a longitudinal section through the heart taken perpendicular to the ventricular septum is often sufficient. Sampling of the conduction system is not routinely done but appropriate techniques have been described.

Tissue fixation is generally with 10% neutral buffered formalin and by immersion of the samples or the entire heart of small animals. Perfusion fixation may be used to optimize fixation quality if ultrastructural studies are to be done. Fixatives such as Trump's solution containing glutaraldehyde and formalin are suitable and are increasingly used for both light and electron microscopic studies. Samples are routinely processed and embedded in paraffin and sections stained with hematoxylin and eosin. Special stains that are often useful to optimally visualize microscopic alterations include phosphotungstic acid hematoxylin (PTAH), Masson's trichrome, periodic acid-Schiff (PAS), and various elastin stains. Application of lipid stains to frozen sections may be of value. Increasingly, investigators are using embedment in water-soluble methacrylate and preparation of semithin 1–4 um sections, or alternatively 1 um sections of blocks prepared for ultrastructural study, for high resolution study of cellular alterations. Also, a variety of enzyme (e.g., acid phosphatase), immunohistochemical (e.g. Factor VIII, vascular endothelial growth factor, endothelin, actin, myosin, desmin), and autoradiography procedures are available for application to cardiac tissue. Several stains have been utilized to demonstrate early ischemic damage to the myocardium. Also, special staining procedures are available to demonstrate apoptosis, altered vascular and cellular permeability, induced proliferation of cardiac cells and to demonstrate *in situ* hybridization.

Ultrastructural Examination

Most cardiac lesions of toxic origin have been studied by transmission electron microscopy to detect the subcellular alterations and to obtain information that may suggest the pathogenesis of the damage. It is important that investigators appreciate the limitations and problems associated with ultrastructural study. Thus, fixation should be optimal (preferably by perfusion), and tissue artifacts should be avoided. Hypercontracted myocytes are often seen at the margin of immersion-fixed tissue blocks; these areas should be avoided in ultrastructural study. Extensive sampling may be necessary if the cardiac alterations are not diffusely distributed. Even under optimal conditions, some cardiotoxicities may not have remarkable alterations since death may have occurred rapidly from functional alterations and morphologic alterations did not have sufficient time to evolve. A variety of techniques have been adapted for use at the ultrastructural level including enzyme- and immunohistochemistry and autoradiography.

Quantitation of Morphologic Alterations

Routine morphologic evaluations at the gross, microscopic, and ultrastructural levels are mainly directed at accurate and thorough descriptions of the observed alterations. Semiquantitation of the microscopic alterations by grading of the severity and distribution of the lesions should be included in evaluations. These scores can be analyzed statistically to identify differences among treatment groups.

Morphometry is being used increasingly to quantitatively evaluate the extent of cardiac damage induced by a wide variety of insults. This technique is especially useful for study of tissues prepared for electron microscopy with optimal fixation and embedding methods to avoid artifacts. By using random sampling and adequate sample sizes it is possible to determine various parameters such as volume density, surface density, and numerical density of an organelle or subcellular component and subsequently analyze this data statistically to detect significant differences among treatment groups.

Biochemical Evaluation of Toxicity

Procuring fresh samples of cardiac tissues, especially myocardium, at the time of euthanasia or by biopsy in living animals and human patients allows use of biochemical analysis to accompany and augment morphologic evaluations. Tissue samples may be assayed for activities of a variety of enzymes, determinations of the concentration of various substrates and endogenous compounds, and various subcellular fractions can be isolated for *in vitro* studies to detect altered biochemical events. Further discussion of these procedures is beyond the scope of this chapter.

Use of Animals as Models

Many experimental animal models of heart failure have been described. No one animal model will mimic all the features of a particular cardiac disease in human patients. However, use of these models to address specific questions regarding the evaluation of the structural, biochemical, or functional alterations in various types of heart failure have been of great value. These models have also provided much needed information on the interaction of etiologic factors, the pathophysiologic alterations, and the efficacy of various therapeutic agents in a variety of cardiac failure syndromes. Use of conscious animals with intact reflexes will tend to maximize the clinical relevance of the obtained data and provide valuable information to supplement the clinical findings on human patients. Although dogs are generally used for safety evaluation of drugs, pigs have been used extensively in experimental studies due to their physiological similarity to humans and their size. Genetically modified mice are also being used for cardiovascular studies. These animals offer the opportunity to study a variety of models of altered cardiovascular development and function.

VESSELS

INTRODUCTION

The vessels, subdivided into arteries, veins, microcirculation (capillaries), and lymphatics, have remarkable adaptations of their structure to achieve required functions. Xenobiotics may provoke vascular alterations that may be unique to the vessels of a particular organ or have tropism for a particular segment of specific types of vessels. A spectrum of morphologic reactions is induced by vascular toxicoses including accelerated atherosclerosis, medial and intimal proliferation, calcification, aneurysms, medial hemorrhagic necrosis, fibrinoid necrosis, microangiopathy, and vasculitis. The outcome of healing of vascular injuries may be dominated by repair processes rather than regeneration and may be complicated by development of thrombosis, aneurysm formation, and vascular rupture.

STRUCTURE AND FUNCTION

Microscopic Anatomy

The vascular system is subdivided into arterial, capillary, venous, and lymphatic segments. The arteries are classified into three types: elastic (conducting) arteries, muscular (distributing) arteries, and arterioles. The venous vessels are termed venules and veins. Interposed between the arterial and venous segments are the capillary beds. Some authors prefer to further define a vascular segment termed the microcirculation that includes arterioles, capillaries, and venules and serves as the major area of exchange between the circulating blood and the peripheral tissues.

The overall design of the blood and lymphatic vessels is similar except that lumenal diameter, wall thickness, and the presence of other anatomic features such as valves will vary between the different segments of the system. The lumenal surface of all vessels is lined by longitudinally aligned endothelial cells lying over a basal lamina. Vascular walls are divided into three layers: intima, media, and adventitia. In general, the intimal layer is composed of endothelium and subendothelial connective tissue; the medial layer of fenestrated elastic laminae with interposed smooth muscle cells and ground substance that is demarcated by the internal and external elastic laminae; and the outer adventitial layer of collagen, elastic fibers, and connective tissue cells (Figure 12.15).

Endothelial cells are flattened and spread out, measuring about 3μm in thickness in their central part. The ablumenal surfaces are invested by a well-defined external lamina, rich in types III and IV collagen. The cytoplasm of endothelial cells, in addition to normal organelles, contains transport vesicles and Weibel-Palade bodies (not present in all species). Weibel-Palade bodies are membrane-bound granules with a dense matrix in which clear tubular spaces

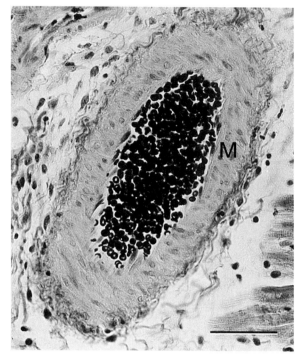

FIGURE 12.15   Selection of normal small atrial epicardial artery of a dog. M, media. Paraffin-embedded, hematoxylin and eosin stain. Bar = 100μm.

20nm in diameter are present. These structures constitute qualitatively specific cytological markers for endothelial cells, von Willabrand factor (factor VIII). Lesions in endothelium may require electron microscopy to be visualized.

The endothelium comprises a single layer of cells that act as a barrier and a thrombosis-resistant surface. Alteration of this monolayer may provoke changes in transendothelial permeability and initiation of thrombosis. The junctions of endothelial cells play an important role in maintaining the functional integrity of the vascular surface. They can be disrupted, with resulting leakage of intravascular content, as the result of direct or indirect effects of various pharmacological agents and other toxicants. The junctions are also subject to dynamic changes, thereby representing another route of transendothelial transport. The patterns of junctions of endothelial cells differ in arterioles, capillaries, venules, and muscular venules. These differences in junctions account for regional variations in endothelial permeability along the microvascular tree.

Physiology and Functional Considerations

Blood Circulation and Tissue Perfusion

The circulatory system can be divided into the pulmonary circulation supplied by the right side of the heart and the systemic circulation supplied by the left side. Blood is ejected from the heart (a modified portion of the vascular system) during systole into large elastic arteries, the aorta and pulmonary arteries, under considerable pressure that causes stretching of elastic tissue in the vessel walls. During diastole, elastic recoil occurs and hydrostatic pressure is maintained to allow blood to be conducted into the muscular (distributing) arteries. To allow distribution to meet the needs of each of the different parts of the body, the muscular arteries and arterioles contract or distend appropriately under the influence of nervous stimulation and autoregulation via local metabolic stimuli. Thus, blood is delivered to the capillary beds in necessary amounts but at low pressure where rapid blood-tissue exchanges occur across the endothelial layer that serves as a thin semipermeable barrier. Blood then enters the venous portion of the circulatory system at low pressure and flows slowly.

Endothelial Permeability

Transvascular exchanges of water and solutes occur mostly by diffusion and less by filtration-absorption processes. Intravascular forces that govern transcapillary exchanges include hydrostatic pressure, osmotic pressure of plasma proteins, and concentration gradients of molecules.

Metabolic Activities in Vascular Cells

In addition to functioning as a semipermeable barrier, the endothelium has a number of metabolic activities that can have both local and systemic ramifications and which vary according to the location in the body. These include a role in hemostasis and thrombosis by production of procoagulant substances (Factor VIII, plasminogen inhibitor) and anticoagulant substances (prostacyclin, plasminogen inhibitor) and anticoagulant substances (prostacyclin, plasminogen activator), a role in the modulation of vascular tone (prostacyclin, angiotensin II, nitric oxide, endothelin), a role in the metabolism of vasoactive substances (angiotensin-converting enzyme; enzymatic degradation of norepinephrine, serotonin and bradykinin); a role in vascular growth and remodelling (transforming growth factor-B, heparin sulfate, glycosaminoglycans, thrombospondin, vascular endothelial growth factor, insulin-like growth factors), a role in inflammatory and immune reactions (nitric oxide, prostacyclin, complement regulatory factors, cytokines, chemokines, adhesion molecules, selectins), secretion of type III and IV collagen to form basal lamina and production of fibronectin, laminin, elastin, glycosaminoglycans,

and blood group antigens A and B. In addition, endothelial cells can secrete matrix-metalloproteinases (MMP) and their specific tissue inhibitors that regulate the turnover of connective tissue proteins and the remodeling of tissues during normal growth and repair of tissue injury. Endothelial cells are able to contract and possess receptors for compounds such as angiotensin and insulin.

Vascular smooth muscle cells are metabolically active and produce type I and III collagen, elastin, and glycosaminoglycans. When stimulated, vascular smooth muscle cells may proliferate, migrate, and assume phagocytic activity. The presence of these smooth muscle cells in the medial portion of the vascular walls of arteries, arterioles, and veins provides the means by which changes in vessel tone can occur. The normal functioning of vascular smooth muscle is dependent on a variety of physiological influences. As a result many factors are responsible for the diverse pharmacologic and toxicologic responses observed in different types of vascular smooth muscle.

Vascular Function

Nervous Influences

Nervous control of the vasculature is exerted mainly by the sympathetic division of the autonomic nervous system. The sympathetic fibers innervate most arteries, arterioles, and veins. These are mostly adrenergic fibers although some vessels receive sympathetic cholinergic fibers. Both alpha and beta adrenergic receptors exist in the same vessels and share the same neurotransmitter (norepinephrine). Whether the smooth muscle constricts or dilates depends on the affinity and numbers of the two classes of adrenergic receptors. Muscarinic cholinergic receptors are present on both smooth muscle cells and endothelial cells. Receptors for histamine, serotonin, ATP and other vasoactive substance are also found in many portions of the vasculature. It has been shown that the nerves do not penetrate the entire thickness of the blood vessels. In small arteries innervation is limited to the adventitia while in larger arteries there are nerve-free regions which include the innermost quarter to half of the smooth muscle layer. As a result there is a significant difference in sensitivity to all common vasoconstrictor substances between those outer portions of the vessel which are innervated and the nerve-free inner layer of muscle. Only the inner layer of muscle is sensitive enough to react to circulating levels of vasoconstrictor hormones (norepinephine, epinephrine) whereas the outer portion of the vessels requires high concentrations of norepinephrine released by sympathetic nerves to provoke a response. Muscle and skin vasculature is controlled by sympathetic innervation. In other tissues, the role of blood vessel control by the autonomic nervous system is less clear, but some studies suggest that autonomic nerves may exert control in renal, cerebral, and coronary blood vessels. In certain situations, adjustment of vascular tone by the autonomic nervous system is less important than other control systems or mediators. It appears that a number of vasoconstrictor and vasodilator substances which act directly on vascular smooth muscle cells also exert an indirect action by altering the release of norepinephrine from sympathetic nerves. Endogenous substances that appear to act at specific presynaptic receptors and decrease norepinephrine release include acetylcholine, adenosine, histamine, dopamine, prostaglandins of the E series, and norepinephrine itself. Other endogenous substances such as angiotensin and prostaglandins of the F series potentiate the release of norepinephrine.

Local Humoral and Environmental Influences

Blood vessels are capable of both synthesizing and metabolizing vasoactive hormones and as a result are not entirely dependent on circulating substances or neurotransmitters for control of vascular tone. The endothelium is the source of many potent endogenous vasoactive substances including the vasodilator nitric oxide and the vasoconstrictor endothelin-1. Endothelial cells also produce prostacyclin, a substance which causes vasodilation and prevents the adhesion of platelets to the vascular endothelium. In addition, the endothelium may contribute to the local control of vascular tone by secreting other relaxing and contracting factors such as angiotensin II and platelet derived growth factor (PDGF). Endothelium-derived relaxing factor, generated by NOS, leads to relaxation of the vascular smooth muscle cells, suppression of platelet activation and decreased adhesion of leukocytes to endothelial cells. Angiotensin II is produced in the lungs and also, to a certain extent, in limb vessels themselves. Regardless of the source, angiotensin II reacts directly with resistance vessels (arterioles) to cause vasoconstriction. PDGF, in addition to its mitogenic properties also acts as a smooth muscle contractile agonist. It is likely that local metabolites (e.g. potassium, ATP, adenosine, oxygen, carbon dioxide) are also available to act on the vascular smooth muscle.

Responses of Blood Vessels to Vasoactive Substances

Blood vessels of different types and from different areas do not react uniformly to the presence of certain drugs and other xenobiotics. Norepinephrine induces uniform contraction of all types of blood vessels but angiotensin exerts more constrictor activity in the resistance vessels than in the veins. Ergot alkaloids, at low doses, demonstrate preferential constrictor activity in veins with little increase in resistance vessel tone. A selectivity of action is also seen with xenobiotics that dilate vessels. Hydralazine mainly relaxes resistance vessels, while glyceryl trinitrate preferentially exerts this action on veins.

Electrical Activity and Intracellular Calcium Responses to Vasoactive Substances

Heterogeneity in smooth muscle responses as a result of exposure to xenobiotics relates in part to the varying patterns of cellular electrical activity and to the variety of mechanisms which are involved in the control of the cytoplasmic concentration of calcium. Smooth muscle cells are characterized by a low resting membrane potential (-40 to $-60\,mV$). The action potential of vascular smooth muscle is mainly driven by an inward flux of calcium ions. Excitation spikes can be detected as calcium enters the cell and the membrane potential becomes more positive. Some types of smooth muscle display phasic activity, an effect which is associated with the generation of spike action potentials. Calcium is also critical to the contractile process. The sarcoplasmic reticulum appears to be the major cellular component for calcium storage; both contraction and relaxation are influenced by the levels of calcium in the cytoplasm. Critical levels of cytoplasmic calcium are achieved by entrance through voltage-dependent membrane channels and through release of the cation from intracellular storage sites. Spontaneous contractile activity as a result of calcium entry in this manner is not present in all smooth muscle; some types develop sustained contractions only in response to agonists such as norepinephrine and angiotensin. Agents that stimulate contraction have the potential to produce greater depolarization and to increase the frequency of spike potentials. However, vascular contractile activity can be induced without membrane depolarization and in these instances alterations in membrane permeability are important. Vascular contraction as a result of changes in membrane permeability appears to involve the movement of calcium through a receptor-operated channel and the subsequent release of additional calcium from intracellular stores. Varying combinations of phasic and sustained contraction are found in the smooth muscle cells from different types of vessels. It has been suggested that entrance of calcium through channels may have limited importance and that agonist-induced contraction may depend entirely on release of calcium from intracellular storage sites. Dependence of the contractile response on calcium influx appears to vary considerably at different points along the vascular tree. The dependence is least in the aorta where contractile responses appear to rely almost entirely on the release of calcium from intracellular storage sites. In contrast, calcium influx is essential for contraction of small resistance arteries. Differences in pharmacologic and toxicologic responses are thought to be related to the varying intrinsic smooth muscle properties found in vessels of different types. The primary action of calcium antagonists such as verapamil and nifedipine on resistance vessels may be related to the greater importance of phasic activity associated with entry of calcium through voltage-dependent calcium channels. In contrast, the preferential action of sodium nitroprusside in veins is an indication of the importance of the receptor-operated sustained contraction mechanism.

Effects of Endothelial Cell Function and Damage on Blood Vessel Activity

Vascular endothelial cells serve as a protective barrier in blood vessel walls and serve as an active source for the synthesis, metabolism, uptake, storage, and degradation of a number of vasoactive substances. Endothelial cell damage has been a factor in several important diseases that affect the vasculature. Endothelial cells from certain arteries and veins seem to be directly involved in the decrease of vascular tone noted in these vessels as a result of exposure to naturally occurring vasodilator substances such as acetylcholine, bradykinin, arachidonic acid, substance P, and ATP. When endothelial cells are destroyed, the vessels lose the ability to relax on exposure to most of these dilator substances. In addition, the loss of functional endothelial cells seems to transform normal vasodilator responses into potent vasoconstrictor activity. A substance which damages or destroys endothelial cells to the extent that vasodilatory responses are altered could conceivably cause significant decreases in blood flow and subsequent tissue damage in certain organs.

MECHANISMS OF TOXICITY

Vasculotoxic Effects of Xenobiotics

Most vasoactive xenobiotics are widely distributed throughout the vascular tree and are therefore capable of system-wide activity. However, rapid metabolism, such as that of acetycholine in the blood, or effective removal, such as that of the prostaglandins of the lung, can lead to limitations of the effects of these substances. Likewise, if a significant amount of a xenobiotic is bound to plasma albumin, as occurs with diazoxide, the concentration of the substance reaching the vessel will be less than expected.

Exposure to certain chemical substances can initiate degenerative or inflammatory alterations in vascular smooth muscle. These toxic effects could occur as a result of excessive pharmacologic activity or by direct reaction of xenobiotics with structural or functional macromolecules in the vascular wall. Ergotamine intoxication leads to sustained arterial vasoconstriction. With continued exposure ergotamine induces occlusive vascular lesions such as intimal proliferation, medial hypertrophy, and hyalinization in some peripheral vessels. Vascular toxicity can also be demonstrated with allylamine. Fibromuscular intimal proliferation in small and medium-sized arteries (such as coronary arteries) occurs in rats given this agent. Metabolism of allylamine yields acrolein, a substance that is capable of denaturing protein and disrupting nucleic acid synthesis. This metabolite is thought to be responsible for other more subtle changes such as medial hypertrophy and proliferation of vascular smooth muscle. Acetylsalicylic acid (aspirin) given to rats produces early alterations in the basement membrane of the endothelial cells of capillaries and postcapillary venules. These changes subsequently may cause small vessel damage in the gastric mucosa. Under certain conditions, sympathomimetic agents are capable of eliciting toxic effects on arterial vasculature. For example, subintimal alterations (medial smooth muscle cell necrosis and calcification) in large and medium-sized arteries have been induced following administration of large doses of norepinephrine. These effects could be due to the excessive stimulation of adrenergic receptors.

Morphologic changes of considerable importance are induced by drugs or chemicals that induce or modify atherosclerotic lesions, either by changes in plasma lipids and lipoproteins or by more direct effects on vascular walls. Carbon monoxide causes direct damage to endothelial cells and smooth muscle cells. This results in increased capillary permeability and hastens plaque formation in animals fed high cholesterol diets. The effect of carbon monoxide might also be due to decreased availability of oxygen, since plaque formation is also accelerated in animals exposed to hypoxic conditions. Tobacco smoke, a complex mixture that includes carbon monoxide, has a direct atherogenic effect due to endothelial damage, change in lipid profiles and proliferation of smooth muscle cells. It also affects platelet function and produces vascular spasm thus facilitating thrombosis. Elevated levels of homocysteine have been associated with thrombotic and arteriosclerotic vascular disease. Homocysteine can react directly with nitric oxide to form highly reactive S-nitroso-thiol compounds that may mediate potentially harmful secondary biochemical effects. Homocysteine appears to induce oxidative injury to endothelial cells and/or smooth muscle cells resulting in a sequence of alterations which includes platelet adhesion, smooth muscle cell proliferation, formation of foam cells, and ultimately loss of the endothelial layer at the site of atherogenic lesions. Vascular changes are also associated with exposure to carbon disulfide. Long-term exposure of industrial workers has been associated with a two- to threefold increase in coronary heart disease. Carbon disulfide has been shown to accelerate the development of atherosclerosis in rabbits maintained on a high cholesterol diet. There are at least two mechanisms by which carbon disulfide might enhance the formation of atherogenic lesions: direct injury to the endothelium and induction of hypothyroidism with resulting alterations in lipid metabolism. Thiocarbamate (thiourea), a potent antithyroid substance, is the principal urinary metabolite detected after exposure to carbon disulfide and may be responsible for the carbon-disulfide-mediated suppression of thyroid glandular activity.

Other toxic substances such as penicillamine and β-aminoproprionitrile can cause vascular alterations by inducing changes in connective tissue, an effect which ultimately results in the formation of nonatherosclerotic aneurysms in the aorta and other large arterial vessels. These agents apparently inhibit specific steps in the connective tissue protein biosynthetic pathway. Chromium seems to have a significant role in maintaining the integrity of the vasculature. Serum cholesterol levels are elevated and the incidence of atheroclerotic plaques increases when chromium is deficient. Long term low dose experimental exposure to cadmium has also resulted in atherosclerosis and hypertension. Recently, exposure to particulate matter in air pollution has been shown to cause endothelial injury and promote atherosclerosis.

Aside from direct toxicity, vasculitis (autoimmune) can result from exposure to sensitizing compounds which act as haptens, presumably combining with the host's own proteins and inducing formation of appropriate antibodies. Usually only small vessels (arterioles, venules and capillaries) are affected, but in some instances the coronary arteries can also develop lesions. Predominant components of the inflammatory reaction include eosinophils and mononuclear cells. The induction of vasculitis is not dose or time dependent and appears related to the deposition of soluble immune complexes in the vessel wall and to the activation of the complement system. Penicillin, sulfonamides, methyldopa, procainamide, quinidine, and a number of other drugs and chemicals have been implicated in causing this reaction in humans.

Vascular Toxicity in Specific Organs

There is increasing evidence that blood vessels vary in their pharmacologic and toxicologic responses to chemical substances. It is known that heterogeneity in response occurs not only between veins and arteries, but also between anatomically similar vessels in different regions of the circulation. A similar spectrum of differences is also reported to exist for microvessels. Some differences in response could be due to external influences such as innervation and the local humoral environment. Other differences may result from internal cellular differences in the receptor subpopulation and composition, differences in endothelial junctions, and the specific processes responsible for cellular electrical activity and the release and uptake of calcium. These and other factors are likely to contribute to the variety of vascular toxicities observed in different organs.

Brain

The blood-brain barrier depends on the metabolic status of the endothelial cells as well as on the effectiveness of their tight junctions. Certain divalent cations, high concentrations of norepinephrine and serotonin, and metrazol-induced convulsions disrupt the junctions leading to increases in cerebrovascular permeability. Hypertonic solutions of various substances (NaCl, urea, mannitol) cause shrinking of vascular endothelium and separation of tight junctions leading to opening of the blood-brain barrier. In newborn rats exposed to lead, widening of tight junctions, increased permeability, and a significant impairment of the blood-brain barrier are known to occur. Inorganic lead can produce changes in arterial elasticity and can also cause sclerosis of renal vessels. These effects are thought to be due to the avid reaction of lead with sulfhydryl groups in critical cellular proteins. Mercury can also disrupt the blood brain barier leading to increased permeability. A variety of chemical substances such as alcohols and other lipid solvents, cobra venom, surfactants, and high concentrations of sulfhydryl reactors increase cerebral vascular permeability. These compounds are disruptive to cell membranes and capillaries. Antineoplastic agents such as cyclophosphamide induce alterations in a number of vascular areas resulting in hemorrhagic lesions in both the cerebral and visceral vasculature. High doses of amphetamine have caused damage to cerebral arteries, possibly as a result of hypertension. Cocaine increases circulating levels of catecholamines causing a generalized state of vasoconstriction that can result in hypertension and cerebral stroke.

Lung

Alveolar capillaries are subject to a variety of insults which may alter permeability and lead to pulmonary edema. This condition can occur following inhalation of irritant substances. Excessive intravenous infusion of fluid can also lead to pulmonary edema. Intravenously administered opiates such as heroin and methadone have produced a delayed pulmonary edema. These opiates may modify central neurogenic influences on pulmonary capillary permeability. Arsenic and hyperoxia also affect the vasculature of the lungs, leading to pulmonary edema. Chronic exposure to ozone causes pulmonary arterial lesions that result in thickening of the arterial walls. Ultrastructural changes in the alveolar capillaries have also been found.

Monocrotaline, a pyrrolizidine alkaloid, causes structural remodeling of pulmonary blood vessels and a delayed pulmonary hypertension in rats. Pulmonary hypertension has been reported in humans following ingestion of pyrrolizidine alkaloid containing plants such as *Crotalaria spectabilis* which is indigenous to the tropics and used in "bush teas". It has also been reported with the appetite suppressant, aminorex, and the antiobesity drugs, phenfluramine and phenteramine. Bacterial endotoxins adversely affect many vascular beds. In the lung, increased vascular permeability and pulmonary hypertension have been reported following exposure to endotoxins. The edema of endothelial cells could be a factor in these actions. Pulmonary veno-occlusive disease has been reported following many antineoplastic drugs such as 5-flourouracil, doxorubicin and mitomysin.

A direct or indirect effect of IL-2 on endothelial cells may damage the vascular endothelium, increase vascular permeability and induce a vascular leak syndrome in the lungs and other tissue. Features of vascular injury in the lungs can include hemoptysis, cough, shortness of breath, wheezing and pleurisy.

Heart

Ergonovine and vasopressin cause marked constriction of coronary arteries. ECG signs such as ST-segment depression indicate that the resulting coronary spasm may lead to myocardial hypoxia. In chronic animal studies, methylsergide has produced coronary intimal proliferation and vascular occlusion. The coronary vasculature is a target site for the toxic effects of bacterial endotoxin. Infusion of endotoxin causes severe coronary artery damage which ultimately results in arterial stenosis. Minoxidil, a long-acting

vasodilating drug, induces a hemorrhagic lesion in beagle dogs and miniature swine which is most consistently present in the atria. A variety of other vasoactive drugs such as phosphodiesterase inhibitors and endothelin-1 antagonists are also capable of inducing coronary artery lesions.

Liver

Liver toxins such as dimethylnitrosamine produce a hemorrhagic necrosis which ultimately leads to complete venous occlusion. Pyrrolizidine alkaloids also cause veno-occlusion (see The Liver, Chapter 9). In this instance the occlusion of veins is preceded by proliferation of endothelial cells and vascular connective tissue. The vascular bed of the liver is altered by bacterial endotoxins. These agents affect the microcirculation by causing swelling of endothelial cells and adhesion of platelets to sinusoid walls. Certain agents causing chronic hepatitis (oxyphenisatin, nitrofurantoin) or cirrhosis (ethanol, arsenicals, methotrexate) ultimately induce portal hypertension.

Kidney

A number of agents causing renal cellular damage also affect renal blood vessels. Any xenobiotic that will cause constriction of preglomerular or relaxation of postglomerular vessels will exert a negative effect on glomerular filtration rate. Inorganic lead causes vasoconstriction of the preglomerular vessels and ultimately sclerosis of these vessels. Renal toxicity caused by lead, cadmium and some analgesics is at times associated with increases in systemic arterial pressure because of alterations in the renal blood pressure regulatory systems. Long-term exposure to cadmium in rats has caused thickening of renal arterioles and diffuse fibrosis of capillaries, alterations which may be responsible for the resulting salt and water retention and hyperreninemia seen after exposure to this agent. Hypersensitivity reactions induced by a number of substances (gold salts and D- penicillamine in humans and mercuric chloride in experimental animals) consistently cause immune-complex deposits on the basement membranes of glomerular capillaries. Hematuria, renal failure, nephrosis and hypertension have all been associated with vascular alterations in the kidney.

RESPONSE TO INJURY

Vascular injuries may be primary or secondary. Secondary lesions develop as an extension of a disease process in surrounding tissues. However, primary vascular diseases are the most frequent type and the lesions may be generalized or regional in distribution. Arteries, the high-pressure segment of the circulatory system, tend to develop significant alterations more frequently than veins, capillaries, and lymphatics. The spectrum of pathologic alterations observed includes degenerative conditions with accumulations of lipid, mineral deposits or fibrous connective tissue; proliferative lesions of the intima, media, or endothelial basal lamina; and inflammatory alterations. The etiology of any of these vascular diseases is multifactorial and is often in part due to aging. Many of these disorders have a slow progressive course and do not become clinically apparent until a secondary event such as thrombosis and subsequent ischemic injury occurs. However, some of the vascular diseases that are initiated by toxic injury, infectious agents, or immunologically mediated mechanisms develop rapidly and may produce widespread lesions.

Regeneration and Repair

Endothelial cells serve a protective role against toxic injury. However overt injury triggers a detrimental cascade leading to activation of intracellular signaling pathways that can result in cell death. Apoptosis is a major pathway for endothelial cell death with similar mechanisms involved as described for cardiomyocyes above.

The consequences of vascular injury are multiple. Most injuries will heal by repair with fibrosis rather than by regeneration to restore normal structure to the affected vessel. Vascular endothelial cells are an exception to this generalization. When the affected area of the vessel is small, the endothelium is repaired by spreading and migration of neighboring endothelial cells. If lesions are extensive, cell proliferation is also required in addition to cell migration to replace irreversible damaged cells and reestablish the continuity of the endothelium. In addition, recently identified circulating bone marrow-derived endothelial progenitor cells play a role in re-endothelialization of vessels following injury. However, residual damage often follows vascular injuries. Damage to the endothelial layer and the other various layers of arterial walls may initiate thrombosis with subsequent regional ischemic injury of the organ in the circulatory field. Other injuries may result in damage to the vessel wall with dilatation and potential rupture of the vessel. Some healed lesions will result in only minor structural and functional alterations of the affected vessels and will be detected only as incidental lesions by microscopic study.

Vessel Alterations

Major vessel alterations are depicted in Figure 12.16. A summary of alterations induced by xenobiotics is given in Table 12.8.

Atherosclerosis

There is epidemiologic evidence in human patients and direct evidence from studies on animal models of atherosclerosis that exposure to certain chemical agents along with the presence of atherogenic risk factors may enhance the development of atherosclerosis. Chemical substances that have been incriminated include goitrogenic agents, carbon disulfide, benz[a]pyrene, dimethylbenz [a]anthracene, homocysteine, carbon monoxide, fluorocarbons, oral contraceptives (especially these containing mainly progestins), combined hydrochlorothiazide and propranolol therapy, cadmium, lead, soft water and particulate matter in air pollution.

The lesions and sequelae of atherosclerosis are well described (Figure 12.17). The vessels with the most severe alterations tend to be the muscular and elastic

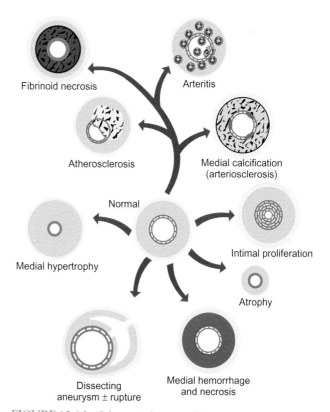

FIGURE 12.16   Schematic diagram of the major arterial diseases. (Redrawn with permission from School of Veterinary Medicine, Purdue University.) From Van Vleet, J. F. and Ferrans, V.J. (2007). Cardiovascular System. In *Pathologic Basis of Veterinary Disease*, 4th ed. (McGavin, M., and Zachary, J.F., eds), Mosby Elsevier, St. Louis, Figure 10-106, p. 608.

TABLE 12.8   Vascular responses to toxic injury with selected examples

Response	Alteration	Xenobiotic
Degeneration and necrosis	Accelerated atherosclerosis	Goitrogens, fluorocarbons, contraceptives, carbon disulfide, carbon monoxide, cadmium, lead, "soft" water
	Medial calcification	Vitamin D or metabolites (food, rodenticides, calcinogenic plants)
	Aneurysm (inhibition of lysyl oxidase)	*Lathyrus* sp (lathyrism), β-aminoproprionitrile, penicillamine, aminoacetonitrile
	Medial hemorrhage and necrosis	Vasodilator drugs (e.g., minoxidil), norepinephrine, epinephrine, theobromine, dopamine, digoxin
	Fibrinoid necrosis	Organic mercury (brain of pigs and guinea pigs), lead (brain of primates and dogs), phenylbutazone (kidney of horses)
	Micro-angiopathy	Cyclophosphamide, cadmium (rat testis)
Inflammation (vasculitis)	Hypersensitivity non-necrotizing vasculitis	Drugs (allopurinal, ampicillin, chloramphenicol, dextran, griseofulvin, indocin, penicillin, sulfonamides, tetracycline), influenza vaccine
		In dogs: itracanazole, ivermectin, ibuprofen, allergy immunotherapy injections
	Toxic necrotizing vasculitis	Arsenic, bismuth, gold, heroin, cocaine, sulfonamides
Non-neoplastic proliferation	Medial proliferation	Ergot alkaloids (ergot and fescue toxicity in cattle, horses), pyrrolizidine alkaloids
	Intimal proliferation	Oral contraceptives, ergotamine, and methylsergide (humans), allylamine
Neoplastic proliferation	Hemangiosarcoma	Analine compounds, vinyl toluene

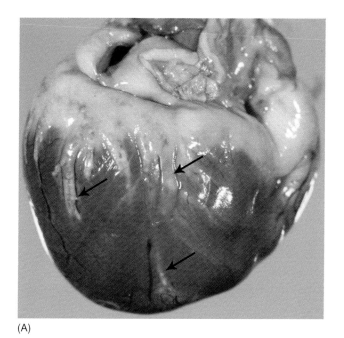

(A)

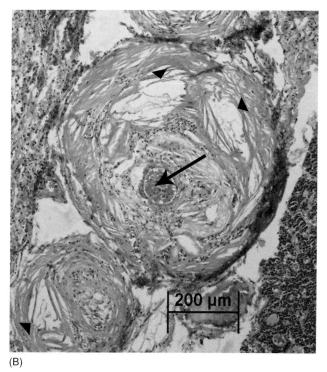

(B)

FIGURE 12.17   Atherosclerosis in a dog with hypothyroidism. (A) Coronary atherosclerosis. Affected coronary arteries (arrows) are prominent and pale, with thickened walls due to atheromatous deposits. (B) The arterial walls are markedly thickened, due to lipid deposits located within the media (arrowheads) and subintimally (lumen identified by arrow). Parathyroid is present on the right. Paraffin-embedded, hematoxylin and eosin stain.

arteries. The pig, rabbit, and chicken are more susceptible to lesion development than the dog, cat, cow, or rat. The initial lesions are fatty streaks (intimal aggregations of foam cells with vacuolated cytoplasm derived from both macrophages and smooth muscle cells) which are most readily detected grossly by application of fat stains such as Sudan IV. The hallmark lesion is the raised intimal atheromatous plaque. The plaque is composed of lipid deposits together with cells (smooth muscle cells, monocytes/macrophages and a few lymphocytes) and connective tissue fibers and matrix. Atherosclerotic lesions may evolve over time into complicated plaques.

Medial Smooth Muscle Hypertrophy and Proliferation

Hyperplasia and hypertrophy of smooth muscle cells in small muscular arteries and arterioles may result from hypertension or exposure to toxins such as ergot alkaloids and pyrrolizidine alkaloids. The chronic vasoconstrictor action of the ergot compounds is the basis for their induction of proliferative lesions. In cattle with ergotism and fescue toxicity, the distinctive clinical feature is ischemic necrosis or dry gangrene of the extremities including the tail, limbs, ears, and nose. These signs are usually present within 10–14 days of exposure to fescue pasture. The ergot alkaloids are produced by *Claviceps purpurea*, a fungus that infects rye and other grains and grasses. Arterioles in the ischemic tissue of the extremities will have prominent medial thickening due to proliferated smooth muscle cells and may also have fibromuscular intimal proliferation. Tall fescue (*Festuca arundinacea*) parasitized by endophytic fungi such as *Neotyphodium coenophialum* (previously *Epichloe typhina* and *Acremonium coenophialum*) will also produce ergot alkaloids. Exposure of pregnant mares results in marked medial proliferation of placental vessels with consequent placental thickening.

Intimal Proliferation

Intimal proliferative lesions of arteries (influx and proliferation of smooth muscle cells, glycosaminoglycan production and endothelial hypertrophy) have been observed with use of estrogen- or progesterone-containing oral contraceptives in women (Figure 12.18), chronic administration of ergotamine and methylsergide maleate in human patients, talc or magnesium silicate exposure in intravenous drug users, and administration of allylamine or phosphodiesterase inhibitors to rats. The intimal lesions produced by ergotamine and methylsergide maleate are primarily fibroblastic in elastic and large muscular arteries but involve fibromuscular hyperplasia in medium and small arteries; similar fibrotic lesions may also occur in

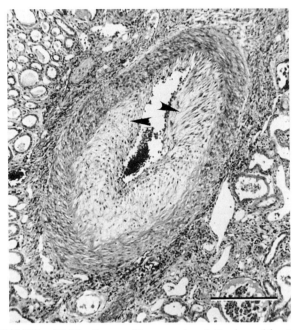

FIGURE 12.18 Severe fibromuscular intimal proliferation (arrowheads) attributed to long-term oral contraceptive use, affecting a renal artery of a woman. Paraffin-embedded, Movat pentachrome stain. Bar = 400 μm. (Courtesy of Dr H. A. McAllister, Jr., St Luke's Episcopal Hospital, Houston, TX.)

cardiac valves and endocardium of affected patients. The pathogenesis of the intimal proliferative lesions is not clear but it is suggested that these agents directly stimulate fibroblastic proliferation or act indirectly via serotonin mediation of the proliferative response.

Calcification

Arterial medial calcification is a frequent lesion in animals. The vascular lesions may involve both elastic and muscular arteries and often have concurrent endocardial mineralization. The toxic etiologies for arterial calcification include calcinogenic plant toxicosis and vitamin D_3 toxicosis. Vitamin D toxicosis may occur acutely as it does in dogs exposed to cholecalciferol-containing rodenticides or from long-term intake of feed containing excessive vitamin D. Affected arteries have a unique appearance grossly as solid dense pipe-like structures or as raised white solid intimal plaques (Figure 12.19A). Microscopically, prominent basophilic granular mineral deposits are present either on elastic fibers of the media of elastic arteries or as a complete ring of mineralization involving the internal elastic lamina and the medial musculature of muscular arteries (Figure 12.19B).

The calcinogenic plants (*Cestrum diurnum, Trisetum flavescens, Solanum malacoxylon, Solanum torvum*) contain the active metabolite of vitamin D_3 (1,25-dihydroxycholecalciferol, calcitriol) or its glycoside. Different names

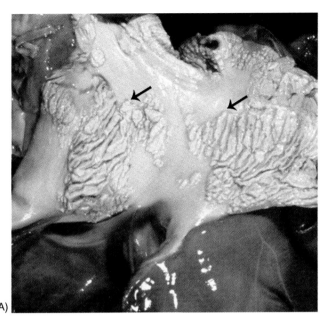

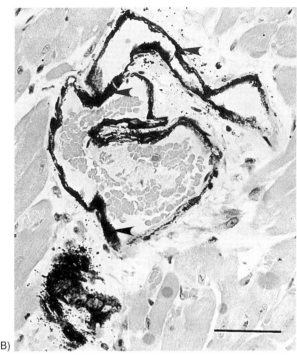

(A)   (B)

FIGURE 12.19   (A) Aortic mineralization in a calf. The surface of the aorta has raised plaque-like lesions due to mineralization; the heart is present below the aorta. (B) Medial calcification (arrowheads) and focal myocyte calcification (bottom left) in the ventricular myocardium of a rat with acute vitamin D toxicosis (1 mg/kg/day dihydrotachysterol orally for three days). Paraffin-embedded, von Kossa stain. Bar = 100 μm.

have been given to these plant-induced syndromes in various areas of the world including "Manchester wasting disease" in Jamaica, "enzootic calcinosis" in Europe, "naahelu disease" in Hawaii, "enteque seco" in Argentina, and "espichamento" in Brazil.

Aneurysms

Localized weakening of the wall of large elastic arteries results in formation of aneurysms. The lesion is produced by administration of *Lathyrus* sp. (termed lathyrism), β-aminoproprionitrile (the active principle of *Lathyrus* sp.), penicillamine or aminoacetonitrile (copper chelators), and copper deficiency. In the turkey model, dissecting aneurysms of the aorta are produced by feeding β-aminoproprionitrile. The mechanisms of lesion production by these compounds is inhibition of lysyl oxidase, a copper-containing enzyme involved in cross-linking of collagen and elastin, which are essential ingredients for normal strength of the walls of elastic arteries.

Medial Hemorrhagic Necrosis

Arterial lesions with necrosis of medial smooth muscle and medial hemorrhage have been observed following treatment with a variety of vasoactive substances including SKF95654, minoxidil, hydralazine, angiotensin, and fenoldopam mesylate (Figure 12.20). Examples are minoxidil, with right atrial vascular damage

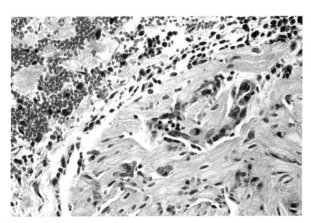

FIGURE 12.20   Epicardial hemorrhage, minoxidil cardiotoxicity, heart, left atrium, pig. Note epicardial hemorrhage (upper left) and prominent small blood vessels with swollen endothelial cells. Paraffin-embedded, hematoxylin and eosin stain. (Courtesy of School of Veterinary Medicine, Purdue University.) From Van Vleet, J. F. and Ferrans, V.J. (2007). Cardiovascular System. In *Pathologic Basis of Veterinary Disease*, 4th ed. (McGavin, M., and Zachary, J.F., eds), Mosby Elsevier, St. Louis, Figure 10-10, p. 565.

and hemorrhage in dogs and left atrial hemorrhage in pigs; hydralazine and nicorandil, with right atrial hemorrhage and medial necrosis and hemorrhage in muscular arteries in dogs; theobromine, which produces right atrial lesions in dogs; diazoxide, which produces left atrial lesions in pigs; digoxin, which produces right atrial and biventricular lesions in dogs; norepinephrine, which produces small disseminated myocardial necroses and more diffuse arteritis involving cardiac, hepatic, and mesenteric vessels in dogs, rabbits, and cats; epinephrine, which produces lesions similar to those of norepinephrine; SK&F 94120 [5-(4-acetamidophenyl)pyrazin-2(1H)-one], an inotrope/vasodilator drug, high doses of which produce necrotizing arteritis in dogs, most frequently in the right atrium; and CI-930, an inotropic compound [4,5-dihydro-6(-4-(1H-imidazol-1-yl)-phenyl)-5-methyl-3(2H)-pyridazinone monohydrochloride], which produces hemorrhages, arterial lesions, and focal myocardial necroses in dogs and monkeys. Medial necrosis of coronary arteries occurred following administration of an endothelin receptor antagonist to monkeys and dogs, and an adenosine agonist antihypertensive to monkeys.

Fibrinoid Necrosis

Accumulation of serum proteins and polymerized fibrin in the wall of small arteries following endothelial damage results in a distinctive eosinophilic homogenous appearance of the media of the affected vessels (Figure 12.21). This lesion has been described in cerebral vessels of pigs and guinea pigs with organic mercury toxicosis, and in those of nonhuman primates and dogs with lead toxicosis.

Fibrinoid necrosis of small veins was considered the primary lesion in horses with phenylbutazone toxicosis; this appeared to be the basis for renal medullary necrosis and oral and gastrointestinal ulceration. The loss of endothelial cells and formation of thrombi may also occur.

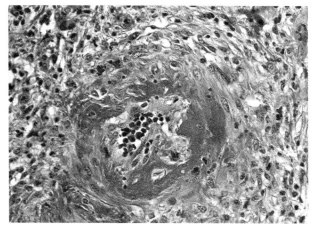

FIGURE 12.21   Fibrinoid necrosis in a myocardial arteriole of a pig. Note the circumferential eosinophilic deposits in the wall of the arteriole. Paraffin-embedded, hematoxylin and eosin stain. (Courtesy of Dr J. Simon, College of Veterinary Medicine, University of Illinois.) From Van Vleet, J. F. and Ferrans, V.J. (2007). Cardiovascular System. In *Pathologic Basis of Veterinary Disease*, 4th ed. (McGavin, M., and Zachary, J.F., eds), Mosby Elsevier, St. Louis, Figure 10-90, p. 602.

Microangiopathy

Cadmium administration to rats results in hemorrhagic testicular necrosis due to selective damage to testicular capillary endothelium. Microthrombosis and hemorrhage have been produced in the heart by administration of cyclophosphamide.

Vasculitis

Vascular inflammatory lesions associated with drugs are divided into hypersensitivity vasculitis, toxic vasculitis and lupus-like syndromes. Drug-induced vasculitis usually affects all 3 layers of mainly small-sized vessels. Medium-sized muscular arteries are occasionally involved, but large arteries and veins are usually not targets of drug-induced vasculitis.

Hypersensitivity Vasculitis

This condition commonly includes the vascular lesions associated with serum sickness, systemic bacterial infections, protozoal infections, reactions to influenza vaccines, and drug-related vasculitides. The lesions are characterized by a predominantly mononuclear leukocytic infiltrate and occasional eosinophils, in the absence of fibrinoid necrosis or necrotizing lesions of the vessel wall. The endothelial lining of involved arterial and venous channels is intact and free of thrombi.

A variety of drugs (see Table 12.7) have been found to induce an immune-mediated vascular injury (ampicillin, procainamide, dextran, hydralazine, penicillin, sulfonamide, tetracycline, propylthiouracil, quinidine, allopurinol, phenylbutazone). This type of drug-induced vasculitis is neither dose- nor time-dependent. The lack of a dose-dependent response and the clinical presentation suggest that this form of drug-related vasculitis is a delayed hypersensitivity phenomenon.

Necrotizing Vasculitis

Inflammation and necrosis are usually limited to small and medium-sized arteries. Acute as well as healing and healed lesions are present. Acute lesions are characterized by focal fibrinoid necrosis of the vessel wall. The associated inflammatory infiltrate is composed primarily of polymorphonuclear leukocytes although eosinophils are occasionally prominent. Occlusive thrombi occur in both acute and healing stages. Lesions are most frequent at sites of bifurcation and in many instances there is aneurysmal dilatation of the defective area of the vessel wall. Certain drugs (methamphetamine, cocaine, heroin, phenylpropanolamine and methylphenidate) have been reported to induce necrotizing vasculitic lesions (see Table 12.7). The etiology of these forms of drug-induced vasculitis is unclear.

Lupus-Like Syndromes

Drug-induced lupus erythematosus occurs among individuals with an intrinsic tendency to the syndrome. The mechanism by which these drugs cause or unmask the lupus-like syndrome is unknown. It is suggested that the drug either modifies nucleoprotein antigenicity or reinforces the antigenicity of circulating DNA which is normally present in small amounts. Many drugs are associated with lupus-like syndromes (see Table 12.7).

Spontaneous Arterial Diseases in the Dog

Detection of drug- induced coronary arterial lesions, such as the hemorrhagic medial necrosis described for minoxidil and other compounds, is complicated in the dog by the occurrence of various spontaneous arterial lesions, some of which are poorly characterized. These spontaneous lesions include idiopathic necrotizing arteritis ("beagle pain syndrome"), idiopathic extramural coronary arteritis, and various degenerative alterations that include arteriosclerosis of intramural coronary arteries, intimal thickening of extramural coronary arteries, excess mucopolysaccharides, atherosclerosis, amyloidosis, hyalinosis, medial calcification, and arterial necrosis associated with uremia.

Neoplasia

Spontaneous neoplasms of the vasculature are uncommon in the rat; hemangiomas of the heart are most common. Hemangiosarcomas have been induced following oral administration of a number of analine compounds as well as inhalation exposure to vinyl toluene. 1,3-butadiene induces hemangiosarcoma in multiple organs following metabolic activation by cytochrome P450 enzymes to toxic epoxide metabolites.

EVALUATION OF VASOTOXIC EFFECTS

Vascular toxicity may be localized to alterations in the blood supply to a particular organ or vascular bed. Studies of the blood supply to specific organs have been carried out using a variety of methods that are, however, applicable to almost all organs. More direct *in vitro* methods further serve to elucidate potential toxic mechanisms. The selection of the method to be used is primarily dependent on which type of vessel is of interest. In a particular tissue, xenobiotics may affect not only arteries or veins but also arterioles and capillaries.

Physiologic Methods for Testing

Blood Flow Measurements

Direct measurement of blood flow can be made by means of electromagnetic flow meters or ultrasonic Doppler flow meters. Use of these instruments is advantageous because the circulation need not be interrupted, since the devices are able to detect flow through the walls of intact blood vessels. In addition, the probes can be chronically implanted so measurements can be made at a later time without the use of anesthetics.

Measurements of organ blood flow can be made with the aid of dilution methods utilizing the Fick principle. All methods use an indicator substance which may be an inert gas, a natural metabolite, a nondiffusible dye, or a radioactive tracer. The indicator substance is injected into the blood and its concentration measured by an appropriate detector at a downstream sampling site. The indicator dilution method is useful for the measurement of mean organ blood flow but may not accurately reflect perfusion of the microcirculation or account for shunting. Other methods such as microspheres, temperature- --pulse decay probes, and gamma-emitting macroaggregates of albumin may serve to measure perfusion over time.

Direct *in vivo* measurement of blood flow is possible by utilizing a semi-isolated dog biceps muscle preparation. The advantage of this preparation is that the principle components (muscle, blood vessels, and nerve) are all part of a single system. Perfusion of isolated hindlimb preparations at a constant rate allows a means of detecting substance-induced alterations in vascular resistance.

Angiography

Alterations in vascular tone can be detected when a suitable contrast medium is injected into the vessel. This technique has allowed identification of substances that possess vasoactive effects. However, it is not possible to determine whether this activity is due to a direct or indirect effect on the vascular smooth muscle.

Direct Observations of Blood Vessels

Direct microscopic observations of microvascular beds can be achieved in easily transilluminated thin membranes. Studies of this type are usually limited to acute experiments in anesthetized animal preparations such as the hamster cheek pouch, the rat and mouse ear, or mesenteric beds. A transparent chamber for use in the rabbit ear considerably lengthens the period for direct observation of substance effects on blood vessels in unanesthetized animals. Microvascular dimensions can be recorded with the aid of an image-splitter television microscope. This technique allows measurement of changes in vessel wall thickness, lumen diameter, and total vessel diameter in both isolated tissues and the intact vascular beds.

In Vitro *Methods for Detecting Vascular Toxicity*

Once the particular vascular effect of a xenobiotic is identified, it may be more useful to examine its action on an isolated system rather than on the entire vascular bed. *In vitro* preparations allow a more controlled analysis of the potential toxic vascular effects. However, it should also be noted that results obtained from isolated or even perfused tissues do not always represent completely the action of the xenobiotic on the vasculature in the intact organism.

In vitro vascular toxicity studies can be conducted on strips or rings obtained from large arteries of laboratory animals such as rabbits and rats. The arterial strip preparation makes it possible to study changes induced in the tone of vascular smooth muscle due to xenobiotics added to the bathing solution.

The use of *in vitro* strip preparations, with and without endothelium, has also provided a means for determining the extent to which endothelial-dependent responses are responsible for the activity of vasoactive xenobiotics.

Cellular Electrophysiological Methods

The actions of some xenobiotics on the vasculature can be mediated by changes in membrane potential, action potential, or contractile activity. Use of an intracellular microelectrode can provide the means for determining the magnitude of the transmembrane potential and whether a substance causes changes in membrane potential. The intracellular microelectrode technique can also be used to determine cell membrane resistance.

Cultured Vascular Smooth Muscle Cells

Methods similar to those described for cultured cardiac muscle cells have produced cultured reaggregates of spontaneously contracting vascular smooth muscle cells which can be used to examine the electrophysiological and toxicologic effects of substances directly on noninnervated vascular smooth muscle cells.

Morphologic Evaluation

Gross Examination

At necropsy, the large vessels, including the large elastic arteries and great veins near the heart, can be grossly examined. Longitudinal incision will expose the intimal surface for inspection and may allow

detection of degenerative lesions of the walls which may be accompanied by mineralization, fibrosis, or lipid deposition. Other grossly apparent lesions include aneurysm formation, thrombosis, and vascular rupture. Indirect evidence of vascular disease may be gained by observation of lesions that accompany vascular damage, including hemorrhage and infarction. However, many vascular lesions will not be detectable by gross examination and intravenous injection of Monastral blue, Evan's blue or horseradish peroxidase prior to necropsy can be utilized to detect sites of compromised vascular permeability. Subsequent screening of these sites by microscopic evaluation can determine the extent and type of injury.

Preparation of Tissues

All isolated vessels, such as aorta, should be sampled by transverse section. Any vessel with gross lesions that indicate either apparent or suspicious vascular damage should be sampled for microscopic evaluation. Microscopic study of the vessels in each of the organs routinely sampled at necropsy will greatly extend the frequency of detection of vascular changes, particularly in small vessels.

Microscopic and Biochemical Evaluation

The evaluation procedures described for the heart may also be used for study of vessels and include light microscopy, electron microscopy, and biochemical analysis. Light microscopic study should include use of special staining procedures for elastic fibers (Verhoeff's elastica), collagen (Masson's trichrome, Movat's pentachrome), and mucopolysaccharides (periodic acid-Schiff). Lipid stains on frozen sections are essential for lipid-containing lesions. Immunohistochemical methods can be utilized for both light and electron microscopic study. Scanning electron microscopy is especially suited for morphologic evaluation of lesions of the lumenal surface.

Use of Animals as Models

Animal models for studies of human vascular disease have mainly centered on research on atherosclerosis and hypertension. Atherosclerosis models are numerous and include those in avians (pigeon, chicken, turkey, and Japanese quail); nonprimate mammals (rabbit, pig, dog, mouse, and rat); and non-human primate mammals (stumptail macaque, rhesus monkey, cynomolgus macaque, pigtail macaque, squirrel monkey, baboon, and African Green monkey). None of these models fulfill all of the requirements of an ideal model of human atherosclerosis. Models of hypertension are the Wistar-Kyoto spontaneously hypertensive rat and the Dahl salt-sensitive rat. The Fawn-hooded rat develops pulmonary hypertension and associated pulmonary vascular alterations.

SKELETAL MUSCLE

INTRODUCTION

Skeletal muscle is a unique tissue functioning to allow support and movement of the body. The mass of the skeletal musculature is large and constitutes 40–50% of the body weight. Recognition of gross pathologic alterations in muscular diseases is complicated by the normal variation in color and consistency observed among the muscles of various animal species and differing ages of animals. Detailed study of the skeletal musculature during routine necropsies generally is not performed. In fact, prosectors often overlook examination of the skeletal muscles in their haste to expose and observe the visceral organs.

Skeletal muscle fibers have unique structural features. Each fiber represents a syncytium formed during myogenesis by fusion of hundreds to thousands of individual myoblasts. The fibers are highly specialized, with approximately 80% of their cell volume occupied by contractile elements. Normal function of these fibers is dependent on normal nervous system function to initiate contraction and further involves intricate control mechanisms to direct movement of calcium ions in and out of the sarcoplasmic reticulum during the contraction-relaxation cycle. Muscle fibers have high-energy requirements, often needed on short notice; this metabolic feature may predispose these cells to injury from certain chemicals and drugs. Use of histochemical staining procedures allows recognition of several fiber types, each with unique metabolic and functional features that may render a specific population of fibers susceptible to certain injurious insults. Critical nutrients needed to maintain the structural integrity of muscle fibers include adequate dietary intake of selenium, vitamin E, and protein. Thus, the skeletal muscle fiber possesses a number of unique metabolic structural features that will influence the pathological reactions observed in muscle diseases.

STRUCTURE AND FUNCTION

Gross and Microscopic Anatomy

Muscles are surrounded and subdivided by connective tissue sheaths. The epimysium envelops entire muscles. Groups of muscle fibers are arranged in fasciculi that are separated by the perimysium, which is contiguous with the epimysium. The endomysium is a delicate network of connective tissue fibers, blood vessels, lymphatic vessels, and nerves which surrounds individual muscle fibers.

Cells of Skeletal Muscle: Biology and Clinical Relevance

Skeletal Muscle Fibers

Microscopic Appearance

Muscle fibers or cells generally extend from tendon to tendon in a muscle and do not branch or form syncytia. In cross-sections, fibers have a polygonal or multifaceted shape in muscle of adults. Many factors such as species, breed, age, weight, sex, plane of nutrition, position and function of the muscle, and exercise influence the diameter of muscle fibers. Measurements of fibers in individual muscles will show variability in fiber size that will be reflected as a bell-shaped curve on a histogram. Differences in fiber size in various species are not directly related to body weight (pig > horse, cow, rabbit > sheep). Fiber size is greater in males than females and tends to increase with age to maturity.

The cellular features of skeletal muscle fibers are best appreciated in longitudinal sections. The fibers are bounded by the plasma membrane or sarcolemma which is covered by an external lamina (stained by periodic acid-Schiff reaction). The thin elongated nuclei are generally positioned beneath the sarcolemma in a spiral pattern spaced 10–50 μm apart. At myotendinous junctions, muscle fibers have numerous centrally located nuclei. Nuclei of satellite cells are positioned between the sarcolemma and the external lamina. Fibers contain hundreds of longitudinally aligned myofibrils composed of repeating sarcomeres. The characteristic transverse striation of skeletal muscle fibers results from parallel alignment of the bands in adjacent myofibrils. The largest bands, termed according to their appearance in polarized light, are A bands (anisotropic or birefringent, appear bright) and I bands (iostropic, appear dark). The I bands, composed of thin myofilaments, are bisected by Z lines (disks, bands) that form the end of each sarcomere; the A bands, composed of thick filaments, are bisected by the less birefringent H bands. The banding pattern, named for the appearance in polarized light, is reversed when studied by light microscopy with phase contrast optics, light microscopy with conventional optics on sections stained with the usual cationic dyes, or transmission electron microscopy.

Application of histochemical stains such as ATPase or NADH-TR to frozen sections of skeletal muscle will allow demonstration of various fiber-type populations that cannot be distinguished in paraffin- embedded sections stained with the usual stains such as hematoxylin and eosin; however, fiber types are recognized by ultrastructural study. The histochemical uniqueness of these fiber types (Types 1, 2A, and 2B) correlates with differences in their physiologic features, such as contraction speed and fatigability; their biochemical and metabolic activities; their gross color; and their structure as revealed ultrastructurally (Table 12.9).

Most muscles will have a mixture of all fiber types to produce the so-called checkerboard pattern of differential histochemical staining. Fibers innervated by the same nerves will have the same fiber type and reinnervated fibers may show reversal of fiber types. Some muscles will have a preponderance of one fiber type, for example, the soleus in birds (red muscle high in type I fibers and capable of sustained action or weight bearing) and the pectorals in birds (white muscle high in type II fibers and capable of sudden action and purposeful motion). The proportions of the various fiber types may vary with species, breed, age, and exercise, and in certain muscular diseases.

Ultrastructural Appearance

The fiber surface is covered by the plasma membrane (sarcolemma) and external lamina. The elongated subsarcolemmal nuclei are surrounded by accumulation of mitochondria, lipid droplets, glycogen granules, elements of sarcoplasmic reticulum and the Golgi apparatus. The fiber contains abundant contractile material that is organized as many myofibrils of 0.5–1.0 μm diameter. Myofibrils are composed of repeating units termed sarcomeres of 2–3 μm length.

Sarcomeres end at dense Z lines that contain α-actinin, actin, and tropomyosin. Thin 60-Å diameter myofilaments containing actin, troponin, and tropomyosin extend on both sides of the Z line to form I bands. The middle half of the sarcomere contains thick (160-Å diameter) myofilaments that are composed of myosin and interdigitate with the adjacent thin filaments. The center of the sarcomere with only thick filaments is the H band and is bisected by the relatively dense M line. Fiber contraction results in shortening of sarcomeres due to sliding of thick and thin filaments over each other to produce narrowed I and H bands. Cross-sections of myofibrils show variable appearance depending on the location in the sarcomere but at the edges of the A band will have thick filaments surrounded by a hexagonal array of thin filaments. The sarcoplasm surrounding myofibrils contains elements of the transverse (T) tubular system and sarcoplasmic reticulum (SR), mitochondria, lipid droplets, glycogen granules, and cytosol. The T tubules are invaginations of the sarcolemma that are often seen at the edge of the I band with two adjacent elements of SR to form a "triad." The T-tubular system functions as a channel to allow rapid spread of an electrical impulse from the motor end plate to the rest of the fiber to elicit release of calcium stored in the SR with subsequent binding to regulatory proteins and interaction of actin and myosin to initiate contraction.

Satellite Cells

Satellite cells are thin cells with a nucleus and a scant amount of sarcoplasm interposed between the sarcolemma of muscle fibers and the external lamina. They are abundant in newborn animals; in muscle of mature animals 3–5% of nuclei in muscle fibers belong to satellite cells. The cells play an important role in

TABLE 12.9   Characteristics of major mammalian skeletal muscle fiber types

	Type 1	Type 2A	Type 2B
Morphologic characteristics			
Natural color	Dark	Dark	Pale
Glycogen content	Low	High	High
Myoglobin content	High	High	Low
Lipid globules	Numerous	Numerous	Few
Mitochrondrial content	High	Intermediate	Low
Physiological features			
Twitch speed	Slow	Fast	Fast
Fatigability	Resistant	Resistant	Susceptible

normal development of fibers and in regeneration of damaged fibers by serving as stem cells that can be activated to undergo mitosis in adult life and subsequently differentiate to myoblasts, myotubes, and eventually mature myofibers.

Motor End Plates

Motor end plates (neuromuscular junctions), generally recognized only by use of special techniques such as metallic impregnation, intravital dyes, histochemical procedures, or electron microscopy, represent a complex and intimate attachment site of the motor nerve fiber on the surface of the skeletal muscle fiber. The end of the nerve fiber is unmyelinated and branches into axon terminals that invaginate into a thickened zone of subsarcolemmal sarcoplasm with numerous nuclei as synaptic clefts. The axon terminal has abundant synaptic vesicles containing the neurotransmitter acetylcholine.

Muscle Spindles

Muscle spindles are fusiform structures 0.5–3.0 mm in length found longitudinally oriented at the edge of muscle fasciculi. The spindle has a thick surrounding fibrous capsule and contains multiple small variably sized intrafusal muscle fibers, nerve fibers, specialized nerve endings, and blood vessels. Muscle spindles have sensory function and serve to maintain muscle tone by responding to stretch.

Connective Tissue

The interstitial connective tissue of muscle is subdivided into the epimysium (surrounds the entire muscle), perimysium (surrounds large angular fascicles divided into primary fascicles of 10 to 100 fibers), and endomysium (surrounds individual muscle fibers). The endomysium contains capillaries, nerve fibers, fibroblasts, and collagen fibrils. Larger amounts of collagen fibrils and large blood vessels and nerves are in the perimysium.

Physiologic and Functional Considerations

The unique structural differentiation of skeletal muscle fibers is closely integrated with their highly developed specialized contractile function for locomotion and maintenance of posture by conversion of chemical energy into mechanical energy. Further specialization in form and function is provided by the differentiation of myofibers into various fiber types each of which is specifically suited for certain physiologic applications.

The functional unit of the neuromuscular system is the motor unit consisting of (1) nerve cell bodies in the ventral horns or brain stem, (2) the axon of these neurons that course to the muscles and terminate as a motor end plate, and (3) the group of specific histochemical type muscle fibers that are innervated by the neuron.

Contraction of muscle is the result of sarcomere shortening with interdigitation of thin and thick myofilaments. According to the sliding filament hypothesis of contraction, the force of contraction is generated by the movement of cross-bridges that project from myosin molecules along actin molecules. The chemical energy for contraction is supplied by high-energy phosphate compounds that are largely generated in type I fibers by mitochondrial oxidative phosphorylation via the electron transport system following the oxidation of fatty acids and glucose via the Krebs cycle, and in Type II fibers by sarcoplasmic anaerobic glycolysis and glycogenolysis. Thus, the metabolic differences of the various fiber types are associated with differences in their functional features, such as speed of contraction and resistance to fatigue.

MECHANISMS OF TOXICITY

The normal structure and function of skeletal muscle can be altered by a variety of chemicals and drugs. Skeletal muscle susceptibility to potential toxicants appears in part related to the specialized metabolism of the tissues and the associated effects on the metabolic process due to the physiologic demands of contraction. In addition, sensitivity to toxic agents may be enhanced because many substances tend to bind to skeletal muscle. Skeletal muscle dysfunction or damage has been induced by both indirect and direct mechanisms. Mechanisms discussed below are listed in Table 12.10.

Altered Neurogenic Function

Muscular atrophy can develop when interruptions occur in peripheral motor nerve function. Usually, not all the motor fibers supplied by the nerve undergo atrophy and some remain relatively normal. A variety of substances are capable of causing or intensifying neuromuscular blockade. No significant morphologic changes appear during neuromuscular blockade and the blockade is usually reversed when the causative substance is removed. In some instances, xenobiotics have induced muscle necrosis by dramatically increasing motor nerve activity or by allowing significant amounts of acetylcholine to accumulate at the myoneural junction. In rats,

TABLE 12.10   Mechanisms of toxicity to the skeletal muscle system with selected examples

Mechanism	Xenobiotic
Altered neurogenic function	Paraoxon, heroin, amphetamine, phenylcyclidine
Altered immunologic function	D-penicillamine, procainamide
Localized damage	Oxytetracycline, meperidine
Cell membrane alterations	Clofibrate, 2,4-dichlorophenoxy acetic acid (2,4-D), monensin, Type A *Clostridium perfringens* toxin
Sarcoplasmic reticulum alterations	Adriamycin
Microtubular alterations	Cholchicine, amiodarone
Myofilament alterations	Plasmocid, emetine
Lysosomal alterations	Chloroquine, amiodarone
Altered intracellular calcium concentration (genetic susceptibility)	Halothane, succinyl choline, nitrous oxide
Altered protein synthesis	Corticosteroids
Altered muscle cell differentiation	6-Mercaptopurine (prenatal exposure)

injection of paraoxon causes a progressive myopathy which ultimately leads to necrosis and phagocytosis of muscle fibers. The myopathy is attributed to excessive concentrations of acetylcholine. Acute rhabdomyolysis is a severe necrotizing myopathy associated with heroin addiction, amphetamine overdoses, and phencyclidine abuse. The muscle damage probably occurs as a result of extreme motor nerve excitation rather than of direct myotoxicity.

Altered Immunologic Function

A xenobiotic may also induce toxicity indirectly by provoking immunologic reactions which lead to generalized muscle weakness. D- Penicillamine induces an inflammatory myopathy which results in clinical dermatomyositis and polymyositis. There is evidence to indicate that autoimmune reactions play a role in the etiology of this myopathy. For example, a form of myositis may develop as part of a drug-induced lupus-like reaction during treatment with procainamide.

Localized Damage

Some xenobiotics may exert localized toxicity when injected into or near the muscle. Focal damage has occurred following intramuscular injection of narcotic analgesics and oxytetracycline. Agents such as pentazocine and meperidine cause a severe fibrotic reaction. Other xenobiotics can produce diffuse damage when given systemically. It is apparent that myopathic effects can occur when a substance directly alters critical structural or functional components of the muscle fiber.

Cell Membrane Alterations

The cell membrane represents an important cellular component which is usually exposed to the highest concentration of a substance. A change in electrical properties can occur if a substance alters the cell membrane. Muscle weakness, which occurs in situations in which the concentration of potassium is reduced, is apparently the result of a decrease in membrane excitability. Severe hypokalemia may lead to muscle fiber necrosis. In contrast, increased membrane excitability is the likely mechanism by which a number of agents (lithium, cimetidine, salbutamol, danazol, and captopril) cause muscle cramping.

The use of clofibrate may also induce muscle fiber necrosis. The precise mechanism by which clofibrate induces muscle fiber necrosis is not known, but there is evidence that clofibrate does affect the cell membrane. Membrane alterations may occur because the drug exerts an inhibiting effect on cholesterol biosynthesis. Other metabolic effects of clofibrate may also contribute to the muscle toxicity.

Dioxocholesterol interferes with the biosynthesis of cholesterol and, as a result, causes accumulation of the cholesterol precursor desmosterol in the serum, the cell membrane, and the sarcoplasmic reticulum. The presence of excessive amounts of desmosterol in the cell membrane leads to excessive chloride permeability and myotonia. Myotonia also occurs following exposure to the herbicidal compound, 2,4-dichlorophenoxyacetic acid (2,4-D). This agent causes metabolic alterations by inhibiting glucose-6-phosphate dehydrogenase, an effect which leads to membrane and subcellular alterations; alterations in ion transport are also provoked. Advanced lesions induced by this agent display vacuolization and muscle fiber necrosis.

Monocarboxylic acids, capable of inhibiting chloride conductance, also produce myotonia. Monensin, a Na^+-selective carboxylic acid ionophore, consistently causes both skeletal and cardiac muscle necrosis in a variety of animals. Evidence suggests that these effects are due to calcium overloading.

Injection of Type A *Clostridium perfringens* toxin induces a unique myopathy. This toxin initially causes alterations in the muscle cell membrane. Subsequently, changes occur in the mitochondria and sarcoplasmic reticulum and ultimately alterations are found in certain contractile components (I and Z bands, A-band filaments).

Sarcoplasmic Reticulum Alterations

Xenobiotics have been found to produce alterations in the sarcoplasmic reticulum. Intraperitoneal injection of adriamycin has caused damage to the diaphragm muscle, an effect which is associated with cytoplasmic vacuolization due to dilatation of the sarcoplasmic reticulum. The vacuolization is similar to that which is well known to be induced in cardiac muscle by anthracyclines.

Microtubular Alterations

There are similarities in the myotoxic effects of colchicine and vincristine, both of which are known to interfere with the function of microtubules. In each instance subsarcolemmal and intermyofibrillar myeloid structures appear and are associated with varying degrees of muscle fiber necrosis. These chemicals cause alterations in one or more other organ systems, particularly the nervous system, an effect which may influence the pathogenesis of the myopathy.

Myofilament Alterations

Myofilamentous degeneration occurs following treatment with plasmocid. This agent caused selective loss of Z and I bands in the rat diaphragm and also in cardiac muscle. Multifocal loss of cross- striations of muscle have been reported to occur in animals treated with emetine. In some areas, loss of oxidative enzyme activity was associated with muscle necrosis. Emetine, a constituent of ipecac, produces a pattern of myotoxicity which is similar to the muscle fiber breakdown seen in certain human myopathies.

Lysosomal Alterations

Certain amphiphilic cationic agents with diverse pharmacologic actions cause a myopathy that includes lysosomal phospholipid accumulation in the form of large masses of concentric lamellae and peculiar structures known as curvilinear bodies. The antimalarial chloroquine is associated with this type of myopathy, as are aminodarone and perhexiline. The myopathy caused by these substances is part of a more general form of intracellular lipid accumulation

which, in addition to skeletal muscle, affects other tissues such as the peripheral and central nervous systems. These agents are both water and lipid soluble and readily diffuse through the plasma membrane. After passing through the cell membrane they become adsorbed onto intracellular membranes and form stable drug-lipid complexes which progressively accumulate within the lysosomes of skeletal muscle cells and other tissues. Apparently they inhibit lysosomal enzymes that degrade phospholipids.

Altered Intracellular Calcium Concentration

A potentially serious drug-induced condition, characterized by muscular rigidity and myoglobinuria, hypermetabolism, and metabolic acidosis, occurs in genetically susceptible individuals undergoing routine surgery. Malignant hyperthermia is commonly precipitated in these individuals by exposure to halothane and succinyl choline. Other halogenated anesthetic agents, nitrous oxide, muscle relaxants, and certain local anesthetic agents may also induce this reaction. A condition similar to the human syndrome has been described in certain strains of pigs. Susceptible pigs are sensitive to stress and develop muscle rigidity, acidosis, and hyperkalemia. Death ensues due to heart failure if these pigs are subjected to stress. These sensitive pigs also react to halothane and depolarizing neuromuscular blocking agents. The malignant hyperthermic reaction appears to be caused by an alteration in muscular control of intracellular calcium levels. Acute increases in this cation cause contracture of muscle fibers, decreased ATP levels, increased metabolism and temperature, and secondary changes in a variety of cellular components.

Altered Protein Synthesis

Prolonged corticosteroid therapy is known to cause a skeletal muscle myopathy. Steroids which are fluorinated in the 9 position (triamcinolone, dexamethasone, and betamethasone) are most likely to be myotoxic, but continuous treatment with any of the corticosteroids will also lead to a myopathy. The clinical syndrome tends to be less severe than the experimentally induced myopathy and usually involves atrophy of type II fibers. The mechanism of steroid-induced myopathy has been explored in a number of animal studies. These hormones are found to alter a variety of myocyte functions. However, the primary mechanism responsible for muscle fiber atrophy appears to be due to a suppression in the rate of protein synthesis.

Altered Muscle Cell Differentiation

Information regarding the possible effect of exposure to xenobiotics during pregnancy on subsequent growth and development of skeletal muscle in the fetus is inconclusive. In tissue culture studies, exposure to some drugs has led to interference with certain aspects of muscle cell differentiation. Prenatal exposure of rats to 6-mercaptopurine has led, after a latent period, to a continuous and progressive atrophic degeneration of muscle cells. These myotoxic effects are not seen when 6-mercaptopurine is administered during the postnatal period.

RESPONSE TO INJURY

Muscle will respond to the numerous insults to which it is exposed by only a limited number of morphologic reactions. In fact, diseases of differing etiologies may exhibit similar types of lesions. Thus, it may not be possible to render a specific etiologic diagnosis even following careful microscopic study of tissues from a given case.

Injury, Regeneration, and Repair

Many injuries of skeletal muscle heal by regeneration. This is especially true for the common monophasic or polyphasic polyfocal myopathies (see subsequent text) such as those associated with nutritional deficiencies, metabolic disorders, and myotoxicities. In these diseases, although extensive muscle fiber necrosis may occur, the scaffolding of external lamina of the muscle fiber and the innervation and blood supply to the damaged muscle are preserved; these permit regeneration which is often virtually complete (Figure 12.22). Regeneration is further promoted in these conditions by the short-term nature of the insult responsible for the muscle injury. This is in contrast to the prolonged expression of insults, such as denervation or genetic derangements, in those muscular diseases with limited effectiveness of regeneration. In severe muscle diseases, extensive disruption of endomysial connective tissues and "tubes" of external laminae of damaged myofibers may occur from trauma, hemorrhage, or infection and the outcome of healing will be limited regeneration accompanied by extensive fibrosis and scarring.

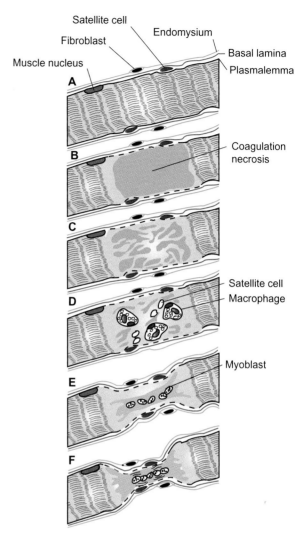

FIGURE 12.22 Schematic diagram of segmental myofiber necrosis and regeneration. (A) Myofiber, longitudinal section. (B) Segmental coagulation necrosis. (C) The necrotic segment of the myofiber has become floccular and detached from the adjacent viable portion of the myofiber. The satellite cells are enlarging. (D) The necrotic segment of the myofiber has been invaded by macrophages, and satellite cells are migrating to the center. The latter will develop into myoblasts. The plasmalemma of the necrotic segment has disappeared. (E) Myoblasts have formed a myotube, which has produced sarcoplasm. This extends out to meet the viable ends of the myofiber. The integrity of the myofiber is maintained by the sarcolemmal tube formed by the basal lamina and endomysium. (F) Regenerating myofiber. There is a reduction in myofiber diameter with central rowing of nuclei. There is early formation of sarcomeres (cross-striations), and the plasmalemma has reformed. Such fibers stain basophilically with H&E. (A–F, Redrawn with permission from Dr M.D. McGavin, College of Veterinary Medicine, University of Tennessee.)

The cellular events of regeneration are well characterized and center around the proliferation of mononucleated myogenic stem cells termed myoblasts, which arise from satellite cells. For unknown reasons, satellite cells tend to be resistant to many insults that destroy mature myofibers. Following selective destruction of skeletal muscle fibers, the sarcoplasmic debris is removed rapidly by invasion of macrophages and phagocytic lysis. The persisting sarcolemmal "tubes" of external lamina rapidly become populated by elongated myoblasts. Myoblasts fuse to form multinucleated cells termed sarcoblasts, which further elongate to form myotubes that rapidly bridge the gap of disrupted sarcoplasm in damaged myofibers. Subsequently, the regenerated muscle fibers may then be indistinguishable from adjacent unaffected fibers.

Skeletal Muscle Alterations

Xenobiotic-induced skeletal muscle alterations consist of degeneration and necrosis, and neurogenic atrophy. In most cases, cardiomyocyte alterations are also present (see Table 12.6).

Degeneration and Necrosis (Myopathy)

Morphologic Changes

Unlike in most tissues, the difference between the reversible sublethal alterations of degeneration and the irreversible lethal changes of necrosis is difficult to detect by microscopic study. Skeletal muscle fibers are large long multinucleated cells and it is often not possible to view the entire length of the fiber in the plane of a tissue section to determine whether the sarcoplasmic damage involves the entire fiber or only a segment of the fiber. It seems likely that segmental degeneration occurs frequently but necrosis of entire fibers is uncommon. In any event, the causes of both degeneration and necrosis are similar.

Specific morphologic types of degeneration have been described. The most common type is so-called hyaline-type or waxy degeneration. Affected muscles may be detected grossly by diffuse pallor or scattered pale streaks, especially if secondary calcification has occurred in damaged fibers (Figure 12.23). Microscopically, affected fibers appear swollen and hypereosinophilic with loss of cross-striations (Figure 12.24 A and B). The altered contractile material frequently becomes fragmented into large blocks or disks scattered along the "tube" of persisting external lamina of the muscle fiber. Within 24 hr, the affected areas will be invaded by an occasional polymorphonuclear leukocyte and numerous macrophages. The "tube" of external lamina persists to guide regenerative events and may be focally disrupted to allow entry of macrophages (Figures 12.25).

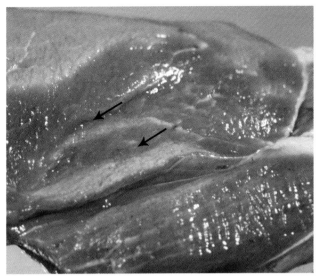

FIGURE 12.23 Acute necrosis (Zenker's necrosis) of skeletal muscle from a sheep, with monensin toxicoses evident as pale areas and streaks (arrows).

Another type of degeneration described in skeletal muscle is granular degeneration. The microscopic appearance differs from hyaline degeneration because the damaged sarcoplasm appears as small basophilic granules that fill the "tube" of external lamina and are identified as mineralized mitochondria by ultrastructural study (Figure 12.26). The causes of granular and hyaline degeneration are similar and include nutritional deficiencies, such as selenium-vitamin E deficiency, various myotoxic drugs and plants, and metabolic disorders such as azoturia and capture myopathy.

The spatial distribution and temporal pattern of lesions of degeneration and necrosis in skeletal muscle have been used to classify reactions as monophasic monofocal, monophasic polyfocal, polyphasic monofocal, and polyphasic polyfocal. Monophasic monofocal reactions result from an isolated single mechanical injury such as external trauma or needle insertion. In monophasic polyfocal reactions, a single insult such as exposure to various myotoxic drugs or chemicals or various metabolic disorders may initiate widespread muscle lesions but all the alterations are in the same phase of injury. Polyphasic monofocal reactions would be the result of repeated localized mechanical injury. Polyphasic polyfocal reactions are frequent in muscular diseases of animals and result from continued insults applied over a prolonged time, for example, from nutritional deficiencies and genetic disorders, as in muscular dystrophies; the lesions are widespread in the musculature and various pathological reactions will occur concurrently including necrosis, leukocytic invasion during resolution, and regeneration (Figures 12.24 C and D, and 12.26).

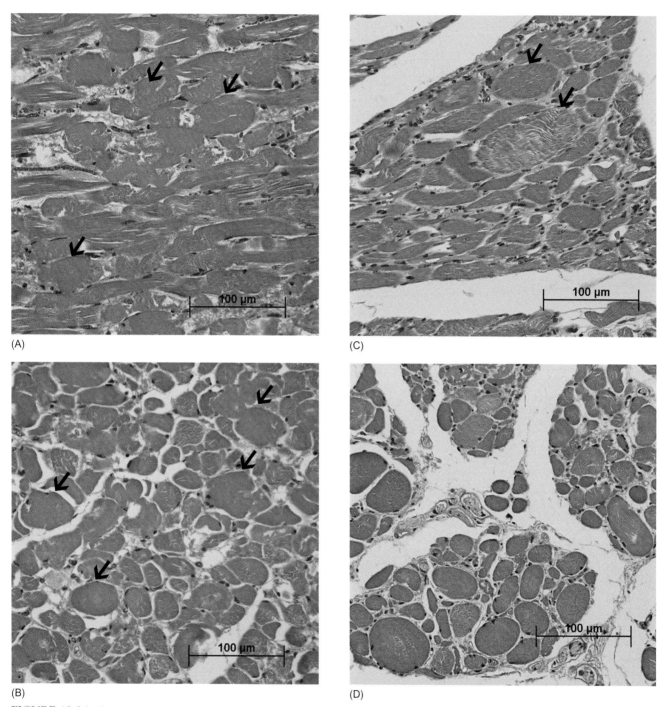

FIGURE 12.24 Segmental myofiber necrosis of skeletal muscle from sheep with monensin toxicosis. Paraffin-embedded, hematoxylin and eosin stain. Acute degeneration: (A) Longitudonal section; (B) Cross-section. Myofibers are segmentally hypercontracted, appearing swollen and hyalinized (arrows), with loss of cross-striations and fragmentation. Subacute degeneration: (C) Longitudinal section; (D) Cross-section. Fascicles are widely separated, due to loss of myofiber mass. Myofibers vary greatly in size, and there is an increase in cellularity between fibers due to an increase in myoblasts and macrophages.

Other less common types of degeneration in skeletal muscle fibers include vacuolar or hydropic degeneration and fatty degeneration. Vacuolar or hydropic type of degeneration occurs with cortisol excess. The affected fibers have vacuolated lacelike areas in the sarcoplasm. Fatty degeneration is uncommon. It is seen as a nonspecific response to injury and results in abundant small spherical lipid vacuoles scattered between myofibrils.

musculature (30–50% of body weight) precludes complete dissection of each individual muscle. Thus, in necropsies of animals without any historical evidence of clinical disease of the skeletal musculature, the prosector should at least inspect the muscles exposed during the necropsy procedure, for example, those of the abdominal wall, diaphragm, proximal portions of the limbs, sublumbar area, neck, and head. In animals with clinical suspicion of muscle disease, a more detailed examination of the musculature should be carried out, with particularly careful inspection of those muscles presumed to be responsible for the clinical signs. Gross alterations in color, shape, size, and consistency should be sought by viewing the surface and cut sections of the muscles. Lesions should be accurately described and, if necessary, photographed. The magnitude of the effort required is increased greatly in the many large animal species presented to a veterinary pathologist. Prosectors should avoid incorrect interpretation of gross findings such as color and size of muscles that may be a function of the normal variation associated with species, age, particular muscle, and state of nutrition seen among animals.

Following somatic death, skeletal muscle will generally remain in relaxation for 2–4 hr until muscle glycogen stores are metabolized and sufficient energy to maintain the relaxed state is no longer present. Rigor mortis then ensues as stiffness of the muscles and immobility of the joints for at least 24–48 hr. Subsequently, rigor will dissipate as autolysis occurs, muscle proteins are denatured, and muscle fibers lose the ability to contract. The onset of rigor mortis will be rapid if the muscle is kept at low pH and high temperature. Abundant muscular glycogen stores at the time of death will lead to delayed onset of rigor. Debilitated animals tend to have weak rigor. Pallor develops in muscles following death, as also seen in necrotic muscle, presumably due to leaching of myoglobin by accumulated lactic acid. The muscles may appear unusually dark following death of debilitated animals with depleted glycogen stores.

Microscopic Evaluation

Analysis of muscle sections can be part of a process that can be used in identifying xenobiotics causing neurogenic or myopathic alterations, specific muscular structural alterations, or specific muscular metabolic alterations. A number of pathologic muscular alterations can be detected in regular paraffin sections of muscle. Cell membrane damage can alter intracellular regulation of calcium, a condition which could cause cell death if severe enough. Ultimately, satellite cells can produce multinuclear myotubes and regeneration

of the muscle fiber. Muscle fiber necrosis and regeneration are common features of myotoxicity. If necrosis is substantial and chronic, regeneration may fail, resulting in progressive fiber loss and replacement by fat and fibrous tissue. Degeneration of muscle fibers without overt necrosis causes structural alteration of myofibrils and sarcoplasm. Pathologic changes could be restricted to one type of fiber in the muscle.

Sample collection must be done carefully to avoid hypercontraction artifacts that are inevitable in fresh muscle collected in biopsy samples and in samples taken from animals soon after death. Each muscle sample should be identified by the muscle involved and the specific location of the sample within the muscle. To prevent contraction artifacts, isolated longitudinal strips of muscle are dissected and clamped or ligated to a strip of wood (e.g., tongue depressor) at isometric length and then excised. Placing the clamped sample in physiologic saline solution for 20 min will further decrease problems with contraction artifacts.

For preparation of tissue sections for routine light microscopy, the clamped sample is fixed in 10% neutral buffered formalin, embedded in paraffin, sectioned, and stained with hematoxylin and eosin. Other stains frequently utilized include Masson's trichrome (connective tissue) and phosphotungstic acid hematoxylin (myofibrils and cross-striations of muscle fibers). Application of lipid stains to frozen sections is useful. Each muscle sample should have longitudinal and cross-sections prepared for microscopic study. For tissue samples to be used for high resolution light microscopy or electron microscopy, the clamped samples are immersed in 3% buffered glutaraldehyde or Trump's universal fixative, postfixed in osmium tetroxide, embedded in either methacrylate or epoxy resins, sectioned, and stained as for other tissues.

Histochemical studies of sections of fresh-frozen muscle can be used to evaluate the dimensions of the muscle fibers, the distribution and quantity of mitochondria, lipid and glycogen content in the cells, myofibrillar enzymes, the profiles of the muscle fibers, and the distribution of the fiber types. Muscle units differ both in size and in certain biochemical properties of their fibers. ATPase stains can identify the two primary types of muscle fibers: type I (fast), which are lightly stained, and type II (slow), which appear darkly stained. Fiber-type differentiation may be useful in evaluating myotoxic effects, since there are instances when one or the other fiber type may be preferentially affected. The neutral fat content of the muscle can be assessed in oil red O stained frozen sections.

For enzyme histochemical study, the samples are frozen in liquid nitrogen and sectioned in a cryostat.

Sections are stained for myosin ATPase activity at three different pH levels, NADH-tetrazolium reductase activity, and succinic dehydrogenase activity. Morphometric evaluation of these sections will allow determination of the percentage of each fiber type and the mean fiber diameters.

Numerous artifacts may be observed in sections prepared either for light or electron microscopy. These artifacts include hypercontracted fibers from improper collection and fixation procedures, mitochondrial vacuolation, distention of elements of sarcoplasmic reticulum and glycogen loss from faulty fixation, and occurrence of knife marks, chatter, and wrinkles from sectioning problems.

Ultrastructural studies of diseased muscle have provided a valuable extension of the resolution limits of the light microscope. There have been some efforts to classify human muscle diseases by alterations in specific organelles resulting in terms such as mitochondrial myopathies or vacuolar myopathies. Such classifications are probably of limited value since it is difficult to identify a specific organelle with primary damage following muscle fiber injury. In addition, these various types of organellar alteration are not specific for particular muscle diseases since muscle fibers have only a limited number of possible morphologic expressions in response to various insults.

Use of Animals as Models

The discovery and laboratory study of specific muscular diseases of animals that provide a suitable animal model for a similar disease in humans have provided much useful information that can be applied to the human disease. Specific models in animals include the various inherited dystrophies, specific conditions such as malignant hyperthermia, myasthenia gravis, myotonia, and storage diseases, as well as multiple examples of myopathies of toxic or nutritional deficiency origin. However, it is highly unlikely to find an animal disease model that possesses all the features of the counterpart disease in human patients. Even with this limitation, animal models provide a great deal of useful information on the pathogenetic mechanisms and natural history of the human disease. This is of particular relevance since the basic types of pathologic reactions in skeletal muscle are similar among species.

FURTHER READING

Acosta, D. Jr (ed.) (2001). *Cardiovascular Toxicology*, 3rd edn. Taylor & Francis, New York, NY.

Ayres, K.M. & Jones, S.R. (1978). The cardiovascular system. In *Pathology of Laboratory Animals* | (Benirschke, K., Garner, F.M. & Jones, T.C. eds), Vol. I, pp. 1–69. Springer-Verlag, New York, NY.

Balazs, T., Ferrans, V.J., Hanig, J. & Herman, E. (1986). Cardiac Toxicity. In *Target Organ Toxicity* | (Cohen, G.H. ed.), Vol. II, pp. 19–43. CRC Press, Boca Raton, FL.

Bishop, S.P. (1999). Necropsy techniques for the heart and great vessels. In *Textbook of Canine and Feline Cardiology* | (Fox, P., Sisson, D. & Moise, N. eds), 2nd edn. Saunders, Philadelphia, PA.

Bishop, S.P. & Kerns, W.D. (1997). Cardiovascular Toxicology. In *Comprehensive Toxicology*, Vol. 6. Elsevier Science, New York, NY.

Carpenter, S. & Karpati, G. (2001). *Pathology of Skeletal Muscle*. Oxford University Press, New York, NY.

Isaacs, K.R. (1998). The cardiovascular system. In *Target Organ Pathology* | (Turton, J. & Hooson, J. eds), pp. 141–176. Taylor and Francis, London.

Kakulas, B.A. & Adams, R.D. (1985). *Diseases of Muscle*, 4th edn. Harper and Row, New York, NY.

Kumar, V., Abbas, A.K., Fausto, N., Robbins, S. & Cotran, R.S. (eds) (2005). *Robbins and Cotran Pathologic Basis of Disease*, 7th edn. Elsevier Saunders, Philadelphia, PA.

Maxie, M.G. & Robinson, W.F. (2007). Cardiovascular system. In *Jubb, Kennedy, and Palmer's Pathology of Domestic Animals* | (Maxie, M.G. ed.), 5th edn, Vol. 3, pp. 1–106. Elsevier Saunders, Philadelphia, PA.

Ramos, K.S., Melchert, R.B., Chacon, E. & Acosta, D. Jr (2001). Toxic responses of the heart and vascular systems. In *Casarett and Doull's Toxicology* | (Casarett, L., Klaassen, C. & Doull, J. eds), pp. 597–651. Macmillan Publishing Company, New York, NY.

Silver, M.D., Gotlieb, A.I. & Schoen, F.J. (eds) (2001). *Cardiovascular Pathology*, 3rd edn. Churchill Livingstone, New York, NY.

Valentine, B.A. & McGavin, M.D. (2006). Skeletal muscle. In *Pathologic Basis of Veterinary Disease* | (McGavin, M.D. & Zachary, J.F. eds), 4th edn, pp. 973–1040. Mosby, Philadelphia, PA.

Van Vleet, J.F. & Ferrans, V.J. (2007). Cardiovascular system. In *Pathologic Basis of Veterinary Disease* | (McGavin, M.D. & Zachary, J.F. eds), 4th edn, pp. 559–611. Mosby Elsevier, Philadelphia, PA.

Van Vleet, J.F. & Valentine, B.A. (2007). Muscle and tendon. In *Jubb, Kennedy, and Palmer's Pathology of Domestic Animals* | (Maxie, M.G. ed.), 4th edn, Vol. I, pp. 185–280. Saunders, Elsevier, New York.

Nervous System

INTRODUCTION

Neurotoxicology is the study of the adverse structural or functional effects on the nervous system following xenobiotic exposure during development and in maturity. A broad range of chemicals may induce neurotoxicity, and it has been estimated that 3% to 28% of all commercial chemicals may be neurotoxic. Neurotoxicants may induce structural or functional changes, and can act on the central nervous system (CNS), the peripheral nerve fibers, the peripheral nerve endings, or muscles or other effector organs. Structural neurotoxic effects are defined as neuroanatomical changes, while functional effects are defined

as neurochemical, neurophysiological, or behavioral changes. Not all neurological alterations observed following chemical exposure are considered adverse; some might be desired responses of neuropharmacological therapies, and others may be transient modifications. In general, however, all chemical-induced structural changes or persistent functional perturbations in behavior, neurochemistry, or neurophysiology of the nervous system are regarded as neurotoxic effects. Reversible effects occurring at doses that could endanger performance in the workplace, or that are associated with a known neurotoxicological mechanism of action are also considered adverse.

In addition to coordinating functions that are commonly associated with the brain (e.g., learning and memory), virtually all physiologic processes are controlled or influenced by the nervous system. A number of factors, including its complexity and limited capacity for repair, predispose the nervous system to toxic insult. Since the many specialized regions of the nervous system are functionally and anatomically interrelated, a localized lesion may have significant effects on more distant parts of the nervous system. The nervous system has a high metabolic rate, and is almost exclusively dependent on aerobic, glucose-dependent metabolic pathways. To support this high metabolic demand, the rat brain receives approximately 15% of the total cardiac output, and consumes 20% of the oxygen capacity of the entire body, although it accounts for only 1.5% to 2% of the total body weight. Thus, the nervous system is extremely sensitive to neurotoxicants that disrupt mitochondrial function and energy metabolism. Elevated concentrations of polyunsaturated fatty acids, and relatively low levels of antioxidant enzymes, also predispose the brain to oxidative damage. The presence of myelin and other lipoproteins enhances the brain's susceptibility to oxidant-induced lipid peroxidation. High brain lipid levels facilitate the absorption and distribution of small molecular weight, lipophilic chemicals throughout the nervous system.

Variable sensitivity to neurotoxicants is a characteristic of different regions of the nervous system. This results from compartmentalization of biochemical or metabolic functions, variations in vascularization and regional blood flows, as well as inherent cellular processes (e.g., regional distributions of neurotransmitters). Some regions of the nervous system, such as peripheral nerves, have a high capacity for regeneration. Other regions (e.g., neocortex) cannot regenerate, and must compensate for neurotoxic damage. Younger individuals appear to have more capacity for both anatomical and functional adaptation (plasticity) than older individuals, suggesting that the aged may be at greater risk from neurotoxic exposure to certain chemicals.

STRUCTURE AND FUNCTION

Macroscopic Structure

The nervous system is divided into various functional domains. The dorsal portions of the brain and spinal cord coordinate incoming impulses, while the ventral regions control effector actions. Major activities include motion, sensation, association ("higher thought"), and control of homeostasis. Somatic components regulate the response to the external environment, while the visceral elements control the internal

milieu. The motor system consists of a somatic motor domain, which conveys impulses to voluntary (skeletal) muscles, and a visceral motor portion, which supplies involuntary (cardiac and smooth) muscles. In like manner, the sensory system is composed of a somatic sensory part, which receives signals from the skin and body wall, and a visceral sensory domain that serves the internal organs. Associative domains integrate signals between lower and higher brain centers.

To a large extent, functional domains are correlated with specific neuroanatomic sites (Figure 13.1). Within these regions, neurons with similar functions are arranged in stereotypical ("somatotopic") patterns that are often, but not always, similar among species. In the mammalian forebrain, the primary somatic centers are typically found in the dorsolateral cerebral cortex, with the motor area located rostral to the sensory area. The spinal cord exhibits a similar functional segregation, with input from the somatic and visceral sensory domains entering the dorsal gray matter, while signals from the somatic motor domain originate in the ventral gray matter. The visceral sensory and motor centers are located in nuclei of the midbrain, brain stem, and intermediate column of gray matter in the spinal cord. The autonomic nervous system is primarily an elaboration of the visceral motor domain. The primary associative center is located in the prefrontal cortex, although white matter cross-connections within and between the hemispheres, and to subcortical centers, provide extensive additional associative capacities. Homeostatic activities usually are regulated at the unconscious level in the many nuclei of the limbic system (especially the hypothalamus), midbrain, and brain stem.

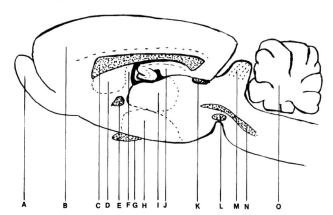

FIGURE 13.1 Longitudinal section of rat brain. (A) Olfactory lobe; (B) Cerebral cortex; (C) Corpus callosum; (D) Caudate-putamen; (E) Anterior commissure; (F) Septum; (G) Optic nerve; (H) Hypothalamus; (I) Thalamus; (J) Hippocampus; (K) Posterior commissure; (L) Substantia nigra; (M) corpora quadrigemina; (N) Lateral lemniscus; (O) Cerebellum.

A defined neuroanatomic structure may, in fact, have multiple subdivisions, each of which may serve a unique function. For example, the apparently homogeneous neuronal populations seen in the corpus striatum and substantia nigra on routinely stained brain sections can be demonstrated to consist of anatomically and chemically distinct compartments using special stains. It is also true that distinct neuroanatomic structures may serve the same function. For instance, the internal division of the globus pallidus (in the diencephalon) and the pars reticulata of the substantia nigra (midbrain) form a single functional unit. Thus, functional domains are more related to specific signal pathways (architectonic units) than to anatomical landmarks.

The mammalian species of toxicologic importance may be divided into rodent (including mouse, rat), carnivore (cat and dog), and primate (monkeys and humans) classes, on the basis of neuroanatomic and functional criteria in the CNS. The most important differentiating features are the degree of brain fissuration, the size of certain spinal tracts, and the prominence of various cortical regions. The arrangement of sulci and gyri varies with both age and species, and within a species it varies between the right and left sides, presumably as a consequence of hemisphere-specific functional needs. In the spinal cord, many white matter tracts, including the dorsal funiculus (the main conduit for transmission of most tactile and proprioceptive sensory impulses) and corticospinal pathways (which mediate cortical control of voluntary motor functions), are largest in primates, of intermediate size in carnivores, and smallest in rodents. In the cerebral cortex, main functional domains have comparable locations in all mammalian species. However, in the carnivore, the primary sensory and motor areas and olfactory cortex account for 80% of the cortex, while these same zones in the primate represent less than 20% of the tissue. The most telling interspecies difference in cortical function is the ratio of paleocortex (which is largely controlled by the limbic system) to that of neocortex (which participates in associative and cognitive activities). Rodent cortex consists almost entirely of paleocortex, while the neocortex accounts for a large proportion of the primate brain.

The chicken, which is occasionally used in neurotoxicology, has a unique neuroanatomical organization. Major anatomic differences relative to the mammalian pattern include the prominent jelly-filled opening (sinus rhomboidalis) in the dorsal midline of the lumbosacral spinal cord, the reduced size of the proprioceptive pathway (the dorsal funiculus and its rostral extension, the medial lemniscus), the greatly enlarged cerebellospinal tract (located just medial to the spinocerebellar tract in the lateral funiculus), and

the absence of the corticospinal tract in the bird. These latter two findings reflect the markedly reduced thickness, the relatively unlaminated nature of the avian cerebral cortex, and extensive subcortical control of avian motor functions by the enormous basal ganglia and the cerebellum.

Microscopic Anatomy

The CNS and peripheral nervous system (PNS) are composed of two main cell classes: neurons and glia (Figure 13.2). Preservation of the normal relationship between neurons and glia is critical to maintaining normal neural function. Neurotoxicants may disrupt this relationship, by selectively or indiscriminately damaging either cell population. An assessment of neuronal and glial integrity is therefore critical to determining whether a chemical is a neurotoxicant.

Neurons are uniquely modified for the generation (excitability), transmission (conductivity), and storage of electrical messages. Neurons are classified using anatomical location (e.g., hippocampal, striatal), primary neurotransmitter (e.g., cholinergic, dopaminergic), morphology (e.g., granule, pyramidal), or function (e.g., motor, sensory). The typical neuron has four morphologically-distinct regions: dendrites; the soma (cell body); axons; and axon terminals. The distal axon has numerous branches, each ending in a presynaptic terminal that contacts the receptive surface of adjacent cells using a chemical or an electrical stimulus. This contact point in the nervous system is the synapse, or in the periphery, the neuromuscular junction or the surface of another effector cell. Morphologic changes in neurons induced by toxicant exposure include cytoplasmic swelling, chromatolysis, accumulation of cytoplasmic filaments, and cell death.

The glia are the predominant cell type in the nervous system, comprising up to 70% of the population. Glial cells have many functions, including neuronal support and maintenance, myelin production, and phagocytosis. Recent research has focused on glia as part of the immune system, with an important role in inflammation via generation of cytokines, as well as their role in modulating neuronal interaction. Three classes of CNS neuroglia have been identified: astrocytes; oligodendrocytes; and microglia. Astrocytes serve support roles, similar to those of connective tissues in other organs, and may be regarded as interstitial cells of the central nervous system. Protoplasmic (type 1) astrocytes are located primarily in cerebral gray matter, while fibrous (type 2) astrocytes are found within white matter tracts. They guide the movements of migratory neurons during development, are required for the formation and maintenance of

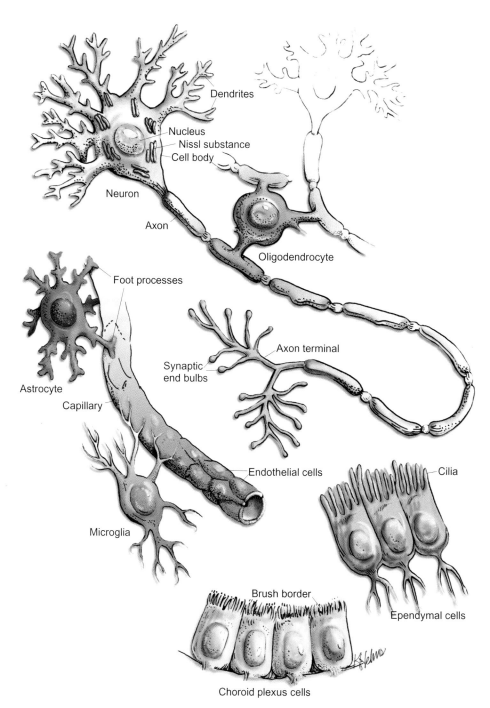

FIGURE 13.2   Cell types in the central nervous system include neurons, astrocytes, oligodendroglia, microglia, ependymal cells, choroid plexus epithelial cells, and vascular endothelial cells. (Courtesy of Dr J.F. Zachary, College of Veterinary Medicine, University of Illinois. Reproduced with permission from Zachary, J.F. (2007). Nervous System. In *Pathologic Basis of Veterinary Disease*, McGavin, M., and Zachary, J.F. eds, 4th edn. Mosby Elsevier, St. Louis. Figure 14-1, p. 834.)

the blood–brain barrier, and play a critical role in the repair process. Astrocytes are also important in glycogen metabolism, scavenge released amino acid and monoamine transmitters, and regulate brain volume by removing potassium and other ions from the extracellular space. Type 2 astrocytes are involved in detoxification of ammonia. Oligodendrocytes in the CNS and their PNS counterparts (Schwann cells) produce myelin, which insulates larger diameter axons and facilitates high-speed nerve conduction

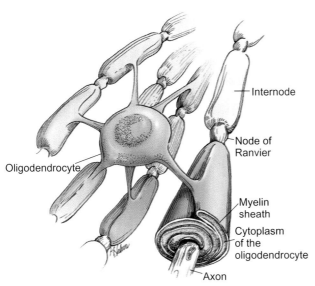

FIGURE 13.3   As depicted in this illustration, each oligodendrocyte sends out numerous cytoplasmic processes that repetitively encircle (myelinate) the portion of an axon between two nodes of Ranvier (internode) on the same and several different axons. Direct or indirect injury to an oligodendrocyte can result in "demyelination" of those internodes myelinated by that oligodendrocyte. This injury will slow the rate of conduction of an action potential, and depending on the site of the lesion may lead to clinical signs of neuronal dysfunction (ataxia, proprioception deficits). (Courtesy of Dr J.F. Zachary, College of Veterinary Medicine, University of Illinois. Reproduced with permission from Zachary, J.F. (2007). Nervous System. In *Pathologic Basis of Veterinary Disease*, McGavin, M., and Zachary, J.F. eds, 4th edn. Mosby Elsevier, St. Louis. Figure 14-14A, p. 845.)

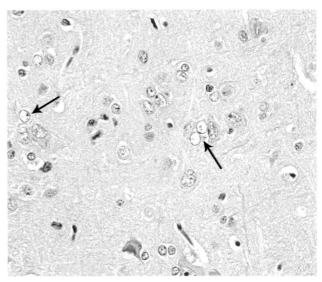

FIGURE 13.4   Formation of Alzheimer type II astrocytes in response to hepatic encephalopathy. Astrocyte nuclei (arrows) are enlarged and vesicular, and often observed in pairs.

(Figure 13.3). Microglial cells have phagocytic actions and act as the CNS macrophage.

Morphologic changes in astrocytes induced by neurotoxic injury include cytoplasmic swelling, hypertrophy, accumulation of glycogen granules, an increased number of cytoplasmic filaments (chiefly glial fibrillary acidic protein, GFAP), and altered arrangement of cellular processes. Interestingly, these astrocytic responses may be observed at sites distant from the area of direct injury. Astrocyte proliferation (astrogliosis) is commonly observed following exposure to kainic acid, 1-methyl-4-phenyl-1,2,3,6-terahydropyridine (MPTP), methamphetamine, trimethyl tin, ethanol, and heavy metals. In experimental lead encephalopathy, astrocytes are swollen and the nuclei may contain electron-dense intranuclear inclusions. The typical oligodendroglial response to toxicants is swelling, while microglia react to toxicant-induced injury by proliferating, enlarging, and altering their cellular proteins to include elements used in their phagocytic activities.

In some species, an acute astrocytic reaction in response to the metabolic disturbance that occurs in hepatic and renal (uremic) encephalopathy is the formation of Alzheimer type II cells (Figure 13.4). The nucleus becomes enlarged and vesicular, and the cytoplasm may swell and become visible. Paired nuclei are often seen. Hepatic encephalopathy occurs due to increased blood ammonia concentration secondary to severe hepatic dysfunction, e.g., with pyrrolizidine hepatotoxicity in cattle and horses.

Specialized Anatomical Features

Blood–Brain Barrier

Protection from some potential toxicants is afforded by the blood–brain barrier (BBB) in the CNS, and a similar blood–neural barrier present in the PNS. The anatomic basis of the blood–brain barrier is thought to reside in specialized microvascular endothelial cells, which decrease the capillary wall permeability due to their tight intercellular junctions, lack of fenestrae, and low endocytotic activity. Astrocytes, whose foot processes encircle the abluminal surfaces of capillaries, are critical for the induction, maintenance, and repair of the blood–brain barrier (Figure 13.5). Transport of xenobiotics to the brain is influenced by the metabolic functions of the blood–brain barrier. For example, D-glucose transporters in the blood–brain barrier actively facilitate transport of glucose to the CNS; comparable carriers also exist for certain amino acids. P-glycoproteins, expressed at the luminal surface of the capillary endothelial cells, impart additional protection by acting as an efflux pump to remove certain xenobiotics from the brain. These include drugs such as avermectins, loperamide, quinidine, cyclosporine A, doxorubicin, and *Vinca* alkaloids.

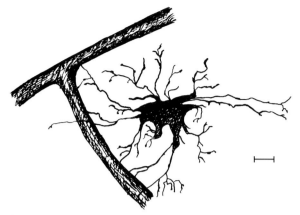

FIGURE 13.5 Fibrous astrocyte in corpus callosum with processes on capillary inducing the blood–brain barrier; four-week-old rat. Golgi stain. Bar = 20 μm.

Dogs, such as collies, that have a multi-drug resistance (MDRI) gene defect, have dysfunctional P-glycoprotein, allowing toxic concentrations of ivermectin to accumulate in the brain. Some drugs (e.g., cyclosporine A, ketoconazole, and tamoxifen) can inhibit p-glycoprotein action, resulting in substrate toxicosis.

Certain neural regions (e.g., spinal and autonomic ganglia, the circumventricular organs) lack a functional blood–brain barrier and may, therefore, be exposed to higher levels of blood-borne neurotoxicants. The blood–brain barrier is incompletely developed at birth, thereby providing access to the infant brain for neurotoxicants that would normally be excluded from the adult brain. Lipophilic toxicants readily cross the blood–brain barrier, while hydrophilic agents cannot.

Under pathologic conditions, such as trauma, ischemia, or following toxicant exposure, an increase in blood–brain barrier permeability may occur that allows plasma constituents to escape into the brain tissue. This "opening" of the blood–brain barrier may, at least in part, be due to a massive release of autacoids, which act as mediators of vasogenic brain edema. Most of the ultrafiltrate released during vasogenic edema accumulates in the white matter, due to the greater physical compliance of this region. Astrocytic swelling also commonly occurs in vasogenic edema. Examples of agents that induce vasogenic edema include triethyl tin, lead, arachidonic acid, and kainic acid toxicity. Grossly, the gyri are flattened and the sulci narrowed, the white matter is moist and swollen. The chief microscopic features are rarefaction of the white matter, and pallor.

Choroid Plexus

The choroid plexus constitutes a barrier between the blood and the cerebrospinal fluid (CSF). It is found along the floor of the lateral ventricles, and on the roof of the third and fourth ventricles. Ependymal cells line the brain ventricles and the neural canal, and facilitate the movement of CSF. The choroid plexus represents approximately 1% of the total brain weight. In spite of its small mass, the choroid plexus has a large surface area (~50% of the blood–brain barrier surface area), which provides for filtration and active production of CSF. The choroid plexus plays a critical role in the transport of many chemicals out of the brain (i.e., from CSF to blood). Many metals (e.g., cadmium, lead, manganese, mercury) accumulate in the choroid plexus at concentrations greater than those found in the CSF and brain tissues. This accumulation of metals may result in both structural and functional changes within the choroid plexus.

Select Functions and Neurotoxicity

The Action Potential

The primary function of the neuron is to generate action potentials, a large depolarizing signal that is the medium of signal conduction. At rest, cytoplasmic potassium levels inside the neuron are high, relative to those of the extracellular milieu. Sodium ion concentrations, however, are higher in extracellular than in intracellular fluids. The action potential is generated in an all-or-nothing fashion by the influx of sodium ions through voltage-dependent sodium channels. Depolarization also results in the opening of voltage-dependent potassium channels, and the efflux of potassium ions. Sodium channels subsequently close, thereby decreasing membrane sodium conductance, and inactivating the action potential. Potassium transfer brings the membrane potential back to its resting state. The original "resting" sodium and potassium equilibrium potentials are re-established, primarily by the action of the energy-dependent sodium and potassium pumps.

The normal functioning of ion channels is thus critical to normal neurophysiology. Many toxicants alter normal transmission of the action potential, including pyrethrin and pyrethroid insecticides, the marine toxins, tetrodotoxin and saxitoxin, and the cyclodiene organochlorine insecticides (e.g., dichloro-diphenyl-trichloroethane (DDT)). For example, the type I pyrethroids (allethrin and tetramethrin) prolong nerve membrane sodium influx, decrease peak sodium current, and decrease steady state potassium efflux. The type I pyrethroids appear to modify sodium channels at their resting or closed states, so that they open more slowly than normal. Agents affecting ion channels often may induce neurotoxicity in the absence of morphologic changes visible by light microscopy.

Among the diverse metabolic activities of the neuron, ATP-dependent ion pumping requires the most energy to maintain the ionic concentration gradients needed for normal neuronal membrane potentials. The most important ion pump in this respect is the sodium-potassium ATPase, which consumes 40% to 60% of all brain ATP. The oxygen consumption rate of neurons is approximately ten-fold greater than that of glia, which likely contributes to the greater sensitivity of neurons to hypoxia-induced damage. Many neurotoxicants poison energy metabolism by targeting mitochondrial cytochrome oxidase or sodium/potassium ATPase. Both hydrogen sulfide and cyanide induce cellular hypoxia by inhibiting cytochrome oxidase and other oxidative enzymes. Following subacute exposure to cyanide, necrotic lesions develop within the striatum and basal ganglia, while some cortical neurons undergo apoptosis. Initially, cyanide acts at the N-methyl-D-aspartate (NMDA) glutamate receptor system to activate a series of intraneuronal signaling cascades, resulting in excessive production of reactive oxygen species and nitric oxide. These products then produce oxidative stress, and eventually cell injury.

Cyanide

Terms such as cyanide, hydrocyanic acid, hydrogen cyanide (HCN), and prussic acid all relate to the same toxic principle. Cyanide is used industrially (electroplating, mirror manufacture), and as a rodenticide and fumigant. Cyanogenic glycosides, which can form HCN by hydrolysis, are present in fruit seeds (apple, apricot, peach, wild cherry, and bitter almond), and some plant species, including *Sorghum* sp and cassava. All animal species are susceptible to cyanide toxicosis. Ruminants are at special risk from cyanogenic glycosides, since hydrolysis can rapidly occur via rumen microorganisms. Acute cyanide poisoning, resulting in death within minutes, is no different from acute fatal CO poisoning. Congestion and petechial hemorrhage are the main lesions. Occasional survivors for 24–36 hours reveal softening of the globus pallidus, based on neuronal necrosis. Chronic cyanide neuropathy may occur in humans following long-term consumption of tropical lima beans and cassava root. In addition to neuronopathies, myelinopathies have also been produced experimentally with cyanide in a number of species including rodents, cats, dogs, and monkeys. The earliest lesions appear within 3–4 hours of exposure, and are florid 2–4 days later.

Mechanisms

The lesions are explained on the basis of histotoxic anoxia or cellular hypoxia, due to inhibition of cytochrome oxidase, the terminal enzyme in the electron transport chain that uses O_2 derived from oxyhemoglobin. The cyanide ion, in combination with ferric (trivalent) iron of the cytochrome oxidase system, blocks electron transport and molecular oxygen transfer from oxyhemoglobin to tissues. This results in a bright red color in venous blood.

Neurotransmitters and Their Receptors

The major form of interneuronal communication is mediated via release of chemical neurotransmitters at synapses. Neurotransmitters are released in a calcium-dependent manner from the presynaptic nerve terminal of a stimulated neuron. They cross the synaptic cleft, and bind to specific membrane receptors on the postsynaptic neuron, thereby inciting a depolarizing or polarizing postsynaptic potential. Synaptic integration of all inhibitory and excitatory postsynaptic potentials on a neuron's membrane determines the timing and strength of the action potential. Neurotransmitters are a diverse group of chemicals, over a hundred in number, including simple amines (e.g., dopamine), amino acids (e.g., δ-aminobutyric acid or GABA), and polypeptides (e.g., enkephalins). Many axon terminals contain more than one neurotransmitter, although each is stored in separate vesicles. Changes in neurotransmitter levels or their receptors may occur as a consequence of, or as compensation for, toxicant exposure. There are a number of sites at which toxicants can effect neurotransmitter synthesis, release, or function.

Depending on the class and relative amounts of the neurotransmitter and receptor, synaptic transmission may result in either depolarization (excitation) or hyperpolarization (inhibition) of the postsynaptic neuron. Excitatory neurotransmitters include acetylcholine, norepinephrine, substance-P, glutamate, and aspartate. Stimulation of excitatory neurotransmission may produce CNS excitation (e.g., acetylcholine-induced tremors), while its inhibition may result in decreased function (e.g., curare-induced paralysis, sodium pentobarbital-induced depression). Inhibitory neurotransmitters include GABA, serotonin, glycine, and β-endorphin. Abrogation of inhibitory neurotransmission may result in CNS stimulation or seizures (e.g., strychnine or penitrem A inhibition of glycine neurotransmission). Conversely, stimulation of inhibitory neurotransmitters may produce CNS depression (e.g., ivermectin-enhanced GABA function).

Acetylcholine

Acetylcholine (ACh) was the first neurotransmitter to be identified. ACh is synthesized from acetyl-CoA

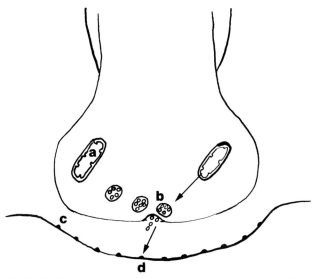

FIGURE 13.6   Neuromuscular junction with acetylcholine liberated from vesicles (b) into synapse (c) to bind to postsynaptic receptors (d). The process requires Ca^{2+} stored in mitochondria (a).

and choline by choline acetyltransferase. Following synthesis, ACh functions at the following sites: (1) all preganglionic nerve terminals of the autonomic nervous system; (2) all postganglionic parasympathetic nerve terminals; (3) the neuromuscular junction (Figure 13.6); (4) the adrenal medulla; (5) the CNS; and (6) the postganglionic sympathetic nerve terminal at sweat glands. Cholinergic muscarinic receptors are linked to second messenger systems via G proteins (so-called metabotropic receptors), and ACh binding causes stimulation of the parasympathetic nervous system. Nicotinic receptors form ion channels (i.e., ionotropic receptors), and are located at the neuromuscular junction of skeletal muscles, at all ganglia of the autonomic nervous system, in the adrenal medulla, and in the CNS. The brief action of ACh in the synaptic cleft is assured by the rapid acetylcholinesterase-catalyzed hydrolysis of ACh into choline and acetate. Along with its potential as a target site for certain neurotoxicants, acetylcholinesterase activity has also been used as a marker for cholinergic neurons. In addition, choline acetyltransferase immunohistochemistry can also be used to visualize chemical-induced damage to cholinergic neurons.

Organophosphorus and Carbamate Insecticides

These are potent inhibitors of acetylcholinesterase, and produce muscarinic (salivation, lacrimation, bronchial secretion, vomiting, diarrhea), nicotinic (tremors, respiratory paralysis), and CNS (seizures, miosis, hyperactivity) effects in all species. Carbamate insecticides are reversible acetylcholinesterase inhibitors, while organophosphorus insecticides bind covalently to the enzyme, resulting in irreversible inhibition. Recovery is therefore dependent on the resynthesis of acetylcholinesterase. Tolerance to some cholinergic effects of cholinesterase-inhibiting compounds may be due to compensatory down-regulation of muscarinic receptors. Measurement of whole blood, brain, or retinal acetylcholinesterase activity is diagnostically useful in cases in which an exposure to an organophosphorus or carbamate insecticide may have occurred.

Interestingly, in addition to the acute effects of organophosphorus insecticides, some compounds (e.g., phosphoramidates, phosphonates) are associated with the development of organophosphate-induced delayed polyneuropathy (OPIDP), characterized by central-peripheral distal axonopathy ("dying back polyneuropathy"). Large diameter myelinated fibers are more susceptible than small diameter fibers which, in turn, are more susceptible than unmyelinated fibers. Hens are particularly susceptible to this condition and, thus, are often used as a test species. The appearance of clinical signs is delayed for several weeks after exposure. When this rare syndrome is encountered clinically, it is characterized by ataxia, hindlimb hypermetria, depressed conscious proprioception, weakness, and an ascending paralysis. Although controversial, the postulated mechanism of action in the development of OPIDP involves the phosphorylation of a second class of esterase, neuropathy target esterase (NTE). Inhibition of NTE is necessary, but not sufficient, evidence of the potential to produce OPIDP.

Botulinum Toxin

Botulism, caused by botulinum toxins (A–G) produced by *Clostridium botulinum*, has been recognized in humans and animals for nearly 200 years. Sources of the toxins include food contaminated by preformed toxin or clostridial spores, contamination of a puncture wound by spores, or ingestion of spores from the environment. In humans, most occurrences follow consumption of contaminated canned food, smoked fish (Japan), and pickled meat. In animals, the disease has been known as "limberneck" in chickens and wild ducks, and "lamsiekte" (South Africa), loin disease, bulbar paralysis, and alkali disease in cattle. The disease is characterized by a progressively increasing flaccid paralysis, starting with visual impairment, weakness, and difficulty swallowing (bulbar paralysis). Death occurs in 3–10 days, and is usually caused by respiratory paralysis. There are no lesions other than those attributable to anoxia.

Mechanisms

Botulinum toxins bind to synaptotagmin, a presynaptic vesicle protein affecting cholinergic synapses by impairing the release of acetylcholine. This action is specifically presynaptic, a blockage of exocytosis of transmitter at active zones. Local administration of acetylcholine is, therefore, able to overcome the effects of botulinum toxin. The CNS is not affected, because the molecule is too large to pass the blood–brain barrier.

Monoamines

The principal catecholamines are norepinephrine, epinephrine and dopamine. These compounds are formed from phenylalanine and tyrosine. Tyrosine is synthesized in the liver, and transported to catecholamine-secreting neurons where it is converted to dopamine. Depending on the neuronal class, dopamine may be used as a neurotransmitter, or further metabolism may occur to form norepinephrine, and finally epinephrine. Catecholamines exhibit PNS excitatory and inhibitory effects, as well as CNS actions such as respiratory stimulation and increased psychomotor activity. Norepinephrine has been identified as the neurotransmitter released by most postganglionic sympathetic nerves (stress, fright, fight, or flight reaction), the adrenal medulla (released in association with epinephrine), and within the CNS. Catecholamine action is terminated by presynaptic uptake and the action of monoamine oxidase (MAO), diffusion from the synapse, and degradation by catecholamine-O-methyltransferase (COMT) present in the synaptic cleft. The catecholamines bind to two different classes of receptors termed the α- and β-adrenergic receptors. The adrenergic receptors are classical transmembrane receptors that couple to intracellular G-proteins. Catecholaminergic neurons may be demonstrated by molecular histology techniques to demonstrate tyrosine hydroxylase (the rate-limiting enzyme in catecholamine synthesis).

Dopaminergic neurons within the substantia nigra play a critical role in the pathogenesis of certain neurological conditions, such as Parkinson's disease and schizophrenia. Dopaminergic neurons primarily synapse with striatal neurons, while additional axons project to the frontal cortex, cingulate cortex, nucleus accumbens, and olfactory tubercle. Aside from controlling movement, dopamine is also involved in feelings of reward, alertness, and purposeful behavior. Many drugs of abuse (e.g., cocaine, heroin, amphetamine, alcohol, and nicotine) elevate synaptic levels of dopamine, and increase locomotor activity in animals. Cocaine increases dopamine concentrations by preventing dopamine reuptake, while amphetamine stimulates dopamine release. There are two major subfamilies of dopamine receptor, D1-like and D2-like, which have different biochemical and pharmacological properties, and mediate different physiological functions. Both D1 and D2 receptor subtypes are G-proteins, but different G-proteins and effectors are involved in their signaling pathways.

Serotonin (5-hydroxytryptamine or 5-HT) is another CNS monoamine neurotransmitter. It is synthesized by the hydroxylation and decarboxylation of L-tryptophan. Serotonin is widely distributed throughout the CNS. Functional roles include the regulation of mood, motor activity, feeding and hunger, thermoregulation, sleep, and possibly some neuroendocrine control mechanisms in the hypothalamus. Multiple 5-HT receptors have been identified, and extensive evidence suggests that 5-HT receptors have a role in learning and memory. The concentration of synaptic 5-HT is controlled directly by its reuptake into the pre-synaptic terminal. Most 5-HT receptors are coupled to G-proteins (metabotropic), however, some are ionotropic.

Gamma-Aminobutyric Acid (GABA)

GABA is the major inhibitory neurotransmitter in the brain. It is formed by the decarboxylation of glutamate, catalyzed by glutamate decarboxylase. GABAergic neurons are located in the substantia gelatinosa of the dorsal horn of the spinal cord, the retina, and multiple brain regions with highest concentrations in the hypothalamus, hippocampus, and basal ganglia. Most GABA receptors are associated with inhibitory interneurons with short axonal processes, although some associated long-axon pathways within the brain are known. If GABA function is impaired, then convulsions, tetany, and spastic disorders may result. GABA exerts its effects by binding to two distinct receptors, GABA$_A$ (ionotropic) and GABA$_B$ (metabotropic). The GABA$_A$ receptors form a chloride ion channel, binding of GABA to the receptor results in increased chloride conductance of presynaptic neurons yielding hyperpolarization. The GABA$_B$ receptors are coupled to an intracellular G-protein, and act by increasing conductance of an associated potassium channel.

Glycine

Glycine is an important postsynaptic inhibitory neurotransmitter in small inhibitory interneurons in the brain stem, and in Renshaw cells of the ventral horn of the spinal cord. Glycine is probably involved in the regulation of spinal and brainstem reflexes. Like the GABA$_A$ receptor, the glycine receptor forms a chloride ion channel and its activation results in hyperpolarization. Strychnine- and penitrem A-induced seizures are mediated through the ability to antagonize glycine. Tetanus toxin induces seizures by inhibiting the release of glycine.

Tetanus Toxin

Tetanus was originally recognized by Hippocrates. Its cause was later defined to be a toxin (tetanospasmin), isolated a century ago, which is produced by *Clostridium tetani*. The toxin is produced in anaerobic wounds infected with *Clostridium tetani*, and binds to myoneural junctions or sensory receptors. It reaches the CNS by retrograde transport along axons within spinal nerves, and binds to axosomatic synapses (presynaptic terminals) in the spinal cord and brain stem. Since the interneuronal synapses are mostly inhibitory, the balance is changed in favor of excitation. Thus, clinical signs are characterized by trismus, tonic spasms, opisthotonus, rigidity, and tetanic seizures. The spasms are precipitated by the slightest sensory stimulations. Mortality in humans is 50–60%. Among domestic animals, horses are the most sensitive species. Causes of death include respiratory failure, aspiration pneumonia, and shock. There are no consistent lesions.

Mechanisms

Tetanospasmin prevents Ca^{2+}-dependent release of glycine, an inhibitory neurotransmitter from CNS neurons, resulting in unopposed excitation of spinal neurons and muscle contraction. Cerebral neurons are spared, because the toxin does not reach cortical neurons by the ascending axonal transport, and does not pass the blood–brain barrier to gain access from the bloodstream. Sympathetic discharges may also be affected, leading to fluctuation in pulse and blood pressure. Unless the condition can be stabilized, death will usually occur within 5–10 days due to the inability of muscles of respiration to relax, and subsequent hypoxia. All species are susceptible, with horses often affected.

Strychnine

Strychnine is a highly-toxic alkaloid, obtained primarily from *Strychnos nux-vomica*. Animal poisonings are usually malicious, and are occasionally caused by exposure to strychnine-containing rodenticides and insecticides. The clinical signs consist of intermittent tonic spasms and seizures precipitated by noise and other external stimuli that can occur within 10–120 minutes of ingestion. The spinal cord shows the most marked stimulation.

Mechanisms

Strychnine binds to glycine receptors of synaptic membranes. It antagonizes the hyperpolarizing action of glycine, a major inhibitory neurotransmitter.

Glutamate

Glutamate is the main excitatory neurotransmitter in the brain. Most brain neurons contain one or more glutamate receptor subtypes, some of which are ionotropic (e.g., NMDA, alpha-amino-3-hydroxy-5-methyl-4-isoxazole propionic acid (AMPA), and kainate subtypes), while others are metabotropic. Glutamate receptors are involved in memory formation. The action of glutamate is terminated by reuptake into the axon terminals and glial cells.

Excess glutamate induces a cascade of effects, leading to increased intracellular calcium concentration, excitotoxicity, and neuronal death. Cerebral ischemia, head and spinal cord injury, and prolonged seizure activity are associated with excessive release of glutamate into the extracellular space, leading subsequently to neurotoxicity. In addition, glutamate-induced excitotoxicity is thought to play a critical role in the development of neurodegenerative conditions, such as Huntington's disease, Parkinson's disease, and amyotrophic lateral sclerosis (ALS). Many neuronal excitotoxins (e.g., quisqualic, domoic, and kainic acids) are glutamate receptor agonists. The regions of the brain affected by glutamate are not protected by the blood–brain barrier.

Systemic administration of high glutamate or aspartate doses to infant mice, rats, or hamsters damages arcuate neurons, yielding a neuroendocrine-hypothalamic deficiency syndrome that includes growth retardation, obesity, and reproductive failure. Many excitotoxins also target brain areas (hippocampus, cerebral cortex, striatum, and cerebellum) that are highly-innervated by glutamatergic afferent fibers. In addition, the hippocampus also has a high density of glutamate receptors, thereby further predisposing it to excitotoxicity. Infant rodents are more vulnerable to excitotoxic damage than are adults, with parenteral administration of these amino acids leading to acute convulsions and retinal damage. In general, administration of NMDA antagonists ameliorates the neurotoxicity.

Domoic Acid

Domoic acid, a glutamate analog, is the cause of amnesic shellfish poisoning (ASP) in humans; it also causes death (acute toxicity) or neurologic disease (chronic toxicity) in marine mammals. It is produced by *Chondria armata* (red macroalgae) and *Pseudo-nitzschia* spp (diatoms), and commonly accumulates in mussels and other shellfish worldwide. Affected mussels off the eastern Canadian coast killed hippocampal neurons in humans. Similar lesions were produced experimentally in nonhuman primates and rodents. The lesions are described as selective injury initially affecting the dendrites, a so-called "dendrosomatotoxic" or "axon-sparing" reaction. The toxin has a high affinity for binding to the kainate receptor (a glutamate receptor subtype), thus exerting its excitatory and cytotoxic effects on hippocampal cells. Neuronal cell death follows the influx of Ca^{2+} ions, and up-regulation of the C-FOS gene.

MECHANISMS OF DISEASE AND CLASSIFICATION OF NEUROTOXIC DISEASES

Toxicological effects are dependent on the concentration of chemicals within the target organ, and on the duration of exposure. Several pharmacokinetic processes (absorption, distribution, metabolism, and excretion) govern chemical disposition in the nervous system. Several unique features of the nervous system further influence disposition, and thus modulate chemical neurotoxicity. For example, the blood–brain barrier limits the distribution of many compounds to the CNS, acting to exclude highly protein-bound and water-soluble agents, while freely passing many lipophilic chemicals. Access to the CNS may be enhanced by transport systems, such as those in the choroid plexus, for many metals. Neural compartmentalization, such as site-specific chemical binding to tissue macromolecules and metabolic processes are other important determinants, especially in instances where xenobiotic metabolites mediate neurotoxicity. The limited metabolic capacity of neural cells for many chemicals often delays xenobiotic elimination. For interspecies extrapolation, determinants important in chemical disposition to and within the CNS must be identified, so that their variation across species and individuals can be measured. Extrapolation of test results between species is aided considerably by toxicokinetic data for a particular agent in multiple species (including humans).

Neurotoxic agents can be classified by their cellular target sites, neuropathologic effects, or mode of action. These classification schemes have certain inherent disadvantages. For example, severe toxicant-induced axonal degeneration may also result in secondary demyelination and neuronal loss. Agents that disrupt vascular integrity may lead secondarily to the development of edema (e.g., mercury). Clearly, no one classification scheme will satisfy all needs. Therefore, we have selected several prototypical neurotoxicants to illustrate common cellular target sites and neuropathologic effects of chemicals. Table 13.1 lists common neurotoxicants and specific targets, while Table 13.2 lists selected toxicants that affect animals, their mechanism and lesions induced.

Neuronopathies

The target site for toxic agents producing neuronopathies is the neuron cell body (Figure 13.7A). Damage to the neuron progresses through various stages, including chromatolysis (Figure 13.7B), and results in cell death and ultimately in axonal and dendritic breakdown. This secondary degeneration of neurites is often referred to as Wallerian degeneration (Figure 13.7C). Nerve terminal degeneration is a very subtle change that may not be detected by routine histopathology, but rather requires silver staining or neurotransmitter-specific immunohistochemistry. Axonal degeneration leads to secondary myelin sheath degeneration. Gliosis may occur in both the CNS and PNS in response to primary neuronal injury. Thus, direct injury to the neuron cell body will produce a cascade of pathological sequelae in many cell processes and cell types. Neuronopathies typically are readily evident on conventionally-prepared material (paraffin sections stained with hematoxylin and eosin, or a special neuronal stain such as Bielchowsky's or cresyl violet). These changes are generally irreversible.

Trimethyltin

One compound that induces relatively selective neurotoxicity is trimethyltin (TMT), a chemical used for various industrial and agricultural purposes, and as an antifungal agent. Humans exposed acutely to TMT develop a limbic-cerebellar neurological syndrome, characterized by hearing loss, disorientation, amnesia, aggressiveness, hyperphagia, disturbed sexual behavior, complex partial and tonic-clonic seizures, nystagmus, ataxia, and mild sensory neuropathy. Animals exposed to TMT develop similar signs. Neuropathologic evaluation of TMT-exposed humans and animals reveals degeneration, both in the granular neurons of the dentate gyrus and in the pyramidal cells in the hippocampus (Ammon's horn) (Figure 13.8). In animals, this lesion demonstrates species- and age-sensitivities, and may also be influenced by the dosage schedule.

Although the hippocampus is the primary site of action, TMT also damages other brain regions, including the neocortex, basal ganglia, cerebellum, brain stem,

TABLE 13.1   Common neurotoxicants and their specific neurological targets

Site of action	Neurotoxic change	Neurotoxic chemical
Neuron cell body	Neuronopathy	Doxorubicin Manganese Methylmercury Quinolinic acid Trimethyltin Vincristine
Nerve terminal	Terminal destruction	1-methyl-4-phenyl-1,2,3,6-terahydropyridine
Schwann cell and/or oligodendroglial myelin	Myelinopathy	Bromethalin Buckthorn neuropathy Carbon monoxide Coyotillo neuropathy Cuprizone® Hexachlorophene Isoniazid Lead Trialklytins
Central axons	Central axonopathy	Clioquinol
Proximal axon	Proximal axonopathy	ß,ß'-Iminodipropionitrile
Central-peripheral distal axon	Distal axonopathy	Acrylamide Carbon disulfide n-Hexane
Astrocytes	Astrocytic swelling (Alzheimer type II astrocytes) Astrocyte dysfunction	Ammonia Lead
Brain capillary	Capillary damage, cerebral edema	Arsenic

spinal cord, dorsal root ganglia, olfactory cortex, retina, and inner ear. TMT is increasingly exploited as a model neurotoxicant in rats to study the impact of chemical-induced altered hippocampal function on behavior.

Mechanism

The mechanism of TMT neuronopathy is not well-understood. Lesions induced by TMT have been proposed to result from neuronal hyperexcitation. Biochemical investigations reveal reductions in glutamate and GABA uptake and synthesis, as well as increased glutamate release in the hippocampus. The neuronal lesions and the targeted regions in TMT neuronopathy resemble those induced by prolonged seizures (e.g., status epilepticus), as well as other excitatory neurotoxicants.

Manganese

Another neuronotoxic agent that demonstrates regional selectivity is manganese. The most commonly recognized effect of this metal is manganism, an extrapyramidal movement disorder resembling Parkinson's disease that results from accumulation of manganese in the basal ganglia. Neurological manifestations of manganism include progressive bradykinesia, dystonia, and gait abnormalities. Severely affected patients often develop progressive, irreversible loss of dopaminergic neurons. Magnetic resonance imaging (MRI) of the brain may reveal signal changes in the globus pallidus, striatum, and midbrain. The primary site of neuropathological damage is the globus pallidus. Significant differences have been widely-documented regarding species-specific sensitivity to manganese neurotoxicity. For example, macaques develop a behavioral syndrome or neuropathological lesion comparable to that seen in manganese-poisoned humans, while rodents do not.

Mechanism

Regional localization of manganese in the basal ganglia of humans and monkeys may reflect the role of transferrin in the transport of manganese to the brain. Regions of highest brain manganese accumulation are efferent to those sites with the highest density of transferrin receptors. Another possible explanation for this primate-selective effect may reside in the high affinity of manganese for neuromelanin, the brain levels of which are low in rodents and highest in primates.

TABLE 13.2 Neuropathology and proposed mechanisms of selected toxicants in domestic animals and wildlife

Target	Agent	Source/use	Disease	Mechanisms	Lesion site/location/type	Other organ systems affected	Species
Neuronal cell body	Doxorubicin	Antineoplastic drug (Adriamycin)		DNA damage, interference with transcription	Sensory root and autonomic ganglia	Heart	Cats especially sensitive
Neuronal cell body	Mercury, organic	Methyl mercury in fish from industrial contamination.	Minimata disease (humans); mercury toxicosis	Binds to sulfhydryl ligands in critical membrane sites or enzyme complexes	Occipital cortex (neurons) and cerebellum (granule cells)	Kidney	Humans, cats
		Organic salts e.g., alkyl mercurial fungicides	Mercury toxicosis		As above Fibrinoid necrosis of leptomeningeal arteries, brain and spinal cord	Kidney, heart (Purkinje fiber degeneration), reproductive	Pigs, horses, sheep cattle, cats, humans
Neuronal cell body	Domoic acid	Some algae and diatom, *Pseudo-nitzschia* spp, accumulated by shellfish	Amnesic shellfish poisoning (ASP, humans), demoic acid toxicosis (wildlife)	Exogenous excitotoxicity due to excessive glutamate receptor activation. Binds to kainate receptor	Limbic system, hippocampus, dentate gyrus (sea lions)	Retina, heart	Humans, marine mammals Rodents experimentally
Neuronal cell body	Repin or other sesquiterpene lactones	Plant: *Centaurea solstitialis* (yellow star thistle) or *C. repens* (Russian knapweed)	Equine nigropallidal encephalomalacia (yellow star thistle poisoning)	Oxidative damage	Globus pallidus and substantia nigra Yellowish discoloration due to coagulation necrosis (malacia)		Horses
Neuronal cell body	Swainsonine (indolizidine alkaloid)	Plant: *Astralagus, Oxytropis* (USA) and *Swainsona* (Australia) spp	Locoism (lysosomal storage disorder)	Inhibition of lysosomal α-mannosidase and Golgi mannosidase II resulting in mannosidiosis	Microvesiculation of neurons and pericytes	Kidney; liver, spleen, macrophages/reticular cells, lymphoid tissue	Ruminants, horses
Neuronal cell body	*Clostridium botulinum* type C	Pasture	Grass sickness, equine dysautonomia		Autonomic ganglia, selected CNS nuclei (e.g., oculomotor, facial, vestibular, dorsal motor nuclei): neuronal necrosis, satellite cell proliferation	Gastrointestinal tract (colic)	Equidae, hares
Neuronal cell body		Plant: *Solanum* spp, e.g., *S. kwebense*	Solanum toxicosis, maldronksiekte		Cerebellar cortex and medulla, brain stem Neuronal (especially Purkinje cell) vacuolation		Cattle, goats
Axons	Vincristine	Antineoplastic drug (periwinkle plant, *Vinca rosea* or *Catharanthus rosea*)	Vincristine neuropathy	Binds to tubulin, disrupts fast axonal transport	PNS	Bone marrow, kidney, gastrointestinal tract	Cats especially susceptible, dogs

(Continued)

TABLE 13.2 (Continued)

Target	Agent	Source/use	Disease	Mechanisms	Lesion site/location/type	Other organ systems affected	Species
Axons	Neurotoxic agents include tullidinol	Plant: *Karwinsia humboldtiana* (Coyotillo, buckthorn)	Coyotillo (buckthorn) polyneuropathy, limber leg	Uncouple oxidative phosphorylation	Peripheral neuropathy		Ruminants, pigs, horses, chickens, children
Axons	Metronidazole	Anti-bacterial/protozoan drug			Vestibulocerebellar axonal swelling and brain stem leukomalacia. Sensory peripheral neuropathy, myelinated fibers		Cats, dogs, monkeys
Axons	Chronic organophosphate exposure (especially triaryl phosphates) e.g., diazinon, leptophos, merphos, malathion, parathion, trichlorphon, triorthocresyl phosphate	Pesticides, herbicides, lubricant oils	Delayed neuropathy (OP-induced delayed polyneuropathy, OPIDP)	Inhibition of neuropathy target esterase (NTE) Actin and tubulin affected. Mediation by acetylcholine	Distal axonopathy Spinal cord and caudal brain stem Long, large diameter ascending and descending axons		Humans, cats, pigs, ruminants, horses, sheep, chickens (used as animal model), ducks, pheasants
Axons		Plant: *Hypochoeris radicata, Taraxacum officinale, Malva parviflora* (Australian or European dandelion, mallow respectively), in some geographic areas	Stringhalt		Peripheral distal axonopathy of longest peripheral nerves	Larynx, muscle (denervation atrophy)	Horses (hindlimb hyperflexion)
Myelin	Arsenic, organic, pentavalent	Arsenicals, feed additives, growth promotants		Uncouple oxidative phosphorylation	Demyelination of optic nerves (arsanilic acid), posterior spinal cord (3-nitro), peripheral nerves		Pigs
Myelin	Hexachlorophene	Historically, antibacterial dermal solution		Uncouple oxidative phosphorylation	Intramyelinic edema		Children, young dogs and cats
Myelin	Bromethalin	Rodenticides (e.g., Assault, Vengeance, Sudden death)		Uncouple oxidative phosphorylation	Intramyelinic edema		Cats especially, dogs

Cell type	Agent	Source	Disease/Syndrome	Mechanism	Lesion	Target organ	Species
Astrocytes	Hyperammonemia	Pyrrolizidine alkaloids, others include lantana, lupinosis, NSAIDs, cycad palms which induce severe hepatotoxicity	Hepatic and renal encephalopathy, colonic dysbacteriosis (horses)	Multifactorial Metabolism of ammonia by astrocytic enzymes, glutamine synthetase and dehyrogenase	Alzheimer type II astrocytosis. Groups of astrocytes with clear swollen nuclei / White matter spongiosis—cytotoxic edema (except horses). See Figure 13.4.	Liver	Horses, ruminants, other
	Thallium (chronic)	Fungicide, pesticide, rodenticide	Thallium toxicoses	Tl^+ binds to K^+ in Na^+/K^+-ATPase or Tl binding to sulfhydral groups	Cerebrum, cerebellum: neuronal changes, edema Axons (?): peripheral and cranial nerves	Gastrointestinal tract, respiratory, skin	
Schwann cells	Lead (chronic)	Contamination of pasture	As above	Schwann cell (peripheral nervous system)	Polyneuropathy, cranial and peripheral nerves		Horses mainly (laryngeal hemiplegia)
Astrocytes and neurons	Lead (acute, subacute)	Car batteries, lead paint, linoleum	Lead toxicosis, plumbism (humans)	Probably multifactorial: dysruption of Ca^{2+} homeostasis, apoptosis, oxidative stress	No change to laminar necrosis of gray matter Cerebral cortex, early changes in tips of gyri	Kidney (intranuclear inclusions), hematopoietic system (anemia), etc.	Cattle mainly, dogs, other
Astrocytes	Sulfur (also sulfates, sulfides)	Feed (plants, corn coproducts) or water	Polioencephalomalacia		As acute lead toxicity, or thiamine deficiency		Cattle
Astrocytes	Thiaminase	Plant: *Aquilinium pteridium* (bracken fern)—experimental	Polioencephalomalacia	Oxidative stress, as thiamine deficiency	As thiamine deficiency		Horses
Astrocytes		Fish diet (cats, farmed foxes and mink; high temperature in feed preparation (dogs); food preservation with sulfur dioxide (cats and dogs)	Thiamine deficiency encephalopathy, Chastek paralysis (fox)	Oxidative stress, as thiamine deficiency	Brain stem nuclei, especially caudal colliculi		Cats, dogs, farmed foxes and mink
Astrocytes	High levels of concentrates, e.g., carbohydrates, molasses, urea	Feed	Polioencephalomalacia	Alteration of rumen microflora altering available thiamine	As thiamine deficiency		Cattle
Astrocytes	Amprolium	Coccidiostat	Polioencephalomalacia	Thiamine antagonist	As thiamine deficiency		Young ruminants
		Plant: *Sorghum* spp, hybrid strain	Equine cystitis ataxia syndrome		Diffuse nerve fiber degeneration in lateral and ventral funiculi of spinal cord and brain stem	Cystitis in horses	Horses, cattle

(Continued)

TABLE 13.2 (Continued)

Target	Agent	Source/use	Disease	Mechanisms	Lesion site/location/type	Other organ systems affected	Species
Astrocyte, Vasculature ?	Sodium chloride	Feed/water: generally indirect toxicosis due to imbalance of salt intake and water availability (water deprivation)	Salt poisoning, water deprivation syndrome	Hyperosmolarity (hypernatremia) due to excessive salt	Laminar necrosis: cerebral cortex (especially dorsolateral cortex) Eosinophil influx (pigs only): perivascular and in leptomeninges		Pigs, occasionally ruminants, children
	Carbon monoxide	Incomplete combustion of heating fuels	Carbon monoxide toxicosis	Binding to hemoglobin, carboxyhemoglobin lacks oxygen-transporting capacity. Histotoxic and anemic anoxia	Cerebral white matter Globus pallidus, substantia nigra and hippocampus	Cardiac dysfunction	Humans, animals
Vasculature ?	Fumonisins	Mycotoxins produced by *Fusarium verticillioides* on corn	Equine leukoencephalomalacia	Vasogenic edema Disruption of sphingolipid metabolism (except in brain)	Brain and spinal cord: perivascular and meningeal edema with minimal inflammation Cerebral white matter: focal malacia	Liver (hepatocyte apoptosis, necrosis, fibrosis), cardiac dysfunction	Equidae only: horse, donkey, mule
Vasculature	Corynetoxins	*Rathayibacter toxicus*, a nematode (*Anguina agrostis*)-vectored gram-positive bacterium	Tremorigenic syndrome: annual ryegrass staggers	Inhibits lipid-linked N-glycosylation of glycoproteins	Brain and meninges: alteration in permeability, edema		Ruminants (mainly sheep), pigs, horses
?	Cyanogenic glycosides (cyanide)	Plants: *Sorghum* sp, some fruit seeds (apple, apricot, peach, wild cherry, bitter almond), flax seed	Cyanide toxicosis (acute)	Inhibition of cytochrome oxidase	No lesion to neuronal necrosis of globus pallidus		Ruminants especially due to rumenal microbial action
?	Lolitrems A, B, C, and D	Mycotoxins from endophyte, *Neotyphodium lolii*, from *Lolium perenne* (perennial ryegrass)	Tremorigenic syndrome: perennial ryegrass staggers	Interfere with excitatory amino acid neurotransmitter release mechanisms	Swelling of Purkinje cell axons		Ruminants (mainly sheep, but includes deer), horses
?	Selenium (as sodium selenite or selenate)	Home mixed feed	Bilateral symmetrical poliomyelomalacia	Nicotinamide or niacin deficiency?	Spinal cord (ventral gray column of cervical and lumbar intumescences) and brain stem: neuropil vacuolation, glial cell degeneration and vascular changes lead to malacia (liquefactive necrosis)		Pigs

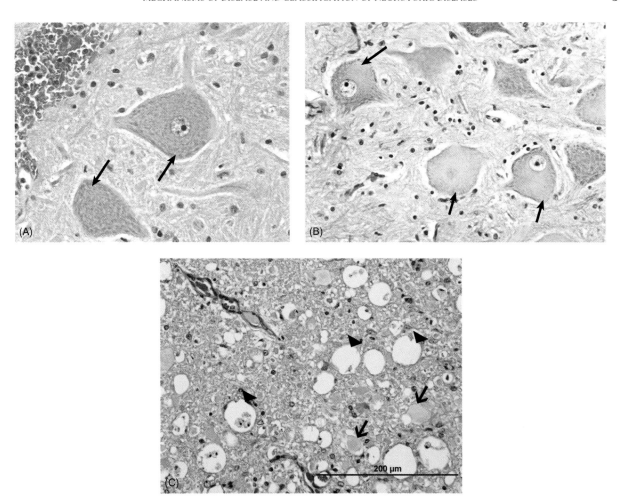

FIGURE 13.7   (A) Neuron structure. The cytoplasm of the neuronal cell body has blue (basophilic (H&E stain)) granular material (rough endoplasmic reticulum) called Nissl substance (arrows). Nissl substance synthesizes proteins, including precursor neurotransmitter proteins and structural proteins (neurofilaments) active in maintaining the integrity (length and diameter) of the axon. (Courtesy of Dr J.F. Zachary, College of Veterinary Medicine, University of Illinois.) (B) Central chromatolysis, neuron cell body, dog. Compare with (A). Affected neurons have eccentric nuclei and pale central cytoplasm, with dispersed Nissl substance (arrows). (Courtesy of M.D. McGavin, College of Veterinary Medicine, University of Tennessee.) (C) Wallerian degeneration, transverse section of spinal cord, horse Trauma and/or severe compression of myelinated nerves can cause a specific sequence of structural and functional changes in the axon and the myelin (distal from the point of injury), referred to as Wallerian degeneration. Axons are initially swollen ("spheroids", arrows), and are eventually removed by phagocytosis to leave clear spaces (arrowheads), which were once the sites of nerve fibers. The cell bodies of affected neurons usually have central chromatolysis (see B), but are metabolically active in an attempt to regenerate the lost portion of the axon (not shown). (A and B courtesy of Dr J.F. Zachary, College of Veterinary Medicine, University of Illinois. Reproduced with permission from Zachary, J.F. (2007). Nervous System. In *Pathologic Basis of Veterinary Disease*, McGavin, M., and Zachary, J.F., eds, 4th edn. Mosby Elsevier, St. Louis. Figures 14-4B, 14-22, 14-23, pp. 837 and 855.)

The putative mechanism for manganese-induced neurotoxicity is induction of oxidative damage in neurons in affected brain regions, due to the synergistic activity of excess manganese with high concentrations of iron and dopamine. Elevated levels of manganese may accelerate the oxidation of dopamine and other catecholamines, while concurrently amplifying the formation of reactive oxygen species.

1-methyl-4-phenyl-1,2,3,6-tetrahydropyridine (MPTP)

The observation that the meperidine analog, MPTP, induced a severe acute Parkinson's-like syndrome in several illicit drug users led to the identification of a novel neurotoxicant that provided one of the few useful animal models for this disease. In both humans and animals, MPTP selectively damages the substantia nigra dopaminergic cells. Astrocytes play a critical role in MPTP neuronal injury through their ability to convert the innocuous MPTP into the toxic pyridinium metabolite, 1-methyl-4-phenylpyridinium (MPP+), by a two-step reaction that requires the enzyme monoamine oxidase B (MAO-B). The toxic product is actively sequestered within dopaminergic neurons by monoaminergic transporters. Rats are relatively insensitive to high doses of MPTP.

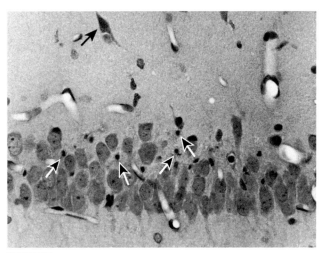

FIGURE 13.8   Large pyramidal neurons of the hippocampus of a rat treated with trimethyltin (TMT) (7.3 mg TMT/kg, po) and killed seven days later to show severe neuronal necrosis of this region (black and white arrows). A dark neuron (black arrow) is also shown; this is a common and well-described artifact that needs to be distinguished from treatment-related effects. H&E stain.

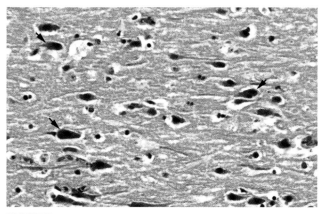

FIGURE 13.9   Cerebrum of a pig with mercury toxicosis. Note the eosinophilic neurons (arrows) with pyknotic nuclei (ischemic cell change) located in the middle to deep lamina of the cerebral cortex. H&E stain.

Mechanism

Inside the neuron, MPP+ poisons mitochondrial metabolism by inhibiting NADH dehydrogenase activity. Dopaminergic neurons are particularly vulnerable, because of their ability to accumulate and retain MPP+ for prolonged periods of time.

Methyl mercury

Mercury is a neuronotoxic waste product of the paper, chloralkali, electrical apparatus, and cosmetic industries. Methyl mercury was first recognized as an environmental health hazard when hundreds of people in the Minamata Bay and Niigata districts of Japan were poisoned in 1950. Although high doses of both inorganic and organic mercury compounds may cause generalized neurotoxicity, low doses exhibit selectivity for certain cell types. This tendency has been demonstrated in rats, pigs, cats, and monkeys, and the distribution and type of lesions are similar to those found in humans exposed to methylmercury.

The lesions in humans and animals have been described as neuronal degeneration progressing to necrosis, with consequent axonal dystrophy and demyelination (Figure 13.9). Methyl mercury preferentially damages granule neurons of layer IV in the visual cortex and the granular cell layer of the cerebellum, as well as sensory neurons in the dorsal root ganglia. The sensitivity of small neurons to this agent has been attributed to extensive binding by cytoplasmic components, particularly ribosomes and rough endoplasmic reticulum, which ultimately inhibits protein synthesis. Brain damage by methyl mercury is amplified by endothelial toxicity that impairs the blood–brain barrier, leading to such sequelae as edema, hemorrhage, perivascular lymphocyte infiltration, and adventitial cell proliferation. In survivors, neural lesions are repaired by proliferation of astrocytes and perivascular mesenchymal cells in essentially irreversible scar formation. Postnatal exposure to methylmercury results in mental retardation, learning deficits, and other neurobehavioral effects in humans, while prenatal exposure results in neural hypoplasia and, rarely, malformations. In veterinary medicine, methyl mercury toxicosis is most likely via ingestion of contaminated fish as a part of the diet, and is most likely to occur in cats.

Mechanisms

A number of biochemical effects have been implicated in methyl mercury neurotoxicity. Effects of the parent compound or its metabolites (mercuric ions and methyl free radicals) may include disruption of the blood–brain barrier, leading to alterations in neural metabolism, inhibition of RNA and protein synthesis, enzymatic dysfunction, and denaturation of cellular proteins and membranes.

Aluminum

No naturally-occurring encephalopathies linked to aluminum exposure have been reported in animals; however, fatal dialysis encephalopathy following 3–7 years of intermittent hemodialysis has been reported in humans. In these cases, an aluminum-containing phosphate-binding gel was used. Brain aluminum levels in these patients were increased. Neurofibrillary tangles were not part of the histologic changes in these cases, but are a specific feature of Alzheimer's disease, a disease also characterized by elevated brain aluminum. The exact role of aluminum, if any, in the pathogenesis of Alzheimer's and other neurodegenerative diseases has not been established. The hypothesis that excessive aluminum incorporation into the brain may play a primary or secondary role in the pathogenesis of Alzheimer's disease is partially based on experiments in animals. Aluminum does appear to play a role in encephalopathy and amyotrophic sclerosis.

It has been shown that subcutaneous, intracranial, and intraventricular injections of aluminum (elemental aluminum, powder, or aluminum salts) induce a neurofibrillary degeneration of motor neurons in the brain and spinal cord in various animal species, particularly cats and rabbits. Changes in perikarya and dendrites are correlated with axonal swellings. Neurofibrillary tangles develop in the cell body, as well as in dilated axons. Axons at both proximal and distal regions are involved. Changes in dorsal roots and sensory neurons are less striking. It has been speculated that aluminum arrests neurofilament transport, by inducing abnormal phosphorylation of neurofilaments in the cell bodies. Aluminum neuronopathy in these experiments primarily involve motor neurons. It should be pointed out that these aluminum-induced neurofibrillary tangles are not identical to the Alzheimer tangles in their ultrastructural configuration; however, the difference may be attributable to species differences between humans and rabbits.

Mechanism

Aluminum crosses the blood–brain barrier and enters the brain by transferrin receptor-mediated endocytosis. It can also enter the brain via the olfactory pathway following inhalation. It deposits mainly in the hippocampus, cortex, and amygdala, areas rich in glutamatergic neurons, as well as in transferrin receptors. Cations, such as calcium, magnesium, and iron are affected by aluminum perturbing neurotransmitter release and systems. Neurons accumulate aluminum, presumably due to their longevity, affecting detoxification of ammonia, phosphorylation of neurofilaments, and other functions.

Locoweed Poisoning

Locoin poisoning (locoism) is related to consumption of loco weeds (genus *Astragalus* and *Oxytropis* in the western United States and Canada, and *Swainsona* in Australia). All species can be affected, but spontaneous disease occurs in sheep, horses, cattle, and wild ruminants that have access to these pastures. Clinical signs include visual impairment, as well as progressive sensory and motor derangements (depression, incoordination, staggering gait, and hyperexcitability). The most prominent microscopic lesion is microvesicular vacuolation of the cytoplasm of cells in many tissues, including kidney (proximal tubular epithelium), liver, endocrine organs, and reticular cells/macrophages throughout the body. In the nervous system, these vacuoles occur in the neurons widely distributed throughout the CNS and PNS, including Meissner's and Auerbach's plexuses. The vacuolization progresses to neuronal necrosis, with resulting axonal degeneration. The material within the vacuoles has been identified as mannose-rich oligosaccharides, making this disease a phenocopy of the inherited lysosomal storage disease α-mannosidosis of Angus cattle.

Mechanism

An indolizidine alkaloid, swainsonine, is the active principle in locoism. It was first isolated from *Swainsona canescens* in Australia, and subsequently from *Astragalus* and *Oxytropis* spp in North America. It now appears that the alkaloid is produced by an endophyte of the plant. The alkaloid inhibits lysosomal α-mannosidase and Golgi mannosidase II, thus preventing hydrolysis of mannose-rich oligosaccharides in cells and accumulation of these oligosaccharides, resulting in cellular dysfunction. In contrast to the inherited mannosidosis, the clinical signs and lesions in locoin poisoning initially are reversible if continued exposure to the plant is avoided.

Yellow-star Thistle Poisoning

Nigropallidal encephalomalacia of horses is caused by the yellow-star thistle, *Centaurea solstitialis*, which grows in dry and weedy pastures of California and other western states, and by Russian knapweed, *C. repens*, which occurs in the inter-mountain region of the western USA and the Great Plains. Horses develop difficulties in eating, drinking, and swallowing after eating this plant. They appear drowsy and walk slowly and aimlessly, while constantly chewing tremulously. The disease has been named nigropallidal encephalomalacia, based on the selective distribution of the lesions. The lesions consist of bilaterally-symmetrical necrosis of the substantia nigra and globus pallidus that grossly appear as yellowish discoloration and even cavitation (malacia) (Figure 13.10).

Histologically, the initial lesion is selective neuronal necrosis. Later, following a rapid progression of the disease, the lesions enlarge, forming circumscribed areas of necrosis at predilection sites. Within 3–6 weeks, mixed scarring and glial encapsulation occurs. The center of the lesion is characterized by

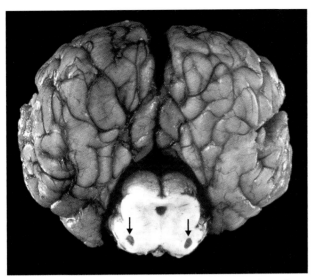

FIGURE 13.10 Equine nigropallidal encephalomalacia, brain, transverse section through the midbrain at the level of the caudal colliculi, horse. This lesion is caused by yellow star thistle poisoning. Note the symmetrically-cavitated (malacia) lesions in the substantia nigra (arrows), resulting from necrosis and phagocytosis by gitter cells. (Courtesy of Dr L. Lowenstine, School of Veterinary Medicine, University of California-Davis, and Noah's Arkive, College of Veterinary Medicine, The University of Georgia. Reproduced with permission from Zachary, J.F. (2007). Nervous System. In *Pathologic Basis of Veterinary Disease*, McGavin, M., and Zachary, J.F., eds, 4th edn. Mosby Elsevier, St. Louis. Figure 14-79, p. 921.)

numerous phagocytic cells and proliferating capillaries. Because of the selective localization of the lesions, nigropallidal encephalomalacia has been compared with Parkinsonism, Hallervorden-Spatz disease, and carbon monoxide (CO) and manganese poisoning in humans.

Mechanism

Several guaianolide sesquiterpene lactones isolated from *Centaurea* species are toxic *in vitro*, with repin, cynaropicrin, and an analog of solstitialin of most interest. In addition, aspartic and glutamic acid (excitatory amino acid neurotransmitters) have also been identified.

At first glance, the lesion resembles an infarct; however, no thrombosis, embolism, or vascular damage is discernible, and selective neuronal loss has been apparent in the absence of vascular changes. Local vasospasms have been considered responsible for the abrupt appearance of necrotic foci. Vasospasms may be induced by local action of vascular smooth muscle, or through vasomotor nerve fibers. This mechanism would require either high local susceptibility of nigropallidal vessels for development of vasospasms, or selective passage and accumulation of the spasmogenic agent into this location.

Doxorubicin (Adriamycin)

Doxorubicin is an antimitotic agent used in cancer therapy. Critical side-effects primarily involve the heart (cardiotoxicity) and bone marrow. Clinical neurological effects attributed to doxorubicin have not been reported in humans; however, typical lesions have been recognized in the dorsal root ganglia in cancer patients at autopsy. The knowledge of the neurotoxicity of doxorubicin has been greatly augmented by experimental work in rats. Since doxorubicin does not pass the blood–brain barrier, the CNS is not affected. The distribution of neuronal degeneration in the PNS is limited to areas in which the blood–neural barrier is absent. While various peripheral ganglia may be affected due to lack of a blood–tissue barrier, the dorsal root ganglia and autonomic ganglia are predilection sites. The lesions consist of reduction of nuclear chromatin, progressing to karyolysis. As nuclear changes progress, chromatolysis, neurofilamentous accumulations, and vacuolization of the cytoplasm enhance cellular degeneration. This degeneration terminates in necrosis and neuronal cell loss.

Mechanism

The neurotoxicity of doxorubicin depends on DNA binding, wherein it intercalates between base pairs of the double helix, which induces breakage of the helical structure and thus interferes with transcription. The selective vulnerability of neurons over other cells may be related to their inherent inability to repair DNA damage.

Cisplatin

Like doxorubicin, cisplatin (*cis*-dichlorodiammine platinum) is an antitumor agent which has chemotherapeutic actions, presumably as a result of binding to DNA. Cisplatin has been shown to produce a marked sensory neuropathy in humans and rats, as well as serious toxicity to other organ systems in both species. The changes in sensory neurons are dose-dependent, and may gradually reverse.

Axonopathies

Axonopathies are diseases in which the primary site of toxicity is the axon. Conceptually, most toxic axonopathies represent a chemical transection of the axon, with points distal to the lesion undergoing degeneration. Disruption of axonal transport appears to be the toxic mechanism for most axonotoxic chemicals. Damage to the axon will result in secondary myelin

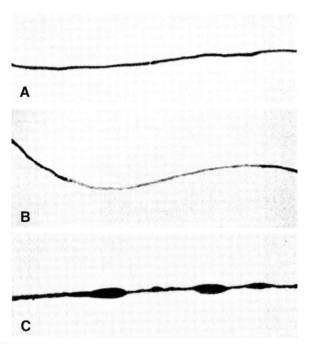

FIGURE 13.11 Teased fibers from (A) control; (B) disulfuram exposed (1% w/w in the feed for five weeks); and (C) CS2-exposed (800 ppm CS2 for 13 weeks, 5 hours per day, 5 days per week) rats. The control fiber has a node of Ranvier in its center. The fiber from the disulfiram-exposed rat exhibits segmental demyelination, while the samples from the CS_2-exposed animals demonstrate characteristic swellings. (Courtesy of Dr William Valentine.)

degeneration, but the neuron cell body will remain intact. Longer axons (e.g., ascending sensory axons and descending motor axons in the spinal cord, PNS axons) are affected first. If the insult is transient, PNS axons can regenerate, but affected CNS axons cannot. A number of chemicals that are associated with axonal injury include acrylamide, β,β'-iminodipropionitrile (IDPN), carbon disulfide, n-hexane, and some dithiocarbamate and organophosphorus compounds.

Axonopathies are generally assessed in screening bioassays, using thin plastic sections of peripheral nerve that have been stained with toluidine blue. However, more specific localization, characterization, and quantification of axonal lesions are best accomplished using teased nerve fiber preparations (Figure 13.11). This specialized technique, while tedious, allows visualization of individual axons and their myelin sheaths.

β,β'-iminodipropionitrile (IDPN)

Chronic administration of IDPN in rodents causes persistent behavioral abnormalities, including lateral and vertical head shakes, random circling, hyperactivity, and increased acoustic startle response (waltzing

syndrome). These behavioral effects are similar to those observed after the acute administration of serotonin or dopamine agonists. High-dose administration of IDPN results in swelling of the proximal axon within several days, primarily affecting large neurons and their axons throughout the neuraxis (Figure 13.12). With time, the initial swelling spreads slowly to the distal axon; however, the lesion differs from that seen specifically with distal axonopathies caused by agents such as hexacarbons (e.g., n-hexane). In contrast, low doses of IDPN confine the swelling more rigidly to the proximal axon. The axonal swelling results from accumulations of intermediate neurofilaments, precipitated by a defect in slow axonal transport. In chronic cases, an irreversible consequence of this proximal axonopathy may be degeneration of motor neurons. IDPN also causes degeneration of the olfactory mucosa in rodents following systemic exposure. IDPN is metabolized to β-aminopropionitrile, cyanoacetic acid, and β-alanine in rats. The molecular mechanism(s) whereby IDPN and/or its metabolites induce the excitatory behavioral syndrome and axonopathy in experimental animals is not completely known.

Acrylamide

Acrylamide, a widely-used vinyl monomer in the polymer and paper industry, reliably induces a progressive peripheral neuropathy. The clinical, neuropathological, and electrophysiological effects documented in exposed humans and animals are comparable. Sensory symptoms occur first in the hands and feet of exposed workers, and in severe cases, the limb muscles become chronically weak and atrophied. These signs accompany selective peripheral and distal central nerve fiber degeneration in the medulla and cerebellum. The characteristic axonopathy of both acrylamide and hexacarbons is characterized by axonal swelling just proximal to nodes of Ranvier as the result of neurofilament, mitochondria, and dense body inclusions (Figure 13.13). However, relative to the hexacarbon lesion, the axonal change caused by acrylamide is less severe, and infrequently leads to paranodal demyelination. Acrylamide affects sensory fibers, particularly the medium and large myelinated fibers, which supply Pacinian corpuscles and primary muscle spindle afferents, respectively. Pacinian corpuscles are affected early. Both humans and macaques develop reduced sensitivity to touch following acrylamide exposure. In addition, monkeys demonstrate electrophysiological evidence of visual dysfunction. Monkeys and rats exposed to acrylamide develop histopathological evidence of optic tract and retinal

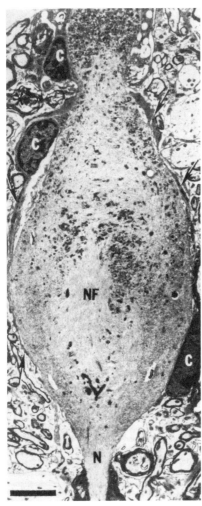

FIGURE 13.12   Axonal swelling proximal to the node of Ranvier (N). Swollen segment is filled with neurofilaments (NF), which are maloriented in the periphery. Myelin sheath is lost in swollen segment. Myelin debris (asterisk, upper left) is visible. Note the ensheathing cells (C) and the processes (arrows) at the margins of the axonal swelling. Bar = 5 μm. (Reprinted with permission from Cork, L. C., Griffin, J. W., Choy, C., Padula, C., and Price, D. L. (1982). *Lab. Invest.*, 46, 89–99.)

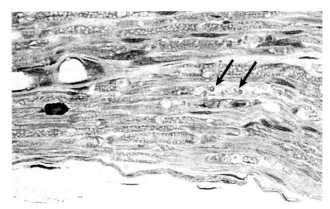

FIGURE 13.13   Tibial nerve from an acrylamide-treated rat to show multiple degenerating fibers with axon loss and myelin debris (arrows), some within digestion chambers. GMA section stained with Lee's Methylene Blue Basic Fuchsin.

ganglion cell degeneration. Rats given acrylamide develop modest decreases (~70% of control values) in tibial motor nerve conduction velocities, a finding mimicked in workers that have been heavily exposed to a mixture of acrylamide and acrylonitrile. The molecular and cellular events leading to acrylamide-induced axonopathy are currently unknown.

Veterinary Drugs Inducing Axonopathy

Vincristine, a vinca alkaloid from the periwinkle plant (*Vinca rosea*), used as an antineoplastic agent, can induce axonal degeneration by binding to tubulin, which disrupts fast axonal transport. Cats appear

especially sensitive. Metranidazole, a nitroimidazole antibacterial and antiprotozoal agent, can result in peripheral sensory neuropathy, as well as CNS effects. The mechanism is unknown, but myelinated fibers are most commonly affected.

Myelinopathies

Destruction of myelin as a primary neurotoxic event may be caused by direct myelin damage, or by selective toxicity to the myelin-producing cells. Many chemicals (e.g., trialkyl tin, hexachlorophene, bromethalin, isoniazid, and biscyclohexanone oxalyldihydrazone-Cuprizone) damage myelin directly, resulting in separation of the myelin lamellae (intramyelinic edema, Figure 13.14). A common mechanism of action has been suggested for these agents, based on the similarity of their lesions. For example, bromethalin, triethyltin, and hexachlorophene are all uncouplers of mitochondrial oxidative phosphorylation; the resulting inhibition of energy production reduces the ability of myelin to segregate fluid from the interlamellar space. Edematous lesions associated with these agents are generally considered to be reversible, and are characterized by marked *status spongiosus* (extensive vacuolization) in white matter tracts (Figure 13.15). Other chemicals result in loss of myelin (demyelination). Agents that primarily target the PNS generally produce symptoms of peripheral neuropathy. A number of histochemical (Luxol fast blue) and immunohistochemical (e.g., myelin basic protein) stains may be used to assess myelin integrity.

Triethyltin (TET)

Organotins are broadly used in industry as stabilizers in plastic polymers, as catalysts in silicon and

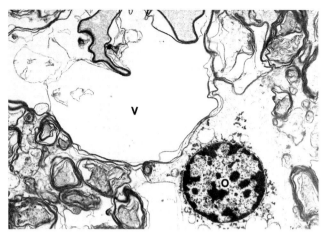

FIGURE 13.14 Transmission electron micrograph of the cerebral white matter of a cat given 1.5 mg bromethalin/kg. Vacuoles in myelin lamellae (V) derived from distorted axons. Contiguous oligodendrocyte (O) is swollen and has edematous cytoplasm. (Reprinted with permission from Dorman et al., 1992.)

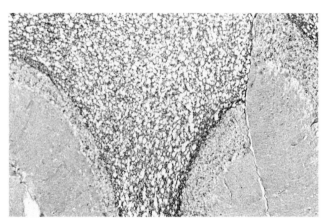

FIGURE 13.15 Severe vacuolization of cerebellar white matter and adjacent gray matter is present in a cat given 1.5 mg bromethalin/kg. H&E stain.

epoxy curing, and as fungicides, bactericides, and insecticides in wood and textile preservation. The most important episode of human TET neurotoxicity occurred in France in the 1950s when a medication for staphylococcal infections (Stalinon) was contaminated with TET during production. Affected humans developed visual disturbances, paraplegia, and increased CSF pressure. Animal studies confirmed that cerebral edema, confined to the CNS white matter, is the characteristic lesion induced by TET. Histologically, edema is most prominent in the corpus callosum, cerebellum, and subcortical white matter, but it can extend into the PNS. Ultrastructurally, vacuoles can be attributed to a lamellar myelin splitting at the intraperiod line. These distended lamellae may rupture in later stages, and the myelin membranes may disintegrate. The edema is nonvasogenic, since the vessels remain intact. Vacuoles also occur in neurons and glial cells. Axons remain intact in the early stages, but degenerate later. Although there is no segmental demyelination comparable to multiple sclerosis, myelin loss of up to 50% has been biochemically established. Oligodendrocyte and Schwann cell bodies are only minimally affected and, together with the more severely affected astrocytes, can recover following TET exposure.

Mechanism

Uncoupling of oxidative phosphorylation and inhibition of mitochondrial ATPase activity within cell membranes is thought to be the mechanism of injury.

Hexachlorophene

Hexachlorophene-induced neurotoxicity in humans has been observed in premature infants and young animals bathed with an antibacterial solution, pHiso-Hex®. The characteristic lesion, intramyelinic edema, is identical to that induced by TET. Excessive exposure may result in severe myelin damage, and secondary axonal degeneration (Figure 13.16). Clinical signs of hexachlorophene toxicosis in humans may include hyperthermia, muscle tremors, apparent blindness, CNS excitation or depression, seizures, ataxia, hypermetria, and paralysis. Experimentally, in rats, lesions are usually most severe in the cerebellum, milder in the spinal cord, and least severe in the brain stem; optic nerve vacuolization, atrophy, and necrosis have also been documented. Retinal ganglion cell layer degeneration was considered secondary to optic nerve damage. Lesions in rats are irreversible in severe cases.

Mechanism

The biochemical basis for hexachlorophene-induced myelin lesions has not been fully elucidated. Hexachlorophene binds to myelin, and a direct correlation between its regional concentration and the degree of myelinopathy has been reported. Neurotoxicity appears to result from uncoupling of oxidative phosphorylation and reduced ATP synthesis in mitochondria.

Bromethalin

Bromethalin is used as a rodenticide, e.g., Assault®, Vengeance®, and Sudden Death®, and is similar to hexachlorophene in toxicity and mechanism of action.

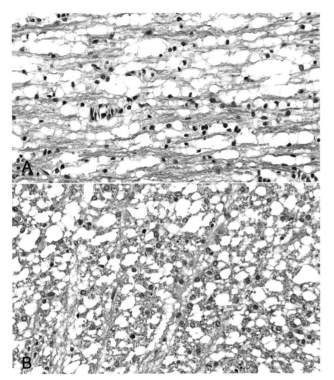

FIGURE 13.16   Intramyelinic edema in the spinal cord of a dog with hexachlorophene toxicosis. (A) Longitudinal section. Myelin sheaths are distended and fragmented along their length, as a result of separation of the myelin lamellae by edema fluid. This lesion is in the early stages, but with time will contain macrophages (gitter cells). (B) Transverse section. Note the distended myelin sheaths. Axons are not apparent, possibly because this stained section is thin ($\approx 3\,\mu m$). Both H&E stain.

Diffuse vacuolation of the white matter of the CNS is found, due to intramyelinic edema (see Figures 13.14 and 13.15). Uncoupling of oxidative phosphorylation results in decreased Na^+/K^+-ATPase activity, weakened ion gradients, and water retention in the myelin lamellae. Cats are more susceptible than dogs, while guinea pigs are resistant, due to their relative inability to metabolize bromethalin into desmethylbromethalin.

Toxicants Affecting Astrocytes and Vascular Integrity

Vessels have three major functions: to deliver oxygen and essential nutrients; clear waste products; and exclude harmful blood-borne substances. A number of agents impair the blood–brain barrier to some degree by increasing vascular permeability (dysoria). Although the vasculature is the primary target for some chemicals, other CNS cells may suffer additional toxic effects once the blood–brain barrier has been impaired.

A growing body of evidence now implicates the astrocyte as a primary target of some toxicants once thought to act directly on the vasculature. Astrocytes play a critical role in the brain including regulation of K^+ levels, inactivation of released neurotransmitters, trafficking of metabolites, and water homeostasis. Experimental studies of thiamine deficiency have identified severe astrocyte dysfunction possibly due to impaired oxidative metabolism. Many alterations have been characterized in astrocytes including changes in glutamate uptake, levels of glutamate and GABA transporters and various proteins. Astrocyte dysfunction can lead to neuronal cell death and edema.

Polioencephalomalacia

Polioencephalomalacia, laminar necrosis of gray matter of the cerebral cortex, is a common neurologic lesion in veterinary medicine, especially in ruminants. Causes of polioencephalomalacia include lead, sulfur, and sodium toxicosis, as well as thiamine deficiency, including thiaminase-containing plants. Bracken fern (*Pteridium aquilinium*) contains the toxin ptaquiloside, a sesquiterpene glucoside. Ingestion by horses can result in thiamine-responsive polioencephalomalacia.

Thiamine (vitamin B_1) is an essential coenzyme for the oxidative decarboxylation of pyruvic acid, and for the transketolase activity in the pentose shunt pathway. Carnivorous animals depend on thiamine intake in their diet, whereas herbivores are capable of synthesizing their own thiamine requirements. Thiamine deficiency is created in carnivorous animals, either by feeding a thiamine deficient diet or by feeding a diet containing thiaminase, as is the case in tunafish meal. Administration of drugs containing substances that interfere with thiamine absorption or activity may also cause thiamine deficiency. In herbivores, thiamine deficiency is more difficult to produce, but natural circumstances of thiamine-related encephalopathy exist and, in some cases, may reach epidemic proportions.

Polioencephalomalacia (PEM) in feed-lot cattle, as well as in sheep and goats on concentrate diets accompanied by a shortage in high-quality roughage, has been recognized as a thiamine-responsive disorder. Administration of thiamine is the only effective therapy. Young animals are more susceptible to developing PEM under these circumstances. The high-concentrate low-forage diet increases the requirement for thiamine pyrophosphate essential for biochemical reactions involved in glucose metabolism. The concentrate diet may lead to reduction of thiamine in the rumen, by reducing thiamine-producing bacteria and instead providing a flora rich in microorganisms (*Clostridium thiaminolyticum*, *Clostridium sporogenes*, or *Bacillus aneurinolyticum*) which synthesize a thiaminase. Treatment with amprolium, a coccidiostat, or with anthelmintic therapeutics, such as thiabendazole and levamisole hydrochloride, may precipitate or exacerbate PEM in borderline cases.

Horses are rarely affected, and thiamine deficiency in that species is mostly traceable to eating plants containing thiaminase, such as bracken fern (*Pteridium aquilinum*), and horse tail (*Equisetum aroena*). In humans, thiamine deficiency causing Wernicke's encephalopathy is generally associated with chronic alcoholism or severe nutritional deficiency, as can be seen in some patients

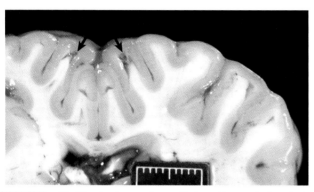

FIGURE 13.17 Acute cerebrocortical polioencephalomalacia, thiamine deficiency, brain, parietal lobe, goat. Note the liquefactive necrosis with varying degrees of tissue separation (arrows) in the deep cortex. Scale bar = 2 cm. (Courtesy of Dr R. Storts, College of Veterinary Medicine, Texas A & M University. Reproduced with permission from Zachary, J.F. (2007). Nervous System. In *Pathologic Basis of Veterinary Disease*, McGavin, M., and Zachary, J.F. eds, 4th edn. Mosby Elsevier, St. Louis. Figure 14-74, p. 912.)

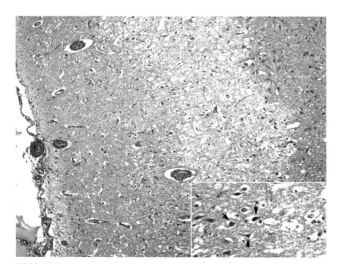

FIGURE 13.18 Polioencephalomalacia in the cerebrum of a cow. At low magnification, a laminar pattern of edema is visible in the middle to deep gray lamina of the cerebral cortex. H&E stain. Inset: At greater magnification, eosinophilic neurons (arrows) with pyknotic nuclei (ischemic cell change) can be seen in the left half of the field, in addition to edema (right field of view). H&E stain.

with stomach carcinoma, chronic gastritis or gastric ulcer, or persistent vomiting as in pernicious anemia.

PEM in cattle and sheep, known in western states as "forage poisoning" or "blind staggers," is certainly the most common form of thiamine deficiency in animals. Neurological signs are tremors, muscular twitching (eyes, ears, and facial muscles), torticollis, opisthotonus, apathy, blindness, and convulsions. Mortality is 50–90%.

The lesions in PEM of ruminants (Figures 13.17 and 13.18) differ in severity, and consist of cerebral edema (deeper cortical layers extending into adjacent subcortical white matter) in mild cases. In severe cases they are best characterized as laminar necrosis affecting the cerebral cortex preferentially around the coronal, suprasylvian, ectosylvian, and lateral calcarine sulci. The deeper layers are preferentially affected. Macrophages are laden with neutral fat (catabolic product of complex lipids) and debris. Astrocytes lose their processes (clasmadodendrosis). Similar lesions may affect the cerebellar cortex, whereas patchy hemorrhage and softening may be recognized in the colliculi, thalamus, and basal ganglia. In surviving animals, proliferating astrocytes participate in scar formation. Areas of malacia may develop where large gaps cannot be filled.

In carnivores (Chastek paralysis in silver foxes, thiamine deficiency in cats and dogs) the lesions are restricted to more archaic parts of the nervous system, preferentially the thalamus, caudate nucleus, inferior colliculi, and central nucleus of the cerebellum. In ruminants these areas may be affected, but to a lesser degree. The lesions consist of edema, vascular dilatation, and hemorrhage with consequential ischemic necrosis. Vascular lesions may be preceded by glial swelling and degeneration which, in turn, may be caused by transketolase deficiency, although this link has not yet been clearly established. Typical lesions of thiamine deficiency were also produced in dogs treated with stilbamidine, a therapeutic agent for systemic blastomycosis.

Mechanisms

There is no doubt that thiamine deficiency is implicated in PEM, and it is definitely the precipitating factor of all lesions described in carnivores. Experimental production of the lesions, with a thiamine-deficient diet in cats and dogs, and the therapeutic effects of thiamine supplementation in all species, attest to the etiologic relationship of thiamine with those conditions. Vascular changes, such as edema and extravasation of serum and blood, are characteristic lesions in carnivores, although it is uncertain whether all or only some parenchymal lesions are consequences of vascular deficiencies, or the direct result of the defective metabolism. As discussed earlier, astrocyte dysfunction may play a critical role in the pathophysiology of these lesions. The laminar necrosis in PEM of ruminants is distinctly different from the lesions observed in carnivores, and may have a unique pathogenesis. The susceptibility of cattle to development of cerebral edema, and the often severe consequences of any volume increase of the brain because of the limited intracranial space, may play a part in the pathogenesis of the disease. Impressions of the calvarian bones are often visible at the cerebral convexity in cattle without obvious signs of edema. In humans, such so-called impressiones digitate are interpreted as an indication of increased intracranial pressure. One is tempted to speculate that edema provoked by thiamine deficiency in cattle may incompletely compress branches of the middle cerebral arteries, leading to impaired circulation at the capillary segment of these vessels, and to a consequential localized ischemia and laminar necrosis.

Sulfur

Administration of inorganic sulfur to sheep and cattle in the presence of adequate thiamine has resulted in the production of an encephalopathy characterized morphologically as PEM at postmortem examination. Subacute exposure to high sulfur levels in the diet or in water may cause neurotoxicity. High dietary sulfur may be due to ingestion of plants that bioaccumulate sulfur. High sulfur content may also be found in barley malt sprouts, and in corn coproducts, since sulfur is added during both the dry and wet milling processes. Ruminants are more sensitive to ingested sulfur, because their ruminal microflora is able to convert sulfur to bioactive species.

Mechanism

The primary mechanism appears to be inhibition of cytochrome c oxidase, which is essential for cellular respiration, by reduction of ingested sulfur to sulfide in the rumen.

Sodium

Excess sodium in feed or water, or deprivation of water may result in sodium toxicosis, commonly known as salt toxicosis. All species are susceptible, but pigs and ruminants are most commonly affected. Clinical signs in pigs include blindness, deafness, head pressing, arching, and later convulsions with a characteristic pattern. The convulsions start with tremors of the snout, extending to clonic spasms of the neck with opisthotonus. This leads to recumbency and generalized convulsions.

The histologic lesions are similar to polioencephalomalacia, consisting of cerebral edema and laminar

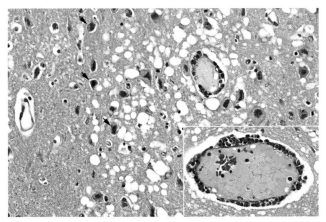

FIGURE 13.19 Hypo-osmotic edema in the cerebrum of a pig with sodium chloride toxicity. Note the region of vacuolation (spongy change) in the neuropil. This lesion is often laminar (middle to deep gray lamina), and accompanied by neuronal necrosis (eosinophilic neurons) (arrows) and astrocytic swelling (evident as vacuolation). Unique to pigs is a perivascular infiltrate of eosinophils and, with longer survival, an influx of macrophages (gitter cells). Inset: Note the eosinophils in the perivascular space of this post-capillary venule. H&E stain.

neuronal loss in the cortex. Additionally, perivascular infiltration of eosinophils (Figure 13.19) within the meninges and brain parenchyma appear to be specific for pigs with salt poisoning. Eosinophils may be replaced by mononuclear cells and so the absence of eosinophils does not rule out salt toxicosis.

Mechanisms

It is necessary to raise and maintain a high sodium chloride concentration in the blood for several days to produce the disease. Hypertonicity initially reduces, but secondarily increases intracranial pressure. This is caused by diffusion of the solute into the brain tissue, and subsequent inibition of fluid when the blood, through renal excretion of sodium, becomes hypotonic relative to the tissue. Sudden access to water following days of deprivation tends to precipitate or aggravate clinical signs of salt poisoning associated with severe cerebral edema. The role of eosinophils in this condition has not been established.

Lead

Common sources of toxic lead concentrations in adult humans are occupational exposures to lead-based paint, battery plates, putty, and asphalt roofing. Similar exposures occur in animals, with cattle most frequently affected. Additional sources of contamination in children are contaminated food, paints, and leaded gasoline. Children and young animals are more susceptible to lead poisoning than adults, and chronic low-level lead exposure has been correlated with impaired cognitive performance. Early neurological signs of lead poisoning (plumbism) include headaches and nausea in humans, and restlessness, hyperesthesia, and head pressing in animals. Later signs are tremors, ataxia, blindness, and convulsions. Horses often exhibit progressive paralysis, with laryngeal paralysis resulting in noisy respiration (roaring). Lesions occur in the CNS (lead encephalopathy), as well as in the PNS (lead neuropathy). The likely primary lesion in acute human lead encephalopathy is breakdown of the blood–brain barrier. Brain capillaries may be dilated, narrowed, necrotic, or thrombosed, and endothelial cells often swell. The consequent extravasation of fluid results in cerebral and cerebellar edema. Accompanying these vascular changes are neuronal necrosis (cerebrocortical and Purkinje cells), with secondary reactive gliosis and astrocytic scar formation. Neuronal lesions may be caused directly by lead, rather than by defective vascular function, since neuronal necrosis without vascular injury has been observed in acute experimental lead toxicity. As discussed above for thiamine toxicity, the astrocyte may play a major role in lead-induced neurotoxicity. Indeed, lead inclusion bodies, if present, are located within astrocytes.

In cattle, lesions of polioencephalomalacia, as described above, are present in acute toxicosis. Early lesions are confined to the tips of the cerebrocortical gyri with a few necrotic neurons, mild astrocytic swelling, and vascular prominence; lesions progress to laminar necrosis. In dogs, vascular damage is more obvious and consistent. It is of interest that thiamine treatment is more beneficial than chelation therapy.

The peripheral nervous system is affected in chronic lead toxicosis. Lead neuropathy in humans and experimental animals is manifested by Wallerian axonal degeneration and segmental demyelination, affecting primarily motor nerves. Lead affects systems other than the nervous system, for example, the hematopoietic, urinary, skeletal, and reproductive systems. The effects on the nervous system are, however, of great concern and have received the most attention.

Equine Leukoencephalomalacia

Leukoencephalomalacia in horses was recognized in the United States in the late nineteenth century, and has been reported worldwide. The fungus, *Fusarium verticillioides*, isolated from corn associated with epizootics of equine leukoencephalomalacia, the causative role of the fumonisin mycotoxins produced by this fungus has been confirmed experimentally.

The clinical signs described are a sudden onset of drowsiness, impairment of vision, weakness, staggering,

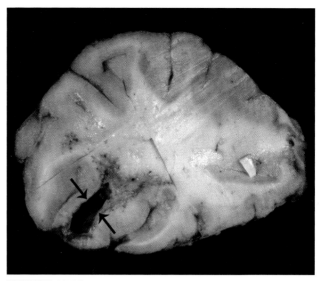

FIGURE 13.20 Leukoencephalomalacia in the left cerebrum of a horse whose diet was contaminated with fumonisins. Focal malacia (necrosis, arrows) is confined to the subcortical white matter.

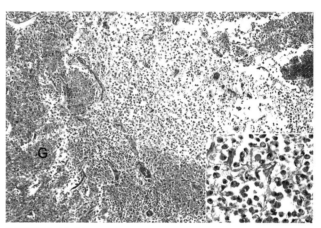

FIGURE 13.21 Leukoencephalomalacia in the cerebrum of a horse. At low magnification, the white matter is severely disrupted (coagulated (liquefactive necrosis)), and there is accumulation of proteinaceous fluid, scattered neutrophils, and abundant macrophages. The interface between the gray (G) and affected white matter contains diffuse edema, perivascular hemorrhage (not shown here), and blood vessels with small leukocytic cuffs. Blood vessel walls are degenerate or necrotic, and some can be infiltrated with neutrophils, plasma cells, and eosinophils. Inset: Note the influx of blood monocytes that mature into tissue macrophages and become gitter cells as they phagocytose necrotic debris. H&E stain.

circling, pharyngeal paralysis, and terminal recumbency. The rate of mortality is high once clinical signs have developed. The most striking lesions consist of large areas, sometimes bilateral, of white matter necrosis (leukoencephalomalacia) (Figures 13.20 and 13.21). Diffuse edema of white matter adjacent to areas of necrosis is readily detectable. The edematous change is not confined to the cerebrum, but extends into the spinal cord. Perivascular infiltration of eosinophils and plasma cells, and many lipid-laden macrophages are present. Thrombosis may also occur and neuronal necrosis, although less characteristic, may be observed in the brain and spinal cord. Fumonisins produce leukoencephalomalacia only in the equine species (horses, donkeys, mules), with different organs targeted in other species. Hepatic injury results from exposure to fumonisins in all species.

Mechanisms

Fumonisins, metabolites or mycotoxins primarily produced by *F. verticillioides* which infects corn, can induce leukoencephalomalacia in horses. Fumonisin B_1 is the most common metabolite, and the most studied. The clinical signs of leukoencephalomalacia have been reproduced in horses by administering fumonisin B_1 intravenously daily over a period of days. The mycotoxin produces vascular injury in the central nervous system, resulting in vasogenic edema followed by necrosis, however, the severe malacia seen in spontaneous cases is rarely found experimentally. Fumonisins alter sphingolipid metabolism in all tissues examined except, interestingly, in brain and spinal cord. Although alteration of sphingolipid metabolism is believed to be the underlying mechanism of fumonisin toxicosis, the pathogenesis of the central nervous system injury in horses is not clear.

Developmental Neurotoxicants (see also Chapter 20)

Like other organ systems, the developing nervous system may be more sensitive to some toxicants. Chemical exposure during the prenatal or early postnatal periods may induce overt malformations, histologic lesions, or persistent behavioral changes as a consequence of neural damage. Toxicants may wreak greater havoc in the developing nervous system because the blood–brain barrier is incompletely formed, and metabolic detoxifying systems are not fully functional. Because different brain regions make neurons and produce myelin at different times, critical developmental periods for the disruption of functional competence exist for each domain during the prenatal and/or postnatal periods (to the time of sexual maturation). Thus, the location and severity of toxic effects will vary with the timing, as well as the degree of exposure.

Many agents act as developmental neurotoxicants. Functional deficits often occur at doses below those at which other indicators of developmental neurotoxicity (e.g., neuropathology) become evident, and at doses with minimal toxicity to adults. Some neurotoxicants yield transient or reversible effects only during early development, while others induce apparently transient effects that re-emerge (with the failure of compensatory mechanisms) as the individual ages. Current dogma states that developmental neurotoxicity in animals is indicative of the potential for altered neurobehavioral development in humans. However, the specific types of developmental defects produced in animals may not be identical to those induced in humans.

Methanol

Methanol is a natural byproduct of normal metabolism, and a major ingredient in the synthesis of organic chemicals, paints, varnish removers, plastics, and coated fabrics. Methanol has also been considered as a major automotive fuel. Acute methanol neurotoxicity in adults has been documented since the early 1900s in people exposed to relatively large doses of methanol (i.e., wood alcohol) through either accidental or intentional ingestion, or inhalation. Acute human exposure results in blindness, CNS depression, weakness, headache, vomiting, and profound metabolic acidosis in adults. Accumulation of formate, a major toxic metabolite of methanol, contributes significantly to the metabolic acidosis and blindness in sensitive species (e.g., adult primates). Adult rodents are relatively insensitive to methanol neurotoxicity, because their detoxification enzymes function more rapidly than those of primates in removing the agent. Rodents in which these metabolic pathways have been inhibited become sensitive to the neurotoxic effects of methanol. Methanol is a rodent teratogen, inducing malformations at multiple sites. Neural tube defects, chiefly exencephaly, occur in mice and rats exposed to methanol during neurulation. The exact mechanisms responsible for the structural anomalies are not known, but one possible explanation includes alterations in the number and proliferative capacity of progenitor (mesodermal and neural crest) cells. Some mesodermal cells undergo degeneration, while certain cell populations (e.g., neural crest) have decreased migration. Other toxic causes of neural tube defects include the mycotoxin fumonisin B_1.

Ethanol

The chief source of ethanol exposure during development is excessive maternal ingestion of alcoholic beverages (binge drinking). High ethanol levels during the period of neurulation (about the third week of gestation in humans, gestational days 8–9 in mice) result in neural tube defects, when the neural folds fail to fuse into the neural tube. High-level exposure to ethanol at later stages of gestation yield micromorphological aberrations, such as neuronal hypoplasia and aberrant neuronal migration. These anatomic changes are associated with behavioral and cognitive abnormalities, a condition in children known as fetal alcohol syndrome (FAS). Comparable changes are found in rodents exposed to high ethanol levels during neurogenesis. The exact mechanisms of neurotoxicity have not been elucidated.

Plant Toxins

A few well-documented neuroteratogenic effects of plants and toxins in animals have been reported. For example, fusion of cerebral hemispheres, hydrocephalus, and cyclopia or anophthalmia (see Figure 20.8) occurs in lambs born following administration of either fresh or dried forms of a range plant, *Veratrum californicum*, to ewes on day 13–14 of gestation. Steroidal alkaloids, such as cyclopamine and jervine, have been isolated from *Veratrum californicum*, and are potent producers of these teratogenic effects.

Neurocarcinogens

Many chemicals induce cancer by either genotoxic (mutagenic) or nongenotoxic mechanisms. Several agents have been shown to induce neural cancers in rats. The most important agents in this respect are acrylonitrile, ethylene oxide and methyl- and ethylnitrosourea (MNU and ENU, respectively). Prenatal or chronic postnatal exposure to these potent DNA-reactive alkylating agents results in the formation of glial tumors in the deep cerebrum. The likely target regions for these agents are the cerebral periventricular zone or subcortical white matter. Both granular cell tumors and malignant reticuloses originating from the cerebral and cerebellar meninges have also been linked with chemical exposure. These tumors likely arise in rats as a consequence of the continued capacity for low-level cell proliferation exhibited by these cell populations throughout adulthood. Cell proliferation occurs in analogous sites in adult mice, monkeys, and humans. It is not known whether or not neurotoxicant exposure is responsible for the preponderance of glial tumors in humans, or which chemical(s) or critical periods of development may be involved.

EVALUATION OF NEUROTOXICITY

Use of Animals as Models

The neurotoxicologist identifies substances that are hazardous to the nervous system, and then obtains information on dose–response relationships, interspecies differences in toxic responses, and mechanisms of action. This information is used to assess and manage risks presented by exposure of humans to chemicals. Conventional *in vivo* rat bioassays remain the principal method for identifying potential human health risks posed by exposure to suspected neurotoxicants. Endpoints of interest often include histopathology to assess morphologic damage, and batteries of functional (neurobehavioral, neurochemical, neurophysiological) tests to examine the operational integrity of the nervous system (Table 13.3).

It may be difficult to determine the most appropriate species in terms of predicting specific effects in humans. There is usually at least one experimental species that mimics the types of effects seen in humans, while in other species tested the neurotoxic effect may be different or absent. For example, certain organophosphate compounds produce OPIDN in hens, similar to that seen in humans, whereas rodents are characteristically insensitive to these compounds. The fact that every species may not react in the same way is probably due to species-specific differences in neural development, neuroanatomy, metabolism, or susceptibility. For risk assessment purposes, it is assumed that the neurotoxic effects seen in animal studies may not be the same as those produced in humans. Consequently, a clear understanding of the pathogenesis and the mechanism of action involved helps to define the relevance of toxic responses in experimental animals to potential responses in humans.

Tests of Nervous System Function

Behavior

Behavior has been defined as the net sensorimotor and integrative processes occurring in the nervous system. It follows that an alteration in behavior might be a relatively sensitive indicator of exposure, since behavior reflects the coordinated function of a large portion of the neural network. Behavioral endpoints are generally noninvasive, and can be used to assess subjects repeatedly during the course of an experiment. Endpoints commonly used in neurotoxicity bioassays include acoustic startle, motor activity, and tests of learning and memory. In addition, the functional observational battery (FOB) is used widely in neurotoxicology. At the present time, there is no clear consensus concerning the routine use of specific behavioral tests to assess chemical-induced sensory, motor, or cognitive dysfunction in animal models. Behavioral tests often lack specificity for the nervous system. Their results must be interpreted within the context of other tests of neurotoxicity and potential

TABLE 13.3 Examples of possible indicators of a neurotoxic effect

Structural or neuropathological endpoints

  Gross changes in morphology, including altered brain weight
  Histologic changes in neurons, glia, or vessels (e.g., neuronopathy, axonopathy, myelinopathy)

Neurochemical endpoints

  Alterations in synthesis, release, uptake, degradation of neurotransmitters
  Alterations in second-messenger-associated signal transduction pathways
  Inhibition and aging of acetylcholinesterase or neuropathy enzyme
  Increases in glial fibrillary acidic protein in adults

Neurophysiological endpoints

  Change in velocity, amplitude, or refractory period of nerve conduction
  Change in latency or amplitude of sensory-evoked potential
  Change in electroencephalographic (EEG) pattern

Behavioral and neurological endpoints

  Increases or decreases in motor activity
  Changes in touch, sight, sound, taste, or smell sensations
  Changes in rate or temporal patterning of schedule-controlled behavior
  Changes in learning, memory, and attention
  Overt clinical signs of neurotoxicity

Developmental endpoints

  Changes in the onset or quality of behaviors during development
  Changes in the growth or organization of structural or neurochemical elements
  Premature onset of behaviors associated with senescence

---

confounders, such as systemic toxicity, with indirect neurological effects (e.g., hepatic encephalopathy).

Neurochemistry

Many neurochemical endpoints have been measured in neurotoxicological studies. Some endpoints have proven particularly useful in understanding neurotoxic mechanisms of action. However, such changes are not necessarily indicative of a neurotoxic effect, unless they induce neurophysiological, neuropathological, or neurobehavioral alterations.

Neurotoxicants can block reuptake of neurotransmitters and/or their precursors, overstimulate receptors, block transmitter release, and inhibit transmitter synthetic or catabolic enzymes. Neuroactive agents may increase or decrease neurotransmitter levels. Typical measures of neurotransmitter systems include neurochemical assays, such as chromatographic determination of transmitter levels, or molecular biological procedures to detect specific elements of a given system.

A common reaction to CNS damage is astrocytic hypertrophy (see Figure 13.4) and enhanced expression of glial fibrillary acidic protein (GFAP), the major intermediate filament protein of astrocytes. Assays quantifying GFAP levels are a sensitive, simple approach for assessing CNS damage. Increases in GFAP may occur in the absence of histopathologic changes, and can also result from events other than neurotoxic injury (e.g., increased corticosteroid levels, normal aging). Methods used to assess GFAP expression include radioimmunoassay, sandwich ELISA, and immunohistochemical techniques. Neurotoxicants known to increase levels of GFAP include trimethyltin, methylmercury, cadmium, MPTP, and 3-acetylpyridine.

Several enzyme histochemical reactions have proven useful in probing the functional integrity of cell membranes and metabolic compartments in toxicologic studies. For example, the visualization of exogenous horseradish peroxidase has been widely-utilized to study chemical-induced damage to vascular endothelium and trace neuroanatomical connections. In a like manner, acetylcholinesterase inhibition induced by organophosphate and carbamate insecticides may be assessed using enzyme histochemical techniques.

Morphologic Evaluation

General

Neuroanatomical changes resulting from xenobiotic exposure are always regarded as adverse. Most neurotoxic changes in structure are detectable only at the light microscopic level, although some agents cause gross changes. Change in brain weight, a commonly used but indiscriminate marker for brain damage, is usually considered a biologically significant effect.

This interpretation is made regardless of changes in body weight, because brain weight is generally protected in adult animals during periods of undernutrition or weight loss. Thus, absolute brain weight analysis is used.

Neuropathology often identifies particularly vulnerable regions or susceptible cell populations in the toxicant-exposed nervous system (see Table 13.1). Lesions can be classified as neuronopathies (alterations in the neuronal body), axonopathies (axonal changes), myelinopathies (abnormal myelin sheaths), dendropathies (dendritic effects), and peripheral neuropathies (aberrations in the peripheral nerves or at the neuromuscular junctions). Within each of these classes of structural alteration, various histologic changes can result from neurotoxicant exposure. For example, changes noted in nerve cell bodies include chromatolysis, vacuolization, and cell death. Axons can undergo swelling, degeneration, and atrophy, while myelin sheaths respond by folding, splitting, and demyelination. Many of these changes result from lesions in specific subcellular components. Examples include the axonal swelling due to neurofilament accumulation during acrylamide toxicity, and myelin splitting caused by edema following triethyl tin exposure. Other changes may represent regenerative or adaptive processes that occur after neurotoxicant exposure, such as the presence of Bunger's bands (aggregates of proliferating Schwann cells) in Wallerian degeneration.

Neuropathological studies require a tiered approach (Table 13.4), and should control for potential differences in the area(s) and section(s) of the nervous system to be sampled; in the age, gender, and body weight of the subject; and in fixation. Methods for fixation include immersion of a tissue block in an excess of fixative, and perfusion, or the replacement of blood by infusing isotonic saline followed by fixative. Perfusion is generally superior to immersion fixation when preserving the CNS, because the aqueous fixatives cannot penetrate the lipid-rich brain tissue at a rapid rate. In addition, perfusion leads to fewer artifacts from postmortem cellular hypoxia, such as dark shrunken neurons and swollen glia. Neuropathology endpoints in conventional neurotoxicity bioassays are performed on perfusion fixed tissues. Brains are removed, blocked in the coronal plane, and embedded in paraffin. Because the brain exhibits major structural changes at both gross and microscopic levels over very short distances and in all three dimensions, careful attention must be given to tissue sampling and sectioning. Fine structures of the peripheral nerves are best observed in specially processed (plastic-embedded) thin sections.

Many special neurohistology techniques have been developed to reveal specific features of neurotoxic damage, including silver staining (to detect degeneration), stereological (morphometric) assessments of cell or organelle size and volume, and novel imaging techniques, such as magnetic resonance imaging. These methods require additional expertise to ensure their proper application and interpretation. Other procedures, such as GFAP stain for astroglial reaction, or assays for apoptosis, may be performed by most reasonably-equipped laboratories. Molecular pathology techniques (e.g., immunohistochemistry or *in situ* hybridization for neural markers) have also become important to obtain functional information in the context of its neuroanatomical location. However, it should be remembered that proteins made in the cell body may be transported into cell processes or terminals, so the results of these specialized studies may not always be correlated at a specific site. Structural changes can often be correlated with altered neurochemistry, behavior, and electrophysiological function. However, many neurotoxicants induce profound functional changes in the absence of any recognizable structural alterations. Thus, reliance on neuropathology as the sole means of identifying neurotoxicants can be misleading.

Diagnostic Neuropathology in Domestic Animals

The cranium should be opened, dura incised, and brain removed intact following transection of the olfactory bulb anteriorly at the ethmoid bone, of the caudal medulla posteriorly, as well as the cranial nerves and internal carotid artery. Minimal handling to avoid artifacts is desirable. In small domestic animals, the spinal canal should be exposed via a dorsal laminectomy, and spinal cord removed with the dura and associated ganglia intact. In large animals, a parasaggital approach using a band saw is helpful. The dura should be incised prior to immersion in fixative to assist in fixation. The spinal cord can be fixed flat, or suspended vertically. Both brain and spinal cord should be examined for abnormalities, including discoloration and lack of symmetry, both prior to and following fixation. Fixation in 10% buffered formalin should be at 10:1 volume of fixative to tissue, and for at least two to three days, preferably a week.

Both the brain and spinal cord should be sliced (0.5 cm thick slices) in the transverse plane, with slices laid out sequentially, rostral to caudal, and examined for abnormalities. Gross examination can reveal the unique topography of lesions in some toxicities, e.g., selenium toxicity in the pig (cervical and lumbar intumescence in spinal cord), or brain hypoxia (caudal colliculi). In diagnostic cases there would not be

TABLE 13.4   Flow chart for morphologic examination of nervous tissue for toxicity

I. Gross examination

External assessment
Brain weight
Internal evaluation (on coronal slabs, approximately 0.5 to 2 cm thick depending on brain size)

   (a) Forebrain
   (b) Midbrain
   (c) Mesencephalom (tectum, tegmentum, colliculi, aqueduct)
   (d) Hindbrain
   (e) Spinal cord

II. Light microscopic examination

A. Central nervous system (detect areas of hemorrhage, neuronal necrosis, vacuolation or gliosis)
1. Paraffin sections (6 μm)–conventional stains (hematoxylin and eosin, silver or cresyl violet for neurons, Luxol fast blue for myelin)

   (a) Forebrain (cerebral cortex, basal ganglia, corpus callosum)
   (b) Midbrain (hippocampus, thalamus, internal capsule, hypothalamus)
   (c) Mesencephalon (substantia nigra, colliculi, tectum, tegmentum)
   (d) Hindbrain (cerebellum, pons, medulla)
   (e) Spinal cord (cervicothoracic, lumbosacral)–emphasizing intumescenses (caudal cervical, caudal lumbar)

2. Plastic sections (1 μm)

   Cellular detail of areas defined in A1.

B. Peripheral nervous system (detect damage to axons, myelin, or end organs of nerves)
1. Plastic or paraffin cross-sections and longitudinal sections

   (a) Sciatic nerve (proximal regional)
   (b) Tibial or peroneal nerve (distal region)

2. Paraffin sections of skeletal muscle to examine end organs

3. If damage is found in B1, look at ventral roots of spinal cord and dorsal root ganglia

III. Ultrastructural examination

A. Site based on light microscopy results
1. Neurons

   (a) Cytoplasmic organelles (especially swelling of mitochondria, RER, and Golgi apparatus; vacuolation)
   (b) Cytoplasmic inclusions (myelin bodies, neurofibrillary tangles)
   (c) Nucleus (distribution of chromatin)
   (d) Nucleolus (fibrillar and granular components)

2. Astrocytes

   (a) Cytoplasmic organelles (swelling, numbers)
   (b) Cytoplasmic inclusions (glycogen granules)
   (c) Nucleus (distribution of chromatin)

3. Oligodendrocytes (myelin sheaths)

4. Microglia (or macrophages)

5. Capillaries (swelling of endothelial cells and pericytes)

B. Site based on light microscopy

1. Examine nerve at axonal swelling (neurofibrillary accumulation)

2. Myelin degeneration (splitting of layers)

3. End organs for degeneration

C. Morphometry or stereology of cytoplasmic details to quantify cytotoxic changes

IV. Special procedures (typically for site-based on light microscopy)

A. Immunohistochemical markers

1. Neurons

   (a) Neurofilament protein (intermediate filament in all neurons)
   (b) Tau
   (c) Cell type specific markers (e.g., neurotransmitters)
   (d) Functional markers (e.g., tyrosine hydroxylase for catecholamine-synthesizing neurons)

(Continued)

TABLE 13.4 (*Continued*)

2. Glia

   (a) Astrocytes–GFAP
   (b) Oligodendroglica–myelin basic protein (MBP)
   (c) Schwann cells–S100
   (d) Microglia

3. Blood vessels

   (a) Permeability assessment–extravasation of horseradish peroxidase
   (b) Endothelium–Factor VIII related antigen

4. Miscellaneous

   (a) Leukocyte markers
   (b) Degenerative cells–apoptosis assessments

B. Enzyme histochemistry

1. Neurons–cytochrome oxidase

2. Glia

C. Morphometric procedures

any controls for comparison so normal, age-matched animals of the same species should be located if possible when subtle lesions are being evaluated. If gross lesions are not observed, sections from 6 to 8 brain areas should be sampled, e.g., frontal lobe, level of optic chiasm, occipital lobe, thalamus, rostral colliculi, cerebellum through cerebellar peduncles and caudal medulla (Summers et al., 1995). Two or three transverse and longitudinally-oriented sections of each region of spinal cord (cervical, thoracic, lumbar, and so on) should be sectioned.

Paraffin embedding with H&E staining is the standard, but special staining e.g., for myelin (Luxol fast blue) and astrocytes (GFAP) can be done. Toxicant-induced changes must be differentiated from non-lesions (e.g., conspicuous germinal cell populations in the young animal), aging (e.g., lipofuscin accumulation in the cytoplasm of neurons), and artifacts. Excessive handling of the brain prior to fixation can result in dark neurons, while prolonged alcohol processing can cause vacuolar white matter change. Autolysis can also induce changes in the nervous system that must be differentiated from toxicant induced change, e.g., increased perivascular space. Electron microscopy on formalin-fixed tissue may be useful in limited situations.

In Vitro Systems

The complex anatomy (including barriers), functions, and compensatory capabilities of the intact brain often serve to complicate interpretation of neurotoxicologic studies in experimental animals. Therefore, less complicated *in vitro* models applicable

to neurotoxicologic research have been developed to investigate specific mechanisms of neurotoxicological relevance. *In vitro* neural systems include whole embryos (including *in ovo* exposure of chicken eggs), whole organs (e.g., dorsal root ganglia), explants (e.g., brain slices), neural micromass or dissociated primary cell cultures, and immortal neural cell lines. *In vitro* models are easily reproduced, and test chemicals or their metabolites may be studied in combination, or individually, to examine direct neurotoxic effects on specific cell populations, including those of human origin. Potential antagonists or other protective agents may be tested as modifiers of a chemical's neurotoxicity. Chemical endpoints (e.g., receptor binding assays, enzyme activity, neurotransmitter release) are preferable for many *in vitro* studies, since they are easily collected and quantified. However, "gross" and histological changes, as well as special stains for cellular function, can be used to perform a "neuropathologic" examination of *in vitro* model systems. Neurotoxicant classes that have been extensively studied via *in vitro* methodologies include metals, solvents, pesticides, pharmaceuticals, and biotoxins.

CONCLUSIONS

Exposure of human populations to a wide variety of chemicals has generated concern about the potential neurotoxicity of new and existing chemicals. Knowledge in the field of neurotoxicology has increased dramatically during the past decade, and continues to do so as advanced imaging modalities, neurochemical, and molecular biological approaches are increasingly applied to basic neuroscience research. Many of these techniques and approaches have only recently been applied to neurotoxicology. Neuropathology will continue to play a critical role in the assessment of chemicals for neurotoxic potential, and this discipline will undergo similar expansion and refinement.

FURTHER READING

Bolon, B., Garman, R., Jensen, K., Krinke, G., and Stuart, B. (2006). A "best practices" approach to neuropathologic assessment in developmental neurotoxicity testing—for today. *Toxicol. Pathol.*, 34, 296–313.

Bolon, B. (2000). Comparative and correlative neuroanatomy for the toxicologic pathologist. *Toxicol. Pathol.*, 28, 6–27.

Broxup, B., Robinson, K., Losos, G., and Beyrouty, P. (1989). Correlation between behavioral and pathological changes in the evaluation of neurotoxicity. *Toxicol. Appl. Pharmacol.*, 101, 510–520.

Chang, L.W., and Slikker, W. Jr. (1995). *Neurotoxicology: Approaches and Methods*. Academic Press, San Diego, CA.

Fix, A.S., and Garman, R.H. (2000). Practical aspects of neuropathology: a technical guide for working with the nervous system. *Toxicol. Pathol.*, 28, 122–131.

Fix, A.S., Ross, J.F., Stitzel, S.R., and Switzer, R.C. (1996). Integrated evaluation of central nervous system lesions: Stains for neurons, astrocytes and microglia reveal the spatial and temporal features of MK-801-induced neuronal necrosis in the rat cerebral cortex. *Toxicol. Pathol.*, 24, 291–304.

Hazell, A.S. (2009). Astrocytes are a major target in thiamine deficiency and Wernicke's encephalopathy. *Neurochem. Int.*, 55(1-3): 129–135.

Krinke, G.J. (1989). Neuropathologic screening in rodents and other species. *J. Am. Coll. Toxicol.*, 8, 141–146.

Krinke, G.J., Classen, W., Vidotto, N., Suter, E., and Würmlin, C.H. (2001). Detecting necrotic neurons with fluoro-jade stain. *Exp. Toxicol. Pathol.*, 53, 365–372.

Krinke, G.J., Vidotto, N., and Weber, E. (2000). Teased-fiber technique for peripheral myelinated nerves: Methodology and interpretation. *Toxicol. Pathol.*, 28, 113–121.

Love, S., Louis, D.N., and Ellison, D.W. (2008). *Greenfield's Neuropathology*, 8th edn. Oxford University Press, Oxford.

McMartin, D.N., O'Donoghue, J.L., Morrissey, R., and Fix, A. S. (1997). Nonproliferative lesions of the nervous system in rats. In: *Guides for Toxicologic Pathology*. Society of Toxicologic Pathology, Washington, DC.

Mitsumori, K., and Boorman, G.A. (1990). Spinal cord and peripheral nerves. In *Pathology of the Fischer Rat* (Boorman, G.A., Eustis, S.L., Elwell, M.R., Montgomery, C.A. Jr., and MacKenzie, W.F. eds), pp. 179–191. Academic Press, San Diego, CA.

Moser, V.C., Aschner, M., Richardson, R.J., and Philbert, M.A. (2008). Toxic responses of the nervous system. In *Casarett and Doull's Toxicology. The Basic Science of Poisons* (Casarett, L., Klaassen, C., and Doull, J. eds), 7th edn, pp. 631–664. McGraw-Hill, New York, NY.

Paxinos, G. (2004). *The Rat Nervous System*, 3rd edn. Academic Press, San Diego, CA.

Paxinos, G. (1995). *The Rat Nervous System*, 2nd edn. Academic Press, San Diego, CA.

Solleveld, H.A., Gorgacz, E.J., and Koestner, A. (1991). Central nervous system neoplasms in the rat. In: *Guides for Toxicologic Pathology*. STP/ARP/AFIP, Washington, DC.

Spencer, P.S., Schamuburg, H.H., and Ludolph, A.C. (2002). *Experimental and Clinical Neurotoxicology*, 2nd edn. Oxford University Press, Oxford.

Summers, B.A., Cummings, J.F., and DeLahunta, A. (1995). *Veterinary Neuropathology*. Mosby, St Louis, MO.

Tilson, H.A., and Harry, G.J. (1999). *Neurotoxicology*, 2nd edn. Taylor and Francis, Philadelphia, PA.

Zachary, J.F. (2007). Nervous System. In *Pathologic Basis of Veterinary Disease* (McGavin, M., and Zachary, J.F. eds), 4th edn, pp. 833–971. Mosby Elsevier, St. Louis, MO.

Bones and Joints

INTRODUCTION

Proper recognition and interpretation of altered morphology in the skeleton depends on understanding normal organ anatomy, histology, and biologic function of bone and joints. In this chapter we highlight the differences among animal species, to aid in establishing the significance of comparable morphologic changes observed in laboratory animals. Pathologic and physiologic mechanisms of toxic bone disease are often not well understood; therefore, discussion of lesions by pathologists is often limited to observable morphologic alterations. The skeletal system can respond to mechanical or biochemical stimuli in a limited number of ways. If the stimulus is small, the response can be considered physiologic and not pathologic in nature, whereas as the stimulus becomes more severe, the reactions are considered pathologic. However, the pathogenesis of the morphologic abnormality may differ significantly from that occurring in normal biologic adaptation.

Methods of examining the skeletal system will highlight gross, histologic, histochemical, and ultrastructural examination, including histomorphometry, which has contributed to a better understanding of static bone morphology. Because laboratory animals are frequently used to determine drug efficacy, animal models for some of the major skeletal diseases of humans will be presented, and their relevance to toxicologic pathology noted.

SKELETAL STRUCTURE AND COMPOSITION

Formation and Development

Bone

Histogenesis of Bone

Mesenchymal tissue arises from the mesoderm during fetal development, and gives rise to connective tissue, bone, cartilage, muscle, and vessels. The mesenchymal cell is the stem cell for all connective tissue cells, with the possible exception of blood cells and osteoclasts. Blood cells are derived from a pluripotential stem cell that is capable of colonizing hematopoietic sites and comprises the colony-forming unit. However, the relationship between the mesenchymal cell and the colony-forming unit is unclear. The chondroclast or osteoclast is a multinucleated giant cell, present in both cartilage and bone. These cells are thought to be identical, remove mineralized bone and cartilage matrix, and to be derived from the same precursor cell as the monocyte.

Chondroblasts, osteoblasts, and fibroblasts secrete procollagen and glycosaminoglycans which form the extracellular matrix. In young cartilage a transition from mesenchymal cells to chondroblasts and chondrocytes can be seen. These secrete matrical components, and surround themselves with secretory product. Osteoprogenitor cells develop into osteoblasts via preosteoblasts (Figure 14.1). Collagen precursor molecules, secreted by osteoblasts, are cleaved enzymatically, form a triple helix, and polymerize as the uncalcified organic matrix osteoid, which contains 95% type I collagen and 5% proteoglycan (percentage dry weight). When osteoblasts are incorporated into bone by surrounding themselves with osteoid matrix, they develop into osteocytes, which occupy spaces (lacunae) in the bone interior and are connected to adjacent cells by cytoplasmic projections that travel in channels (canaliculi) through mineralized matrix.

Limb Bud Development

Limb buds develop from the unsegmented mesoderm (somatopleure) of the lateral body wall during

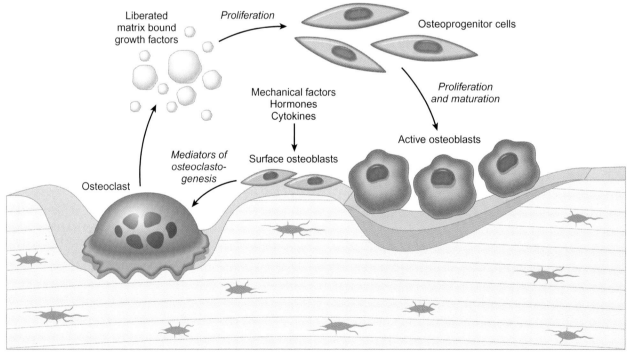

FIGURE 14.1   Bone resorption and formation are coupled processes that are controlled by systemic factors and local cytokines and growth factors, some of which are deposited in the bone matrix. Cytokines, growth factors, and signal-transducing molecules are key to the communication between osteoblasts and osteoclasts (From Rosenberg, A.E. (2005). Bones, joints, and soft tissue tumors. In: *Robbins and Cotran Pathologic Basis of Disease*, Kumar, V., Abbas, A.K., and Fuasto, N. eds, 7th edn. Elsevier Saunders, New York. Figure 26-4, p. 1277).

the early embryonic period. The precise developmental time is dependent on the gestation period of the species. Regardless of the timing, each bud consists of an ectodermal sheath and a mesodermal core, the development of which is dependent on the apical ridge ectoderm. Rapid cell division within the center of the limb bud results in condensation of the primitive totipotent mesenchymal cells; cells that form any skeletal structure, as well as skeletal musculature, tendons, blood vessels, and fat.

Many teratogenic agents, such as thalidomide, phenytoin, and radiation, which interrupt epithelial development, can alter or even arrest further skeletal development from the mesenchyme. Inhibition of DNA synthesis, localized cell death, and reduced proliferation are causative factors in teratogenesis, whereas the timing of cell death in relation to the stage of limb development is critical in the production of some malformations.

Bone Formation and Maturation

Mesenchymal cells within the limb bud condense in the presumptive bone, forming sites that include the primitive joint spaces. At most sites, the cells secrete matrix, forming a cartilaginous model surrounded by a mesenchymal cell layer. Bone is formed from the cartilage model by endochondral bone formation, a process that includes all activities responsible for formation of most weight-bearing bones. At a few locations (skull vertex, facial bones, mandible, clavicle), bone is formed by direct transformation from fibrous stroma, via intramembranous bone formation. However, a sleeve of osseous tissue (ring of Ranvier) is formed in long bones around the central portion of the cartilage model, by direct transition from the surrounding mesenchymal tissue layer (intramembranous ossification). Cartilage within the center of the primitive cartilage model (primary ossification center) undergoes a sequence of changes, repeated throughout bone growth in the secondary ossification centers and in growth plates. Cells in the central portion proliferate, secrete matrix, and undergo hypertrophy, whereas matrix dehydration, mineralization, and chondrocyte death (necrobiosis or planned cell death) is seen in outer layers. Vessels invade the zone of chondrocyte necrosis and matrix mineralization, following which mesenchymal cells differentiate into osteoblasts, osteoclasts, fat cells, and vessels. Following mineralization, cartilage is removed from the center of the diaphysis to make room for the expanding marrow cavity. The sleeve of bone increases in size, forming the primitive bone cortex. As the primary ossification center progresses toward the bone end, osseous tissue is deposited on remnants of cartilage matrix within the marrow cavity at the growth plate metaphyseal junction, forming primary trabeculae. By

birth, most of the long bones of mammals have been ossified throughout a major portion of their bone length.

Following the formation of a perichondrial bone cylinder in the diaphysis and creation of a medullary cavity by the resorption of cartilage, the bone end is still cartilaginous. Secondary ossification centers appear within the cartilaginous epiphyses at various times, depending on specific bone and species. Most of the long bones have at least three ossification centers: a primary center and two secondary centers in the epiphyses. Development and expansion of the secondary ossification center continues until the majority of the cartilage is replaced by bone, cartilage remaining only as an articular surface or as a disk or plate between the epiphysis and diaphysis (Figure 14.2). Complete expansion of the epiphyseal secondary ossification center forms an end plate of cancellous bone on the epiphyseal side, juxtaposed to the growth plate cartilage. Within the metaphysis, a trabecular framework of lamellar bone gradually replaces mineralized bars of the primary spongiosa. This process gradually makes space for the expanding bone marrow.

Removal and reshaping of the primary trabeculae, bone modeling begins as a process by which osteoclasts and osteoblasts function independently. Osteoclasts

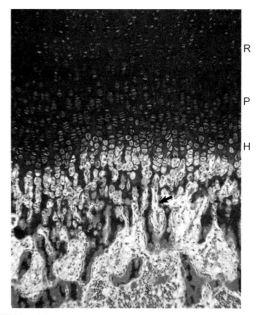

FIGURE 14.2 Growth plate, long bone, dog. Resting (R), proliferating (P), and hypertrophic (H) zones of the growth plate are visible. Apoptotic chondrocytes are released from their lacunae by invading vessels and chondroclasts, leaving only the longitudinal septa (arrow) as a base on which bone will be deposited to form primary trabeculae. H&E stain. (Courtesy of Dr S.E. Wesibrode, College of Veterinary Medicine, The Ohio State University.) (From Weisbrode, S.E. (2007). In *Pathologic Basis of Veterinary Disease*, McGavin, M., and Zachary, J.F., eds, 4th edn. Mosby Elsevier, St. Louis. Figure 16-16, p. 1050.)

reduce the number and width of longitudinal calcified cartilage bars of the primary spongiosa, while osteoblasts lay down woven bone on the cartilage surface. Soon modeling changes to remodeling, and osteoclastic resorption is followed at the same location by osteoblastic activity; net accretion of bone on the trabecular surface occurs. The result of metaphyseal bone modeling and remodeling is decreased numbers and orientation of trabeculae, with an expansion of marrow space and an increased trabecular width resulting in the adult spongiosa.

Since the metaphyseal bone in the region of the growth plate is wider than the diaphysis, the outside contour of the metaphysis must undergo continual change as the bone grows in length. At the border of the metaphysis where it joins the epiphysis, the periosteum of the cortex merges into the surrounding perichondrium. A reduction in metaphyseal diameter as the metaphysis progressively becomes part of the narrower diaphysis gives the metaphysis a funnel shape. In order to bring about a change in width of the bone, osteoclastic resorption occurs on the external surface, while deposition of endosteal bone occurs on the internal surfaces. This extensive osteoclastic activity on the lateral surface, which results in narrowing of the metaphysis, is called the "cut-back zone."

Longitudinal and lateral bone growth produces more spongiosa and cortical bone. As longitudinal bone growth increases the bone length and mass, the cortical diameter increases as a result of intramembranous bone formation. There is lateral growth from the bone shaft in the subperiosteal area of the diaphysis. Vessels are incorporated into the bone structure during periosteal or endosteal bone growth in a manner which differs among species. One of the most common types of vascular canals is the primary canal that can run longitudinally or transversely (Volkmann's canal) through the bone (Figure 14.3). At a very constant age for each ossification center, cellular replication within the growth plate cartilage ceases, the growth plate is remodeled, and the trabecular meshwork of the epiphysis joins the meshwork of the metaphysis. The process by which growth plate closure occurs differs among growth plates, and among species. As union approaches, new cartilage is added to the epiphyseal surface of the growth plate by chondrification of the epiphyseal marrow. During growth plate closure, the orientation of the trabeculae undergoes restructuring (modeling and remodeling) to meet mechanical demands. In fact, the bone is continually adapting to changing mechanical demands; modeling and remodeling is a skeletal maintenance function that continues throughout life.

Joints

Synovial Joints

Most movable articulations are synovial joints (diarthroses), although some are amphiarthroses (intervertebral discs). Synovial joints are formed early in the process of limb bud differentiation where shortly after the limb bud appears, there is axial condensation of the mesenchyme by cell aggregation to form a blastema. After mesenchymal chondrification of future bone, synovial mesenchyme begins to form in the peripheral portion of the interzone between the two bones. This potential joint in the developing limb now consists of two cellular mesenchymal layers, surrounding the adjacent chondrifying limbs, and a loose mesenchymal interzone. Cavitation begins centrally in the interzone, and is complete in all large synovial joints early in the fetal period.

Intervertebral Joints

Controversy exists regarding early development of the axial skeleton; in particular, whether the intervertebral disc and adjacent vertebrae develop from the same sclerotome during segmentation in early development. The intervertebral disc can be observed initially as the perichondrial disc, a band of densely cellular tissue that surrounds the notochord. The *annulus fibrosus* is self-differentiating, developing from the peripheral part of the perichondrial disc. The *nucleus pulposus* is first represented by an aggregation of notochord cells in the intervertebral region, growing very rapidly in lumbar discs during late fetal life. Defects in the development of the vertebral bodies may be due to an early defect in the migration and development of the vertebral body and intervertebral disc.

Blood Supply and Nerves

The epiphyseal artery supplies the epiphyseal secondary ossification center. Here vascular channels, called cartilage canals, course through the hyaline cartilage of the epiphysis, and within the growth cartilage zone beneath the region that will develop into articular cartilage (Figure 14.4). Two independent vascular networks anastomose with each other and supply the bone of the adult. Blood vessels enter the medullary cavity by way of the nutrient canal. In the adult, the final position of the nutrient canal relative to the bone end is dependent mainly on the rates of growth of the respective ossification centers. The nutrient artery branches within the cavity of the cortex to supply the entire spongiosa after growth plate closure. Branches of the nutrient artery nourish the

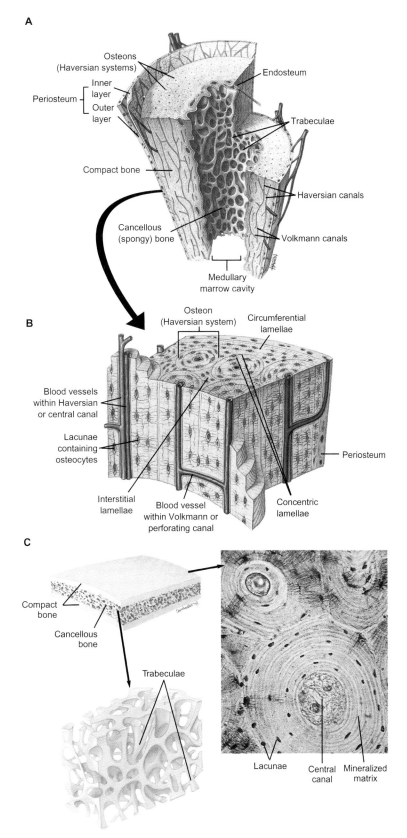

FIGURE 14.3   Schematic diagram of the structure of compact and cancellous bone. (A) Longitudinal section of a long bone, showing both cancellous and compact bone. (B) A magnified view of compact bone. (C) Section of a flat bone. Outer layers of compact bone surround cancellous bone. Fine structure of compact and cancellous bone is shown to the right. (A, B, and C, from Thibodeau, G.A., and Patton, K.T. (2003). *Anatomy and Physiology*, 5th edn. Mosby, St Louis.)

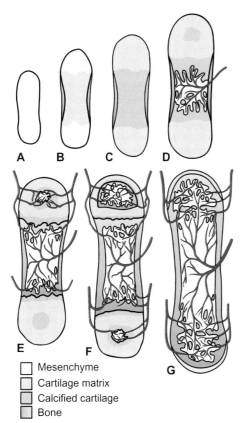

☐ Mesenchyme
☐ Cartilage matrix
☐ Calcified cartilage
☐ Bone

FIGURE 14.4   Correlation of long bone development and vascularization. (A) The primitive mesenchyme that makes up the skeletal primordia has no blood vessels. (B and C) This mesenchyme condenses and undergoes mineralization, and a bony collar forms in the periosteum of the diaphysis. (D) The nutrient artery enters the mineralized cartilaginous tissue in the diaphysis, bringing osteogenic and osteoclast precursors, enabling endochondral ossification to occur (primary center of ossification). (E) Similarly, the epiphyseal arteries bring these cells to the secondary centers of ossification in the epiphyses. (F and G) Extensive anastomoses develop as the bone continues to develop, and as the growth plates close. (From Bank, W.J. (1993). *Applied Veterinary Histology*, 3rd edn. Mosby, St Louis.)

entire cortex of rodents, but in large mammals such as the dog, the nutrient artery furnishes only the endosteal half of the cortex. The corticoendosteal arteries freely anastomose with numerous vascular branches that supply the periosteum and external cortical bone. The periosteum is also supplied with lymph vessels and numerous nerves. Unmyelinated nerve fibers have been identified ultrastructurally within cartilage canals in the developing epiphyses. Thus, pain impulses are readily elicited if the periosteum is damaged or stretched.

Composition of Bone

The extracellular matrix of bone is composed of mineral, collagen, water, noncollagenous proteins, and other organic compounds. The proportion of these constituents is fairly constant in all bones, although there are some differences with varying species, age, and disease state. Bone mineral is an imperfect type of hydroxyapatite, which is calcium deficient and contains carbonate. Mineralization of bone matrix takes place in several distinct steps. Since osteoid does not mineralize immediately after it is deposited by osteoblasts, the first step in bone mineralization is the creation of a matrical environment conducive to mineralization. There are certain post-translational chemical modifications, and certain structural features in the packing arrangement of molecules in the bone collagen fibril, that distinguish it from collagen fibrils in the unmineralized soft tissues. The formation of initial mineral crystals (nucleation) is the second aspect of the mineralization process. Prior to the formation of hydroxyapatite, calcium phosphate intermediates are first produced. Growth of the hydroxyapatite crystal, secondary nucleation, and multiplication to form additional crystals constitute the third step, and organization of these collagen matrices determines the orientation of the bone mineral crystal.

Collagen is the major organic component of osteoid, accounting for about 70% of bone matrix. The collagen precursor molecule, procollagen, is formed by osteoblasts, where important modifications, including disulfide bond formation, hydroxylation, and glycosylation for helical stabilization occur within the osteocytic rough endoplasmic reticulum (RER) and Golgi apparatus. After transport and secretion, enzymatic cleavage produces soluble tropocollagen.

Noncollagenous proteins within the bone matrix play an important role in bone metabolism. Noncollagenous proteins account for 5% of the weight of osteoid. Major noncollagenous proteins synthesized by bone cells and unique to bone include bone phosphoproteins, osteonectin, osteopontin, osteocalcin (bone gla-protein), bone proteoglycan, bone morphogenetic protein, bone sialoprotein, and bone proteolipid.

Species Differences in Composition and Changes with Age

The timing of ossification during the prenatal period, the postnatal appearance of various bones, and the size and shape of particular bones differ among the animal species. The occurrence of secondary centers of ossification in the bones at birth divides laboratory animals into two large groups. Swine, goats, guinea pigs, cattle, and horses have many secondary centers at birth, whereas nonhuman primates, dogs, cats, rabbits, mice, and rats do not. In rabbits, the bony sutures of the skull remain throughout life. In addition, some laboratory animals have additional bones that are not present in other mammals. The size, shape, and vascularity of the secondary centers of ossification differ among the laboratory animals. Cartilage canals are absent in the epiphyses of monotremes, mice, and rats; a distinct difference from other young mammals. The degree of maturation of the skeleton at birth differs greatly among species, e.g., it is very mature in guinea pigs, which can run soon after birth.

Contrary to the usual accepted textbook explanations of how Haversian systems are formed, Haversian-type vascular channels are not formed before birth in the femora and other bones of mammals, including humans. Comparative studies of the femoral diaphysis of mammals suggest that Haversian systems are normally found as a characteristic vascular canal in adult mammals that have a relatively thick diaphyseal cortex. However, the Haversian-type channel is usually not found in femora where the cortex is relatively thin. Mice, rats, gerbils, and hamsters display low levels of Haversian-type bone. Since secondary osteons, which make up Haversian bone, represent remodeling activity within cortical bone, bone remodeling in these species is found in bone trabeculae and when induced by strong anabolic agents or stressful metabolic conditions.

The development of the vertebral body of nonhuman primates is similar to that of humans. In contrast, secondary ossification centers develop in the centrum during embryonic development in other mammals. A longitudinal section of the vertebral centrum of a young animal appears similar to a long bone with growth plates and secondary ossification centers at both ends. Intervertebral discs in most mammals are similar to those of the child, but an exception is seen in equine animals, which do have a nucleus pulposus at birth. The nucleus pulposus undergoes spontaneous degeneration at an early age in chondrodystrophic dogs, including the beagle. Chondroid metaplasia of the notochord-type mucous-producing cells predisposes these dog breeds to herniation of the disc.

BONE PHYSIOLOGY AND FUNCTION

Modeling and Remodeling of Bone

Modeling incorporates all architectural changes that occur during growth, including changes in gross contour, orientation in space, and size of bony, cartilaginous, and fibrous tissue structures. Modeling should be distinguished from growth, repair, and turnover (remodeling). Adaptation of the bone diameter to an increased load during growth occurs because of appositional cartilage growth at the perichondrial ring. Bone can also change shape during growth, through selective bone resorption and formation at specific separate locations. Osseous modeling activity takes place principally on the periosteal and endosteal surfaces, leading to transitional change in the bone shape from the epiphysis to the diaphysis. Lamellar bone responds to mechanical stress by bone modeling that causes the bone surface to move through tissue space to minimize bone strain.

Remodeling is the mechanism by which microscopic packages, called the basic multicellular unit of old or damaged bone, i.e., bones with microcracks, are removed and replaced with new bone, without alteration in the bone's shape. Thus the skeletal architecture is maintained, but a constant turnover of osseous tissue is possible. Skeletal growth and modeling results in peak bone mass and strength being attained in the young adult. Thereafter, physiologic mechanisms attempt to maintain skeletal mass, but in most species a gradual decline occurs during aging. Remodeling activity affects all bone envelopes and takes the morphologic form of an osteonal-remodeling unit; as a rule, remodeling units adjacent to marrow results in net bone loss.

Biomechanics

Physical forces acting on the skeleton constitute a major extrinsic influence on development during embryonic and postnatal periods. Changes in the physical forces acting on bone cause bone deformations and skeletal disease. The cartilage thickness in a mature joint is also the result of the local stress environment created by physical activity. That biomechanics can affect bone architecture was appreciated before the turn of the century when it was stated as such in Wolff's Law: bone responds to an applied force (stress) by undergoing an architectural deformation, and the bone strain is a measure of that deformation.

Bone can undergo deformation because collagen in bone imparts tensile strength, whereas the hydroxyapatite mineral crystals impart compressive strength. However, stress may produce sufficient strain to fracture the bone, or be sufficient to induce secondary alterations in bone growth, modeling, or remodeling. Flexural stress of a sufficient magnitude will cause a bone to bend, with a compressive strain developing along the concave surface, and a tensile strain along the convex surface.

In the growing animal, mechanical force can cause longitudinal bone growth to increase bone size, and cause modeling to influence both bone size and shape. On the other hand, the effects of biomechanically-induced strain on remodeling do not serve to greatly increase bone mass in the adult, but serve to control net losses in existing trabecular and endocortical bone.

Increasing vigorous exercise depresses the recruitment of new remodeling units, but increasing mechanical usage makes the change in bone per basic multicellular unit less negative, even positive in certain locations. Acute disuse derepresses the formation of new remodeling sites that result in remodeling-dependent bone loss. In the context of drug action and toxicity, the suggestion that mechanical usage could mediate the effects of circulating agents, genetics, drugs, and disease on bones (and *vice versa*) is important.

Mineral Homeostasis

Blood calcium concentrations are normally maintained within a very narrow range by a very sensitive negative feedback mechanism. Three major organs—kidney, gut, and bone—and three major hormones—vitamin D, parathyroid hormone (PTH), and calcitonin (CT)—are involved. When blood becomes slightly hypocalcemic, the parathyroid glands respond with an increased rate of secretion of PTH into the peripheral circulation. When calcium reaches a normal or above-normal level, the rate of PTH secretion declines; thyroid parafollicular cells secrete CT. These two agents work in an opposing manner to control serum calcium concentrations.

Parathyroid hormone is thought to act by increasing the flow of calcium ions into cells. It promptly stimulates renal tubular calcium reabsorption, increased renal phosphate secretion, and mobilizes calcium from bone, an action dependent on adequate concentrations of 1,25-dihydroxy vitamin D_3. Parathyroid hormone has a trophic effect on the 1-hydroxylase enzyme system within the renal tubular epithelium, stimulating the synthesis of the hormonal form of vitamin D. Calcitonin is hypocalcemic in action, and its secretion is controlled by negative feedback; an increase in the calcium ion concentration affects the CT-containing cells located principally in the thyroid gland. Calcitonin reduces serum calcium by reducing calcium efflux from bone, which can occur without vitamin D.

The unique organization of the organic matrix and mineral phase of bone means that only a small percentage of the mineral (1–5% depending on age and rate of bone turnover) is available for rapid physicochemical exchange with ions of the extracellular fluid. Mammals may respond to changes in concentration of extracellular fluid ions, hormones, and drugs by either adding or removing ions from the bone mineral phase, without significant concurrent bone resorption or formation. Because the extracellular fluid contains ionized calcium and phosphate at concentrations supersaturated with respect to hydroxyapatite, there is a gradient of calcium from blood to bone proportional to the phosphate concentration in the extracellular fluid. The rate of loss of calcium to bone is usually greater than the rate of absorption of calcium from the intestinal tract. Therefore, a continuous return of calcium from bone to extracellular fluid is necessary. The return of calcium and phosphate from bone to serum is under the control of PTH. Hence, a fall in the calcium concentration of extracellular fluid occurs when PTH is absent. On the other hand, the overall loss of control of blood calcium levels is negligible when CT is absent, although there may be a decline in fine control.

Cellular activity is required for the mobilization of large amounts of mineral ions from the skeleton to the extracellular fluid, or for the deposition of large quantities of mineral ions. The altered morphology of bone seen in metabolic bone diseases represents extreme alterations in bone remodeling undertaken to maintain a normal serum concentration of calcium.

Regulation of Bone Cell Function

Determining the molecular basis for development, maintenance, and repair of the skeleton is the aim of modern bone biology. This science is in its infancy, but certain significant contributions have been made. Hormones that act systemically, or locally regulate bone cells, include cytokines, growth factors, and prostaglandins.

Systemic Factors Regulating Bone Cell Function

Parathyroid hormone, in addition to being a potent stimulator of bone resorption, causes the appearance of increased numbers of both osteoclasts and osteoblasts. Thus, PTH is a major activator of bone turnover. Abnormalities in the secretion of PTH are usually associated with osteopenia. In primary hyperparathyroidism there is an increase in both resorptive and formative surfaces, a decrease in the depth of osteoclastic resorption, and decreased mean wall thickness. In contrast PTH, under certain circumstances, may have a stimulatory effect on bone formation, so patients with hyperparathyroidism may occasionally develop osteosclerosis. Increased cancellous bone mass has been observed as part of intermittent administration of low doses of PTH (amino terminal, 1–34) in animals. Although the major effect of PTH on bone involves an osteoclast-mediated function, this effect is probably indirect, since PTH or 1,25-dihydroxy vitamin D_3 receptors have not been demonstrated on osteoclasts. The way in which PTH-sensitive osteoblasts communicate with PTH-insensitive osteoclasts may be by paracrine interaction, or by physical contact.

Calcitonin is a potent inhibitor of osteoclast function *in vivo* and *in vitro*. Osteoclasts have CT receptors. Neither a deficiency nor an excess of CT appears to alter bone mass significantly, but decreased activation frequency has been shown in patients with hypercalcitoninism (medullary carcinoma of the thyroid). Calcitonin also inhibits intestinal absorption of calcium and phosphorus, and increases the renal excretion of calcium. However, since this was shown at high doses, the physiological meaning is uncertain.

1,25-Dihydroxy vitamin D_3 is the active hormonal form of vitamin D_3. After vitamin D_3 is ingested, or made biosynthetically in the skin by the action of ultraviolet light, it is transported to the liver where it is hydroxylated at the 25 position. 25-hydroxy vitamin D_3 is transported to the kidney, where again it is hydroxylated at the 1 or 24 positions to form 1,25- or 24,25-dihydroxy vitamin D_3 respectively. The active hormone is of major importance in maintaining normal serum and tissue concentrations of calcium, and in the mineralization of bone.

Originally 1,25-dihydroxy vitamin D_3 was thought to be the major hormone causing bone mobilization, but now it is recognized that the *in vivo* hormone effect differs, depending on the dietary calcium level. The *in vivo* role of the various vitamin D metabolites needs to be defined further. Although 1,25-dihydroxy vitamin D_3 is considered the most potent metabolite, some consider 24,25-dihydroxy vitamin D_3 to be essential for normal bone formation and mineralization. Specific cytosolic receptors for the 1,25 form have been demonstrated in osteoblasts and preosteoblasts, but not in osteoclasts. The hormone acts via a nuclear mechanism characteristic of other steroid hormones. It stimulates the synthesis and secretion of bone glaprotein (osteocalcin).

Patients with glucocorticoid excess are known to develop osteoporosis. Glucocorticoids have complex effects on bone, and probably operate through their effect on protein metabolism. Decreased bone formation is the most important effect of glucocorticoid excess *in vivo*. In cancellous bone, decreased activation, decreased mean wall thickness, and an increased remodeling period may be seen. Long-term effects of corticosteroid excess may also involve somatomedin

(SM), since glucocorticoids are necessary for the release of SM by the liver, and are known to impair the effect of SM on cartilage growth.

Insulin is a regulator of cartilage and bone growth. Animals with experimental diabetes show decreased bone and cartilage formation, and impaired bone mineralization. Some of insulin's effects are due to insulin regulation of SM release from the liver. Insulin also has direct stimulatory effects on cartilage and bone formation. Cartilage has specific insulin receptors responsible for its stimulatory effect on proteoglycan synthesis.

Growth hormone is one of the major growth-regulating hormones, and has direct effects on longitudinal bone growth and muscle. It has no direct effects on cartilage or bone formation, but SM mediates its effects. Somatomedins are a family of insulin-like peptides with growth-promoting activity in a variety of tissues. Growth hormones act through changes in the production of insulin-like growth factor 1 (IGF-1), or somatomedin C, a potent stimulator of skeletal growth, acting via multiple pathways at multiple sites. Growth hormone modulates IGF-1 activity by regulating IGF-binding proteins. Somatomedin A is closely related to multiplication stimulating activity (MSA), which has growth-promoting activity for a variety of tissues.

Sex steroids, such as estrogens and androgens, are important in skeletal maturation of growing individuals, and in the prevention of bone loss associated with aging. The principal effects of estrogen and androgen withdrawal are an increase in bone resorption with a smaller increase in bone formation (increased activation), and a consequent decrease in bone mass. Progestins and prolactin may also be involved in bone metabolism.

Several growth factors have been isolated from serum and many tissues. Some of the factors have SM-like activity, while others are mitogenic. Three of these growth factors have been tested for their *in vitro* effects on bone. Epidermal growth factor (EGF) is a single polypeptide chain that has growth stimulatory activity on various ectoderm-, endoderm-, and mesoderm-derived cells, including chondrocytes. Fibroblast growth factor (FGF) is a peptide isolated from bovine pituitary gland, which stimulates cell replication in mesodermal cells including chondrocytes, but inhibits the synthesis of cartilage proteoglycans. Platelet-derived growth factor (PDGF) stimulates collagen and noncollagen protein synthesis by smooth muscle cells. It is released from platelets, and cortisol enhances its stimulatory effect on bone. Platelet-derived and fibroblast growth factors may be important in the acute phase of fracture healing.

Local Factors Regulating Bone Cell Function

A number of growth factors isolated from bone or produced by bone marrow stromal cells affect bone marrow proliferation and differentiation or bone cell activity. A group of glycoprotein growth factors, collectively known as colony-stimulating factors, stimulate marrow progenitor stem cells (PSG) to form colonies of cells that mature along distinct hemopoietic lineages. These factors are defined by the major colony they produce. For example, the macrophage colony-stimulating factor stimulates osteoclasts. Studies with the osteopetrotic mouse (op/op) suggest that a colony-stimulating factor plays a major role in the formation of osteoclasts.

Transforming growth factors have the ability to induce normal cells to form colonies in soft agar. These colonies are categorized according to their relationship with EGF. Transforming growth factor β (TGF-β) is a prototype factor that controls proliferation, differentiation, and other functions in many cell types. The abundance of TGF-β in bone suggests that this factor functions as a local regulator of bone metabolism.

Bone matrix is a rich source of nontransforming growth factors, substances that promote the proliferation or function of bone cells. Terminology for these substances is confusing. Substances isolated from human bone, such as human skeletal growth factor, and from rat bone cultures, such as bone-derived growth factor, seem to be identical. This is one of the factors that triggers the proliferation and activation of adjacent cells to form new bone matrix (coupling, i.e., the coupling of bone formation to bone resorption) following bone remodeling. Bone morphogenic protein is an 18 kDa protein derived from bone matrix that can induce bone formation in subcutaneous and skeletal sites. This ossification process involves a cascade of events, including proliferation and differentiation of perivascular mesenchymal cells to form bone by a process that simulates fracture repair, and includes endochondral ossification and eventual transformation into mature bone with marrow.

Cartilage contains a peptide, cartilage-derived growth factor, with SM-like properties. It appears to be a local regulator of cartilage growth, since it stimulates proteoglycan synthesis and cell replication of cultured chondrocytes.

Cytokines are factors produced by mononuclear leukocytes. Bone resorbing activity (osteoclast-activating factor) has been found in the supernatants of cultured peripheral blood mononuclear cells stimulated by mitogen or antigen. The principal product of phytohemagglutin-stimulated leukocytes has been identified as interleukin 1β. Interleukin 1α and tumor necrosis factors α and β (lymphotoxin) are potent leukocyte-derived stimulators of bone resorption *in vitro*, as well as potent stimulators of prostaglandin production in bone. Cytokines are considered to be important in the pathogenesis of periodontal disease and other bone or joint inflammatory processes. Although most cytokines stimulate bone resorption *in vitro*, interferon γ is an inhibitor of resorption. Multifocal osteolytic lesions occurring in multiple myeloma are induced, in part, by the local production of lymphotoxin.

Prostaglandins (PG) are a group of unsaturated, oxygenated fatty acids synthesized from arachidonic acid via a cyclooxygenase mechanism. Prostaglandins are made by a variety of cells, appear to have a local regulatory function, and are rapidly degraded. Prostaglandins with the greatest skeletal effects include PGE_1, PGE_2, and PGI_2. The chronic *in vivo* administration of PGE_2 increases cancellous and cortical bone mass, and the result is some regional differences in the skeletal response. It activates bone modeling and increases formation, and it increases activation frequency of remodeling. There is an imbalance during bone remodeling in favor of bone formation. Prostaglandin has been used to induce new bone formation in the osteopenic skeleton. Prostaglandins have been implicated in some hypercalcemias of malignancy; humoral hypercalcemia in these models responds to inhibitors of PG synthesis. Local bone loss in periodontal disease and in inflammatory arthritis has been associated with increased production of PGE_2.

MECHANISMS OF TOXICITY

Bone Toxicity

Primary Toxicity

Although the skeletal system is exposed to circulating xenobiotics, it is not known to have a significant role in biotransformation of such substances. Agents reported to have a direct toxic effect on bone or cartilage are somewhat limited. It may be that we have not yet learned to evaluate the early primary toxic effects of drugs, chemicals, or other environmental agents on hard tissues. A list of agents and mechanisms causing skeletal pathology are given in Table 14.1.

Alcohol or the injection of corticosteroids may cause aseptic necrosis of the femoral head; however, it is unlikely that the drugs themselves directly cause necrosis of osteocytes. In contrast, cyclophosphamide, a cancer chemotherapeutic agent, influences mitotic division of bone cells, thereby inhibiting bone formation and growth. Antibiotics of the quinolone class, for example, nalidixic acid and ciprofloxacin, have been shown to cause chondrolysis. So, it can be seen that chemicals can induce cell degeneration and death in skeletal tissues, just as they do in other body systems.

It has long been thought that Kashin–Beck disease has an environmental cause. This disease is an endemic osteoarticular disorder affecting millions of individuals in the region where Siberia interfaces with

TABLE 14.1   Mechanisms of bone and joint toxicity[a]

Physiologic mechanism	Morphologic change	Biological mechanism	Agent
Hyperparathyroidism	Fibrous osteodystrophy	High serum phosphorus depresses serum calcium	Excess dietary phosphorus; low dietary calcium: phosphorus ratio; elevated serum phosphorus associated with renal disease
		Skeletal resistance to PTH/renal calcium loss	Gallium
Excessive absorption of calcium	Soft tissue mineralization; sometimes increased bone	Increased serum level of 1,25-dihydroxy vitamin D_3	Vitamin D intoxication; ingestion of plants containing vitamin D metabolites
		Increase in dietary osmolarity	Lactose and certain polymers increase calcium absorption
		Direct effect on membrane	Filipin, ionaphore A23187
Reduced absorption of calcium	Rickets, osteomalacia	Chelation of dietary calcium	Oxalate
		Reduction in active absorption	Agents that induce renal disease or otherwise interfere with synthesis of 1,25-dihydroxy vitamin D_3, such as cadmium, vanadium, lead, tin, and strontium; anticonvulsants considered to induce hepatic microsomal enzymes which catabolize vitamin D or its metabolites
		Direct effect on membrane cation transport	Anticonvulsants
Reduced absorption of phosphorus	Rickets, osteomalacia	Interference with intestinal transport	Aluminum sulfate; high dietary calcium:phosphorus ratio
Induction of cartilage cell growth	Cartilage hyperplasia	Increased numbers of cartilage cells	Growth hormone (somatotropin) dose-related growth response; somatomedin; diethylnitrosamine (indirect)
Decreased cartilage matrix	Chondromalacia	Lysosomal release of enzymes or production of local factors	Vitamin A; polyene antibiotics cause lysosomal instability
		Inhibition of proteoglycan or collagen synthesis or inhibition of collagen cross-links	Cadmium inhibits chondroitin sulfate synthesis; thallium inhibits production of acid mucopolysaccharides; cyclophosphamide and methotrexate cause matrix degradation; zinc, cadmium, beta-amino-proprionitrile, semicarbizide, and copper antagonists (molybdenum, sulfate) inhibit lysyl oxidase
Decreased bone matrix	Osteopenia, osteoporosis	Reduced synthesis/increased remodeling period	Glucocorticoids, aluminum
		Interference with collagen cross-links	See "Decreased cartilage matrix"
		Unknown	Heparin
Decreased matrix mineralization	Rickets, osteomalacia	Interference with collagen cross-links	See "Increased cartilage matrix"
		Inhibition of matrix mineralization	Fluoride, aluminum, tetracycline, metal ions (strontium, manganese), acid/base balance, bisphosphonates 1,25-dihydroxy vitamin D_3, phenytoin, cadmium
Net bone resorption	Osteopenia	Increased osteoclasts	Pasteurella type D toxin causes resorption of turbinates in swine

(Continued)

TABLE 14.1   (*Continued*)

Physiologic mechanism	Morphologic change	Biological mechanism	Agent
		Reduced bone mass	Occurs with primary or secondary hyperparathyroidism, such as ethylene-glycol-induced oxalosis; vitamin A and related retinoids also induced fractures
		Disuse	
Decreased bone resorption	Osteosclerosis (metaphysis during growth)	Inhibition of osteoclast function	Bisphosphonate, calcitonin, actinomycin, gallium, mithra-mycin, lead, yellow phosphorus, thionaphthene-2-carboxylic acid
		Decreased solubility of bone crystals	Bisphosonate, fluoride
Accelerated longitudinal bone growth	Giantism increased growth plate width	Increased numbers of proliferating cells	Growth hormone (somatotropin), somatomedin, androgens, calcitonin; insulin and thyroid hormones have indirect effects
Decreased longitudinal bone growth	Growth retardation	Decreased cell proliferation	Inanition, tetracycline (premature infants), methylphenidate, furosemide, prostaglandin E_2, corticosteroids, cyclophosphamide, and methionine
		Interference with cartilage metabolism	Premoline produces growth retardation in children
		Premature closure of growth palate	Quinolones, warfarin, vitamin A
Increased activation frequency	Reversible bone loss	Increased numbers of active osteons	Thyroid hormone or drugs that induce hyperthyroidism; parathyroid hormone, fluoride
Decreased activation frequency	Maintenance of bone volume	Decreased numbers of active osteons	Estrogens, calcitonin, non-physiological levels of glucagon, protamine, nonsteroidal anti-inflammatory drugs
Increased formation of bone matrix	Hyperosteoidosis	Osteonal bone formation greater than resorption	PTH (1-34), estrogens, bone marrow depression (see "Fibrosis")
		Bone formation without significant prior resorption	Fluoride, aluminum, prostaglandin E_2, and E_1; also possibly 1,25-dihydroxy vitamin D_3, and *Solanum malacoxylon*
Marrow fibrosis	Osteomyelofibrosis and sclerosis	Anemia (increased circulating levels of erythropoietin); see "Increased formation of bone matrix"	Toxic substances that cause chronic bone-marrow depression, such as benzene, lead acetate, and bone-seeking radionuclides
Tumor induction	Osteosarcomas most common	DNA damage Unknown	Bone-seeking radioisotopes Beryllium salts, bisphosphonates, methylcholanthrene, cupric-chelate N-hydroxy-2′-acetylaminofluorene
Joint degeneration	Loss of articular cartilage	Causes cartilage cell necrosis	Quinolone antibiotics (nalidixic acid, ciprofloxacin, ofloxacin), Mg deficiency
		Causes matrix degeration/lack of synthesis	See "Decreased cartilage matrix"; corticosteroids, immunosuppressive drugs
Joint inflammation	Synovial inflammation/ hypertrophy	Induces immune-mediated arthritis	Numerous drugs, including penicillin
		Nonimmune mechanisms	Lysosomal membrane destabilizers (streptolysin S, filipin); charged molecules (poly-D-lysine, dextran sulfate); enzymes (collagenase, papain); other (zymosan, double stranded polyriboinosinate-polycytidylate, 6-sulfanilamidoindazole) perfluorocarbon contrast agents
	Deposition of urate crystals	Causes hyperuricemia	Cytotoxic drugs, diuretics, ethambutol, nicotinic acid, pyrazinamide, salicylates
Tendon degeneration	Necrosis of cells/ matrix	Causes tendon rupture	Quinolone antibiotics

[a]These represent a characterization of actions that have been studied. There is a wide divergence in the way many agents produce their effects, which can be observed at different organizational levels (e.g., molecular to whole animal)

China. Many environmental agents have been considered to be of pathogenetic importance, but few have stood the test of time. Mycotoxins from *Fusarium* species have been the agents most recently in favor. It is interesting that fusarchromanone, a water soluble mycotoxin derived from *F. roseum* "Graminearum," has been reported to cause avian tibial dyschondroplasia. This statement is not made to support the notion that Kashin–Beck disease is caused by a mycotoxin, but to indicate the importance of toxicologic mechanisms in osteo-articular disorders.

There are numerous agents that are teratogenic, and some affect the embryonic development of bone. Agents may have specific effects on skeletal morphogenesis, or cause abnormalities by inhibiting musculoskeletal movement. Congenital arthrogryposis is considered to develop because of lack of proper fetal movement. It can be induced by ingestion of alkaloids from certain plants such as burley or wild tree tobacco, lupines, or poison hemlock, all of which cause sustained uterine contraction. The mesenchyme, which later forms the bones and cartilage, condenses into a recognizable shape early on in embryonic development. During this process, the apical ectodermal ridge (the epithelial cells are thought to serve a paracrine function) and the polarizing region play an important role in the outgrowth of the limb bud. Later, growth is controlled by cell-to-cell communication that includes autocrine, paracrine, and endocrine signals. These signals include classical hormones, local inducing factors, and growth factors. Interferences with these and other processes, including matrix synthesis, can lead to congenital skeletal anomalies. However, several teratogenic compounds have generalized cell toxicity, and induce skeletal disorders merely because they are administered during the critical period of limb bud differentiation.

Circulating chemicals have complete access to bone surfaces and surface-lining cells. For example, tetracycline is uniformly deposited in all mineralizable bone matrices throughout the skeletal system. In contrast, the only contact that buried osteocytes and matrix have with extracellular fluid is through the osteocyte–canalicular system. However, although bone is not as well-supplied with blood vessels as some organs, osteoblasts and osteoclasts lie within a fraction of a millimeter of a blood capillary.

Skeletal matrix uptake and release of foreign materials are essentially surface chemistry phenomena; exchange takes place between the bone surface and the extracellular fluid. The exchange takes place at the hydroxyapatite crystals, chiefly on the vascular and canalicular surfaces. Thus, bone with a high rate of turnover would accumulate more exchangeable ions. The newly-formed crystals contain imperfections in crystal structure and are greatly hydrated, which allows ready exchange of ions in and out of the crystal by diffusion. Many ions, particularly those of the actinide series and the transuranic elements, also bind to organic components of the matrix, for example, glycoproteins. The bulk of the intracrystalline ions are soon deeply buried by continued bone formation, so only the recently formed ions are in contact with the circulation and able to undergo exchange. More than half of the known elements can be found in osseous tissue, a reflection of their distribution in nature. Once the element is absorbed into the circulation and presented to the bone surfaces, the extent to which it will be taken up depends on its physical properties.

Fluoride and lead are two elements that are ubiquitous in our environment, create an occupational hazard, and have a primary effect on bone. The principal source of fluoride is from food and water. It is rapidly absorbed from the gastrointestinal tract, and then partly deposited in bone and developing teeth, and partly excreted in urine. Fluoride in the extracellular fluid enters the hydration shell of the hydroxyapatite crystal, penetrating to the crystal surface. Because of similarities in size and charge, F^- readily replaces OH^- in the crystal lattice structure, by an exchange and adsorption reaction.

When the content of fluoride in bone reaches 2500 ppm, major pathological changes begin to occur (Figure 14.5). Mottled osteons appear, characterized by hypomineralization, enlarged peripheral osteocyte lacunae, tangled canaliculi, and increased numbers of peripheral osteocytes, with loss of osteocytes in the remainder of the osteon. Excessive fluoridation reduces the biomechanical properties of the bone, increases resorption and remodeling activity, which is observed as enlargement of the marrow cavity, converts the inner cortex to cancellous bone, and accelerates development of resorption cavities in the outer cortical laminar zone. If activation of the resorption occurs too rapidly, the cortex becomes osteoporotic, and may become reinforced by periosteal new bone formation. Any bone formed during exposure to a high concentration of fluoride in extracellular fluid is histologically altered, and has a hematoxylinophilic matrix. Severe osteomalacia may result. In humans, moderate oral doses of sodium fluoride with dietary calcium appear to stimulate bone formation either by direct deposition, or by increasing the incremental volume following remodeling.

Lead poisoning results from accidental ingestion or occupational exposure. Principal sites of lead deposition are red cells, the liver, and the skeleton. Lead is readily incorporated into the mineral phase of bone.

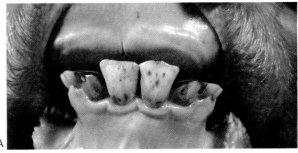

A

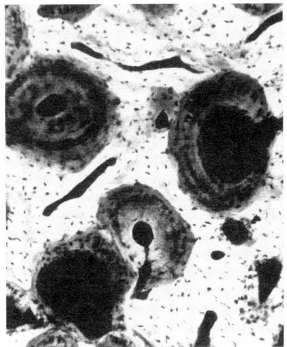

B

FIGURE 14.5   (A) Dental fluorosis, calf born to a fluoride-intoxicated cow. Brown discoloration of enamel and enamel hypoplasia are present. (Courtesy of Dr L. Krook, College of Veterinary Medicine, Cornell University.) (B) Microradiograph of cortical bone from a pig demonstrates several osteons, with increased numbers of peripheral osteocytes, enlarged osteocyte lacunae, and hypomineralization.

The amount of lead accumulated in bone represents 90% of the body burden, because there is a relatively low level of exchange in bone. Although it is likely that Pb^{2+} exchanges with Ca^{2+} in the bone crystal lattice, conflicting reports can be found in the literature. When bone which contains lead is resorbed by osteoclasts, ultrastructural cellular alterations and lead inclusions that are morphologically similar to those produced in other body organs are observed. When lead-containing matrix is taken up by the osteoclast, there is interference with osteoclastic degrading function. In growing animals, lack of adequate osteoclastic resorption of metaphyseal trabeculae leads to osteosclerosis and transverse lines of increased radiodensity, so-called lead lines (Figure 14.6).

Secondary Toxicity

Since skeletal tissues do not play a major role in biotransformation or elimination of potentially toxic substances from the body, most exogenous chemicals exert their effects on the skeleton via secondary mechanisms. It has been suggested that toxic effects may be mediated by alterations in blood flow within the skeleton. Increased oxygen tension is thought to stimulate bone resorption locally, while decreased oxygen tension causes bone to accumulate. The close similarity of some drug-induced tissue reactions to those observed in spontaneous diseases mediated by a vascular reaction supports the argument for a vascular pathogenetic mechanism. Conversely, such reactions could be a manifestation of the limited number of ways in which skeletal tissues can respond to injury.

An example of a tissue reaction which might be mediated by a vascular response is the subperiosteal formation of new bone in dogs following the administration of PGE_2. The drug-induced gross and microscopic lesions are nonspecific, but are very similar to those observed in hypertrophic (pulmonary) osteo(artho)pathy (Figure 14.7). In hypertrophic pulmonary osteopathy, it is hypothesized that space occupying lesions in the chest lead to reflex vasomotor changes (mediated by the vagus nerve), and increased blood flow to the extremities. The increased arterial pressure to the limb leads to hyperemia and edema of the periosteum. New bone formation and thickening of the limb may progress rapidly, but will regress following vagotomy or if the primary lesion is removed.

Substances inducing secondary skeletal changes are usually hormones, vitamins, or minerals, or affect metabolism of skeletal-regulating agents. Our understanding of the pathogenesis of most bone toxicants is incomplete, but as our knowledge of general skeletal biology continues to advance, so will our understanding of toxicant effects. For example, many agents affecting skeletal tissues were said to cause bone formation or bone resorption, yet our modern understanding of bone biology recognizes that resorption and formation are coupled processes in remodeling. When such agents were chronically given to animals, no major change in skeletal mass was observed. Therefore, many agents that induce bone resorption cause bone formation at a later time, so there may be little change in bone mass.

The long-term effects of PTH, corticosteroids, somatotropin, CT, bisphosphonates, and vitamin D and its metabolites on bone resorption and formation are similar, but vary in magnitude. When new remodeling units are activated to increase bone turnover (PTH, thyroid hormone), the initial bone resorption enlarges the remodeling space, so there is a temporary nonprogressive bone loss. Conversely, agents that

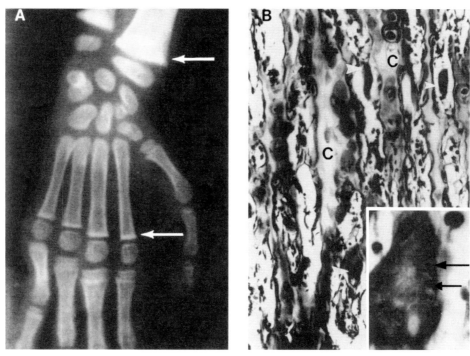

FIGURE 14.6   Lead intoxication. (A) Radiograph of a three-month-old Celebes ape (*Cynopithecus niger*) illustrates radiodense metaphyseal regions (lead lines) adjacent to the growth plates (arrows). (B) Microscopically, the lead line consists of persistent thick cartilaginous trabeculae (C) thinly lined with bone. Numerous osteoclasts can be seen (arrowhead). (From Zook et al. (1973), Am J Physiol Anthropol 38:414–423, with permission.) Inset: intranuclear acid-fast inclusions (arrows) in osteoclast, undecalcified section. (From Hsu et al. (1973), Science 181:447–448, with permission.)

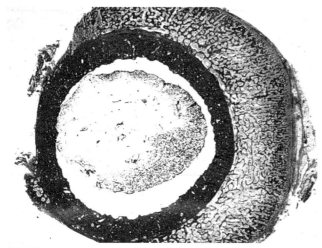

FIGURE 14.7   Hypertrophic pulmonary osteopathy, cross-section of long bone, dog. Extensive new bone formation is present subperiosteally. (Courtesy Dr L. Krook, College of Veterinary Medicine, Cornell University.)

depress activation (CT, increased dietary calcium and vitamin D intakes, estrogens, nonsteroidal anti-inflammatory agents, and some bisphosphonates) reduce resorption first, leading to a small nonprogressive net gain in bone.

Some agents act on several, or all, of the sequential remodeling stages (corticosteroids, PTH), whereas others act on only one particular stage (estrogen decreases activation frequency). This will determine whether a specific modality of timed drug delivery is effective in eliciting a skeletal response. Since bone remodeling events represent a sequence of different biological activities, treatment with intermittent, sequential, brief, or continuous delivery with the same agent may give different skeletal responses. The response might also differ if drug administration followed xenobiotic or otherwise induced synchronization of a population of basic metabolic units, so they pass through a particular stage of the remodeling sequence simultaneously, referred to as coherence treatment.

Skeletal responses to pharmacologic agents diminish with time, particularly if the agent is administered continuously, i.e., tolerance may develop. For example, the diminution of the skeletal response is seen with continual usage of bone anabolic agents. The response will plateau, because the additional bone will activate the negative mechanical usage feedback loop to rid the skeleton of unneeded bone. One probable factor responsible for different drug doses causing varied biological responses is the differential action of drugs on the modeling and remodeling stages. For example, a very small dose of 1,25-dihydroxy vitamin D_3 reverses the endochondral growth abnormality associated with vitamin D deficiency, but higher doses induce severe metaphyseal hyperosteoidosis.

It is important to recognize that skeletal cell-to-cell and cell-to-matrix interactions involve both bone cells and cells of the bone marrow, and are controlled by both systemic and local factors. Therefore, the measurement of cell functional activities, or cellular interactions, really represents the final common pathway of toxic action, rather than a basic mechanism of toxic action. Circulating agents, such as hormones, influence the local events, but the effects of circulating agents are also determined by local factors, such as mechanical usage. In addition, the processes that cause disease need not necessarily be the same processes operating in physiologically normal states.

For example, in severe hyperparathyroidism, excessive remodeling occurs. However, resorption also leads to bone loss by broad removal of cortical bone from the endosteal surface, perforation of trabeculae, and the occurrence of numerous resorption bays in unusual locations, such as the middle of trabeculae. Resorption of large amounts of compact bone is associated with fibrous repair and replacement with new woven bone trabeculae. Thus, the process extends far beyond the physiological range where there is merely an increased resorption space. In severe cases, a return to normal PTH levels cannot be expected to restore normal bone morphology.

Certain diseases appear to affect one bone envelope (periosteal, Haversian, endocortical, or trabecular) more than another. In general, the trabecular bone envelope is more reactive and responsive than the Haversian envelope, because there is greater surface and higher bone turnover. Surface-to-volume ratio and turnover rate is three times higher in trabecular bone than cortical bone, in both human and dog. Drugs also appear to affect certain envelopes, and there are also species differences. For example, PGE_2 administration in the human and dog causes greater subperiosteal proliferation than endosteal proliferation of woven bone. In contrast, in the rat endosteal proliferation is greater. Mice and quail treated with estrogen produce much more marrow cancellous bone than other animals. Osteopenia following ovariohysterectomy in rats is greater than in dogs.

Age also affects the responsiveness of the skeletal system. It is well-recognized that fracture healing is less vigorous in old than in young individuals. The same is true concerning the response of the skeleton to circulating agents. The modeling and remodeling processes present beneath the growth plates of growing animals respond to xenobiotics to a greater extent

than those in cortical or cancellous bone of older animals. In chronic studies, drug toxicity may influence, or be influenced by, the incidence and severity of spontaneous lesions occurring in the animal strain being used. For example, chronic studies with nitrofurazone show a drug-related effect that greatly increases the severity of age-related degenerative cartilage changes and the lesion distribution in rats.

Joint Toxicity

The underlying biochemical mechanisms involved in immune-mediated and nonimmune articular reactions to drugs are similar, since the production of local factors can lead to chondromalacia, or degradation of articular cartilage. Systemic administration of small molecular weight peptidoglycans can induce acute polyarthritis by a nonimmune-mediated process, an inflammatory response probably mediated by mast cell degranulation. Development of immune-mediated arthritis with peptidoglycans or other antigens requires the antigenic material to be deposited in the joint, and the development of delayed hypersensitivity.

Non-immunoglobulin T-cell-derived molecules (lymphokines) that bind specifically to antigen are the effector molecules. One such protein has been designated arthritogenic factor, because of its ability to sustain proliferative synovitis when instilled into the joint cavity. The joint lesion that develops following a single injection of arthritogenic factor persists for at least four weeks, and does not require complement.

The chronicity of antigen-induced arthritis depends on the persistence of a sufficient amount of antigen, and the retention is mediated by antibody-dependent trapping. Electronic charge of the antigen also appears to determine the development of arthritis, because antigen penetration into cartilage matrix depends both on molecular weight and charge. Immune complexes trapped in joint collagenous tissue provoke an inflammatory response. The pathologic role of sequestered antigen in the maintenance of the chronic inflammatory response lies in long-lasting leakage of antigen into surrounding tissue. Immune complexes can be phagocytosed by macrophages or synovial cells, with the production of interleukin 1. Alternatively, immune complexes with the production of C3a and C5a components activate complement, and these are known to induce interleukin 1 secretion.

Degradative changes in articular cartilage leading to subchondral bone erosion are a feature of both inflammatory and degenerative joint disease (Figures 14.8 and 14.9). Loss of articular cartilage may result, since normal matrix degeneration continues in the face

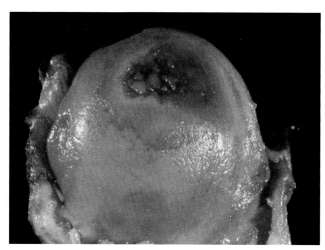

FIGURE 14.8 Advanced osteochondritis dissecans (OCD, osteochondrosis), articular cartilage, humerus, proximal end, dog. Cartilage is focally ulcerated, with roughening of the underlying subchondral bone.

of decreased synthesis. Lysosomal enzymes, including collagenase, cathepsins, elastase, and arylsulfatase, are present in inflammatory, synovial, bone, and cartilage cells. Their release may cause degradation of proteoglycan, as is seen in papain-induced or hypervitaminosis A conditions. Enzymatically generated superoxide (O_2^{2-}) or peroxide can depolymerize polysaccharides, and degrade synovial fluid and cartilage. Synovial lining cells from rats with adjuvant arthritis generated H_2O_2 constitutively, whereas cells from corresponding areas in control rats did not.

The cartilage catabolic process also involves aggrecanase or neutral metalloproteases, which act on connective tissue macromolecules (collagenases, proteoglycanases). Synoviocytes and chondrocytes produce these enzymes. Their secretion is induced by peptidic factors released from cells of the immune system. Among these mediators, interleukin 1 plays an important role. Since synovial cells also produce

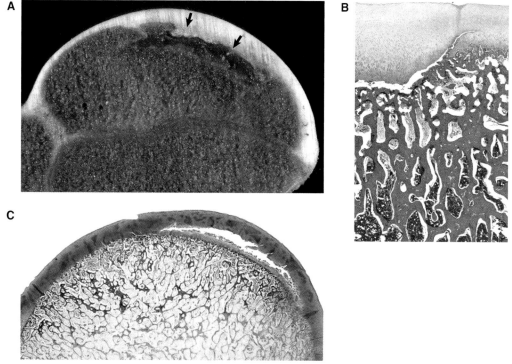

FIGURE 14.9 Dysplasia of the articular-epiphyseal (AE) complex, osteochondritis dissecans (osteochondrosis), bone. (A) Humerus, pig. The retained cartilage has separated from the subchondral bone (arrows), but a fissure has not formed to the articular surface. (B) AE complex, femur, distal end, horse. A linear fissure between the dysplastic AE complex and underlying (subchondral) bone is extending into adjacent normal (right) articular cartilage. H&E stain. (C) Humerus, horse. Note the fissure within the region of the AE complex. A pre-existing dysplasia is not obvious. H&E stain. (A and B, courtesy of Dr S.E. Weisbrode, College of Veterinary Medicine, The Ohio State University. C, courtesy of Dr C. Bridges, College of Veterinary Medicine, Texas A&M University and Dr J. King, College of Veterinary Medicine, Cornell University.) (From Weisbrode, S.E. (2007). In *Pathologic Basis of Veterinary Disease*, McGavin, M., and Zachary, J.F., eds, 4th edn. Mosby Elsevier, St. Louis. Figure 16-49, p. 1069.)

interleukin 1, an inflammatory condition does not seem to be necessary for it to be secreted. Degradation of articular cartilage does not necessarily require an exogenous source of enzymes arising from synovial cells or from neutrophils within synovial fluid. Neutral metalloproteases can be released from cartilage cells themselves as latent enzymes requiring activation, probably by serine proteases, such as plasminogen activator. Interleukin 1 induces the synthesis of cartilage neutral metalloproteases, stimulates the production of plasminogen activator, and promotes the destruction of matrix macromolecules. Tissue inhibitors of metalloproteases (TIMPs) are expressed constitutively in cartilage to prevent over-activity of the proteases. Catabolic states within cartilage are characterized by inactivation of TIMPs, resulting in activation of metalloproteases.

RESPONSE OF THE SKELETON TO TOXIC INJURY

Bone

The number of ways bone can respond to injurious agents is limited, and is exemplified by the various types of reactions that occur during fracture healing (Figure 14.10). After a bone becomes fractured, six principal responses occur. First, tissue disruption leads to hemorrhage and necrosis of cortical bone, extending a variable distance from the fracture site. Second, the injured region becomes a special sphere of influence, where normal physiologic processes are accelerated (this has been termed a general metabolic shift, or regional acceleratory phenomenon (RAP)). Third, there is acute inflammation, organization of the initial hematoma, and formation of granulation tissue. This process may progress to fibrosis in the case of a nonunion. Fourth, a fracture callus forms, which is a process that repeats bone growth during fetal development. On the periosteal surface at the end of the retracted periosteum, an initial ball of mesenchymal tissue is formed. Cell proliferation, differentiation of mesenchymal cells into fibrous tissue, and hyaline cartilage of the external and internal calluses ensue; later, there is endochondral ossification. Next, bone remodeling occurs, based on the basic multicellular unit of the injured and necrotic original cortical bone, and the newly-produced woven bone. Last, there is macromodeling, a process of much greater intensity in children than in adults, where resorption and formation drifts straighten crooked bones.

All the bone toxicology responses to exogenous chemical substances represent either a normal reparative response that may be observed during fracture healing, or a pathologic condition in which there is an interruption of the normal healing process. Chemicals causing metabolic bone disease alter normal bone remodeling, whereas formation of periosteal or endosteal new bone is similar to the process observed in the formation of a fracture callus. Even neoplasia can be considered a disruption in the normal process of cell proliferation and differentiation.

Necrosis

Bone necrosis is seen as a spontaneous lesion in laboratory animals. Assignment of this lesion as a treatment effect must be done with regard to the location and natural prevalence of the lesion in the species being studied. Zones of necrotic bone may be encountered in which there is very little response in the surrounding tissue. Age-related idiopathic osteocyte necrosis was observed in normal bone from healthy rhesus monkeys. It is virtually absent in young animals, and present to some degree in mature individuals. In one rodent study, bone necrosis was observed in 4.6% of the mice examined. Considerable variation was observed among mouse strains, but the condition was more common in females. Lesions in mice were usually quite circumscribed, and limited in extent. Large areas of necrosis in the head of the femur occurred rarely. Bony portions of the menisci of the knee are necrotic in a large proportion of aged rats and mice. Bone necrosis occurs as part of Legg–Calve–Perthes disease of the femoral head in immature small breed dogs. Drugs which cause severe anemia, occlusive vascular disease, thrombosis, or pancreatic release of lipolytic enzymes, may lead to aseptic bone necrosis (Figure 14.11).

Bone necrosis as a toxicity reaction is most frequently encountered following external or internal irradiation. In radiation osteopathy, necrosis arises directly from radiation, and indirectly from vascular injury. Microscopic changes include Haversian canal plugs, atypical fibro-osseous response, and atypical filling of the resorption cavity, which obliterates the vascular supply and causes individual osteonal necrosis.

Regional Acceleratory Phenomenon

Whenever bone is subjected to a regional noxious stimulus of sufficient magnitude, normal physiologic defense and healing processes accelerate in that area. The size of the region affected, and the magnitude of the response, varies with the individual and the intensity

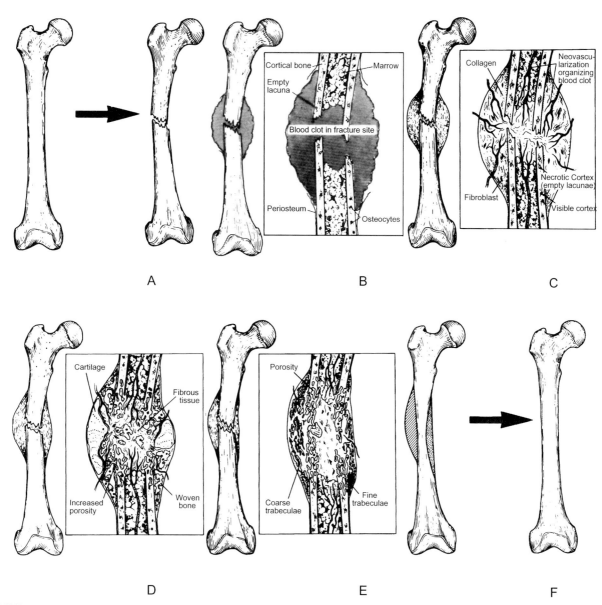

FIGURE 14.10 Reaction to injury, fracture healing. (A) Injury. Break in continuity of the bone and periosteum. The moment a fracture occurs, the stage is set for repair, and all physiologic processes, including bone remodeling, are accelerated (regional acceleratory phenomenon, RAP). (B) Hematoma phase. The degree of soft tissue injury, the amount of the hemorrhage, and the amount of cortical bone necrosis depend on the severity of the injury. (C) Inflammatory phase: vascular dilation and exudation of fluid and leukocytes are followed by organization of the blood clot by neovascularization, and formation of granulation tissue. (D) Reparative phase: pluripotential mesenchymal cells from the soft tissue, periosteum, and bone marrow form a callus composed of fibrous tissue, cartilage, and bone. The callus becomes consolidated, and continuity between fragments is restored by fusion of osteogenic layers on either side of the callus. (E) Remodeling phase: the size of the callus is reduced, as newly-formed woven bone is gradually converted to lamellar bone. The necrotic cortex is removed by accelerated remodeling (RAP), as cutting cones remove necrotic bone and give the cortex a trabecular appearance. (F) Modeling phase: in the young animal, a malunion up to 30° will straighten completely by a process of disproportionate osteoclastic resorption (hatched), and bone formation (stippled).

of the stimulus. When the regional acceleratory phenomenon (RAP) has been evoked, most vital tissue processes are accelerated above their normal value. These processes include, but are not limited to, bone tissue perfusion, modeling, and remodeling. RAP has been observed in association with numerous diseases, such as trauma, denervation, burns, bone infections, and neoplasms. An example of RAP is the acceleration of the remodeling process following a bone biopsy. Unfortunately, the RAP means serial biopsies of the same bone cannot be used to make comparisons of pre- and post-treatment effects. Normally, only moderate

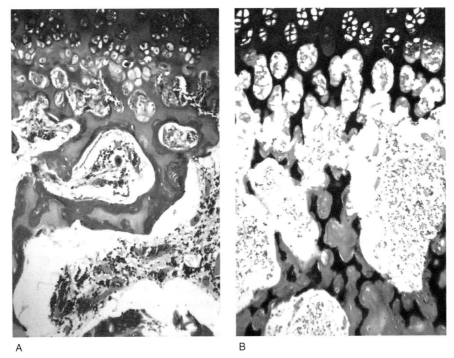

A   B

FIGURE 14.11   Femoral head, necrosis (experimental) bone, femur, pig. Necrosis was produced experimentally by a ligature placed around the femoral neck. Several days after the procedure, the only difference between the control (A) and the infarcted bones (B) is the coagulation necrosis of the marrow and bone cells. The hard tissue of the cartilage and bone remains unaffected. H&E stain. (A and B, courtesy of Dr S.E. Weisbrode, College of Veterinary Medicine, The Ohio State University.) (From Weisbrode, S.E. (2007). In *Pathologic Basis of Veterinary Disease*, McGavin, M., and Zachary, J.F., eds, 4th edn. Mosby Elsevier, St. Louis. Figure 16-63, p. 1083.)

bone turnover occurs in the mandible, but following osteomyelitis and osteoperiostitis, the remodeling process is accelerated, permitting the formation of multiple cement lines which give the bone a mosaic pattern. Note that RAP also involves soft tissue. RAP can often accelerate longitudinal bone growth following a fracture, denervation, tumor, or a surgical procedure such as periosteal stripping.

Inflammation and Repair

Acute inflammation, formation of granulation tissue, and fibrous repair are reactions to injury that occur in all tissues; the processes in the skeletal system do not differ from those seen in other systems. Since one of the major functions of the skeleton is biomechanical support, diseases that weaken or reduce skeletal strength can lead to a pathologic fracture. Therefore, adaptive reconstruction and reparative processes often predominate in the morphologic picture. It is frequently necessary to study the progression of a particular lesion, and to examine early stages, in order to fully understand the pathogenesis of the condition. Fibrous tissue is sometimes deposited as a substitute for bone when disease prevents normal ossification.

The fibrosis associated with hyperparathyroidism probably represents more than the fibrosis of chronic injury (Figure 14.12). Fibrous tissue is closely applied to bone trabeculae, particularly at resorptive sites, in hyperparathyroidism. The distribution of fibrils, identified by reticulum stains, is pathognomonic for this condition. In addition, fibrosis is a part of the disease complex of osteosclerosis and myelofibrosis associated with myeloproliferative disorders in humans. Since marrow fibrosis can be induced in the dog by administering erythropoietin, this too probably differs from simple reparative fibrosis.

Growth and Mineralization

Longitudinal bone growth is determined by the rate of cell division in the proliferating zone and enlargement caused by cell hypertrophy, and production of interstitial matrix in the maturing cartilage zone. Enlargement in metaphyseal diameter is accomplished by cell division and apposition at the perichondrial ring. Any drug that causes inanition or negative nitrogen balance can reduce longitudinal bone growth. Whenever longitudinal growth slows and the growth plate begins to close, focal degradative changes may be observed in the cartilage, and the

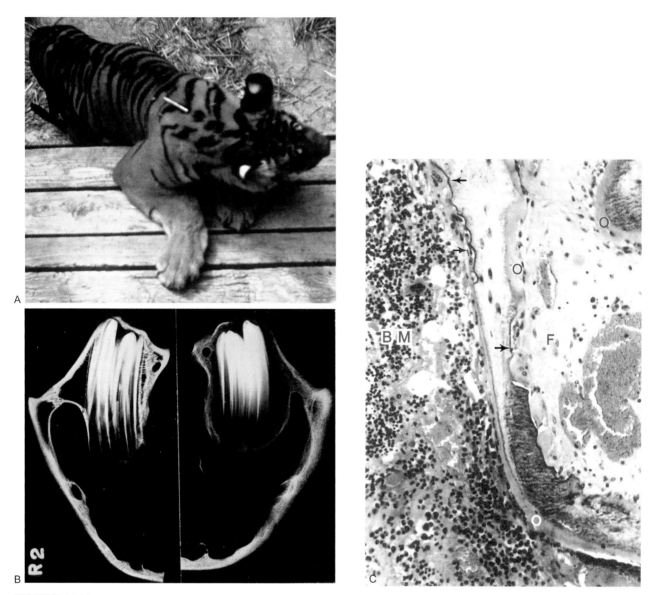

FIGURE 14.12 Nutritional secondary hyperparathyroidism. (A) Tiger from zoo. A meat-only diet resulted in low calcium, high phosphate. Note distortion of the joints. (B) X-ray, mandible, horse. Normal mandible (right) and affected mandible (left), due to high dietary phosphate. There is distortion of the mandible, due to fibrous osteodystrophy. (A and B Courtesy of Dr Krook, College of Veterinary Medicine, Cornell University.) (C) Horse, bone. Increased bone resorption (arrows) and bone formation, osteoid (o). Normal bone marrow on left (BM), and fibrotic marrow on right (F). Undecalcified section.

trabeculae in the metaphysis appear thicker because the slowing of longitudinal growth permits osseous tissue to be deposited on the trabecular surface over a longer period. When cessation of growth is severe enough, there may be an attempt at growth plate closure, and a lateral plate of bone, termed transverse bridging, is formed beneath the growth plate. If growth is reinitiated, these transverse bone plates will be left behind in the metaphysis as the growth cartilage moves away from them (Figure 14.13). When they are visualized radiographically or in bone specimens, they are termed Harris growth-arrest lines. The line

is eventually remodeled. Early growth plate closure is seen in vitamin A toxicity in rats, and also in pigs and calves. The growth plate depth is reduced, and there is focal growth plate closure (Figure 14.14) after administration of excessive amounts of vitamin A. When the bone content of osteocalcin or bone gla-protein is reduced by treatment with warfarin, growth plate closure also occurs.

Normally, longitudinal and transverse growth is coupled, but different factors affect growth at these two sites. Growth hormone governs growth rate at both locations indirectly, and a deficiency (dwarfism)

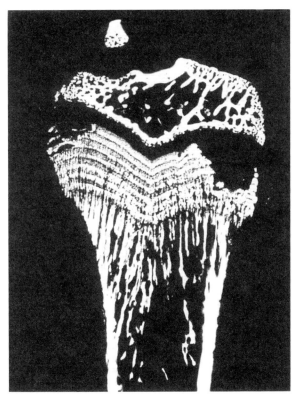

FIGURE 14.13 Growth arrest lines. Microradiograph of rat tibia with peripheral growth plate enlargement (rickets). The radiodense metaphyseal regions are growth arrest lines, and are related to the daily injection of a bisphosphonate. (From Miller et al. (1985), Toxicol Appl Pharmacol 77:230–239, with permission.)

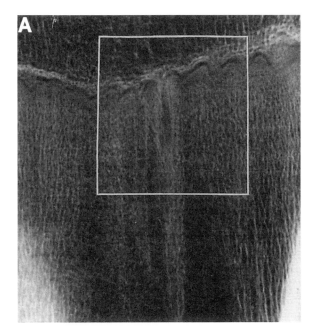

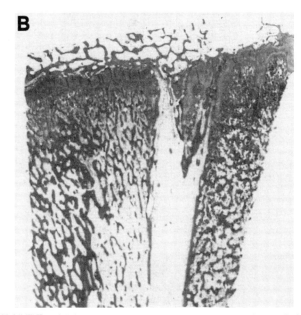

FIGURE 14.14 Bovine vitamin A intoxication. Radiograph (A) and histologic section (B) illustrate focal growth plate closure.

or excess (giantism) causes a proportional change in the bone width and length. However, drugs have the potential to alter the growth at each site differentially. If longitudinal growth is inhibited more than transverse appositional growth, then the bones will be short, but have a more normal diameter. Compounds that induce rickets or induce changes similar to osteochondrodysplasia would produce such changes. If transverse growth is inhibited more than longitudinal growth, the bone becomes long and thin.

Bones with this characteristic feature are seen in vitamin A toxicity in rats, where pathologic fractures occur in the thin cortices. Vitamin A toxicity first causes an alteration in growth plate cartilage similar to that seen following the injection of papain, but the rate of longitudinal growth is not inhibited as much as transverse growth. The changes are considered to result from the release of lysosomal enzymes, and can be prevented by the injection of cortisone. Longitudinal growth rate determines the age and amount of trabecular tissue in different metaphyseal zones. A faster longitudinal growth rate results in an increased amount of cancellous bone of a lesser age,

whereas a slower growth rate gives less bone of a greater age. Since altered longitudinal bone growth rate changes the dynamics of metaphyseal bone modeling and remodeling, studying a drug that alters the quantity of metaphyseal bone in a young animal should determine whether there is an effect on longitudinal bone growth.

Drugs affecting calcium:phosphorus ratio homeostasis may interfere with cartilage or bone matrix mineralization, hence causing abnormal endochondral ossification. These lesions are broadly grouped as rickets, but differences in the growth-cartilage morphology and tissue chemistry of calcium deficiency-, phosphorus deficiency-, and bisphosphonate-induced rickets have been described (Figure 14.15). The pathogenesis of drug-induced malfunctions in endochondral ossification may differ similarly.

Abnormal mineral homeostasis in the adult leads to an increased mineralization lag time and osteomalacia. Osteomalacia is defined as replacement of normal lamellar bone by unmineralized lamellar bone. This is due to a defect in bone mineralization, where normal bone matrix is not properly mineralized.

Hyperosteoidosis may occur because of increased numbers of formation surfaces, increase in the thickness of osteoid because of a mineralization defect, or increased rate of osteoid production. In some cases, osteoid is not mineralized properly, because the matrix

is abnormal. Fluorosis, *Solanum malacoxylon* toxicosis, and internal irradiation are examples. Pharmacologic doses of 1,25-dihydroxy vitamin D_3 cause increased osteoid formation, but impaired mineralization of matrix, despite a high calcium:phosphorus product. Bone fluorosis is also characterized by abnormal mineralization of the matrix. This is best seen in microradiographs (Figure 14.16), where mottling of the osteons can be observed. When bone undergoes necrosis, mineralization of the tissue increases, because canaliculi and osteocyte lacunae may become filled with mineral, an event termed micropetrosis.

Hyperostosis is an abnormal increase in the ossification of the skeleton. Osteosclerosis is a special type of hyperostosis, in which increased bone density occurs without alteration in the shape of the affected bone. Exostosis and enostosis are other examples in which

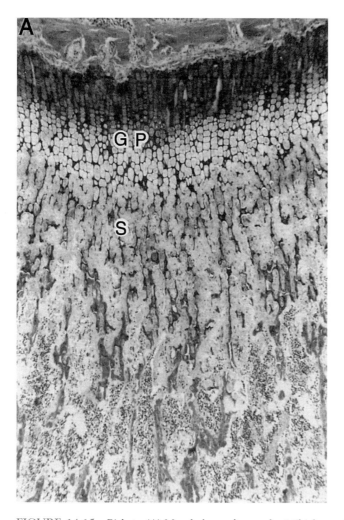
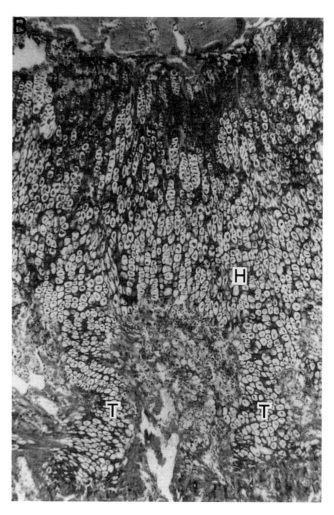

FIGURE 14.15 Rickets. (A) Morphology of normal rat tibial growth plate (GP) and primary spongiosa (S). (B) Abnormal endochondral ossification induced by bisphosphonate is characterized by increased depth of the zone of hypertrophic chondrocytes (H) and irregular vascular invasion that leaves irregular tongues of cartilage (T). (C) Region of abnormal vascular invasion: vessels (V) irregularly penetrate hypertrophic cartilage (H). There is irregular diminution of the cartilage matrix on the right (H_2), compared with the dark staining (metachromatic) cartilage on the left (H_1).

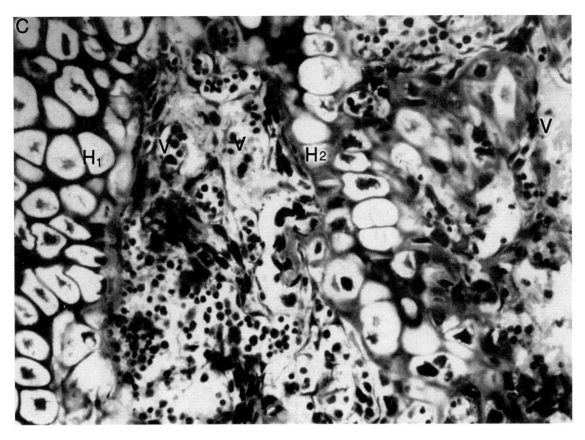

FIGURE 14.15   (Continued)

bone forms on the periosteal, endocortical, or trabecular envelopes. Under physiological conditions, as an adaptive response, or in disease, adult bone increases in amount by increasing the incremental difference between resorption and formation during osteonal remodeling. An example of this type of hyperostosis occurs in osteosclerosis with myelofibrosis (Figure 14.17), a condition that follows persistent bone marrow depression, and has been reported to follow radiation injury or administration of toxic chemicals, such as benzene or lead acetate. In the adult, reactivation of formation modeling drifts may also be seen, as occurs during the formation of marginal osteophytes in osteoarthritis (Figure 14.18). Under pathologic conditions, bone can be produced by the deposition of woven bone. Woven bone can be produced on the periosteal, endocortical, or trabecular surfaces following administration of fluoride, PGE_2, and aluminum, or as a pathologic response to compressive loading.

Evaluation of cellular production of new bone in toxicity studies must consider species-related spontaneous occurrence of hyperostotic lesions. In laboratory rodents, two spontaneous lesions associated with

increased intramedullary bone have been recognized. The first is an increase in the amount of cancellous bone in aged rats. This type of hyperostosis in rats is uncommon, but occurs as a generalized condition, affecting long bones, sternum, and vertebrae. The other condition is seen commonly in old female mice of certain strains (Figure 14.19), but it is rarely seen in males. It can be seen in the sternum, facial bones, and long bones, where hyperostosis begins as a partial replacement of the marrow cavity with mesenchymal cells and matrix. Osteoblasts, osteoclasts, and fibroblasts can be recognized in the lesion, as can fibrous tissue, osteoid, and woven bone.

Murine strains with hyperostotic lesions have, in addition, a high incidence of ovarian cysts and cystic adenomatous hyperplasia of the uterus. Long-term administration of high doses of a synthetic PGE_1 analog enhanced the occurrence of the spontaneous hyperostosis. The high incidence of hyperostosis in female mice, the concomitant occurrence of reproductive lesions associated with estrogenism, and the known relationship between hyperostosis and estrogens in mice suggest that hyperostotic lesions have a hormonal basis. Dietary estrogens have been shown to

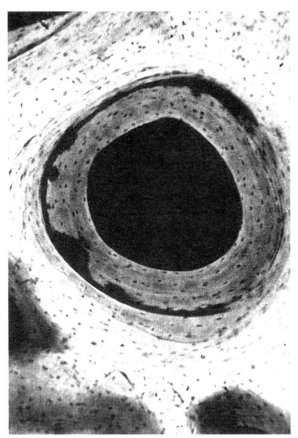

FIGURE 14.16   Hypervitaminosis D. *Solanum malacoxylon* intoxication. Microradiograph demonstrates actively-forming osteon, with incomplete mineralization of the peripheral matrix.

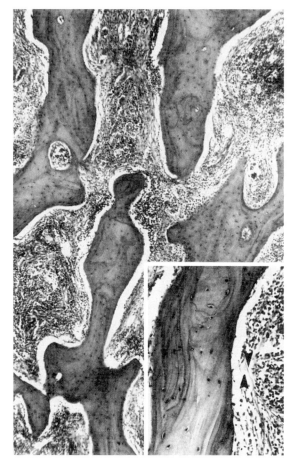

FIGURE 14.17   Osteosclerosis. Diaphyseal bone marrow from a dog with anemia illustrates increased number and width of trabeculae of lamellar bone. Inset: numerous cement lines and fine collagen fibers (arrows), myelofibrosis, adjacent to bone.

hasten the development of hyperostosis, and are considered to serve as one of many factors predisposing C3H mice to the development of osteosarcoma. In C3H mice following [226]Ra administration, an accentuation in the appearance of spontaneous hyperostotic lesions has been reported; some were thought to be preneoplastic.

Neoplasia can be considered cell proliferation without adequate differentiation and control. In general, primary bone neoplasia in laboratory animals is similar to the phenomenon in humans, except that a few morphologic tumor forms have not been recognized, e.g., osteoid osteoma. The vast majority of primary malignant bone neoplasms are osteosarcomas, 85% in the dog (Figure 14.20), the remaining scattered among the other connective tissue cell types. Alkaline phosphatase enzyme reaction can be used to distinguish primary spindle cell osteosarcomas from fibrosarcomas; however, chondrosarcomas often contain this enzyme. Osteomas containing C-type particles may be found in mice. Chordomas are uncommon axial skeleton neoplasms that arise from residual foci of primitive notochord anywhere along the vertebral column, but most commonly involve the cranial and caudal portions. They are slow growing, but highly infiltrative, producing bony destruction and frequently extending into soft tissue. They have been reported in humans, rats, mice, dogs, ferrets, cats, and mink.

Studies have shown that radiation-induced tumors in laboratory animals are of a similar type to those occurring spontaneously in that species. For example, neoplasms induced by internal irradiation in the cat had a higher incidence of primary bone tumors that were not osteosarcomas than was observed in the dog, and an example of an osteocalstoma was seen among the induced tumors. Similar experiences have been observed in spontaneously-arising feline bone tumors. The distribution of the tumors produced by internal irradiation in the dog is somewhat different, since neoplasms of the axial skeleton are more common, and spontaneous osteosarcomas occur more commonly in long bone metaphyses. It is interesting to

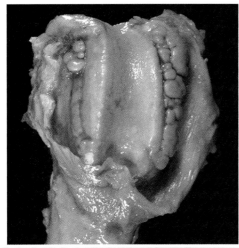

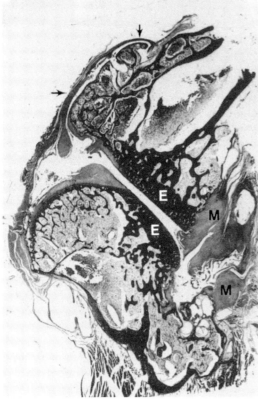

FIGURE 14.18   Osteophytes. (A) Degenerative joint disease, distal femur, dog. Note the marked formation of osteophytes (arrows) at the lateral and medial margins of the trochlear ridges. (Courtesy of Dr H. Liepold, College of Veterinary Medicine, Kansas State University, and Noah's Arkive, College of Veterinary Medicine, The University of Georgia.) (From Weisbrode, S.E. (2007). In *Pathologic Basis of Veterinary Disease*, McGavin, M., and Zachary, J.F., eds, 4th edn. Mosby Elsevier, St. Louis. Figure 16-38, p. 1061.) (B) Rabbit, shoulder joint. Mature osteophyte (arrow) on rim of scapula, eburnation (E) of articular surface of scapula and humerus, and cartilaginous metaplasia (M) of synovium.

note that the Saint Bernard dog has an earlier appearance of radiation-induced neoplasm than the beagle. In the natural disease process, the Saint Bernard has a higher incidence of bone tumors. This is possibly

due to the fact that the bone surface-to-volume ratio is higher, and the bone turnover is greater, in large breed dogs. *Chondroma rodens*, or multilobular osteoma, is a somewhat unusual neoplasm that has a greater prevalence in the dog than other species; its incidence does not appear to be increased by radiation.

Bone Modeling

Bone modeling as a process occurs principally during growth, but continues to a small extent throughout life. Bone modeling-dependent toxicity reactions affect compact bone, and lead to insufficient or excess accumulations of bone, or to mechanically inappropriate architecture.

Substances causing bone modeling abnormalities include chemicals that cause angular limb deformities. For example, maternal ingestion of excessive iodine results in foals with congenital hypothyroidism and angular limb deformity. Some bisphosphonates interfere with osteoclastic resorption of bone, causing an abnormal metaphyseal contour (Figure 14.21). The reactivation of modeling drifts can occur in adult animals, e.g., the formation of marginal osteophytes, in association with degenerative arthropathy. Another example of abnormal bone modeling is acromegaly, where growth hormone causes reactivation of growth plate endochondral ossification and articular cartilage chondrocyte proliferation. Also, anabolic agents, such as PTH and PGE_2, add bone mainly by modeling dependent bone gain or by formation drifts. The production of woven bone in the adult, or the resorption of bone in association with neoplasia, can be considered modeling activities. Osteoclastic-mediated bone resorption may occur because T-lymphocytes secrete a lymphokine, osteoclast-activating factor, in response to products of sensitized macrophages.

Bone Remodeling

Bone remodeling is an ongoing process under the influence of many different factors, both systemic and local. It is the process by which microdamage induced by mechanical activity can be repaired. Remodeling is responsible for maintaining mineral homeostasis when the capacity of the bone surface–canalicular system is overextended. Remodeling-dependent reactions to injury occur in growing animals as the spongiosa is remodeled, and in the adult after modeling has slowed.

In the growing bone, once the primary spongiosa is formed, the number of trabeculae is reduced and their thickness increased by remodeling. The scalloped chondroid cores and reversal cement lines within metaphyseal trabeculae are evidence of this activity. If osteoclastic resorption of the metaphyseal trabeculae

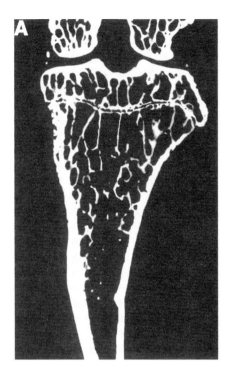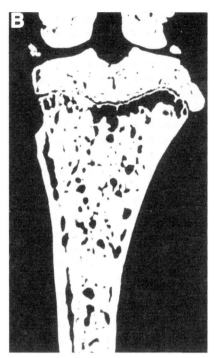

FIGURE 14.19   Spontaneous hyperostosis of mice. (A) Microradiograph of two-year-old, control Fischer mouse. (B) Osteosclerotic female mouse from same control group as (A). (Courtesy of Dr P.H. Long, Proctor and Gamble Company.)

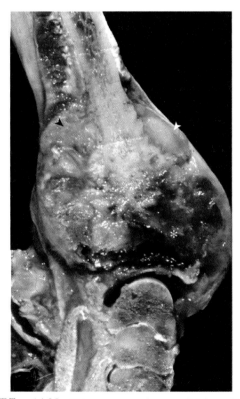

FIGURE   14.20 Osteosarcoma, bone, distal radius, dog. Osteosarcoma has lysed and replaced normal bone. There is reactive periosteal bone formation (arrowheads), and a large area of hemorrhage and necrosis(*). (Courtesy of Department of Veterinary Biosciences, The Ohio State University, and Noah's Arkive, College of Veterinary Medicine, The University of Georgia.) (From Weisbrode, S.E. (2007). In *Pathologic Basis of Veterinary Disease*, McGavin, M., and Zachary, J.F., eds, 4th edn. Mosby Elsevier, St. Louis. Figure 16-73, p. 1089.)

is inhibited, metaphyseal sclerosis results, since the remodeling process normally leads to net tissue loss. Metaphyseal sclerosis associated with bisphosphonate, yellow phosphorus, and lead toxicities are examples (Figure 14.22). Also, the amount of bone may be increased within the metaphysis following increased biomechanical loading, or by administering anabolic agents that cause an imbalance that favors formation over resorption, so there is a net increase in bone at the end of the remodeling cycle.

Usually, agents that reduce bone turnover give a transient bone gain. Since there is a normal loss in the amount of cancellous bone during metaphyseal remodeling, any drug that increases the turnover rate causes osteopenia. In the rat increased metaphyseal turnover following ovariohysterectomy leads to osteopenia, an event that can be inhibited by bisphosphonate. In order to prove that the loss or gain in metaphyseal cancellous bone within a growing animal is remodeling-dependent, one must show that the change is not related to growth modeling events.

In adults, drugs can cause remodeling-dependent bone reactions that include losses or gains in the amount of bone, improper distribution of trabeculae, or bone of abnormal quality. Osteoporosis has been defined in the past as a pathologic reduction in bone mass, in which the remaining bone is structurally normal. However, it is becoming increasingly evident as the material and architectural quality of bone

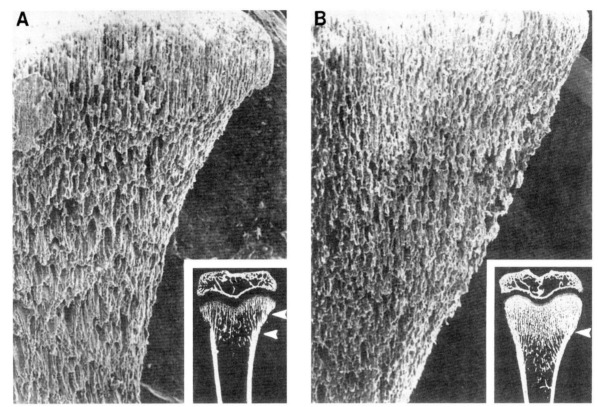

FIGURE 14.21   Abnormal metaphyseal contour. (A) Scanning electron micrograph (SEM) of the lateral periosteal surface of the proximal tibial metaphysis from a control rat. Extensive resorption occurs at the surface, cut-back zone, during normal modeling of the metaphysis associated with longitudinal bone growth. Inset: microradiograph of frontal section of proximal tibia; arrowheads delineate periosteal surface viewed in the SEM micrograph. (B) SEM of proximal tibial metaphyseal periosteum from rat treated with a bisphosphonate. Surface differs from (A) in that it is slightly convex. Inset: microradiograph of a frontal section of the proximal tibia from bisphosphonate-treated animal; widening of the metaphysis bone is greatly increased compared with (A). (From Miller and Jee (1979), Anat Rec 193:439–462, with permission.)

is examined more closely, that the remaining bone is not normal. Osteopenia refers to the state in which overall bone mass is reduced, but in which remaining bone is qualitatively normal. Reversible osteopenias arise when the remodeling space is increased, through activation of osteoclastic resorption or a prolonged remodeling period. For example, in the osteopenia of thyrotoxicosis or hyperparathyroidism there is increased activation. Drugs that depress activation can prevent reversible osteopenias.

Irreversible bone loss is the result of absolute bone volume deficits that usually arise on the trabecular and endocortical surfaces. During aging, the amount of bone removed during remodeling declines, but the amount of bone that refills the resorption bay declines even more; therefore, there is accelerated bone loss, even though there is decreased bone resorption. Any event enhancing the deficit would cause an irreversible osteopenia. Examples causing irreversible osteopenia include malnutrition, adrenal cortical steroids, and chronic metabolic acidosis. Although hormones were considered to be the agents responsible for the

coupling of bone resorption to formation, local growth factors may be better candidates. Any agent that affects the production of coupling factors could cause irreversible bone loss, because of a failure to recruit new mesenchymal cells during the bone formation phase of bone turnover, an imbalance where resorption is greater than formation.

Joints

Non-neoplastic Changes

The synovial membrane is a thin vascular lining covering the inner surface of the articular capsule and intra-articular ligaments and tendons. It is usually composed of two layers: a thin internal surface layer two to three cells deep; and a deeper subintimal, loose or fibrous connective tissue layer. Synovial cells are of two types: Type A (M) cells that have a prominent Golgi apparatus, prominent vesicles, and little rough endoplasmic reticulum; and type B (F) cells that have a well-developed rough endoplasmic reticulum, but

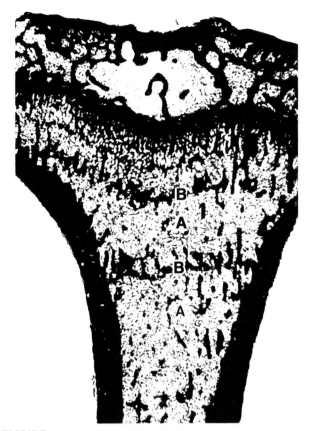

FIGURE 14.22 Effect of longitudinal bone growth and bone turnover on the quantity of the metaphyseal cancellous bone. Ovariectomy in the rat increases bone turnover, and reduces the quantity of metaphyseal trabeculae (zone A). Periodic administration of a bisphosphonate inhibits longitudinal bone growth, reduces bone turnover, and increases the metaphyseal bone during the periods of drug administration (Zone B). (Courtesy of Dr Wronski, University of Florida.)

a poorly-developed Golgi apparatus. Synovial cells with an intermediate type of morphology also exist.

Synovial villi project into the joint at specialized regions, such as niches between the large fat folds. These are nearly always nonvascular protrusions, and are usually so small that they are only visible microscopically. Scanning electron microscopy characteristics of normal synovial cells show only a smooth surface interrupted by raised nuclear prominences, but transmission electron microscopy demonstrates filopodia, which are surface membrane ruffles or folds involved with phagocytosis. In rats, rabbits, and calves, when the synovial cells become closely packed, cell junctions are apparent.

In acute synovitis, periarticular edema, fibrin deposition within the synovial membrane or joint space, and an inflammatory infiltrate composed principally of neutrophils can be seen. With acute exudative reactions, edema and fibrin deposition may be considerable, with only a limited inflammatory cell infiltrate.

Polymorphonuclear leukocytes migrate quickly through the synovium into the joint space; thus, synovial fluid may contain many more neutrophils than are apparent in a synovial biopsy. Even minor joint disturbances, such as saline flushing or instilling the joint with contrast agents, causes an acute inflammatory response with alteration in the surface lining cells. As acute inflammation subsides, the synovial inflammatory infiltrate changes character, and becomes composed of mononuclear cells, with macrophages predominating. A lymphoplasmocytic infiltrate characterizes the immune-mediated arthritides—germinal centers are rarely seen.

With all joint inflammations there is a reaction of the synovial lining cells. An increase in the intermediate-type cell and type B-cells is seen in arthritis. Therefore, in inflammatory conditions leading to increased phagocytic activity and lysosome production, a hypertrophy of the rough endoplasmic reticulum occurs to meet the demand for the production of lysosomal acid hydrolases.

Synovial cells can also undergo hyperplasia and hypertrophy (Figure 14.23). When this occurs, the lining cells increase in numbers, become plump and rounded, and have numerous surface filopodia (Figure 14.24). The synovial membrane has a tremendous capacity to undergo villous proliferation as a feature of low-grade inflammation. In the various joint diseases, these villi vary widely in size, shape, and composition. In part, this is a reflection of their development. Fibrin deposited within the joint space can become organized, much like an organizing thrombus.

Initially, villi which develop by this mechanism appear avascular and hypocellular. Later, they become vascularized, looking like the hypercellular villi seen with any immune-mediated or nonimmune chronic arthritis. With, or because of, synovial inflammation, there is destruction of the articular cartilage (Figure 14.25). Fragments of articular cartilage that break off, or are eroded from the joint surface, lodge in synovial crevices and may become incorporated as part of villous proliferation. These cartilage fragments gradually lose their proteoglycan staining ability, and supposedly provoke continued inflammation and articular cartilage destruction, an immune response mounted against the liberated proteoglycan or type II collagen.

In addition to joint inflammation and villous proliferation, there may be secondary responses within the synovial membrane. In rare instances, osteochondral nodules develop in association with chronic inflammation. Considerable deposition of hemosiderin pigment within synovial lining cells, or within macrophages of the synovial membrane or articular capsule may be seen. Fibrosis and articular capsular hypertrophy occur in chronic arthritis. There may also

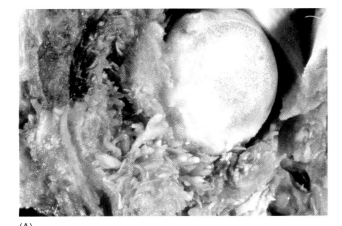

(A)

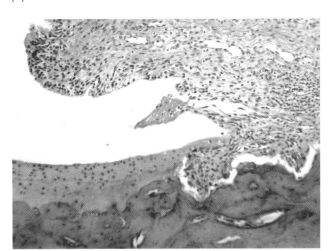

(B)

FIGURE 14.23 (A) Marked synovial villous hyperplasia, hip dysplasia, coxofemoral joint, articular capsule, and femoral head, dog. The extent of this proliferation is unusually severe for hip dysplasia. Microscopically, this hyperplasia is routinely accompanied by variable lymphoplasmacytic inflammation that is independent of the cause of the articular damage. (B) Pannus, rheumatoid-like arthritis (experimentally-induced), articular cartilage, tibia, distal end, rat. Pannus originating from the synovium (right) is invading and destroying the articular cartilage and bone. H&E stain. (A and B courtesy of Dr S.E. Weisbrode, College of Veterinary Medicine, The Ohio State University.) (From Weisbrode, S.E. (2007). In *Pathologic Basis of Veterinary Disease*, McGavin, M., and Zachary, J.F., eds, 4th edn. Mosby Elsevier, St. Louis. Figures 16-34, p. 1060 and 16-37, p.1061.)

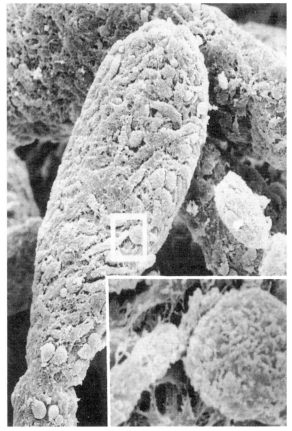

FIGURE 14.24 Scanning electron micrograph of synovial villi in inflammatory arthritis. Inset: surface filopodia are characteristic of hypertrophic synovial cells.

be mineralization within the synovial wall and joint capsule. In humans, drugs that induce hyperuricemia cause gout tophi to form. Chondroid, collagen, and osteoid have an affinity for uric acid salts, and these salts deposit in sheaths of sharp-pointed crystals, and induce a granulomatous inflammatory response.

Too much pressure, or a lack of sufficient contact on the bone end, leads to alteration in articular cartilage. In the former case, cells in the superficial cartilage zone become necrotic, with loss of matrix staining.

In the latter case, the cartilage matrix becomes fibrillated (Figure 14.25). Deformation of articular cartilage can lead to cartilage creep. Microscopically, this can be observed as a disorientation of the chondrocytes.

Chondromalacia is the macroscopic term used to describe rubbery articular cartilage. By hematoxylin and eosin staining and light microscopy, chondromalacic cartilage often appears normal; however, a loss of cartilage matrix can be identified microscopically by special staining techniques with cationic dyes, such as safranin-O or toluidine blue.

Cartilage cell necrosis can be determined if the number of cartilage cells or the number of empty lacunae per unit area is quantified. In other examples, chondrocyte necrosis may be easily visualized, using light microscopy to visualize pyknotic nuclei. Loss of intercellular matrix follows degeneration of chondrocytes. This process begins as a loss of the articular cartilage surface, termed *lammina splendens*, and continues as the quantity of cartilage and the metachromatic staining properties of its matrix are lost. Normal collagen fibrils within the cartilage matrix become more prominent by light microscopy. Cracks and crevices develop,

Normal   Fibrillation   Eburnation

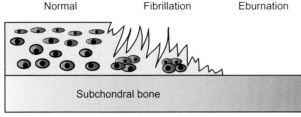

(A)

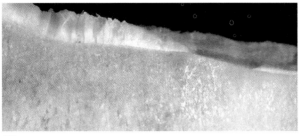

(B)

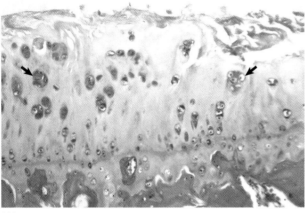

(C)

FIGURE 14.25 Degenerative joint disease, fibrillation, and ulceration of articular cartilage. (A) Schematic diagram showing fibrillation and eburnation of articular cartilage overlying subchondral bone which has increased density. (B) Tibia, proximal articular cartilage, sagittal section, bull. To the left, the cartilage is frayed (fibrillation). To the right is an ulcer. Note that the cartilage is missing from the bed of the ulcer in the plane of the section, but the edge of the ulcer with a rim of normal cartilage is visible at its back. The cartilage to the right of the ulcer is very thin, indicating erosion. (C) Femoral head, articular cartilage, dog. The superficial cartilage is fibrillated and hypocellular (necrosis), with clusters of chondrocytes (arrows) representing an ineffectual attempt at repair. H&E stain. (B and C courtesy of Dr S.E. Weisbrode, College of Veterinary Medicine, The Ohio State University.) (From Weisbrode, S.E. (2007). In *Pathologic Basis of Veterinary Disease*, McGavin, M., and Zachary, J.F., eds, 4th edn. Mosby Elsevier, St. Louis. Figures 16-30(A), 16-31(B), 16-32(C), p. 1059.)

and fragment the remaining cartilage into longitudinal clefts. In some cases, superficial portions of cartilage may become dislodged, and develop into loose bodies or "joint mice." In the case of drug toxicities, as seen with the quinolone class of antibiotics, the distribution

of necrotic chondrocytes is unique. Necrosis usually occurs only in animals in which the articular cartilage is still in the process of growth, beginning within the zona intermedia of the articular cartilage. An exception is ofloxacin, which can produce the lesion in articular cartilage of skeletally-mature dogs. Necrosis of cartilage cells, and subsequent matrix lysis, produces a cleft seen grossly as a blister on the articular surface which quickly ruptures (see Figure 14.23).

Whenever there is cartilage cell necrosis, or loss of the superficial cartilage layers, the remaining cartilage cells undergo cell division, producing daughter cells, clusters, cell clones, or chondrones. The ability of articular cartilage to replace itself following injury is limited, but a significant amount of regeneration can occur, more than was previously appreciated. Cartilage cells can reproduce sufficiently in certain pathologic states to recreate functional articular surfaces. Under normal circumstances, surface cartilage is worn away by friction, and small cartilage clones develop in the middle zone, appearing to migrate toward the surface to be shed into the joint space. The deep margin of cartilage is slowly transformed into chondroid bone. Progressive tidemarks of calcified cartilage form a historical marker of changes in the osteochondral border.

In certain disease conditions of the adult, this normally slow bone modeling process is exaggerated to such an extent that the bone contour is altered. This process has been divided into progressive, regressive, and circumferential reactions. In the progressive reaction, there is initial interstitial proliferation of cartilage, and increased thickness of the articular cartilage. The base of the cartilage becomes progressively mineralized, and there is conversion into bone. Occasionally, vascular invasion of the thickened cartilage and conversion into bone produces a new subchondral plate. Since the initial reaction represents a growth process, remodeling of the tissue follows. Progressive changes are particularly apparent in acromegaly following growth hormone stimulation of cartilage growth.

Regressive changes can be seen whenever loss of the cartilage surface, and a subsequent loss of bone, changes the bone contour. The cause is unknown, but may be related to mechanical overloading. This change happens during the process of eburnation. Occasionally, cartilage regenerates over the bone surface. Marginal osteophytes are circumferential modeling alterations due to periosteal bone formation, ossification of tendons or ligaments, or upward and lateral growth of cartilage with progressive transformation into bone.

The response of articular cartilage to trauma is dependent largely on the depth of the injury. Superficial lacerations evoke only a short-lived metabolic and enzymatic response, failing to provide sufficient numbers of cells or matrix to repair the smallest injury. However, when the injury penetrates the osteochondral border, the response is similar to that occurring in other vascularized tissues. The reaction in this region is typically a granulation tissue response, similar to that described in fracture repair, except that bone proliferation stops at the margin of the cartilage–bone junction, leaving fibrous tissue to unite the cartilage wound edges. The fibrous tissue undergoes progressive hyalinization and chondrification to produce a fibrocartilaginous mass. Continuous passive motion has been shown to assist conversion of fibrocartilage to a more hyaline-type of cartilage.

Not only does the vascular reaction occur within the subchondral marrow, but synovial vessels may also become stimulated. When this occurs, a fibrovascular membrane, or pannus, originating from the synovium becomes attached to and infiltrates the cartilage defect. The response of the subchondral osseous trabeculae is probably due to altered biomechanical stresses and strains. Trabeculae undergo more vigorous remodeling, and become thicker. When the trabecular thickness becomes excessive, central Haversian-like canals develop, and the subchondral bone acquires an appearance more like compacta. The chondrification of fibrous tissue filling the marrow may be deficient, and the tissue is more characteristic of myxomatous connective tissue. There may be focal bone resorption, surrounding trabeculae may form a wall around the myxomatous reactive tissue, and the lesion develops into a pseudocyst.

Neoplasia

Fibrosarcomas rarely develop in the periarticular tissues, and must be distinguished from the more common spindle cell appearing synovial sarcomas. Synovial sarcomas typically have a biphasic cell population. However, one must examine numerous samples to appreciate the characteristic features, which include slit-like spaces or a pseudoglandular pattern. Using immunohistochemical techniques, cells within synovial cell sarcomas show a biphasic pattern with spindle cells containing vimentin-positive intermediate filaments, and epithelial-like cells staining for cytokeratin. Fibrosarcomas fail to stain for cytokeratins.

EVALUATION OF SKELETAL TOXICITY

Most drug toxicity protocols are not designed to examine the effects of chemical agents on the skeletal system. Although bone and its marrow are examined during toxicity testing, evaluation is sometimes limited to the sternum. If one does not examine the growth plate and mid-shaft mataphysis of the growing animal, the evaluation of the major bone activities—longitudinal bone growth and modeling—is forfeited. Whenever a test agent is suspected of having an action on the skeleton, the toxicity protocol should be modified so the effect the agent has on the skeleton can be measured. In a separate group of animals, bone fluorescent markers can be employed to determine tissue dynamic changes, and longitudinal and radial bone growth.

Radiologic examination is a valued addition to gross evaluation. Ideally, one should examine a sagittal section of the femoral-tibial joint; a frontal section through the tibia to include the secondary ossification center, growth plate, and metaphysis; and a cross-section through the tibia near the tibio–fibular junction.

Comparison of various types of joints, including small joints on the paws, major joints of the limbs, and the intervertebral joints with adjoining bone, may be necessary. In addition to trying to determine adverse reactions that various chemicals might have on bone and joints, studies may be designed to determine the mechanism of action. Also, animal models of bone or joint disease may be used to determine drug effectiveness.

Testing for Skeletal Toxicity

In Vivo Studies

Skeletal maintenance requires the coordinated efforts of cellular destruction and reconstruction of osseous tissue. These activities are controlled by systemic and local biomechanical and mechanical factors, many of which remain unknown. It is unlikely that in vitro systems will replace the whole animal in determining drug action on remodeling systems dependent on cooperative activities of multiple organs. Since most agents affecting bone operate on precursor cells, or indirectly modulate cell production and function, bone toxicity studies must be designed to evaluate these effects. Although humans are the ideal experimental animals, preliminary studies must first be conducted in laboratory animals, in a cost-effective way. Even though rodents do not normally have secondary osteons in cortical bone, they can still be used to examine bone development, growth, modeling, and cancellous and endocortical bone remodeling.

Cortical bone is used to study the reaction of the periosteal and endocortical envelope, and the metaphysis is used for the trabecular envelopes. The study of intracortical bone remodeling cannot be undertaken in rodents, but dogs, primates, or large domestic animals such as sheep are satisfactory. Cancellous bone remodeling in the rodent can be examined in the secondary spongiosa of long bones or vertebrae, including coccygeal vertebrae. Studies of cancellous remodeling in the rodent must consider the effects of growth on the age of the metaphyseal cancellous bone. Rodent long bones continue to grow to a small extent even in the adult (5 μm/day at six months). Furthermore, mechanical loaded and unloaded skeletal sites should be surveyed, because biomechanical factors can modify the skeletal response. Teratogenic studies determine the effects of agents on bone development, while major adverse reactions on longitudinal bone growth, bone modeling, or joint structure can be determined in subacute, subchronic, or chronic toxicity studies.

In Vitro *Studies*

Bone metabolism may be studied in isolated bone cells, or in organ cultures. These systems permit study of the direct actions of agents on bone isolated from the homeostatic and biomechanical control mechanisms. Organ cultures of fetal long bones, neonatal calvaria, or fetal metatarsals show a disruption in skeletal development, possibly because of the absence of systemic trophic factors.

Systems to study coupling of resorption and formation are actively being sought. Cultures of mature osteoclasts have been described; however, except for those obtained from birds, these are not obtained in sufficient numbers to allow extensive studies. Two types of *in vitro* methods for studying bone resorption have been used. One method consists of treating the whole animal with an agent suspected to alter resorption. Collagen and calcium deposition or release is analyzed by short-term incubation of bone fragments. In the other method, chick embryos are used, or bones from fetuses or young animals can be maintained for long periods in suitable media. Unfortunately, one cannot be certain that all the calcium released from bone was the result of osteoclastic resorption.

Chick embryos also are used to study the effects of agents on cartilage and joints, or wing bud tips can be established as an organ culture. In addition, chondrocyte from nasal septum or costal cartilage, and chondrocytes or synovial cells from normal or rheumatoid joints, can be cultured. An agent can be added to the organ culture media, so that increased bone resorption, or release of proteoglycans from cartilage, can be quantified by the release of radioactive calcium and matrix markers into the media. Sources of error include bone formation and redeposition of released radioisotopes, as well as physicochemical exchange of radioactive and stable calcium.

Usually, the *in vivo* and *in vitro* effects are thought to be similar, although the initial findings with prostaglandins (PGs) are a notable exception. *In vitro* studies with PGs showed bone resorption, whereas PG caused formation of woven bone when administered to intact rats or dogs. *In vitro* methods have been, and will continue to be, used successfully to test the response of bone cells to local factors, and to investigate specific biochemical mediator mechanisms. On the other hand, *in vitro* methods cannot accurately predict the skeletal response to circulating agents. Long-term skeletal toxicity or response to pharmacologic agents is determined by their effect on mediator mechanisms that require an intact whole organism.

Morphologic Evaluation

Radiological Examination

Radiology is an essential component in examining the skeleton. Radiographs may be used to survey the skeleton, or may be selectively used on bone slabs taken from specific lesion sites. Radiobisphosphonate bone scans following the administration of 99^m-technetium-labeled ethylene diphosphonate may be advantageous. Bone scintigraphy reveals enhanced radiobisphosphonate deposition, due to changes in blood flow or increased osteoblastic activity. Whatever the method, the role of radiological examination is to locate and characterize the disease process.

Because it may not be practical to examine all the bones of the body thoroughly, radiographs can be used to localize lesions that would otherwise be missed. Radiographs are useful in determining whether a lesion causing clinical signs of local lameness is part of a systemic disease process. They are also helpful in deciding which bone locations should be examined histologically to characterize the disease process.

A radiograph of a bone tumor, particularly when interpreting a biopsy, is as essential as the histologic slide in making a final diagnosis. The radiograph can give information concerning the extent of the lesion, its distribution within the bone, areas of bone formation and destruction, the quantity of periosteal reactive bone, and the location of the tissue specimen. Factors to be considered in viewing the radiograph are alterations in bone density, alterations in geometry, lesion location and distribution, periosteal reactions, and soft tissue changes.

Gross Examination

The detail with which examination of the skeletal system is carried out will differ, depending on the objectives of the necropsy procedure. At a minimum, the rib bones should be isolated and examined grossly for breaking strength and irregularities of the costochondral junction. The rib is easily handled, represents high turnover cortical bone, and can be trimmed easily to examine the growth region. Five major joints, in addition to those opened during the necropsy procedure, should receive open inspection. Longitudinal saw cuts should be made through the middle of at least two long bones. The examination of the limb bones is best accomplished by removing the muscular attachments surrounding the joint. The joint can then be opened using a pair of serrated shears or scissors, being careful not to let the tips touch articular cartilage. Do not use a knife or scalpel. Local congestion and autolysis can alter the gross appearance of synovial fluid, the synovial membrane, and articular cartilage. Hemolysis of blood can cause synovial fluid and articular cartilage to be stained red. The synovial fluid is normally viscid, and has a clear to yellow color.

Grossly, normal articular cartilage appears white, milky, and opaque in the thicker areas. In thin areas overlying bone marrow, the cartilage may be translucent and slightly blue. On cut section, the thickness of the articular cartilage is variable, not only from joint to joint within an individual, but also from region to region within a given joint. There is a wide range of articular cartilage thickness between animal species.

Synovial fossae are normal anatomical structures that appear as nonarticulating depressions in the joint surface. They are absent at birth, but the time of appearance, size, shape, and persistence of any given fossa varies. It is important to recognize synovial fossae and linear grooves as normal anatomical structures, so they can be distinguished from areas of articular collapse or lesions of osteoarthritis. Also, the gross color and transparency of menisci and articular discs are regionally variable, and reflect the thickness and composition of the structure. Thin portions of menisci and discs are translucent and have a blue-gray color. With increasing thickness, there is increased opacity and a gradual change in color, which becomes whiter.

Most ligaments grossly appear white and have a fibrous texture, although ligaments containing a significant amount of elastic tissue, such as the *ligamentum nuchae*, have a yellow color. The synovial lining of the joint capsule is pink, usually smooth, and glistening. Synovial villi are particularly prominent in certain places, such as a joint out-pouching or cul de sac. They are larger and more regularly spaced in animals than in humans, and they are more prominent in large domestic animals, such as the horse.

A frequent mistake made in examining the skeletal system is the superficial inspection of the joint by making a simple incision to expose the joint surface. Beginning osteophyte lesions of osteoarthritis or osteochondrosis lesions cannot be observed in this manner. It is necessary to completely expose the joint, so the articular margins and bone grooves through which ligaments pass can be closely inspected. The formation of small osteophytic excrescences at locations where muscle tension pulls on ligamentous insertions may indicate joint disease before visual inspection of the joint cartilage surface shows significant alterations. It is sometimes advantageous to macerate the specimen by boiling in detergent to reveal such lesions.

Visual inspection of the articular surface alone is insufficient to recognize many cartilaginous lesions. For example, the early changes of osteochondritis dissecans can be visualized on bone sagittal sections prior to the appearance of surface lesions. The use of radiographs as an aid to the examination of articular cartilage is advantageous, as the articular cartilage is radiolucent, and the radiographic interface between two joint surfaces actually represents the mineralized cartilage and the subchondral bone of each surface. Thus, bone fractures or bipartite sesamoid bones, which might otherwise be overlooked, can be detected.

Radiographs of sagitally-sliced slabs are also useful in examining the trabecular patterns within the bone metaphysis. The amount of cortical and trabecular endosteal bone can be observed directly. It is useful to compare the gross appearance of a bone slab with its counterpart from the opposite limb. Differences would indicate a potential lesion. Conversely, symmetrical alteration would suggest a systemic or metabolic disease.

Gross specimens may be macerated by boiling, using meat-eating beetles or exposing the specimen to enzymes; then statistical comparisons can be made of distances between surface features. Measurements made on each bone can be transformed to represent approximations of the bone's shape. Stepwise discriminate analysis has been used to show increased variation in mice following exposure to γ-radiation and environmental chemicals. Fourier analytic procedures can be used to describe complex morphologic shapes.

Bone may be extracted with lipid solvents in a Soxhlet's apparatus, and the fat-free dry weight determined. Bone volume and mean specific density, weight per unit volume, is determined by using Archimedes' principle. Bone ash is obtained after specimens are heated at 600°C, and calcium content can be quantified by atomic absorption analysis. Because of marked variation within bone locations, results are more meaningful if expressed as a function of the whole bone. However, values for trabecular bone and cortical bone should be reported separately. Neutron activation analysis can be used simultaneously to obtain calcium, phosphorus, sodium, and chloride content.

Newer methods for estimating bone mass or mineral content include X-ray densitometry, single or dual photon absorptiometric measurements, or computer assisted tomography mineral determinations. All of these techniques give method-specific differences in the bone mass among groups of animals. Certain parameters, such as the mean specific density, must be used with caution as a bone mass determination when there is osteomalacia. Accumulation of osteoid may lead to an increase in dry weight, with a disproportionate reduction of mineralized bone.

Microscopic Examination

Preparation of Tissues

Unfortunately, obtaining high-quality tissue sections of bone and cartilage is more an art than a science! Each laboratory has its preferred methods for tissue preparation and staining. How each tissue specimen is handled depends on the information that needs to be obtained. One of the major problems encountered in the preparation of bone in many laboratories is inadequate fixation of hard tissues. All fixatives penetrate bone poorly; therefore, it is imperative that bone be cut so fixative can penetrate the cortex. Fixatives do not penetrate even the bones of small rodents quickly. For example, cancellous bone specimens should not be more than 0.5 cm thick.

A convenient way to prepare the tibia of a rat is to shave off the tibial crest with a razor blade, so that a flat cancellous bone surface of the full metaphysis can be seen. Care must be taken not to fracture the growth plate artifactually. The use of large sections of whole bone or joints has the advantage of maintaining anatomic integrity, and allows one to separate major pathological features from reactive processes. If higher resolution is required of specific regions, the large paraffin blocks can be trimmed to a suitable size for further sectioning.

Formalin fixation is adequate for preserving the morphology of most skeletal tissue. However, if fluorescent bone labels have been given, the acid environment will decalcify the outer surface and cause label to be lost after 24 hours. A practical substitute for formalin is an alcohol–formalin solution made with 10 mL formaldehyde and 90 ml 70% ethanol. Since the solution is nonpolar, tetracycline labeling is maintained, and cell morphology is superior to that when using alcohol alone. Formalin- or alcohol-fixed tissues may be treated with cyanuric chloride and N-methyl morpholine for osteoid staining of decalcified tissues. The use of Bouin's solution, or B5 fixative, results in slightly superior hematoxylin and eosin staining of bone and marrow cells. Since Bouin's solution is acid, partial decalcification occurs during the fixation period.

Decalcification with ethylenediaminetetracetic acid (EDTA) is gentle to the tissues, and can be used to preserve enzymatic activity. There are many acid decalcification solutions that act much faster than EDTA, most appearing to work satisfactorily as long as the specimen is removed from the solution immediately after decalcification is complete. Radiographic determination of decalcification endpoints is helpful for inexperienced technicians.

Dehydration and infiltration of bone with paraffin is more difficult than for soft tissue. Modification of the standard embedding schedule is usually required. Three major points must be followed to obtain quality histologic sections: first, vacuum embedding should be employed; second, the dehydration and embedding times should be thorough, but kept as short as possible to prevent hardening of collagenous tissues (a three-day schedule with an automatic processor is sufficient for very large blocks); and third, a sharp microtome knife must be maintained.

To section undecalcified cancellous bone specimens, embedding in methyl methacrylate with plasticizer is desirable. Sections of 3–15 μm can be obtained with a tungsten carbide, D-profile knife. These can be stained using a variety of techniques, such as fluorochrome labels to highlight mineralized tissue, osteoid, or cellular details. One of the advantages of plastic embedding is the avoidance of much of the tissue shrinkage that usually affects histomorphometry.

Sections of undecalcified cortical bone are very difficult to make, and best results are obtained with ground sections. Tissues are embedded by standard methods in methyl methacrylate. A plasticizer is not required. Sections 200–250 μm in thickness are obtained with a diamond wafering blade, milling machine with jeweller's saw blade, or other suitable apparatus, then ground using an automatic lapping machine, or by hand. The thick sections are glued to plastic slides with cyanoacrylic glue, and the surfaces are polished to remove scratches. Because the staining solution only penetrates a few micrometers of the exposed surface, the morphology is similar to that of a thin section stained with toluidine blue for osteoid, cells, or cement lines.

Alternatively, sections may be placed in 14% EDTA overnight, before staining for cement lines using toluidine blue at basic pH. Other toluidine blue stains at various pHs are useful for demonstration of cells or osteoid. If thick sections are ground to 100 μm they can be used to make microradiographs. Microradiographs allow bone density of microscopic regions to be visualized, and are especially useful in identifying mineralization defects (see Figure 14.1). Sections should be ground to approximately 20 μm for visualization of fluorescent labels.

Histologic Examination

Ideally, in the standard toxicology protocol, sections are obtained through a joint, so that synovium and articular cartilage may be observed. A section through a long bone growth plate and metaphysis should also be made, so that growth, modeling, and remodeling parameters may be assessed. Since researchers frequently use frontal sections of the rat tibia, normal values for growth rates and cartilage cell division and maturation can be found in the literature. Sections from this location can be used to examine the growth plate, metaphyseal cortical surface, spongiosa, maturation of the secondary ossification center, bone cells, and marrow. It is important to recognize that, in acute toxicity studies where only a single dose of a test agent is given, the bone immediately beneath the growth plate may not have been formed under the influence of the test drug. The intrinsic cellular properties in rapidly growing animals include bone elongation, and baseline values of bone elongation and associated remodeling. These properties are very strong, and they may overshadow the effects of drug treatment.

The mineralizing front, the basophilic line between the surface osteoid and mineralized bone, is difficult to see in woven bone or in specimens that have been subjected to excess acid. An accurate assessment requires the use of special techniques to differentiate between mineralized and unmineralized collagen. It is important to examine the quantity and width of osteoid, because this is increased in chemically-induced osteomalacias.

The amount of surface osteoid of the spongiosa of growing rat trabeculae is not reliably identified in decalcified hematoxylin- and eosin-stained sections. Except for the metaphysis of a growing bone, roughly 20% of cancellous bone surfaces should be covered with osteoid, and less than 2% of the bone should be made up of osteoid. Osteoid thickness should not exceed 15 μm, and only a small percentage of the osteoid surface should be covered by plump osteoblasts.

Except for the initial bone laid down, woven bone is not normally seen in tissue sections and, when found, should be explained by appropriate pathology studies. Juxtaposed bone is the deposition of woven bone on pre-existing viable or necrotic bone, and may be seen under some conditions. A classic example of the above is creeping substitution of dead bone, but juxtaposed bone may be seen in toxic osteopathies, such as fluorosis. It indicates a sudden disruption of normal surface bone remodeling process by an overpowering insult or inciting agent.

Fibrosis may be seen in primary disorders of bone and marrow. It occurs as a diffuse deposition of reticulum fibers in myelofibrosis, and is seen in a juxtatrabecular location in renal osteodystrophy and hyperparathyroidism. Metastatic tumors also elicit exuberant myelo-fibroblastic responses.

Ultrastructural Examination

Ultrastructural studies of bone and joint tissues remain primarily a research tool. The very diverse nature of skeletal structure and function precludes ultrastructural changes being the sole basis of examination. Both scanning and transmission electron microscopy can play important roles in tissue evaluation under specific circumstances. Ruthenium red fixation and freeze-substitution methods have improved the preservation of matrix so that it closely approximates the native state. As our knowledge of the properties of bone and cartilage matrix advances, ultrastructural studies of these components will become more important.

The ultrastructure of specific bone cells gives evidence of their functional activities, and these characteristics may be used to study the effects of drugs on cells in growing and modeling systems. One of the better-known endpoints of osteoclastic activity is the demonstration of a ruffled border. The use of special techniques, such as X-ray diffraction, back scatter imaging, or energy dispersive X-ray microanalysis will continue to contribute to toxicologic evaluations.

Histochemical Examination

Histochemical methods have always been very valuable in studying bone biology and pathology. Chemically-different matrix components can be specifically stained using the periodic acid-Schiff reaction, toluidine blue, and alcian blue at critical electrolyte concentrations. Safranin O stains glycosaminoglycans in a semiquantitative manner. Von Kossa's technique for identification of phosphate groups has been used to distinguish mineralized bone matrix from osteoid. Histochemical stains for iron and aluminum have been used in the study of their toxic effects. Tartrate-resistant acid phosphatase isozyme is generally accepted as a cytochemical marker for osteoclasts and their immediate precursors. The acid phosphatase isoenzyme of monocyte and macrophages is sensitive to tartrate. Osteoblasts and preosteoblasts stain intensely for alkaline phosphatase activity, a cytochemical marker for the osteoblast phenotype. Lectin histochemistry can be used to localize carbohydrate groups in cartilage, and specific antibodies to matrix macromolecules have been developed recently for immunohistologic use. The development of monoclonal antibody technology offers the promise that the effects of drugs on osteoprogenitor cells can be studied in the future. Antibodies can be used to demonstrate cytoplasmic components, such as cytokeratins, intermediate filaments, or cell surface antigens that may suggest common cell lineage.

Morphometric Analysis

Bone toxicology studies can have two different objectives. The first is to detect any drug-induced adverse tissue reactions, and the second is to determine the mechanism of drug action on osseous tissue. Although quantitative morphologic differences that escape visual examination may be detected by bone histomorphometry, the major value of this method is to determine the mechanisms of drug action on bone. The techniques and methods are well worked out, and are not overly difficult, but they are exceedingly time-consuming. The histologic methods give excellent morphologic preparations and have a certain value, even if sections are not quantified. For example, morphology of bone and marrow cells is superior in plastic sections to determine the width of osteoid seams. Any histomorphometric methods should include dynamic measurements obtained following bone fluorochrome double labeling.

Quantitative morphology can be used to measure several cellular activities associated with bone and cartilage growth and maintenance. These include measurement of longitudinal bone growth, morphology of the long bone metaphysis, bone modeling activities, cortical bone remodeling, cancellous bone remodeling, and morphology of articular cartilage. The definitive method for classifying metabolic bone disease is histomorphometry of undecalcified bone sections. The purpose of using histomorphometric analysis is to obtain precise measurements of the amount of bone tissue or osteoid, and to quantify rates and duration of activity. To determine the effect an agent has on the remodeling cycle, it must be administered long enough to go through several remodeling periods. A three-month-long toxicity study would be adequate for the rat, but too short for the dog. Stained sections are used to measure "static" parameters, such as cancellous bone volume and fluorochrome labels from which "dynamic" rate parameters are derived. Static parameters can be measured manually, semi-automatically, or obtained with a quantitative television

microscope. Comparisons of the Merz grid determination of cancellous bone volume with computerized morphometry shows that both methods yield essentially the same results. The quality of the histologic preparation and the skill of the individual making the analysis govern the reliability of the data generated.

Biochemical Evaluation

Clinical chemistry evaluation can be of assistance in determining whether drugs affect the skeletal system. Serum calcium levels are under homeostatic control mechanisms and, therefore, are usually within normal range, unless there is a very serious disturbance in the homeostatic mechanisms.

Since half of serum calcium is bound to protein, ionized calcium should be measured, otherwise total serum calcium concentrations must be corrected for serum protein levels. Elevations of serum protein or pH increase the protein-bound fraction, and produce a false hypercalcemia, which masks a true hypocalcemia. Serum phosphorus levels fluctuate more readily than serum calcium, depending on dietary intake, release from bone, and urinary excretion. Elevated phosphorus levels temporarily depress serum calcium, and lead to PTH secretion. Radioimmunoassays for serum levels of PTH, CT, and vitamin D metabolites can be accomplished in several species of laboratory animals. The determination of acid–base balance is a valuable part of the clinical chemical profile.

Elevated serum levels of the bone isozyme of alkaline phosphatase are seen in conditions in which there is increased osteoblastic activity. Elevations may indicate an increased level of bone turnover, rather than a change in bone balance.

The major vitamin K-dependent protein of bone, osteocalcin, or bone gla-protein (BGP), is a specific product of the osteoblast. A small fraction of the amount synthesized does not accumulate in bone, but is secreted directly into the bloodstream. For most bone disorders, increases in the serum levels of bone BGP closely parallel serum increases in bone alkaline phosphatase. Bone gla-protein released from bone matrix undergoing osteoclastic resorption is degraded, and not detectable in serum assays. Radioimmunoassay for this protein is of value in toxicology studies, but laboratory assays for serum BGP give a reasonably consistent picture of bone mineral metabolism only if results are expressed as a percentage of serum BGP levels in control animals.

Another marker of bone formation is the intact form of the C and N terminal propeptide of type I collagen (PICP, PINP). They reflect osteoblastic activity, but also some collagen degradation. However, their measurements are not widely used.

If an animal is uniformly labeled with [^{3}H] tetracycline prior to an experiment, the release of label from bone and appearance in serum and urine is a measure of osteoclastic resorption. This method is superior to radiocalcium labeling, because tetracycline is rapidly excreted in the urine whereas the kidney reabsorbs most of the calcium. Several points need to be made about the use of this technique. First, administration of [^{3}H] tetracycline to a growing animal does not lead to uniform skeletal deposition, because of the bone modeling process. Second, while release of label indicates bone resorption, this does not necessarily indicate a change in bone balance or mass. Third, results will obviously depend on the rate at which the tracer is being redeposited in the skeleton.

Increases in serum or urinary hydroxyproline have been interpreted to indicate increased bone resorption rate if collagen and elastin breakdown in the rest of the body remains constant. Hydroxyproline is not used as an amino acid during protein synthesis; therefore, there is very little reutilization of this molecule. Measurements of urinary and blood hydroxyproline are probably an unreliable measure of bone resorption, since 90% of hydroxyproline is oxidized and only a small portion is excreted in the urine. More specific measures of collagen degradation in bone are urinary N-terminal cross-linked telopeptides of type I collagen (NTX), pyridinolone (PYD), deoxypyridinolone (DPD), and for osteoclastic activity by tartrate-resistant acid phosphatase (TRAP). The DPD is more specific for bone collagen than PYD. The TRAP assay reflects osteoclastic activity, but must distinguish the enzyme activity from prostate, blood cells, and pancreas.

All bone markers have been developed for humans, but have been modified for animal use. Measurement of urinary excretion of substances should be measured relative to creatinine (Cr), and expressed in the concentration ratio as mg/dl (substance/Cr). Calcium and phosphorus excretion relative to the glomerular filtration rate can be obtained by multiplying the Ca:Cr or P:Cr concentration ratios by the plasma creatinine. Tubular reabsorption can be derived using appropriate nomograms, and expressed as the tubular maximum (TM) resorptive capacity relative to glomerular filtration rate (GFR) (TM/GFR). Calcium balance studies may be desirable under very special circumstances.

Animal Models of Skeletal Disease

Skeletal dysplasias in animals, as in humans, represent a heterogeneous group of disorders that manifest themselves as generalized defects in cartilage and bone growth and development. An international nomenclature of constitutional diseases of bone was developed to assist in the classification of the diseases in humans. Five major divisions were defined: osteochondrodysplasias; dysostoses; idiopathic osteolyses; chromosomal aberrations; and primary metabolic abnormalities. The best-defined bone dysplasias in animals that make useful models for disease processes in humans include proportionate and disproportionate dwarfism, multiple cartilaginous exostoses, osteogenesis imperfecta, and osteopetrosis. Ideally, animal models should closely mimic the human disease in induction, progression, and pathology.

Excellent animal models are available for most of the metabolic bone diseases, including rickets, osteomalacia, osteitis fibrosa—usually identified as fibrous osteodystrophy in animals, scurvy, lathyrism, and hypercalcemia of malignancy. There also are good models for osteopenia in laboratory animals, but none are exact counterparts for type I postmenopausal osteoporosis of women.

Osteoarthritis in humans has multifactorial patterns of joint failure; thus, different models may be useful for studying various aspects of the condition. Joint laxity in laboratory animals, whether it occurs through genetic predisposition or is surgically-induced, initiates a sequence of events in articular and meniscal cartilage that cause degenerative changes similar to osteoarthritis in humans. Animals with inflammatory joint disease have been sought, mainly as models for rheumatoid arthritis, a systemic disease in humans. However, none of the induced or spontaneous animal models unequivocally meets the requirements of a model with the complete spectrum of lesions found in human rheumatoid arthritis. Most notably, many of the animal models do not have the characteristic systemic features of this disease, such as disseminated arteritis, chronic pericarditis, subcutaneous nodules, or lymphoproliferative changes in salivary glands. In addition to the lesions of chronic synovitis with formation of synovial villi, joint lesions should show destruction of articular cartilage by invasion of granulation tissue from the synovial margins and from subchondral bone marrow. Even though there may not yet be a precise model for human rheumatoid arthritis, certain models, e.g., adjuvant arthritis, may be used to screen anti-inflammatory agents. It must be recognized, however, that the results of drug action on the model and on human patients may be different.

SUMMARY

Acute toxicity tests are designed to determine the LD$_{50}$ dose and pathologic changes associated with acute toxicity. Test substances must produce profound skeletal alterations for bone lesions to be detected by this procedure. Since only a small amount of osseous tissue is produced or turned over during the acute toxicity test, examination of the metaphysis of a fast-growing bone will give the greatest opportunity to determine a drug-related effect. During subacute or subchronic toxicity tests, there is a greater opportunity for the test compound to have a demonstrable skeletal effect.

Many chemical agents affect the skeletal system indirectly, via mediator action on cell differentiation or modulation of cell function. Therefore, skeletal effects may be reflected in the rates at which cells function. In the growing animal, any study of skeletal cell function in the metaphysis must distinguish between possible drug action on longitudinal bone growth, and metaphyseal cancellous remodeling. Although bone histomorphometry can detect quantitative differences that might be missed by a less rigorous histologic assessment, this methodology has its greatest value in determining mechanisms by which skeletal alterations have occurred.

Animal disease processes can be used as models for human disease. Conflicting opinions regarding bone cell biology result from inappropriate extrapolation from an experimental model to other animals and humans. It is true that knowledge of disease pathogenesis and development of preventive or therapeutic agents develops much more rapidly when there is an appropriate animal model. In order to screen drugs, there is a requirement for inexpensive animal models. Understanding the utility and limitations of each system will help separate fact from fiction. It is important to recognize that, if the model is not a good counterpart to the human condition, the drug, when used in humans, may not show similar therapeutic effectiveness.

Because laboratory rodents show little cortical bone Haversian systems, they have been considered inappropriate models for the study of bone remodeling processes. However, it has been shown that cancellous bone of laboratory rodents, either in the vertebra or metaphyses of long bones, undergoes a similar remodeling process as cancellous bone of humans. Furthermore, it is the loss of endocortical bone, cortical bone adjacent to marrow, which will mainly reduce cortical bone mass and strength, and not intracortical bone remodeling. Rodents, therefore, can be used as inexpensive laboratory animals to screen the effects of drugs on the modeling and remodeling process (tissue level responses), as long as one takes precautions to ensure that one accounts for the changes in longitudinal bone growth. After drug efficacy has been determined, drug effects on cortical bone remodeling can be determined in other types of laboratory animals, such as the beagle dog.

FURTHER READING

Adams, M.E., and Billingham, M.E.J. (1982). Animal models of degeneration of degenerative joint disease. *Curr Topics Pathol.*, 71, 265–297.

Bain, B.J., Clark, D.M., Lampert, I.A., and Wilkins, B.S. (2001). *Bone Marrow Pathology*, pp. 1–499. Blackwell Science, Oxford.

Baron, R., Tross, R., and Bignery, A. (1984). Evidence of sequential remodeling in rat trabecular bone: Morphology, dynamic histomorphometry and changes during skeletal maturation. *Anat. Rec.*, 208, 137–145.

Bilezikian, J., Raisz, L., and Martin, T.J. (eds) (2008). *Principles of Bone Biology*, 3rd edn. Academic Press, Elsevier, San Diego, CA.

Bullough, P. (2003). *Orthopaedic Pathology*, 4th edn. Mosby, Elsevier, New York, NY.

Carter, D.R., Orr, T.E., Fyhrie, D.P., and Schurman, D.J. (1987). Influences of mechanical stress on prenatal and postnatal skeletal development. *Clin. Ortho. Rel. Res.*, 219, 237–249.

Enlow, D.H. (1966). Osteocyte necrosis in normal bone. *J. Dent. Res.*, 45, 213.

Enlow, D.H. (1963). *Principles of Bone Remodeling*. Thomas, Springfield, IL.

Erlich, G.E. (1985). Animal models of osteoarthritis: Implication for pathogenesis and treatment. *Ration. Drug Ther.*, 19, 1–5.

Frost, H.M. (1973). *Bone Modeling and Skeletal Modeling Error.* Thomas, Springfield, IL.

Frost, H.M. (1976). Histomorphometry of trabecular bone. In *Bone Histomorphometry. Second International Workshop* (Meunier, P.J. ed.), pp. 361–370. Laboratorie de Recherches sur l'Histodynamique Osseuse, Lyon, France.

Kember, N.F. (1983). Cell kinetics of cartilage. In *Cartilage: Structure, Function and Biochemistry* (Hall, B.K. ed.), Vol. I, pp. 149–180. Academic Press, New York, NY.

Khurana, J.S. (2009). *Bone Pathology*, pp. 1–360, 2nd edn. Humana Press, Totowa, NJ.

Kimmel, D.B. (1996). Animal models for *in vivo* experimentation in osteoporosis research. In *Osteoporosis* (Marcus, R., Feldman, D., and Kelsey, J. eds). Academic Press, New York, NY.

Magaki, G. (1982). Compendium of inherited metabolic diseases in animals. In *Animal Models of Inherited Metabolic Diseases* (Desnick, R.J., Paterson, D.F., and Scarpelli, D.G. eds), pp. 473–501. Liss, New York, NY.

Mankin, H.J. (1981). Cartilage healing. In *Pathophysiology in Small Animal Surgery* (Bojrab, M.J. ed.), pp. 557–567. Lea and Febiger, Philadelphia, PA.

Pearce, A.I., Richards, R.G., Milz, S., Schneider, E., and Pearce, S.G. (2007). Animal models for implant biomaterial research in bone: a review. *Eur. Cell Mater.*, 13, 1–10.

Rasmussen, H., and Bordier, P. (1973). The cellular basis of metabolic bone disease. *N. Engl. J. Med.*, 289, 25–32.

Recker, R.R. (ed.) (1983). *Bone Histomorphometry: Techniques and Interpretation*. CRC Press, Boca Raton, FL.

Risneck, D., and Niwayama, G. (eds) (1981). *Diagnosis of Bone and Joint Disorders*. Saunders, Philadelphia, PA.

Rosenberg, A.E. (2005). Bones, joints, and soft tissue tumors. In *Robbins and Cotran Pathologic Basis of Disease* (Kumar, V., Abbas, A.K., and Fausto, N. eds), 7th edn, pp. 1273–1324. Elsevier Saunders, New York, NY.

Sokoloff, L. (1984). Animal models of rheumatoid arthritis. *Int. Rev. Exp. Pathol.*, 26, 107–144.

Stern, P.H. (1980). The D vitamins and bone. *Am. Soc. Pharmacol. Exp. Ther.*, 32, 47–80.

Teitelbaum, S.L., and Bullough, P.G. (1979). The pathophysiology of bone and joint disease. *Am. J. Pathol.*, 96, 283–354.

Thompson, K. (2007). Bones and joints. In *Jubb, Kennedy, and Palmer's Pathology of Domestic Animals* (Maxie, M.G. ed.), 5th edn, Vol. I, pp. 1–184. Saunders, Elsevier, New York, NY.

Vigorita, V.J. (2007). *Orthopaedic Pathology*, 2nd edn. Lippincott, Williams & Wilkins, Philadelphia, PA.

Weisbrode, S.E. (2007). Bone and joints. In *Pathologic Basis of Veterinary Disease* (McGavin, M., and Zachary, J.F. eds), 4th edn, pp. 1041–1105. Mosby Elsevier, St. Louis, MO.

Wold, L., Unni, K.K., Sim, F., and Sundaram, M. (2008). *Atlas of Orthopedic Pathology*. Saunders, Elsevier, New York, NY.

Immune System

INTRODUCTION

A major focus of immunotoxicology is the detection and evaluation of undesired effects of substances on the immune system. Toxic response may occur when the immune system acts as a passive target of chemical insults, leading to altered immune function. Alternatively, toxicity may arise when the immune system responds to the antigenic specificity of the chemical as part of a specific immune response (i.e., hypersensitivity or allergy). Chemically-induced toxicity, in which the immune system is the target, can result in an increased incidence of infectious diseases, as well as the development of allergies, autoimmune diseases, or neoplasia.

FUNCTION AND STRUCTURE OF THE IMMUNE SYSTEM

Function of the Immune System

The immunological defense of the body against pathogens from the environment is a finely-tuned interplay between various cell types and soluble mediators secreted by these cells (Table 15.1). The defense can be roughly divided into specific responses, in which the reaction is directed to one specific determinant (antigenic determinant or epitope), and nonspecific responses. Specificity is based on recognition by specific receptors on lymphocytes or by antibodies; the nonspecific response involves effector cells, such

TABLE 15.1   Compartments, cells, and functions of lymphoid tissues

Organs and compartments	Cells	Functions
Bone marrow	Hematopoietic cells organized as islands within fatty tissue, mature leukocytes, plasma cells	Differentiation of stem cells into cells of the erythroid, myeloid-monocytoid, platelet and lymphoid lineage. Antibody synthesis. Memory cells
Thymus		
Cortex	Fine reticular epithelium, macrophages, immature T-cells	Generation of T-cell competence: T-cell receptor rearrangement, positive selection (MHC restriction), negative selection, autoreactive cells, phenotypic changes
Medulla	Plump reticular epithelium, macrophages, dendritic cells, T-lymphocytes	T-cell competence generation (negative selection); thymic hormone synthesis. Antigen presentation
Corticomedullary zone (CMZ)	Immature and mature lymphocytes	Entrance of bone-marrow derived stem cells, exit of T-cells having undergone intrathymic maturation
Epithelial-free areas (EFA)	Immature T-cells, macrophages	T-cell proliferation, function unknown
Lymph node and spleen		
Paracortex (lymph node) and PALS (spleen)	Interdigitating cells, T helper and T suppressor cells	Lymphocyte entry through high endothelial venules (HEV, lymph node) or central arteriole (spleen), antigen presentation to T helper cells, T-cell proliferation–differentiation–regulation (T-suppressor cells)
Primary follicles, follicle mantle of secondary follicles	Dendritic cells (subtype of follicular dendritic cells), dendritic macrophages, B-cells, small number of T-cells	Storage of (virgin/memory) B-cells, recirculating B-cells (surface IgM^+ IgD^+)
Germinal center	Follicular dendritic cells, dendritic macrophages (starry sky macrophages), B-cells (centrocytes, centroblasts), T helper cells	T-cell-dependent B-lymphocytes, differentiation, antigen presentation in the form of immune complexes (with/without complement C3)
Medulla (lymph node), red pulp (spleen)	Plasma cells, T effector cells, reticular cells, polymorphonuclear granulocytes	Termination of antigen-specific reaction: antibody synthesis and immune complex-mediated clearance, reactions of T-delayed type hypersensitivity and cytotoxic cells
Marginal zone (spleen)	Marginal zone macrophages, marginal metallophilic cells, marginal zone B-cells	T-cell-independent B-lymphocyte proliferation–differentiation, e.g., to bacterial polysaccharides, B-cell memory (surface IgM^+ IgD^- cells)
Mucosa-associated lymphoid tissue		
Organized lymphoid tissue (Peyer's patches, NALT, BALT)		
Covering epithelium	M (microfold) cells, lymphocytes	Transport (uptake of exogenous substances, mainly particles), initiation of immune responses including IgA response
Follicles	See lymph node and spleen	
Interfollicular area	Mainly small T-cells, interdigitating cells	Lymphocyte entry through high endothelial venules, antigen presentation to T-cells
Single cells		
Epithelium	Epithelial cells, T cytotoxic cells, NK cells, T γδ cells	First line of defense, synthesis of cells, extrathymic maturation of lymphocytes, secretory component, transport of IgA (IgM) to lumen
Lamina propria	Plasma cells, macrophages, lymphocytes	Synthesis of IgA antibody, phagocytosis and killing

as macrophages and granulocytes, and mediator systems, including the complement system. The classical reaction to bacterial infection, resulting in antibacterial antibody formation and destruction of the pathogen mediated by these antibodies, still occurs, but represents only a portion of the intrinsic capacities of the system. Some further general designations attributed to the system are summarized in the following sections.

Antigen Presentation and Recognition

The initiation of an immune response requires adequate recognition of the pathogen. This recognition often occurs immediately after entry into the body (Figure 15.1). The first defense includes inactivation in a nonspecific way, for example, by nonspecific killer cells, granulocytic leukocytes, and cells of the mononuclear phagocyte system (MPS). It also includes antigen processing and presentation to T-cells, which are able to generate a specific response. During major histocompatibility (MHC) assembly, antigen presenting cells, such as dendritic cells and macrophages, incorporate peptides from various processed antigens into their MHC molecules, which are subsequently presented to T-cells. Antigens which have been processed by endocytosis are presented predominantly by MHC class II molecules, whereas endogenous antigens are presented predominantly on MHC class I molecules. The T-cell subset that can be activated by these peptide–MHC complexes recognizes these molecules, by dual recognition: their T-cell receptor binds to the MHC peptide complex and their CD4 or CD8 molecules bind to nonpolymorphic regions of MCH class II, or MHC class I, respectively, on the antigen presenting cell. So, this dual recognition has the functional consequence that viral antigens and tumor-associated antigens are predominantly recognized by CD8+ T (T_C) cells, whereas exogenous antigens are recognized predominantly by CD4+ T (T_H) cells.

Specificity

The system has the capacity to distinguish one particular determinant in an immense spectrum of putative determinants. The discrimination between "self" and "non-self" is an example of this specificity. Lymphocytes are central to antigen specificity, as they express receptors for a single, distinct, antigenic determinant on their surfaces. For B-cells, this antigenic determinant is essentially an antibody (immunoglobulin) molecule. The size of an antigenic determinant or epitope is about ten amino acids; the antigen can also be made of carbohydrates or lipids. The antigen-binding fragment of both the surface receptor, and the secreted antibodies, produced after differentiation of B-cells into plasma cells, has a virtually identical structure. However, B-cell surface immunoglobulin, and the immunoglobulin product of plasma cell progeny, can differ in the constant part of the heavy chain. On virgin B-cells, the surface receptor is an IgM or IgD molecule; however, after class switching occurs, IgG, IgA, and IgE molecules can be synthesized by the resultant plasma cell.

For T-cells, the antigen receptor is a heterodimeric molecule (either an α–β heterodimer, or a γ–δ heterodimer) which has a constant and a variable part similar to that of immunoglobulin molecules. To enable transmembrane signaling after antigen contact, this heterodimer is linked to a tripeptide molecule (CD3) on the cell surface. Structural differences between the T-cell antigen receptor (TCR) and the B-cell receptor (immunoglobulin) find their basis in the different gene segments encoding the receptors. It is thus not surprising that T-cells recognize other determinants on the antigenic compound than B-cells do. For large antigens, such as proteins, distinct T-cell and B-cell epitopes can be identified. T-cells of the helper–inducer population (T_H) and delayed-type-hypersensitivity population (T_{DTH}) (see subsequent text) recognize the antigenic determinant only when it is presented together with the individual's own (self) determinant of class II major histocompability complex (MHC). This phenomenon is called MHC class II restriction. T-cells of the suppressor population (T_S) and cytotoxic population (T_C) are MHC class I restricted. B-lymphocytes, on the other hand, do not function in an MHC-restricted manner. The total repertoire of antigen-recognition specificities is about 10^7 for antibodies, and somewhat lower for the T-cell receptor.

Choice of the Effector Reaction

After activation of CD4+ T_H cells, the system makes its choice of effector reactions to enable the optimal destruction or inactivation of the antigen or pathogen. A rough division is made into the humoral (antibody-mediated) and cellular (cell-mediated) arms.

In the humoral arm, CD4+ T_H cells together with antigen activate specified B-cells to become antibody-producing plasma cells. The antibodies produced mediate the subsequent inactivation of the foreign substance in a number of ways. When present in the form of immune complexes, IgG and IgM activate the complement system, and induce complement-mediated cytotoxicity, or activate secondary effects. These secondary effects include: (1) vasodilation, increased vascular permeability, and attraction of granulocytes with subsequent release of lysosomal proteolytic enzymes (i.e., components of acute inflammation); (2) IgG-mediated antibody-dependent cellular cytotoxicity (ADCC), in which the antibody forms the antigen-specific bridge between killer cell (a macrophage binding the Fc fragment of IgG) and target; (3) IgG- and IgM-induced opsonization and ingestion by phagocytic cells (granulocytes, macrophages), with involvement of receptors for immunoglobulin Fc

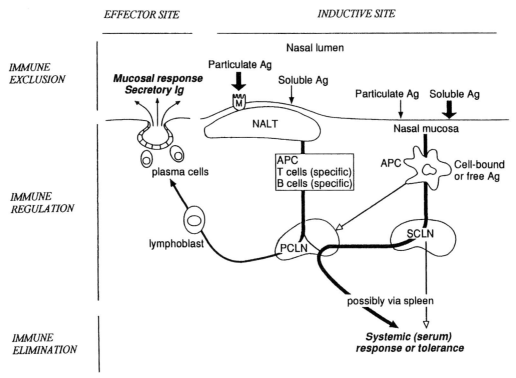

FIGURE 15.1   Schematic presentation of hypothetical pathways eliciting local and systemic immune responses via the respiratory mucosa. Ag, antigen; APC, antigen-presenting cell; Ig, immunoglobulin; M. microfold epithelial cell; PCLN, posterior cervical lymph node; SCLN, superficial cervical lymph node. Adapted from Kuper et al. (1992). *Immuno. Today* **13**, 219–224.

and complement-split product C3; and (4) IgE bound to IgE receptors on the surface of mast cells and basophilic granulocytes, inducing degranulation with mediator release after antigen binding.

In the cellular arm, CD4+ T_H cells activate precursors of CD8+ T_C cells, which subsequently differentiate and kill the target via antigen-specific recognition; also, precursors of lymphokine-producing cells (e.g., T_{DTH} cells) can be activated, the lymphokines subsequently secrete activated macrophages to kill the target. *In vitro* studies on CD4+ T_H cells have revealed the existence of two different subtypes of T_H cells, the T_{H1} and T_{H2} cells, which originate from pluripotent precursor T_{H0} cells. After activation of antigen presenting cells by interleukin (IL)-12, mature T_{H1} cells synthesize Il-2, interferon-γ, and other cytokines, as well as providing help to B-cells (especially IgG2a synthesis) and initiating delayed-type hypersensitivity. T_{H2} cells predominantly secrete the interleukins Il-4, IL-5, and IL-13, as well as providing major help to B-cells (in IgM, IgG1, IgA and IgE synthesis), but they play no role in the initiation of delayed-type hypersensitivity.

Cytokines from either subset are mutually inhibitory. Il-4 is inhibitory to T_{H1} cells, and interferon-γ is inhibitory to T_{H2} cells. The functional consequences are considerable. Repetitive clonal expansion of either subset will lead to a shift in the overall cytokine profile of all T-cells, and inadequate regulation of T-cell responses. This phenomenon, called T-cell "skewing," frequently results in severe immunopathology responses. The capacity of the T-cell compartment for T_{H1} or T_{H2} skewing after repetitive T-cell activation is determined genetically which, by inference, has a significant impact on individual susceptibility to immune-mediated reactions.

Finally, it should be noted that the immune system exerts other responses that do not involve the activation of T_H cells. These include the T-cell-independent activation of B-cells, mostly when antigens consist of repeating polysaccharide units (present on bacteria such as *Escherichia coli* and *Pneumococcus*). They also include the direct activation of T-killer cells, which bear antigen-specific receptors comprising the α–β heterodimer.

Immunologic Memory

A special feature of the immune response is the generation of memory after initial contact with the antigen. The first response includes activation and amplification of antigen-specific T- or B-cells in exerting effector reactions. It also ends with the return of antigen-recognizing cells to the normal resting state (small lymphocytes). The second contact with the antigen causes recruitment of more antigen-specific cells. This recruitment gives a higher signal, and a more efficient elimination of the antigen or pathogen. Not only is there a better signal, but there is also a faster response and a stronger binding of antibody to antigen.

The memory effect for the humoral arm is evident by isotype switching of B-cells between primary and secondary immune responses. The first response only manifests the IgM class antibody, but antibodies of other immunoglobulin classes (especially IgG in the internal system) are generated after subsequent contact.

The cellular basis of immunologic memory is evident within the T-cell population by phenotypic changes between virgin and memory T-cells. Ater antigen encounter, T-cells demonstrate a rearranged isoform of the leukocyte common antigen CD45. They lose the expression of CD45RA, while the expression of CD45 R0 becomes detectable. Simultaneously, the expression of the lymphocytic homing receptor CD44 is increased. In contrast to the B-cell population, T-cell memory is long-lasting, and is associated with stimulatory activity of the antigen in germinal centers of secondary lymphoid tissue. The generation of memory is the basis for vaccination.

Immunoregulation

The induction of the effector reaction involves a finely-tuned interplay between cells and soluble mediators. On the one hand, cell–cell contact is required; for instance, between the antigen-presenting cell with (processed) antigen on its surface and the T_H cell. On the other hand, mediators influence cell function at a distance.

Examples of mediators influencing immune reactions in a positive way are IL-1, which is secreted by the antigen-presenting cell and stimulates T_H cells; IL-2, which is secreted by T_H cells and stimulates a variety of T-cells in amplification of the response; and a number of B-cell stimulatory and growth factors. Surface receptors for such interleukins are present on certain immune cells (and also in neuroendocrine tissue), or can become expressed during activation. For instance, IL-2 receptors become expressed on T-cells

as part of the activation process, and their expression is used in the assessment of the state of cell activation.

For down-regulation after stimulation of T_H cells in the initiation of the response, precursors of T_S cells are activated. These subsequently inhibit the T_H cells from further amplifying the response (by direct cell–cell contact or by secretion of soluble inhibitors). Immunoregulatory circuits have also been documented at the antibody level, where the first antibody generates a second antibody, directed against itself. The relevance of this antibody-anti-antibody network, the "anti-idiotype" network, remains a subject of speculation. The immune system is in a continuous state of homeostatic balance. The introduction of an antigen (pathogen) disturbs the balance, due to activation of antigen-specific cell clones (of T- and/or B-lymphocyte origin). The system not only allows the proliferation and amplification of relevant clones to cope with the antigen, but also searches for (and reaches) a state of newly-defined homeostasis.

Unresponsiveness of the immune system to an antigen can result from clonal deletion of T_H cells by a subset of T-cells, called "suppressor cells" or T_{H3} cells, leading to a state of tolerance. After activation via their antigen receptor, these cells have been reported to be nonantigen specific in their effector phase by production of the immunosuppressive cytokine TGF-β1. By consequence, polyclonal expansion of T_{H3} cells after exposure to certain toxic compounds can lead to an immunosuppressive state with an increased susceptibility to opportunistic infections.

Communication with other homeostatic mechanisms in the body is an important aspect of immunoregulation. IL-1, generated by antigen-presenting cells, affects the temperature regulatory center (induction of fever) and sleep regulatory center (induction of slow-wave sleep) in the hypothalamus. Communication with the clotting system and kallikrein system by communication with the central nervous system (CNS) and the endocrine system is another effect (see later).

Neuroendocrine System–Immune System Interactions

The neuroendocrine and immune systems communicate and cooperate intricately for the maintenance of physiological homeostasis (Figure 15.2). These systems interact bi-directionally by a common language, consisting of a shared molecular network of ligands and receptors. Most of the influence of the brain on the immune system seems to be exerted by hormones released by the neuroendocrine system; most of the influence of the immune system on the

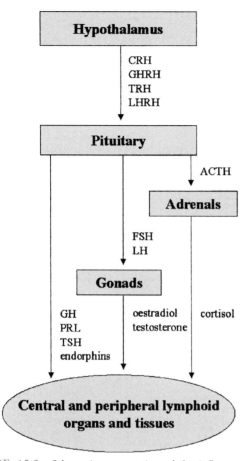

FIGURE 15.2 Schematic presentation of the influence of the neuroendocrine system on the immune system. ACTH, adrenocorticotropic hormone; CRH, corticotropin-releasing hormone; FSH, folic-stimulating hormone; GH, growth hormone; GHRH, growth hormone-releasing hormone; LH, luteotropic hormone; LHRH, luteinizing hormone-releasing hormone; PRL, prolactin; TRH, thyrotropin-releasing hormone; TSH, thyroid-stimulating hormone.

brain seems to be exerted by cytokines. Indeed, receptors for hormones have been detected on cells of the immune system, whereas receptors for cytokines have been detected in the endocrine glands and brain. It is also noteworthy that almost all lymphoid tissues are innervated, although the role of this neuroregulatory pathway is largely unknown.

The hypothalamus–pituitary–adrenal (HPA) axis represents the major pathway in the communication between the CNS and the immune system. Synthesis of glucocorticoid hormones by the adrenal gland, induced by adrenocorticotropic hormone (ACTH) from the pituitary gland, results in the suppression of immune responses. Other mechanisms are those mediated by the direct action of neuropeptides, such as opioid peptides, on immune cells; these are either stimulatory or down-regulatory. Cells of the immune

system carry receptors for a number of hormones, neuropeptides, and neurotransmitters, such as CRH, ACTH, prolactin (PRL), β-endorphin, growth hormone (GH), and sex steroids. In addition, cells of the immune system produce inflammatory cytokines, specifically tumor necrosis factor-α (TNF-α) and interleukins (IL-1 and IL-6), that act on the central components of the HPA axis and the sympathetic system.

One biological activity of the thymus that is under neuroendocrine control is the secretion of thymic hormones. The secretion of thymulin, a nonapeptide strictly produced by thymic epithelial cells, is modulated by GH and PRL.

Structure of the Immune System

Primary lymphoid development first begins in the thymus, with subsequent development in other tissues, generally similar for both mammals and birds. Thymic development from the third and fourth pharyngeal pouches is an early event in all species, occurring at 6–7 days of embryogenesis in the chickens, 10 days in the mouse, 31 days in the pig, and 40 days in the human. In all species, the rudimentary thymus is colonized rapidly by large lymphocytes, shortly after formation of the rudimentary organ. The splenic rudiment appears at day 13, and lymphopoiesis begins within a week. Lymph nodes develop from outpouches of endothelial ducts concurrently with the spleen, and become active sites of lymphopoiesis in the mouse embryo at 18 days, 52 days in the pig, and 70–100 days in the human.

Overview

Components of the immune system are present throughout the body (Table 15.1). The T-cell and B-cell compartments are lodged in lymphoid organs. From there, cells can move to sites of infection or inflammation. Phagocytic cells of monocyte–macrophage lineage, called the mononuclear phagocyte system (MPS), occur in lymphoid organs and also at extranodal sites, such as the liver (Küpffer cells), lung (alveolar macrophages), kidney (mesangial macrophages), and brain (glial cells). Polymorphonuclear leukocytes (PMNs) are mainly present in blood (and bone marrow); they accumulate at sites of inflammation.

Lymphoid organs can be roughly classified in two ways. In one classification, primary or "central" (antigen-independent) and secondary or "peripheral" (antigen-dependent) lymphoid tissues are distinguished, based on the antigen-dependence of lymphoid cell proliferation and differentiation. Bone marrow and thymus are central lymphoid organs. Peripheral lymphoid organs in the body include lymph nodes, spleen, and lymphoid tissue along secretory surfaces, such as in the gastrointestinal and respiratory tracts. It should be kept in mind that the classification of organs and tissues into lymphoid and nonlymphoid organs and tissues is somewhat artificial. For example, the liver plays an important role in lymphopoiesis in the fetus, in the clearance of immune complexes (by Küpffer cells), in IgA transport, and in the regulation of immune responses in the intestines. In this chapter, the traditional classification into lymphoid and nonlymphoid organs and tissues is maintained.

The bone marrow is both a primary and a secondary organ. Located here are pluripotent hemopoietic stem cells that differentiate to progenitors of myeloid cells (which differentiate into polymorphonuclear granulocytes, mast cells, monocytes, and platelets) and lymphoid progenitors. The common lymphoid progenitor cell subsequently differentiates into T- and B-lymphoid progenitors. Progenitor T-cells then move to the thymus for further maturation. B-lymphoid progenitors mature via the pre-B-cell stage into virgin B-cells, which then leave the bone marrow microenvironment and lodge in the periphery. In birds, B-cell maturation is accomplished in the Bursa of Fabricius, an epithelial organ located adjacent to the termination of the gastrointestinal tract.

The bone marrow also functions as a secondary lymphoid organ, because terminal antigen-induced lymphoid cell differentiation can occur in its microenvironment. For instance, bone marrow cells include the memory lymphocyte pool and the major plasma cell population contributing to the intravascular immunoglobulin pool. Normally, plasma cell differentiation follows antigen presentation at peripheral sites, and then stimulated B-cells subsequently migrate to the bone marrow for final differentiation into plasma cells. Other peripheral lymphoid organs in the body include lymph nodes, spleen, and lymphoid tissue along secretory surfaces such as the gastrointestinal and respiratory tract.

A second classification is based on the location of lymphoid organs. In this system, lymphoid organs are divided into internal organs (some lymph nodes and spleen, in addition to thymus and bone marrow), and external organs (lymphoid tissue along secretory surfaces, and lymph nodes draining the mucosa-associated lymphoid tissue, MALT). These two lymphoid compartments behave somewhat independently in host defense. Immunoglobulin synthesis is a good example of this independence. The main function of the external or secretory immune system is to produce secretory IgA antibody. IgE synthesis in the body is also along secretory surfaces. The extent of the secretory immune system should not be underestimated. About half of the body's lymphocytes are located in the secretory immune system, and the capacity for immunoglobulin synthesis is about 1.5 times that of the internal system. The internal immune system, on the other hand, produces IgG or IgM.

Another, sometimes unappreciated, immune organ is the skin. The skin does not contain lymphoid tissue *per se*, but is drained by lymph nodes. However, there are Langerhans cells in the epidermis. These are a special cell subtype of the MPS. They are adapted to process antigen, and transport it to the associated draining lymph node. Within the node, these cells "interdigitating cells," present the antigen to lymphocytes.

Immune cells and cellular products are transported between lymphoid organs by blood and lymph vessels. For example, Langerhans cells on their way from the skin to a lymph node are present in lymph as "veiled macrophages." The blood only contains a minor part of the body's total pool of lymphocytes (estimated at about 1%), and only a selected population at that, namely, the recirculating lymphocyte pool. Therefore, assessment of only the blood lymphoid compartment does not give a complete inventory of the body's immune system, since it ignores the activities of the non-recirculating cells.

Apart from conventional histologic features, expression of cell surface markers (immunological phenotype) needs to be emphasized. The typing of cells in the T-lymphocyte lineage is a good illustration of immunological phenotyping. Subsets with a different function (e.g., T_H, T_S, T_C, or T_{DTH} activity) normally cannot be identified by conventional cytology or histology, but they can be recognized by immunological phenotyping. For example, T-cells with a helper–inducer function are labeled by monoclonal antibodies in the CD4 cluster, and cells with a suppressor function are labeled by monoclonal antibodies in the CD8 cluster. However, not all CD4+ cells are helper–inducer cells; some T-cells in the delayed-type hypersensitivity subset and in some macrophage populations are also CD4 + . CD8+ T-cells can also be subdivided into the suppressor cell subset or the cytotoxic cell subset.

Thymus

The thymus is a bilobed organ located in the mediastinum, anterior to the major vessels of the heart. It is located in the neck region in the guinea pig. The two independent lobes, attached to each other only by thin connective tissue, and surrounded by a thin fibrous capsular membrane, consist of smaller lobules which are also separated from each other by thin fibrous tissue septa. These have basically the same architecture, with subcapsular and outer cortical areas, a cortex, occupying the outer two-thirds of the lobule, and a medulla occupying the central one-third (Figure 15.3A, B). Its anatomic location complicates *in vivo* thymectomy; complete removal of the thymus is difficult.

Blood vessels enter the lobules at the cortico-medullary junction, and extend radially into the cortex. Nerves course along the blood vasculature (Figure 15.3A). Fenestrated capillaries are very infrequent in the cortex. The thymus is unique among the lymphoid organs in mammals, because its microenvironment consists of reticular epithelium (Figure 15.3C); in birds, the Bursa of Fabricius also has an epithelial framework. Macrophages derived from the bone marrow occur in the cortex and medulla as a transient population. Dendritic cells located within the medulla (Figure 15.3D) are specialized macrophages, have a major function in antigen presentation, and strongly express MHC class II antigen.

T-cell Maturation

T-cells reside in the thymus during their maturation from progenitor cells to immunocompetent T-cells. The gland has a privileged function in promoting the maturation process. The process of T-cell maturation includes a number of steps that are associated with different microenvironments. The most immature cells enter the lobules by the blood vasculature at the cortico-medullary junction, and move to the outer subcapsular cortex, where they appear as large lymphoblasts. They then pass through the cortex, where the cells become densely-packed small lymphocytes with scant cytoplasm. Finally, the cells move to the medulla, where they appear as medium-sized lymphocytes. These translocational stages in development are monitored on the basis of the immunologic phenotype. Consider the CD4 and CD8 phenotypes: cells progress from CD4 − CD8− (double negative) at a very immature stage to a CD4 − CD8+ stage, into a CD4 + CD8+ (double-positive) phenotype, which makes up almost all lymphocytes in the cortex. In the medulla, by contrast, T-cells have the phenotype of mature T-cells, being larger, with more abundant cytoplasm, with distinct CD4 + CD8+ (about 70%) and CD4 − CD8+ (about 30%) populations.

This phenotypic change is accompanied by a crucial aspect of intrathymic T-cell maturation. The genesis of the T-cell receptor (TCR) consists of the α–β heterodimer. After surface expression of the TCR, the cell undergoes a process unique to T-cells, namely, specific selection on the basis of recognition specificity.

First, the cell is examined for affinity to its own MHC (self-restriction). T-cells with an intermediate affinity for self-MHC peptides are allowed to expand (positive selection). Second, T-cells with a high affinity for self-MHC are deleted (negative selection). Current theories of negative selection state that this step is not possible for all putative autoantigens in the body, rather it applies to a selection of potentially-harmful specificities (in particular MHC antigens). In this way, the random pool of antigen recognition specificities of T-cells is adapted to the host's situation.

Function of the Microenvironment in Maturation

It is generally accepted that the epithelial microenvironment of the thymic cortex plays a major role in positive selection. This microenvironment expresses MHC class I and class II products, and ultrastructurally is characterized by close interactions with lymphocytes. This close interaction is reflected in the complete inclusion of lymphocytes inside the epithelial cytoplasm, which functions as a thymic nurse cell. Negative selection has been ascribed to both the medullary epithelial compartment and medullary dendritic cells. The different processes occurring in early (cortical), and late (medullary), maturation are associated with differences in the microenvironment. For example, epithelial cells in the cortex and medulla differ in antigen expression, ultrastructural characteristics, and capacity to synthesize thymic hormones, such as thymulin, thymic humoral factor, thymosin, or thymopoietin. These hormones have a major function late in intrathymic T-cell maturation; hence, they are produced mainly by the medullary epithelium.

The thymic cortex can be considered a primary lymphoid organ because of its antigen-free microenvironment and blood–thymus barrier. In contrast, antigens can move relatively freely into the thymic medulla, where they can encounter antigen-presenting dendritic cells, as well as antigen-reactive T-cells. Thus, the medulla has properties of a secondary lymphoid organ.

Growth and Involution

Thymic changes can occur secondarily to peripheral antigenic stimulation, thus in some ways resembling the bone marrow. For example, although the thymus is fully-developed early in ontogeny (day 17 in the mouse), it grows considerably immediately after birth. This growth is caused by the immense postnatal antigen stimulation; at that time, large numbers of mature T-cells are required. On the other hand, the thymus typically starts to involute after adulthood is reached.

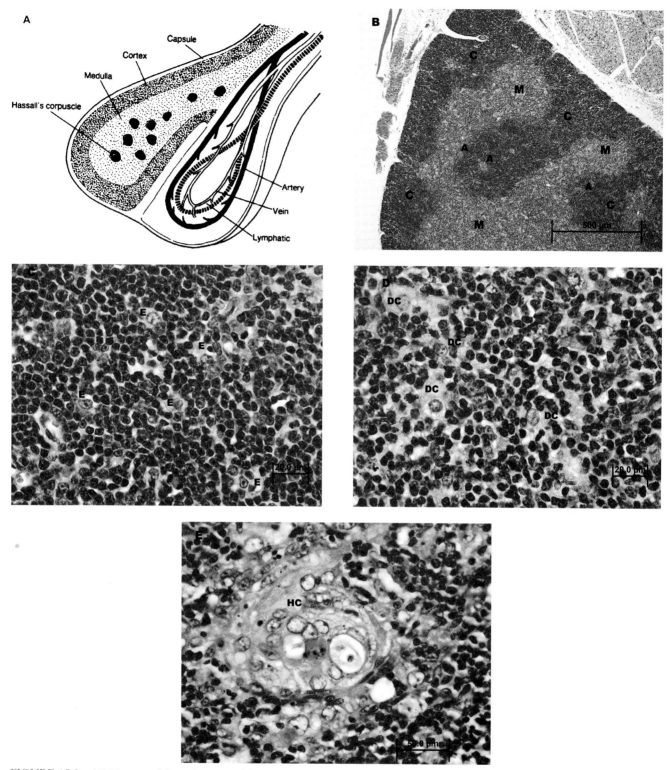

FIGURE 15.3 (A) Diagram of the architecture of the thymus. One lobule is shown with the capsule, cortex, and medulla. Hassall's corpuscles are characteristic epithelial structures in the medulla that are present in the human, but generally not in rodent thymus (depending on the strain). Also shown is the organization of the arterial and venous blood supply, and efferent lymphatic vessels. (Reproduced from Sell (1987). *Immunology, Immunopathology, and Immunity*, 4th edn. Elsevier Science, with permission.) (B) Normal thymus from a mouse, showing the T-lymphocyte rich cortex (C) and less densely populated medulla (M). Numerous arteries (A) radiating from the cortico-medullary junction, are present. (C) High magnification image of thymic cortex from a normal mouse, illustrating the dense lymphocytic population surrounding and closely apposed to thymic epithelium (E). (D) High magnification image of thymic medulla from a mouse, illustrating numerous dendritic cells (DC) around which are clustered medium-sized lymphocytes. (E) Hassall's corpuscle (HC) from the thymus of a cat. See text for details about the structure of Hassall's corpuscles.

The underlying mechanisms are not fully understood, but may be related to changes in the hormonal status of the individual; circulating thymic hormone is at very low levels in adults. Apparently, the persistent generation of new antigen-recognition repertoire in the T-cell population of adults is not needed; instead, the body can defend itself using the established repertoire and extrathymic self-renewal of T-cells.

It should be emphasized that the basic architecture of the thymus does not exist as a fixed histologic entity; morphologic features vary, depending on the age and stress-hormone status of the individual. A "normal" architecture can only be expected during the late gestational period until young adulthood, prior to the start of age-associated involution. This phenomenon has important implications in age-selection of rodents for immune function studies, and in the interpretation of immunological toxicologic pathology.

Lymph Nodes

Lymph nodes are connected by lymph vessels. The basic anatomic features are cortex and medulla (Figure 15.4A, B). The cortex is the site of antigen encounter and initiation of immune reactions. The products of an immune response (activated cells, effector lymphocytes, inflammatory-mediators) are generated in the medulla. The cortex consists of follicles, mainly just underneath the lymph node capsule (Figure 15.4B), and interfollicular areas which often extend to the medulla, and therefore are also designated as paracortex. An anatomical reversal of this arrangement is present in the pig. The follicles contain mostly B-cells, while T-cells are the major lymphocyte population in the paracortex. The paracortex is easily distinguished by the presence of blood vessels (Figure 15.4B, C). The arterial blood supply, entering the node at the medulla, ends in the paracortex as arteriolar capillaries. These feed venules that are lined by high endothelial cells (Figure 15.4D). Lymphocytes migrate through these high endothelial venules, following adherence to the endothelium by specific receptor–ligand interactions. The specificity of these receptor–ligand interactions is different between lymph nodes of the internal and the external lymphoid system. Therefore, by using the same transport system (blood circulation), lymphocytes "belonging" to one of these systems can specifically access the internal or external lymphoid tissue. After migration into the parenchyma, the cells move to their microenvironment in follicles or interfollicular areas.

Reactions after Antigen Contact

The major route of entry for antigens and pathogens is by the afferent lymph flow, which ends in the subcapsular area in all animals except the pig, in which the flow ends in the medulla. From there, antigens, either free or processed by macrophages ("veiled macrophages" in the afferent lymph), move to the paracortex. The subcapsular area is also rich in macrophages (sinus macrophages) that can phagocytose free antigen. In the paracortex, antigens are presented to immune T_H lymphocytes for the initiation of the immune response. The main antigen-presenting cell population consists of interdigitating cells, which are a special type of MPS cell, closely related to Langerhans cells in the skin, and veiled macrophages in the afferent lymph. These cells are often surrounded by CD4+ T_H cells. The antigen-presenting cells express MHC class II antigens in high density, enabling the T_H cells to recognize the antigenic determinant with their α–βTCR, and the polymorphic ("self") MHC class II molecule. The CD4 molecule, by which T_H cells are recognized, has functional significance in this process. It acts as a receptor for the nonpolymorphic determinant of MHC class II molecules; by binding this determinant, it reinforces the binding between antigen-presenting cell and T_H cell. In this cellular interaction, the immune response starts with synthesis of cytokines such as IL-1 and IL-2. For down-regulation, T_S cells are present. These cells are located near, but not immediately surrounding, the interdigitating antigen-presenting cell. How this subset is activated is not completely understood.

For B-cell activation, the process proceeds in the lymphoid follicle (Figure 15.4C). Two types of follicles exist. Primary follicles are aggregates of small resting (surface IgM+ IgD+) virgin B-cells in a microenvironment of follicular dendritic cells. During B-cell activation these change into secondary follicles, consisting of a germinal center surrounded by a mantle (Figure 15.4C). These are easily distinguished in conventional histologic staining. The mantle contains small B-cells at high density, similar to primary follicles, whereas the germinal center contains larger B-lymphoblasts that are designated as centrocytes and centroblasts. Histologically, the mantle stains densely basophilic, while the germinal center is paler. Active germinal centers also manifest phagocytic cells, visible as "starry-sky" macrophages. In the germinal center, antigens are presented to B-cells in the form of immune complexes trapped in cytoplasmic extensions of follicular dendritic cells, which form the framework of the microenvironment. CD4+ T_H cells,

A

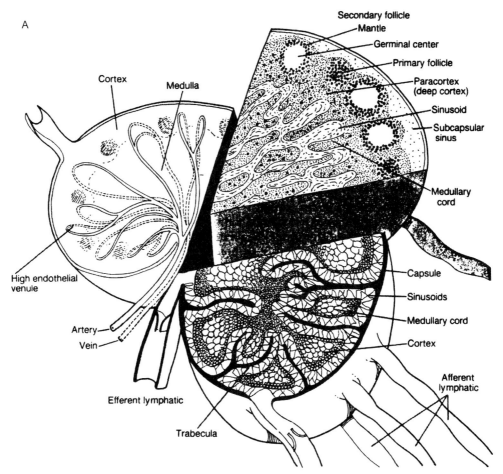

Secondary follicle
Mantle
Germinal center
Primary follicle
Paracortex
(deep cortex)
Sinusoid
Subcapsular
sinus
Medullary
cord
Capsule
Sinusoids
Medullary cord
Cortex
Afferent
lymphatic

Cortex   Medulla

High endothelial
venule

Artery
Vein

Efferent lymphatic

Trabecula

FIGURE 15.4   (A) Diagram of the normal lymph node. The basic structure comprises the cortex, with primary and secondary follicles (B-lymphocyte areas) and paracortex (T-cell area), and the medulla with medullary cords. Afferent lymphatics enter the node at the capsule, and drain through the cortex around the follicles into medullary sinusoids. The main artery entering at the hilus divides into capillaries; veins follow the trabeculae and exit at the hilus. Note the high endothelial venules, the site where lymphocytes migrate between the blood circulation and tissue parenchyma. (Reproduced from Sell (1987). *Immunology, Immunopathology, and Immunity*, 4th edn. Elsevier Science, with permission.)

normally present at relatively high density in the germinal center, assist in B-cell activation; CD8+ cells are almost absent at this location. Complement-split products in the immune complexes, such as C3b, may have an accessory function in antigen presentation.

The activation and proliferation of B-cells in the germinal center is accompanied by an isotype switch of the immunoglobulin class synthesized by the B-cell. The route of entry of antigens into the follicular parenchyma is not fully-established; some authors claim transport by immune (T) cells. Because antigen can remain in the follicular microenvironment for a long time, it causes a persistent activation of B-cells, and so contributes to immunological memory within the B-lymphocyte compartment. After antigen disappearance, immunologic memory in the B-cells is

short-lived, and is taken over by the T-cell population. The centrocytic–centroblastic B-cell differentiation in follicles is accompanied by plasma cell differentiation. Plasma cells are few in the periphery of the germinal center, but numerous in medullary cords.

The major site of effector immune reactions in most species is the medulla (Figure 15.4E). Medullary cords contain macrophages, polymorphonuclear granulocytes, and plasma cells. In addition, one may find activated effector cells at this location, depending on the type of response initiated in the cortex. Among these are CD8+ T_C cells, bearing an α–βTCR that recognizes antigen in the context of the polymorphic determinant of MHC class I molecules. The CD8 molecule has an accessory function in this process, since it binds the nonpolymorphic class I determinants. Antigen

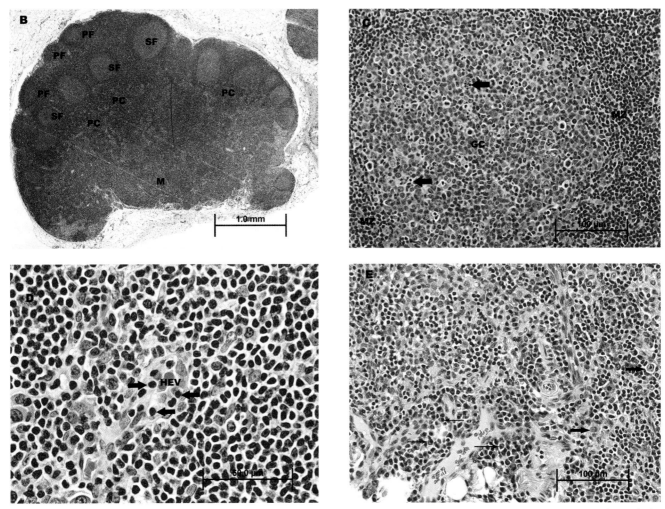

FIGURE 15.4   (Continued) (B) Low magnification image of a rat lymph node. PF indicates primary follicles in the cortex just beneath the capsule; SF indicates secondary follicles which lie deeper in the cortex, while PC indicates the paracortex; M indicates the medulla. (C) High magnification image of a secondary follicle in the cortex of a rat lymph node. GC indicates the germinal center populated by large B-lymphoblasts; MZ indicates the mantle zone of small lymphocytes; arrows point to "starry-sky" cortical macrophages replete with apoptotic B-lymphocytes. (D) High endothelial venule (HEV) in the paracortex; lymphocytes (arrows) can be seen migrating through the vessel wall lined by columnar endothelium. (E) High magnification of medulla from the lymph node of a rat. Plasma cells (thin arrows), macrophages (thick arrows), and an assortment of small lymphocytes are present.

recognition by T_C cells is thus fundamentally different from that by T_H cells. T_{DTH} cells, synthesizing a variety of lymphokines, also occur in the medulla. The reaction products leave the lymph node from the medulla via the efferent lymph or blood circulation for other sites in the body. For instance, plasma cell precursors home to the bone marrow, which supplies the major portion of intravascular immunoglobulins.

Growth and Involution

The lymph node architecture just described should be considered a dynamic, rather than a static, feature. The "normal" lymph node is very small, being a storage site for virgin T- and B-cells; most follicles are primary. After stimulation (e.g., infection in the area drained by the lymph node), the organ increases in size in a relatively short time, showing high proliferative activity of lymphocytes, for example, germinal center formation. After termination of the reaction, or transfer of the reaction to the next draining node, it returns to its original size. Thus, passenger lymphocytes lodge in different parts of the lymph node in the proper microenvironment. The phenomenon is illustrated by the accumulation of lymphocytes at extranodal sites, particularly in cases of chronic inflammation. In such situations, not only is lymphoid infiltration observed, but often a microenvironment resembling that of the lymph node

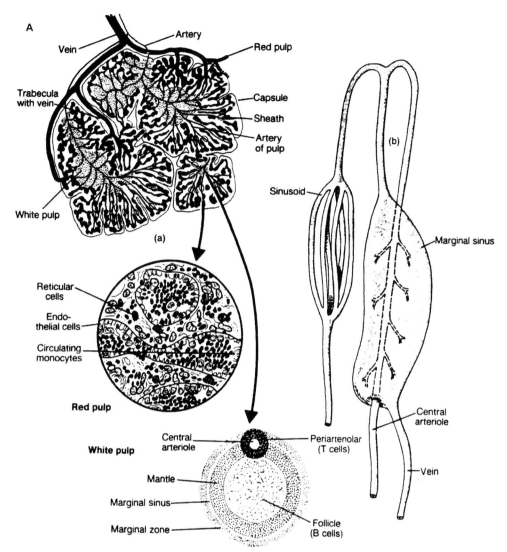

FIGURE 15.5 (A) Diagram of the spleen. The red pulp (a) is composed of sinusoidal channels filled mainly with red blood cells. This site performs its main function in phagocytosis, and the destruction of old red blood cells. The white pulp (b) comprises a T-cell area directly around the central arteriole (the periarteriolar lymphocyte sheath, PALS). B-cells occur in follicles and the marginal zone. There are no lymphatic vessels in the spleen. Blood entering the spleen by the central arteriole supplies either the white pulp or the sinusoids in the red pulp. Both branches drain separately into the splenic vein. (Reproduced from Sell (1987). *Immunology, Immunopathology, and Immunity*, 4th edn. Elsevier Science, with permission.)

is generated, with the formation of follicles comprising follicular dendritic cells, and interfollicular areas containing interdigitating cells. Distinct cell populations can be recognized by special antibodies using immunohistochemistry. This type of response underlies the close interaction between lymphoid cells and microenvironment that is necessary for proper cell function.

Spleen

The spleen consists of two main compartments, the red pulp and the white pulp (Figure 15.5A, B). The red pulp consists of blood-filled sinusoids and cords of

Billroth (Figure 15.5), containing macrophages, lymphocytes, and plasma cells. Macrophages in the red pulp perform a major function in red blood cell clearance and in phagocytosis, especially of nonopsonized particles. This high-volume blood filter function is made possible by two factors: direct unobstructed contact between phagocytic cells and blood-borne particles; and large blood supply (estimated at about 5% of the total blood volume per minute). The phagocytic function is especially important in early intravascular bacterial infection, before antibody formation and subsequent opsonization occurs. Splenic macrophages and the hepatic phagocytic system together synthesize

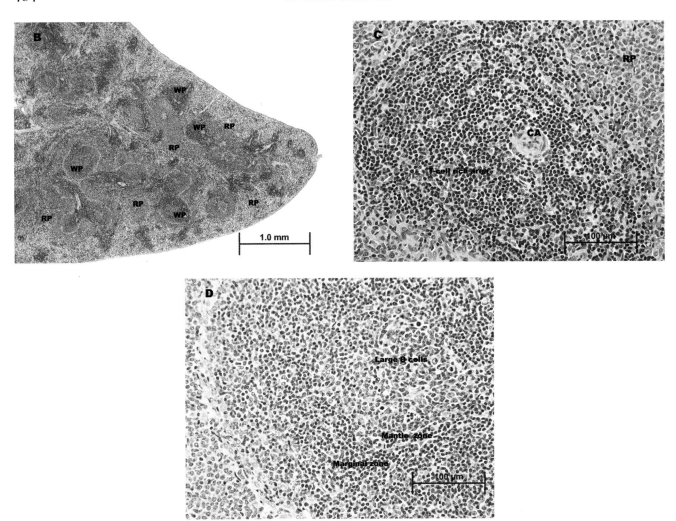

FIGURE 15.5 (Continued) (B) Low magnification of a mouse spleen showing red pulp (RP) filled with red blood cells and white pulp (WP), oriented around central arterioles. (C) A splenic PALS from a mouse without an associated follicle. The small T-lymphocytes surrounding a central arteriole (CA) are present. Adjacent red pulp (RP) can also be seen. (D) Splenic PALS with associated follicle in a mouse spleen, showing the larger B-lymphocytes within the center of the follicle, and the small B-lymphocytes in the surrounding mantle zone, in turn surrounded by small T-lymphocytes in the marginal zone.

the majority of complement components involved in the classical complement cascade. In most species, the red pulp also contains nests of extramedullary hemopoiesis, characterized histologically by megakaryocytes and normoblasts.

White Pulp

The spleen contains about a quarter of the body's total lymphocyte population; during lymphocyte recirculation, more cells pass through the spleen than through all the lymph nodes. Lymphocytes in the spleen reside in the white pulp, which consists of central arterioles surrounded by the periarteriolar lymphocyte sheaths (PALS), a T-lymphocyte-rich structure.

The outer PALS contain B-lymphocytes and, after antigenic stimulation, plasma cells. Adjacent follicles contain B-cells. Around each PALS and follicles is a corona containing B-cells called the marginal zone; this region is easily distinguished, especially in rats. The PALS have a microenvironment and passenger leukocyte content that is similar to that of the lymph node paracortex. Some sources claim that the spleen is a rich source of T_S cell activity, exceeding that of lymph nodes. The spleen performs a major function in humoral immunity by the synthesis of IgM class antibodies, especially against blood-borne antigens.

The marginal zone has a microenvironment that is unique to the spleen. Histologically, B-cells at this site are of medium size; they are larger and paler than

B-cells in primary follicles and the follicular mantle of secondary follicles. In addition, they do not show the morphology of centrocytes or centroblasts found in germinal centers. Their phenotypic expression (surface IgM+ IgD−) indicates that marginal zone B-cells are a separate B-cell population. The microenvironment of the marginal zone is unique, due to the presence of special macrophage types; the marginal zone macrophages, and marginal metallophilic macrophages. Marginal metallophilic macrophages are located at the periphery of the white pulp and along the inner border of the marginal sinus. They can be stained by silver impregnation.

The marginal zone retains B-lymphocyte memory. Second, the marginal zone features humoral responses that do not directly involve T-cells. These T-independent responses are elicited by polysaccharide antigens of encapsulated bacteria; these antigens are present in repeating units on the microorganism, and are presented to the B-cells by marginal zone macrophages. Antibodies generated are mainly of IgM class, since T-cell help is required for an isotype switch.

In conclusion, the main immunological function of the spleen is to guard the body's vascular compartment. It does so by generating T-cell-independent IgM-antibody responses to bacterial polysaccharides, and by exerting an enormous phagocytic power. Loss of this function occurs following splenectomy. In such cases, reduced nonspecific phagocytosis of non-opsonized particles, lowered serum IgM levels, and increased susceptibility to infections by encapsulated bacteria have been documented.

Mucosa-Associated Lymphoid Tissue (MALT)

Mucosa: The First Line of Defense

The secretory epithelial surfaces of the body form a major route of entry for potentially pathogenic substances. These surfaces include the epithelium of the gastrointestinal, upper and lower respiratory, and urogenital tracts. The host response at such locations ranges from physical (epithelial barrier, gastrointestinal motility, and respiratory mucociliary "escalator") or chemical (low gastric pH, mucus, lysosomal and digestive enzymes) responses, to antigen-specific immune responses.

T-cells disseminated in the epithelium and lamina propria of the gastrointestinal tract form the body's largest single T-cell pool. Together with the T-cells in organized mucosal lymphoid sites, such as Peyer's patches and draining mesenteric lymph nodes, these T-cells play a crucial role in the host's defense, and

carry out specialized tasks in the initiation and achievement of responses to antigens present in the intestinal lumen. The cells can leave their local sites after antigen-driven activation and join the systemic circulation, where they may contact cells from the systemic immune system. Thereafter, they may migrate back to mucosal surfaces. The epithelium of the gastrointestinal tract is possibly a lymphocyte-generating organ, analogous in some ways to the thymic epithelium. In the case of γδ-TCR+ intraepithelial lymphocytes (IEL), extra thymic maturation clearly exists.

Nonspecific killer (NK) cells are especially important in the epithelium of the gastrointestinal tract. In addition, lymphocyte-like epithelial cells have been found; these can kill pathogens, presumably without prior sensitization.

Lymphoid Tissue

Lymphoid tissue occurs just underneath the secretory epithelium, as seen in Peyer's patches in the duodenum and jejunum (Figure 15.6), the appendix of the large intestine, and as lymphoid aggregates along bronchi and in the oro- and nasopharyngeal region. These mucosal lymphoid tissues share structural and functional characteristics, and are strongly interrelated. Therefore, the common designation "mucosa-associated lymphoid tissue" (MALT) is used to cover bronchus-associated (BALT), gut-associated (GALT), and (oro)nasal-associated (NALT) lymphoid tissues. In humans and domestic animals, the large NALT in the pharyngeal region are called tonsils. The organization of MALT is similar to that of lymph nodes, with B-cell-containing follicles and T-cell-containing interfollicular areas. Afferent lymph vessels are lacking, because pathogens can enter these tissues through the covering epithelial layer. Epithelial cells (M, or microfold, cells) at these locations are often thinner than those at other secretory sites, in order to enable the efficient passage of pathogens for immune sampling. Stimulated lymphoid tissue in GALT and tonsils in humans often feature prominent follicles with germinal centers. In contrast, germinal centers are scarce in stimulated BALT and NALT in rodents. This paucity of follicles may be ascribed to the fast transfer of the immunological reaction to the draining cervical lymph nodes in rodents. It should also be noted that medullary areas, like those in lymph nodes, are absent in MALT.

The homing specificity of lymphocytes into MALT has the advantage that the same circulatory pathway (i.e., the blood) is used by both the secretory and internal immune system (with the possibility of mutual contact). In addition, the antigen message received at one distinct secretory site is followed by

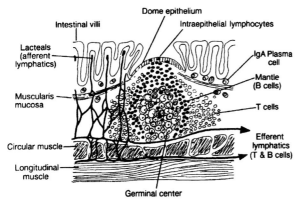

FIGURE 15.6   Diagram of a Peyer's patch in the gastrointestinal tract. Follicles and interfollicular areas occur just underneath the mucosal epithelium. Note the absence of medullary cords, and direct drainage in efferent lymph vessels. The epithelium covering this lymphoid structure (dome epithelium) is thin, to enable the efficient penetration of pathogens (M or microfold cells). Lymphocytes occur in the dome epithelium and epithelium of the villi. In mouse, these cells are characterized as T-cells with the γ-δ T-cell receptor. (Reproduced from Sell (1987). *Immunology, Immunopathology, and Immunity*, 4th edn. Elsevier Science, with permission.)

the generation of effect at all secretory surfaces. Thus, after antigen presentation in the gastrointestinal tract, effector cells can be found not only at the site of stimulation, but also at other secretory sites (e.g., the respiratory tract).

Secretory IgA-antibody Response

The immune response in MALT differs from that in other sites in the body, being especially devoted to the generation of an IgA response. Thus, MALT contains precursors of IgA plasma cells. In addition, MALT contains populations of T-cells capable of promoting the B-cell immunoglobulin isotype switch into IgA-producing B-cells/plasma cells after local antigen presentation, by trafficking lymphocytes homing to a specific site. Precursors move through draining lymph nodes into the blood and from there to the targeted secretory surface, where they lodge and differentiate into IgA plasma cells in the lamina propria. Homing phenomena exist by which these cells are able to specifically select final mucosal destination.

In contrast to IgA produced by the bone marrow and circulating in blood, IgA synthesizd by plasma cells of MALT consists of dimeric immunoglobulin subunits. The two monomers are linked together by a polypeptide called the J chain (about 15 kDa). These IgA antibodies have their main effect outside the body proper (e.g., salivary and gastrointestinal secretions). Transport from the site of synthesis

across the epithelial barrier is specifically adapted for dimeric IgA and, to a lesser extent, for pentameric IgM. Epithelial cells express a receptor for these immunoglobulins called secretory component (SC, a polypeptide of about 70 kDa). After binding to this receptor, the molecule is transported through the epithelium, possibly through its cytoplasm, and excreted on the lumenal surface. During this process, SC is attached covalently to the immunoglobulin molecule; the composite molecule comprising dimeric IgA, J chain, and SC is called secretory IgA. In rodents, a similar SC-mediated transport occurs in the liver. Here, SC on the hepatocyte surface mediates the passage of dimeric IgA from the sinusoids to the bile canaliculi. In this way, dimeric IgA entering the liver by the portal vein recirculates efficiently to the bile, and from there into the gastrointestinal lumen. Secretory IgA is more resistant to lumenal conditions (especially proteolytic enzymes) than dimeric IgA, and is thus better able to function there.

IgA lacks the effector reactivity of IgM and IgG for complement activation by the classical cascade. IgA also performs poorly in opsonization, phagocytosis, and ADCC. This may be related to the absence of effector systems (complement, phagocytes) in secretory fluid. The main function of IgA is to prevent the entry of potentially pathogenic substances into the body, by coating the epithelium with "antiseptic paint."

Immunologic Tolerance Induction

A final feature of MALT is its power to generate immunological tolerance. After antigenic priming at secretory surfaces, subsequent systemic antigenic challenge often results in nonresponsiveness. After local immunization, suppressor T-cells have been found in the spleen and suppressor factors in the circulation. This induction of tolerance primarily pertains to dead microorganisms or inactivated proteins that come in contact with the MALT. Therefore, vaccination via the MALT should be done with vaccines containing live organisms. The mechanism of tolerance induction and differing responses to live and dead microorganisms is not completely defined, but is important in tolerance to food antigens, and the development of food allergies.

Because MALT can function independently of the internal immune system, blood analysis alone may not provide complete information on MALT function. Instead, analysis of secretory fluids, such as saliva (for IGA antibody), or direct investigation of the tissue itself is more appropriate.

COMPARATIVE MECHANISMS OF IMMUNE TOXICITY

Introduction

Because the primary function of the immune system is to recognize exogenous agents and neutralize them, it interacts with many chemicals in an antigen-specific fashion. Obviously, this holds true for larger molecules, such as (glyco)proteins, but it also holds for small molecular weight compounds against which immune responses may develop, especially if such compounds bind to larger protein structures present in the host itself. Usually, immune responses to exogenous agents are beneficial to the host. There are those instances, however, where immune responses to chemical agents (or to host structures altered because of interaction with chemical agents), have a greater impact than the actual toxic effects of the chemical compounds themselves. In these cases, the undesired responses are designated as allergic or autoimmune. In addition, chemical compounds may interact with the immune system in an antigen-nonspecific fashion. In those cases, the chemical agent exerts direct toxicity to components of the immune system. This can either lead to malfunctioning of the system as a whole, or to the disruption of regulatory systems, which in turn my give rise to exaggerated responses.

Nonantigen-specific Interactions

With regard to direct toxic actions of chemicals on the immune system, it should be mentioned that the dynamic nature of the immune system renders it especially vulnerable to toxic influence. This applies in particular to the bone marrow and thymus. The "stromal" framework of the immune system is relatively resistant to the action of toxic substances. Toxicity to these stationary stromal components mainly affects its supportive functions (e.g., the secretion of biologically-active mediators, or the cell–cell interactions by specific surface ligands). In contrast, nonstromal, immature T-cells (thymocytes) are especially susceptible to the action of toxic compounds. This is due to the fragile composition of these cells, and to the delicate interactions between these cells and their stromal microenvironment.

The dynamic processes of lymphocyte function are associated with gene amplification, transcription, and translation. Many toxic compounds exert their toxicity by affecting these processes. The disappearance of lymphoid cells from blood and tissue is often the first sign of toxicity. This also applies to the "passenger cells" contributing to stromal interactions (e.g., tissue macrophages or interdigitating cells). Stromal components may respond to the disappearance of these passenger cells by degeneration, ending in atrophy and fibrosis of the affected lymphoid organ(s). Also, persistence of regulatory passenger cells with functional inhibition properties can occur, leading to atrophy. Conversely, a phenomenon that is quite the opposite is polyclonal B-cell activation, which may result from chemical exposure, leading to inadvertent antibody deposition in places such as the joints and the renal glomeruli.

Despite its susceptibility to toxic damage, the dynamic nature of the immune system provides it with a great regenerative capacity. In principle, the white blood cell population is generated by a single pluripotent progenitor cell in the bone marrow. For the thymus, single thymocyte precursors have an enormous capacity for expansion. Thus, even after exposure to xenobiotics that destroy the functional arm of the immune system, regeneration can occur in a relatively short time. For example, original architecture of lymphoid tissue is restored 3–4 weeks following involution due to irradiation, or treatment with glucocorticoids or organotin compounds.

Antigen-specific Interactions

Adverse specific responses of the immune system to chemicals are consequences of inadvertent sensitization. Following the classification of Gell and Coombs, four types of hypersensitivity can be distinguished (Table 15.2). The type I reaction is the immediate type, mediated by IgE antibodies, and resulting in mediator release by mast cells and basophils. The type II reaction represents IgM or IgG antibody responses to cell-bound antigen. The type III reaction is the immune complex type, with vascular lesions as the major consequences. Type IV reactions are of the delayed type, mediated either by lymphokines of T_{DTH} cells, with granuloma formation, or by T_C cells and macrophages.

The elicitation of an immune reaction strongly depends on the capacity of the compound to form immunogenic hapten-carrier conjugates with endogenous proteins. This conjugate formation involves either the parent molecule itself, or its reactive metabolites. In the subsequent immune response, the compound in native, unconjugated form serves as the target. Immune response to these compounds can be documented both at the antibody level, with *in vitro* lymphocyte stimulation tests, and by *in vivo* skin tests.

The manifestations of inadvertent sensitization vary widely, and include systemic anaphylaxis, hemolytic anemia, serum sickness, vasculitis, urticaria, contact

TABLE 15.2   Overview of the four types of antigen-specific reactions

Type of reaction	Principal mechanisms leading to tissue injury	Predominant morphology of inflammation
I. Anaphylactic type	Specific cytotrophic (e.g., IgE) antibody binds to receptors on mast cells and basophils and reacts with antigen. This results in activation of the mast cells and basophils and release of granule products and synthesis of inflammatory mediators	Vascular congestion, edema, degranulation of mast cells and basophils, influx of eosinophils, neutrophils, platelet aggregation, goblet cell hyperplasia
II. Cytotoxic type	Cytotoxic (IgG, IgM) antibodies formed against antigens on (target) cells surfaces or in connective tissues. Binding of antibodies to target cells leads to cell death by complement or via macrophages. Binding may also lead to physiologic changes in target cells. Binding of antibody to connective tissue antigen leads to direct or indirect damage	Generally, inflammation is organ specific; macrophages, NK cells, granulocytes, necrosis
III. Immune complex type	Antibodies (IgG, IgM, IgA) formed against exogenous or endogenous antigens. Deposition of antigen–antibody (immune) complexes from the circulation in the tissues evoke an inflammatory response at the site of deposition, involving complement activation and macrophages	Generally, inflammatory is not organ specific; vasculitis, immune complex deposition; neutrophils, edema, hemorrhage, fibrinoid necrosis, macrophages, granuloma
IV. Cell-mediated type	Antigen-elicited cellular immune reaction that results in tissue damage without requiring participation of antibodies. Antigen-specific T-cells and macrophages are involved	Delayed-type hypersensitivity; lymphocytes, monocytes, macrophages, and fibroblasts, evolving into a granulomatous reaction when the stimulus persists. T-cell or natural killer cell-mediated cytotoxicity; target cell lysis, lymphocytes

dermatitis, hepatitis, and nephritis, depending on the mechanism that is active. In certain instances, different mechanisms may be active. Hemolytic anemia, for example, results from mechanisms such as the attachment of certain drugs (e.g., penicillin and cephalosporins) to erythrocyte surfaces, with subsequent antibody binding and activation of complement, attachment of drug–antidrug immune complexes to C3b receptors on the erythrocyte (e.g., phenacetin and quinine), and modification of self-antigen with autoantibody generation and fixation to the cell (e.g., the Rh antigen modified by methyldopa).

Responses may also occur that are reminiscent of specific immune response, when in reality they are not. For example, in a large number of individuals with acute urticaria, mast cell degranulation is the result of direct action by the irritant. These irritants include drugs (e.g., codeine), physical stimuli (cold, heat, pressure), or other potentiating agents (e.g., plasma protein products, gelatin, starch, and dextran). This type of "pseudo allergy" can also be mediated by complement components following activation by the alternative pathway, especially by C3b, because mast cells and basophils have C3b receptors. Such IgE-independent responses are quite similar in manifestation to antigen specific type I reactions. A more detailed list of mechanisms of immunotoxicity is presented in Table 15.3. Agents shown to, or suspected to, cause lesions via these mechanisms are also presented.

Examples of Immunotoxic Agents

Steroid Hormones

Sex Hormones and Hormone Receptors

Sex steroid hormones have a profound influence on immune reactivity. In general, male sex hormones are considered immunostimulatory, and female sex hormones are considered immunosuppressive. Considerable changes are seen in lymphoid organs during pregnancy, and increased serum 17β-estradiol levels during pregnancy correlate with lymphopenia and suppression of cellular immunity. The balance between male and female sex hormones (e.g., estradiol and testosterone) influences the degree of immune responsiveness. Autoimmune diseases, such as systemic lupus erythematosis (SLE) and rheumatoid arthritis, are linked to sex hormonal imbalance. These diseases occur more frequently in females; the course of disease is often exacerbated when the sex hormone ratio shifts toward a higher estrogen to androgen ratio, such as during menarche, pregnancy, or ingestion of estrogen-containing oral contraceptives. The basis of enhanced antibody-synthesizing capacity on the part of B-lymphocytes has been related to a depressed T_S activity, which in turn is associated with the presence of cytosolic estrogen receptors in lymphocytes, especially in CD8+ cells.

Estrogen receptors have also been documented in the thymus, both in thymocytes and in epithelial cells.

TABLE 15.3 Mechanisms of toxicity with selected examples of xenobiotics associated with or implicated in injury to the immune system

Mechanism	Xenobiotic
● Receptor-mediated immunosuppression	Cyclosporin A, diethylstilbestrol, female sex hormones (estrogens), glucocorticosteroids, halogenated aromatic hydrocarbons, o,p9-DDT, mycotoxins, TCDD, Δ^9-tetrahydrocannabinol
● Receptor-mediated immunostimulation	Male sex hormones (androgens)
● Direct immunosuppression	Alkylating agents (e.g., cyclophosphamide, nitrogen mustard, nitrosoureas), antifungal agents (e.g., griseofulvin), anti-inflammatory agents (e.g., NSAIDs), antimetabolites (e.g., azathioprine, 5'-fluorouracil, methotrexate), asbestos, benzene, cytochalasin A, glucocorticosteroids, heavy metal ions (esp. lead), irradiation, L-asparaginase, organotin compounds, oxidant air pollutants (O_3), p-benzoquinone, triazenes
● Direct immunostimulation	Hexachlorobenzene (rat)
● Direct immunologic reaction (Hypersensitivity)	
Type I	Antibiotics (e.g., penicillin), beryllium, ethylenediamine, food additives, (e.g., BHT), isocyanates, nickel and nickel salts, plasticizers (e.g., trimetallic anhydride), platinum compounds, pesticides, resins
Type II	Antimicrobials (e.g., penicillin), mercurials
Type III	Gold, mercuric chloride, sodium aurothiomalate
Type IV	Antibiotics, antimicrobials (e.g., parabene, EDTA), beryllium, chromium, formaldehyde, pesticides, plasticizers, resins
● Autoimmunity	Mercury, silica, therapeutic drugs (halothane, hydralazine, isoniazid, procainamide), vinyl chloride

Thymocytes also have androgen receptors. Therefore, sex hormones affect thymic physiology, and can produce histologic changes.

Evidence shows that immunotoxicity and thymotoxicity correlate, for the most part, with estrogenicity. The mechanisms responsible for these effects are complex, probably mediated through a direct chemical interaction with lymphoid (thymus) cells, as well as effects on nonlymphoid thymic epithelial cells. These altered interactions result in the release of soluble immunoregulatory factors by the thymic epithelial cells, probably through binding to estrogen receptors or receptor-like structures.

Glucocorticosteroids

The second group of steroid hormones consists of glucocorticosteroids, either of adrenal–cortical origin, or administered therapeutically. Their immunosuppressive action is well-known. The inhibitory effect on processes of activation and proliferation forms the basis of their use in anti-inflammatory therapy, for example, in autoimmune diseases and transplant rejection.

Glucocorticosteroids have their main action inside the cell, as a hormone–receptor complex bound to DNA. At the transcriptional level, antigen presentation is inhibited by corticosteroids via down-regulation of MHC class II expression on antigen-presenting cells. Effector reactions are blocked by down-regulation of cytokines like IL-1, interferon-γ, and tumor necrosis factor-α (TNF-α). Thus, dexamethasone-treated rats have decreased production of TNF-α in lipopolysaccharide-induced inflammatory reactions; IL-2 receptor synthesis is also diminished. Finally, glucocorticosteroids may modulate IL-2 receptors on the cell surface, thereby interfering in the binding of IL-2 to its receptor. Thymocytes treated with glucocorticosteroids *in vitro* undergo apoptosis; this same process occurs *in vivo* (Figure 15.7).

Glucocorticosteroid hormones have a pivotal position in the homeostasis of the immune system. They serve as messengers between the central nervous system and the immune system. Adrenocorticotropic hormones released by the pituitary induce the synthesis of glucocorticosteroids by the adrenal cortex and the subsequent suppression of the immune system. This often leads to lymphopenia. Glucocorticosteroids belong to the family of so-called stress hormones. Histologically, the thymus is the first organ affected by these hormones. In acute stress induced experimentally by exercise, there are thymic alterations, whereas chronic stress also results in reduction of the peripheral T-cell compartment.

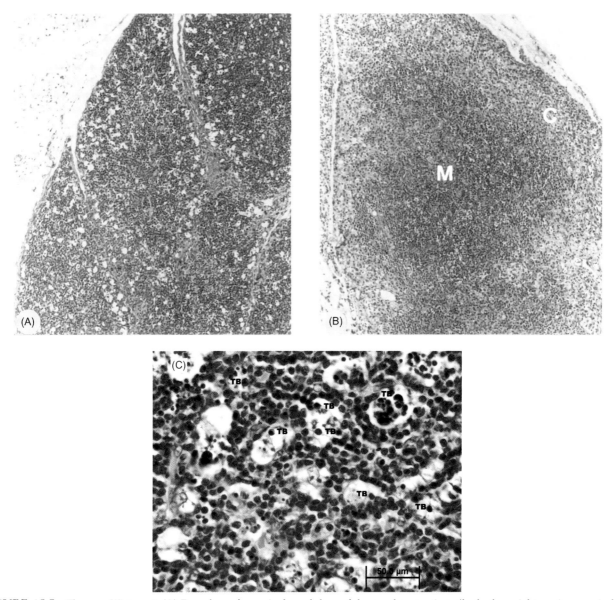

FIGURE 15.7   Thymus, Wistar rat. (A) Four days after a single oral dose of dexamethasone, 6 mg/kg body weight, an increase in lymphophagocytosis (starry-sky macrophages) in the cortex is seen. (B) After a seven-day period with daily oral administration of dexamethasone, 0.3 mg/kg body weight, there is a lymphocyte-depleted cortex, with inverse density of lymphocyte populations in cortex (C) and medulla (M). Hematoxylin and eosin stain; 90X. (C) Color high magnification image of thymic cortex from a cat showing numerous tingible bodies (TB).

It is not known why the thymus is so susceptible to acute stress. It has been postulated that the temporary shut-down of thymic function in inflammatory stress responses is beneficial to the individual. Generation of potentially autoreactive cells, which may contribute to the inflammatory process, is prevented due to this short-term involution. In any case, the toxicologic pathologist should be aware of stress-associated thymic involution in rodents, in order to correctly interpret the effects of xenobiotics in short-term high-dosage toxicity studies.

Xenobiotics with Estrogenic Activity

A number of xenobiotics manifest potential estrogenic activity. These include chlorinated hydrocarbons like the pesticide $o,p9$-dichlorodiphenyltrichloroethane ($o,p9$-DDT), the mycotoxin zearalenone, 9-tetrahydrocannabinol, and the nonsteroidal synthetic estrogen, diethylstilbestrol (DES).

DES has been extensively studied for its action on the immune system. Short-term (5-day) subcutaneous administration at dosages of 0.2–8 mg/kg/day in mice results in increased splenic weight and reduced thymic weight. Lymphocyte depletion is observed in the thymic cortex and splenic PALS. In addition to binding to the cytosolic estrogen receptor, DES shares with other catechol estrogens the ability to interfere directly with the cytoskeleton in the cell and on the cell surface, by binding nucleophilic sulfhydryl groups on molecules such as tubulin and actin. This binding blocks redistribution events ("capping") immediately after cell surface receptor and intracellular reactions.

Apart from thymus involution discussed earlier, the main effects of DES are the increased activation of the monocyte–phagocyte system, suppression of cell-mediated immunity, and reduction of natural killer cell activity. Natural killer cell activity especially is sensitive to DES action. Apparently, this effect is mediated by an effect on the cyclooxygenase pathway of prostaglandin synthesis, since indomethacin and aspirin prevent the effect.

Studies performed in laboratory animals demonstrate numerous immune alterations following *in utero* exposure to DES, including abnormal B-cell and T-cell responses, and diminished natural killer cell activity. Most of the immune effects following *in utero* exposure persist for the lifetime of the animal, and some even become more severe with age. Limited data are available on long-term immune effect in humans following *in utero* DES exposure. Hence, the relevance of these findings to possible health consequences in humans is unknown.

2 3,7,8-Tetrachlorodibenzo-p-dioxin and Related Compounds

Polychlorinated dibenzo-p-dioxins (PCDDs), dibenzofurans (PCDFs), and biphenyls (PCBs) elicit a wide spectrum of toxicologic effects, which are dose-related and species- and organ-specific. One group comprises the structurally-related 2,3,7,8-substituted PCDFs and PCDDs, and some nonortho and mono-ortho-substituted PCBs that have a planar configuration, which exhibit binding to a soluble cytosolic protein—the aryl hydrocarbon (Ah) receptor. Most of the toxic responses of PCDDs, PCDFs, and planar PCBs are thought to be mediated via the Ah receptor, including immunotoxicity. Of these compounds, the effect of TCDD has been studied in greatest detail. In rodents, short-term daily oral dosing, using about 5μg/kg per day TCDD, results in significant reductions of thymic and splenic weights. Cell-mediated response, such as *in vitro* lymphocyte proliferation after mitogen stimulation, delayed type hypersensitivity, T_C activity, and T_H activity in antibody responses, are especially reduced. The effects on antibody synthesis after primary and secondary immunization are variable. Natural resistance mechanisms and phagocytosis are

less sensitive to TCDD action than the more specific immune reactivities.

As a result of TCDD induced immunosuppression, particularly of T-cell-mediated responses, host resistance to various infectious agents is impaired. Using different mouse models, TCDD has been shown to suppress resistance to *Salmonella bern*, *Salmonella typhimurium*, *Streptococcus pneumoniae*, herpes II, influenza, *Plasmodium yoelli* (malaria), and *Trichinella spiralis*. TCDD-exposed mice also have marked susceptibility to endotoxin from gram-negative bacteria. A TCDD-induced increase in the production of TNF-α may be responsible for the endotoxin hypersensitivity in dioxin-treated animals. Similarly, lowered serum complement levels can explain the decreased resistance to *S. pneumoniae*. The sensitivity of the immune system to TCDD appears to be an age-related phenomenon, as TCDD causes more severe immunotoxic effects after perinatal administration than after administration in adulthood.

Many studies have been performed to investigate the mechanism of TCCD-induced thymic atrophy. In mice it has been established that susceptibility to TCDD treatment is determined genetically. Susceptibility segregates with the locus encoding the cytosolic receptor mediating aryl hydrocarbon hydroxylase activity. TCDD has a high affinity for the Ah receptor. Because thymic atrophy is Ah-receptor-mediated, this response has been studied to develop toxic equivalence factors (TEFs) for TCDD congeners. The TCDD effect on the thymus may be due to its action on epithelial cells, as has been substantiated by *in vitro* studies on both cultured mouse and human epithelial cells, as well as *in vivo* studies with susceptible and nonsusceptible mice and rat strains. For example, the enhanced lumphoproliferative capacity of thymocytes after coculture with thymic epithelial cells is reduced when the latter are pretreated with TCDD.

Investigations of persons exposed to TCDD in Missouri suggest an association between TCDD exposure and the hormone secreting activity of thymic epithelium, as the mean serum level of the thymic peptide thymosin-a1 was significantly lower when compared to a control group. Thus, TCDD-induced thymic atrophy may be explained by the inability of epithelial cells to provide the support needed to induce T-cell maturation and differentiation. Also, a direct action of TCDD on bone marrow stem cells has been proposed. This has been substantiated by the finding that bone marrow cells of TCDD-treated donors manifest a reduced capacity to populate the thymus of irradiated hosts. In addition to an effect on the thymus, and hence on thymus-dependent immunity, TCDD also affects B-cells, as manifested by suppressed antibody responses to thymus-independent antigens. This suppression, which occurs at higher concentrations, also appears to be Ah-receptor-mediated. Impaired B-cell maturation is thought to be due to the direct inhibition of late events in B-cell maturation and, unlike the effects on cell-mediated immunity, is less dependent on the age of the animals.

A number of accidents involving exposure to halogenated aromatic hydrocarbons have been reported in humans. From these studies, it can be concluded that TCDD and related compounds cause immune alterations, particularly of the thymus-dependent immunity. The findings in humans correlate in qualitative terms with the findings in experimental animals, including the sensitivity of the developing immune system, thus illustrating the relevance of studies in laboratory animals. However, exposure data on these mixtures of contaminants are virtually lacking for those individuals in which immune parameters were investigated, and there is remarkable inter-species variation in the toxicity of TCDD. Hence, assessment of the risk of these chemicals on the immune system of humans remains difficult in quantitative terms.

Hexachlorobenzene

The effects of hexachlorobenzene (HCB), a fungicide, on the immune system are highly species-dependent. In mice, reduced levels of serum immunoglobulins and secondary antibody responses have been reported. However, in rats, prominent changes include an increase in weights of spleen and lymph nodes, increased total serum IgM levels, and increased peripheral granulocyte and monocyte counts. The spleen shows increased extramedullary hemopoiesis in the red pulp, and hyperplasia of B-cells in marginal zones and follicles. In lymph nodes there is an increase in high endothelial venules, indicative of activation. Oral HCB exposure of rats also results in inflammatory skin and lung lesions. In the lung, high-endothelial-type venules and accumulation of macrophages in BALT are observed. Inflammatory changes of the skin are characterized by epidermal hyperplasia, activated deep dermal vessels, and inflammatory infiltrates. Functionally, cell-mediated DTH reactions and humoral immunity (primary and secondary IgM, and IgG responses to tetanus toxoid) are enhanced, and the developing immune system appears particularly vulnerable following perinatal exposure.

The mechanism by which HCB affects skin, lungs, and immune system is still unclear. HCB-induced lung lesions are strain- and thymus-independent, and do not correlate with parameters of immune modulation.

Therefore, an autoimmune or allergic etiology resulting from the binding of HCB or its metabolites to macromolecules in the body is probably not involved in HCB-induced lung lesions; however, the induction for skin lesions in the rat is highly strain-dependent. Thymus-dependent T-cells do not seem essential for the induction of the skin lesions, but enhance the rate of induction and progression of the lesions in the Brown Norway rat. Moreover, in HCB-treated rats there was no deposition of immune complexes in the skin, and no autoreactive antibodies to skin proteins could be detected in the serum. Therefore, it is concluded that the induction of skin and lung lesions by HCB is probably not due to binding of HCB or its reactive metabolites to macromolecules in the body.

Polycyclic Aromatic Hydrocarbons

Exposure to polycyclic aromatic hydrocarbons (PAHs) such as anthracene, benzanthracene, benzo[a]pyrene, dimethylbenz[a]anthracene, and methylcholanthrene is mainly by polluted air, for example, through exposure to exhaust fumes from burning fossil fuel. These compounds are immunosuppressive, and especially affect humoral responsiveness. T-cell-mediated effector functions are diminished, as shown by increased susceptibility to *Listeria monocytogenes* infection and suppression of T_C cell induction. This is in line with the thymotoxic effect of benzo[a]pyrene observed in the rat. Thymotoxicity and suppression of thymus-dependent immunity may involve the cytoplasmic *Ah* gene complex. Like TCDD, benzo[a]pyrene binds to the Ah receptor, and Ah receptor antagonists can block the immunosuppressive activity on human T-cells. For 7,12-dimethylbenz[a]anthracene, the *in vivo* and *in vitro* immunosuppressive effects in mice appear to be independent of the *Ah* locus. Alkylation of diol-epoxide metabolites has been proposed as a possible mechanism of toxic action.

The main property of the PAH compounds is their carcinogenicity. Besides a direct action of the compounds in inducing neoplasia, it is speculated that induction of neoplasia is also related to their immunosuppressive effects. This immunosuppression causes a reduction of natural immunosurveillance for tumor cells. The cells mediating immune surveillance include natural killer cells.

Organotin Compounds

Organotin compounds are widely applied as pesticides; as preservatives of wood, paper, textiles, leather, and glass; in heat/light protection of PVC plastics; and in antifouling paints. The use of dialkyl-tin compounds can cause hepatotoxicity, whereas tri-alkyltin compounds can cause neurotoxicity. Toxicity is greater for substances with alkyl groups of shorter chain length.

The effect of organotins on the immune system has been evaluated for di- or trialkyltin compounds, either in the form of oxides or chlorides. Rats treated daily with oral tri-n-butyltinoxide (TBTO) for 4–6 weeks or longer develop lymphopenia, and have reductions in weights of thymus and spleen. This immunosuppression is accompanied by reduced T-cell-mediated immune responses, including delayed-type hypersensitivity reactions, graft-versus-host reactivity, and T_H activity in antibody formation after immunization with immunogens like ovalbumin. *In vivo*, resistance to the nematode *Trichinella spiralis* is decreased. Serum IgG concentrations are decreased, but increased serum IgM levels have been noted. Natural killer cell activity is decreased, and macrophage phagocytosis is also affected by di-n-octyltindichloride (DOTC), dipropyl-tinchloride, and TBTO.

Other toxic effects of organotin compounds, primarily on the developing immune system, indicate a primary effect on the thymus. For both short-term and long-term exposures, 1-year-old rats require higher doses of TBTO than 4- to 6-week-old animals to manifest similar systemic effects, such as decreased resistance to *Trichinella spiralis* and *Listeria monocytogenes*.

Rats are more susceptible than mice and guinea pigs to the toxic action of organotin compounds on the thymus. Adrenalectomy has no effect on organotin-induced thymic involution, and growth hormone treatment after hypophysectomy has no effect on recovery after organotin-induced thymic atrophy. These data provide additional evidence for the absence of a glucocorticosteroid-mediated mechanism. Thymic atrophy is observed for both tri- and diorganotin compounds. Since TBTO and tri-n-butyl-tinchloride (TBTC) are rapidly dealkylated after oral administration, the atrophy may in fact be induced by the dialkyl metabolite.

In vitro and *in vivo* studies have both shown that tri-organotin compounds directly inhibit thymocyte viability and proliferation. Bone marrow seems unaffected. The antiproliferative effect is associated with a reduction in the capacity to form rosettes with sheep erythrocytes. This rosetting capacity is mediated by the CD2 molecule on the thymocyte surface, which has a transmembrane signaling function in early thymocyte activation (with leukocyte function-associated molecule LFA-3 on the stroma as the ligand). Another factor involved in early thymocyte activation is Il-2, the synthesis of which is down-regulated at the mRNA level by DOTC. These data indicate that a blockade of intrathymic T-cell maturation is induced by organotin compounds.

The presence of organotin compounds as pollutants in the aquatic environment has initiated some toxicity studies in fish species. In *Poecilia reticulata* (guppy), the thymus is among the organs most sensitive to TBTO (exposure to water levels above 0.03 μg/liter during 1–3 month exposure studies) and DBTC (at levels of 320 μg/liter or higher). The thymic atrophy is species-dependent; it is present in the guppy, but not in *Oryzias latipes* (medaka). Additional studies show that TBTO also affects the thymus of *Platichthys flesus* (flounder), as shown by morphometric analysis.

A number of mechanisms have been suggested to explain the effects just mentioned. The toxic effects of dialkyltin substances can be reversed or prevented by dithiol compounds, which points to the possible involvement of sulfhydryl groups in toxicity. These groups are pivotal in membrane-related functions, such as secretion, phagocytosis, transport, cytoskeletal function, cell-to-cell contact, and transmembrane signaling. It is, therefore, not surprising that the immune system, especially the thymus, is very susceptible to sulfhydryl-reactive compounds, which include p-benzoquinone, cytochalasin A, heavy metals, and organotin compounds. Other proposed mechanisms of toxicity include interference with mitochondrial metabolism and glycolytic pathway, and decreased cAMP production. Synthesis of both RNA and protein is also inhibited by organotin compounds. The increased sensitivity of thymocytes over hepatocytes may be related to the unfavorable pattern of purine metabolic enzymes in immature thymocytes, making these cells prone to "suicide" after activation.

Irradiation

It is well-known that ionizing radiation has a profound influence on the individual, especially on proliferating cell populations. Ionizing radiation is commonly used as therapy for cancer. Of the body's constituents, the hemopoietic system is particularly sensitive to irradiation; when the pluripotent stem cell is affected, the regenerative activity is lost. Therefore, after intensive chemotherapy and whole-body irradiation as cancer treatment, destroyed hemopoietesis has to be restored, for example by bone marrow transplantation. Other systems destroyed by this treatment, like the intestinal epithelium, have an intrinsic self-renewal capacity, and do not need replacement therapy.

Whole-body irradiation of rodents with doses of 0.5 Gy (1 Gy = 100 rad) or higher causes severe lymphocyte depletion of lymphoid organs, blood, and lymph within 1–2 days. The various lymphoid constituents of the immune system differ in radiosensitivity. Peripheral T-lymphocytes are more radioresistant than B-cells. Cell-mediated immune reactions are less affected by ionizing irradiation than are antibody responses. Within the T-cell population, T_S cells are more radiosensitive than T_H cells. Depending on the dose, a radiation-induced augmentation of immune reactivity (e.g., higher antibody levels and higher T-cytotoxic activity to tumor cells) can be observed. Mature lymphocytes, including effector T-cells, memory T-cells, and plasma cells, are less sensitive to ionizing irradiation. Finally, secondary immune responses are more radioresistant than primary immune reactions. Macrophages and macrophage function in antigen-processing are relatively radioresistant.

Regeneration of the immune system after irradiation depends on the dose of irradiation. The restoration of individual organs can occur by two mechanisms: either by repopulation from bone marrow stem cells; or by proliferation of locally remaining radioresistant lymphocytes. The second mechanism makes a greater contribution in the case of a lower irradiation dose (e.g., whole-body irradiation of doses up to 5 Gy). In this situation, the T-cell compartment shows a more rapid repopulation than the B-lymphoid population, which may take more than 30 days.

The thymus is very sensitive to irradiation. Within the medulla, a refractory population (about 20–30%) is present, but most cells are radiosensitive (D_0 about 0.7 Gy). The capacity of thymic stroma to support precursor T-cell processing is very radioresistant. After irradiation, the recovery of the original architecture follows a biphasic pattern. The first peak probably reflects the proliferation of the remaining intrathymic precursor cells, and the second peak marks the influx of newly-generated precursor cells from the bone marrow.

The acute effects following irradiation are lymphocyte depletion followed by regeneration. In addition to cell depletion, lymphocyte recirculation is affected at doses of 0.5 Gy. This phenomenon suggests radiosensitivity of high endothelial venules, or of the expression of cell surface molecules involved in lymphocyte migration through these venules.

The sensitivity of lymphocytes to ionizing irradiation cannot be solely ascribed to the susceptibility to cell death during cell proliferation. Cells in the resting state disappear after irradiation, which does not correspond to their fate due to the physiological half-life. Apparently, cell death of lymphocytes occurs in phases between cell division. This phenomenon is designated as interphase death, which is apparently a

distinct entity of lymphocytes, and makes the immune system sensitive to irradiation. Thus, the immune system is a very sensitive indicator of radiation exposure.

Ultraviolet B Radiation

Both ionizing and ultraviolet (UV) radiation interfere with immune function. Most effective in this sense is UVB radiation in the wavelength range of 200–315 nm. Interest in UVB arises from the fact that exposure to UVB at the earth's surface increases as the amount of ozone in the stratosphere decreases. In addition, exposure to sunlight and artificial UV sources may contribute to increased UV exposures in the population. Although UV has positive effects, such as Vitamin D_3 synthesis, its well-known damaging effects include sunburn, snow blindness, and cataracts of the eyes. In addition, UVB causes DNA damage, and is carcinogenic. Apart from the genotoxicity of UVB, part of its carcinogen effect is due to the suppression of immune defense against tumor cells. UVB-induced tumors show increased growth after transfer into animals that have been pretreated with UVB radiation. UVB radiation is not required at the site of tumor inoculation, indicating that UVB radiation has a systemic effect on the immune system. It is not clear how UVB exposure in the skin leads to system suppression of a variety of immune mechanisms. The migration of Langerhans cells in the epidermis to draining lymph nodes after UVB exposure, as well as altered interleukin patterns, may play a role. Both keratinocytes and Langerhans cells are affected by UVB; keratinocytes show altered immunologically active cytokine profiles, and Langerhans cells disappear from skin. Their antigen-presenting abilities are also affected. As a result, contact hypersensitivity reactions cannot occur in skin exposed to UVB. In addition, natural killer activity in the circulation has been shown to be affected by UVB irradiation. Transfer of splenic or thymic lymphocytes from animals after UVB irradiation or bearing UVB-induced tumors to naive recipients also results in a diminished response to UVB-induced skin tumors. Apparently, suppressor cells that inhibit this response are evoked by UV irradiation. Even though there are many lines of evidence, the precise mechanisms of induction of immunosuppression by UVB are still being clarified.

Heavy Metals

Direct Effects

Metals have profound but diverse effects on the immune system. Some, as trace elements, serve to enhance immune responses, a phenomenon best exemplified by zinc. Zinc (Zn) deficiency is associated with immune deficiency. The thymic hormone thymulin depends on the presence of zinc in the molecule to become biologically active. Aluminum (Al) is used in the form of aluminum hydroxide [Al(OH)3] as an immunologic adjuvant.

Most heavy metal ions are toxic to immune system components at dosages below those resulting in general toxicity. As an example, the addition of lead to drinking water at concentrations above 0.4 mM for 4–10 weeks results in decreased resistance to *Listeria monocytogenes* infection in mice. Inhibitory effects of metals on the *in vitro* plaque-forming humoral response to sheep red blood cells are mercury (Hg^{2+}) > copper (Cu^{2+}) > manganese (Mn^{2+}) > cobalt (Co^{2+}) > cadmium (Cd^{2+}) > chromium (Cr^{3+}); and zinc (Zn^{2+}) > tin (Sn^{2+}). Lead (Pb^{2+}) and nickel (Ni^{2+}) have a potentiating effect, whereas no effect is observed for Fe^{2+}. Two mechanisms of this metal ion effect have been documented: Ni^{2+} treatment of red blood cells alters their immunogenicity; and Pb^{2+} has a direct effect on effector lymphocytes. A decrease in antibody formation can be noted in mice after excess (2 g/kg) zinc is added to the diet, especially when this is done during gestation.

Various mechanisms have been proposed to explain the effect of metal ions on immune reactions. Divalent ions, such as Pb^{2+} and Cd^{2+}, directly interfere by competition with or displacement of calcium (Ca^{2+}) in the activity of essential Ca^{2+}-binding proteins, such as calmodulin. Thiol-related components may also be directly involved, especially following Hg^{2+} exposure, which manifests its toxicity by binding to cellular sulfhydryl groups. This may result in a net increase in helper–inducer activity for T-lymphocyte subsets, because CD4+ cells are less susceptible to thiol-blocking agents than CD8+ cells. Pb^{2+} has a lower binding capacity for sulfhydryl groups, but may activate lymphocytes by binding to phosphatidylcholine and modulating membrane phospholipids. Both Pb^{2+} and Cd^{2+} modulate intracellular glutathione. In addition, heavy metals affect lipid peroxidation, thereby altering the redox state of the cell and/or modulating prostaglandin synthesis. This interference may underlie the inhibitory effect of some metals on phagocytosis and tumoricidal activity by macrophages, on natural killer activity *in vivo* and *in vitro*, and on cell-mediated cytotoxicity and antibody-dependent cell-mediated cytotoxicity. Enhanced immune responses have also been observed. For example, Pb^{2+} and Hg^{2+} *in vivo* enhance antibody production. Thymocytes from mice after a 6-week treatment with 10 mM Pb^{2+} in the drinking water show an enhanced proliferative response to IL-2, and increased antibody synthesis by splenic cells *in vitro*. Both Pb^{2+} and Cd^{2+}

increase the phagocytic activity of peritoneal macrophages. Intermediate dosages of Pb^{2+} enhance, and high dosages suppress, *in vitro* responsiveness. Because of the varying mechanisms by which heavy metals interfere with leukocyte function, it is not surprising that the net effect of heavy metal exposure can be either enhancement or suppression. Xenobiotic interactions complicate things further, since combined treatment may cause synergism or inhibition. For example, Zn^{2+} and Cd^{2+} show an additive effect on immunologic cytotoxic responses, but Zn^{2+} has no effect on Cd^{2+}-induced inhibition of primary antibody responses. However, Zn^{2+} inhibits the stimulatory effects of low-dose Cd^{2+} in the plaque-forming cell assay, and on lymphocyte proliferation *in vitro*.

Toxicity caused by excessive intake of heavy metals has been noted in humans, and mirrors experimental data from laboratory animals. Addition of 150 mg elemental Zn^{2+} twice daily for six weeks (a dose about 20 times the normal intake) causes impaired immunologic reactivity, as assessed by *in vitro* lymphocyte proliferation and phagocytic activity. Lowered complement C3 levels have been reported for workers exposed to lead, whereas blood lymphocyte subsets remain unaltered.

Immunomodulating Effects

In addition to a direct toxic effect on cells of the immune system, heavy metals can indirectly induce tissue damage. For example, the effect of Pb^{2+} on the immune system may be mediated through sex hormones.

Metal ions can also initiate hypersensitivity reactions. Metals including Ni^{2+}, Co^{2+}, Hg^{2+}, Pb^{2+}, and Cr^{3+} commonly cause human contact hypersensitivity. For example, Ni^{2+} in jewelry often causes cutaneous sensitization. The delayed-type hypersensitivity response apparently reflects a T-lymphocyte response towards the metal salt, which acts as a hapten and becomes immunogenic after coupling to endogenous protein. Ni^{2+}-specific T-lymphocyte reactivity has been documented in sensitized (allergic) individuals. Another example is occupational exposure to beryllium, which can result in a hypersensitivity pneumonitis with pulmonary granuloma formation (berylliosis). The granulomatous hypersensitivity reaction reflects a T_{DTH} reaction to the metal, which has been documented in the lymphocyte transformation assay and in skin tests.

Mercuric-chloride-induced Glomerulopathy

Hypersensitivity reactions induced by heavy metals can also be of the immune-complex type. Such a reaction has been documented for renal disease resembling immune-complex glomerulonephritis induced by Cd^{2+} or $HgCl_2$ exposure in Brown Norway or Wistar rats. Polyclonal B-cell activation, with loss of T_S activity, most likely contributes to this hypersensitivity.

$HgCl_2$ can also induce a true autoimmune phenomenon. In susceptible rats, $HgCl_2$ administration results in the genesis of antibodies to the glomerular basement membrane, with the subsequent development of severe membranous glomerulopathy. The mechanism of this autoimmunity has been ascribed to abnormal T_H activity, presumably with reactivity to the individual's own MHC class II molecules.

Mercury is not the only metal that causes the glomerular immune-complex type of hypersensitivity. Kidney glomerular and tubular lesions have been found after sodium aurothiomalate administration in rats. It is also known that gold therapy in patients with rheumatoid arthritis can be associated with membranous immune-complex glomerulonephropathy. Interestingly, in these patients, this type of hypersensitivity is related to the HLA-DRw3 haplotype.

Airborne Pollutants

Airborne pollutants may enter the respiratory tract as gas, as liquid droplets, or as particulate matter. The subsequent interaction with the local defense systems may result in specific or nonspecific local and systemic responses. Epidemiological studies have established the association of air pollution with compromised health status in industrialized areas. There is a wealth of evidence in a variety of human situations, linking air pollution, particularly NO_2, SO_2, and O_3 gases, to decreased respiratory immune function.

Impaired resistance to respiratory infections has been observed frequently in animal studies. After NO_2 or O_3 inhalation, there is an increased susceptibility to airway infection, for example by *Klebsiella pneumoniae*, influenza virus, and *Listeria monocytogenes* in the rat. In such experiments, the concentration of oxidant gases had a greater impact than the duration of exposure. The reduced resistance to respiratory infection is explained by the decreased phagocytic function of alveolar macrophages, despite increased influx of these cells. Other cell types of the host defense system may be affected. These include natural killer cells, whose activity is stimulated at low exposures, and suppressed at higher concentrations of inhaled O_3. A further illustration is provided by changes in the lymphoid component of host defenses. After O_3 inhalation and pulmonary *Listeria* infection, T-cell-mediated responsiveness is impaired. Thus, oxidant gas inhalation not only has

profound effects on the mucosal immune system, but may also suppress the systemic immune system.

With respect to particulate matter, a number of epidemiological studies have shown associations between exposure, impaired lung function, and prevalence of allergy, but it is unclear which mechanisms play the primary role. Asymptomatic atopics show clinical symptoms following combined exposure to both allergen and pollutant. It is assumed that air pollution alone does not affect the subjects, but in combination with allergens may swing them into an atopic state. It is speculated that irritation of the lung parenchyma by air pollution triggers cytokine release, which may not only orchestrate the detrimental actions of inflammatory cells such as eosinophils, mast cells, and lymphocytes, but may also affect the T_{H1}/T_{H2} balance in favor of a T_{H2} response. In experimental studies, a combined exposure of animals to diesel exhaust particles (DEP) plus ovalbumin or pollen, or exposure to house dust mites, increased antigen specific IgE titers compared to stimulation by the allergen alone, indicating the adjuvant activity of air polluting components. Studies in healthy subjects show a significant increase in IgE, but no IgG, IgA, or IgM, following nasal challenge with DEP. Subjects with hay fever responded with a higher pollen-specific IgE titer induced by costimulation with DEP. Particles and irritating gases increased production of the proinflammatory cytokines IL-6 and IL-8, and inducible NO synthase (iNOS), in bronchial asthmatics exposed to high levels of ozone or traffic-related air pollution, increased IL-8 in nasal lavage fluid (NALF), and increased NO in expired air were shown. Apparently, environmental air pollutants induce cellular damage and evoke cytokine production, and may thus be capable of shifting the T_{H1}/T_{H2} balance to a T_{H2} response.

Several airborne pollutants may induce specific antigen-mediated inflammatory responses in the respiratory tract. Large proteinaceous molecules from spores, pollens, bacteria, and laboratory animals can induce antigen-specific inflammation. Workplace examples of antigenic low molecular weight chemicals are acid anhydrides, diisocyanates, and reactive dyes. The type of response and the sites of the respiratory tract affected by these compounds are determined mostly by the physiochemical nature of the inducing agent, the genetic predisposition of the exposed individual/animal, and lifestyle factors.

Cyclosporin

Cyclosporin A is one of the most powerful immunosuppressive drugs. It is a neutral lipophilic cyclic peptide consisting of 11 amino acids (MW 1203) isolated from the fungus *Tolypocladium inflatum*. The main application of the drug is in transplantation medicine, i.e., prevention of transplant rejection, and prevention of graft-versus-host reactions in bone marrow transplants. The drug is also used as therapy for autoimmune diseases.

The major complication of cyclosporin use is its nephrotoxicity. This can even begin at therapeutic dosages, and frequently occurs at somewhat higher levels. In its immunosuppressive action cyclosporin does not affect resting lymphocytes, but blocks events following stimulation, particularly the metabolism of lymphokines, including IL-1 and IL-2, and IL-2 receptors. The synthesis of IL-1 by antigen-presenting cells and the synthesis of IL-2 by T_H cells are inhibited. In addition, the synthesis of interferon-γ and tumor necrosis factor-α and -β is blocked. These events probably occur inside the cell at the transcriptional level. The response of precursor cytotoxic cells to IL-2 is also inhibited. In this way, effector reactions mediated by T-lymphocytes (DTH responses, cytotoxic responses) are blocked. The generation and activity of T_S cells seems unaffected. After passively diffusing through the cell membrane, cyclosporin binds to two ubiquitous intercellular proteins, cytophilin and calmodulin, and inhibits calmodulin-dependent (Ca^{2+}-dependent) enzyme activation. Inside the nucleus, the drug–receptor complex interferes in the transcription of messenger RNA encoding lymphokines. The immunomodulation by cyclosporin also involves the polyamine biosynthetic pathway. This pathway is generally activated in proliferating cells, and results in the synthesis of di- or polyamines (putrescine, spermidine/spermine), depending on the state of cell differentiation. It is initiated by ornithine decarboxylase, the induction of which is blocked by cyclosporin.

An interesting feature of cyclosporin is its specific action on the thymus. The thymus is reduced in weight after cyclosporin treatment. Histologically there is a decrease in medullary area. The development of CD4+ CD8− or CD4− CD8+ thymocytes from CD4+ CD8+ precursors is decreased by cyclosporin, and the process of negative selection involving deletion of potentially autoreactive T-cells apparently does not occur. The medullary stroma manifests a decrease of MHC class II expression after cyclosporin treatment, which indicates a loss of dendritic cells. These cells normally contribute to the negative selection process. The auto-reactive T-cells may even attack the medullary epithelium. Remarkably, cyclosporin itself has a stimulatory effect on thymic epithelium, both *in vitro* (human) and *in vivo* (mouse).

RESPONSE OF THE IMMUNE SYSTEM TO TOXIC INJURY

Weight and gross morphology of lymphoid organs are the first parameters studied in toxicity assessment. Response to injury is often expressed as a change in tissue size and weight. Hyperplastic lymphoid tissue may be characterized by white nodules and increased organ pallor, with the white areas representing lymphoid follicles with lymphocyte proliferation. Neoplastic proliferation is characterized by enlargement of the lymphoid organs, and a homogeneous white or paler appearance. The pallor in this scenario is due to proliferation of neoplastic lymphocytes. It is often difficult, however, to differentiate hyperplasia from neoplasia. Involution of lymphoid tissue is characterized by decreased organ size, and increased similarity of the affected tissue color to that of surrounding tissues.

Conventional histopathology enables the evaluation of the effects of xenobiotics on main cell subsets by assessing their distinct cytomorphology or tissue location. In this way, the effects on lymphocytes of T- and B-lineage or, on components of the supporting stroma can be evaluated. Necrosis, hyperplasia, or neoplasia can be detected. The evaluation of effects on distinct subpopulations is not always possible using conventional histology, but immunohistochemistry techniques help differentiate the subpopulations. The sensitivity of histopathologic assessment can be increased by quantitative methods, such as morphometry, organ cell counts, and flow cytometry.

The primary limitation of histopathology is that a tissue section represents a static time point in a dynamic process. Therefore, the dynamics of the immune system should be carefully considered in histopathologic assessment of immunotoxicity. For example, the histologic appearance of the thymus depends on the age and stress state of the animal at sampling. The histologic structure of lymph nodes is highly dependent on (local) antigenic stimulation. Normally, mesenteric lymph and superficial lymph nodes are in a state of chronic stimulation (draining, respectively, the antigen-rich gastrointestinal tract and the oronasopharynx). In the nonimmunized animal, they contain a well-developed paracortex, considerable numbers of macrophages in the sinuses and paracortex (mesenteric lymph nodes), prominent secondary follicles or germinal centers, and abundant medullary cord plasma cells. Both lymph node groups are part of the secretory immune system; therefore, histologic assessment only gives information concerning this part

TABLE 15.4   Histopathological changes in lymphoid organs and tissues[a]

Organs and compartments	Semiquantitative changes
All organs, all compartments	Increased or decreased size
	Increased or decreased cellularity (lymphocytes, plasma cells, blast cells)
	Increased numbers of cells otherwise not present or in low numbers
	Tingible body macrophages ("starry-sky appearance")
	Phagocytizing or pigmented macrophages
	Mast cells and granulocytes
	Apoptotic cells
	(Micro)granulomata or macrophage aggregates
Thymus	Altered cortex:medulla ratio
	Effects on number and size of epithelium-free areas
	Increased epithelial cords and tubules
Lymph nodes, spleen, and mucosa-associated lymphoid tissue	Increased or decreased germinal center development
Lymph nodes and mucosa-associated lymphoid tissue	Prominent high endothelial venules
Lymphatics and lymph nodes	Lymphatic ectasia

[a]Adapted from Kuper et al. (2000)

of the immune system (similar to Peyer's patches). In the unstimulated experimental animal, splenic histology is preferred for assessment of lymphoid organs of the internal immune system, since these are directly associated with blood. However, spleen weight does not allow discrimination between the effects on white pulp (lymphoid portion) or red pulp.

Morphology is a powerful technique in immunotoxicity assessment. The present state of knowledge regarding the relationship between structure and function of lymphoid organs is such that often a preliminary hypothesis of the possible mechanisms of toxicity to the lymphoid system can be formulated following histologic examination. However, different mechanisms of tissue injury can yield similar histopathologic features. The following sections discuss histopathologic changes that occur with immunotoxic injury. The mechanisms of toxicity for the compounds mentioned have been described in the preceding section.

The International Collaborative Immunotoxicity Study has developed an approach to study lymphoid organs in 28-day toxicity studies using the Organization for Economic Cooperation and Development (OECD)-407 guidelines. Two aspects are emphasized. First, morphologic alterations are reported per compartment, because immunotoxic compounds may have an effect on one compartment and leave others unaffected. Information on the affected compartment is of interest for the evaluation of the mode of action of a compound, because distinct compartments within a lymphoid organ have one or more specific functions, and each houses lymphoid and nonlymphoid cells of different lineages, in varying ratios. Second, the terminology to describe morphologic disturbances may be better-described in quantitative rather than qualitative terms (e.g., altered cellularity instead of atrophy, involution and hyperplasia (Table 15.4)). One of the problems in the detection of alterations is the discrimination from "normal" morphology. The spectrum of "normal" in lymphoid organs is wide, due to the dynamic nature of the immune system. Therefore, it should be established whether the morphologic spectrum of lymphoid organs either of all control animals, or a majority, is considered "normal." This implies that so-called "blind scoring" of the tissue sections cannot be done right from the beginning of the morphologic evaluation, but it can be helpful at a later stage of the evaluation.

Decreased Cellularity

Morphology

When a semiquantitative term like decreased cellularity is used to describe a decrease in certain cells in one or more lymphoid compartments, it should be established whether it refers to a decrease in cell density or a decrease in compartment size. Moreover, there may be a decrease in one type of cell (e.g., lymphocytes), but a concomitant increase in a different cell type (e.g., tingible body macrophages), as in corticosteroid-related thymic involution. Therefore, we propose to restrict the term "decreased cellularity" to decreased cell density of lymphocytes, blast cells, and plasma cells that are normal constituents of a given compartment. When the number of these cells is decreased, the size of the compartment may change rather than the cell density, because the stroma of most compartments is rather flexible and will shrink or expand as cell numbers require. In that case, we propose to record the changes as decreased size rather than decreased cellularity.

Atrophy in a lymphoid organ can result from selective or nonselective lymphoid cell death. The death pathway involved can be nonprogrammed, and is called oncotic necrosis. If the programmed cell death pathway is followed, this is called apoptotic necrosis. Oncotic necrosis is almost always accompanied by acute inflammation, whereas apoptotic necrosis usually is not, unless it is a massive event. The discrimination between apoptotic necrosis and oncotic necrosis can help determine the mechanism of action of an agent.

Effects on Non-thymic Organs: Irradiation

A severe and rapid depletion of lymphocytes in all lymphoid organs, blood, and lymph occurs after whole-body irradiation. The acute effects are cell death during cellular proliferation, as well as interphase death. Mature resting lymphocytes in peripheral organs are most resistant. Degeneration and cell death is particularly visible at sites of lymphoproliferation such as the thymus and secondary lymphoid follicles (Figure 15.8A). Depending on the dose of irradiation, areas containing plasma cells are the final refuge of lymphoid cells. The framework constituents of lymphoid tissues are much more radioresistant than the lymphoid components (Figure 15.8B). These constituents are affected during the chronic phase that occurs at least one month after exposure. Lymphoid tissue is atrophic, due to damage of the vascular system, with ensuing reduced migration of lymphocytes into the tissue parenchyma. The atrophic state can be associated with fibrosis, which represents a nonspecific response following persistent lymphoid cell depletion. Finally, a long-term effect of irradiation is the increased occurrence of lymphoid neoplasms. This may be a consequence either of direct radiation-induced damage of surviving cells (which escape interphase death), or of decreased natural resistance against tumor growth (immune surveillance).

After total lymphoid irradiation (TLI), the thymus shows a reduction of the medullary stroma, including both epithelial cells and dendritic cells; macrophages also disappear from the tissue. However, CD4+ CD8− or CD4− CD8+ single-marker positive thymocytes of

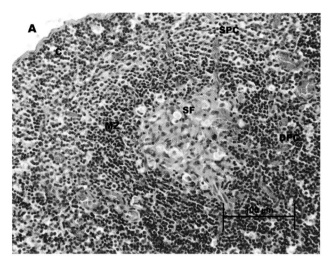

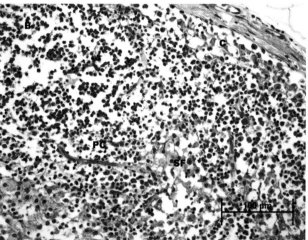

FIGURE 15.8 (A) Lymph node from a cat showing depletion of lymphocytic populations mimicking irradiation. Large B-lymphocytes in the secondary follicle (SF) are virtually absent, with only the larger meshwork of supporting fixed macrophages present. Areas in the cortex (C) and superficial paracortex (SPC), where active B-lymphocytes and active T-helper lymphocytes are located, respectively, show moderately depletion. Areas in the mantle zone (MZ) and deep paracortex (DPC), where small B-lymphocytes and small T-lymphocytes reside, respectively, are not depleted at all. (B) Lymph node from a dog with severe depletion of all lymphocyte populations, as would be seen with severe irradiation. Lymphocytes are severely depleted from the cortex (C), paracortex (PC), and secondary follicle (SF); the remnant population of more radioresistant dendritic macrophages is now quite prominent.

medullary phenotype persist, and apparently lodge in the cortex. During the recovery phase after TLI, the peripheral lymphoid organs show an excess of B-cells in the presence of persistent T-lymphocytopenia. In addition, large lymphoid cells that do not bear T- or B-lymphocyte markers are found in the circulation and spleen.

A severe and rapid depletion of lymphocytes in all lymphoid organs, blood, and lymph occurs after whole-body irradiation. The acute effects are cell death during cellular proliferation, as well as inter-phase death. Mature resting lymphocytes in peripheral organs are most resistant. Degeneration and cell death is particularly visible at sites of lymphoproliferation, such as the thymus and secondary lymphoid follicles. Depending on the dose of irradiation, areas containing plasma cells are the final refuge of lymphoid cells.

Thymocyte Susceptibility

The susceptibility of thymocytes, especially cortical thymocytes, is related to the fragile composition of these cells, and to the delicate interactions between these cells and their microenvironment. Therefore, a decrease in size or involution of the organ can be the first manifestation of toxicity. Generally, the main result is disappearance of a distinct thymocyte population, resulting in involution of the organ. As a consequence, the peripheral T-cell population can be affected. The close connection between the thymus and the adjacent parathymic lymph nodes can become particularly evident in sections of the involuted thymus.

Effect on Immature Thymocytes

Precursor (immature) T-cells find a protected environment for receptor gene rearrangements and selection in the thymic cortex (e.g., the "blood–thymus barrier" separating cortex from circulating blood). Apparently, the protection in the cortex is not absolute, and toxic substances can enter and affect the cortical thymocytes. The effect of toxic substances can vary; in the histologic section, adjacent thymic lobes can show a variable extent of involution, which might be related to the different extent of penetration by the toxic compound.

Glucocorticosteroid hormones have their main effect on cortical CD4+ CD8+ double positive thymocytes. This effect is associated with the relatively abundant expression of glucocorticosteroid receptors in these cortical thymocytes. The effect is very fast. Within a few days, histologic cortical changes progress from increased apoptotic necrosis of cortical thymocytes, which is easily-visualized by increased tingible body macrophages (Figure 15.7C) containing ingested apoptotic thymocytes, to lymphocyte depletion. The cortical depletion can be such that a reversed pattern of lymphocyte density exists temporarily, in which a higher lymphocyte density is observed in the medulla (Figure 15.9A, B). Lymphocytes within thymic nurse cells persist longer than cortical thymocytes outside these complexes. The experimentally-induced depletion of cortical thymocytes is identical to thymic involution in humans and virtually all other mammalian species in

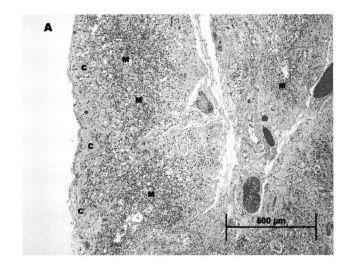

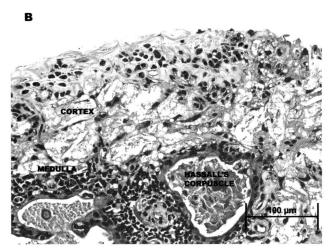

FIGURE 15.9   Thymus from a monkey with severe radiation sickness, illustrating the depletion of both cortical and medullary lymphocytes, and "collapse" or condensation of remaining epithelial and dendritic cell stroma. (A) Low magnification image illustrating the depletion of lymphocytes from both cortex and medulla, with condensation of the stroma. A reversal of the usual lymphocyte "gradient" is evident, with more lymphocytes present in the medulla than in the cortex. (B) High magnification image of a thymic lobule showing the condensed reticular epithelial cells in the cortex, remnant lymphocytes in the medulla, collapse of medullary stroma, and dilated Hassall's corpuscles.

conditions of acute stress. This is due to the increase in glucocorticosteroid synthesis by the adrenal cortex.

Radical but reversible changes are caused by the natural alteration of the sex hormone balance during pregnancy. After an initial rise in thymic weight in early pregnancy, involution starts with lymphocyte depletion of the cortex. Histologically, cell death is observed as apoptotic bodies and lymphocyte phagocytosis by macrophages ("starry-sky" macrophages). Remarkably, large lymphoblasts in the outer cortex remain relatively unchanged, as do lymphocytes in thymic nurse cells. Xenobiotics with estrogenic activity affect the thymus in a similar way. DES administration in mice causes lymphocyte depletion of the thymic cortex; it also reduces peripheral T-cells in splenic PALS.

Some organotin compounds affect the lymphoblast population in the outer cortex, presumably by inhibition of cell division. The loss of cortical thymocytes is manifested as an inverse pattern of lymphocyte density in cortex and medulla. Tingible body macrophages are not prominent, unlike in glucocorticosteroid-induced thymic atrophy. Adrenalectomy has no effect on organotin-induced thymic involution, and growth hormone treatment after hypophysectomy has no effect on recovery after organotin-induced thymic atrophy. These data provide additional evidence for the absence of a glucocorticosteroid mechanism. The rat thymus shows an increase of immature CD4+ CD8− OX44+ cells, which represent cells in a maturation stage prior to that of intrathymic proliferation.

Cytostatic agents, such as azathioprine, affect DNA synthesis, and hence cell proliferation that normally occurs mainly in the outer cortex. The same holds for irradiation. In these cases, cell death is not by apoptotic necrosis; thus, a clear increase in tingible body macrophages is not evident after exposure to either cytostatic agents or ionizing radiation. After prolonged exposure to these agents, a decrease in the number of peripheral T-cells occurs, observable, for example, in blood as lymphopenia. Decreased T-cells in the PALS, in the spleen and paracortex of lymph nodes, manifest as reduced organ weights.

During experimentally-induced depletion of lymphocytes from the thymic cortex, epithelial-free areas frequently disappear, and the epithelial stroma condenses to some extent, because the spongy matrix of the reticular epithelium is no longer filled with lymphocytes (Figure 15.9B).

Generally, a large, pale-staining epithelium remains after lymphocyte depletion; the cells often have vacuolated cytoplasm. After completion of cortical lymphocyte depletion, macrophages, in particular tingible body macrophages, are no longer evident. The thymic stromal components can recover their original status when new precursor lymphocytes immigrate to the depleted organ.

A major function of the thymus is T-cell repertoire generation during fetal and early postnatal life. The susceptibility of this function to disruption by toxic compounds, and the subsequent effect on cell-mediated immunity are most prominent during these periods of life. Apart from the age-associated effect, the extent of toxic damage may also depend on the gender and nutritional status of the individual.

Effects on Mature Thymocytes

Lymphocytes in the medulla are more resistant to thymotoxic compounds than cortical cells. Lymphodepletion of the medulla, if it occurs, mainly follows lymphodepletion of the cortex, depending on the experimental conditions. There are no reports showing preferential lymphodepletion of the medulla with maintenance of the architecture and cellular composition in the cortex. Interestingly, in conditions where the thymus becomes extensively depleted of lymphocytes in cortex and medulla, perivascular spaces can be quite prominent, and filled with leukocytes to a higher density than in the thymic epithelial microenvironment.

Effects on Stromal Cells

Some compounds affect the stromal components of the thymus. An example is TCDD, which specifically affects the epithelium of the cortex (Figure 15.10). Typical of the TCDD-effect are the aggregation of epithelial cells, and the expression of marker molecules that normally occur either on subcapsular and medullary cells or on cortical epithelium. These epithelial cells have been claimed to represent a thymic epithelial precursor cell. Histologically, depletion of cortical thymocytes is observed. This depletion gives the impression of an inverted thymic architecture, with higher lymphocyte density in the medulla than in the cortex. Lymphophagocytosis is not as obvious as in glucocorticosteroid- or stress-hormone-induced thymic changes, and overt signs of lymphocyte destruction are not observed.

Macrophages in the cortex are affected by the food additive 2-acetyl-4(5)-tetrahydroxybutylimidazole, or THI, as documented by the disappearance of immunolabeling with the macrophage antibody ED2. In addition, THI treatment results in a decrease in the size of the cortex, and an expansion of the medulla. There are decreased numbers of recent thymic emigrants, which suggests that ED2+ macrophages are indispensable for the processing of T-cell precursors.

The immunosuppressive drugs cyclosporin and FK-506 affect the thymic medulla. This is ascribed to the disappearance of the stroma, in particular the population of the interdigitating dendritic cells, as manifested by a decrease in MHC class II expression. As a secondary phenomenon, medullary thymocytes disappear. The development of CD4+ CD8− or CD4− CD8+ thymocytes from CD4+ CD8+ precursors is decreased by cyclosporin. The depletion (or reduced MHC class II expression) of medullary interdigitating cells may be of consequence for the negative selection of thymocytes, as the process of negative selection involving the deletion of potentially-autoreactive

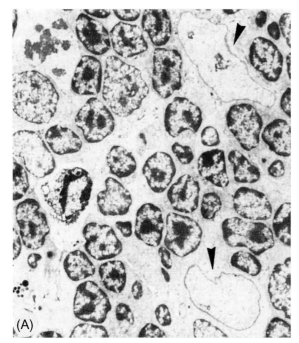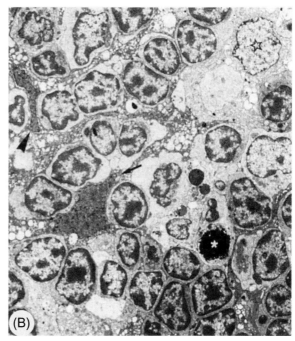

FIGURE 15.10   Thymus, Wistar rat. (A) Electron micrograph of noninvoluted thymus cortex, showing electron-lucent "pale-type" epithelial cells (arrowheads) and lymphocytes (2500 ×). (B) Ten days after a single oral intubation of 2,3,7,8-tetrachlorodibenzo-*p*-dioxin, 150 µg/kg body weight, the cortex shows an increase in electron-dense "intermediate-type" (arrow) and "dark-type" (arrowhead) epithelial cells. Also a "pale-type" cell is indicated (open star). Note the extensive vacuolation in epithelial cell cytoplasm. A pyknotic nucleus (apoptotic figure) is indicated (*) (2500×). (Courtesy of E. De Waal, National Institute of Public Health and Environmental Protection, Bilthoven, The Netherlands.)

T-cells apparently does not occur with cyclosporin treatment. Only some medullary epithelial cells remain, the outer medulla becomes populated by small-sized cortical lymphocytes, and thus resembles cortex. This gives the impression of a markedly-reduced medullary compartment, although the blood vessel architecture indicates that the original cortex–medulla boundary remains largely intact. The process of "cortification" of the medulla is reversible, and the original thymic medulla is restored after discontinuation of treatment. However, during regeneration, areas can be observed that lack a medullary stromal microenvironment, and are filled with medium-sized lymphocytes of medullary lymphocytic phenotype. Such areas have not been described so far in the normal thymus, but similar areas exist in the thymus of autoimmune diabetes-prone BB rats. The disturbed thymus, after FK-506 and cyclosporin exposure, represents a unique situation where potential autoreactive cells can be exported, resulting in autoimmune symptoms and syngeneic graft-versus-host disease in the periphery. T-dependent areas in peripheral lymphoid organs of cyclosporin-treated animals appear normal to slightly depleted in histologic sections. However, immunophenotyping of lymphocytes in these areas has shown the presence of markedly-increased numbers of CD4+ DC8+ double positive immature T-cells.

Effects on Mucosal Surfaces and Skin

Immunotoxic compounds may affect single intraepithelial and lamina proprial lymphocytes (IEL and LPL, respectively). Examination of the local immune system in toxicology is generally focused on Peyer's patches, BALT, and NALT, and the regional lymph nodes. However, the IEL and LPL differ markedly from T-cells in the organized lymphoid tissues in terms of phenotype, origin, and function. It is therefore questionable whether effects of toxic compounds on organized lymphoid tissues are representative of effects on the single T-cell pool. Unfortunately, the diffuse localization of this lymphocyte pool hampers sampling and examination. The lack of reports on effects on Peyer's patches may be partly due to the selection of patches for microscopic examination. For example, the immunosuppressive drug azathioprine reduces the number of macroscopically visible patches, but the patches selected at necropsy and examined microscopically are normal. UVB light influences the skin immune system, and a

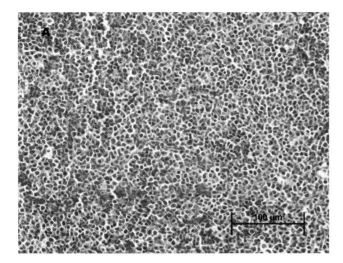

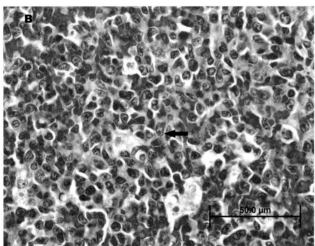

FIGURE 15.11 Spleen, Wistar rat. (A) Effacement of splenic parenchyma by sheets of neoplastic lymphoid cells characteristic of large granular cell leukemia cells. (B) High magnification image of the neoplastic cells. The cell in the middle of the field (arrow) contains minute basophilic cytoplasmic granules characteristic of this type of neoplasm.

systemic effect may be induced by the disappearance of the antigen-presenting Langerhans cells from the skin.

Regeneration

The dynamic nature of the immune system provides it with a great regenerative capacity. In principle, the white blood cell population is generated by a single pluripotent progenitor cell in the bone marrow. For the thymus, single thymocyte precursors have an enormous capacity for expansion. Thus, after exposure to xenobiotics that destroy the immune system, regeneration occurs in a relatively short time. The original architecture is restored 3–4 weeks following

the involution due to irradiation, or treatment by glucocorticosteroids, or organotin compounds. This restoration process can occur in waves, depending on the differential sensitivity of the precursor T-cell in the thymus and bone marrow.

Thymus weight, as well as function, decreases with age. It is therefore conceivable that the thymus becomes less sensitive to toxic insults with age and, if affected, that the toxic effects on the thymus have less functional impact, and subsequent regeneration of the affected thymus is less effective. Decreased sensitivity has been demonstrated in the few immunotoxicity studies performed with older animals. However, the components are still present in healthy aged animals, and they are able to function, as shown by reconstitution studies. Therefore, a decreased sensitivity to toxic compounds may not be a general property of the age involuted thymus, and regeneration of the affected thymus and of related extrathymic lymphocytes may occur, although recovery may not be complete and may be more prone to abnormalities than in young animals.

Relation to Autoimmune Disease

Decreased cellularity in an entire lymphoid organ, or in compartments of it, may point to the development or presence of autoimmune inflammation in other nonlymphoid organs. For example, thymic atrophy may accompany autoimmune disease in the autoimmune prone *Praomys* (*mastomys*) *nataliensis* and (NZBxNZW)F1 mouse, although thymic hyperplasia occurs more often. Thymectomy- and cyclosporin-induced partial thymus depletion in young animals can result in autoimmune (like) diseases. Therefore, certain forms of thymic depletion may be considered as possible early indicators of autoimmune disease. Moreover, particular substances can display immunosuppressive properties in certain animal species or strains under certain conditions, but produce autoimmune diseases in other sensitive animals. For instance, mercuric chloride induces autoimmune nephropathy and Sjogren's Syndrome-like adenitis in the lacrimal and salivary glands of Brown Norway rats, while it has immunosuppressive properties in Lewis rats. In addition, oral exposure to vomitoxin (deoxyvalinol) can both suppress and stimulate immunity, depending on the dose, gender, and animal species tested. Functional immunosuppression is not necessarily reflected morphologically by lymphoid depletion. Still, a substance-related depletion in so-called insensitive animal strains can be used as an indication for further research into deranged autoimmunity. Inappropriate, massive apoptotic necrosis has been proposed as the underlying mechanism for the development of systemic lupus.

Increased Cellularity

Morphology

In addition to agents such as vaccines, which stimulate lymph nodes and spleen intentionally, only a few compounds have been reported to cause morphologically-observable increased cellularity, hyperplasia, and/or germinal center development. Macrophage accumulation has been reported more often, especially in lymph nodes draining lungs that are loaded with particulate material. The limited data available include (increased) development of germinal centers in the thymus and spleen, lymph node enlargement with germinal center development, increased size of paracortex, and/or increased numbers of macrophages or granulomas Stimulated lymph nodes (i.e., increased cellularity in paracortex and/or well-developed germinal centers), can be observed at sites draining skin exposed to compounds with allergenic properties, such as dinitrochlorobenzene (DNCB) and trimetallic anhydride (TMA), and at site draining footpads injected subcutaneously with a number of drugs with immunomodulatory potential. The increase in lymph node weight during such reactions forms the basis of the auricular and popliteal lymph node (ALN and PLN, respectively) assays.

Hyperplastic responses as an expression of toxicity are exemplified by the effects of HCB on spleen, Peyer's patches, and mesenteric lymph nodes. Hyperplasia of the B-cell system is observed as an increase in the number of follicles, and in the thickness of the marginal zone of the spleen. HCB also induces increased numbers of high endothelial venules in T-cell-dependent areas of the lymph nodes and Peyer's patches. In addition, HCB interacts with the MPS. Following oral administration, rosette formation of erythrocytes with macrophages in the sinuses of mesenteric lymph nodes, and macrophage accumulations in the alveolar lumens of the lungs, are observed.

An example of expansion of the thymus, with an increase in thymocyte numbers, occurs in old animals after exposure to luteinizing hormone releasing hormone, resulting in enlargement of the thymus. The expansion of a thymic compartment without a major change in the size or weight of the whole organ also can occur after exposure to low dose of the immunosuppressive drug cyclosporin, which induces an increase in the cortex:medulla ratio, or the food additive THI, which induces an expansion of the medulla at the cost of the cortical compartment. After higher doses

of cyclosporin, the thymus is reduced in weight, and medullary reduction is observed as a decrease of medullary dendritic cells and lymphocytes of the CD4+ CD8− or CD4− CD8+ phenotype.

Mucosal Surfaces and Skin

Reported hyperplastic/stimulating effects of xenobiotics on lymphoid tissues and cells of mucosal surfaces and skin are even scarcer than hyperplastic/stimulating effects on thymus, spleen, and lymph nodes, with the exception of DTH reactions. DTH reactions are an example of local T-cell-dependent immune responses that are characterized microscopically by an accumulation of mononuclear inflammatory cells. These reactions have been studied mostly in skin, although they are also reported in oral mucosa and lungs.

Neoplasia

Tumors of lymphoid tissues include leukemias (lymphocytic neoplasms originating in bone marrow and manifesting themselves in the blood) and lymphomas (solid tumors of lymphocytic origin in lymphoid organs or extranodal tissues), as well as "parenchymal" tumors, such as thymoma (thymic epithelial cell tumors). "Stromal" tumors include hemangioma/lympangiomas or hemangiosarcomas/lymphangiosarcomas (endothelial cell origin), histiocytomas, and histiocytic sarcomas (macrophage origin).

The existing classifications of hematopoietic neoplasms are mainly based on histologic or cytological criteria. A number of proposed classifications are useful in assessing the grade of malignancy. Some of these are based on the resemblance of tumor cells to their counterparts in normal cell differentiation, for example, the Kiel non-Hodgkin's lymphoma classification. A comparative evaluation of six major classifications of human non-Hodgkin's lymphoma has resulted in the definition of the so-called "Working Formulation," used mainly to determine the grade of malignancy.

In addition to the morphologic classification, immunological phenotyping of malignant hemopoietic cells has been introduced. This phenotyping can be of value in differentiating hemopoietic cell tumors from other kinds of tumors, such as carcinomas, and in distinguishing lymphomas from reactive proliferations (e.g., monotypic immunoglobulin light chain expression in B-cell neoplasms). It can also be used in assessing the leukocyte subset lineage, and in determining the stage of maturation and differentiation, as well as the stage of proliferation and activation, of the tumor cells. For example, using this approach, non-Hodgkin's lymphomas of follicle center origin are almost exclusively

TABLE 15.5 Classifications of hemopoietic neoplasms in mouse and rat

Mouse: Pattengale–Frith–Taylor classification	Rat: Harleman–Jahn classification
Lymphoma	Lymphoma
Lymphoblast (B, T-cell)	Large granular cell
Small lymphocyte (B, T-cell)	Lymphocytic
Immunoblast (B-cell)	Lymphoblastic
Plasma cell (B-cell)	Pleomorphic
Follicular center cell: small, large, and mixed type	Plasmacytic
Leukemia (granulocytic, erythrocytic, megakaryocytic)	Not otherwise specified
Histiocytic sarcoma	Leukemia (granulocytic, erythrocytic, megakaryocytic, not otherwise specified)
Mast cell tumor	
	Mast cell tumor

B-lymphocyte in origin (Table 15.5); immunoblastic and lymphoblastic lymphomas can be either of B- or T-cell sublineage, with the phenotype of either immature or fully-mature cells. A strict correlation between the morphologic classification and immunological phenotype is not apparent, however. A good example of immunological phenotyping is the large granular lymphocyte leukemia in the rat (Figure 15.11), in particular the Fischer 344 rat. In nearly all cases, leukemic cells express the OX8 (CD8) marker normally present on T_S and T_C cells, and on cells with natural killer cell activity. Leukemic cells also express the asialo-GM1 marker normally found on natural killer cells.

A number of chemicals induce lymphoma and leukemia. Examples include methylcholanthrene in mice; the antitumor drug 4(5)-(3,3-dimethyl-1-triazeno)imidazole-5(4)-carboxamide, and the immunosuppressive drug azathioprine in Sprague–Dawley rats; and alkyl-nitrosourea compounds and alkylbenz[a]anthracene in Sprague–Dawley and Fischer rats. Urethane induces thymoma in Buffalo and Fischer rats. A magnesium-deficient diet has been associated with thymic lymphomas in Sprague–Dawley rats. This deficiency may underlie the genesis of lymphoma by the alkyl-nitrosamine compounds. The final example of induced lymphoproliferative disease comes from atypical immunological reactions, such as (pseudo)-graft-versus-host disease, in which there is lymphocyte stimulation under conditions of a marginally functional immune system. Since developing T-cells undergo proliferation in the thymus during generation of immune competence, this type of induced lymphoid neoplasm has a predilection for the thymus.

Inflammation in Nonlymphoid Tissues

The classical lymphoid organs are not the only sites where cells of the immune system reside. Subsets of macrophages reside in almost every organ, and there are even more macrophages in lungs and liver than in thymus and spleen. Lymphocytes are found throughout the mucosal surfaces, the skin, and the liver in large numbers. Moreover, antigen-specific deranged processes, such as autoimmune disease and allergy, lead to tissue damage, protein (immune) complex deposits, and/or inflammatory cell infiltrates, predominantly in nonlymphoid organs. Well-known nonlymphoid target sites are the vasculature, kidneys, synovial membranes, thyroid, skin, liver, and lungs.

The morphologic hallmark of autoimmune (like) disease and allergy is inflammation. Unfortunately, at present there are no morphologic criteria to identify antigen-mediated inflammation, let alone criteria to discriminate between allergic and autoimmune inflammation. Autoimmune inflammation in nonlymphoid organs includes changes such as granulocytic and lymphocytic cell infiltrates, granulomas, oncotic necrosis, and fibrosis. These changes are also common in other types of inflammation, and therefore their interpretation is difficult. Changes such as vasculitis, interface dermatitis, fibrinoid necrosis of blood vessel walls, and expansion of extracellular matrix are more suggestive of an allergic- or autoimmune-related inflammation. Various textbooks describe in detail the morphology of autoimmune diseases.

The histology of clinically-manifested inflammatory reactions, which are antigen-specific, depends on the type of reaction according to the Gell and Coombs classification (Table 15.2). It should be kept in mind that an antigen induces almost always more than one type of reaction, which is reflected by the morphology of the inflammation.

The type IV reactions, which reflect T-effector cell-mediated immunopathology, manifest as infiltrations of the target tissue(s) by lymphocytes and macrophages. Many autoimmune (like) diseases, such as rheumatoid arthritis, autoimmune diabetes, chronic thyroiditis, and autoimmune hepatitis, are characterized morphologically by mononuclear cell infiltrates in the affected tissues. However, mononuclear cell infiltrates are also present in other disease, such as allergy, viral and bacterial infections, and even neoplasia.

When lymphokine secretion is the main factor in inflammation, the inflammatory cells can organize into granulomas. Granulomas are typical not only of type IV (and sometimes type III) reactions, but also of nonimmunological reactions to poorly-degradable material. Whereas the type of granuloma induced is highly-defined by the inducing agent, host factors play a role as well, as exemplified by inhalation studies with beryllium (Be) in dogs and rats. So-called immune granulomas can be induced in dogs exposed to Be and are considered to be the result of persistent antigenicity of the compound. The immune granulomas are complex, discrete, and tightly-organized, with a central region of epithelioid-type macrophages surrounded by significant numbers of lymphocytes and a few multinucleated giant cell macrophages of Langhan's type. Lymphocytes in the lungs of dogs with Be-induced immune granulomas contain Be-specific T-cells. Be-specific cells cannot be detected in rats, however. Be-induced granulomas in the rats are considered to be solely the result of persistent irritation by the compound and can be denoted as foreign body granulomas. The foreign body granuloma is simpler in rats, organized more loosely than the immune granulomas in dogs, and contains only enlarged and vacuolated macrophages and multinucleated foreign body giant cells. Few to no lymphocytes are present in the lesions.

In silicosis, crystalline silica may continue to be mobilized from relatively fixed stores (i.e., macrophages and granulomas), in the lung and draining lymph nodes, even long after exogenous exposure to the silica, producing progressive lesions. In these lesions, alterations in extracellular matrix with fibrinoid necrosis are the characteristic features. Silica may disseminate via lymph and blood, leading to granulomas in organs outside the respiratory tract and its local lymph nodes. The continuous stimulation and degradation of inflammatory cells by silica has been associated by some authors with autoimmune (like) diseases, such as antineutrophil cytoplasmic antibodies (ANCA), associate glomerulonephritis, and vasculitis.

TESTING FOR IMMUNOTOXICITY

In Vivo and *In Vitro* Approaches

A wide array of methods to assess immune function is available for most species that serve as targets for toxic compounds (Table 15.6). In humans, most of these assays pertain to blood analysis (serum or plasma for humoral substances like immunoglobulins/antibodies and blood mononuclear cells for subset composition and function). These assay panels are

TABLE 15.6   Tiered approach of testing immunotoxicity in the rat

Tier one: Screening assays

Conventional hematology (differential white blood cell counts)

Serum IgM, IgG, and IgA concentrations

Bone marrow cellularity

Organ weights (thymus, spleen, lymph nodes)

Histopathology (thymus, spleen, lymph nodes, mucosa-associated lymphoid tissue in intestinal and respiratory tract)

Optional: immunohistochemistry and cytofluorography of lymphoid tissues

Tier two: Functional assays

Cell-mediated immunity	*In vivo* sensitization to T-cell-dependent antigens (e.g., ovalbumin, tuberculin, *Listeria*) and the delayed-type hypersensitivity response
	In vitro lymphoproliferative response to specific antigens (*Listeria*) and T-cell mitogens (concanavalin A, phytohemagglutinin)
Antibody-mediated immunity	Serum IgM, IgG, IgA, and IgE antibody concentration after sensitization to T-cell-dependent antigens (ovalbumin, tetanus toxoid, sheep red blood cells, *Trichinella spiralis*)
	Serum IgM antibody to T-cell-independent antigen (*Escherichia coli* lipopolysaccharide)
	In vitro lymphoproliferative response to B-cell mitogen (lipopolysaccharide)
Monocyte/ macrophage function	*In vitro* phagocytosis and killing of the gram-positive bacterium *Listeria monocytogenes* by adherent splenic and peritoneal macrophages
	In vitro cytolysis of YAC-1 lymphoma cells by adherent splenic and peritoneal macrophages
Natural killer cell activity	*In vitro* cytolysis of YAC-1 lymphoma cells by nonadherent splenic, peritoneal, and pulmonary cells
Host resistance and autoimmunity	*In vivo* challenge with *T. spiralis* (muscle larvae counts and worm expulsion)
	In vivo challenge with *L. monocytogenes* (clearance in spleen and lung)
	In vivo model of adjuvant arthritis

regularly revised by national and international committees, and will not be discussed in detail here.

Testing for Direct Immunotoxicity

In evaluating the immunotoxicity of a compound, regulatory authorities in most industrialized countries require, in addition to acute testing, the multidose 28-day (acute) or 90-day (subchronic) toxicity studies.

At least three dose levels, ranging from a low dose (aimed at no observable effect) to a high dose (inducing overt toxicity), must be used, and these systems have been standardized. For this evaluation, a tiered approach to immunotoxicity testing in the rat has been developed by the OECD in their 407 Guidelines.

Chemicals found to be positive in the first screening are subject to second-tier function studies. Third-tier investigations include special studies on the mechanism of action of the compound. In such studies, *in vitro* assays are of great value, for example, to elucidate the pathophysiological behavior of cells in suspension under influence of the toxic compound or the interactions with humoral mediators of the immune system. Such studies are currently being extended by the inclusion of molecular biological techniques, to evaluate the effect on gene expression at the RNA level.

In vitro tests are receiving increased attention. This is mainly due to the workload and expense associated with the large number of toxicity studies that are currently required, and the ethical issue of limiting *in vivo* animal experiments. *In vitro* experiments have not been used extensively for screening purposes. The complexity of the immune system's function *in vivo* makes it almost impossible to mimic *in vitro*. The main value of *in vitro* assays is in studies on the mechanisms of toxicity. *In vitro* studies also enable immunotoxicologists to evaluate toxicity in humans. *In vivo* studies, as well as *ex vivo* and *in vitro* studies in humans, are virtually restricted to cases of accidental exposure.

Interlaboratory validation using model toxic compounds is an absolute prerequisite for adequate immunotoxicity evaluation. This standardization has been accomplished for some test methods in the mouse, and has been initiated for the rat. The use of validated methods and parameters of study is particularly important for risk evaluation. In risk assessment, the no-effect level can be based on tier-one and tier-two parameters determined in relevant models, such as host resistance assays and *in vivo* assessment of hypersensitivity and antibody production. Usually a factor of 10 is applied in the extrapolation of data in experimental animals to the human situation, and an additional factor of 10 for differences in susceptibility between individuals. A further safety factor can be used to compensate for the high sensitivity of the developing immune system *in utero*, in cases where data are not available on peri- or postnatal animal exposure.

Testing for Induction of Allergy and Autoimmunity

Reliable and predictive experimental animal models are not available for the detection of chemical- or drug-induced hypersensitivity or autoimmunity, apart from tests for skin allergy. Experimental models to predict the potential of a chemical to induce allergy in the respiratory, and especially gastrointestinal, tracts need to be developed and validated. Chemical- or drug-induced autoimmunity is even more difficult to predict, because of the complex interactions with and within the immune system during the development of such a response.

Chemically-induced autoimmunity shares a number of features with hypersensitivity responses. The cells play a crucial role in both immunopathological phenomena. The popliteal lymph node assay is useful to predict the immunogenicity of chemical and drugs for T-cells. Data generated by this assay show a good correlation with the capacity of drugs and chemicals to cause hypersensitivity in humans. The assay needs further evaluation and validation.

Morphologic Techniques

For conventional histology, fixation of tissue in buffered 10% formalin, followed by paraffin embedding and staining of 6 μm thick sections with hematoxylin and eosin (HE), is the most widely-used technique. It is standard in most histology laboratories, and is suitable for assessing lymphoid tissue. The specimens can be fixed without preparation, except for gut-associated lymphoid tissue (GALT). The gastrointestinal tract is first processed into a so-called swiss-roll before fixation. This processing includes cutting the gastrointestinal segment longitudinally, and rolling it around a (wooden) stick with a lumenal side toward the center. An alternative fixative in routine histology is sublimate formalin, which is suitable for immunohistochemical assessment of cell markers, mainly intracellular antigens. Some membrane markers of the T- or B-cell lineage can be analyzed on sections of formalin-fixed tissue, due to the recent development of antibodies that react to formalin-denatured antigens. An alternative stain in routine histology of lymphoid organs is the Giemsa stain, which provides a better cytomorphologic discrimination of distinct leukocyte subpopulations. For better cytomorphologic detail, semi-thin sections (about 1 μm) can be prepared using harder embedding media than paraffin, for example, plastic (glycol methacrylate). This embedding medium is routinely used for the assessment of bone marrow specimens after decalcification of the tissue.

For immunohistochemistry, frozen tissue sections are still the best. To avoid artifacts, tissues should be frozen immediately after removal in liquid nitrogen (avoid direct contact with the liquid to prevent damage due to boiling of the nitrogen). Mild acetone or methanol fixation permits the preservation of both tissue architecture and antigenicity of the markers to be analyzed. As stated earlier, some cell markers can be analyzed using antibodies reacting with formalin-denatured antigens, but for most cell membrane markers only antibodies reacting to frozen tissue sections are available. A wide variety of immunohistochemical procedures use enzymatic detection reactions, or gold, or fluorochromes, as labeling substances. Immunoperoxidase methods using a (monoclonal) antibody in the first incubation, followed by an enzyme-conjugated second antibody and an enzyme-substrate detection reaction are widely used. Horseradish peroxidase is most often used as the marker enzyme, with 3,3-FT-diaminobenzidine tetrahydrochloride or 3-amino-9-ethylcarbazol as the chromogen substrate. To increase the sensitivity, a three-step procedure using a third antibody directed to the second one or the avidin-biotin complex reaction can be used. Kits are commercially available for the latter reaction.

Electron microscopy can be used to study subcellular morphology. This method of visualization requires rapid fixation of tissue in a special fixative, such as a mixture of glutaraldehyde and paraformaldehyde. To achieve rapid penetration of the fixative, the specimen should be sectioned (quickly) into small pieces (1–2 mm^3) before fixation; in vivo perfusion with the fixative is recommended.

The study of lymphoid cells in suspension enables analysis in functional assays, and the quantitative assessment of subsets in flow cytometry. Lymphoid cells are isolated from tissues simply by cutting tissue specimens, or forcing them through a sieve. Enzymatic digestion by collagenase or dispase can be used for the isolation of cells that adhere more to the tissue matrix, such as macrophages. This method may also allow isolation of matrix cells themselves. When working with cells in suspension, the investigator should watch for artifacts resulting from selective isolation, and should take into account the selective loss of subpopulations due to the isolation procedure. For instance, proliferating and dividing cells are easily lost, whereas resting cells in the G_0 phase are more resistant to damage during isolation. Cells of the macrophage lineage easily adhere and form aggregates during isolation; this can be partly prevented by working in a calcium-free medium. For immunophenotyping of cells in suspension, cytofluorography combines the simultaneous detection of cell size and (one or more) immunolabeling signals, and thereby provides the quantitative supplementation to the histologic location of particular subpopulations in tissue-section analysis.

Hybridohistochemistry or in situ hybridization can be performed on tissue sections using DNA or RNA segments complementary to the gene segment under study (probes) with immunochemical and/or enzymatic detection. DNA segments can be analyzed in formalin-fixed tissue sections, whereas RNA is visualized on frozen tissue sections. With special precautions, RNA analysis is also possible on formation-fixed tissue sections. In cases where localization is not required, DNA and RNA segments can be detected with greater sensitivity from tissue digests using spot blots. Also, Southern and Northern blots can be used for the detection of DNA and RNA, respectively, allowing the detection of the size of segments after restriction enzyme digestion. Finally, the polymerase chain reaction is achieving increasing importance; this technique encompasses the strong amplification of the segment to be analyzed using DNA polymerase, and primers complementary to the DNA segment of interest. The manipulations for RNA detection require special conditions during the phase of tissue preservation or cell isolation. These conditions are necessary to avoid denaturation following the action of RNAse, an enzyme which is practically ubiquitous.

In the evaluation of immune status, DNA analysis by the Southern blotting technique is performed to detect rearrangements of genes encoding T-cell receptor chains or immunoglobulin chains (related to lymphoid cell maturation). RNA analysis is used, for example, in studies of the capacity of interleukin mediator synthesis between transcription and translation. Interference by toxic substances in such processes has been demonstrated for steroid hormones and organotin compounds.

Animal Models

Most immunotoxicity studies are performed in rodents (i.e., the mouse or the rat). In vivo studies using spontaneously-occurring mutants or artificially-constructed laboratory animals are of value. For investigations concerning the role of immune lymphocytes in the effects observed, congenitally athymic (nude) animals are useful. They allow the direct effect on B-cells to be studied without interference by T-cells. A number of single gene animal models of immunodeficiency are now available to extend such studies for the evaluation of effects on specific arms of the immune system. An interesting model of immune deficiency in this respect is the mouse with the scid mutation, which shows severe combined immunodeficiency. The lack of immunocompetent T- and B-cells in this mutant is related to a defective recombinase function. Due to this enzyme defect, the appropriate rearrangement of genes encoding the T-cell receptor and immunoglobulin molecules cannot occur. An immune system can be constituted in this animal by grafting human fetal lymphoid tissues: the *scdihu* mouse presents an interesting model for the *in vivo* study of immunotoxicity on human lymphocytes.

Finally, genetically-modified animals represent a new generation of laboratory animal constructs. Gene overexpressing mice are generated by the injection of DNA segments of interest, linked to an appropriate promoter, into fertilized mouse eggs, and the subsequent implantation of these eggs into foster mothers. Offspring with the "transgene" integrated into the genome can be studied for biological activity of the injected DNA and its transcription or translation product (i.e., the protein encoded by the transgene). In order to generate gene "knockout" mice, in which a specific gene has to be deleted, a neomycin cassette is inserted between the promoter and the first exon, which results in a truncated expression, and absence of a functional gene product. If evaluation of specific toxicity to distinct proteins or genomic segments is indicated in tier three studies, either transgenic or knockout animals may constitute a valuable *in vivo* model.

SUMMARY

Toxicity to the immune system may arise from the direct action of toxic chemicals on components of the immune system. Compounds causing injury to lymphoid organs include glucocorticosteroids (stress hormones), halogenated aromatic hydrocarbons (e.g., TCDD and HCB), nonhalogenated (polycyclic) aromatic hydrocarbons, organotin compounds, heavy metals, immunosuppressive drugs (e.g., cyclosporin), and cytostatic agents. Also, ionizing and UVB radiation, as well as oxidant air pollutants, cause injury to components of the immune system. The morphologic response can be involution of lymphoid organs (the thymus being very susceptible to toxic injury), and also hyperplasia (e.g., HCB in rats) and neoplasia (e.g., nonhalogenated aromatic hydrocarbons). In lymphoid organs, the passenger (lymphoid) population generally is more susceptible to toxic damage than the stationary components. Toxicity also arises as the result of immunological reactions to the toxic chemical or dysregulation of immunological reactions by toxic insult. This response is classified as hypersensitivity or autoimmunity. In this type of toxicity, the target of toxicity can be found at multiple sites of the body, depending on the presence and specificity of the hypersensitivity or autoimmune reaction. Compounds giving this type of toxicity are, for example, certain drugs and heavy metals.

FURTHER READING

Burns-Naas, L.A., Meade, B.J., and Munson, A.E. (2001). Toxic responses of the immune system, Chapter 12. In *Cassarett and Doull's Toxicology: The Basic Science of Poisons* (Klaasen, C.D. ed.), 6th edn, pp. 419–470. McGraw-Hill, New York, NY.

Dean, J.H., Luster, M.I., Munson, A.E., and Amos, H. (eds) (1994). *Immunotoxicology and Immunopharmacology*, 2nd edn. Raven Press, New York, NY.

Dutton, R.W., Bradley, L.M., and Swain, S.L. (1998). T cell memory. *Annu. Rev. Immunol.*, 16, 201.

Environmental Health Perspectives Supplements (1999). "Linking Environmental Agents to Autoimmune Disease. *Environmental Health Perspective Supplement*. 102, Suppl. 5.

Golden, R.J., Noller, K.L., Titus-Ernstoff, L., Kaufman, R.H., Mittendorf, R., Stillman, R., and Reese, E.A. (1998). Environmental endocrine modulations and human health: An assessment of the biological evidence. *Crit. Rev. Toxicol.*, 28, 109–227.

Gopinath, C. (1996). Pathology of toxic effects on the immune system. *Inflamm. Res.*, 45, S74–S78.

Kuper, C.F., Haleman, J.H., Richter-Reichman, H.B., and Vos, J.G. (2000). Histopathological approaches to detect changes indicative of immunotoxicity. *Toxicol. Pathol.*, 26, 454–466.

Kuper, C.F., de Heer, E., Van Loveren, H., and Vos, J.G. (2002). Immune System, Chapter 39. In *Handbook of Toxicologic Pathology* (Haschek, W.M., and Rousseaux, C.G. eds), Vol. 2, pp. 585–646. Academic Press, San Diego, CA.

Kuper, C.F., Schuurman, H.J., Bopr-Kuijpers, M., and Bloksma, N. (2000). Predictive testing for pathogenic autoimmunity: The morphologic approach. *Toxicol. Lett*, 112–113, 433–442.

Lawrence, D.A. (1997). Toxicology of the Immune System. In *Comprehensive Toxicology*, Vol. 5. Pergamon Press, New York, NY.

Schuurman, H.J., de Weger, R.A., Van Loveren, H., Krajne-Franken, M.A.M., and Vos, J.G. (1990). Histopathological approaches. In *Principles and Practice of Immunotoxicology* (Turk, J., Nicklin, S., and Miller, K. eds). Blackwell Scientific, Oxford.

Society of Toxicologic Pathologists (2006). A monograph on histomorphologic evaluation of lymphoid organs. *Toxicologic Pathology*, 34(5), 409–696.

16

Hematopoietic System

INTRODUCTION

Toxic responses in humans and animals may involve the hematopoietic system directly or indirectly through injury to other body systems. Thus, examination of the blood and bone marrow is a standard procedure of dose-response studies utilizing laboratory species, as well as in human and animal clinical situations where systemic toxicities are the suspected cause of disease. Primary or direct effects on hematopoietic cells may occur as with myeloid hyperplasia in response to lithium; secondary or indirect effects may be due to toxic injury to a major organ system. In a similar manner, a direct toxic effect on erythropoiesis by heavy metals may result in anemia, whereas anoxia of various causes may have the indirect result of causing erythrocytosis. In all considerations of the hematopoietic system where perturbations of a toxic nature are suspected, it is important to consider blood and bone marrow in a product and precursor relationship,

in which they are examined together and interpreted in the light of changes occurring in blood and tissues.

Phylogeny

Phylogeny refers to the developmental history of a given species. The development of intracellular recognition systems is present in some single cell organisms, but specific antibody defenses associated with T- and B-lymphocyte differentiation are not found in invertebrates. Circulating cellular defenses are present in starfish and earthworms, which are able to form leukocytes in their coelemic cavities. The thymus is present in cartilaginous fish, including sharks and rays; these species also have blood granulocytes and mononuclear cells, and are capable of cell-mediated immunity. Fishes with bony skeletons have beginnings of bone marrow, whereas amphibians, reptiles, birds, and mammals have both a thymus and bone marrow. Thus, in development from primitive fishes to

491

mammals, the full range of immune and defensive cells, organs, and functions become present and active.

Ontogeny

Ontogeny refers to the development of the individual organism and, for this chapter, the development of the hematopoietic system within an individual of a given species. Hematopoietic development in mammals appears to mimic that of the chick embryo. In birds, transitory structures known as the blood islands form in the yolk sac and contain the primordial blood cells. With the development of the circulation, which links the blood islands to the circulatory system, blood cells populate parenchymal organs and migrate to marrow cavities as soon as these appear within the cartilaginous framework of fetal bones. It has been suggested that a separation of primordial blood cells from the rest of the embryo on the surface of the yolk sac is a means of separating these hematopoietic stem cells from the army of inductive cytokines operative in the developing embryo, which might induce inappropriate differentiation in stem cells of pluripotent potential. A major difference between birds and mammals is that hematopoiesis is concentrated in the liver of embryonic mammals, whereas in birds the blood islands of the yolk sac continue to be a source of blood cell production until much later in embryonic development.

In early postnatal development blood production becomes rapidly centered in bone marrow, but foci of hematopoiesis are still present in the liver of pigs at birth, and such foci persist in the spleen of mice and, to a lesser extent, rats, throughout life. In other mammals, hematopoiesis may return to the spleen under conditions of prolonged demand for increased cellular production.

STRUCTURE AND FUNCTION

Gross and Microscopic Anatomy

Hematopoiesis organs include the bone marrow, spleen, lymph nodes, and thymus. All of these tissues are characterized by an architecture in which there are very light stromal structures with delicate reticulin fibers arborizing on the surface of small vessels, and distributed sparsely in the intervening parenchyma. In addition, the vessels are thin-walled, permitting cellular egress from the bone marrow, and "homing" to specific sites in other areas of the body. (Figure 16.1A, B).

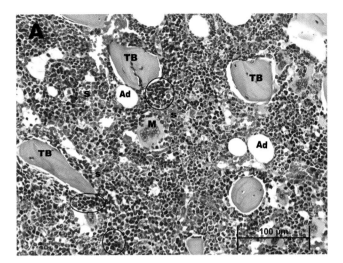

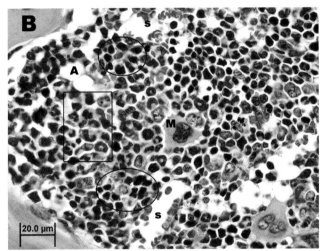

FIGURE 16.1 Normal bone marrow from the sternum of a mouse. (A) Low magnification image of marrow showing islands of erythropoiesis (ellipses and circle) among normal marrow adipose cells (Ad). A megakaryocyte (M) is present among the islands of erythropoiesis and myelopoiesis. Spicules of trabecular bone (TB) that support the marrow are also present. (B) High magnification image showing vascular sinusoids (s) near which are islands of erythropoiesis (ellipses). In these islands, the intensely basophilic erythroid precursor cells surround a paler eosinophilic nurse cell. Further away from the sinusoids are areas of myelopoiesis (rectangle) containing myeloid precursor cells that have more abundant more eosinophilic cytoplasm, and "cleaved" or reniform nuclei. Megakaryocytes (M) and adipose cells (A) are also present.

In the bone marrow, there is a confluence of small blood vessels on the endosteal surface of bones, which then permeates in a centripetal manner to the central venous sinus of the marrow. Under normal circumstances, most hematopoiesis occurs within 200 um of bone, or directly under the endosteal surface where this bone-to-marrow portal system appears to be most conducive to stem cell maintenance and proliferation. Erythropoiesis, for the most part, occurs adjacent to the sinusoids, where mature erythrocytes can be released directly into circulation. Erythroid precursors are clustered tightly around a modified macrophage (nurse cell) that provides the appropriate cytokines, as well as iron, to the maturing erythrocytic cells. Myelopoiesis, on the other hand, occurs closer to endosteal surfaces, where the appropriate cytokines are produced. Unlike erythropoiesis, myelopoiesis is not confined to "islands" of developing precursors. The compound venous drainage system of the marrow also provides the basis for marrow regeneration in fatty areas; hematopoietic tissue gradually thickens in depth if the need for additional cells continues. If the process of marrow hyperplasia persists for months or years, the reddening will increase in depth in a centripetal manner that will surround the residual bone marrow fat in a tubular cuff. It is important to note that these changes occur slowly, and visible evidence of hematopoietic regeneration on gross examination indicates that the process has been in effect for weeks or months.

In assessing marrow activity on gross examination, it must be remembered that the bone marrow cavity is a closed chamber with a constant volume from which the maturing cells constantly egress. If the marrow has been hyperplastic for some months and then is terminally depleted of cells, or if a normal marrow is severely damaged by a myelotoxic agent, the loss of volume from the interstitial areas of the bone marrow will be made up by dilation of the sinuses. Thus, a marrow that appears very red grossly may, on histological examination, turn out to be hypocellular as far as hematopoietic cells are concerned (Figure 16.2).

The spleen as a hematopoietic organ consists of a fibromuscular capsule enclosing a complex vascular system designed to act as a physical filter for foreign or infectious agents present in the blood. Athletic animals, including most predators, members of the dog and cat family, as well as horses, have a splenic capsule that is largely muscular, permitting contraction and infusion of additional blood into the circulation for periods of rapid pursuit or escape. In contrast, the splenic capsule of ruminants and most laboratory species is largely connective tissue; hence, the spleen may be distended over a period of time, but is not capable of large and rapid changes in volume. For spleens possessing either type of capsule, any prolonged enlargement with congestion of the filtering system will lead to proliferation of the supporting stroma that impedes subsequent contraction to a more normal state.

The spleen receives antigen only through the blood, and has no afferent lymphatics. The major arteries of the spleen arborize into small muscular arterioles, which are sheathed with a dense cuff of lymphocytes

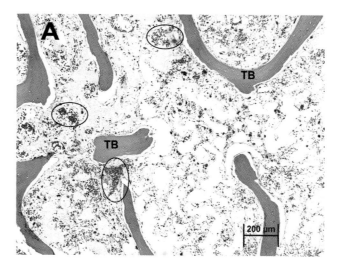

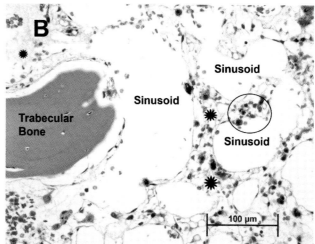

FIGURE 16.2 Bone marrow from a monkey exposed to ~700 Gy of ionizing radiation. (A) Low magnification image showing a virtual complete depletion of erythroid and myeloid precursors and stem cells, with dilation of sinusoids (ellipses) among the spicules of trabecular bone (TB). (B) High magnification image of depleted marrow showing the depleted hematopoietic regions (asterisks) and dilated sinusoids. Encircled is a remnant hematopoietic islet.

of which the immediate inner lining lymphocytes are of the T-cell type, with an outer sheath of bone-marrow-derived lymphocytes. Collectively, this complement of lymphocytes is known as the periarteriolar lymphoid sheath (PALS). Tertiary branches from these muscular arterioles deliver antigen to the dendritic cells of the splenic germinal centers. Other arterioles terminate in a multiple array of small or penicillary venules that deliver blood into the venous sinuses and filtering system. Under normal circumstances, most of the blood delivered to the spleen passes directly through and re-enters the blood vascular system without filtration, whereas about 3% of the blood enters the sinus-filtering system, where foreign material and aged cells are removed. Thus, the entire blood volume passes through the filtering system of the spleen at least once each day. Large macrophages attached to the fenestrated walls of the venous sinuses have highly folded or ruffled plasma membranes, this is ideally suited to the entrapment of aged blood cells. In the slow flow areas of the splenic red pulp, there is decreased blood glucose, pH, and cholesterol, all of which are hazardous to in-transit blood cells, particularly erythrocytes. Prolonged sojourn in a distended splenic filtering area with these chemical alterations results in a process known as "conditioning," whereby the red cells may be aged prematurely and withdrawn from the circulation by macrophages. The net result is increased red cell destruction, and a "splenic anemia" that may be without immune overtones.

Understanding the microscopic anatomy of the spleen assists the interpretation of gross morphology. For example, an acutely enlarged spleen removed from a freshly dead animal that underwent barbiturate anesthesia prior to death will continue to contract and exude blood during gross examination. However, a spleen that has been enlarged chronically, and has increased cellularity of the sinus areas, will maintain a relatively dry cut surface shortly after death. The splenic germinal centers may become grossly obvious in a B-cell lymphoma of the follicular type, whereas proliferative areas are focal, and may be confined to the areas of pervious germinal centers. They may also be visible in amyloidosis, which usually involves the spleen in a focal manner centered on

the germinal centers, giving rise to visible waxy foci, "sago spleen," on the cut surface of the fresh organ. Alternatively, in cachectic animals, the spleen may be very thin and relatively bloodless, with the interior of the spleen appearing relatively dry and fibrous on a cut surface. Extramedullary hematopoiesis is a common normal finding in the spleen of some species (e.g., the mouse), but less common in species such as rat or dog. In humans, extramedullary hematopoiesis ceases at birth, and only reappears in spleen (as well as the liver, lymph nodes and sometimes thymus, adrenal, and lung) if the bone marrow is producing insufficient red cell mass to meet the oxygen need of the body. In many species, an increase in the extramedullary hematopoiesis above background suggests inadequacy of the marrow (Figure 16.3).

Hematopoiesis

Superimposed on the supporting vascular structures there is a cascade of cells produced by the bone marrow that through trilineage differentiation produces the granulocytes, macrophages, platelets, and red cells that populate the hematopoietic organs and the blood vascular system (Figure 16.4). The stem cells themselves, which for many years remained a theoretical concept and a morphologic enigma, have been defined on a functional basis, first through the spleen colony technique in mice (colony-forming unit spleen (CFU-S), and colony-forming unit culture (CFU-C). Stem cells are found most frequently in bone marrow in subendosteal areas of red marrow, and circulate at low levels in the peripheral blood. They may be increased in the blood in conditions of hematopoietic stress, and are found at high levels in fetal circulation and in fetal umbilical cord blood. The differentiation of hematopoietic stem cells is dependent on: (1) their inherent genetic capability; and (2) environmental forces, consisting of succeeding stimuli from some two dozen cytokines that lead cellular proliferation through several irreversible branch points into a final pathway of differentiated product asP myeloid (granulocytic/monocytic), erythroid, megakaryocytic, or lymphoid lineages. The number of divisions that take place between a pluripotent stem cell and an identifiable hematopoietic precursor is unknown. However, for both myeloid and erythroid systems, a morphologically-identifiable stem cell goes through three generations of mitosis, and at least three levels of morphologic differentiation, to become either a neutrophil or a red blood cell. Some minor expansion of the proliferating compartments may be obtained in order to gain additional output from a single stem cell; however, this level of adaptation

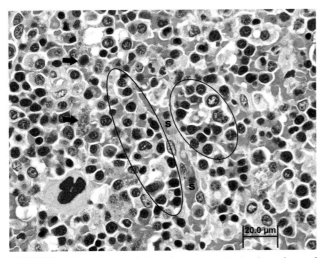

FIGURE 16.3 Extramedullary hematopoiesis in the spleen of a dog with prolonged blood loss secondary to hemolytic anemia. The hematopoietic tissue is less organized than that of the marrow. Areas of erythropoiesis are encircled. Arrows point to macrophages containing hemosiderin, the source of iron for the developing erythroid cells.

is small, and appears to be limited to about 10% of increased final product. Thus, it is apparent that an understanding of the kinetics of production and differentiation of the pluripotent cells, and their progeny, is the key to understanding responses of the hematopoietic system to various toxicoses.

Cellular Kinetics

In performing their functions, hematopoietic cells have markedly differing lifespans and fates. The production time of hematopoietic cells of mammals appears to be largely governed by the average cell cycle, or generation time, which appears to be about 24 hours for most cellular lineages that are in continuous proliferation. The most variability occurs in lymphocytes, which vary from cell populations with high proliferation and high death rates, such as occurs in germinal centers to long-lived memory cells, which may live for years. Myeloid and erythroid systems have three morphologically recognizable cellular

divisions, followed by three maturation stages to produce a mature neutrophil or red cell (Figure 16.4). Neutrophil production time is six days in the calf, with mature cells appearing in the blood after a further day or maturation. Production times are somewhat shorter in the cat and dog, and somewhat longer in humans. In almost all mammals, red cell production is complete within four days, which requires the cell cycle time of the erythroid precursors to be shorter than that of the myeloid series. Progeny of the neutrophil series are short-lived, with granulocytes replaced three to four times a day, representing a peripheral blood circulation time in the range of 6 to 8 hours. Granulocytes which exit the blood vascular system do not re-enter the circulation, but are utilized and removed *in situ*. The red cell lifespan varies remarkably in species—as short as 30 days in mice and chicken, 150 days in cattle and horses, close to 120 days in dogs and humans, 70 days in cats, and about 50 days in rats. Platelets have the same production time as red cells, with the first two days of

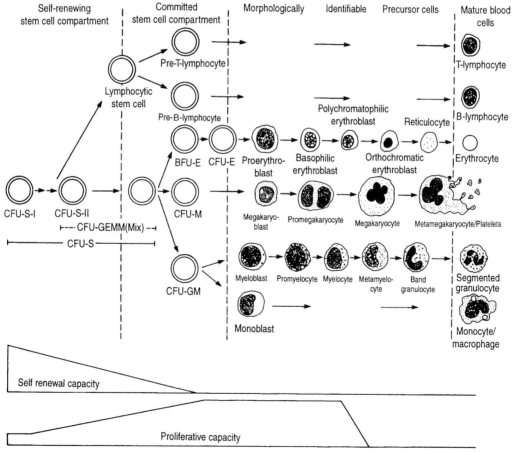

FIGURE 16.4   Schematic diagram of hematopoiesis, showing the relationship between proliferation and self-renewal in the stem cell and precursor cell compartments.

thrombopoiesis involved in a series of nuclear divisions to a level of 16 to 32N of ploidy, followed by two days of cytoplasmic maturation. The cytoplasmic volume tends to vary with the nuclear ploidy and with increased hormonal stimulation, higher levels of ploidy may occur, followed by an increased cytoplasmic volume. It is believed that platelet production is based on approximately 50 platelets per nuclear unit, with a peripheral lifespan of approximately 7–9 days in most of the larger species, and approximately 3–5 days in rabbit and rats, respectively.

All hematopoietic lineages are driven by a series of cytokines, of which erythropoietin and granulocyte or granulocyte/macrophage cytokines are in now being used clinically in humans, though rarely in animals. Similar systems drive the other cell lines, with some cytokines acting at the primitive levels and influencing the direction of differentiation, and others stimulating subsequent growth and development.

COMPARATIVE MECHANISMS OF TOXICITY (TABLES 16.1 AND 16.2)

Toxic effects on the hematopoietic system from pharmaceuticals or chemicals may occur from accidental or intentional overexposure, the latter invariably in preclinical safety assessment studies, or through idiosyncrasy. Accidental or occupational exposure may also occur with marketed compounds. Bone marrow toxicity (myelotoxicity), or toxicity of lymphoid organs, may result from the direct action of a drug or chemical on hematopoietic tissues (e.g., oncolytic agents), or it may require bioactivation of the agent in the liver, as in the case of cyclophosphamide.

Idiosyncratic Reactions

Idiosyncratic toxicity is characterized by a sudden, severe decrease in circulating blood cells, and may rarely also involve the marrow. An idiosyncratic reaction usually affects one or two animals in a study or population, and occurs most often in dogs. It involves neutrophils, erythrocytes, or platelets, singly or in combination, with one cell type often being much more affected than other cell types in an affected individual. The phenomenon is named for the cell that is most affected (e.g., idiosyncratic neutropenia, or idiosyncratic thrombocytopenia); if red cells are affected the syndrome would be referred to as idiosyncratic hemolytic anemia. Idiosyncratic cytopenias have many of the characteristics of an immune-mediated

process, such as rapid clearance or premature removal of affected cells from the circulation, rapid recovery when the drug is withdrawn, shortening of induction time upon re-exposure to the drug and, in many instances, reinduction of the cytopenia with a lower dose than the inciting dose. The formation of drug-dependent antibodies and/or immune complexes has been implicated in the pathogenesis of these cytopenias, and induction of a neoantigen by the interaction of the drug with the cell membrane of the affected cell has also been postulated as causal. Nonimmune etiologies (e.g., reactive metabolites) have also been proposed.

In idiosyncratic, drug-induced anemia the onset is abrupt, and frequently the hematocrit plunges precipitously. In the dog, for example, if the hematocrit declines by half or more than half in 30 days or less and there is no evidence of hemorrhage, hemolytic anemia is present because the normal 120-day lifespan of the erythrocyte in the dog has been reduced to one quarter of what is normal. If the dog in question is the only one affected, or is one of a few dogs affected in a study or group, then the hemolytic anemia is idiosyncratic, and likely immune-mediated. Spherocytosis and agglutination may be observed on peripheral blood smears if the blood sample is obtained when cells are being removed from the circulation rapidly. The reticulocyte count is normal to increased, and the direct antiglobulin test may be positive. Erythropoiesis is normal or increased in bone marrow if time sufficient for a regenerative response (i.e., 4–7 days) has elapsed. Erythrophagocytosis may also be prominent. The absence of one or more of these laboratory features does not preclude the diagnosis of idiosyncratic immune-mediated anemia, especially if erythropoiesis is normal or increased in the marrow.

The characteristics of idiosyncratic neutropenia are similar. A single or occasional dog is affected, a graded dose-response is absent, neutrophil counts are decreased markedly, a neutrophil "left shift" is not present unless infection supervenes, and the bone marrow is normo- or hypercellular at the nadir of the neutropenia. Also, neutrophil counts return to normal rapidly following cessation of drug treatment, and there is no decrease in CFU-GM (granulocyte macrophage) cloning activity in bone marrow cell cultures, indicating intact neutrophil stem cell proliferative capacity. Laboratory evidence for the immune-mediated destruction of neutrophils is difficult to provide. Ideally, specific laboratory confirmation requires the demonstration of either a drug-dependent antineutrophil antibody test, or a similar drug-dependent test for immune complexes. Such tests are available, but they are technically complex and frequently provide

TABLE 16.1 Mechanisms of toxicity to blood and bone marrow with selected examples

Mechanism Circulating cells	Xenobiotic
Erythrocytes	
• Oxidative hemolysis	
• Methemoglobinemia (oxidation of heme iron)	Aliphatic esters of nitrous acid (N-hydroxylamines), aliphatic esters of nitric acid (glyceryl trinitrate), amyl and butyl nitrite, local anesthetics (e.g., lidocaine), nitrate-contaminated water, nitrite, nitroaromatics (nitrobenzene, phenylhydroxylamine, dinitrotoluene), plants (Brassicaceae, capeweed, pigweed, sorghums, Tribulus, variegated thistle), potassium chlorate
• Sulfhemoglobin, with or without Heinz body formation	Acetaminophen, aniline, chlorate salts, hydroxylamine, dimethyl disulfide, methylene blue (in G-6-PD deficient individuals), naphthalene, nitrobenzenes, phenols, primaquine, sulfites, sulfonamides
• Membrane damage	Acetaminophen, arsine, copper, dapsone, primaquine, ribavirin, snake venom (vipers)
• Metabolic antagonist or mechanism unknown	Aminopterin, lead
• Immune-mediated damage	Cephalosporins, α-methyldopa, penicillins, phenacetin, quinidine, sulfonamides
• Act as hapten	Penicillin
• Alter membrane antigenicity	Quinidine, quinine, sulfonamides
• Trigger true autoimmunity	α-Methyldopa
Leukocytes	
• Altered granulocyte adherence and motility	Colchicine, dextran, ethanol, glucocorticoids, iron oxide, rifampicin
• Oxidant damage	Clozapine
• Immune-mediated	Aminopyrine, ampicillin, clozapine, dicloxacillin, gold, levamisole, lidocaine, phenothiazine, phenytoin, procainamide, quinidine
• Unknown or undefined	Allopurinol, flurazepam, opiates, phenothiazine, radiocontrast agents (e.g., iohexal and ioxaglate), rifampicin
Platelets and coagulation factors	
• Immune-mediated thrombocytopenia	Estrogen, halothane, heparin, local anesthetics (lidocaine, procainamide), penicillins, phenothiazine, quinidine, quinine, sulfonamides, xanthine diuretics (caffeine, theophylline)
• Altered function	
• Unknown or undefined	Ristocetin (agglutination), heparin (transient thrombocytopenia), myelosuppressive agents (cytosine arabinoside, busulfan)
• Inhibition of prostaglandin synthesis	NSAIDs
• Blockage of membrane receptors	β-lactam containing antibiotics (e.g., penicillin, ampicillin, cephalosporins)
• Blockage of calcium channels	β-blocker cardiac drugs (e.g., propranolol)

(Continued)

TABLE 16.1   (*Continued*)

Mechanism Circulating cells	Xenobiotic
Bone marrow cells	
• Damage to resting and proliferating stem cells (i.e., phase-specific agents)	Busulfan, nitrosoureas
• Damage to proliferating stem cells	Cyclophosphamide
• Altered stem cell regulation	Benzene, busulfan, ionizing radiation
• Damage to proliferating cells of any type (i.e., cycle-specific agents)	Benzene, bichloroethylamines, chlorambucil, melphalan, nitrogen mustards
• Interference with microtubule assembly (G2/M arrest)	Benzene, colchicine, methotrexate, *vinca* alkaloids
• Interference with RNA or DNA synthesis	Cytosine arabinoside, methotrexate (folate antagonist), 6-mercaptopurine and 5-fluororacil (inhibitors of purine or pyrimidine synthesis)
• Interference with thiamine-dependent reactions	Thiaminase (bracken fern)
• Unknown or undefined	Azathioprine, chloramphenicol, ptaquiloside (bracken fern toxin), isoniazid, phenytoin

TABLE 16.2   Selected examples of xenobiotics which cause lesions in hematopoietic tissues

Lesion/alteration Circulating cells	Xenobiotic/agent	Species commonly affected
Anemia		
Hemolytic (nonimmune-mediated)	Acetaminophen	Mainly cats, dogs
	Benzocaine/lidocaine	Mainly cats, dogs
	Methylene blue	Cats
	Propylene glycol	Cats
	Allium species: onions, leeks, garlic, chives	Cats, dogs, cattle, horses
	Potentiated sulfonamides	Dogs
	Copper	Sheep
	Cruciferous plants: rape, kale, turnip	Cattle, sheep, goats
	Phenothiazine	Horses
	Crude oil	Marine birds and reptiles
	Lead	All species
Hemolytic (immune-mediated)	Penicillin	dogs, horses
	Cephalosporins	dogs
	Sulfonamides	dogs and horses
	Propylthiouracil	cats
Hemorrhagic (not due to thrombocytopenia)	Warfarin and related compounds	Dogs, cats, horses, pigs
	Dicoumarol (moldy sweet clover)	Cattle, pigs
Granulocytopenia		
Thrombocytopenia	Acetaminophen	Cats
	Aspirin	Cats

(*Continued*)

TABLE 16.2 *(Continued)*

Lesion/alteration Circulating cells	Xenobiotic/agent	Species commonly affected
	Levamisole	Dogs
	Penicillin	Horses
	Sulfisoxazole	Dogs
Pancytopenia	See below	See below
Bone marrow		
Megaloblastic anemia	Methotrexate	Cats, dogs
	Phenytoin	Cats, dogs
	Potentiated Sulfonamides	Dogs, horses
	Lead	All species
Cytopenias		
Granulocytopenia	Furazolidine	Pigs
Thrombocytopenia	Bracken fern (thiaminase and/or ptaquiloside)	Cattle, sheep, pigs
	Penicillins	Horses
Aplastic anemia	Cephalosporins	Dogs
	Chloramphenicol	Cats
	Cyclophosphamide	Cats, dogs
	Estrogen	Cats, ferrets, dogs
	Ionizing radiation	All species
	Phenylbutazone	Dogs, horses (rarely)
	Ptaquiloside (bracken fern toxicity)	Cattle, sheep, pigs
	Potentiated sulfonamides	Dogs
Myelofibrosis	Cephalosporins	Dogs
	Colchicine	Dogs
	Estrogen	Dogs
	Ionizing radiation	Dogs
	Phenobarbital	Dogs
	Phenylbutazone	Dogs
	Phenytoin	Dogs
Myelodysplasia	Cephalosporin	Dogs
	Chloramphenicol	Dogs
	Vincristine	Dogs

false negative results. The demonstration of leukoagglutinin has also been considered as evidence for the immune-mediated destruction of neutrophils, but the test lacks specificity. Therefore, the diagnosis is generally made on the basis of the clinical and hematologic features described earlier.

Idiosyncratic thrombocytopenia also has similar characteristics: rapid decrease in platelet counts in a single or few treated animals, coupled with normal to increased thrombocytopoiesis in the bone marrow; normal CFU-Meg (megakaryocyte) cloning activity in *in vitro* cell culture; and rapid return of platelet counts to normal on the withdrawal of drug. Laboratory confirmation, utilizing the platelet-associated immunoglobulin test, gives inconsistent results. Idiosyncratic thrombocytopenia, which is compound-related, should be distinguished from pseudothrombocytopenia, a spurious finding that occurs when the EDTA anticoagulant exposes neoantigens on platelet membranes as blood samples cool in the laboratory prior to analysis.

Direct Damage

Direct damage by toxicants is most often manifested in the peripheral blood, where the cells are in direct contact with xenobiotics in the plasma. Bone marrow cells, in contrast, are somewhat more sequestered by supporting stromal cells and less prone to direct damage, even though they are much more sensitive to agents which affect cell cycle (see below). Red cells, being anucleate, have limited capacity for repair or regeneration; hence, when their antioxidant defense systems (e.g., glutathione, glutathione peroxidase, and glutathione reductase) are damaged or overwhelmed, their ability to compensate is virtually nil. Therefore, the list of agents that can damage red cells is much longer than that for leukocytes in general. Granulocytes, having cytoplasm well-stocked with organelles, are in a somewhat better position to resist damage, and high levels of antioxidant enzymes are protective while the cells are in circulation. Macrophages and lymphocytes tend to be the most resistant of all to the direct action of cytotoxic agents, although there are numerous agents that can significantly alter their functions in inflammation and immunity.

Damage to Erythrocytes

Oxidative Damage

Since red cells are basically large, membrane-bound containers of tetrameric hemoglobin, oxidative damage to hemoglobin is a prime mechanism of toxicity in red cells. Oxidation of Fe^{+2} to Fe^{+3} in the hemoglobin molecules results in the formation of methemoglobin, which imparts a brownish color to the molecule, and renders it incapable of carrying oxygen, as well as decreasing the affinity for oxygen of other hemoglobin molecules within the tetramer. Methemoglobin that forms as a byproduct of normal metabolism is normally maintained below 1% of total hemoglobin, but certain oxidizing agents (Table 16.1) can facilitate the oxidation of heme to metheme, and increase methemoglobin concentrations substantially. Methemoglobin levels of more than 20% are clinically relevant. In domestic animals, specifically grazing animals, high nitrite and nitrates in water supplies are prime causes of methemoglobinemia; however, plants such as those of the Brassicaceae family (mustards, kales, turnips, cabbages, etc.), sorghum, variegated thistle (Silybum), pigweed (Amaranthus), capeweed (Cryptostemma), and Tribulus, which contain variable but sometimes high concentrations of nitrate may also be causal. Cattle are more susceptible than sheep and horses. Potassium chlorate, a herbicide, can also cause methemoglobinemia in grazing animals that ingest contaminated plants.

A variety of therapeutic drugs and environmental chemicals have also been shown to induce methemoglobin formation, or have been associated with enhanced methemoglobin formation experimentally. These include aminobenzenes, nitrobenzenes, aniline dyes, amyl and butyl nitrate, potassium chlorate, and nitrotoluenes. Also implicated in humans have been amino ester local anesthetics (e.g., lidocaine), dapsone, primaquine, sulfonamides, silver nitrate, and nitroglycerine.

In addition to oxidation of iron at the heme core of hemoglobin, oxidative damage can occur to the protein (globin) part of the molecule itself. Oxidation of vital free (and exposed) cysteine residues to form disulfide linkages, leads to sulfhemoglobin, a denatured nonfunctional form of the parent molecule. Aggregation and precipitation of this denatured hemoglobin, often near the cell membrane, is the basis of Heinz body formation. Removal of Heinz bodies by the mononuclear phagocyte system in organs such as spleen can lead to abnormally-shaped erythrocytes named "bite cells" or "blister cells." Heinz body anemia secondary to oxidative damage to hemoglobin has been identified in domestic animals after ingestion of fava beans, rape and kale (cattle), red maple (Acer rubrum) by horses, consumption of onions (cattle, horses, and dogs) and treatment with phenothiazine or acetaminophen (cats).

Hemoglobin is not the only molecule prone to oxidative damage. Erythrocyte membranes are also prone to damage. Oxidative damage to the cell membrane often results in cross-linking of phospholipids and subsequent "stiffening" of the membrane, leading to decreased flexibility (needed to pass through narrow capillary beds), and enhanced fragility. Severe membrane damage may lead to impaired ability to maintain ion gradients, leading to swelling and even bursting of the damaged erythrocyte. Erythrocytes with damaged membranes may be removed by organs, such as the spleen, if damage is slowly evolving, or may lyse within the bloodstream if membrane damage is severe and fulminating. Copper is notoriously damaging to erythrocyte membranes, especially in sheep, which are extremely sensitive to damage by this element. Snake venom, especially from the viper group, also causes membrane damage, as do arsine (arsenic hydride), a byproduct of certain industrial processes, and the aniline-based drugs, dapsone and primaquine. Recently, the antiviral drug ribavirin has been shown to cause not only membrane damage, but also decreased Na^+-K^+ membrane pump function and methemoglobin formation.

Immune-mediated Reactions

The list of drugs that have been reported on a sporadic basis to produce immune-mediated hemolytic anemia is very long indeed, and these reactions can often be difficult, if not impossible, to distinguish clinically from idiosyncratic reactions. However, some classes of drugs seem to produce these reactions on a somewhat more consistent basis. Drugs associated most often with autoimmune hemolytic anemia in multiple species, including humans, dogs, and horses, include the penicillins, cephalosporins, and sulfonamides. Propylthiouracil-induced autoimmune hemolytic anemia occurs in cats being treated for hyperthyroidism, while phenacetin, quinidine, and α-methyldopa, among numerous others, have been reported to cause autoimmune hemolytic anemia in humans.

In general, there are three mechanisms that have been identified in drug-induced autoimmune hemolytic anemia. In the first type, seen with penicillin, the prototype for this class is the binding of the drug as a hapten to the surface of the erythrocyte; hence the antibodies bind only red cells to which drug has been bound. In the second type, typified by quinidine, the drug causes a change in the membrane itself, such that the erythrocyte membrane *per se* now becomes foreign to the immune system. The third type, in which α-methyldopa has been implicated, is induction of true autoimmunity against erythrocytes, resembling idiopathic autoimmune hemolytic anemia.

Damage to Leukocytes

Direct toxicity to leukocytes is typically associated with neutropenia, neutrophils being the most labile and easily depleted leukocyte type. Toxic neutropenia may be immune-mediated or nonimmune-mediated. Immune-mediated neutropenia is difficult to detect and to assess, due to inherent properties of the neutrophil itself, such as nonspecific binding of immunoglobulins and complement via F_c and C_3 receptors, respectively, and their tendency to adhere to one another *in vitro*.

As with autoimmune hemolytic anemia, numerous agents have been associated with, or linked to, impaired neutrophil function leading to neutropenia, but only a few have clear-cut and consistent associations. Among these are glucocorticoids in virtually all species, while the antipsychotic clozapine, opiates (especially heroin), radiocontrast agents (e.g., ioxaglate), aminopyrine, and zinc salts have been implicated in humans.

A large number of agents can alter neutrophil function. This may lead to premature neutrophil death and neutropenia; however, impairment of function is not often manifested morphologically in the blood, but rather at the tissue level where the effectiveness of the inflammatory reaction may be drastically affected. A wide variety of agents have been shown to alter adherence, mobility, and/or chemotaxis, for example, glucocorticoids, iron oxide, rifampicin, colchicine, and dextran, while drugs such as the antipsychotic clozapine appear to produce oxidant damage, resulting in premature death.

Damage to Platelets

As with erythrocytes and leukocytes, direct toxin-induced damage to platelets includes both immune-mediated and nonimmune-mediated mechanisms. In most cases, the ultimate effect is increased platelet consumption leading to thrombocytopenia. In immune-mediated thrombocytopenia, mechanisms of are similar to those for erythrocytes—hapten formation, modification of membrane constituents to make them immunogenic, or induction of true autoimmunity. In all three cases, opsonization by antibodies and/or complement leads to increased clearing of the coated platelets by fixed macrophages in spleen and other lymphoid organs. Compounds such as the sulfonamides, penicillins, quinidine, quinine, and a host of others can produce thrombocytopenia by such mechanisms. Immune complex disease leading to platelet aggregation and consumption via thrombosis can occur when antibodies form against the heparin–Platelet Factor 4 complexes in patients treated for prolonged periods with heparin.

A rather large number of drugs can affect platelet function directly, without the intervention of the immune system. Severity of platelet damage by these drugs is highly variable, and generally not only species-dependent, but also very dependent on individual susceptibility to the particular drug. Nonsteroidal anti-inflammatory drugs (NSAIDS) are perhaps the best known class of drugs to affect platelet function, exerting their effects by inhibiting prostaglandin synthesis, vital for proper platelet function. Other drugs, like many antibiotics, interfere with membrane receptors essential for activation, while still others interfere with Ca^{+2} flux necessary for platelet aggregation (e.g., calcium channel blockers). For many drugs, however, the mechanism of interference with function is unknown. Because they affect function, rather than impair production or induce destruction, chemical agents that alter function produce no visible alterations in platelet morphology or number. The impairment of function itself is often not clinically manifest unless a second underlying platelet defect (such as von Willebrand's disease) is also present.

Myelotoxicity

Bone marrow toxicity is most often manifested as suppression, the most frequent side-effect of many cancer chemotherapeutic agents. Rapidly-proliferating bone marrow cells demonstrate unique susceptibility to certain cytotoxic agents compared with their non-proliferating counterparts. Although many agents are selectively toxic to rapidly-dividing cell populations, there can be considerable variation in the response of proliferating precursor, progenitor, and stem cell populations to a toxic agent.

Some agents show specificity for stem cell populations that favor self-renewal. Potent alkylating agents, such as busulfan or the nitrosoureas, target resting pluripotent stem cells as well as proliferating cells, leading to severe and prolonged bone marrow damage with delayed recovery. Cyclophosphamide, by contrast, preferentially affects stem cells with low self-renewal potential and high proliferative activity.

Other alkylating agents, such as actinomycin D, classified as cycle-specific agents, target cycling cells in any phase. Bichloroethylamines, melphalan, chlorambucil, and nitrogen mustards are examples of compounds that are cycle-specific. These agents typically produce a dose-dependent bone marrow suppression that is often followed by protracted recovery.

Some compounds, such as colchicine, the vinca alkaloids, and methotrexate, target cells in a specific phase of the cell cycle, and produce a plateau type dose-response curve. Colchicine and the vinca alkaloids interfere with microtubule assembly and mitotic spindle formation, which results in an arrest at G2/M. Susceptibility, therefore, is confined to cells in late S and early G2 phase at the time of exposure. Since only a proportion of asynchronously-dividing marrow cells are in this part of the cycle at any given time, increasing the dose of a phase-specific cytotoxic agent beyond an effective threshold does not increase the number of affected cells.

For cycle- or phase-specific agents, the frequency and duration of exposure can be an important factor in determining toxicity, because altering the timing of exposure relative to cell cycle (e.g., varying the interval between doses) can lead to synchronization of the cell cycle, with subsequent alteration of the number of cells susceptible to toxicity at any one time. For example, a single therapeutic dose of cyclophosphamide can result in a transient depression in circulating leukocytes, whereas multiple dosing at two-week intervals may result in severe leukopenia, aplastic anemia, and death.

Benzene appears to share characteristics with both cycle-specific and phase-specific agents. It causes an arrest of cycling cells in G2/M. This arrest is seen as an initial increase, followed shortly by a decrease in bone marrow cell turnover, suggesting a defect in the maturation of precursor cells. Hydroquinone and its terminal oxidation product, p-benzoquinone, have been implicated as the benzene metabolites responsible for the effects of benzene on proliferating cells. These compounds arrest cycling cells in G2/M by inhibiting microtubule assembly, thereby interfering with sulfhydryl-dependent GTP binding to the

tubulin dimer. The effects of benzene are, however, not entirely restricted to cells in G2 or M phases of the cell cycle. At noncytotoxic concentrations, the quinone metabolites of benzene can inhibit the entry of resting cells into cycle, thus modulating the dose-response relationship between responding cells and proliferative stimuli. Direct effects on the cytoskeleton and interference with RNA synthesis have been hypothesized to explain these effects.

Nitrosourea-induced bone marrow toxicity has been reproduced in a wide variety of animal models; however, relative differences in species susceptibility to these compounds exist. Mice and cats appear to be particularly susceptible to the effects of nitrosourea compounds on bone marrow, whereas rats, guinea pigs, and sheep appear to be somewhat resistant.

Myelotoxicity involving the granulocyte cell lineage alone can occur, either as an antibody-mediated process, or as a cytotoxic effect often mediated by reactive metabolites. The administration of recombinant granulocyte colony stimulating factor (rG-CSF) or recombinant erythropoietin to a heterologous species, for example, may result in selective granulocytic or erythroid neutropenia or anemia in that species, due to the induction of a neutralizing antibody cross-reacting with the endogenous growth factor. Myelotoxicity due to an impaired maturation of megakaryocytes, neutrophil precursors, or erythroid precursors (ineffective hematopoiesis) may also occur. For example, in lead poisoning there is ineffective erythropoiesis and granulopoiesis, but anemia and leukopenia are uncommon.

Myelotoxicity may occur after exposure to a number of mycotoxins, usually ingested through the inclusion of moldy grain in human and animal feedstocks. While a variety of toxic effects may result with the different toxins, the trichothecenes have primary effects on the bone marrow, and may cause aplastic pancytopenia in both humans and animals, in particular horses and cattle, ingesting feed contaminated with the mold *Stachybotrys*, which produces the trichothecene toxins. The mechanism(s) for these effects is at this point undefined.

Ingestion of bracken fern is another example of a "naturally occurring" cause of aplastic cytopenia in cattle, sheep, and horses, although the effects can also be reproduced experimentally in rats. The mechanisms for the hematotoxicity are not yet firmly established, but to some extent are related to thiaminases in the plant that degrade thiamine, producing a thiamine deficiency. This deficiency produces pathological changes in other systems as well (e.g., the central nervous system), the exact manifestations being somewhat species-dependent; however, all suffer some degree of myelosuppression leading to pancytopenia. Recently, another toxic principle associated with the cancer-causing effects of bracken fern (ptaquiloside, a sesquiterpenoid), has been linked to the pancytopenia associated with toxicity. Ptaquiloside is an alkylating agent, and hence has effects similar to other alkylating agents known to cause myelosuppression and pancytopenia.

As with idiosyncratic reactions in general, there is a long list of drugs that have been implicated as causing myelosuppression and pancytopenia, mostly on a sporadic basis. Myelosuppression associated with azathioprine, isoniazid, and phenytoin have been reported more frequently than most others, however, suggesting something more than an idiosyncratic response. The mechanisms behind these particular drug-induced pancytopenias are not yet defined.

Occupational exposure to a wide variety of compounds may result in myelotoxicity related to a single cell lineage, or may cause panmyelosis. Recently-introduced substitutes for the chlorofluoro-carbons, 2-bromopropane and hydrochlorfluoro-carbons, resulted in pancytopenia with markedly hypoplastic marrow in exposed Korean plant workers. Associated toxicities involved both ovarian and testicular malfunction. Compounds developed for therapeutic use in humans and animals may have narrow safety margins, or may be recognizably toxic but used as treatments of last choice. The immunosuppressive agent, azathioprine, used to treat immune-mediated diseases, such as thrombocytopenia and hemolytic anemia, has been found itself to cause thrombocytopenia or pancytopenia in a number of cases. Similarly, carboplatin has been linked to thrombocytopenia and mild non-regenerative anemia.

Because myelotoxicity is usually a consequence of the effects of toxic doses of ionizing radiation or cytotoxic chemicals that typically affect rapidly-dividing cells generally, it is usually accompanied by lymphoid, gastrointestinal, and testicular toxicity. Therefore, it is incumbent on the toxicologic pathologist to examine these organ systems as well, to determine if the toxic effect is specifically hematopoietic in nature or more generalized in its effects.

RESPONSES OF HEMATOPOIETIC TISSUES TO TOXIC INJURY

Changes in Blood

General Considerations

Hematologic changes observed most frequently in toxicological studies are physiological responses of the bone marrow to changes/lesions elsewhere in the body. Common examples include chronic nephritis or pneumonia causing anemia or leukocytosis, respectively. In short-term (30 to 90 days) or long-term (90 days or longer) studies, the hematologic system is usually not affected in a primary manner. In these situations, the changes found in blood tend to be mild, and reflect part of a general pattern of injury to other body organ systems. Therefore, a consideration of the changes in all tissues is essential, to confirm primary effects on the bone marrow or other hematopoietic organs. However, specific and crucial information may be obtained from microscopic evaluation of blood smears, and from the results of complete blood cell counts.

Brown blood, for example, is compatible with methemoglobinemia and/or sulfhemoglobinemia, resulting from exposure to oxidizing agents. The brown color can be an indicator of oxidative injury to hemoglobin and/or red cell membrane proteins. "Eccentrocytes," "bite cells," and irregularly-condensed and densely-staining erythrocytes (pyknocytes) on blood smears also indicate oxidative injury to hemoglobin and/or red cell membranes. Heinz bodies, condensed inclusions composed mainly of damaged and precipitated hemoglobin, are not frequently seen in oxidative injury to erythrocytes in toxicity studies, however common they may be in certain clinical situations (e.g., Heinz body anemia secondary to acetaminophen toxicity in the cat). The finding of spherocytes (small, dark, round red cells) in the absence of poikilocytosis (irregular red cell shapes), on the other hand, is compatible with immune-mediated anemia. If both spherocytes and poikilocytosis are present, however, fragmentation hemolysis is present, indicating a different pathogenesis for the injury. Fragmentation hemolysis is frequently accompanied by an increase in Activated Partial Thromboplastin Time (APTT) and/or Prothrombin Time (PT), and a decreased platelet count, whereas in oxidative hemolysis APTT, PT, and platelet counts are normal.

Dose-related neutropenia, lymphopenia, and reticulocytopenia are characteristic of bone marrow toxicity from cancer chemotherapeutic agents, whereas neutropenia and/or thrombocytopenia or anemia in a single individual is more suggestive of idiosyncratic cytopenia. Dose-related decreases in fibrinogen or platelets are associated with the administration of thrombolytics or antiplatelet agents, respectively, but decreases in both may occur with thrombolytics, with the decrease in fibrinogen proportionately greater than that of the platelet count. A rapid decline in hematocrit in the absence of overt hemorrhage is compatible with hemolytic anemia.

Specific Responses

Hemolytic Anemia

Acquired hemolytic anemia is among the most frequently reported drug reactions in humans, but is usually of minor severity. Decreased lifespan of circulating erythrocytes defines hemolytic anemias. This type of anemia can range from subtle red cell membrane changes resulting in premature removal from circulation, to life-threatening hemolysis.

Intravascular hemolysis is dramatic and often life-threatening, due to the sudden drop in hematocrit and oxygen-carrying capacity of the blood, as well as the release of cell contents. This type of hemolysis is typified by hemoglobinemia, hemoglobinuria, and hyperbilirubinemia. Signs of regeneration (i.e., reticulocytosis, see below) are often not present, due to the rapid progression of the condition to death. Intravascular hemolysis associated with toxicity is most often immune-mediated in origin, typically due to a type II reaction. Antibiotics, such as penicillin and cephalosporins, are notorious for inducing this type of anemia in domestic animals. Toxic agents may also induce intravascular hemolysis directly, the prototypical example being acute copper toxicity in sheep.

Extravascular hemolysis, on the other hand, is often less dramatic and more insidious in its presentation. As with intravascular hemolysis, this type of reaction can be immune-mediated, and is commonly induced by antibiotics, such as the penicillins, cephalosporins, and sulfonamides. These reactions may be type II in mechanism, with nonlytic fixation of complement, or type III in nature, with immune–complex formation and removal of the coated erythrocytes by the mononuclear phagocytic cells in the spleen, liver, and lymph nodes. Erythrocytes damaged directly by hematotoxic agents without assistance from the immune system are removed in a similar fashion by these cells. Since affected erythrocytes are not lysed within the vascular space, hemoglobinemia and hemoglobinuria are not observed, and hyperbilirubinemia is variable, depending on the rate of hemolysis. Hemolytic anemias that occur extravascularly are often accompanied by a regenerative response manifested by hyperplasia of the bone marrow and increased circulating reticulocytes, which may increase mean corpuscular volume (MCV), since reticulocytes are larger than mature erythrocytes. The peripheral blood smear may show morphologic evidence of erythrocyte destruction, including schistocytes and spherocytes, and occasionally Heinz bodies, depending on the pathogenesis of the anemia.

Splenomegaly is frequently encountered in chronic hemolytic anemias, because of sequestration of damaged erythrocytes by fixed macrophages within the red pulp. These cells can hypertrophy, and can become quite large and prominent and give the spleen a solid "meaty" appearance grossly. The presence of widespread and marked extramedullary hematopoiesis adds to this change. Extensive splenic extramedullary hematopoiesis occurs in species secondary to anemia, blood loss, or hypoxia (Figure 16.3). Numerous clusters of erythroid precursor cells may be found in the red pulp, along with hemosiderin-laden macrophages (siderophages). In severe cases, the entire red pulp may be occupied by erythroid precursors. The presence of basophilic and polychromatic erythroblasts can usually be discerned on routine histologic sections.

One other cause of anemia should perhaps be mentioned in association with toxicity, although its mechanism is not due to erythrocyte destruction but to loss of blood via hemorrhage. This type of anemia, which becomes regenerative if the animal survives, in the context of toxicologic pathology is typically the result of impaired hemostasis, leading to uncontrolled hemorrhage. This can be due to impairment of platelet production in the marrow, impaired platelet function by the action of the toxic agent, or by alterations in the function of coagulation factors. Agents altering platelet function are discussed below. Among the agents affecting hemostasis, the most commonly encountered in clinical settings include warfarin and related compounds (bromodiolone, brodifacoum, chlorofacinone, difacinone, pindone), dicoumarol (in moldy sweet clover hay), and coumarol; these are Vitamin K antagonists, and hence inhibit the action of clotting factors II, VII, IX, and X, leading to impaired hemostasis.

Cytopenias/Cytoses

A number of xenobiotics that alter granulocyte adherence are known to markedly alter the equilibrium between the circulating and marginated compartments of the leukocyte pool. Ethanol, colchicine, and epinephrine can rapidly increase the circulating granulocyte pool, by inducing demargination of mature granulocytes from the vascular endothelium. Histamine, iron oxide, and dextran produce an apparent granulocytopenia by increasing the size of the marginated pool.

Because of the short lifespan of the neutrophil in the circulation, neutropenia is usually the earliest detectable sign of myelotoxicity in the peripheral blood, occurring as early as 1–3 days, especially if high doses of alkylating agents are administered, and somewhat later (7–14 days) with lower doses of alkylating agents and with other agents. Anemia is not seen because of the long lifespan of the erythrocyte, but reticulocytopenia may be detected as early

TABLE 16.3 Summary of adverse marrow changes[a]

Conditions	Morphology of change		Kinetics of change	
	Marrow	Blood	Marrow	Blood
Myeloid hyperplasia	Synchronous myelopoiesis; increased M/E[b]	Normal or increased WBC, often with left shift	Increased stem cell input and granulocyte output	Lesion-related increase in granulocyte consumption
Myeloid metaplasia	Late asynchrony; increased M/E	Normal or increased WBC, often with left shift	Increased stem cell input and granulocyte output	No apparent target tissue or lesion
Myeloid hypoplasia	Late asynchrony; decreased M/E	Leukopenia; neutropenia; minimal left shift	Decreased stem cell input and granulocyte output	Shortened granulocyte $t_{1/2}$ due to tissue deficit
Dysmyelopoiesis	Early asynchrony; M/E variable	Normal or reduced WBC, minimal left shift	Adequate stem cell input with impaired maturation	Tissue deficit due to leukopenia and/or impaired migration
Megakaryocytic hyperplasia	Synchronous thrombopoiesis; hyperdiploidy	Usually thrombocytopenia with platelet immaturity	Increased stem cell input and platelet output	Shortened $t_{1/2}$ due to increased consumption
Megakaryocytic hypoplasia	Early asynchrony; hypodiploidy	Thrombocytopenia; small pale platelets without immaturity	Decreased stem cell input and platelet output	Normal or shortened platelet $t_{1/2}$ with reduced turnover
Dysthrombopoiesis	Normal or increased ploidy with reduced cytoplasmic volume and maturation	Variable level of small, pale and poorly granulated platelets	Adequate stem cell input with impaired maturation	Usually reduced platelet $t_{1/2}$ and turnover
Erythroid hyperplasia	Synchronous erythropoiesis; decreased M/E	Increased or decreased red cells with immaturity; anisocytosis	Increased stem cell input and red cell output	Normal red cell $t_{1/2}$ (hypoxic) or reduced (hemolysis); increased turnover
Erythroid hypoplasia	Late asynchrony; increased M/E	Normochromic normocytic anemia without immaturity	Decreased stem cell input and red cell output	Normal red cell $t_{1/2}$; reduced turnover
Dyserythropoiesis	Early asynchrony with binucleation, micronuclei, and late-stage mitoses	Normochromic normocytic anemia without immaturity	Adequate stem cell input with impaired maturation	Normal red cell $t_{1/2}$ reduced turnover

[a]The changes listed here may be caused by toxic, immune, or idiopathic mechanisms. Reprinted by permission from ILSI, Valli et al. (1990)
[b]Myeloid/erythroid ratio

as 2–3 days if automated counting techniques, with their high accuracy and precision, are used. However, decreases in reticulocytes need to be interpreted with caution, as they can occur nonspecifically, probably as a sequel to diminished erythropoiesis in inflammation. Because there is an overlap in values between decrease in reticulocyte counts due to cytotoxic agents or inflammation, additional data are needed to determine the predictive value of reticulocytopenia in the early detection of myelotoxicity associated with oncolytics and other cytoablative agents.

Thrombocytopenia occurs following increased destruction, consumption, aggregation, or sequestration of platelets. Xenobiotics can bind to platelets and act as haptens, or promote the binding of immune complexes to their surfaces by other means. Antibody binding to platelets can trigger direct complement-mediated lysis or sequestration and phagocytosis of platelets coated by C3 and immunoglobulin by cells of the mononuclear phagocyte system. Agents suspected to act directly on platelets include the antibiotic ristocetin, which induces agglutination, and heparin.

Changes in Bone Marrow (Table 16.3)

General Considerations

In interpreting bone marrow responses, a number of factors need to be considered, including the proportions and density of cells from each of the trilineage patterns of differentiation. In histologic examination, normal bone marrow is generally about 50% fat and

50% hematopoietic tissue in cats, dogs, rabbits, and larger animals, while 70–80% hematopoietic tissue is more common in rats and mice (Figure 16.1). In young beagle dogs, the amount of hematopoietic tissue normally present in sternal bone marrow may approach that of rodents, whereas in femoral bone marrow the amount of hematopoietic tissue is highly variable and can range from 20–80%. In marrow functioning under homeostatic conditions, there is tight packing of the differentiating cells in hematopoietic areas, with deviation from the norm indicating a rapid exit of cells of particular lineage from the marrow, or reduction in overall production (Figure 16.2). Because blood cells are produced in a pipeline fashion, any recent changes in the health of the animal must be considered in interpreting bone marrow cellularity. In most species, for cells in continuous proliferation, the cell cycle takes about 24 hours, which dictates that the proliferating cascade of three to four divisions will take at least that many days for blood cells to reach a functional stage for release into the peripheral blood. Marrow assessment should also consider the myeloid:erythroid (M:E) ratio, which generally has a mild myeloid predominance in most species. They should also consider the proportions of cells of each lineage in proliferation and maturation phases. In the early stages of marrow hyperplasia, there may be increased proportions of proliferative phase cells, but if the stimulus for increased production persists, there will be an expansion of marrow, with the proportions of proliferation to maturation phase cells returning to normal while maintaining peripheral blood leukocytosis (myeloid hyperplasia) (Figure 16.5).

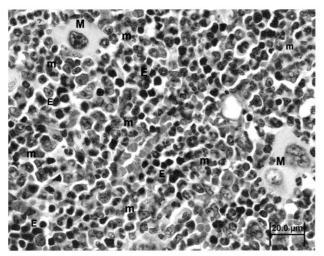

FIGURE 16.5   Sternal bone marrow from a mouse with myeloid hyperplasia, showing extensive areas of myelopoiesis (m). Islands of erythropoiesis (E) are still present, but decreased in number relative to areas of myelopoiesis. Megakaryocytes (M) are also present.

In normal mammals with bone marrow production and release under steady state conditions, the proportion of proliferating-to-maturing marrow cells remains close to a 1:4 ratio. The kinetic basis for this relationship has been determined by the autoradiographic labeling of bone marrow cells in a number of species, including humans. The stage in the process of pipeline cell development of proliferating and maturing cells can be determined, because they both pass through a series of morphologic changes. In this manner, the output of a single committed stem cell in the myeloid series produces 1 myeloblast, 2 promyelocytes, 4 myelocytes, and 8 metamyelocytes. These 8 metamyelocytes then mature to 8 band neutrophils, and 8 segmented neutrophils. There are some additional divisions, likely at the myelocyte stage, which occur to produce about 10 rather than 8 maturing cells. Collectively, a myeloblast plus 2 promyelocytes and 4 myelocytes constitute 7 proliferative phase cells. With second divisions of some myelocytes, the 10 progeny of 10 each of metamyelocytes, band, and segmented neutrophils constitute a marrow granulocyte reserve of 30 cells. These 7 proliferative phase cells, plus the 30 maturation phase cells, constitute the typical 1:4 relationship of normal marrow in synchronous proliferation and maturation. A similar system is present in the erythroid series, where 1 erythroblast produces 2 prorubricytes and 4 basophilic rubrictyes. The maturing progeny of this 1 erythroblast constitutes 8 to 10 polychromatic, normochromic, and metarubricytes, with a similar proportion of proliferating to maturing cells as for the myeloid system. For convenience, the maturation index, as calculated in Table 16.2, is expressed as a fraction in which the numerator and the denominator are the sum of the proliferating and maturing cells, respectively (e.g., $8/30 = 0.23$). This index in rats studied at four months, one year, and in pregnancy, is remarkably consistent, with maturation indices varying from 0.21 to 0.30. If good marrow aspirates are obtained, and the smears are prepared so that marrow cells can be counted differentially with a minimum of peripheral blood dilution, the maturation index constitutes a sensitive yardstick for detecting deviations from normal marrow proliferation and maturation.

Deviations from normal in the synchrony of cellular maturation are one of the most important clues to toxic effects on bone marrow. Well-defined deviations from normal maturation occur in iron deficiency anemia, where there is late asynchrony due to an increased proportion of late stage rubriblasts that are delayed in release from the marrow, due to an insufficient level of cytoplasmic hemoglobin saturation. In contrast, in megaloblastic anemia associated with a deficiency of vitamin B12 and folic acid, there is early asynchrony of all cell lines, with increased numbers of proliferative phase cells, which have larger nuclei due to delays in mitoses as a result of impaired nucleotide synthesis for DNA production and mitosis. The resulting progeny are, therefore, deficient in numbers but larger in both nuclear size and cytoplasmic volume, due to skipped divisions. These types of changes may occur in dyshematopoiesis of a variety of causes, including toxic inhibition of cellular maturation. In contrast, agents such as cell-cycle-dependent chemotherapeutic drugs will impair stem cell production and differentiation, resulting in rapid and trilineage marrow hypoplasia (Figure 16.2). In most circumstances, careful examination of marrow histology and cytology must be made to determine if there is an altered pattern of cellular maturation, which would in turn justify differential counts of bone marrow cells to better define the nature of the hematopoietic defect. This approach has led to the development of tabular data on bone marrow to define a proliferative or maturation effect more specifically. A tabular summary of adverse marrow changes is presented in Table 16.1.

Dysplastic changes can be detected morphologically in all three lineages. Changes associated with dysmyelopoiesis include the presence of an increase in proliferative phase cell plus numerous metamyelocytes with "donut" shaped nuclei. Morphologic characteristics of dyserythropoiesis include the presence of late stage binucleated rubricytes with marked variation in nuclear size, micronuclei, or budding projections from the nuclei of early stage rubricytes. In the megakaryocyte system, assessment of dysplastic changes is more challenging. The earliest stage of megakaryocytic production can be recognized as binucleated cells that otherwise have the characteristics of an erythroblast. These cells then go through a period of symmetrical nuclear multiplication to 2, 4, and 16 nuclei over the first two days of growth, followed by the fusion of nuclei, and a further two days in which cytoplasm increases rapidly in volume and in granulation and decreases in basophilia. Increased hormonal pressure (thrombopoietin) on megakaryocyte production results in the differentiation of an increased number of blast cells for this series, as well as increased numbers of nuclear divisions to hyperploidy in the range of 64N. Synchronous maturation in this series constitutes an increase in cytoplasmic volume in proportion to the nuclear ploidy. Dysplastic changes can be detected in the process of thrombopoiesis by morphologic changes, including failure of nuclear aggregation and fusion, insufficient cytoplasmic volume for the size of the nucleus, and insufficient cytoplasmic development with deficient granulation and pyknosis of the nucleus. The result is death of the cell before there is completion of cytoplasmic maturation and release of platelets. Under these circumstances, the presence of increased numbers of megakaryocytes may be associated with ineffective thrombopoiesis and reduced numbers of platelets in the peripheral blood. This may reduce the normal peripheral blood lifespan.

Specific Responses Resulting from Marrow Suppression

A huge number of examples can be given that result in the specific responses discussed briefly below. The literature in humans, and to a lesser degree experimentally in rodents and other laboratory species, is vast. Clinically, however, the number of hematotoxic agents clearly associated with bone marrow suppression is much smaller. Table 16.3 is a partial list of responses to some better-known hematotoxic agents in domestic animals.

Megaloblastic Anemia

Erythrocytes are less susceptible than leukocytes to numerical alterations resulting from interference with hematopoiesis, since they have a long lifespan relative to leukocytes. Therefore, frank anemia is usually a late manifestation of bone marrow suppression, even though erythropoiesis *per se* may be more sensitive to chemical disruption than granulopoiesis. Bone-marrow suppression-related anemias rarely occur in the absence of accompanying cytopenia(s) and maturational or "megaloblastic" changes in circulating blood cells. Xenobiotics that interfere with RNA or DNA synthesis, or produce disturbances in cell division, frequently produce a megaloblastic anemia. Such agents include folate antagonists (methotrexate), inhibitors of purine or pyrimidine synthesis (6-mercaptopurine and 5-fluorouracil), and pentose sugar analogs, such as cytosine arabinoside. Lead can also cause anemia, but this anemia is typically microcytic in nature, and thought to be related to its inhibitory effects on the initial, rate-limiting step in heme synthesis. Either macrocytic or microcytic erythrocytes can be present in megaloblastic anemias that arise from bone marrow suppression. Distinctive morphologic changes can be seen as discussed above.

Cytopenias

Reductions in the number of circulating platelets, granulocytes, or lymphocytes are the most common manifestations of bone marrow suppression. Thrombocytopenias are the most frequent blood dyscrasias reported secondary to xenobiotic exposure.

A wide variety of drugs have been implicated in immunomediated thrombocytopenia in humans, including quinine and heparin, but animal models are not well-defined.

Thrombocytopenia, with or without leukopenia, is often encountered following exposure to myelosuppressive agents. Species differences exist in the outcome of toxicity. Cytosine arabinoside and busulfan are extremely effective in inducing experimental thrombocytopenia in a wide variety of species, but clinical reports are rare or nonexistent. On the other hand, cyclophosphamide administration to BDF1 mice has been reported to produce a marked depression in the number of bone marrow megakaryocytes and CFU-M, with only a slight decrease in blood platelets. In contrast, administration of a single low dose of vincristine to BALB/c mice has been reported to result in thrombocytosis without prior thrombocytopenia, whereas high doses of vinblastine, but not bleomycin, produce a transient thrombocytopenia in rats. Dogs appear to be sensitive to estrogen-induced thrombocytopenia, presumably mediated through decreased megakaryocytopoiesis, although an immunomediated mechanism has been suggested for diethylstilbestrol-induced thrombocytopenia in this species.

Granulocytopenia may be a useful indicator of myelotoxicity; however, fluctuations in granulocyte numbers frequently occur in experimental animals, independent of drug-induced bone marrow suppression. Nonspecific stresses or systemic chemical toxicity can transiently alter cell cycle kinetics in proliferating bone marrow populations, producing wide fluctuations in circulating granulocyte numbers. Rodents and rabbits are especially susceptible to stress-induced leukopenias.

Aplastic Anemia

Aplastic, or non-regenerative, anemia is a syndrome associated with bone marrow failure, characterized by anemia, pancytopenia, and varying degrees of bone marrow hypocellularity. It is distinguished from other diseases producing pancytopenia, such as leukemia, infiltrating malignancies, or myeloproliferative disease, by histologic examination of the bone marrow. Histologically, hematopoietic precursor cells may be almost totally replaced by fat, leaving a few mature hematopoietic cells interspersed throughout (Figure 16.2).

Aplastic anemia is classified as idiopathic or secondary, depending on whether its onset can be attributed to known causes, for example, ionizing radiation, drug, or chemical exposure. The syndrome carries a grave prognosis, because in the absence of successful bone marrow transplantation, approximately 40% of all affected humans die within six months of diagnosis. Aplastic anemias arising secondarily to chemotherapy or xenobiotic exposure carry an even more dismal prognosis.

Aplastic anemia is a disorder of stem cell regulation. Aplastic anemia has been suggested as a disorder of pluripotent stem cells which, either through exhaustion of numbers, or a defect in differentiation, are unable to recapitulate blood cells. Stromal cell defects may also play an important role in chronic bone marrow failure. In some of these cases there is evidence to support a clonal origin for aplastic anemia. Animal models of aplastic anemia are relatively few, and have been largely restricted to those induced by viruses, busulfan, irradiation, or benzene.

The bone marrow has long been recognized as particularly susceptible to radiation-induced aplastic anemia in many species, including dogs, monkeys (Figure 16.2), and mice. Dogs have been used as models for radiation-induced aplastic anemia, figuring prominently in models used for bone marrow transplantation. Radiation produces both transient and prolonged bone marrow suppression, depending on the dose, dose rate, and exposure conditions. Local irradiation of rats with 2000 rad results in a transient hypoplasia and recovery. This pattern of suppression followed by regeneration is also present in other species (Figure 16.6). Twice the dose results in a transient hypoplasia with a latent period, followed by a prolonged hypoplasia. Aplastic anemia resulting from either busulfan treatment or irradiation is characterized by a marked reduction in most proliferating cell populations in mice.

Clinically, phenylbutazone therapy in dogs and prolonged exposure to estrogen in cats, ferrets, and dogs, has been associated with severe suppression of all three cell lineages. Chemotherapeutic drugs, such as cyclophosphamide and other antimitotic, agents have a similar, if somewhat more sporadic association (i.e., affecting one, two or all three cell lineages, depending on species and individual susceptibilities) that in some cases is a direct toxic action, apparently idiosyncratic in other cases, and autoimmune in still others.

Myelofibrosis

Primary myelofibrosis is now classified as a myeloproliferative disease in humans; it is rarely reported in animals, usually in the dog. Secondary myelofibrosis, however, is more frequently reported, often as a result of marrow necrosis followed by replacement with fibrous connective tissue (i.e., "scar tissue"). This

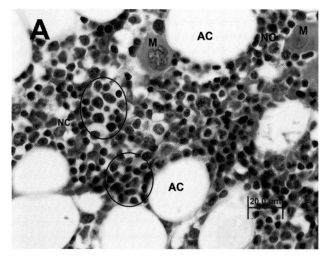

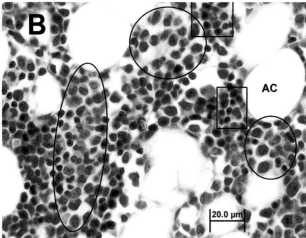

FIGURE 16.6 Generalized hyperplasia of bone marrow in a monkey recovering from ~700 Gy of ionizing radiation. (A) Section of hypercellular marrow with increased erythropoiesis, showing erythroid islets (encircled) with a predominance of intensely basophilic early erythroid forms. The expanded marrow has impinged on resident adipose cells (AC). Megakaryocytes (M) are also present with a predominance of intensely basophilic early erythroid forms and associated nurse cells (NC). (B) An area of enhanced myelopoiesis (enclosed by ellipses) with a predominance of eosinophilic early myeloid forms with large reniform or folded nuclei. An erythroid islet is enclosed within a rectangle.

reaction may become progressive, resulting in virtual total replacement of hematopoietic precursor cells with inactive fibrous tissue (Figure 16.7), probably as a result of interference with bone marrow blood supply. Hematologic findings vary considerably, depending on the species and the severity of the lesion; however, the spleen is usually enlarged and myeloid metaplasia is a predominant feature. Extramedullary hematopoiesis in other tissues, such as spleen, liver, and lung has been observed in association with this condition. Secondary myelofibrosis associated with drug or toxin exposure has been most frequently reported in

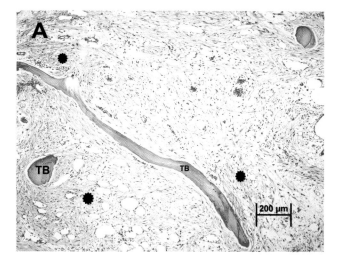

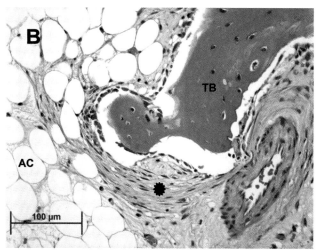

FIGURE 16.7 Myelofibrosis in the marrow of a dog with disseminated neoplasia. (A) Low magnification image illustrating the extensive replacement of hematopoietic tissue by loosely woven fibrous tissue * between trabecular bone (TB) spicules and remaining sinusoidal vasculature. (B) High magnification image illustrating the replacement of hematopoietic tissue by fusiform fibroblasts within a sparsely collagenous matrix (asterisks) near a spicule of trabecular bone (TB). Resident adipose cells (AC) are also present.

the dog, with drugs or toxins that frequently produce generalized myelosuppression (e.g., estrogen) being the most frequently implicated (Table 16.3).

Specific Responses Associated with Increased Proliferation (Clonal Hemopathies)

Myelodysplastic Syndromes

Leukemia, primarily acute myelogenous leukemia, is often preceded by a "preleukemic" or prodromal state of chronic bone marrow insufficiency. This phenomenon occurs with alarming frequency in leukemias arising secondarily to previous cancer therapy, and is termed myelodysplastic syndrome. Myelodysplastic syndrome can be manifested as either bone marrow insufficiency, or a proliferative disorder. Insufficiency is associated with varying degrees of anemia, usually accompanied by macrocytosis and leukopenia, or thrombocytopenia. Histologically, the bone marrow is usually hypocellular or, alternatively, an excessive proliferation of one or more cell lineages can be observed. The rate of progression from myelodysplastic syndrome to frank leukemia in humans appears to be particularly high in cases arising secondary to chemotherapy or benzene exposure. Studies using cytogenetic or biochemical markers to identify the clonal origins of abnormal cell populations have revealed that clonal abnormalities may be present for years prior to the clinical onset of leukemia. Myelodysplastic syndrome carries a grave prognosis with reported mortalities of 30–84%.

Leukemias

Leukemias are among the most widely-recognized and feared malignancies in humans. Derived from bone marrow, they are usually disseminated via the blood at some time during their development. In general, leukemias can arise as abnormal cell populations from any cell lineage, although there is some predisposition to one or more cell types, depending on the method of induction and the species or strain studied. Leukemias in humans that are associated with chemical or drug exposure are predominantly of the acute myeloid type. Although there are exceptions, leukemias consisting predominantly of immature or blast cells tend to proliferate rapidly and be aggressive, whereas those in which a more differentiated phenotype prevails tend to take a more protracted course. Reports that clearly link treatment with drugs to induction of leukemias of hematopoietic lineage in domestic animals are exceedingly rare, although myelodysplasias have been reported with somewhat more frequency (see above).

A common feature of hematologic malignancies in both experimental animals and humans is their clonal nature; that is, they are derived from a single cell. Lymphoid and myeloid stem cells are consistently involved as the targeted cell compartment in leukemias of lymphoid and myeloid origin. Leukemogenesis is a multifactorial process that cannot be modeled or simulated as a function of a uni- or bimolecular event. Therefore, it is not surprising that no initiation/promotion paradigms have been established for chemical leukemogenesis in experimental animals.

The distinction between lymphoma, a malignancy involving primarily the thymus, lymph nodes, or splenic white pulp, and leukemia, a malignancy involving primarily the bone marrow, spleen, or blood is often difficult or unwarranted. Mouse lymphoid neoplasms form space-occupying lesions, yet spread in a leukemoid manner, rendering the distinction difficult. Granulocytic neoplasms usually present as blood-borne neoplasms in most species, whereas they exhibit a significant tendency to spread as solid tumors in rodents. While these distinctions may be of little biological significance, they can be important considerations in the interpretation of tumor incidence data derived from animal studies in which different classification schemes are used.

HEMATOPOIETIC ASSESSMENT

Most toxicological studies involve terminal collection of blood and bone marrow, and in rodents these are usually the only collections performed. If the material under test is evaluated in dogs or primates, or is expected to have a primary effect on the hematopoietic system in any species, additional serial collections of blood are taken, but marrow is still collected terminally. In instances where idiosyncratic cytopenias have occurred unexpectedly, marrow core biopsies and/or aspirates are obtained to assist in profiling the cytopenia during the in-life phase of the study. Blood is preferably obtained from large veins, although other sites (e.g., retroorbital sinus, heart, abdominal aorta) may also be used. Using the retroorbital sinus site in the rat may result in a sample that is unsuitable for the critical assessment of erythrocyte morphology or the performance of coagulation screening assays, such as APTT, PT, and thrombin clotting time (TCT). Samples from this site are not ideal for platelet counts, because of the activation of hemostasis during specimen collection with subsequent platelet clumping and spurious reductions in platelet counts. In collecting and interpreting blood for hematologic examination, it is important to recognize that, under normal circumstances, peripheral blood leukocytes are in constant transit between margination and adherence to the endothelium of small blood vessels and detachment to enter axial flow. Thus, the true leukocyte cohort in the peripheral blood is approximately twice that which is apparent from the total leukocyte count. Neutrophils, being more adhesive than lymphocytes, tend to have a greater proportion of marginated cells. Stress, excitement, and problems with restraint during blood collection tend to cause increased numbers of leukocytes to enter axial flow, and result in increased leukocyte counts. In contrast, conditions of toxemia or hypotension will tend to increase the number of cells adhered to endothelium, and result in a leukocyte count lower than the actual number of cells in the peripheral circulation. Also, ethylenediaminetetraacetic acid (EDTA) can occasionally cause spurious decreases in total leukocyte counts by decreasing neutrophil counts. Stress, excitement, and restraint will also spuriously increase red blood cell counts in dogs, as a result of splenic contraction. Platelets may be spuriously decreased in dogs in an idiosyncratic fashion (pseudothrombocytopenia) by EDTA anticoagulant when the blood sample sits at room temperature. Similarly, autoagglutination of red cells on cooling will cause a spurious decrease in the red cell count, and a spurious increase in mean cell volume. Frank hemolysis, on the other hand, spuriously elevates mean corpuscular hemoglobin concentration.

Marrow is typically collected at necropsy for histopathologic assessment. It is best to perform the primary histopathological evaluation of marrow on a section from an axial site (e.g., sternum or rib), although both axial and peripheral marrow (e.g., femoral marrow) samples are usually collected and processed for examination. Of these sites, the sternum and rib are more physiologically relevant, since the axial marrow is hematopoietically active regardless of the age of the animal, making it more representative of the hematopoietic state of the animal. Although histopathologic assessment can give a good overall qualitative view of bone marrow changes, its sensitivity is somewhat limited, and substantial changes in cell populations on the order of 80% may have to occur before becoming noticeable histologically. Cytological preparations and techniques, such as flow cytometry, can increase sensitivity substantially although collection and preparation are more difficult, time-consuming, and expensive.

Marrow should be collected without delay at necropsy, and, if cytological assessment is also desired, smears made within two or three minutes of death (before clotting occurs). For cytologic smears, marrow can be obtained from the exposed surface of the cut sternum or rib, using a sable brush moistened with homologous serum to which EDTA has been added. To extrude the marrow from the rib or sternum, the cut bone is squeezed gently with pliers to cause a drop of marrow to well up. The tip of the brush is rolled gently into the exposed marrow, and several stripes of marrow are made on glass slides. Repeating the process with a cleaned brush after dipping it in additional homologous serum can be employed where additional slides are needed for special staining. Particularly where quantitative cytologic counts are to be made, it is preferable to prepare marrow cells in the trailing edge of a spreader slide as for blood films, or with a brush as just described, rather than the "crush technique" with marrow granules flattened between two glass slides. The spreader slide method provides a "granule trail" of cells where differential counts can be made, with a minimum of peripheral blood dilution. If marrow is to be examined by flow cytometry, this marrow should be collected into serum containing EDTA, as described below.

Flow cytometry can be used to differentiate between major hematopoietic populations in marrow, and to provide a bone marrow differential that is broadly similar to, but potentially more accurate and reproducible, than a microscopic differential count. The M:E ratio and maturation indices can also be calculated when utilizing this procedure. The procedure has been validated in the dog, and in the rat. The procedure for the rat, with appropriate modifications of sampling technique, can be used in primates and other species. Marrow is flushed from the femur, tibia, or both, with fetal bovine serum, and centrifuged to fat and debris. The resulting pellet of marrow cells is dispersed with gentle agitation, and resuspended in phosphate buffered saline (PBS), to give a total nucleated cell count, which on further dilution in PBS yields a nucleated cell count that gives an optional fluorochrome-to-cell ratio (determined during validation of the procedure) for flow cytometric analysis. Dilutions of the PBS/marrow cell suspensions are incubated with the dye 2′,7′-dichlorodihydrofluorescein diacetate, which detects peroxidase activity in granulocytes, or with rat-specific T- and B-lymphocyte antibodies. Then, by appropriate gating to exclude non-nucleated cells (mature erythrocytes and reticulocytes), nucleated marrow cells are resolved into early and late myeloid cells, early and late erythroid cells, lymphocytes, and megakaryocytes. Early and late myeloid cells correspond to the proliferating and maturing marrow pools, respectively. Early erythroid cells also correspond to proliferating pool cells (rubriblasts, prorubricytes, and larger rubrictyes); late erythroid cells correspond generally to maturing cells, but in addition to a preponderance of maturing cells (metarubricytes), the separated fraction also contains some proliferating cells (smaller rubrictyes). Nevertheless, flow cytometry provides a relative bone marrow differential, from which the absolute bone marrow differential is calculated by multiplying the percentages of the various cell types by the total nucleated cell count. Relating late myeloid or erythroid fractions to the corresponding early fractions results in a maturation index.

Hematological changes should also be interpreted in conjunction with standard reference ranges for various cell types, especially in dogs and primates. In addition, statistical analysis of data is necessary, statistical analysis being the most efficient way to detect trends and variability in hematology data, as well as providing the most effective means to identify differences among groups. It must be cautioned, however, that to achieve perspective on the toxicological relevance of compound-related changes, one must study reference ranges for the parameters in question. Reference ranges help in determining if a biologically significant toxicological change is present, and in assigning perspective to that change. In rodents, reference ranges are also useful, despite the fact that statistical analyses are more powerful in these species, because larger group sizes are typically used in studies.

For reference ranges to have maximum usefulness, each laboratory should derive its own set of reference ranges for the species studied commonly in that laboratory. Nonparametric statistics (percentile ranking of data) that make no assumptions about the distribution characteristics of the data being analyzed should be used whenever possible in deriving reference ranges. Only clinically healthy animals, stratified by age and sex, should be used, and animals administered vehicles or subjected to other confounding procedures should not be included in the general reference range population. For each parameter, 95% limits of the values should be included, unless the population is less than 50, in which case the upper and lower values define the limits. Outliers should be excluded by objective statistical testing, such as Dixon's range test.

SUMMARY

With all the sophistication in molecular and cellular biology, there is still a need for strong morphologic skills in interpreting changes in hematopoietic cells and tissues. It is important for professionals working in toxicology to be able to look at a blood film and recognize that a cell counting system is producing spurious results.

Nevertheless, it must be stated that the older concept of a marrow with tremendous reserves of cells ready to respond has not met the test of quantification. Instead of a huge reserve pool of cells in the marrow, it appears that marrow granulocyte reserves at least are no larger than the cohort normally present in the peripheral blood. Therefore, it is important that professionals learn to assess the subtle morphologic changes in blood that suggest that the hematopoietic system is under stress before cellular levels are above or below normal ranges. Furthermore, development of newer systems of blood analysis to detect and quantify subtle morphologic changes with increasing precision is needed.

FURTHER READING

Boggs, D.R., and Winklestein, A. (1981). The phagocytic system. In *White Cell Manual*, 4th edn, pp. 29–59. Davis, Philadelphia, PA.

Cronkite, E.P. (1985). The regulation and structure of hematopoiesis: Its application in toxicology. In *Toxicology of the Blood and Bone Marrow* (Irons, R.D. ed.), pp. 17–38. Raven Press, New York, NY.

Farr, S., and Dunn, R.T. (1999). Concise review: Gene expression applied to toxicology. *Toxicol. Res.*, 50, 1–9.

Lee, G.R. (199). Anemia: A diagnostic strategy. In *Wintrobe's Clinical Hematology* (Williams and Wilkins, eds), 10th edn, Vol. I, pp. 897–907. Baltimore, MD.

McGrath, J.P. (1993). Assessment of hemolytic and hemorrhagic anemias in preclinical safety studies. *Toxicol. Pathol.*, 21, 158–163.

Metcalf, D., and Moore, M.A.S. (1971). *Hematopoietic Cells*. North-Holland, Amsterdam, The Netherlands.

Perkins, S.L. (1999). Examination of blood and bone marrow. In *Wintrobe's Clinical Hematology* (Williams and Wilkins, eds), 10th edn, Vol. I, pp. 9–35. Baltimore, MD.

Pisciotta, A.V. (1990). Drug induced agranulocytosis: Peripheral destruction of polymorphonuclear leukocytes and their marrow precursors. *Blood Rev.*, 4, 236–237.

Ragan, H.S. (1999). Comparative hematology. In *Wintrobe's Clinical Hematology* (Williams and Wilkins, eds), 10th edn, Vol. II, pp. 2749–2763. Baltimore, MD.

Valli, V.E.O., and McGrath, J.P. (1997). Comparative leukocyte biology and toxicology. In *Comprehensive Toxicology* (Bloom, J.C. ed.), pp. 201–215. Pergamon, Elsevier Science, New York, NY.

Weiss, D.J., Blauvelt, M., Sykes, J., and McClenahan, D. (2000). Flow cytometric evaluation of canine bone marrow differential cell counts. *Vet. Clin. Pathol.*, 29, 97–104.

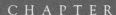

CHAPTER

17

Endocrine System

INTRODUCTION

A review of the literature of chemically-induced lesions of the endocrine organs indicates that the adrenal glands are most commonly affected, followed in descending order by the thyroid, pancreas, pituitary, and parathyroid glands.

ADRENAL CORTEX

Structure and Function

Gross and Microscopic Anatomy

In mammals, the adrenal or suprarenal glands are flattened bilobed organs located in close proximity to the kidneys. A midsagittal section of the adrenal glands

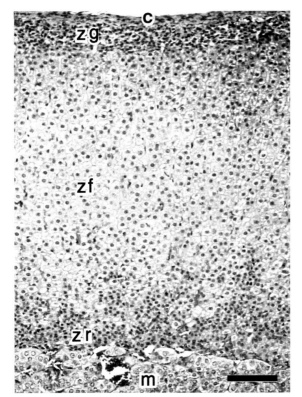

FIGURE 17.1   Adrenal cortex from a normal rat. The distinct capsule (c), zona glomerulosa (zg), zona fasciculata (zf), and zona reticularis (zr) are clearly distinguishable from the medulla (m). Bar: 100 μm. From Yarrington et al. (1985), Fundam Appl Toxicol 5:370 with permission.

reveals a clear separation between the cortex and the medulla. The cortex is firm and yellow, and occupies approximately two-thirds of the entire cross-sectional diameter of the organ. In contrast, the medulla is soft, and has a prominent gray-tan coloration. The ratio of cortex to medulla is approximately 2:1 in healthy animals. Defined zones, consisting of the *zona glomerulosa*, *zona fasciculata*, and *zona reticularis*, histologically characterize the cortex. These zones are not always clearly delineated, as illustrated in the normal rat adrenal cortex (Figure 17.1).

The mineralocorticoid-producing *zona glomerulosa* occupies 15% of the cortex, and contains cells aligned in a sigmoid pattern in relationship to the capsule. Loss of this zone, or the inability to secrete mineralocorticoids, e.g., aldosterone, may result in death due to the retention of excessive levels of potassium in association with an excessive loss of sodium chloride and water. The largest zone is the *zona fasciculata*. Cells in this zone occupy 70% of the cortex and are arranged in long anastomosing cords or columns, separated by small capillaries. They are responsible for the secretion of glucocorticoid hormones, e.g., corticosterone or cortisol, which promote the elevation of blood glucose, in addition to many other effects. The innermost portion of the cortex is the *zona reticularis*, occupying 15% of the cortex. This zone secretes minute quantities of adrenal sex hormones.

Physiological and Functional Considerations

All hormones produced by the adrenal cortex are steroids that are synthesized from cholesterol. Once in the circulation, the steroid hormones (e.g., cortisol or corticosterone) are bound to plasma proteins (e.g., transcortin, albumin). Under normal conditions, 10% of the glucocorticoids are in a free unbound state. The unbound steroid is free to interact with target cells, either to exert metabolic effects or to be transformed into an inactive metabolite. A complex shuttling of steroid intermediates between mitochondria and endoplasmic reticulum characterizes specific synthetic processes. Glucocorticoid hormones increase glucose production with a concomitant breakdown of proteins for purposes of gluconeogenesis, and also suppress inflammation in association with the attenuation of fibroplasia and immunological responses.

The common biosynthetic pathway from cholesterol is the formation of pregnenolone, the basic precursor for the three major groups of adrenal steroids (Figure 17.2). In the *zona fasciculata*, pregnenolone is first converted to progesterone by two microsomal enzymes. Three subsequent hydroxylation reactions occur resulting in cortisol, which is the major glucocorticoid in teleosts, hamsters, dogs, nonhuman primates, and humans. Corticosterone is produced in a manner similar to the production of cortisol. In the *zona glomerulosa*, on the other hand, pregnenolone is converted to aldosterone by a series of enzymatic reactions in the *zona glomerulosa*.

The adrenal cortex also produces small amounts of sex steroids, including progesterone, estrogens, and androgens. In the presence of liver disease, the turnover of steroid hormones, particularly cortisol, may be decreased, and can result in abnormal adrenal function tests in patients or animals without adrenal cortical lesions. Occasionally, peripheral tissues may activate steroid hormones, e.g., testosterone to dihydrotestosterone, or, as in the case of cortisol, convert the steroid to other less active forms of the hormone.

Mineralocorticoids, e.g., aldosterone, are the major steroids secreted from the *zona glomerulosa* under the control of the renin-angiotensin II system.

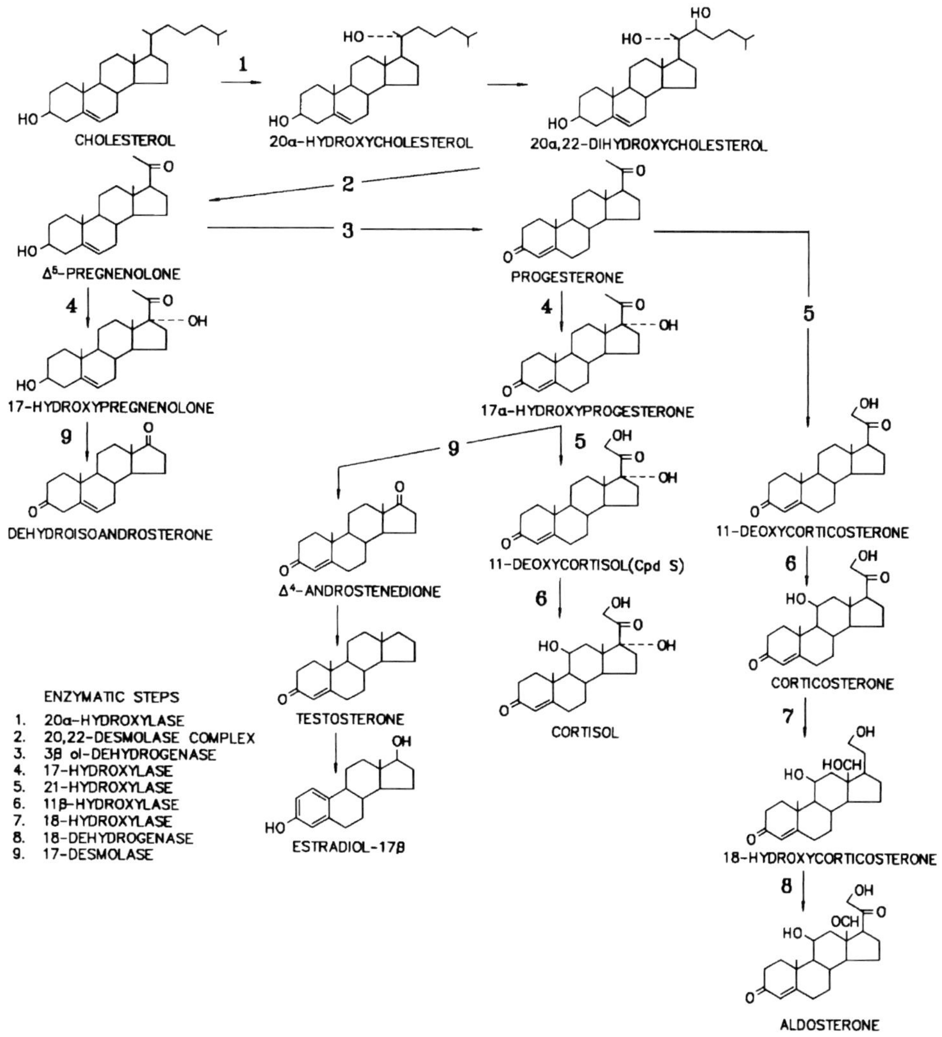

FIGURE 17.2 Adrenal steroid biosynthetic pathways. From Temple and Liddle (1970), Annu Rev Pharmacol 10:199–218 with permission.

Mineralocorticoids have their effects on ion transport by epithelial cells, particularly renal cells, resulting in the conservation of sodium chloride and water with loss of potassium. In the distal convoluted tubule of the mammalian nephron, a cation exchange exists that promotes the resorption of sodium from the glomerular filtrate and the secretion of potassium into the lumen under conditions of decreased blood flow or volume. The enzyme renin is released into the circulation at an increased rate by cells of the juxtaglomerular apparatus of the kidney, and is associated with potassium loading or sodium depletion. Renin in the peripheral circulation acts to cleave angiotensinogen to angiotensin I. By means of an angiotensin-converting enzyme (ACE), angiotensin I is subsequently hydrolyzed to angiotensin II, which

acts as a trophic hormone to stimulate the synthesis and secretion of aldosterone. Some of the angiotensin II undergoes further enzymatic modification to form angiotensin III. Angiotensin III appears to be nearly as active as angiotensin II in stimulating aldosterone secretion.

Adrenocorticotropin (ACTH) is the principal control for the production of glucocorticoids. ACTH release is largely controlled by the hypothalamus through the secretion of corticotropin-releasing hormone (CRH). An increase in ACTH production normally results in an increase in circulating levels of glucocorticoids, although it can also cause weak stimulation of aldosterone secretion. Negative feedback control normally occurs when the elevated blood levels of cortisol act on the hypothalamus, anterior pituitary, or both, to cause a suppression of ACTH secretion. In contrast to the normal negative feedback mechanism, abnormally high corticosteroid levels in the plasma above physiological levels causes marked ACTH suppression. If the suppression is prolonged, secretory cells in the *zonae fasciculata* and *reticularis* will undergo atrophy, with a corresponding decrease in the synthesis and secretion of corticosteroid hormones. However, when corticosteroid levels are subnormal, ACTH release from the pituitary gland is increased markedly, in an attempt to enhance hormonal output from the adrenal cortex.

Mechanisms of Toxicity

The *zonae reticularis* and *fasciculata* appear to be the principal target of xenobiotic chemicals. The adrenal cortex is predisposed to toxic effects due to adrenocortical cells storage of lipids, which enables lipophilic compounds to accumulate, and they have enzymes, including many enzymes of the cytochrome P450 family capable of the biotransformation of xenobiotic chemicals. Depending on the toxicant, the biotransformation may result in increased or decreased toxicity. Classes of chemicals known to be toxic for the adrenal cortex include short chain aliphatic compounds, lipidosis inducers, and amphiphilic compounds. These compounds frequently produce necrosis, particularly in the *zonae fasciculata* and *reticularis* (e.g., acrylonitrile, 3-aminopropionitrile, 3-bromopropionitrile, l-butanethiol, and 1,4-butanedithiol), and lipidosis (e.g., aminoglutethimide, amphenone, and anilines). Biologically-active cationic amphiphilic compounds, such as chloroquine, triparanol, and chlorphentermine, tend to produce a generalized phospholipidosis that primarily involves the *zonae reticularis* and *fasciculata.*

Hormones, particularly natural and synthetic steroids, also affect the adrenal cortex by causing functional inactivity and morphologic atrophy during prolonged exogenous use. However, other steroid hormones have been reported to cause proliferative lesions in the adrenal cortex of laboratory animals.

The final class of compounds represents a miscellaneous group of chemicals including o,p'-DDD and α-(1,4-dioxido-3-methylquinoxalin-2-yl)-N-methylnitrone (DMNM) that affect hydroxylation and other functions of the organelles mitochondrial and microsomal fractions. Many of the chemicals that cause morphologic changes in the adrenal glands can also affect adrenal cortical function (Table 17.1).

Chemically-induced changes in adrenal gland function result either from blockage of the effects of the adrenocorticoids at peripheral sites, or from inhibition of steroidogenesis. Most chemicals affecting adrenal function appear to do so by altering steroidogenesis.

Response to Injury

Disorders of Hyperfunction and Hypofunction

Spontaneous pathologic conditions, such as ACTH-secreting pituitary tumors or glucocorticoid hormone-producing adrenal cortical tumors, can give rise to changes in the functional status of the adrenal cortex. Primary hypoadrenocorticism (Addison's disease) is visualized as destruction of all three zones of cortical parenchyma of both adrenals. Secondary hypoadrenocorticism, with atrophy only of the *zonae fasciculata* and *reticularis*, is caused by destructive lesions or neoplasms in the pituitary, which result in a loss of ACTH production.

Chemicals can also produce functional alterations of the adrenal cortex. Prolonged use of exogenous glucocorticoids can mimic a syndrome of excess adrenal cortical function. Abrupt cessation of steroid use may cause a patient to develop secondary adrenal cortical insufficiency, because of the prolonged suppression of ACTH production and the subsequent trophic atrophy of cells in the adrenal cortex. The toxic effects of many chemicals result in primary adrenal cortical hypofunction, best characterized in the dog.

Exogenous glucocorticoid hormone therapy often mimics naturally-occurring cases of hypercortisolism, e.g., Cushing's syndrome. Clinical observations include polyuria, polydipsia, an enlarged pendulous abdomen, muscular wasting, alopecia and thinning of the skin with cutaneous pigmentation and mineralization, and hepatomegaly. Significant laboratory findings include an increase in alkaline phosphatase, an eosinopenia with marked lymphopenia, and leukocytosis due to the increased formation of neutrophils. Dogs with hypercortisolism infrequently develop significant alterations in serum concentrations of sodium, potassium, or chloride, in contrast to those electrolyte imbalances frequently seen in humans with Cushing's syndrome. Urinary and plasma levels of 17-hydroxycorticosteroids or metabolites are often increased modestly in resting nonstimulated patients. The use of stimulation and suppression tests, including evaluation of the cortisol response to exogenous ACTH and low- and high-dose administration of dexamethasone, is helpful in establishing a diagnosis and in determining whether the primary lesion is pituitary or in the adrenal cortex. During the prolonged use of exogenous glucocorticoids, ACTH administration results in an inadequate

TABLE 17.1 Examples of pharmacological inhibition of adrenal steroid biosynthesis, secretion, or function[a]

Compound	Steroid or conversion site inhibited	Mechanism of action
Aminoglutethimide	Cholesterol to pregnenolone	Competitive inhibition of 20 α-hydroxylase
o,p'-DDD	Cholesterol to pregnenolone; 11-deoxycortisol to cortisol	Partial 11 β-hydroxylase inhibition
DMNM	Cholesterol to pregnenolone?	Unknown
Triparanol	Desmosterol (24-dehydrocholesterol) to cholesterol	Inhibited reduction of 24, 25 bond
Cyanoketone	δ^5-3β-ol steroids to δ^4-3-oxo steroids	3β-Hydroxysteroid dehydrogenase inhibition
Trilostane	Δ^5-3β-ol steroids to Δ^4-3-oxo steroids	3β-Hydroxysteroid dehydrogenase inhibition
Su-9055	Cortisol; aldosterone	Inhibition of 17 α-hydroxylase; interference of oxidation at Cl8
Su-8000	Cortisol; aldosterone	Inhibition of 17 α-hydroxylase; interference of oxidation at Cl8
Metapyrone	11-Deoxycortisol to cortisol	Inhibition of 11 β-hydroxylase; inhibition of other hydroxylation reactions depending on species
SKF 12185	11-Deoxycortisol to cortisol	Inhibition of 11 β-hydroxylase
Carbon tetrachloride	Nonspecific inhibition	Inhibition of cytochrome P450 portion of microsomal enzymes 17α- and 21-hydroxylases
Cadmium	Nonspecific inhibition	Inhibition of NADPH-cytochrome P450 reductase portion of 21-hydroxylase; other microsomal as well as mitochondrial hydroxylases may also be affected
Amphenone	Nonspecific inhibition	Inhibition of 20α-, 11β-, 17α-, and 21-hydroxylases?
Cortexolone (11-deoxycortisol)	Competitive binding to glucocorticoid receptors	Diminished translocation of glucocorticoid-receptor complex to nucleus of target cell
R01–8307/heparinoids	Aldosterone	Inhibition of 18-oxidation
Spironolactone	Aldosterone	Competitive inhibition of peripheral receptor sites, resulting in sodium diuresis; possible direct effects on synthesis and secretion
Captopril	Aldosterone; inactivation of rennin–angiotensin system	Inhibition of angiotensin-converting enzyme
Triaryl phosphate	Cholesterol ester to cholesterol	Neutral cholesterol ester hydrolase inhibitor
PD 132301–2	Esterification of cholesterol	Inhibition of acyl-CoA; cholesterol acyltransferase
2, 3, 7, 8- Tetrachlorodibenzo-*p*-dioxin	Cholesterol side chain cleavage	Bioactivation via Cytochrome P450s

[a]From Yarrington (1983). Reprinted, in part, courtesy of Springer-Verlag

release and blunted increase in blood levels of cortisol. Additional findings include an abnormal electrocardiogram, with spiked T-waves and flattening of the P-wave. These electrocardiographic alterations appear to be due to the prominent increase in serum potassium in dogs with hypoadrenocorticism and subnormal secretion of aldosterone. Plasma and urinary 17-hydroxycorticosteroids are often at low levels in the resting state.

Effects during Embryogenesis

It is well-documented that synthetic and naturally-occurring corticosteroids are potent teratogens in laboratory animals, e.g., adrenal aplasia occurred in 8 of 81 and 1 of 13 white Danish rabbits when the dams were given thalidomide. Indirect effects of chemicals on the development and function of the fetal adrenal cortex are illustrated by the syndrome of prolonged gestation in sheep, due to the consumption of the plants *Veratrum californicum* or *Salsola tuberculata*. *V. californicum* may also produce giant fetuses that have cyclopian deformities. Common to both plant toxicities is the presence of hypoplastic adrenal cortices in the affected fetuses. The pituitary, although developed, lacks the normal neural and vascular connections with the hypothalamus, due to extensive central nervous system malformations. The hypoplastic fetal adrenal cortices fail to induce the 17α-hydroxylase in the placenta that is necessary to synthesize increased estrogens near term in preparation for partuition.

In *S. tuberculata* intoxication, the pituitary is small with a lack of normal granulation of the trophic hormone-secreting cells of the adenohypophysis. In both plant toxicities there is a loss of functional activity of the hypothalamic–pituitary–adrenal cortical axis that is necessary for the normal induction of parturition in the ewe. It has been suggested that the plant *S. tuberculata* contains chemicals that inhibit fetal hypothalamic-releasing hormones.

Morphologic Alterations

Macroscopic lesions of chemically-affected adrenal glands are characterized by enlargement or reduction in size that is often bilateral, such as seen in medullary hyperplasia or pheochromocytoma or atrophy. Midsagittal longitudinal sections of the glands will reveal a disproportionately wider cortex relative to the medulla or *vice versa*, resulting in an abnormal cortical:medullary ratio.

Nodular lesions that distort and enlarge one or both glands suggest that a neoplasm is present in the cortex. A single well-demarcated nodular lesion suggests an adenoma, whereas widespread incorporation of the entire gland by a proliferative mass is suggestive of carcinoma, especially if there is evidence of local invasion into periadrenal connective tissues, or into adjacent blood vessels and the kidney.

Non-neoplastic Lesions

Histologically, non-neoplastic lesions of the adrenal cortex induced by chemical agents are characterized by changes ranging from acute progressive degenerative

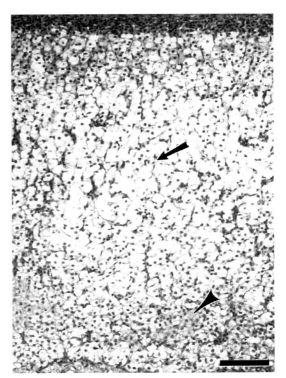

FIGURE 17.3 Vacuolar (arrow) and granular (arrowhead) degeneration in the adrenal cortex of a rat treated with 100 mg/kg/day of DMNM for 31 days. Bar: 100 μm. From Yarrington et al. (1985), Fundam Appl Toxicol 5:370 with permission.

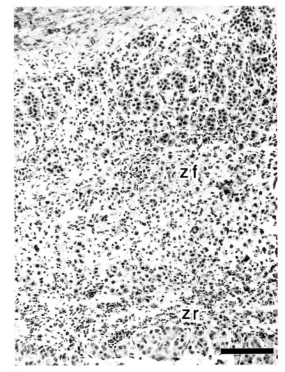

FIGURE 17.4 Necrosis of the zona fasciculate (zf) of the zona reticularis (zr) in the adrenal cortex of a monkey given 75 mg/kg/day of a hematinic compound (MDL 80,478). Bar: 1 μm. From Yarrington et al. (1985), Fundam Appl Toxicol 5:370 with permission.

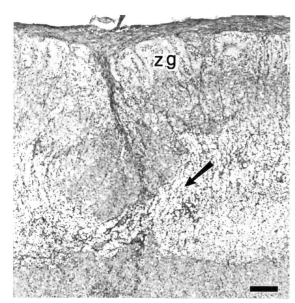

FIGURE 17.5 Hypertrophy of the zona glomerulosa (zg) and vacuolar degeneration of the remainder of the cortex (arrow) in a dog given 75 mg/kg/day of MDL 80,478. Bar: 100 µm. From Yarrington et al. (1985), Fundam Appl Toxicol 5:370 with permission.

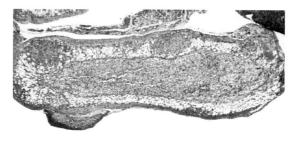

FIGURE 17.6 Atrophy, vacuolar degeneration, and nodular hyperplasia (arrows) of the adrenal cortex from a rat treated with 50 mg/kg/day of DMNM for 90 days. Bar: 100 µm. From Yarrington (1985), Fundam Appl Toxicol 5:370 with permission.

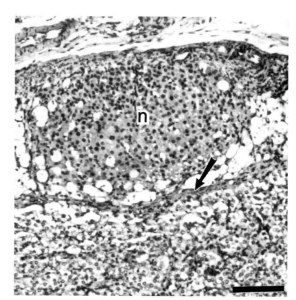

FIGURE 17.7 Higher magnification of Fig. 17.9 Prominent area of nodular hyperplasia (n), thin cortex, and mild fibrosis (arrow) of the zona reticularis in a rat receiving 50 mg/kg/day of DMNM for 90 days. Bar: 100 µm. From Yarrington et al. (1985), Fundam Appl Toxicol 5:370 with permission.

to reparative in nature. Vacuolar degeneration is a reflection of impaired steroidogenesis, resulting in excess storage of unmetabolized steroid precursors (Figure 17.3). More destructive lesions may be observed in the form of hemorrhage and/or necrosis (Figure 17.4), often in association with an inflammatory response. At the same time, one area of the cortex (e.g., the zona glomerulosa) may undergo hypertrophy, while another area has degenerative lesions, e.g., vacuolar degeneration of the zona fasciculata (Figure 17.5). If the zona glomerulosa remains functional, and there are no clinically-significant signs of hypoadrenocorticism, chronic regenerative changes may subsequently develop. Usually the adrenal cortex will be shrunken or atrophic, with fibrosis and areas of multinodular hyperplasia (Figures 17.6 and 17.7). Occasionally, the effect of a chemical is limited to a specific zone of the adrenal cortex, and may be species-specific, e.g., administration of PD 132301-2 to monkeys induces a narrow band of degeneration or necrosis in the mid to outer zona fasciculata, while all three cortical zones are affected in the adrenal glands of dogs treated with this compound (Table 17.2). The zonae reticularis and fasciculata typically are most severely affected, although eventually the lesions involve the zona glomerulosa. These alterations may be classified as follows: endothelial damage (e.g., acrylonitrile); mitochondrial damage (e.g., DMNM, oJ-DDD, amphenone); endoplasmic reticulum changes (e.g., triparanol); lipid aggregation (e.g., aniline);

lysosomal phospholipid aggregation (e.g., chlorophentermine); and possible secondary effects due to embolization by medullary cells (e.g., acrylonitrile).

Mitochondrial damage with vacuolization (Figure 17.8) and accompanying changes in the endoplasmic reticulum and autophagocytic responses appear to be among the most common ultrastructural changes observed following chemical injury in the adrenal cortex. Similarly, increased lipid droplets (Figure 17.9)

TABLE 17.2   Examples of chemically induced microscopic and ultrastructural changes of the adrenal cortex[a]

Compound	Initial predilection site	Histology	Ultrastructure
Nafenopin	Zona fasciculata	Hypertrophy	SER[b] and peroxisome proliferation
Acrylonitrile	Zona reticularis	Hemorrhage	Damage to vascular endothelium; embolization of medullary cells and cell fragments of capillaries
Aminoglutethimide	All zones; more marked in outer zona fasciculata	Vacuolar degeneration; increased lipid	Mitochondrial hypertrophy and cavitation
o, p'-DDD	Zona reticularis and fasciculata	Vacuolar degeneration; cytotoxic cellular atrophy	Mitochondrial vacuolization; SER dilation
α-(l,4-Dioxido-3-methylquinoxalin-2-yl)-N-methylnitrone	Zona reticularis and fasciculata	Granular and vacuolar degeneration; cytotoxic cellular atrophy	Mitochondrial vacuolization; SER dilation
Triparanol	All zones; most marked in zona fasciculata	Increased eosinophilia and inclusions	Decreased lipid droplets; mitochondrial alterations; SER hypertrophy; lysosomal formation
Cysteamine (1-mercaptoethylamine)	Zona reticularis and fasciculata	Hemorrhage and necrosis	Retrograde emboli of medullary cells
Amphenone	Zona reticularis and fasciculata	Fatty degeneration	Mitochondrial alterations
7,12-Dimethylbenzanthracene	Zona reticularis and fasciculata	Necrosis; hemorrhage; calcification	Mitochondrial alterations, including variation in size
Corticosteroids, (e.g., prednisolone, dexamethasone)	Zona reticularis and fasciculata	Atrophy	Increased lipid droplets surrounded by membranous "whorls"; increased myelin figures and lysosomes
Propylthiouracil	Zona reticularis	Ceroid degeneration	Lipid and mitochondrial degeneration
Carbon tetrachloride	Zona reticularis and fasciculata	Necrosis	Swelling of SER
Tamoxifen	Zona reticularis and fasciculata	Degeneration and necrosis; lipid droplets	Necrosis; lipid droplets in macrophages; few lysosomal inclusions
Spironolactone	Zona glomerulosa	Hypertrophy and inclusions	Lipid droplets surrounded by whorls of SER ("spironolactone bodies"); mitochondrial alterations
Hexadimethrine bromide (polybrene)	Zona glomerulosa	Necrosis and infarction	Protein-containing vacuoles and hyalin bodies; microthrombi
R01-8307, a sulfated mucopolysaccharide	Zona glomerulosa	Condensation	
Captopril	Zona glomerulosa	Atrophy	Decreased mitochondria and SER
1,1'-Thio-diethylidene-ferrocene (MDL 80, 478)	All zones	Granular and vacuolar degeneration; hyperplastic zona glomerulosa	Mitochondrial vacuolation; increased lipid droplets
Aniline	All zones	Hypertrophic cortical cells laden with lipid droplets	Increased lipid droplets; hypertrophic SER; mitochondrial degeneration
Chlorophentermine	All zones	Nothing remarkable	Increased lysosomal alterations in the form of lamellated cytoplasmic inclusions
Triaryl phosphate	All zones	Cytoplasmic lipid droplet	Increased number/size cytoplasmic droplets
PD 132301–2	Zona fasciculata	Coarse vacuolation	SER aggregation; changes of autophagosomes

[a]From Yarrington (1983). Reprinted, in part, courtesy of Springer-Verlag. For mechanism of action, see Table 1

[b]Smooth endoplasmic reticulum

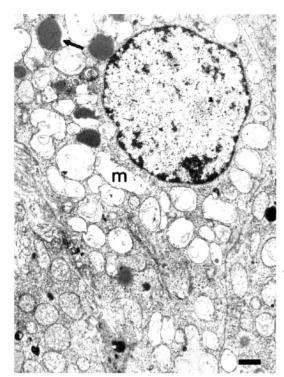

FIGURE 17.8   Cell of the zona fasciculata of the adrenal cortex of a rat treated with 100 mg/kg/day of DNMN for 21 days. Note vacuolated mitochondria (m) and some lipid droplets undergoing lipolysis (arrow). Bar: 1 μm. From Yarrington et al. (1985), Fundam Appl Toxicol 5:370 with permission.

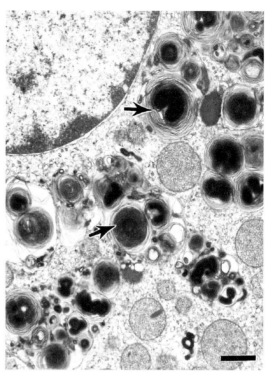

FIGURE 17.10   Large myeloid bodies (arrows) compatible with lysosomal phospholipidosis in an adrenal cortical cell of a rat treated with a cationic amphiphilic compound. Bar: 1 μm.

and lysosomal phospholipidosis (Figure 17.10) are compatible with altered steroid biosynthesis as a result of chemical inhibition of steroid precursors, e.g., cholesterol. The increased accumulation of lipid and severe mitochondrial vacuolization appear to correspond to light microscopic findings of marked cytoplasmic vacuolar and granular degeneration. More severe ultrastructural injury may result, and some parenchymal cells of the cortex have an electron-dense cytoplasm, chromatolysis, and disruption of the plasma membranes (Figure 17.11). Frequently, macrophages containing cholesterol clefts, numerous lipid droplets, and membranous debris can be observed among the necrotic cells.

Proliferative Lesions

Less frequently reported are chemically-induced proliferative lesions of the adrenal cortex consisting of hyperplasia, adenoma, or carcinoma. Unlike the diffuse hyperplasia associated with the adrenal cortical response to excess ACTH stimulation, chemically-induced hyperplasia is usually nodular in type, and often multiple. Each nodule is an oval-to-spherical lesion of variable size consisting of enlarged normal or vacuolated cells (Table 17.3).

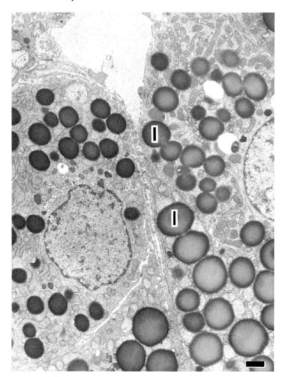

FIGURE 17.9   Numerous lipid droplets (1) in the cytoplasm of cells of the zonae fasciculata and glomerulosa from a rat treated with 500 mg/kg/day of MDL 80,478. Bar: 1 μm. From Yarrington et al. (1985), Fundam Appl Toxicol 5:370 with permission.

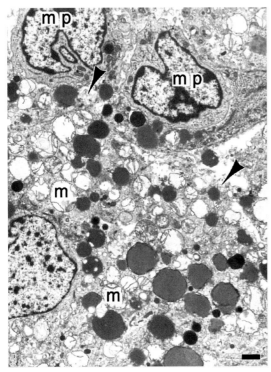

FIGURE 17.11　Necrotic cell of the zona reticularis in a dog treated with 22.5 mg/kg/bid of DMNM for 21 days. Many degenerative mitochondria (m) and numerous lipid droplets are present in cytoplasm with disruption of the plasma membrane (arrowheads). Two macrophages (mp) are present. Bar: 1 μm. From Yarrington et al. (1985), Fundam Appl Toxicol 5:370 with permission.

Most of the reported tumors tend to be benign (adenoma), although an occasional one may be malignant (carcinoma). The *zonae reticularis* and *fasciculata* are more prone to develop tumors, whereas the *zona glomerulosa* is spared unless invaded by an expanding tumor in the adjacent zones of the cortex. Tumorigenic agents of the adrenal cortex appear to have a diverse chemical nature and use (Table 17.3).

Cortical adenomas may be partially encapsulated by a thin band of fibrous connective tissue. Adrenal cortical carcinomas are composed of large polyhedral or pleomorphic cells, with an eosinophilic or vacuolated cytoplasm. Tumor cells have prominent nucleoli and variable numbers of mitotic figures, and form different histologic patterns, including sheets, lobules, and cords. The invasive nature of the malignant cells is also apparent by penetration through the capsule, obliteration of the normal architecture of the affected gland, and metastasis to distant sites. Blood-filled spaces and localized areas of necrosis are common in cortical carcinomas.

Spontaneous proliferative lesions may be found in all zones of the adrenal cortex in most species. Naturally-occurring adrenal cortical tumors are found infrequently in domestic animals, except adult dogs and castrated male goats. Adrenal tumors are being recognized with greater frequency in ferrets, as they

TABLE 17.3　Examples of compounds producing tumors of the adrenal cortex[a]

Compound	Chemical properties	Type of lesion	Animal affected
Aflatoxin/stilbesterol	Fungal metabolite/steroid	Adenoma and hyperplasia	Rat
Cholesterol	Steroid	Microadenomas	Rabbit
Dibromochloropropane	Soil fumigant	Adenoma	Rat
7, 12-Dimethylbenzanthracene	Organic solvent	Adenoma; eosinophilic and basophilic foci	Rat
Estrone, estriol, diethylstilbesterol	Natural and synthetic estrogens	Adenocarcinoma	Rat
Formic acid 2-[4-(5-nitro-2-furyl)-2-thiazolyl]hydrazide	Antimicrobial	Adenoma	Hamster
Parathion	Insecticide	Adenoma; carcinoma	Rat
Tetrachlorovinphos	Insecticide	Adenoma	Rat
Testosterone	Hormone	Adenoma	Hamster
Urethane	Organic solvent; intermediate in organic synthesis	Adenoma	Rat
Linoleic acid	Unsaturated fatty acid	Carcinoma	Rat

[a]Predilection sites are zona reticularis and fasciculata

are being kept as household pets and living to a more advanced age.

Evaluation of Toxicity

Provocative testing for the evaluation of adrenal cortical functional reserves is essential to determine the extent of any cortical damage. The most commonly used provocative test is the administration of ACTH to human patients or animals. When assessing adrenocortical function, it is noteworthy to consider the effects of aging on both steriodogenesis and the response to ACTH. Comparative studies of young and adult rats and dogs have revealed that basal levels of circulating corticosteroid and the response to ACTH may be different at different ages. *In vitro* studies may be useful in determining the specific cellular consequences of xenobiotic exposure on steroidogenesis. In many instances, the results of these *in vitro* assessments are helpful in correlating the development of adrenocortical degeneration to an inhibited pathway of steroidogenesis.

Diagnostic imaging such as ultrasound and computed tomography has now become a more practical technology to access, in a noninvasive way, morphologic alterations of the adrenal cortex caused by xenobiotics. Newer technologies that appear to have the potential to visualize the adrenal glands better include magnetic resonance imaging (MRI) and single-photon emission computed tomography (SPECT).

Morphologic evaluation of the adrenal cortex commences with macroscopic observation of the adrenal glands to detect changes in size, color, or structure, e.g., nodularity. In addition to hematoxylin and eosin staining and evaluation, special stains such as Congo red (amyloid), or histomorphometric analysis to assess subtle differences in cell size, width of the different cortical zones, and cortical:medullary ratio may define the alterations further. Transmission electron microscopy is an important tool for detecting changes in the internal architecture of adrenal cortical cells, especially when this is performed in association with morphometric analysis, cytochemistry, and immunocytochemistry procedures.

ADRENAL MEDULLA

Structure and Function

Anatomy

The medulla constitutes approximately 10% of the volume of the adrenal gland. The bulk of the medulla is composed of chromaffin cells, which are the sites of synthesis and storage of catecholamines. Ultrastructurally, norepinephrine-containing granules appear highly electron dense, whereas epinephrine granules are less dense with finely granular matrices. In addition to chromaffin cells, the adrenal medulla contains variable numbers of ganglion cells. A third cell type has also been described, and has been designated the small granule containing (SGC) cell or small intensely fluorescent (SIF) cell. These cells morphologically appear intermediate between chromaffin cells and ganglion cells. They may possibly function as interneurons. Adrenal medullary cells also contain serotonin and histamine, but it has not been determined if these products are synthesized *in situ* or are taken up from the circulation.

Mechanisms of Toxicity

Proliferative lesions of the medulla have been reported to develop as a result of a variety of different mechanisms. Some data are available on the relationship of anterior pituitary hormones to the development of adrenal medullary lesions. For example, the long-term administration of growth hormone is associated with the development of pheochromocytomas, as well as tumors in other sites. Some authors have suggested that prolactin-secreting pituitary tumors may play a role in the development of proliferative medullary lesions.

Evidence for a role of pituitary hormones in the development of medullary lesions is provided by data suggesting that hypophysectomy eliminates the development of these lesions. Although not all animals with adrenal medullary lesions have concurrent pituitary abnormalities, at least some with histologically normal pituitaries might have hypothalamic defects, resulting in the decreased dopaminergic inhibition of prolactin release. It is also possible that certain neuroleptics increase prolactin by decreasing dopamine release. Several drugs have been reported to increase the incidence of adrenal medullary proliferative lesions, including reserpine, zomepirac sodium (a nonsteroidal inflammatory drug), isoretinoin (a retinoid), and gemfibrozil (a hypolipidemic drug). However, the mechanisms responsible for the stimulation of adrenal medullary proliferation by these drugs are unknown.

Response to Injury

Characteristics of Proliferative Lesions

The adrenal medulla undergoes a series of proliferative changes ranging from diffuse hyperplasia

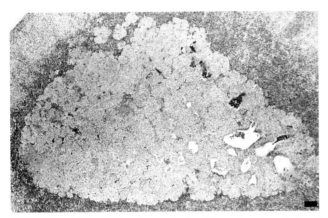

FIGURE 17.12   Diffuse hyperplasia of the adrenal medulla of an old male Long-Evans rat. Serial sections failed to reveal the presence of nodular lesions. Bar: 1 μm.

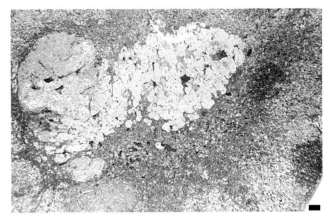

FIGURE 17.13   Focal hyperplasia of adrenal medullary cells (upper left portion of the field) in an old male Long-Evans rat. Although there is some compression of the cortex, the nodule blends imperceptibly into the adjacent medulla. Morphometric analyses also revealed diffuse hyperplasia of the medulla. Bar: 100 μm. From Tischler et al. (1985), Lab Invest 53:486–498 with permission.

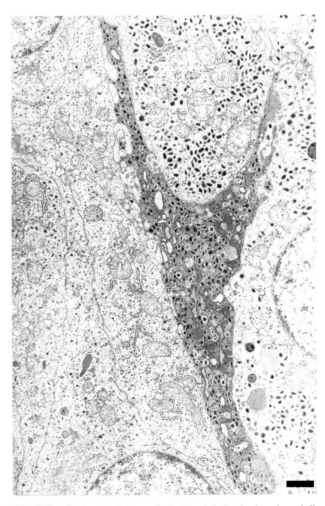

FIGURE 17.14   Focal hyperplasia ("nodule") of adrenal medulla from an old male Long-Evans rat. Cells comprising the nodule (left) have few small secretory granules compared to the larger and more pleomorphic granules of the adjacent medullary cells. Bar: 1 μm. From Tischler and DeLellis (1988), J Am Coll Toxicol 7:23–44 with permission.

to benign and malignant neoplasia. Diffuse hyperplasia is characterized by symmetric expansion of the medulla, with maintenance of the usual sharp demarcation of the cortex and the medulla (Figure 17.12). The medullary cell cords are often widened, but the ratio of norepinephrine to epinephrine cells is similar to that of normal glands. Focal hyperplastic lesions are often juxtacortical, but may occur within any area of the medulla. The small nodules of hyperplasia, in general, are not associated with compression of the adjacent medulla (Figure 17.13); however, the larger foci are often associated with medullary compression. Foci of adrenal medullary hyperplasia are typically composed of small cells with round to ovoid nuclei and scanty cytoplasm. The classification of such lesions has engendered considerable controversy in the literature. According to some authors, the lack of a chromaffin reaction in such nodules has been said to preclude the diagnosis of pheochromocytoma. However, the chromaffin reaction is quite insensitive, and catecholamines, particularly norepinephrine, can be demonstrated by biochemical extraction studies and by formaldehyde- or glyoxylic acid-induced fluorescence methods.

At the ultrastructural level, the cells composing these focal areas of hyperplasia contain small numbers of dense core secretory granules resembling the granules of SIF or SGC cells (Figure 17.14). Larger adrenal medullary proliferative lesions are generally accepted as pheochromocytomas, with lesions composed of relatively small cells similar to those found in smaller proliferative foci. Alternatively, they may be composed of larger cells or a mixture of small and large cells (Figure 17.15). Even in larger medullary lesions, the chromaffin reaction is often equivocal, but catecholamines may be demonstrated both biochemically

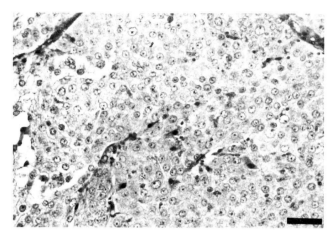

FIGURE 17.15 Pheochromocytoma from an old male Long-Evans rat. The tumor compressed the adjacent cortex and medulla. Bar: 100 μm.

and histochemically. Invasion of the capsule of the adrenal with or without distant metastases occurs in malignant pheochromocytomas.

Neuroblastomas also may occur infrequently in the adrenal medulla in rodents. Neuroblastomas develop as a centrally-located expansive mass that compresses the surrounding cortex, and are composed of small cells with round to ovoid hyperchromatic nuclei and scant cytoplasm. Cells comprising neuroblastomas resemble lymphocytes and tend to form pseudorosettes. Neurofibrils or unmyelinated nerve fibers can usually be demonstrated in neuroblastomas.

Ganglioneuromas are usually small benign tumors arising in the medulla and compressing the surrounding cortex. They are composed of multipolar sympathetic ganglion cells and neurofibrils with a prominent fibrous connective tissue stroma. Neoplastic cells in medullary tumors occasionally differentiate along two lines, resulting in adjacent pheochromocytomas and ganglioneuromas in the same adrenal gland.

Evaluation of Toxicity

Morphologic Evaluation

A variety of techniques may be used for the demonstration of catecholamines in tissue sections. The chromaffin reaction is the oxidation of catecholamines by potassium dichromate solutions, and results in the formation of a brown to yellow pigment that may be seen both grossly and microscopically. The chromaffin reaction, as performed traditionally, possesses a very low level of sensitivity and should not be used for the routine demonstration of catecholamines. Similarly, both argentaffin and argyrophil reactions, which have been used extensively in the past for the demonstration

of chromaffin cells, also possess low sensitivity and specificity. Fluorescence techniques using formaldehyde or glyoxylic acid represent the methods of choice for the demonstration of catecholamines at the cellular level. These aldehydes form highly fluorescent derivatives with catecholamines, which can be visualized by ultraviolet microscopy. Immunohistochemistry provides an alternative approach for the localization of catecholamines in chromaffin cells and other cell types. Antibodies are now available that permit epinephrine- and norepinephrine-containing cells to be distinguished, even in routinely fixed and embedded tissue samples. Catecholamine biosynthetic enzymes may also be demonstrated by immunohistochemical procedures. Antibodies to chromogranin A can be used for the demonstration of this protein constituent in chromaffin cells by immunohistochemistry.

PITUITARY GLAND

Structure and Function

Anatomy

The pituitary gland develops from a dorsal evagination of the oropharyngeal ectoderm (Rathke's pouch or craniopharyngeal duct) for the adenohypophysis, and a ventral downgrowth of diencephalic neuro-ectoderm for the neurohypophysis. The pituitary gland, also known as the hypophysis, may be divided into two major compartments: the anterior adenohypophysis composed of the *pars distalis, pars tuberalis,* and *pars intermedia*; and the posterior neurohypophysis, which includes the *pars nervosa* or infundibular process, infundibulum, infundibular stem, and *tuber cinereum.* In most animals and in human fetuses, the thin cellular zone between the adenohypophysis and neurohypophysis is referred to as the *pars intermedia* or intermediate lobe.

The pituitary lies within the *sella turcica* of the sphenoid bone, and receives blood via the posterior and anterior hypophyseal arteries, which originate from the internal carotid arteries. Arteriolar branches penetrate the pituitary stalk, lose their muscular coat, and form a capillary plexus near the median eminence. These vessels drain into the hypophyseal portal veins, which supply the adenohypophysis. This hypothalamic–hypophyseal portal system transports hypothalamic-releasing and release-inhibiting hormones directly to the adenohypophysis for interactions with their specific target cells.

The neurohypophysis is joined to the hypothalamus via the infundibular stalk, and is composed of densely-packed bundles of nonmyelinated axons and capillaries that are supported by modified glial cells or pituicytes.

Both oxytocin and vasopressin (antidiuretic hormone (ADH)) are synthesized in supraoptic and paraventricular nuclei as large precursor molecules, which contain both active hormones and their associated neurophysins. As the biosynthetic precursor molecules travel along the axons in secretion granules from the neurosecretory neurons, the precursors are cleaved into the active hormones and their respective neurophysins. These secretory products can be detected immunocytochemically.

Functional Cytology

The adenohypophysis represents the largest portion of the pituitary gland. Here the cells are responsible for the synthesis of growth hormone (GH), prolactin (PRL) or luteotropic hormone (LTH), and adrenocorticotropin (ACTH), follicle-stimulating hormone (FSH), luteinizing hormone (LH), and thyroid-stimulating hormone (TSH) or thyrotropin.

Cells of the anterior lobe, viewed microscopically using hematoxylin and eosin staining, include acidophils, basophils, and chromophobes, constituting approximately 40%, 10%, and 50% of the total cell population, respectively. The growth hormone-secreting acidophils (somatotrophs) constitute approximately 50% of the total cell population in the *pars distalis* (Figure 17.16). These cells are distributed throughout the adenohypophysis, and are generally round to ovoid in shape. The growth hormone-producing cells stain positively with orange C and eosin, and these cells typically have numerous secretory granules, which have an average diameter of 300 nm. Occasional growth hormone-containing secretory granules may measure up to 500 nm in diameter.

Although most of the growth hormone-synthesizing cells correspond to acidophils, some may be chromophobic, when they are in an actively synthesizing phase of the secretory cycle. At the ultrastructural level, actively synthesizing cells have few secretory granules, but abundant granular endoplasmic reticulum and Golgi complexes. Prolactin-secreting acidophils (luteotrophs) compose 15–25% of the total cell population. They tend to be concentrated in the dorsocephalic region of the adenohypophysis.

Prolactin cells, particularly those with larger granules, stain positively with erythrosine and carmoisine. However, the sparsely-granulated cells with smaller granules often fail to stain with these dyes, and appear chromophobic. ACTH-producing cells (corticotrophs)

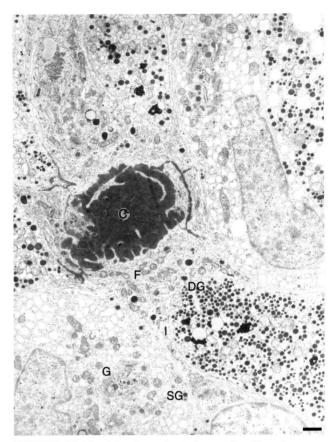

FIGURE 17.16 Adenohypophysis from a dog. Densely granulated acidophils (DG) are in the storage phase and contain numerous secretory granules. Sparsely granulated acidophils (SG) have few mature secretory granules but many dilated cisternae of granular endoplasmic reticulum and well-developed Golgi regions (G). Follicular (stellate) cell, F; colloid, C. Bar: 1 μm. From Capen and Koestner (1967), Vet Pathol 4:326–347 with permission.

are round to ovoid, may be chromophobic or lightly basophilic (in humans), and can stain weakly positive with PAS. These cells are widely distributed within the *pars distalis*, and form the bulk of the *pars intermedia*.

Thyrotropin-producing (TSH) basophils or thyrotrophs account for about 5% of the cells of the adenohypophysis. These cells tend to occur in small clusters within the *pars distalis*, and have a stellate to polygonal shape. They may be basophilic or chromophobic and are also PAS positive. Hypertrophy and hyperplasia of TSH cells under these conditions are due to a lack of negative feedback by T_3 and, to a lesser extent, T_4 on the hypothalamus and thyrotrophs.

Gonadotropin-producing (GTH) basophils or gonadotrophs are relatively large round to oval cells, and account for approximately 10% of the cells concentrated in the dorsocephalic region in the *pars distalis*. These cells are responsible for the production of FSH and LH. Immunoperoxidase stains have revealed that some cells contain both FSH and LH, whereas others contain only LH or FSH. Gonadotroph cells undergo a series of changes following castration, resulting in the formation of "gonadectomy cells." In some cells, a single large vacuole occupies most of the cytoplasm, producing cells with a "signet ring" appearance. Ultrastructurally, gonadectomy cells contain abundant dilated cisternae of endoplasmic reticulum, well-developed Golgi complexes, and few secretory granules.

In addition to specific hormone-secreting cells, a population of supporting cells is also present in the adenohypophysis, called stellate (follicular) cells, which stain selectively with antibodies to S-100 protein. Stellate cells typically have elongate processes and prominent cytoplasmic filaments (Figure 17.16). These cells appear to provide a phagocytic or supportive function, in addition to producing a colloid-like material.

The hypothalamus serves as the major regulator of the adenohypophysis. Each cell type within the adenohypophysis is under the control of a corresponding releasing hormone that is synthesized within nerve cell bodies of the hypothalamus. The releasing hormones are transported via axonal processes to the median eminence, where they are released into capillaries and are carried by the hypophyseal portal system to trophic hormone-producing cells in the adenohypophysis. Specific releasing factors have been identified for TSH, FSH and LH, ACTH, and GH. Prolactin secretion is stimulated by a number of factors, the most important of which appears to be thyrotropin-releasing hormone (TRH). TRH stimulates the release of prolactin with many of the same dose-response characteristics as the stimulation of TSH release.

Multiple influences contribute to the control of adenohypophyseal hormone secretion. Dopamine serves as the major prolactin inhibitory factor by suppressing virtually all aspects of prolactin secretion, and also inhibits cell division and DNA synthesis of this cell type. Dopamine also suppresses ACTH production by corticotrophs in the *pars intermedia* of some species. A second hypothalamic release-inhibiting hormone is somatostatin (somatotropin release-inhibiting hormone, or SRIH), which inhibits the secretion of both growth hormone and TSH. In some situations, SRIH also inhibits the secretion of PRL and ACTH. The control of pituitary hormone secretion is also affected by negative feedback loops resulting from the interaction of end organ hormones, adenohypophyseal hormones, and corresponding hypothalamic-releasing and release-inhibiting hormones.

Mechanisms of Toxicity

Induction of Pituitary Tumors

Pituitary tumors can be induced readily by sustained uncompensated hormonal derangements leading to increased synthesis and secretion of pituitary hormones, where the absence of feedback inhibition of the pituitary cell may lead to its unrestrained proliferation. This effect can be potentiated by the concurrent administration of ionizing radiation or chemical carcinogens.

Response to Injury

Non-neoplastic Lesions

Pituitary cysts developing spontaneously from remnants of Rathke's pouch are usually of microscopic size, but occasional larger cysts may develop from these remnants. The cysts are either confined to the adenohypophysis, or may be joined to the lumen of the craniopharyngeal duct, are typically lined by a ciliated cuboidal to columnar epithelium, and may be uni- or multilocular. Squamous epithelium may also line the cysts, which typically occur in the *pars distalis* and pars *intermedia*, and rarely in the neurohypophysis.

Pituitary dwarfism in dogs is usually associated with a failure of the oropharyngeal ectoderm of Rathke's pouch to differentiate into trophic hormone-secreting cells of the *pars distalis*. This results in a progressively enlarging, multiloculated cyst in the *sella turcica* and an absence of the adenohypophysis. Juvenile panhypopituitarism occurs most frequently in German shepherd dogs, but it has been reported in Spitz, toy pinscher, and Carelian bear dogs. The dwarf pups appear normal from birth to about two months of age. Subsequently, the slower growth, retention of puppy hair coat, and lack of primary guard hairs gradually become evident. A bilaterally symmetrical alopecia develops gradually, and often progresses to complete alopecia except for the head and tufts of hair on the legs. There is also progressive hyperpigmentation of the skin until the skin is uniformly brown-black over most of the body.

Neoplastic Lesions

Craniopharyngioma

The craniopharyngioma is an uncommon naturally-occurring neoplasm arising from the craniopharyngeal duct epithelium of Rathke's pouch that is composed of nests and cords of squamous cells with areas of cyst formation. As these tumors enlarge, they may extend into the adjacent brain; however, the tumors rarely metastasize. Craniopharyngiomas are often large and grow along the ventral aspect of the brain, where they can surround several cranial nerves. In addition, they extend dorsally into the hypothalamus and thalamus.

Microscopically, craniopharyngiomas have alternating solid and cystic areas. The solid areas are composed of nests of epithelial cells (cuboidal, columnar, or squamous) with focal areas of mineralization. The cystic spaces are lined by either columnar or squamous cells, and contain keratin debris and colloid. It has been proposed that some pleomorphic neoplasms in the suprasellar region of younger dogs be classified as primary germ cell tumors rather than craniopharyngiomas, based on a midline suprasellar location, presence within the tumor of several distinct cells, and positive staining for α-fetoprotein.

Pituicytoma

Primary neoplasms of the *pars nervosa* are extremely uncommon. The tumors that have been reported to occur at this site have been designated as pituicytomas. These naturally-occurring tumors are composed of small, closely-packed, spindloid cells arranged in cords and bundles. Most pituicytomas are quite small, but larger tumors may extend into the adenohypophysis and into the adjacent brain tissue; however, metastases have not been reported. Occasionally, the larger tumors may be impossible to distinguish from gliomas or meningiomas of the brain.

Proliferative Lesions of the Adenohypophysis

The histopathological separation among nodular hyperplasia, adenoma, and carcinoma is often more difficult in endocrine glands, such as the pituitary, than in most organs of the body. However, criteria for their separation should be established and applied in a uniform manner in the evaluation of proliferative lesions in endocrine glands, as there appears to be a continuous spectrum of proliferative lesions between diffuse or focal hyperplasia and adenomas derived from a specific population of secretory cells. Prolonged stimulation of a population of secretory cells predisposes to the subsequent development of a higher-than-expected incidence of tumors.

Focal ("nodular") hyperplasia usually appears as multiple small areas that are well demarcated but not encapsulated from adjacent normal cells. Cells making up an area of focal hyperplasia in the adenohypophysis closely resemble the cells of origin; however, the cytoplasmic area may be slightly enlarged, and the nucleus more hyperchromatic than in normal cells.

Adenomas are usually solitary nodules that are larger than the multiple areas of focal hyperplasia. They are sharply demarcated from the adjacent normal pituitary glandular parenchyma, and there is often a thin, partial to complete, fibrous capsule. The adjacent parenchyma is compressed to varying degrees, depending on the size of the adenoma. Cells composing an adenoma may closely resemble the cells of origin morphologically and in their architectural pattern of arrangement; however, there are often histological differences, such as multiple layers of cells lining follicles and vascular trabeculae, or solid clusters of secretory cells subdivided into packets by a fine fibrovascular stroma.

Carcinomas are usually larger than adenomas in the pituitary, and usually result in a macroscopically-detectable enlargement. The separation between adenoma and carcinoma of an endocrine gland is often difficult using only morphologic criteria. Histopathological features that are suggestive of malignancy include extensive intraglandular invasion, invasion into adjacent structures (e.g., dura mater, sphenoid bone), formation of tumor cell thrombi within vessels, and particularly the establishment of metastases at distant sites. The growth of neoplastic cells subendothelially in highly vascular benign tumors should not be mistaken for vascular invasion. Malignant endocrine cells are often more pleomorphic than normal, but nuclear and cellular pleomorphism are not consistent criterion to distinguish adenoma from carcinoma in the adenohypophysis of rodents. Mitotic figures may be frequent in malignant cells, but the significance of this criterion can vary considerably with the degree of background stimulation of the endocrine gland. Many neoplasms derived from parenchymal cells of the pituitary are functionally active, secrete an excessive amount of hormone either continuously or episodically, and result in clinical syndromes of hormone excess.

Morphologically, an endocrine tumor can often be interpreted as endocrinologically active if the rim of normal tissue around the tumor undergoes trophic atrophy, due to negative feedback inhibition by the elevated hormone levels or an altered blood constituent. In response to the autonomous secretion of hormone by the tumor, these non neoplastic secretory cells, especially the cytoplasmic area, become smaller than normal, and eventually the number of cells is decreased. Functional pituitary neoplasms secreting an excess of a particular trophic hormone (e.g., ACTH or prolactin) will be associated with striking hypertrophy and hyperplasia of target cells in the adrenal cortex (e.g., *zonae fasciculata* and *reticularis*) or mammary gland (ductal hyperplasia, galactocele formation, and increased incidence of mammary tumors) in chronic rodent studies.

Adenoma of Pars Intermedia

Adenomas of the *pars intermedia* are uncommon, and may vary considerably in size. Larger adenomas may compress the adenohypophysis and neurohypophysis, whereas smaller lesions may be of microscopic dimensions. These tumors are nonencapsulated, but do compress the adjacent normal tissue. The cells often have faintly basophilic cytoplasm with round to ovoid nuclei. In contrast to the relative rarity of adenomas derived from cells of the *pars intermedia* in the rat, these tumors are common neoplasms in the horse and dog. Adenomas derived from cells of the *pars intermedia* are the most common type of pituitary tumor in horses, the second most common type in dogs, infrequent in nonhuman primates, and rare in other species. They develop in older horses, with females affected more frequently than males. Nonbrachycephalic breeds of dogs develop adenomas in the *pars intermedia* more often than brachycephalic breeds. Two cell populations have been identified in the *pars intermedia* of normal dogs by immunocytochemistry: the predominant A- and B-cells. B-cells may account for the high bioactive ACTH concentration found in the *pars intermedia* of dogs, and may produce unique corticotroph (ACTH-secreting) adenomas of the *pars intermedia* in dogs with the syndrome of cortisol excess.

Pituitary Carcinoma

Pituitary carcinomas are uncommon neoplasms compared with adenomas. They are usually endocrinologically inactive, but can cause significant functional disturbances by destruction of the *pars distalis* and neurohypophyseal system, leading to adult onset panhypopituitarism and *diabetes insipidus*. Carcinomas are large and invade extensively into the overlying brain, along the ventral aspect of the cranial cavity incorporating cranial nerves (II, III, IV), and locally into the adjacent sphenoid bone of the *sella turcica*, where they may cause osteolysis. Metastases occur infrequently to regional lymph nodes, or to distant sites such as the spleen or liver. Carcinomas are highly cellular, and often have large areas of hemorrhage and necrosis. Giant cells, nuclear pleomorphism, and mitotic figures are encountered more frequently than in adenomas.

Functional Characteristics of Pituitary Adenomas

The vast majority of pituitary adenomas in humans and rodents have been described as chromophobic

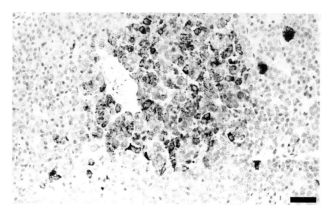

FIGURE 17.17   Pituitary adenoma in an old male Long-Evans rat. The section was stained for the β chain of luteinizing hormone. Occasional cells have intense immunoreactivity whereas others have only moderate to weak immunoreactivity. Bar: 100 μm. From Lee et al. (1982), Lab Invest 47: 595–602 with permission.

in type; however, many of these tumors have been found to stain for prolactin by immunohistochemistry. Occasionally, prolactin cells within adenomas may be admixed with FSH/LH-, TSH-, or ACTH-positive cells. Infrequent adenomas composed of populations of ACTH or FSH/LH cells have also been reported (Figure 17.17). Functional (endocrinologically-active) neoplasms arising in the pituitary gland of dogs most likely are derived from corticotroph (ACTH-secreting) cells in either the *pars distalis* or the *pars intermedia*. These neoplasms induce a clinical syndrome of cortisol excess (Cushing's disease), and are encountered most frequently in dogs, particularly in adult to aged boxers, Boston terriers, and dachshunds. The pituitary gland is consistently enlarged; however, neither the occurrence nor the severity of functional disturbances appears to be directly related to the size of the neoplasm.

Because the *diaphragma sella* is incomplete in the dog, the line of least resistance favors dorsal expansion of the gradually enlarging pituitary mass, with extension into the overlying brain. This results in invagination into the infundibular cavity, dilatation of the infundibular recess and the third ventricle with eventual compression or replacement of the hypothalamus, and possible extension of the neoplasm into the thalamus.

Bilateral enlargement of the adrenal glands occurs in dogs with functional corticotroph adenomas. This enlargement is due to cortical hypertrophy/hyperplasia, primarily of the *zonae fasciculata* and *reticularis*. Nodules of yellow-orange hyperplastic cortical tissue are often found outside the capsule, as well as extending down into and compressing the adrenal medulla.

Pituitary corticotroph adenomas are composed of well-differentiated, large or small, chromophobic cells supported by fine connective tissue septa. Hormone-containing secretory granules can be demonstrated by electron microscopy in functional corticotroph adenomas of dogs.

Spontaneous Pituitary Adenomas

The high frequency of spontaneous pituitary adenomas in laboratory rats is a well-recognized phenomenon that must be considered in any long-term toxicological study. The incidence of these tumors is determined by many factors, including strain, age, sex, reproductive status, and diet. Rapid body growth rates and high levels of conversion of feed to body mass in early life, or high protein intake in early adult life, predispose any strain of rat to the development of pituitary adenomas.

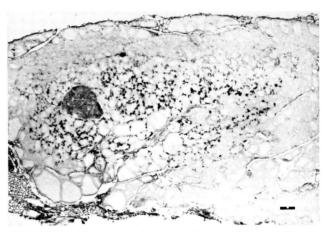

FIGURE 17.18 Distribution of C-cells in thyroid gland from a young male Long-Evans rat stained for calcitonin with the peroxidase-antiperoxidase method. C-cells are concentrated around the parathyroid gland (P), which has slight nonspecific staining. Bar: 100 μm. From DeLellis et al. (1979), Lab Invest 40: 140–154 with permission.

Evaluation of Toxicity

Morphologic Evaluation

Immunohistochemical evaluation is an extremely important approach for the functional and morphologic analysis of normal and abnormal pituitary glands. For most routine toxicological studies, formalin fixation provides adequate preservation of the pituitary hormones for immunohistochemical studies; however, some authors have recommended Bouin's fixation for immunohistochemical staining of the pituitary, because this fixative produces more precise localization of the hormones at the light microscopic level.

Many immunohistochemical procedures have been used to study pituitary hormones, including direct and indirect peroxidase conjugates, peroxidase antiperoxidase (PAP), and avidin–biotin–peroxidase complex (ABC) methods. In most studies, PAP and ABC methods have been found to have greater sensitivity than indirect peroxidase conjugate procedures. Recent studies have employed *in situ* hybridization techniques for the identification of messenger RNAs encoding the hormonal peptides.

THYROID C-CELLS

Structure and Function

C-cells or parafollicular cells of the thyroid gland, named after their major secretory product (calcitonin),

are located either within the thyroid follicles between the basal regions of the follicular cells and the basement membrane of the follicle, or in an interfollicular location. In addition to calcitonin, C-cells contain a variety of other peptides, including somatostatin and bombesin. These cells tend to be concentrated within the central regions of the lobes, and are most prominent at the levels of the parathyroid glands (Figure 17.18). By light microscopy, C-cells often have a clear or light appearance; however, variable numbers of membrane-bound secretory granules in which calcitonin is stored can be visualized ultrastructurally. Although the secretory granules of normal C-cells have considerable heterogeneity in terms of size and density, all of the granules have calcitonin immunoreactivity.

C-cell hyperplasia, nodular aggregations of calcitonin-producing C-cells, in dogs should be diagnosed only when there is a definite increase in C-cell numbers throughout each thyroid lobe. Both thyroid lobes should be sectioned longitudinally in a consistent manner for microscopic evaluation, so as to minimize the prominent regional differences of C-cells in the thyroid glands of normal dogs that can result in the overinterpretation of these focal aggregations of C-cells as a significant lesion. C-cells in focal aggregations have an abundant, lightly-eosinophilic, finely-granular cytoplasm, and a spherical-oval nucleus. There are occasional colloid-containing follicles within the focal accumulations of C-cells along the course of vessels within the thyroid lobe, or in the connective tissues of the thyroid hilus in dogs.

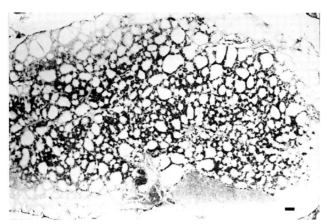

FIGURE 17.19 Diffuse C-cell hyperplasia in a thyroid gland from a 2-year-old male Long-Evans rat stained for calcitonin with the peroxidase-antiperoxidase method. The number of C-cells is increased markedly compared to those in a young rat from the same strain (Fig. 18). Bar: 100μm. From DeLellis et al. (1979), Lab Invest 40: 140–154 with permission.

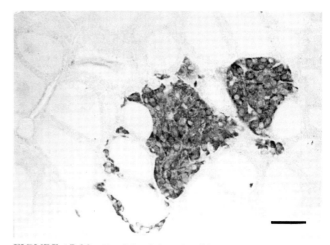

FIGURE 17.20 Focal "nodular" C-cell hyperplasia partially filling a thyroid follicle. Thyroid gland from an old male Long-Evans rat stained for somatostain with the peroxidase-antiperoxidase technique. In serial sections the same proliferating C-cells also stained positive for calcitonin.

Mechanisms of Toxicity

Radiation administered to newborn rats is followed by a striking reduction in the numbers of C-cells. The number of C-cells increases after one year, but their distribution within the gland was often patchy, suggesting a clonal regrowth. Further studies have demonstrated conclusively that the incidence of C-cell tumors increased after irradiation, but high calcium levels in drinking water did not appear to potentiate the carcinogenic effect of irradiation in C-cells. However, it has been noted that a significant increase in C-cell tumor incidence has been associated with excess vitamin D_3. These findings have suggested that vitamin D or one of its metabolites may affect C-cell growth directly. It is known that certain vitamin D metabolites can stimulate calcitonin secretion in vitamin D-deficient pigs.

Response to Injury

Proliferative Lesions of C-cells

Hyperplasia of C-cells is not usually associated with any macroscopic abnormality of the thyroid gland. Two types of C-cell hyperplasia are evident microscopically: diffuse and focal (nodular). In diffuse hyperplasia, the number of C-cells is increased throughout the thyroid lobe, to a point where they may be more numerous than follicular cells (Figure 17.19). The relationship of C-cells to follicular cells in cases of diffuse hyperplasia is similar to that noted in juvenile thyroid glands. Focal (nodular) hyperplasia of C-cells often occurs concurrently with diffuse hyperplasia in the thyroid glands of rats. The follicles

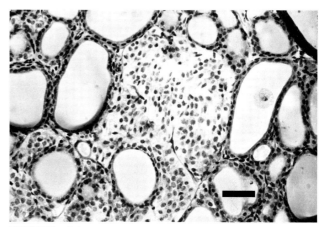

FIGURE 17.21 Focal ("nodular") C-cell hyperplasia in thyroid gland from an old male Long-Evans rat. Bar: 100μm. From DeLellis et al. (1979), Lab Invest 40: 140–154 with permission.

become progressively enlarged with increasing numbers of C-cells. Follicular cells adjacent to the proliferating C-cells are often compressed and atrophic, with prominent supranuclear accumulations of lipofuscin.

At later stages of development, C-cell-filled follicles often assume irregular, twisted, and elongate configurations (Figures 17.20 and 17.21). Occasional colloid-filled follicles are entrapped among the proliferating C-cells. The histologic distinction between focal hyperplasia and adenoma of C-cells is often difficult and somewhat arbitrary. Cell boundaries are often indistinct, and hyperplastic C-cells within the basement membrane may compress individual thyroid follicles.

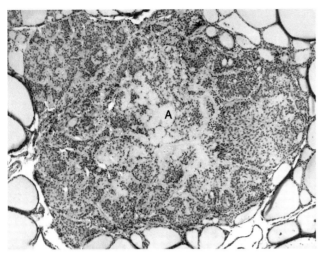

FIGURE 17.22   C-cell adenoma in thyroid gland from a 2-year-old Sprague–Dawley rat. The adenoma is sharply demarcated from the adjacent thyroid follicles that are partially compressed. Amyloid (A) deposits are present within the adenoma.

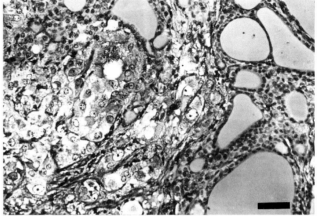

FIGURE 17.23   C-cell carcinoma in thyroid gland from an old male Long-Evans rat with extensive intrathyroidal invasion. Tumor cells have large nuclei, abundant cytoplasm, and resemble ganglion cells. Bar: 100 μm. From DeLellis et al. (1979), Lab Invest 40: 140–154 with permission.

C-cell adenomas are discrete, expansive masses or nodules of C-cells larger than five average colloid-containing thyroid follicles (Figure 17.22). Adenomas are either well circumscribed, or partially encapsulated from adjacent thyroid follicles that often are compressed to varying degrees. C-cells have an abundant cytoplasmic area that stains lightly-eosinophilic, and a round-to-oval nucleus with finely stippled chromatin, and may be subdivided by fine connective tissue septae and capillaries into small neuroendocrine packets. Occasional capillaries are distended considerably with blood. Some C-cell adenomas are composed of larger cells with amphophilic cytoplasm, large nuclei with coarsely clumped chromatin, and prominent nucleoli. These cells bear a histologic resemblance to ganglion cells (Figure 17.23). Occasional amyloid deposits may be found both in nodular hyperplasia and in adenomas.

C-cell carcinomas show evidence of extensive proliferation and infiltration of C-cells, often with macroscopic enlargement of one or both thyroid lobes. There is evidence of intrathyroidal and/or capsular invasion by the proliferating C-cells (Figure 17.23), often with areas of hemorrhage and necrosis within the neoplasm. Malignant C-cells are more pleomorphic (cuboidal, oval, spindle shaped) than those comprising benign proliferative lesions with indistinct boundaries of the lightly-eosinophilic cytoplasmic area and mitotic figures that may be numerous. Amyloid production is consistently associated with medullary thyroid carcinoma in humans, and has also been reported in certain other endocrine tumors. Amyloid in C-cell tumors is present between tumor cells (Figure 17.22), around vessels, and in the interstitium of laboratory rats, dogs, horses, and bulls, but in amounts that vary (minimal to substantial) from case to case.

Spontaneous C-cell Lesions

C-cell proliferative lesions occur commonly in rat strains, but are uncommon in the mouse, where there is a striking correlation between the age of the animal and the presence of the entire spectrum of C-cell proliferative lesions.

THYROID FOLLICULAR CELLS

Structure and Function

Organogenesis

The thyroid gland originates as a thickened plate of epithelium in the floor of the pharynx. It is intimately related to the aortic sac in its development, and this association leads to the frequent occurrence of accessory thyroid parenchyma in the mediastinum. This accessory thyroid tissue may undergo neoplastic transformation as, for example, in the adult dog. The ultimobranchial bodies fuse with the lateral extensions and deliver C-cells (neural crest origin) to each thyroid lobe. A portion of the thyroglossal duct may persist postnatally and form a cyst, due to the accumulation of proteinic material secreted by the lining epithelium.

Thyroglossal duct cysts develop in the ventral aspect of the anterior cervical region. Their lining epithelium may undergo neoplastic transformation and give rise to papillary carcinomas in dogs. Accessory thyroid tissue is common in the dog, and may be located anywhere from the larynx to the diaphragm. About 50% of adult dogs have accessory thyroids embedded in the fat on the intrapericardial aorta. These nodules are usually 1–2 mm in greatest dimension, and may number from one to five. They are completely lacking in C-(parafollicular) cells, which secrete calcitonin, but their follicular structure and function are the same as that of the main thyroid lobes.

Thyroid Histology

The thyroid gland is the largest of the organs that function exclusively as endocrine glands. The basic structure of the thyroid is unique for endocrine glands, consisting of follicles of varying size (20–250 μm) that contain colloid produced by the follicular cells. Follicular cells are cuboidal to columnar, and their secretory polarity is directed toward the lumen of the follicles. An extensive network of inter- and intrafollicular capillaries provides the follicular cells with an abundant blood supply. Follicular cells have long profiles of rough endoplasmic reticulum, and a large Golgi apparatus in their cytoplasm for the synthesis and packaging of substantial amounts of protein that are transported into the follicular lumen. The interface between the lumenal side of follicular cells and the colloid is modified by numerous microvillar projections.

Thyroid Hormone Synthesis

The biosynthesis of thyroid hormones is also unique among endocrine glands, because the final assembly of the hormones occurs extracellularly within the follicular lumen. Essential raw materials, such as iodide, are trapped efficiently by follicular cells from plasma, transported rapidly against a concentration gradient to the lumen, and oxidized by a thyroid peroxidase in microvillar membranes and colloid to iodine (I_2) (Figure 17.24). The assembly of thyroid hormones within the follicular lumen is made possible by thyroglobulin synthesized by follicular cells. Iodine is bound to tyrosyl residues in thyroglobulin at the apical surface of follicular cells to form, successively, monoiodotyrosine (MIT) and diiodotyrosine (DIT) (Figure 17.25). The resulting MIT and DIT combine to form the two biologically-active iodothyronines: thyroxine (T_4) and triiodothyronine (T_3). Other tissues, such as the salivary gland, gastric

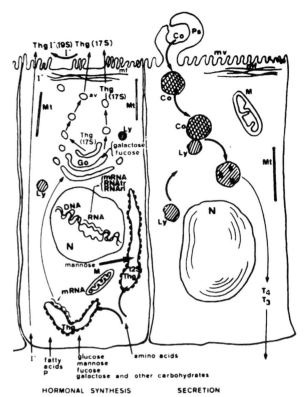

FIGURE 17.24 Normal thyroid follicular cells illustrating two-way traffic of materials from capillaries into the follicular lumen. Raw materials, such as iodine, are concentrated by follicular cells and are transported rapidly into the lumen (left). Amino acids (tyrosine and others) and sugars are assembled by follicular cells into thyroglobulin (thg), packaged into apical vesicles (av), and released into the lumen, iodination of tyrosyl residues occurs within the thyroglobulin molecule to form thyroid hormones in the follicular lumen. Elongation of microvilli and endocytosis of colloid by follicular cells occur in response to TSH stimulation (right). Intracellular colloid droplets (Co) fuse with lysosomal bodies (Ly) and the active thyroid hormone is cleaved enzymatically from thyroglobulin, and free T_4 and T_3 are released into circulation. From Bastenie et al. (1975), In: Molecular Pathology (R.A. Good, ed.), Charles C. Thomas, Springfield, pp. 243–261 with permission.

mucosa, and lactating mammary gland, also have the capacity to actively transport iodide, albeit at a much lower level than the thyroid.

Species Differences in Thyroid Hormone Economy

Long-term perturbations of the pituitary–thyroid axis by various xenobiotics or physiologic alterations, such as iodine deficiency, partial thyroidectomy, and natural goitrogens in food, are more likely to predispose the laboratory rat to a higher incidence of proliferative lesions, e.g., hyperplasia and adenomas of cells, in response to chronic TSH stimulation than in the human thyroid. This is particularly true in the male rat, which has higher circulating levels of TSH than female rats. The greater sensitivity of the rodent

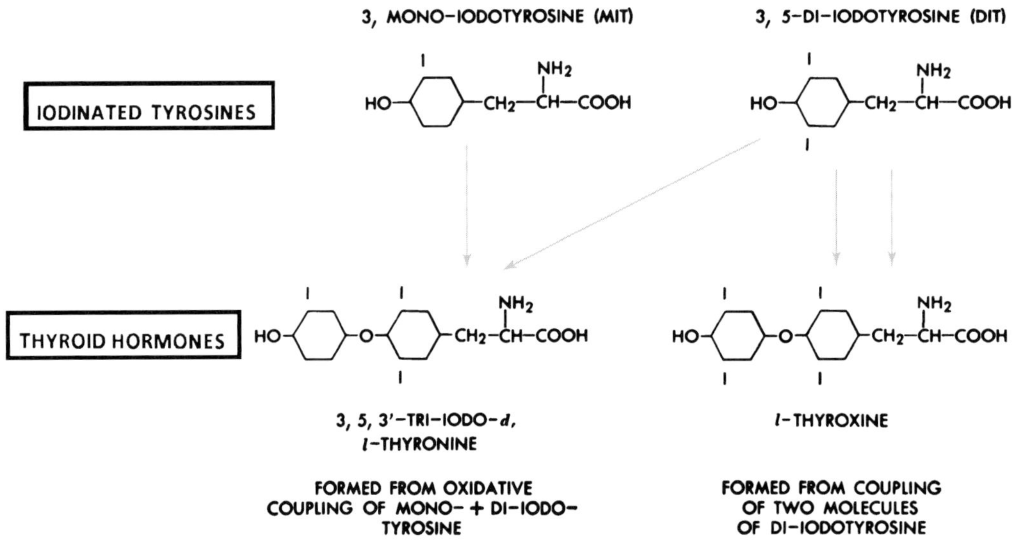

FIGURE 17.25   Formation of thyroid hormones (3,5,3'-triiodothyronine,l-thyroxine) from iodinated tyrosines (MIT and DIT) within the follicular lumen of the thyroid gland. From Capen and Martin (1989), Toxicol Pathol 17:266–293 with permission.

thyroid to derangement by drugs, chemicals, and physiologic perturbations is also related to the shorter plasma half-life of T_4 than in man, due to the considerable differences between species in the transport proteins for thyroid hormones.

In human beings and monkeys, circulating T_4 is bound primarily to thyroxine-binding globulin (TBG), but this high-affinity binding protein is not present in rodents, birds, amphibians, or fish (Table 17.4). The percentage of unbound active T_4 is lower in species with high levels of TBG than in animals in which T_4 binding is limited to albumin and prealbumin. Therefore, a rat without a functional thyroid requires about 10 times more T_4 for full substitution than an adult human. Triiodothyronine is transported bound to TBG and albumin in human beings, monkey, and dog, but only to albumin in mouse, rat, and chicken (Table 17.5).

Thyroid Hormone Secretion

The elongation of microvilli and the formation of pseudopods on follicular cells initiate the secretion of thyroid hormones from stores within lumenal colloid, and are increased by pituitary TSH. They extend into the follicular lumen and indiscriminatingly phagocytize a portion of adjacent colloid by endocytosis (Figure 17.26). Colloid droplets within follicular cells fuse with numerous lysosomal bodies that contain proteolytic enzymes and release thyroxine and triiodothyronine, which diffuse out of the follicular cells and enter interfollicular capillaries. Iodinated tyrosines (monoiodotyrosine (MIT) and diiodotyrosine

TABLE 17.4   Thyroxine (T_4) binding to serum proteins in selected vertebrate species[a,b]

Species	T_4-binding globulin	Postalbumin	Albumin	Prealbumin
Human	++	−	++	+
Monkey	++	−	++	+
Dog	+	−	++	−
Mouse	−	++	++	−
Rat	−	+	++	+
Chicken	−	−	++	−

[a]Modified from Döhler et al. (1979) Pharmacol Ther 5:305–318
[b]Degree of T_4 binding to serum proteins: + or + + . Absence of binding of T_4 to serum protein: −

TABLE 17.5   Triiodothyronine (T_3) binding to serum proteins in selected vertebrate species[a,b]

Species	T_3-binding globulin	Postalbumin	Albumin	Prealbumin
Human	+	−	+	−
Monkey	+	−	+	−
Dog	+	−	+	−
Mouse	−	+	+	−
Rat	−	−	+	−
Chicken	−	−	+	−

[a]Modified from Döhler et al. (1979) Pharmacol Ther 5:305–318
[b]Degree of T_3 binding to serum proteins: + or + + . Absence of binding of T_3 to serum protein: −

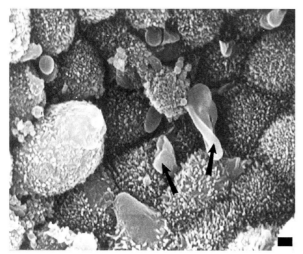

FIGURE 17.26 Scanning electron micrograph of the lumenal surface of thyroid follicular cells following TSH stimulation. Note the numerous expanded cytoplasmic processes (arrow) extending into the follicular lumen. Bar: 1μm. From Capen and Martin (1989), Toxicol Pathol 17:266–293 with permission.

(DIT)) released from the colloid droplets are deiodinated enzymatically, and the iodide generated under normal conditions is either recycled to the lumen to iodinate new tyrosyl residues in thyroglobulin, or is released into the circulation.

Negative feedback control of thyroid hormone secretion is accomplished by the coordinated response of the adenohypophysis and certain hypothalamic nuclei to circulating and local tissue levels of T_3. In the rat, 50% or more of the pituitary content of T_3 is generated locally from circulating T_4 by a 5'-deiodinase (type II). A decrease in thyroid hormone concentration in plasma is sensed by groups of neurosecretory neurons in the hypothalamus that synthesize and secrete thyrotropin-releasing hormone into the hypophyseal portal circulation. This hormone binds to isoreceptors on the plasma membrane of thyrotrophic basophils in the adenohypophysis, and activates adenylate cyclase resulting in the formation of cyclic AMP. Intracellular accumulation of cyclic AMP in thyrotrophic basophils results in an inflow of calcium ions that leads to the contraction of microfilaments and peripheral movement, and the discharge of TSH-containing secretion granules into pituitary capillaries. Thyroid-stimulating hormone is conveyed to thyroid follicular cells where it binds to the basilar aspect of the cell, activates adenylate cyclase, and increases the rate of the biochemical reactions involved in the synthesis and secretion of thyroid hormones.

One of the initial responses by follicular cells to TSH is the formation of numerous cytoplasmic pseudopodia, resulting in the increased endocytosis of colloid and the release of preformed hormone stored within the follicular lumen (Figure 17.26). If the secretion of TSH is sustained for hours or days, thyroid follicular cells become more columnar and follicular lumens become smaller, due to the increased endocytosis of colloid.

Numerous PAS-positive colloid droplets are present in the lumenal aspect of the hypertrophied follicular cells. Conversely, in response to an increase in circulating levels of thyroid hormones, there is a corresponding decrease in circulating pituitary TSH. Thyroid follicles become enlarged and distended with colloid, due to the decreased TSH-mediated endocytosis of colloid. Follicular cells lining the involuted follicles are low cuboidal and have few endocytic vacuoles at the interface with the colloid.

Thyroid hormones are degraded primarily by conjugation with glucuronic acid in the liver. A wide variety of drugs and chemicals can influence thyroid hormone metabolism by inducing one or more classes of hepatic microsomal enzymes that increase the degradation of thyroid hormones. Chemicals such as FD&C Red No. 3 (erythrosine) and amiodarone disrupt thyroid hormone metabolism by inhibiting the 5'-deiodinase in liver (type I enzyme), thereby inhibiting the conversion of T_4 to T_3, thus resulting in increased circulating levels of TSH that leads to the development of follicular cell hyperplasia (goiter), and predisposes to a greater incidence of thyroid tumors.

In dog plasma, T_4 is bound to albumin and three globulin fractions, and T_3 is bound to albumin and one globulin fraction, but the overall binding affinity of the plasma proteins for T_4 is lower in dogs than in humans. Most importantly, the affinity of the canine inter-α-globulin fraction for T_4 is much less than that of the human thyroxine-binding globulin (TBG). As a result of this weaker binding, as well as an efficient enterohepatic excretory mechanism, total T_4 concentration is lower, and thyroid hormone turnover is more rapid in dogs than in humans. The ratio of T_4 to T_3 in canine plasma is about 20:1, even though they are produced by the thyroid at a ratio of about 2:1. The peak concentration T_3 and T_4 usually occurs at about midday and the minimum at about midnight. Both the overall rates of turnover and the loss of hormone in the feces are much higher in dogs than in humans. Fecal wastage substantially reduces the efficiency of hormone utilization, but also explains the remarkable tolerance of the dog for excess thyroid hormone.

Biological Action

The overall effects of thyroid hormones are to: increase the basal metabolic rate; increase the availability to meet the elevated metabolic demands by increasing glycolysis, gluconeogenesis, and glucose absorption from the intestine; stimulate new protein synthesis; increase lipid metabolism and conversion of cholesterol into bile acids and other substances, activate lipoprotein lipase, and increase the sensitivity of adipose tissue to lipolysis by other hormones; stimulate the heart rate, cardiac output, and blood flow; and increase neural transmission, cerebration, and neuronal development in young animals. The overall functions of T_4 and T_3 are similar, although much of the biological activity is the result of monodeiodination of T_4 prior to interaction with target cells (Figure 17.27). Under certain conditions, such as in protein starvation, neonatal animals, liver and kidney disease, and febrile illness, thyroxine is preferentially monodeiodinated to 3,3',5'-triiodothyronine (reverse T_3) (Figure 17.28). Because this form of T_3 is biologically inactive, monodeiodination to reverse T_3 provides a mechanism to attenuate the metabolic effects of thyroid hormones. Certain xenobiotics selectively block 5'-deiodinase, resulting in the conversion of most of T_4 to reverse T_3, leading to subnormal T_3 and a compensatory increase in TSH secretion by the pituitary gland to form T_3.

The administration of thyroxine will increase the heart rate by a direct effect on heart muscle cells. Normal function of the central nervous system (CNS) is dependent on the normal output of thyroxine. During periods of deficient thyroxine levels, the central nervous system fails to function in the normal fashion and the animal is lethargic, dull, and mentally deficient. Myelin in the fiber tracts is decreased, cortical neurons are smaller and fewer, and vascularity of the CNS is reduced.

The neurons are permanently damaged by a deficiency of thyroid hormones in a young growing animal fed a severely iodine-deficient diet. However, an excess of thyroid hormone production, as occurs in a hyperthyroid animal or human patient, stimulates CNS activity to the extent that the animal is nervous, irritable, and hyperactive. The subcellular mechanism of action of thyroid hormones resembles that of steroid hormones, because free hormone enters into target cells and binds to a cytosol-binding protein (Figure 17.27).

Mechanisms of Toxicity

Direct Thyroid Effect

Inhibitors of Thyroid Hormone Synthesis

Blockage of iodine uptake. A number of anions act as competitive inhibitors of iodide transport, e.g., perchlorate (ClO_4), thiocyanate (SCN-), and pertechnetate (Figure 17.29). Blockage of the iodide-trapping mechanism has a disruptive effect on the thyroid–pituitary

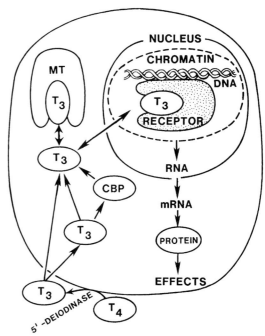

FIGURE 17.27 Subcellular mechanism of action of thyroid hormones in target cells. Primarily free triiodothyronine (T_3) enters target cells, as most thyroxine (T_4) undergoes monodeiodination in the liver or elsewhere in the periphery to form T_3. Free cytosolic T_3 binds to cytosolic-binding proteins (CBP), to high-affinity receptors on the inner mitochondrial (MT) membrane and activates oxidative phosphorylation, or to nuclear receptors in target cells. In the nucleus, T_3 increases the transcription of mRNA, which returns to the cytoplasm to direct the synthesis of new proteins. The increased synthesis of new proteins (structural or enzyme) carries out the multiple biologic effects of the thyroid hormones. From Capen and Martin (1989), Toxicol Pathol 17:266–293 with permission.

axis similar to the effect of iodine deficiency. The blood levels of T_4 and T_3 decrease, resulting in a compensatory increase in the secretion of TSH by the pituitary gland. The hypertrophy and hyperplasia of follicular cells following sustained exposure result in an increased thyroid weight and the development of goiter.

Inhibition of thyroid peroxidase. A wide variety of chemicals, drugs, and other xenobiotics affect the second step in thyroid hormone biosynthesis (Figure 17.29). Classes of chemicals that inhibit the organification of thyroglobulin include thionamides such as thiourea, thiouracil, propylthiouracil, methimazole, carbimazole, and goitrin; aniline derivatives and related compounds such as sulfonamides, p-aminobenzoic acid, p-aminosalicylic acid, and amphenone; substituted phenols such as resorcinol, phloroglucinol, and 2,4-dihydroxybenzoic acid; and miscellaneous inhibitors such as aminotriazole, tricyanoaminopropene, and antipyrine and its iodinated derivative, iodopyrine.

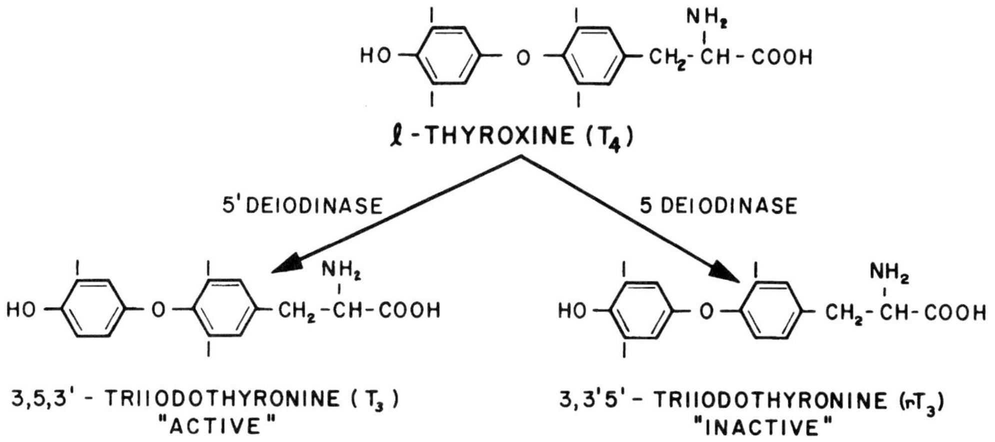

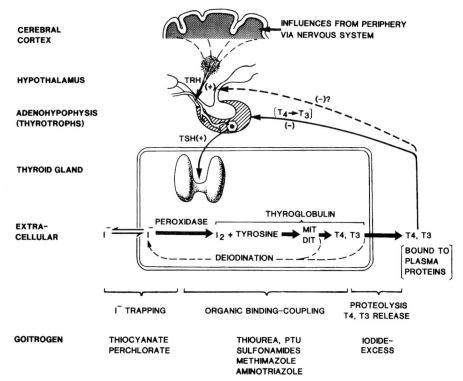

FIGURE 17.28 Monodeiodination of thyroxine to form either active T_3 (left) or inactive (reverse) rT_3 (right) depending on the need for the metabolic actions of thyroid hormone. From Capen and Martin (1989), Toxicol Pathol 17:266–293 with permission.

FIGURE 17.29 Mechanism of action of goitrogenic chemicals on thyroid hormone synthesis and secretion. Goitrogens affect iodide trapping, organic binding-coupling, or proteolysis of colloid and release of T_4 and T_3. From Capen and Martin (1989), Toxicol Pathol 17:266–293 with permission.

Many of these chemicals exert their action by inhibiting thyroid peroxidase, which results in a disruption both of the iodination of tyrosyl residues in thyroglobulin and of the coupling reaction of iodotyrosines to form iodothyronines—T_3 and T_4. It is not surprising that the sensitive species (e.g., rat, mouse, and dog) are much more likely to develop follicular cell hyperplasia and thyroid tumors after long-term exposure to sulfonamides than resistant species (e.g., nonhuman primate, human, guinea pig, and chicken).

Inhibitors of Thyroid Hormone Secretion

Blockage of thyroid hormone release by excess iodide and lithium. Relatively few chemicals selectively inhibit the secretion of thyroid hormone from the thyroid gland (Figure 17.29). An excess of iodine inhibits the secretion of the thyroid hormone, and occasionally can result in goiter and hypothyroidism in animals and human patients. High doses of iodide have been used therapeutically in the treatment of patients with hyperthyroidism, to lower circulating levels of thyroid hormones.

Several mechanisms have been suggested for this effect of high iodide levels on thyroid hormone secretion, including a decrease in lysosomal protease activity (human glands), inhibition of colloid droplet formation (mice and rats), and inhibition of TSH-mediated increase in cAMP (dog thyroid slices).

Xenobiotic- (or Metabolite-) Induced Thyroid Pigmentation or Colloid Alteration

The antibiotic minocycline produces a striking black discoloration of thyroid lobes in laboratory animals and humans with the formation of brown pigment granules within follicular cells, and administration of the antibiotic at a high dose to rats for extended periods may result in a disruption of thyroid function and the development of thyroid enlargement or goiter. The pigment granules stain similarly to melanin, and are best visualized on thyroid sections stained with the Fontana–Masson procedure. Electron-dense material first accumulates in lysosome-like granules and in the rough endoplasmic reticulum.

Brown to black pigment granules may be present in follicular cells, colloid, and macrophages in the inter-thyroidal tissues, resulting in a macroscopic darkening of both thyroid lobes. Serum T_4 and T_3 are decreased, serum TSH levels are increased by an expanded population of pituitary thyrotrophs, and thyroid follicular cells undergo hypertrophy and hyperplasia. Similar thyroid changes or functional alterations usually do not occur in dogs, monkeys, or humans.

Inducers of Hepatic Microsomal Enzymes

Hepatic microsomal enzymes play an important role in thyroid hormone economy, because glucuronidation is the rate-limiting step in the biliary excretion of T_4, and sulfation by phenol sulfotransferase is the rate-limiting step in the excretion of T_3. Long-term exposure of rats to a wide variety of different chemicals induces these enzyme pathways, and results in chronic stimulation of the thyroid by disrupting the hypothalamic–pituitary–thyroid axis. Xenobiotics that induce liver microsomal enzymes and disrupt thyroid function in rats include central nervous system drugs, e.g., phenobarbital, benzodiazepines; calcium channel blockers, e.g., nicardipine, bepridil; steroids, e.g., spironolactone; retinoids; chlorinated hydrocarbons, e.g., chlordane, DDT, TCDD; and polyhalogenated biphenyls, e.g., PCB, PBB.

Secondary Mechanisms of Thyroid Oncogenesis

Understanding the mechanism of action of xeno-biotics on the thyroid gland provides a more rational basis to extrapolate findings, from long-term rodent studies to safety assessment of a particular compound for humans. Many chemicals and drugs disrupt one or more steps in the synthesis, secretion, and peripheral metabolism of thyroid hormones, resulting in subnormal levels of T_4 and T_3, associated with a compensatory increased secretion of pituitary TSH (Figure 17.30). When tested in highly-sensitive species, such as rats and mice, these compounds result early in follicular cell hypertrophy/hyperplasia, and increased thyroid weight, and in long-term studies an increased incidence of thyroid tumors by a secondary (indirect) mechanism. In the secondary mechanism of thyroid oncogenesis in rodents, the specific xenobiotic chemical or physiologic perturbation evokes another stimulus, e.g., chronic hypersecretion of TSH, which initially promotes hypertrophy and hyperplasia, and subsequently the development of follicular adenomas and infrequently carcinomas.

The relative resistance to the development of thyroid cancer in humans with elevated plasma TSH levels is in marked contrast to the response of the thyroid gland to chronic TSH stimulation in rats and mice. The human thyroid is much less sensitive to this pathogenetic phenomenon than rodents, so prolonged stimulation of the human thyroid by TSH will induce neoplasia only in exceptional circumstances, and possibly acting together with some other metabolic or immunologic abnormality.

Response to Injury

Histopathological Criteria of Proliferative Lesions

Follicular Cystic Hyperplasia

Follicular cystic hyperplasia is a nodule, or nodules, in the thyroid formed by the coalescence of adjacent colloid-distended follicles. The follicular wall is lined by 1–2 layers of low cuboidal epithelium with hyperchromatic nuclei that occasionally form papillary projections (Figure 17.31). Adjacent thyroid follicles are normal, with minimal evidence of compression and no encapsulation by fibrous connective tissue.

Focal or Multifocal Hyperplasia of Follicular Cells

Focal or multifocal areas of hyperplasia of thyroid follicular cells usually only enlarge the affected lobe slightly. The areas of focal hyperplasia are not encapsulated, and the adjacent thyroid parenchyma is not compressed. Hyperplastic nodules are composed of irregularly-shaped, usually colloid-filled follicles, lined by more basophilic cuboidal follicular cells. The multiple nodules of follicular cell hyperplasia may coalesce to form macroscopically-observable thyroid

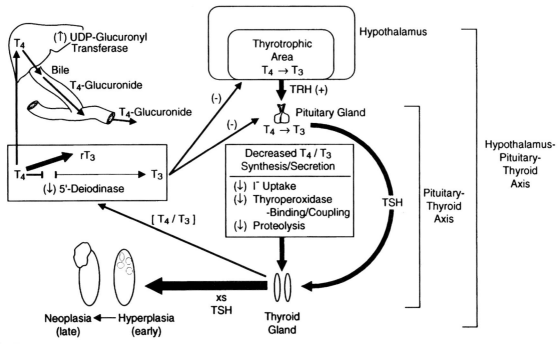

FIGURE 17.30 Multiple sites of disruption of hypothalamic-pituitary-thyroid triad by xenobiotic chemicals. Chemicals can exert direct effects by disrupting thyroid hormone synthesis or secretion and indirectly influence the thyroid through an inhibition of 5′-deiodinase or by inducing hepatic microsomal enzymes (e.g., T_4-UDP glucuronyl transferase). All of these mechanisms can lower the circulating levels of thyroid hormones (T_4 and T_3), resulting in a release from negative feedback inhibition and a compensatory increased secretion of TSH by the pituitary gland. The chronic hypersecretion of TSH predisposes the sensitive rodent thyroid gland to develop an increased incidence of focal hyperplastic and neoplastic (adenomas) lesions by a secondary (epigenetic) mechanism.

adenomas. Focal hyperplasia is different from the diffuse (TSH-mediated) type of follicular cell hyperplasia observed with iodine deficiency and also with a wide variety of xenobiotic drugs and chemicals that disrupt thyroid hormone economy to result in an increased secretion of TSH.

Follicular Cell Adenoma

An adenoma is a well-circumscribed, usually solitary, benign tumor formed by the autonomous proliferation of follicular cells within the thyroid lobe (Figure 17.32). Adjacent thyroid follicles are compressed to varying degrees, depending on the size of the adenoma. Adenomas usually do not have a complete fibrous capsule, but larger adenomas may be partially encapsulated by a thin layer of fibrous connective tissue. Neoplastic cells are often more hyperchromatic than the surrounding normal follicular cells, and form variably sized colloid-containing follicles, line large cystic spaces, or form solid sheets. Neoplastic cells may form papillary structures extending into larger cysts, with cells varying from cuboidal to low columnar; the nucleus to cytoplasm ratio is often high. There is no evidence of vascular invasion. Endocrinologically-active thyroid adenomas result in the colloid involution of follicles in the rim of the

surrounding thyroid, due to the inhibition of TSH secretion by elevated blood T_4 and T_3 levels.

Follicular Cell Carcinoma

A carcinoma is an extensive proliferation of neoplastic follicular cells with evidence of intrathyroidal, capsular, or vascular invasion that often enlarges the affected thyroid lobe considerably. Malignant follicular cells form colloid-containing follicles of varying size, papillary projections extending into cystic spaces, or solid sheets of cells. The cells are pleomorphic, and nuclei are hyperchromatic with occasional mitotic figures. A prominent desmoplastic reaction often accompanies the infiltration of neoplastic cells into the thyroid capsule. The perithyroidal connective tissue, as well as adjacent trachea and cervical muscles, may be invaded by larger carcinomas (Figure 17.33).

Disorders of Thyroid Function

Hypothyroidism

Hypothyroidism is a well-recognized clinical entity in dogs and occurs in many purebred and mixed breed dogs. Doberman pinschers, golden retrievers, beagles, and Irish setters, appear to be more commonly affected. Hypothyroidism may also develop

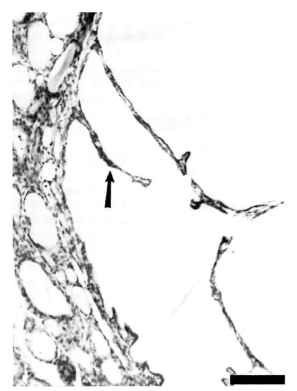

FIGURE 17.31   Follicular cystic hyperplasia in a male Sprague–Dawley rat exposed to FD&C Red No. 3 *in utero* and fed at the 4% level for a lifetime of 30 months. There is a coalescence of adjacent colloid-distended follicles that are lined by cuboidal epithelium with hyperchromatic nuclei with occasional papillary projections into the cyst (arrow). Adjacent thyroid follicles are only minimally compressed and there is no evidence of encapsulation. Bar: 100μm. From Capen (1983), with permission.

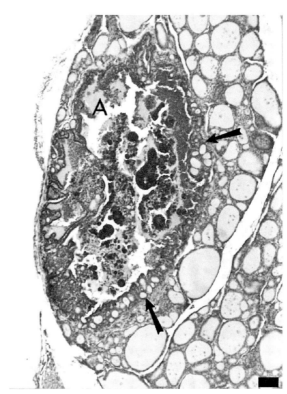

FIGURE 17.32   Thyroid follicular cell adenoma (A) in a male Sprague–Dawley rat exposed to FD&C Red No. 3 *in utero* and fed at the 4% level for the lifetime of 30 months. The adenoma is well circumscribed (arrows) and adjacent follicles are slightly compressed. Hyperchromatic neoplastic cells line a cystic space and form papillary projections into the lumen. Bar: 100μm. From Capen (1983), with permission.

secondary to long-standing pituitary or hypothalamic lesions that prevent the release of either TSH or thyrotropin-releasing hormone. Subnormal function of the thyroid is recognized less frequently as a naturally-occurring entity in other animal species. However, a large number of drugs, chemicals, dietary deficiencies, or excesses can disrupt one or more steps of thyroid hormone biosynthesis, secretion, metabolism, or degradation and result in subnormal blood levels of thyroid hormones (see Figure 17.29).

Hypothyroidism is often the result of primary diseases of the thyroid gland, especially idiopathic follicular atrophy and immune-mediated lymphocytic thyroiditis. In follicular atrophy there is a progressive loss of follicular epithelium, and replacement by adipose connective tissue with a minimal inflammatory response. The remaining follicles are small, lined by columnar follicular cells, and contain small amounts of irregularly clumped colloid. Nests of unaffected thyroid C-cells are present in the thyroid gland, especially near the hilus.

Hypertrophy and hyperplasia of TSH-secreting basophils occur in the *pars distalis* of dogs with follicular

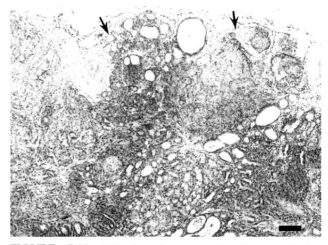

FIGURE 17.33   Follicular cell carcinoma in a Sprague–Dawley rat with capsular invasion and growth of neoplastic cells in the perithyroidal connective tissues (arrows). Tumor cells form follicles of varying size and colloid content plus solid areas. Hematoxylin and eosin. Bar: 100μm.

atrophy and hypothyroidism. Lymphocytic thyroiditis in dogs, Buffalo rats, OS strain of chickens, and marmoset monkeys resembles Hashimoto's disease in humans, and appears to be genetically conditioned, at least in certain breeds. Although the exact mechanism in the dog is not well-established, evidence suggests a polygenic pattern of inheritance similar to that observed in the human disease. The immunological basis for the development of chronic lymphocytic thyroiditis in both humans and dogs appears to be through the production of autoantibodies directed against thyroglobulin, a microsomal (thyroid peroxidase) antigen, TSH receptor protein, nuclear antigen, and a second colloid antigen. Histopathological alterations in the thyroid glands consist of either a diffuse or a nodular infiltration of lymphocytes, plasma cells, and macrophages. Many of the remaining thyroid follicles are small and lined by tall columnar follicular cells, reflecting the long-standing stimulation by TSH in an attempt to compensate for the low blood levels of thyroid hormones. Ultrastructurally, numerous lymphocytes and macrophages are observed within the follicular basement membrane extending between follicular cells into the lumina of follicles.

Hyperthyroidism

Hyperthyroidism is uncommon in animals, except in adult to aged cats. Follicular cell adenomas, often developing in a thyroid with multinodular hyperplasia, are encountered more commonly than malignant thyroid tumors. Neoplastic cells release both T_4 and T_3 at an uncontrolled rate, resulting in markedly elevated blood levels of both hormones. Follicles in the rim of the thyroid around a functional adenoma are enlarged markedly, and distended by the accumulation of colloid with low cuboidal and atrophic follicles with little endocytotic activity in response to the elevated levels of thyroid hormones. Thyroid tumors in the dog only occasionally secrete sufficient thyroid hormone to produce clinical signs of hyperthyroidism. The likelihood of developing clinical hyperthyroidism associated with thyroid neoplasms in animals depends on the capability of tumor cells to synthesize T_4 and T_3, and the degree of elevation of circulating levels of T_4 and T_3, which depends on a balance between the rate of secretion of thyroid hormones by the tumor and the rate of degradation of thyroid hormones.

Hyperplasia of Follicular Cells ("Goiter")

Mechanisms of goitrogenesis. Non-neoplastic and non-inflammatory enlargement of the thyroid, called goiter, develops in all laboratory animals, domestic mammals, birds, and submammalian vertebrates. Certain forms of thyroid hyperplasia, especially nodular, may be difficult to differentiate from adenomas. The major pathogenic mechanisms responsible for the development of thyroid hyperplasia include iodine-deficient diets, goitrogenic compounds that interfere

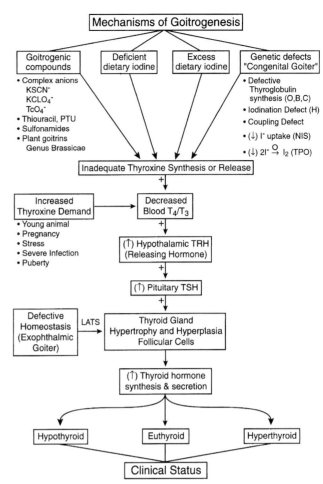

FIGURE 17.34 Mechanisms of goitrogenesis. Multiple pathogenic factors (goitrogenic compounds, deficient and excess dietary iodine intake, and genetic enzyme defects) result in inadequate thyroxine (T_4)/triiodothyronine (T_3) synthesis and lead to the long-term stimulation of thyroid follicular cells by an increased secretion of pituitary TSH. LATS (long-acting thyroid stimulator) is an autoantibody that directly stimulates follicular cells by binding to the TSH receptor on follicular cells of the human thyroid gland.

with thyroxinogenesis, dietary iodide excess, and genetic enzyme defects in the biosynthesis of thyroid hormones (Figure 17.34). All of these seemingly divergent factors result in inadequate T_4 and T_3 synthesis, and decreased blood levels of thyroid hormones.

Diffuse hyperplastic (iodine-deficient) goiter. Iodine deficiency in the diet resulting in diffuse thyroid hyperplasia was common in many goitrogenic areas throughout the world before the widespread addition of iodized salt to animal diets. Presently, marginal iodine-deficient diets containing certain goitrogenic compounds, such as thiouracil, sulfonamides, anions of the Hofmeister series, and a number of plants from the genus Brassica, result in thyroid follicular cell hyperplasia and clinical evidence of goiter with hypothyroidism. These goitrogenic substances include those shown in Figure 17.29.

Both lateral lobes of the thyroid are enlarged uniformly in animals with diffuse hyperplastic goiter. Enlargements may be extensive and result in palpable swelling in the cranial cervical area, and the affected lobes are firm and dark red, because an extensive interfollicular capillary network develops under the influence of long-term TSH stimulation. The thyroid enlargements are the result of intense hypertrophy and hyperplasia of follicular cells, often with the formation of papillary projections into the lumens of follicles or multiple layers of cells lining follicles. Endocytosis of colloid usually proceeds at a rate greater than synthesis, resulting in the progressive depletion of colloid.

Under long-standing TSH stimulation, thyroid follicles become smaller than normal, and there may be a partial collapse of follicles due to the lack of colloid. Hypertrophic-lining follicular cells are columnar with a deeply eosinophilic cytoplasm and small hyperchromatic nuclei that are often situated in the basilar part of the cell. Either single or multiple layers of hyperplastic follicular cells that, in some follicles, form papillary projections into the lumen, line the follicles. Similar proliferative changes are present in ectopic thyroid parenchyma in the neck and mediastinum.

Colloid goiter. Colloid goiter represents the involutional phase of diffuse hyperplastic goiter in young adults. The markedly hyperplastic follicular cells continue to produce colloid, but the endocytosis of colloid is decreased, due to diminished pituitary TSH secretion in response to the return of blood T_4 and T_3 to the normal range. Both thyroid lobes are enlarged diffusely, but are more translucent and lighter in color than with hyperplastic goiter. The differences in macroscopic appearance are the result of less vascularity in colloid goiter and the development of macrofollicles distended with colloid. Colloid goiter may develop either after sufficient amounts of iodide have been added to the diet, or after the requirements for T_4 have diminished in an older animal. Blood thyroid hormone levels return to the normal range, and the secretion of TSH by the pituitary gland is decreased correspondingly. Follicles are progressively distended with densely eosinophilic colloid, due to diminished TSH-induced endocytosis. Follicular cells lining the macrofollicles are flattened and atrophic. The interface between the colloid and the lumenal surface of follicular cells is smooth, and lacks the characteristic endocytic vacuoles of actively secreting follicular cells. Some involuted follicles in colloid goiter have remnants of the papillary projections of follicular cells extending into their lumen.

The changes in diffuse hyperplastic and colloid goiters are consistent throughout the diffusely enlarged thyroid lobes.

Iodide-excess goiter. Although seemingly paradoxical, an excess of iodide in the diet can also result in thyroid hyperplasia in animals and humans. The thyroid glands of the young are exposed to higher blood iodide levels than those of the dam, because of the concentration of iodide; first by the placenta and subsequently by the mammary gland. High blood iodide interferes with one or more steps of thyroxinogenesis, leading to lowered blood thyroid hormone levels and a compensatory increase in pituitary TSH secretion. Excess iodide appears primarily to block the release of T_3 and T_4 from thyroglobulin, by interfering with the proteolysis of colloid by lysosomes.

Nodular goiter. Multinodular hyperplasia, or goiter, in thyroid glands of old animals appears as white-to-tan nodules of varying sizes in one or both lobes. The affected lobes are moderately enlarged and irregular in contour. Nodular goiter in most animals, except cats, is endocrinologically inactive, and encountered as an incidental lesion at necropsy. However, thyroid hormone-secreting adenomas in old cats with hyperthyroidism often develop in a gland with multinodular hyperplasia.

Nodular goiter consists of multiple loci of hyperplastic follicular cells that are sharply demarcated from the adjacent thyroid parenchyma, but are not encapsulated, and result in minimal compression of adjacent parenchyma. Some hyperplastic cells form small follicles with little or no colloid. Other nodules are formed by larger irregularly-shaped follicles lined by one or more layers of columnar cells that form papillary projections into the lumen. These changes appear to be the result of alternating periods of hyperplasia and colloid involution in the thyroid glands of old animals. The areas of nodular hyperplasia may be microscopic or grossly visible, causing modest enlargement of the thyroid.

Congenital (dyshormonogenetic) goiter. An inability to synthesize and secrete adequate amounts of thyroid hormones beginning before or at birth has been documented in several animal species, and in human infants. The more prevalent forms of inherited goiter in humans include defects in the iodination of tyrosines, deiodination of iodotyrosines, synthesis and proteolysis of thyroglobulin, coupling of iodotyrosines to form iodothyronines, and transport of iodide from the blood to the follicular lumen.

A congenital dyshormonogenetic goiter in animals, as inherited by an autosomal recessive gene, has been documented in sheep (Corriedale, Dorset Horn, Merino, and Romney breeds), Afrikander cattle, and Saanen dwarf goats. Thyroid glands are symmetrically enlarged at birth, due to an intense diffuse hyperplasia of follicular cells. Tall columnar cells line thyroid follicles, but they often have collapsed because of lack of colloid resulting from the marked endocytotic activity. Numerous long microvilli extend into the follicular lumen. The lack of thyroglobulin in the most common form of congenital goiter in animals appears to be due to a defect in thyroglobulin mRNA, leading to aberrant processing of primary transcripts or aberrant transport of the mRNA from the nucleus to the endoplasmic reticulum.

Evaluation of Toxicity

Thyroid Function Tests

Thyroid Hormones

The most sensitive and accurate method for measuring blood T_4 and T_3 levels is radioimmunoassay (RIA). The advantages of measuring free T_4 over total T_4 include a higher correlation with thyroid secretory function, less overlap of hypothyroid and euthyroid levels, and slower decrease with nonthyroidal illness. The range of values given for serum T_4, T_3, and reverse T_3 should be considered only as general guidelines.

Thyroid-stimulating Hormone

Thyroid-stimulating hormone—TSH or thyrotropin—is a glycoprotein synthesized by thyrotrophic basophils in the adenohypophysis. The hormone circulates primarily in the free (unbound) form, and has a short plasma half-life. In the evaluation of potential thyroid toxicity of various xenobiotics, an accurate quantitation of circulating levels of TSH is essential, in order to determine whether proliferative lesions of follicular cells are mediated by a chronic hypersecretion of TSH. Xenobiotics that disrupt thyroid hormone synthesis, secretion, or peripheral metabolism often result in prompt increases in circulating TSH levels.

Morphologic and Morphometric Evaluation of Thyroid

Morphologic and morphometric evaluations of the follicular cells are sensitive indicators of potential toxic effects of xenobiotics on the thyroid gland. Fixation of the thyroid lobes attached to the adjacent trachea in buffered formalin is the best procedure for routine studies. After 24 hours of fixation, each thyroid lobe is dissected carefully from the perithyroidal connective tissue, preferably by one person, blotted gently with filter paper, and weighed individually. The combined weight of the right and left thyroid lobes can be expressed as a ratio to total body or brain weight.

Changes in thyroid weight are a sensitive overall indicator of the effects of relatively mild goitrogenic chemicals on thyroid structure. Bouin's fixation of thyroid tissue, plus staining with the periodic acid-Schiff procedure, are useful when high quality photomicrographs are required to document a particular histologic change. Immunohistochemical procedures are particularly helpful with selected proliferative lesions to determine whether they are of follicular cell (thyroglobulin-positive) or C-cell (calcitonin-positive) origin.

Morphometric evaluation of thyroids is a valuable adjunct to histopathologic evaluation and determination of thyroid weights to detect and quantitate subtle changes in follicular cells. Ultrastructural evaluation of thyroids of selected animals from control and experimental groups is often helpful in documenting early or subtle changes induced by xenobiotics. Rapid fixation of thyroid tissue is essential, due to the high concentration of lysosomal enzymes in follicular cells.

Histologic examination of a biopsy of the thyroid is a useful and reliable aid in the diagnosis of thyroid disease in larger animals when either the results of serum assays for T_4 and T_3 are equivocal, or a nodule is palpated in the thyroid area. Removal of the caudal quarter of either lobe of the thyroid for histologic examination is a simple surgical procedure without significant risk.

Hematology

A moderate normocytic normochromic anemia is often associated with subnormal function of the thyroid in dogs. This anemia has also been observed in humans and in experimental animals, and is known to be of a non-regenerative type. The stained blood smear characteristically has little or no evidence of active erythrogenesis such as anisocytosis, polychromasia, or nucleated red cells. Leptocytosis may be especially prominent. The hemogram is characteristic of anemia associated with a variety of chronic diseases, including neoplasia and chronic infection.

PARATHYROID GLAND

Introduction

Phylogenetically, parathyroids first appear in amphibians, coincident with the transition from an aquatic to a terrestrial life. Since the calcium ion plays a key role in many fundamental biological processes, the precise control of calcium ions in extracellular fluids is vital to the health of humans and animals. To maintain a constant concentration of calcium, endocrine control mechanisms primarily consist of the interaction of parathyroid hormone (PTH), calcitonin, and vitamin D.

Structure and Function

Embryology and Macroscopic Anatomy

Parathyroid glands in most animal species consist of two pairs of glands situated in the anterior cervical region. In the dog and cat, both external and internal parathyroids are close to the thyroid gland. Rats are the exception, because they have a single pair of parathyroid glands that are located close to the thyroid. Embryologically they arise from the third and fourth pharyngeal pouches, in close association with the primordia of the thymus (Figure 17.35). The entodermal bud that forms the thyroid gland arises on the midline at the level of the first pharyngeal pouch. This gives rise to the thyroglossal duct that migrates caudally.

Functional Cytology

Chief Cells

Parathyroids contain a single type of secretory cell, chief cells, concerned with the elaboration of a single hormone. They are seen in different stages of secretory activity, from the inactive chief cell to active oxyphil cells in certain species (Figure 17.36). Chief cells are cuboidal and have interdigitations between contiguous cells. The relatively electron-transparent cytoplasm contains poorly-developed organelles and infrequent secretory granules. The cytoplasm often has either numerous lipid bodies and lipofuscin granules, or aggregations of glycogen particles. Chief cells in the active stage of the secretory cycle occur less frequently in the parathyroid glands of most species.

Oxyphil Cells

The significance of oxyphil cells in the pathophysiology of the parathyroid glands has not been elucidated completely. They are observed either singly or in small groups interspersed between chief cells (Figure 17.36). They are absent in parathyroids of the rat, chicken, and many species of lower animals. They are larger than chief cells, and their abundant cytoplasmic area is filled with numerous large, often bizarre-shaped, mitochondria, but they do not have an

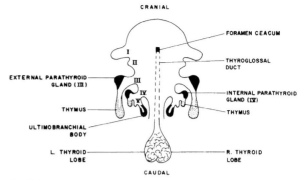

FIGURE 17.35 Embryology of thyroid and parathyroid glands. The thyroid gland develops from a midline primordia (thyroglossal duct), whereas parathyroid glands develop from the cranial portions of the third and fourth pharyngeal pouch in association with the thymus.

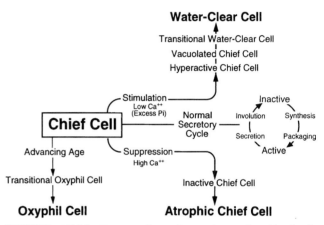

FIGURE 17.36 Functional cytology of parathyroid glands under normal and pathologic conditions. From Capen and Rosol (1993), In: Pathology of the Thyroid and Parathyroid Gland: An Update (VA LiVolsi and RA DeLellis, eds), pp 1–33, Williams and Wilkins, Philadelphia with permission.

active function in the biosynthesis of parathyroid hormone. Oxyphil cells have been shown histochemically to have higher oxidative and hydrolytic enzyme activity than chief cells. Some cells are observed with cytoplasmic characteristics intermediate between those of chief and oxyphil cells. Therefore, oxyphil cells do not appear to be degenerate chief cells as previously thought, but are metabolically active cells, derived from chief cells as the result of aging or some other metabolic derangement.

Parathyroid Hormone

Biosynthesis and Chemistry

A larger biosynthetic precursor of parathyroid hormone, preproparathyroid hormone, (pre-proPTH) is the initial translation product (Figure 17.37). Pre-proPTH is then rapidly converted to proparathyroid hormone (proPTH). Enzymes cleave a hexapeptide

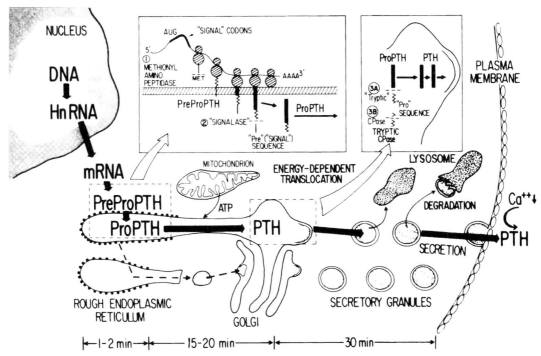

FIGURE 17.37   Subcellular compartmentalization, transport, and cleavage of precursors of parathyroid hormone (PTH). Preproparathyroid hormone (pre-proPTH) is the initial translation product from ribosomes of the rough endoplasmic reticulum, which is converted rapidly to proparathyroid hormone (proPTH). The hydrophobic sequence on the amino-terminal end of the pre-proPTH facilitates penetration of the leading portion of the nascent peptide into the lumen of the endoplasmic reticulum. ProPTH is transported to the Golgi apparatus where it is converted enzymatically by a carboxypeptidase (CPase) to biologically active PTH. A major portion of the biosynthetic precursors and active PTH is degraded by lysosomal enzymes and is not secreted by chief cells under normal conditions. Parathyroid secretory protein (PSP) may function as a binding protein for PTH during intracellular storage in secretion granules and be released with PTH into the extracellular space. From Habener and Potts (1979), Endocrinology 104:265–275 with permission.

from the biologically-active end of the molecule, forming active parathyroid hormone, which is packaged into secretory granules in the Golgi apparatus for subsequent storage in chief cells.

Under certain conditions of increased demand, PTH may be released directly from chief cells without being packaged into secretory granules. Molecular fragments of PTH are formed in the peripheral circulation and in the liver. The immunoheterogeneity created by the multiple circulating fragments of PTH has caused significant problems in the development and application of highly-specific radioimmunoassays to diagnostic problems in human patients and animals.

Biological Actions

Parathyroid hormone is the principal hormone involved in the fine regulation of blood calcium in mammals. It exerts its biological actions by directly influencing the function of target cells, primarily bone and kidney, and indirectly influencing cells in the intestine to maintain plasma calcium at a level sufficient to ensure the optimal functioning of a wide variety of body cells. The action of PTH on bone is

the mobilization of calcium from skeletal reserves into extracellular fluids. The increase in blood calcium results from an interaction of PTH with osteoblasts and osteoclasts in bone, along with increased tubular reabsorption of calcium in the kidney.

Osteoclasts appear to be primarily responsible for the catabolic action of PTH on bone by increasing resorption. PTH has been known for some time to stimulate an increased activity of preformed osteoclasts; however, recent findings have failed to demonstrate receptors for PTH on osteoclasts, but receptors were present on osteoblasts. Isolated osteoclasts respond to PTH only with the concurrent presence of osteoblasts. The mechanisms by which binding of PTH to osteoblasts results in the stimulation of osteoclasts are not completely understood, but appear to include direct effects on the osteoblast, as well as release of secretory products by osteoblasts which are capable of stimulating osteoclastic bone resorption. Osteoclasts appear to be primarily responsible for the long-term actions of PTH on increasing bone resorption and overall bone remodeling.

Parathyroid hormone has a rapid and direct effect on renal proximal convoluted tubular function, leading

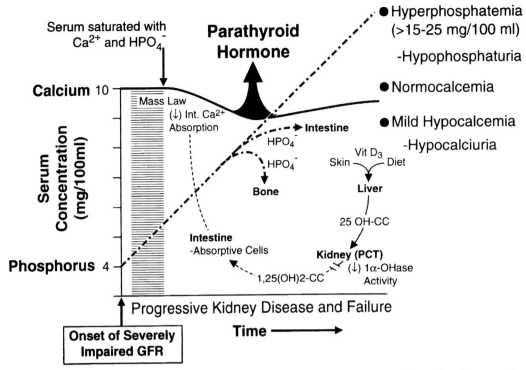

FIGURE 17.38   Alterations in levels of serum calcium and phosphorus during the pathogenesis of secondary hyperparathyroidism associated with chronic progressive renal failure.

to decreased reabsorption of phosphorus and phosphaturia. PTH binds to a receptor on the basolateral aspect of renal epithelial cells, stimulates adenylate cyclase, increases intracellular cAMP, and inhibits phosphorus reabsorption across the brush border through the actions of protein kinases. The kidney is also a major organ for the degradation and excretion of PTH.

Mechanisms of Toxicity

Agents Influencing the Development of Proliferative Lesions

Irradiation significantly increases the incidence of parathyroid adenomas in rats, and the incidence can be modified by feeding diets with variable amounts of vitamin D. Parathyroid adenomas have been encountered infrequently in rats following the experimental administration of a variety of chemicals such as rotenone.

Modification of Parathyroid Function Associated with Metabolic Disorders

Secondary hyperparathyroidism as a complication of chronic renal failure is a metabolic state characterized by an excessive, but not autonomous, rate of PTH secretion. Parathyroid stimulation associated with chronic renal disease can be attributed directly to hypocalcemia. The secretion of hormone by the hyperplastic parathyroid gland usually remains responsive to fluctuations in blood calcium. When the renal disease progresses to the point at which there is a significant reduction in the glomerular filtration rate, phosphorus is retained and progressive hyperphosphatemia develops (Figure 17.38). Although the concentration of blood phosphorus has no direct regulatory influence on the synthesis and secretion of PTH, when elevated it contributes to parathyroid stimulation by virtue of its ability to lower blood calcium levels.

Nutritional hyperparathyroidism is a compensatory mechanism directed against a disturbance in mineral homeostasis induced by nutritional imbalances. The disease occurs in dogs, cats, monkeys, laboratory rodents, and others fed improper diets. Dietary mineral imbalances of etiologic importance in the pathogenesis are a low content of calcium, excessive phosphorus with normal or low calcium, and inadequate amounts of cholecalciferol (vitamin D_3) in New World nonhuman primates housed indoors without exposure to sunlight. The significant end result is hypocalcemia, which results in parathyroid stimulation (Figure 17.39). In response to nutritionally-induced hypocalcemia, all parathyroid glands undergo cellular hypertrophy and hyperplasia.

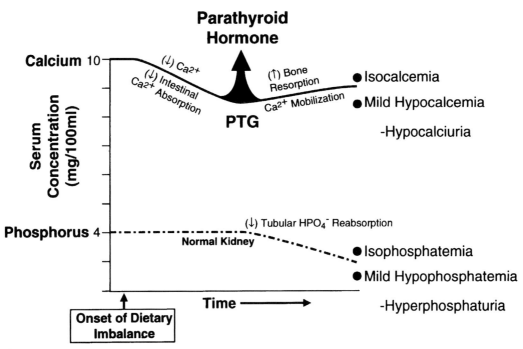

FIGURE 17.39 Alterations in serum calcium and phosphorus in the pathogenesis of nutritional secondary hyperparathyroidism caused by feeding a diet low in calcium or deficient in cholecalciferol but with normal amounts of phosphorus.

Hypoparathyroidism is a metabolic disorder in which either subnormal amounts of PTH are secreted by pathologic parathyroids, or the hormone secreted is unable to interact normally with target cells. Hypoparathyroidism is often associated with diffuse lymphocytic parathyroiditis, resulting in the extensive degeneration of chief cells and replacement by fibrous connective tissue. In the early stages of lymphocytic parathyroiditis there is infiltration of the gland with lymphocytes and plasma cells, and nodular regenerative hyperplasia of the remaining chief cells. Lymphocytic parathyroiditis appears to develop by immune-mediated mechanisms, as a similar destruction of secretory parenchyma and lymphocytic infiltration has been produced experimentally by repeated injections of parathyroid tissue emulsions. The functional disturbances of hypoparathyroidism primarily are the result of increased neuromuscular excitability and tetany. Bone resorption is decreased because of a lack of PTH, and blood calcium levels diminish progressively (Figure 17.40).

In primary hyperparathyroidism, PTH is produced in excess by a functional tumor in the gland, and the normal control of PTH secretion by blood calcium is lost. A prolonged increased secretion of PTH results in accelerated bone resorption, and increased renal production of 1,25-dihydroxycholecalciferol. The lesion in the parathyroid gland responsible for the excessive secretion of PTH is usually an adenoma composed of active chief cells.

There are three mechanisms by which tumors can induce hypercalcemia: local destruction of bone by hematologic cancers; solid tumors can widely metastasize to bone and result in local bone loss associated with the tumor metastases; and humoral hypercalcemia of malignancy (HHM), in which solid tumors that have no or few metastases to bone induce their effects distant from the site of the tumor by the elaboration of one or more factors.

Humoral hypercalcemia of malignancy is a syndrome associated with diverse malignant neoplasms in canine and human patients. Characteristic clinical findings with HHM include hypercalcemia, hypophosphatemia, hypercalciuria, increased fractional excretion of phosphorus, increased nephrogenous cAMP, and increased osteoclastic bone resorption. Humoral effects on bone, kidneys, and possibly the intestine induce hypercalcemia. Malignant neoplasms that are commonly associated with HHM in animals include the adenocarcinoma derived from apocrine glands of the anal sac in dogs, some T-cell lymphomas of dogs, and miscellaneous carcinomas that induce HHM sporadically.

Response of Parathyroid Chief Cells to Injury

Small cysts are observed frequently as naturally-occurring lesions within the parenchyma of the parathyroid, or in the immediate vicinity of the glands in

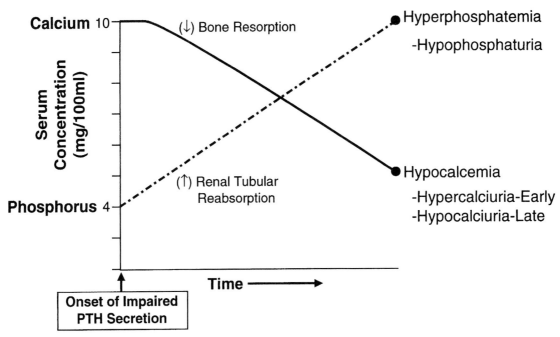

FIGURE 17.40 Alterations in serum calcium and phosphorus in response to an inadequate secretion of parathyroid hormone (hypoparathyroidism). There is a progressive increase in serum phosphorus and a marked decline in serum calcium to levels that result in increased neuromuscular excitability and tetany.

rats, dogs, and occasionally in other animal species. They are usually multiloculated, lined by a cuboidal to partially-ciliated columnar epithelium, and contain a densely-eosinophilic proteinic material. Some parathyroid (Kürsteiner's) cysts develop from a persistence and dilatation of remnants of the duct that connects the parathyroid and thymic primordia during embryonic development (see Figure 17.35).

Proliferative Lesions of Parathyroid Chief Cells

Incidence

Proliferative lesions of the parathyroid gland include diffuse and focal hyperplasia, adenomas, and carcinomas. Neoplasms of the parathyroid glands are uncommon in all species of laboratory and domestic animals, but occur in low incidence in rats, Syrian hamsters, dogs, and rarely, mice. Parathyroid hyperplasia may be primary or secondary, and may be functional or non-functional, depending on their ability to secrete PTH.

Chief cell hyperplasia may affect the parathyroid in a distinctly focal or multifocal distribution (Figure 17.41). The focal area(s) of chief cell hyperplasia is poorly demarcated, and not encapsulated from adjacent parenchyma. Chief cells within the nodules have a relatively uniform composition with a high cytoplasm:nucleus ratio, and a slightly more hyperchromatic nucleus than adjacent normal chief cells. There

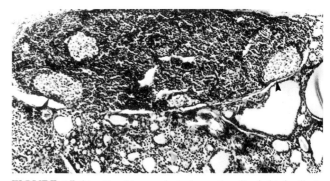

FIGURE 17.41 Focal hyperplasia (arrowhead) of chief cells in parathyroid glands of a Long-Evans rat. The focal areas of increased cellularity are poorly demarcated and not encapsulated from adjacent parathyroid parenchyma. Bar: 100 μm. From Rosol and Capen (1989), Toxicol Pathol 17:346–356 with permission.

may be slight compression of adjacent chief cells around larger focal areas of hyperplasia.

Focal chief cell hyperplasia is often difficult to separate from a chief cell adenoma using only morphologic criteria. The presence of multiple nodules of varying sizes and uniform cellularity in one or both parathyroids with minimal compression and no encapsulation is more compatible with an interpretation of focal hyperplasia than chief cell adenoma.

Diffuse parathyroid hyperplasia, as is seen with chronic renal failure and long-term dietary imbalances, results in a uniform enlargement of all parathyroid

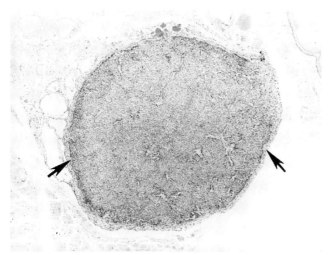

FIGURE 17.42 Diffuse hyperplasia of chief cells with overall enlargement of parathyroid gland in a F344 rat. There is a uniform increase in cellularity due to hypertrophy and hyperplasia of chief cells. Arrows indicate parathyroid capsule. Bar: 100μm. From Rosol and Capen (1989), Toxicol Pathol 17:346–356 with permission.

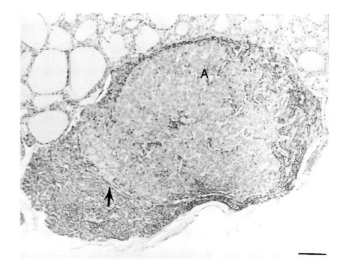

FIGURE 17.43 Chief cell adenoma (A) illustrating sharp demarcation and partial encapsulation (arrow) from adjacent parathyroid parenchyma in a Fischer rat. Chief cells in the adenoma have a larger cytoplasmic area than those in the compressed rim of the parathyroid gland. Bar: 100μm. From Rosol and Capen (1989), Toxicol Pathol 17:346–356 with permission.

glands. The uniform enlargement of parathyroid glands in diffuse hyperplasia is due to both hypertrophy and hyperplasia of chief cells. There is no peripheral rim of compressed atrophic parathyroid parenchyma as seen around a functional adenoma, but there is a uniform population of hyperplastic chief cells extending to the capsule of the gland (Figure 17.42). Chief cells are packed together closely, often with indistinct cell boundaries. The expanded cytoplasmic area of chronically-stimulated chief cells is lightly eosinophilic, with occasional distinct vacuoles. A more prominent fibrovascular stroma in some diffusely hyperplastic parathyroids may result in a lobulated appearance (Figure 17.42). In other hyperplastic parathyroids, chief cells form distinct acinus-like structures in the gland.

Parathyroid adenomas vary from microscopic in size to unilateral nodules several millimeters in diameter, located in the cervical region by the thyroids, or infrequently in the thoracic cavity near the base of the heart. Tumors of parathyroid chief cells do not appear to be sequelae of long-standing secondary hyperparathyroidism of either renal or nutritional origin. The unaffected parathyroid glands may be atrophic if the adenoma is functional, normal if the adenoma is non-functional, or enlarged if there is concomitant hyperplasia. Adenomas are solitary nodules that are sharply-demarcated from adjacent parathyroid parenchyma by a partial fibrous capsule (Figure 17.43). Adenomas are usually non-functional in rats, but may be functional in dogs, cats, and humans. Chief cells in non-functional adenomas are cuboidal or polyhedral

and arranged in a diffuse sheet, in lobules, or in acini with or without lumens. Nuclei are round to oval, often vesicular, and mitotic figures may be present; however, they are usually infrequent. Chief cells from functional adenomas are often closely packed into small groups by fine connective tissue septae. Chief cells are cuboidal, and the cytoplasm stains lightly-eosinophilic. The cytoplasmic area varies from normal size to an expanded area. There is a much lower density of cells in functional parathyroid adenoma than in the adjacent rim with atrophic chief cells. Occasional oxyphil cells, water-clear cells, and transitional forms may be distributed throughout the adenoma.

Chief cell carcinomas are rarely encountered in rodents and domestic animals. Parathyroid carcinomas are often more fixed in position than chief cell adenomas, due to invasion of either the adjacent thyroid lobe or adjacent cervical skeletal muscle. Some of the enlargement may be due to central necrosis and hemorrhage in the carcinoma. Malignant chief cells are arranged in solid sheets subdivided into lobules by a fibrovascular stroma, as palisade along blood sinusoids, or form acinar structures. There is usually complete incorporation of the affected gland and evidence of invasion through the parathyroid capsule. Evidence of vascular invasion and formation of tumor cell emboli are infrequently observed. Malignant chief cells may be more pleomorphic than those that constitute adenomas, but mitotic figures are infrequent. The cytoplasmic area stains lightly-eosinophilic, and boundaries of adjacent chief cells are indistinct.

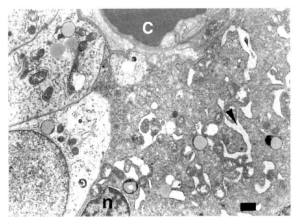

FIGURE 17.44 Syncytial ("giant") cell (right) and adjacent inactive chief cells (left) in the parathyroid gland from a dog. The large cytoplasmic area of the syncytial cell is formed by the fusion of adjacent chief cells following the disruption of plasma membranes. The multiple nuclei in the syncytial cell are smaller and more electron dense than in the normal chief cells (N) (left) and have condensed chromatin. Some mitochondria are swollen with disruption of cristae, and profiles of endoplasmic reticulum are distended in syncytial cells (arrowhead). C, capillary. Bar: 100μm. From Capen and Rosol (1989), Toxicol Pathol 17:333–345 with permission.

Parathyroid glands of dogs and rats occasionally develop unique multinucleated syncytial giant cells more numerous near the periphery of the parathyroid gland, but this is variable between animals, and considerable numbers can be present in the more central portions of the gland. The number of syncytial cells often varies considerably between parathyroids in the same animal, but may account for up to half the parenchyma of the gland. These cells appear to form by the fusion of the cytoplasmic area of adjacent chief cells. The cytoplasm of syncytial cells is densely eosinophilic and homogeneous, and the plasma membranes between adjacent cells often are indistinct (Figure 17.44). Nuclei are smaller, more hyperchromatic, and more oval than those in adjacent chief cells. The electron-dense cytoplasm of syncytial cells often has organelles with early degenerative changes. Membrane-limited secretory granules are observed infrequently in the cytoplasm. The mechanism by which syncytial cells form is uncertain, but it does not appear to be related to improper fixation of the parathyroid. They usually do not occur in numbers sufficient to interfere with parathyroid function.

Evaluation of Toxicity

Morphologic Evaluation

The parathyroid gland is infrequently injured directly by the acute or chronic administration of xenobiotics. However, parathyroid function may be altered by a wide variety of chemicals that either elevate or lower the blood concentration of calcium ions. In response to hypocalcemia, chief cells undergo hypertrophy and eventually hyperplasia.

The expanded cytoplasmic area is lightly-eosinophilic and vacuolated, compared with chief cells in normal animals. Perivascular spaces are narrow in a hyperplastic parathyroid, and there are few fat cells in the interstitium. In response to hypercalcemia, the cytoplasmic area of chief cells is decreased and more densely-eosinophilic, often with a widening of intercellular and pericapillary spaces. If the hypercalcemia is prolonged, there is an overall reduction of glandular parenchyma, with increased fibrous or adipose connective tissue in the interstitium.

Ultrastructural evaluation of chief cells is a sensitive means of assessing morphologically whether a particular drug or chemical affects the parathyroid gland. Perfusion of the thyroid–parathyroid area with glutaraldehyde-based fixatives followed by postfixation with osmium tetroxide results in the best retention of structural detail in parathyroids of animals. Morphometric studies at the ultrastructural level can be used to quantitate total cytoplasmic area and area occupied by a particular organelle, e.g., secretory granule. Secretory granules accumulate initially in response to an elevation in blood calcium, but subsequently decrease due to degradation by lysosomal enzymes. Atrophic chief cells develop in response to sustained or more severe hypercalcemia. Their cytoplasm is more electron-dense and irregularly shrunken, with widened intercellular spaces. Cytoplasmic organelles are poorly-developed, and may have early degenerative changes suggested by mitochondrial vacuolation with disruption of cristae, and distention of endoplasmic reticulum, with loss of ribosomes.

Assay of Circulating Parathyroid Hormone

The metabolism of PTH and the formation of multiple circulating forms of PTH have made the development of clinically useful immunoassays challenging. Early immunoassays for PTH were single-site radio-immunoassays for C-terminal peptides. These assays were suboptimal, as the biologically-active form of PTH was not measured. Intact serum PTH concentrations are best measured by two-site immunoradiometric assay (IRMA) or N-terminal RIA. Serum-intact PTH can be measured in dogs and cats, with assays developed for human PTH due to the cross-reactivity of the antisera used in the assays.

FURTHER READING

Anderson, M.P., and Capen, C. (1978). The endocrine system. In *Pathology of Laboratory Animals* (Benirschke, K., Garner, F.M., and Jones, T.C. eds), pp. 423–508. Springer-Verlag, Berlin, Germany.

Arnaud, C.D., and Pun, K. (1992). Metabolism and assay of parathyroid hormone. In *Disorders of Bone and Mineral Metabolism* (Coe, F.L., and Favus, M.J. eds), pp. 107–122. Raven Press, New York, NY.

Barsoum, N.J., Morre, J.D., Gough, A.W., Sturgess, J.M., and de la Iglesia, F.A. (1985). Morphofunctional investivations on spontaneous pituitary tumors in Wistar rats. *Toxicol. Pathol.*, 13, 200–208.

Biancifiori, C. (1979). Tumours of the thyroid gland. In *Pathology of Tumours in Laboratory Animals* (Turusov, V.S. ed.), Vol. 2, pp. 451–468. International Agency for Research on Cancer, Lyon, France.

Capen, C.C. (1996). Functional and pathologic interrelationships of the pituitary gland and hypothalamus in animals. In *Endocrine System* (Jones, T.C., Capen, C.C., and Mohr, U. eds), 2nd edn, pp. 3–32. Springer-Verlag, Berlin, Germany.

Capen, C.C. (1996). Pathobiology of parathyroid gland structure and function in animals. In *Endocrine System* (Jones, T.C., Capen, C.C., and Mohr, U. eds), 2nd edn, pp. 293–327. Springer-Verlag, Berlin, Germany.

Capen, C.C., DeLellis, R.A., and Yarrington, J.T. (2002). Endocrine system. In *Handbook of Toxicologic Pathology* (Haschek, W.M., Rousseaux, C.G., and Wallig, M.A. eds), 2nd edn. Academic Press, New York.

Capen, C.C., and Martin, S.L. (1982). Diseases of the pituitary gland. In *Textbook of Veterinary Internal Medicine* (Ettinger, S.J. ed.), 2nd edn, pp. 1523–1529. Saunders, Philadelphia, PA.

Colby, H.D. (1988). Adrenal gland toxicity: Chemically induced dysfunction. *J. Am. Coll. Toxicol.*, 7, 45–69.

Curran, P.G., and DeGroot, L.J. (1991). The effect of hepatic enzyme-inducing drugs on thyroid hormones and the thyroid gland. *Endocr. Rev.*, 12, 135–150.

Gilbert, G., Gillman, J., Loustalot, P., and Lutz, W. (1988). The modifying influence of diet and the physical environment on spontaneous tumor frequency in rats. *Br. J. Cancer*, 12, 565–593.

Gilbert, G., Gillman, J., Loustalot, P., and Lutz, W. (1988). The modifying influence of diet and the physical environment on spontaneous tumor frequency in rats. *Br. J. Cancer*, 12, 565–593.

Goodman, D.G., Ward, J.M., Squire, R.A., Chu, K.C., and Linhart, M.S. (1979). Neoplastic and non-neoplastic lesions in aging F344 rats. *Toxicol. Appl. Pharmacol.*, 48, 237–248.

Hallberg, E. (1990). Metabolism and toxicity of xenobiotics in the adrenal cortex, with particular reference to 7,12-dimethybenz(a) anthracene. *J. Biochem. Toxicol.*, 5, 71–90.

Hornsby, P.J. (1989). Steroid and xenobiotic effects on the adrenal cortex: Mediation by oxidative and other mechanisms. *Free Radic. Biol. Med.*, 6, 103–115.

La Perle, K.M.D., and Capen, C.C. (2007). Endocrine system. In *Pathologic Basis of Veterinary Disease* (McGavin, M., and Zachary, J.F. eds), 4th ed., pp. 693–741. Mosby Elsevier, St. Louis.

Mallette, L.E. (1994). Parathyroid hormone and parathyroid hormone-related protein as polyhormones. In *The Parathyroids* (Bilezikian, J.P., Levine, M.A., and Marcus, R. eds), pp. 171–184. Raven Press, New York, NY.

McClain, R.M. (1994). Mechanistic considerations in the regulation and classification of chemical carcinogens. In *Nutritional Toxicology* (Kotsonis, F.N., Mackey, M., and Hjelle, J. eds), pp. 273–304. Raven Press, Ltd., New York, NY.

Moriello, K.A., Fehrer-Sawyer, S.L., Meyer, D.J., and Feder, B. (1988). Adrenocortical suppression associated with topical optic administration of glucocorticoids in dogs. *J. Am. Vet. Med. Assoc.*, 193, 329–331.

Nakagami, K. (1967). Comparative electron microscopic studies of the parathyroid glands. II. Fine structure of the parathyroid gland of the normal and the calcium chloride treated mouse. *Arch. Histol. Jpn.*, 28, 185–205.

Ottenweller, J.E., and Hedge, G.A. (1982). Diurnal variations of plasma thyrotropin, thyroxine, and triiodothyronine in female rats are phase shifted after inversion of the photoperiod. *Endocrinology*, 111, 509–514.

Randolph, J.F., Center, S.A., Reimers, R.J., Scarlett, J.M., and Corbett, J.R. (1995). Adrenocortical function in neonatal and weanling beagle pups. *Am. J. Vet. Res.*, 56, 511–517.

Rhodin, J.A. (1971). The ultrastructure of the adrenal cortex of the rat under normal and experimental conditions. *Ultrastruct. Res.*, 34, 23–71.

Ribelin, W.E. (1984). The effects of drugs and chemicals upon the structure of the adrenal gland. *Fundam. Appl. Toxicol.*, 4, 105–119.

Rosol, T.J., and Capen, C.C. (1997). Calcium-regulating hormones and diseases of abnormal mineral (calcium, phosphorus, magnesium) metabolism. In *Clinical Biochemistry of Domestic Animals* (Kaneko, J.J., Harvey, J.W., and Bruss, M.L. eds), 5th ed., pp. 619–702. Academic Press, New York.

Rothuizen, J., Reul, J.M., Fijnberk, A., Mol, J.A., and de Kloet, E.R. (1991). Aging and the hypothalamuspituitary-adrenocortical axis, with special reference to the dog. *Acta Endoerinol.*, 125 (Suppl.), 73–76.

St. Germain, D.L. (1988). Dual mechanisms of regulation of type I iodothyronine 5'-deiodinase in the rat kidney, liver, and thyroid gland. *J. Clin. Invest.*, 81, 1476–1484.

Strandberg, J.D. (1989). Focal hyperplasia, adrenal cortex, rat. In *Endocrine System. Monographs on Pathology of Laboratory Animals* (Jones, T.C., Mohr, U., and Hunt, R. eds), pp. 37–41. Springer-Verlag, Berlin, Germany.

Tischler, A.S., and DeLellis, R.A. (1988). The rat adrenal medulla I. The normal adrenal. *J. Am. Coll. Toxicol.*, 7, 1–21.

Tischler, A.S., and DeLellis, R.A. (1988). The rat adrenal medulla II. Proliferative lesions. *J. Am. Coll. Toxicol.*, 7, 23–44.

Wong, G.L. (1986). Skeletal effects of parathyroid hormone. In *Bone and Mineral Research* (Peck, W.A. ed.), pp. 103–129. Elsevier Science, Amsterdam, The Netherlands.

Yarrington, J.T., and Reindel, J.F. (1996). Chemically induced adrenocortical degenerative lesions. In *Endocrine System* (Jones, T.C., Capen, C.C., and Mohr, U. eds), 2nd edn, pp. 467–476. Springer-Verlag, Berlin, Germany.

Zbinden, G. (1988). Hyperplastic and neoplastic responses of the thyroid gland in toxicological studies: The target organ and the toxic process. *Arch. Toxicol. Suppl.*, 12, 98–106.

INTRODUCTION

The male reproductive tract comprises the testes where the continuous process of gamete production (spermatogenesis) occurs and where testosterone is produced; the epididymus, an excurrent duct system for transport, maturation, and storage of the sperm; accessory glandular organs that produce the seminal fluid and secrete complex molecules into the final ejaculate; and the penis, which provides an erectile organ for the penetration and delivery of the gametes into the female reproductive tract (Figure 18.1). Production, release, and maturation of spermatozoa all depend on specialized functions of the testicular cells and epididymal epithelium. An equally varied morphology and ultrastructural composition reflect these varied functions.

Integration and control of these diverse functions necessitate specialized cellular interactions and hormonal control mechanisms. Many of these interactions are incompletely understood, but include endocrine control through the hypothalamic-pituitary-testicular axis and paracrine regulation between neighboring cell types, as well as autocrine or self-regulation of individual cells. Development of the male reproductive

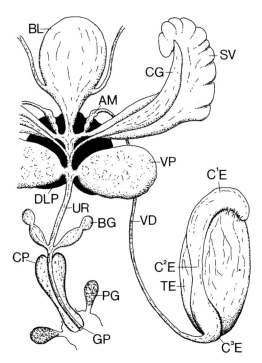

FIGURE 18.1 Anatomical arrangement of the testes, excurrent ducts, and secondary sex organs in the rat. BL, bladder; AM, ampulla; CG coagulating gland; SV, seminal vesicles; VP, ventral prostate; DLP, dorsolateral prostate; UR, penile urethra; BG, bulbourethral glands; VD, vas deferens; CP, corpus penis; GP, glans penis; PG, preputial gland; TE, testis; C1/C2/C3E, caput/corpus/cauda epididimis. Reproduced with permission from Creasy (1998).

tract and imprinting of male sexual behavior and other male phenotypic characteristics are dependent on androgen and estrogen exposure during critical windows of fetal and neonatal development. If hormonal status is disturbed during these critical periods, male reproductive development and/or subsequent fertility of the adult can be altered dramatically

The complexity of structure, physiology, and regulatory control of male reproductive function provides enormous potential for toxicologic disturbance at very many sites, both in the adult and in the neonate. It therefore presents an interesting challenge to the toxicologic pathologist to gain sufficient understanding of reproductive biology in order to investigate and evaluate the pathological basis of male reproductive toxicity.

STRUCTURE AND CELL BIOLOGY

Embryological Derivation of the Reproductive Tract

The primordial gonad develops as the genital ridge, which grows along the coelemic surface of the mesonephros. Primordial germ cells migrate from the yolk sac endoderm and combine with somatic (Sertoli)

cells from the mesonephros to form the seminiferous (medullary) cords. Once these cords are formed the fetal Leydig cells begin differentiating from mesenchymal cells, which are present in the interstitial tissue between the cords. This differentiation is thought to be under the control of the Sertoli cells. Fetal Leydig cells secrete testosterone during the fetal and neonatal period. Testosterone is responsible for the masculinization of various processes and systems, including the central nervous system and sexual behavior. Fetal Leydig cells regress and are replaced by a different generation of adult Leydig cells, which also differentiate from interstitial mesenchymal cells. There is no proliferation of existing cells. Proliferation of precursor mesenchymal cells is regulated by paracrine and endocrine factors, whereas the differentiation of precursors to adult type Leydig cells is luteinizing hormone (LH) dependent.

The excurrent duct system, comprising the rete testis, efferent ducts, epididymis, and the vas deferens, develops from the degenerating Wolffian duct system. The seminal vesicles develop from lateral buds of this duct. However, the prostate and bulbourethral glands, along with the urethra and external genitalia, have a different embryological origin, developing from the urogenital sinus and urogenital tubercle.

Structure of the Testes

Gross Structure

In most adult mammals each testis is enclosed in a scrotal sac that lies outside the abdominal cavity. At puberty, the testes descend through the inguinal canal, remaining connected to the internal inguinal ring by the cremaster muscles. The mechanism and timing of descent vary between species but the passage through the inguinal ring is androgen dependent and involves a structure called the gubernaculum. The swelling and migration of the gubernaculum through the inguinal canal precede the testis and force open the inguinal ring, allowing the testis to move passively into the scrotum. Once this function is served, the gubernaculum regresses. The spermatic cord, which comprises the internal cremaster muscle, the vessels, and the nerves that supply the testis and the vas deferens, links the testis to the abdominal cavity. The testicular parenchyma is composed of seminiferous tubules separated by interstitial tissue and enclosed in a capsule that has three layers: the outer tunica vaginalis, the middle tunica albuginea, and the innermost layer, the tunica vasculosa.

The seminiferous tubules are long, highly convoluted tubes that empty at both ends into the rete testis. In the rat there are approximately 30 separate tubules, folded to form about 12 m of tubule per gram of testis. In man, there are many more tubules, forming between

15 and 25 m per gram of tissue. The tubules are lined by the seminiferous (or germinal) epithelium and are bounded by the tunica propria. This multilayered peritubular capsule is composed of an inner basement membrane surrounded by a layer of myoid peritubular cells, a noncellular layer, and an endothelial layer, which, in some species, forms the lining of the interstitial lymphatic spaces. The seminiferous epithelium lies on the basement membrane and is composed of somatic supporting cells called Sertoli cells and a differentiating population of germ cells in various stages of maturation (Figures 18.2 and 18.3). The only cells in contact with the basement membrane are the Sertoli cells and the spermatogonia; the more mature germ cells lie within recesses of the Sertoli cell surface. As the germ cells mature, they move toward the lumen where they are finally released and transported along the tubule into the rete testis. The process whereby primitive stem cell spermatogonia develop to form highly specialized spermatozoa is termed spermatogenesis. Interstitial tissue surrounds the tubules; it is composed of loose connective tissue containing Leydig cells, macrophages, fibroblasts, blood vessels, and lymphatic channels.

The testis is supplied by the internal spermatic artery, a highly coiled tortuous vessel. The spermatic artery gives off the superior and inferior epididymal branches, which supply the cauda and corpus epididymis, and continues as the testicular artery to supply the testis. This vessel divides into radiate arteries, which in turn give rise to intertubular arterioles. These supply the capillary network of the tubules, which comprises the intertubular and the peritubular capillaries. The capillary endothelium is nonfenestrated and is surrounded by ensheathing perivascular cells. The lymphatics form a labyrinth of channels between the Leydig cells and the peritubular cells of the seminiferous tubules. The venous return from the testis enters the pampiniform plexus, a system of venous channels that closely surround the incoming spermatic artery, acting as a countercurrent heat-exchange system.

In most mammals the testes are situated outside the abdominal cavity because the temperature at which spermatogenesis proceeds normally is a few degrees below normal body temperature. However, the temperature differential and temperature sensitivity are species dependent. To maintain and control this temperature differential, a thermoregulatory mechanism has developed through a specialized arterial supply and venous return, and through the cooling properties of the scrotum.

Histology and Cell Biology

Sertoli Cells

Sertoli cells, also known as sustentacular cells, provide the supporting framework in which the germ

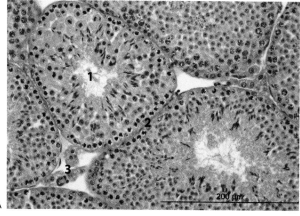

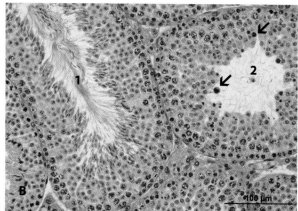

FIGURE 18.2 Testicular parenchyma, seminiferous tubules and interstitium, normal spermatogenesis, mouse. (A) Seminiferous tubules have a central lumen (1) and are surrounded by a basement membrane (2). Interstitial tissue (3) contains Leydig (interstitial) cells, macrophages and lymphatics. (B), Spermatozoa are present in the lumen of one tubule (1), while residual bodies (arrows) are prominent in another tubule (2). Davidson's fixative, paraffin embedded, H & E stained.

cells are embedded. The Sertoli cell is irregularly columnar in shape and its basal aspect is attached to the basement membrane by hemidesmosomes. The size and shape of the Sertoli cell is difficult to appreciate in conventional sections viewed by light microscopy. The apical portion of the cell extends to the lumen, forming sheet-like processes termed apical or lateral processes that separate and envelop each germ cell (Figure 18.3). The Sertoli cell is connected to the germ cells by a variety of cell junctions, some of which are unique to this cell type. Adjacent Sertoli cells are joined at their basal aspect by specialized occluding junctions, which form the major component of the barrier.

In all species, Sertoli cells have a limited period in which they divide. In the rat, division ceases after 18 to 21 days of age. During this period, the Sertoli cell also undergoes significant maturational changes in

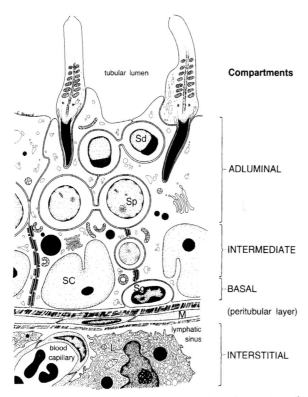

FIGURE 18.3 Diagrammatic representation of a portion of a seminiferous tubule with its associated interstitial tissue showing cellular organization and testicular compartments. L, Leydig cell; SC, Sertoli cell; Sg, spermatogonium; Sp, spermatocyte; Sd, spermatid; M, myoepithelial cell. Adjacent Sertoli cells are separated by occluding junctional complexes, which open and reform around the developing germ cells to allow movement from the basal to the adlumenal compartment, so forming a temporary intermediate compartment. Reproduced with permission from Foster (1988a).

its function and its regulation. Sertoli cell functions are central to the integrity of the seminiferous epithelium. These functions include regulation of spermatogenesis, structural and metabolic support of the germ cells, sperm release, secretion of tubular fluid for sperm transport, and maintenance of a permeability barrier between interstitial and tubular compartments. Disturbance of any of these functions is likely to impair sperm production.

Spermatogonia

Spermatogonia represent the stem cell population of the germ cells. They lie on the basement membrane but are not attached to it. There are three classes of spermatogonia: stem cell spermatogonia, proliferative spermatogonia, and differentiating spermatogonia. Stem cell and proliferative spermatogonia are responsible for renewing their own cell number and producing a pool of spermatogonia that are committed to differentiation. Multiple mitotic divisions of these differentiating

spermatogonia result in the main expansion of the spermatogonial population. Within this group of differentiating spermatogonia, four successive generations of type A spermatogonia have been described: A1–A4. Each is derived by mitotic division from the preceding generation. The A4 spermatogonia divide to produce intermediate spermatogonia, which in turn give rise to type B spermatogonia. Type A (and earlier spermatogonia) are distinguished by a pale staining nucleus with a fine "dusty" distribution of heterochromatin throughout the nucleus (Figure 18.4). Type B cells have dense clumps of heterochromatin around the periphery of the nucleus, whereas intermediate spermatogonia have an appearance somewhere between the two. As the cells undergo mitosis, cytokinesis is incomplete, leaving the descendant population of spermatocytes linked together in a syncytial arrangement. This is maintained throughout spermatogenesis and may play an important role in the synchronized development and differentiation of the individual populations of cells.

Spermatocytes

Spermatocytes are formed from the final mitotic division of the type B spermatogonia. The cells then undergo meiosis, passing through preleptotene, leptotene, zygotene, pachytene, and diplotene stages, diakinesis, and the first meiotic division to produce secondary spermatocytes. The second meiotic division follows rapidly to produce the haploid spermatid. As the spermatocytes pass through meiotic prophase they become larger and the appearance of the nuclear chromatin alters, reflecting the condensation and movement of the chromosomes as they prepare for meiotic division. Preleptotene spermatocytes produced by the dividing B spermatogonia are almost identical to their parent cell, but have a slightly smaller nucleus. During preleptotene, DNA synthesis occurs and the cells move away from the basement membrane and pass through the tight junctional complex between the Sertoli cells. During leptotene, the chromosomes condense to form thin delicate filaments, coming together in zygotene as homologous pairs that form characteristic tripartite structures in the nucleus called synaptonemal complexes (Figure 18.4). During the pachytene phase, the chromosomes become shorter and thicker and split into two chromatids joined by the centromere. Pachytene is a lengthy phase, lasting about 12 days in the rat; during this time there is a marked increase in cellular and nuclear volume. As the cells enter diplotene and diakinesis, the chromosomes begin to separate and condense further while synaptonemal complexes disappear. Diakinesis and the two meiotic divisions occur in rapid succession; a single

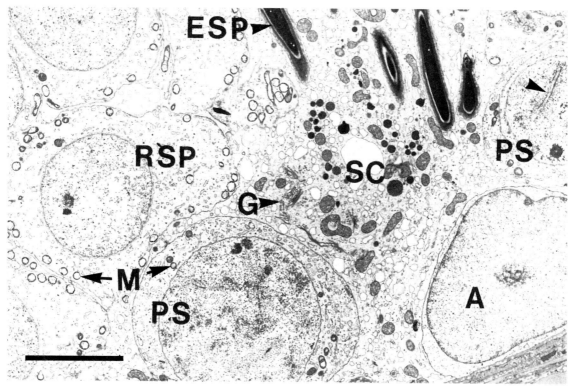

FIGURE 18.4   Basal area of a rat seminiferous tubule. Basement membrane and peritubular cell (bottom right), Sertoli cell cytoplasm (SC) with multiple Golgi (G), type A spermotogonium (A), pachytene spermatocytes (PS), round spermatid (RSP), and elongating spermatid (ESP). Note the differences in mitochondrial (M) morphology of the different cell types. Synaptonemal complexes (arrowheads) are visible in the nuclei of pachytene spermatocytes. Bar = 5μm.

cross section of tubule will often contain diakinetic spermatocytes, spermatocytes in the first and second stages of division, secondary spermatocytes (from the first division), and the newly formed spermatids from the second division.

Spermatids

The second meiotic division of the spermatocytes results in the formation of the haploid spermatid, which is almost identical to the secondary spermatocyte but the nuclear diameter is reduced. During the course of its differentiation into a spermatozoon, the nucleus and cytoplasm undergo a number of extremely complex morphological modifications. An acrosome [visible in periodic acid-Schiff (PAS)stained histological sections] develops over the highly condensed inactive nucleus while the cytoplasm and organelles are totally rearranged to form a motile tail section. To some extent these changes are species specific, but the general features are similar.

The acrosome is required for the sperm to penetrate and fertilize the oocyte. During the early formation of the acrosome, the Golgi apparatus and the chromatoid body appear to have a close association with the

developing acrosome and are thought to be involved in its synthesis. Nuclear condensation occurs to such an extent that all the chromatin exists as heterochromatin (Figure 18.4); the chromatin is therefore totally inactive during the rest of the life of the cell. Because there is a negligible capacity for metabolic or synthetic activity on the part of the spermatid cytoplasm, most of the organelles of the cell are redundant.

Because the 19 steps of spermiogenesis in the rat have been described previously, only a brief outline of the major changes will be given. Spermatid development is conveniently divided into a number of phases: Golgi phase, cap phase, acrosome phase, and maturation phase.

During the Golgi phase, the proacrosomic granules formed in the Golgi region coalesce to form a single acrosomic granule within a membrane-bounded vesicle closely applied to the lumenal aspect of the nucleus. The cap phase begins as an extension grows out from the acrosomic vesicle to form an acrosomic cap that spreads out to cover over one-third of the anterior pole of the nucleus. The chromatoid body migrates to the position of the two centrioles; from here the flagellum develops.

During the acrosome phase, the acrosomic region of the nucleus is orientated through 180° to face the base of the tubule and the nucleus undergoes elongation and condensation to form the head of the spermatozoon. The cytoplasm of the cell is redistributed to the lumenal pole of the cell, away from the acrosome, thus forming an elongated cell with the nucleus at one end and cytoplasmic tail at the other. Within this lumenal cytoplasm develops the manchette, a cylindrical sheath of microtubules attached to the nucleus and surrounding the initial segment of the flagellum. The flagellum forms the neck and tail regions of the spermatozoon; it develops from the distal centriole and is surrounded by nine longitudinally oriented coarse fibers. Mitochondria migrate to form a sheath around these fibers from the neck region to the annulus, a ring-like structure part of the way down the tail. The region encircled by mitochondria is termed the midpiece; distal to this the nine coarse fibers are enclosed by a fibrous sheath.

In the final maturation phase of spermiogenesis, the cytoplasmic volume of the spermatid is greatly reduced by Sertoli cell phagocytosis. There is relatively little alteration in the structure of the acrosome or the nucleus during this phase, but cellular remodeling of the spermatid results in many of the redundant organelles being deposited in the residual body, which is shed at the time of spermiation. One metabolic function retained by the spermatozoa is energy production by the sheath of mitochondria enveloping the tail; this is an obvious requirement for the motile phase of the gamete. Most of the other metabolic requirements of the mature spermatid within the testis are met by the Sertoli cells; outside the testis, the spermatozoon is sustained by the complex mixture of fluids secreted by the epididymis and secondary sex organs.

Peritubular Cells

The elongated flattened peritubular or myoid cells lie between layers of loose collagen fibers and form an overlapping layer surrounding the tubules. These cells contain large numbers of actin filaments that impart contractile properties; contraction of this peritubular layer is thought to be largely responsible for propulsion of the sperm along the tubules to the rete testis and to occur in response to oxytocin secretion from the Leydig cell. Evidence shows that peritubular cells also play an important role in regulation of the testis, responding to testosterone from the Leydig cells and modulating Sertoli cell function (e.g., production of androgen-binding protein).

Leydig Cells

Interstitial tissue between the seminiferous tubules is composed of a loose connective network containing Leydig cells, precursor Leydig cells, macrophages, fibroblasts, blood vessels, and lymphatic channels. Leydig cells (sometimes called interstitial cells) form clusters of cells that are intimately associated with the blood and lymph vessels (Figure 18.3); however, the precise anatomical localization is species specific. Their size, position, and activity may also vary during the spermatogenic cycle.

Leydig cells are rounded or polyhedral in shape and, by light microscopy, are strongly eosinophilic. Ultrastructurally the cells are typical of steroid-synthesizing cells, with a predominance of smooth endoplasmic reticulum and mitochondria. As part of their functional role in regulating spermatogenesis, they are able to adapt to altered demands for secretion. For example, where spermatogenesis is disrupted, the Leydig cells will be subjected to increased gonadotropin stimulation and will increase testosterone output. This is often visible as a hypertrophy or a hyperplasia of the Leydig cell population.

Testicular Macrophages

Macrophages are estimated to constitute 25% of the cells in the interstitium of the rat; other species have not been examined in detail. Although macrophages and Leydig cells can be distinguished easily at the ultrastructural level, they may be confused at the light microscopic level unless special stains such as acid phosphatase are used. They may also be distinguished in PAS stained sections by their increased staining relative to Leydig cells. A major function of the testicular macrophage is phagocytosis. Cell death within the testis rarely elicits an inflammatory cellular infiltrate (see below). Instead the macrophage population increases and is largely responsible for phagocytizing cellular debris from the interstitial compartment.

Physiology and Functional Considerations of the Testis

Spermatogenesis

The process of spermatogenesis comprises a series of successive mitotic divisions by the spermatogonial population, meiosis by the spermatocytes, and extensive cellular remodeling and differentiation throughout the haploid spermatid development (spermiogenesis) (Figure 18.5). Four generations of cells develop simultaneously within the seminiferous epithelium of the rat; their synchronous development gives rise to specific cellular associations that follow each other in a precisely defined sequence. One unit of repetition of the sequence of cellular associations is termed a cycle

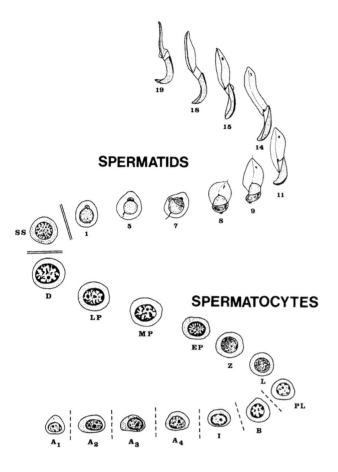

SPERMATIDS

SPERMATOCYTES

SPERMATOGONIA

FIGURE 18.5 Spermatogenesis: the process of cell division and maturation whereby primitive spermatogonial stem cells develop into highly specialized haploid spermatozoa. Spermatogonia undergo numerous mitotic divisions from type A (A) through intermediate (I) to type B (B) spermatogonia. The final division produces spermatocytes, which undergo the long prophase of meiosis passing through the stages of preleptotene (PL), leptotene (L), zygotene (Z), early, mid, and late pachytene (EP, MP, LP), and diplotene (D). This is followed by the first division to produce secondary spermatocytes (SS) and the second division to produce the haploid spermatid (1). The complex differentiation of the spermatid (spermiogenesis) can be separated into 9 different steps using morphological criteria.

of the seminiferous epithelium (often abbreviated to spermatogenic cycle), whereas individual cell associations are referred to as stages of the cycle.

Cycle of the Seminiferous Epithelium

Using the widely accepted scheme of Leblond and Clermont, classification of the rat spermatogenic cycle into stages is largely based on the developing morphology of the spermatid acrosome, which is visualized using periodic acid-Schiff stain. In the rat, the

scheme defines 19 different steps of spermiogenesis, which are denoted by arabic numerals (1–19). The presence of these cells is used as a marker to identify 14 different cellular associations (or stages), referred to by roman numerals (I–XIV) (Figure 18.6). In the rat, mouse, dog, and rabbit, tubular cross sections only contain a single cell association, allowing ready identification of the stage of spermatogenesis (Figure 18.7), whereas in some higher primates, including man, cell associations are arranged in a helical pattern within the tubule, making staging more complex. In some species, such as the dog, cell associations for individual stages are synchronized much less strictly than in rodents, and defined steps of spermatid elongation and nuclear condensation may be present over one or two stages. The release of sperm (spermiation) also occurs over more than one stage, whereas in the rat and mouse it always occurs in a single defined stage. In rodents, the entire process from stem cell spermatogonium to spermatozoal release spans 4.5 cycles. As each cycle is completed, another generation of spermatogonia divides and becomes committed to maturation (Figure 18.6). The duration of the cycle and thus of spermatogenesis is constant for a given species and strain of animal (Table 18.1), although age has a slight influence on the kinetics. The number of stages into which the cycle is divided is arbitrary and depends on the classification criteria used by the originator of the particular scheme. Maps similar to the one depicted in Figure 18.4 have now been devised for most of the common laboratory species. Although the duration of a particular stage cannot be measured directly, it is proportional to the frequency with which that stage occurs in cross sections of tubules, i.e., the longer a stage lasts, the more frequently tubules in that stage are encountered This is remarkably constant between individual rats within a given strain.

Wave of the Seminiferous Epithelium

The cycle of the seminiferous epithelium occurs over a period of time at a given point in the tubule. If a length of tubule were to be examined at a single point in time, the stages of the cycle would be arranged in consecutive order along the tubule, forming a wave (Figure 18.8). Occasionally this order reverses for a short distance and then reverts back again. Such irregularities are termed modulations of the cycle. A wave contains all 14 stages of the cycle, as well as any modulations that may be present in that segment of the tubule. In the dog, the sequential progression of stages along the tubule is less well defined, with large numbers of modulations occurring and nonsequential stages occurring next to one another.

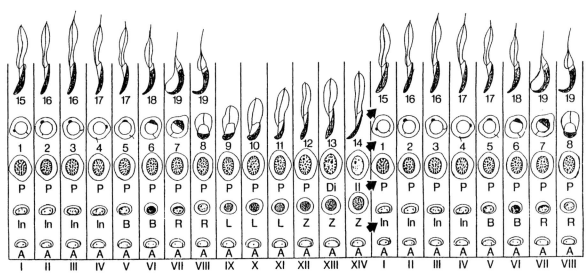

FIGURE 18.6 Diagram illustrating the cellular composition of the 14 stages of the cycle of the seminiferous epithelium where each column represents a stage (denoted by roman numerals I–XIV). The stages are defined by the step of development of the accompanying spermatid. Spermatid development is subdivided into 19 steps (denoted by arabic numerals 1–19) according to the appearance of the acrosome structure, which can be demonstrated using the periodic acid-Schiff-hematoxylin technique. In a given area of tubule, cellular associations succeed one another in time, proceeding from the left to the right of the diagram. Stage XIV is followed by stage I to begin another cycle. One complete sequence of the 14 cellular associations constitutes one cycle of the seminiferous epithelium, whereas the developmental sequence of spermatogonia through spermatocytes to spermatids constitutes the process of spermatogenesis. This is also illustrated in the diagram where, with succeeding cycles (beginning bottom left), type A spermatogonia (A) divide mitotically and differentiate into intermediate type spermatogonia (In) and type B spermatogonia (B). These give rise to spermatocytes, which proceed through the various phases of meiosis: preleptotene or resting (R), leptotene (L), zygotene (Z), pachytene (P), and diakinesis (Di). Meiotic division gives rise to secondary spermatocytes (II) and then to haploid spermatids, which undergo the steps of spermiogenesis (1–19). As the cells proceed through spermatogenesis, they move up through the epithelium and are replaced by another generation of cells so four generations of cells develop in synchrony. The mature step 19 spermatid is finally released into the tubular lumen during stage VIII. Reproduced with permission from Foster (1988).

Structural Support and Movement of Germ Cells

The process of spermatogenesis involves the continual movement of germ cells from the base to the lumen of the tubule. Although the precise mechanism of this process is incompletely understood, it is thought to be largely mediated by conformational changes in the Sertoli cell plasma membrane and changes in the specialized junctions between the two cell types. The Sertoli cell changes shape easily; this is reflected by the well-developed cytoskeleton. The Sertoli cell shape and the profile of its plasma membrane may be important aspects of Sertoli – germ cell interaction, as disruption of the cytoskeletal filaments and retraction of the lateral processes that surround germ cells are associated with premature exfoliation of germ cells into the lumen.

Phagocytic Activity

Phagocytosis is an important function of the Sertoli cell. During spermiogenesis, the cytoplasmic volume of the spermatid is reduced by up to 70%, and a large proportion of its organelles is discarded. This is accomplished by formation of the residual body, which contains redundant organelles and cytoplasm; it is shed from the spermatozoon at the time of spermiation, phagocytized by the Sertoli cell, and transported down to the basal Sertoli cell cytoplasm, where it is digested. The autophagic vacuoles are readily apparent by light microscopy in all stage IX–XI tubules and must not be confused with degenerating germ cells. Apoptotic germ cells, which are a normal feature of spermatogenesis, as well as a result of toxic injury, are also removed rapidly by phagocytosis.

Formation of the Blood-Tubule Barrier and Compartmetalization of the Seminiferous Epithelium

The main exclusion barrier is formed by the basal occluding cell junctions between adjacent Sertoli cells, situated at a level above the spermatogonia and below the spermatocytes with capillary endothelial cells and peritubular cells serving as partial barriers. By virtue of the peritubular cell layer and the inter-Sertoli cell tight junctions, the testis can be divided into a number of physiological and toxicologic compartments (Figure 18.3),

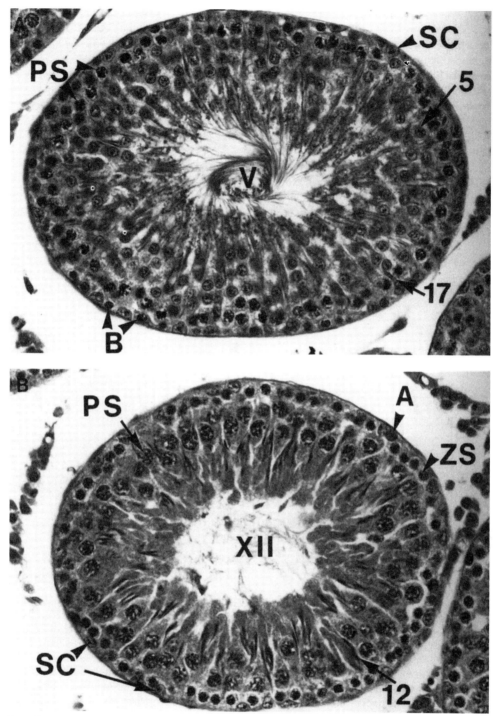

FIGURE 18.7 Typical appearance of rat seminiferous tubules in paraffin sections showing the different cellular associations. Stage V tubule (A), stage XII tubule (B). SC, Sertoli cell; ZS zygotene spermatocyte; PS, pachytene spermatocyte; A, type A spermatogonia; B, type B spermatogonia; 5, 12, and 17, spermatids at respective steps of spermiogenesis. Bar = 50 μm.

i.e., the interstitial, basal, and adlumenal compartments. The interstitial compartment is exposed to all substances transported through the capillary endothelium, including toxicants. Although the peritubular cells may exclude some large molecules, the basal compartment, which contains the spermatogonia, is also readily accessible to blood-borne substances. In contrast, the adlumenal compartment, which contains all meiotic and postmeiotic cells, is only exposed to blood-borne substances that have been transported

TABLE 18.1   Species differences in aspects of spermatogenesis and the spermatogenic cycle

Species	Sperm produced/g testis/day $\times 10^6$	No. stages in the cycle	Duration of one cycle (days)	Duration of spermatogenesis (days)	Epididymal transit time (days)
Rat	17	14	13	51.6	11
Mouse	54	12	8.6	34.5	7–10
Dog	20	8	13.6	54.4	10
Rabbit	25	8	10.9	51.8	9–10
Human	4	6	16	64	12

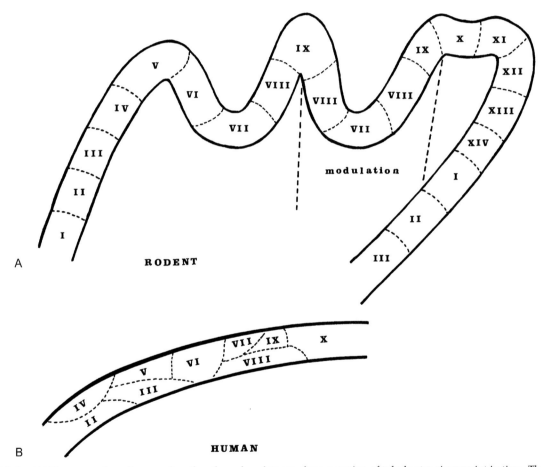

FIGURE 18.8   (A) The spermatogenic wave describes the order of stages along a section of tubule at a given point in time. The stages generally run in consecutive order, but may reverse for short distances (modulations). A wave includes all 14 consecutive stages plus any modulations. (B) The arrangement of stages in the seminiferous tubule of man is different from that in most other species. The patchwork of stages is arranged in a helical pattern so a single cross section contains cells from more than one stage.

through the Sertoli cell. This provides some protection against genetic damage or death of the gamete by toxicants. These junctions begin to develop 15–18 days after birth in the rat.

Testosterone Synthesis

Leydig cells are the major site for the synthesis of the predominant male steroid hormone, testosterone. Cholesterol is the obligatory intermediate in the synthesis of testosterone and is supplied to the Leydig cell either by receptor-mediated endocytosis of lipoprotein or by *de novo* synthesis from acetate. The rate-limiting step in testosterone synthesis is the metabolism of cholesterol to pregnenolone by the side chain cleavage enzyme complex. This is a cytochrome P450-containing enzyme located in the mitochondria. The remainder of the process occurs outside the mitochondrion, principally on the smooth endoplasmic reticulum. Following secretion from the Leydig cell, testosterone is metabolized further in the liver, androgen-dependent tissues, and a variety of peripheral tissues (Figure 18.9).

Endocrine Regulation

Overall hormonal control of the testis is maintained by the hypothalamic-pituitary axis and is mediated by the gonadotropins, luteinizing hormone and follicle-stimulating hormone (FSH) (Figure 18.9). These major hormones are overlaid by paracrine control mechanisms, which "fine tune" or modulate the endocrine effects (Table 18.2).

Follicle-Stimulating Hormone

Follicle stimulating hormone is produced and exported from the pituitary to act principally on the Sertoli cells, although interstitial testicular macrophages may also respond. FSH is a glycoprotein hormone containing two subunits. It is secreted in a pulsatile manner in response to luteinizing hormone-releasing hormone (LHRH), also referred to as gonadotropin-releasing hormone (GnRH), from the hypothalamus. Inhibin, secreted by the Sertoli cell, is involved in a feedback loop from the testis to the pituitary to inhibit FSH production (Figure 18.9). FSH is believed to exert the majority of its effects via a classical cAMP second messenger system. The action of FSH on immature and mature animals is profoundly different. FSH is often considered to be the hormone of puberty, as rising levels of FSH act as a trigger for testicular growth and initiate spermatogenesis and the expansion of the seminiferous tubules. Once this has occurred, the Sertoli cell switches its responsiveness from FSH to testosterone and many of the FSH-regulated functions in the immature animal are taken over by testosterone in the adult. The mode of action of FSH in the adult is virtually unknown, although its importance seems to vary between species. Suppression of FSH in the adult rat has a negligible effect on spermatogenesis, whereas in nonhuman primates it results in the considerable suppression of spermatogenesis and sperm output. In the rat, FSH appears to have a

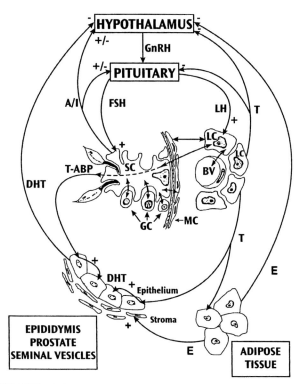

FIGURE 18.9 Major endocrine and paracrine pathways regulating male reproductive function. The main hormone testosterone (T) secreted by the Leydig cell ([C) in response to luteinizing hormone (LH) from the pituitary, which is under the control of the gonadotropin-releasing hormone (GnRH) secreted from the hypothalamus. The follicle-stimulating hormone (FSH), which acts on the Sertoli cell (SC), also has a permissive role in the maintenance of spermatogenesis and is positively regulated by activin (A) and negatively controlled by inhibin (I) secreted by the Sertoli cell. In response to testosterone, the Sertoli cell secretes a variety of proteins (androgen-regulated proteins), which modulate germ cell (GC) development. One of these proteins, androgen-binding protein, binds and acts as a transport protein for testosterone within the seminiferous tubule fluid (T-ABP). Androgen receptors on the blood vessels (BV) and peritubular myoid cells (MC) also enable testosterone to regulate blood flow and vascular permeability as well as tubular contractility. The regulation is a two-way process with factors being secreted by the target cells back to the Leydig cells. Testosterone enters the peripheral circulation and is also transported by the seminiferous tubule fluid to the secondary sex tissues where it is converted to dihydrotestosterone (DHT) and to peripheral tissues such as adipose tissue where it is converted into estradiol (E). DHT and estradiol maintain secondary sexual characteristics and provide regulatory feedback to the hypothalamic-pituitary axis. Reproduced with permission from Creasy (1999).

modifying effect on the number of differentiated spermatogonia entering meiosis but has little effect on the mitotic expansion of the undifferentiated and differentiating population. In primates, FSH appears to be important in the regulation of the expansion of undifferentiated stem cell spermatogonia.

TABLE 18.2   Endocrine and paracrine regulation of male reproduction[a,b]

Hormone	Origin	Site of action	Effect
GnRH	Hypothalamus	Pituitary	Controls release of gonadotropins LH and FSH
	Sertoli cell	Leydig cell	Increases/decreases T production
LH	Pituitary	Leydig cell	Stimulates steroidogenesis
FSH	Pituitary	Sertoli cell (prepubertal)	Stimulates estrogen production, stimulates tight junction formation between Sertoli cells, initiates spermatogenesis
		Sertoli cell (adult)	Helps maintain spermatogenesis, stimulates secretion of regulatory proteins and intermediary metabolites
		Spermatocytes	Acts with T to stimulate meiotic conversion to spermatids
		Spermatogonia	Acts with T to stimulate conversion to spermatocytes, stimulates mitotic proliferation
Thyroid hormones	Thyroid	Sertoli cell (prepubertal)	Inhibits proliferation and promotes maturation
Prolactin	Pituitary	Prostate	Enhances androgen uptake and regulates secretory activity, role in prostatic development.
		Seminal vesicles	Regulation of secretory activity
		Leydig cell	Maintenance of LH receptor numbers (rat only)
Inhibin	Sertoli cell	Pituitary	Inhibits FSH secretion
Activin	Sertoli cell	Hypothalamus/pituitary	Increases FSH secretion
Testosterone	Leydig cell	Sertoli cell	Stimulates secretion of tubular proteins including ABP, controls secretion of seminiferous tubule fluid
		Spermatids	Promotes/permits conversion of round spermatids to elongate spermatids
		Testicular vasculature	Controls blood flow and interstitial fluid volume
		Prostate	Prohormone for conversion to DHT
Oxytocin	Leydig cell	Peritubular cells	Induces contractility of seminiferous tubules
	Pituitary neurohypophysis	Epididymis	Modulates epididymal sperm transport
Androstenedione	Adrenal cortex	Prostate (human)	Promotes growth in situations of adrenal hyperfunction
Aldosterone	Adrenal cortex	Epididymis	Involved in fluid-epithelial ion transport, regulating sperm concentration
Estrogen	Sertoli cell (neonate)	Leydig cell	Inhibits testosterone production
	Adipose tissue (by aromatization of circulating T and androstenedione)	Pituitary	Inhibits LH secretion
	Leydig cell (converted from T by aromatase)	Leydig cell	Inhibits testosterone production
	Leydig cell T converted in MPOA (neonate)	CNS neurons	Sexual differentiation of male CNS
Dihydro-testosterone	Leydig cell T converted in epididymis	Epididymis	Acquisition of fertilizing ability in sperm, regulates storage of caudal sperm
	Leydig cell T converted in sex accessory tissue	Prostate and seminal vesicles	Regulates growth, differentiation and secretory function.
	Leydig cell T converted in MPOA (neonate)	CNS neurons	Sexual differentiation of male CNS
Insulin	Pancreas	Sertoli cell	Regulates glucose uptake

[a] Modified with permission from Creasy (1999)
[b] T, testosterone; LH, luteinizing hormone; FSH, follicle-stimulating hormone; DHT, dihydro testosterone; ABP, androgen-binding protein; CNS, central nervous system; MPOA, medial preoptic area

Follicle stimulating hormone appears to be the major regulatory hormone in seasonally breeding animals, producing expansion of the Leydig cell population and reinitiating spermatogenesis in response to a stimulatory photoperiod. Prolactin probably also plays an important role in these species by modifying the responsiveness of the Leydig cell to LH by altering LH receptor numbers..

Luteinizing Hormone

Luteinizing hormone (LH), like FSH, is a glycoprotein hormone secreted in a pulsatile fashion by the pituitary under LHRH control. It acts exclusively on Leydig cells in the testis and is the primary regulator of testosterone secretion, which is also secreted in a pulsatile fashion (LH pulses occurring before testosterone). Circulating plasma testosterone (or its metabolites) complete the feedback loop to the pituitary to modulate LH secretion (Figure 18.9). The Leydig cell response to the binding of LH to its receptor is mediated through a number of transducing systems, including a cAMP cascade, a phosphoinositol-diacyiglycerol, and an arachidonic acid-prostaglandin mechanism. Thus, a number of potential modifiers of LH action control the overall function of the Leydig cell (Figure 18.10). Prolactin modifies LH-stimulated testosterone secretion in the rat by increasing the number of LH receptors on the Leydig cell. Pulses of LH increase at puberty, both in amplitude and in frequency. LH is involved in the control of Leydig cell development, as differentiation of Leydig cells fails to occur in the absence of LH, but the primary impetus for their development appears to be via the FSH surge.

Testosterone

The major androgenic steroid testosterone is synthesized by the Leydig cells and has both intratesticular effects (on spermatogenesis) and peripheral effects (on accessory sex organs as well as nonreproductive organs such as muscle, bone, and skin). The concentration of testosterone within the testis is very much greater than in the systemic circulation. For example, levels of the steroid in the testicular interstitial fluid can be up to 100-fold higher than in the plasma, and the concentrations in the two compartments are not directly proportional to one another. Therefore, sampling plasma levels of testosterone does not provide a measure of testicular testosterone levels. Although these high intratesticular testosterone levels may be required to quantitatively maintain maximum spermatogenic potential, qualitatively normal spermatogenesis can be maintained with much lower intratesticular concentrations.

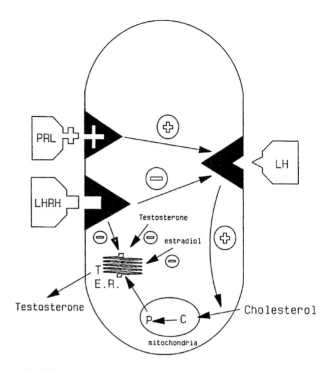

FIGURE 18.10 Diagrammatic representation of a Leydig cell and the hormonal control of steroidogenesis. LH, luteinizing hormone; PRL, prolactin; LHRH, luteinizing hormone-releasing hormone; C, cholesterol; P, pregnenolone; T, testosterone; ER, endoplasmic reticulum. Reproduced with permission from Foster (1988b).

Testosterone is not stored within the Leydig cell, it is secreted into the interstitial fluid as it is synthesized. From here it is bound to the androgen-binding protein, which is secreted by the Sertoli cell and transported through the seminiferous epithelium into the seminiferous tubule fluid and on into the epididymis and the secondary sex organs (Figure 18.9). Testosterone is also transported from the interstitial fluid into the interstitial capillaries and on into the peripheral circulation where it has wide-ranging effects on other tissues of the body, as well as effects on the central nervous system that control aggression, libido, and sexual behavior. Feedback inhibition of LH and LHRH is mediated through circulating levels of testosterone and its metabolites, dihydrotestosterone and estradiol, but the relative importance of the various molecules is species dependent. In the rat, androgens are the main feedback molecule, whereas estrogen feedback is more important in the dog, monkey, and man. Aromatization of testosterone to estradiol largely takes place in peripheral tissues such as adipose tissue, whereas conversion to other androgens is a function of androgen-dependent tissues such as the epididymis, prostate, and seminal vesicles. In those species regulated by circulating levels of estrogen, the aromatization of testosterone also occurs in the central nervous system. In these species, the administration of aromatase inhibitors, which prevent the conversion of testosterone to estradiol, results in increased LH secretion and stimulation of the Leydig cells.

Inhibin

Inhibin is a protein secreted by both testis and ovary that will decrease FSH but not LH secretion by pituitary cells. The protein is a dimer composed of an subunit and one of two different 3 subunits. In the male, inhibin is secreted by Sertoli cells and appears to have both endocrine (via its effect on the pituitary) and paracrine (other effects on cells within the testis) properties. During the isolation of inhibin, a number of new proteins were found that possess FSH-stimulating activity in pituitary cells. These compounds, now termed activins, appear to be similar in structure to inhibin, but are dimers with two subunits.

Paracrine Regulation of Testicular Function

As already discussed, testosterone is the major regulatory hormone within the testis, but its secretion is modified by a variety of substances produced by the Sertoli cell, the blood vessels, the peritubular cells, interstitial macrophages, and by the Leydig cells themselves. These paracrine and autocrine hormones provide a faster response time and allow more sensitive control of testosterone secretion as well as providing a cascade of cell-to-cell chemical communication. The list of these secreted "hormones" is growing continuously and rapidly and includes glycoprotein and steroid hormones, peptide growth factors, cytokines, proopiomelanocortin (POMC) derivatives, and neuropeptides (Table 18.2). The receptors for most of these molecules have been identified *in vitro*, although for most, their physiological function and significance are unknown, but the production of such a variety of pharmacologically potent molecules within the testis has obvious potentially important toxicological implications.

Structure and Function of the Epididymis and Excurrent Ducts

When sperm are released from the seminiferous epithelium into the tubular lumen, they are transported rapidly into a common collecting duct within the testis, termed the rete testis. Sperm then pass into a number of efferent ducts that lead into a single highly coiled duct to form the epididymis (Figure 18.11).

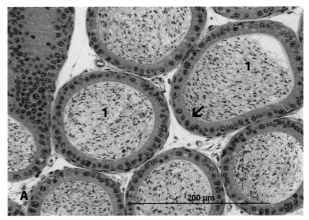
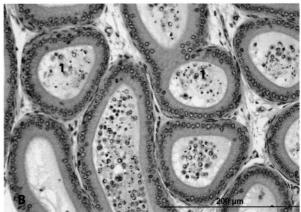

FIGURE 18.11   Epididymis, mouse. (A) With normal spermatogenesis, the lumen of the epididymal duct (1) is filled with spermatozoa and lined mainly by columnar epithelial cells (principal cells, arrow). (B) With abnormal spermatogenesis, as shown here, the lumen of the epididymal duct (1) contains small numbers of sloughed spermatids and debris. Examination of the epididymis can be very helpful in evaluating spermatogenesis. Davidson's fixative, paraffin embedded, H & E stained.

This structure, largely surrounded by adipose tissue and closely applied to the surface of the testis, is divided into three major parts: the caput (head), corpus (body), and cauda (tail) epididymis. The coiled epididymal duct leads into a straight portion termed the ductus or vas deferens, which extends through to the urethra. Various glands empty their secretions into this duct. Smooth muscle cells surround the ductal epithelium; the layers increase in thickness until, in the vas deferens, there is a very thick muscle coat. A loose connective tissue network consisting of fibroblasts and collagen and containing capillaries and small nerves separates adjacent convolutions of the duct from each other.

Rete Testis

The rete testis comprises a single or series of interconnected channels lined by simple cuboidal or columnar epithelium into which the seminiferous tubules open and which leads into the efferent ducts. In some species, such as the rat and mouse, the rete is situated in a subcapsular position at the cranial pole of the testis, but in other species, including the dog and rabbit, it forms a series of ducts running through the center of the testis. The rete testis serves as a collecting reservoir for sperm within the testis. It is also the site of inhibin reabsorption from the testis into the circulation and the first site of seminiferous tubule fluid reabsorption. Tubuli recti, which are lined only by Sertoli cells, form the junction between the seminiferous tubules and the rete and can sometimes be mistaken for atrophic seminiferous tubules. Both ends of a seminiferous tubule empty into the rete, and the probable function of the Sertoli cell lining in the tubuli recti is to act as a one-way valve for the passage of sperm and fluid into the rete, opening only when the pressure in the tubule rises above that in the rete and efferent ducts.

Efferent Ducts

The efferent ducts (ductuli efferentes) arise from the extratesticular rete and extend through the epididymal fat to empty into the initial segment of the epididymis. The number of ducts varies (6–15) depending on the species. In most species, the epithelium of the efferent ducts is composed of two cell types, although in some species, including man, up to six cell types have been described. In the rat, the principal cell forms the bulk of the epithelium but it is interspersed with ciliated cells that possess long cilia and have a lumenally positioned nucleus. Surrounding the duct is one to three layers of smooth muscle. This part of the duct is largely concerned with the propulsion of the sperm from the rete to the epididymis. In addition, the efferent ducts reabsorb a large proportion of the seminiferous tubular fluid secreted by the Sertoli cells.

Epididymis

The initial segment of the caput epididymis is richly vascularized, and its reddish color is grossly visible. The transition between the epithelial cells of the efferent ducts and the epididymis is abrupt; ciliated cells give way to basal cells, apical cells, and much taller principal cells, producing a marked increase in the height of the epithelium. There is no sharp anatomical or histological demarcation between the end of the caput and the beginning of the corpus. The corpus is the narrow portion of the epididymis between the caput and the cauda. The cauda forms a grossly distinct structure due to dilatation with stored sperm.

The basal cells are more numerous than in the caput or corpus. The principal cells are cuboidal, have a more compact microvillous border, and contain basal lipid droplets. Clear cells are frequently seen. These cells have a basal pale nucleus, and the cytoplasm contains varying numbers of large clear vacuoles, lipid droplets, and dense granules.

Epithelial cells of the epididymis synthesize and secrete many macromolecules, including a number of glycoproteins; reabsorb more than 90% of seminiferous tubular fluid; and are involved in the active transport of ions and protein across the epithelium. The major part of the synthetic and reabsorptive role of the epididymis is carried out in the caput and corpus by the principal cells, whereas the larger diameter cauda serves as a storage receptacle for the mature motile sperm prior to ejaculation. Depending on the species and the frequency of ejaculation, sperm reach the cauda 1–2 weeks after release from the seminiferous tubule. Sperm production is a continuous process: if the stored sperm are not removed by frequent ejaculation, they are voided in the urine.

During the passage of sperm through the epididymis, changes in sperm morphology and metabolism occur. Excess cytoplasm in the form of the residual cytoplasmic droplet is shed from the sperm and there are changes in the structure of the acrosome and midpiece and different surface antigens are expressed. Associated with these events is the acquisition of the ability to fuse with, and fertilize, an oocyte. There are many potential sites for the direct toxicologic disturbance of epididymal function. In addition, many of the functions are androgen dependent, making them secondarily susceptible to toxic effects on the testis.

As with the testis, there is a barrier protecting the lumenal sperm from the immunologically competent cells of the blood. This barrier is formed by the apical tight junctions between adjacent ductular cells. However, these tight junctions are not as robust as the Sertoli-Sertoli occluding junctions in the seminiferous epithelium and are damaged and breached more easily. Also, the barrier is not as restrictive to molecules as that in the testis and will allow more substances into the ductular fluid, providing the potential for direct toxicity to the sperm.

Vas Deferens

The vas deferens (ductus deferens) is a thick-walled convoluted tube that is continuous with the tail of the epididymis and extends to the prostatic urethra. In most species, the final part of this tube is dilated to form the ampulla, which joins the duct of the seminal vesicle to become the ejaculatory duct.

The histological transition between the epididymis and the vas is abrupt; this is largely due to the development of a thick smooth muscle coat around the latter. The epithelium is pseudostratified with long microvilli (stereocilia) on the apical surface. The ejaculatory duct is lined by transitional epithelium as it approaches the urethra. The vas deferens transfers the sperm, which have been stored in the epididymis, to the urethra, where additional secretions are added to produce the semen. The very thick fibromuscular coat that surrounds the duct is innervated by the sympathetic nervous system and, when stimulated, contracts to provide rapid propulsion of the sperm along the tract during ejaculation.

Structure and Function of Accessory Sex Organs

The accessory sex organs in rodents are the seminal vesicles, prostate, coagulating gland, bulbourethral gland, and preputial gland. They are located along the route of the urethra as it relays sperm from the vas deferens out through the penis. The glands secrete a variety of complex fluids that transport and sustain the sperm during their lengthy journey out of the male and through the female genital tract. Their structure is typical of active exocrine secretory glands, although the characteristics of the individual secretions are markedly different. Because the secretory activity of the accessory sex glands is extremely sensitive to androgen levels, weight change and altered cellular activity in the prostate and seminal vesicle can be used as a good, and relatively rapid, indicator of altered circulating androgen levels. There are major species differences in the complement of secondary sex glands (Table 18.3).

Prostate

The prostate forms multiple lobes around the urethra. It is a compound tubuloalveolar gland that secretes a colorless serous fluid into the urethra through a number of ducts. In the rat, a discrete pair of ventral lobes and a smaller group of dorsal and lateral lobes are situated at the neck of the bladder. A pair of anterior lobes, otherwise known as the coagulating glands, is situated closely adjacent to the seminal vesicle. The glandular acini are lined by a simple columnar epithelium. The prostatic fluid secretion constitutes 15–30% of the ejaculate. It is a colorless fluid rich in proteolytic enzymes (e.g., acid phosphatase). The fluid also contains relatively high levels of zinc, inositol, transferrin, and citric acid.

Seminal Vesicles

The seminal vesicles are paired elongated hollow organs filled with a yellowish-white viscous fluid. They are situated distal to the ampulla of the vas deferens and empty via the ejaculatory duct into the urethra. The mucosa has a honeycombed structure formed by complex folding to produce irregular anastomosing channels that communicate with the central cavity; thin primary folds of the mucosa also extend out into the vesicle lumen. The epithelium is composed of pseudostratified columnar cells in the mouse and a simple columnar epithelium in the rat. The seminal vesicle fluid is a viscous secretion constituting 50–80% of the ejaculate. The fluid is alkaline, which is thought to neutralize the acid pH of the vagina; it contains citric acid as the major component, as well as fructose and lactoferrin. Lactoferrin is one of the sperm-coating antigens and, as its name suggests, is also involved in iron binding.

TABLE 18.3   Presence of accessory sex glands in man and various species

Species	Ampulla	Prostate	Seminal vesicles	Bulbourethral gland	Preputial gland
Man	+	+	+	+	−
Rat	+	+	+	+	+
Mouse	+	+	+	+	+
Rabbit	+	+	+	+	+
Dog	+	+	−	−	−
Cat	−	+	−	−	−
Cattle	+	+	+	+	−
Sheep	+	+	+	+	−
Horse	+	+	+	+	−
Pig	−	+	+	+	−

Bulbourethral Glands

Bulbourethral glands (Cowper's glands, Mery glands) are paired compound tubuloalveolar glands that secrete a mucoid material into the penile urethra. The epithelial cells are pyramidal to columnar with a microvillous surface. The bulbourethral glands secrete a small quantity of clear, viscous fluid, which, in rodents, is secreted immediately after ejaculation of the sperm, along with fluid from the coagulating gland, to form a copulatory plug in the vagina, preventing loss of sperm and further copulation.

Preputial Gland

Preputial glands are paired sebaceous glands located in the subcutaneous tissue near the tip of the penis in the mouse and along the ventral midline in the inguinal region of the rat. Ducts leading from the sebaceous acini are lined by squamous epithelium. The gland is a holocrine gland releasing its secretion by rupture of the acinar cells. The ductular secretion and the intracellular secretory granules are intensely eosinophilic, resembling keratin in appearance. Secretion from the preputial gland contains pheromones (aliphatic alcohols) and β-glucuronidase.

TABLE 18.4 Functions of reproductive tract tissues

Tissue	Major reproductive function
Testis	Production of sperm from stem cell spermatogonia
	Production of testosterone from Leydig cells
Epididymis	Maturation of sperm surface antigens enabling fertilization
	Storage of sperm prior to ejaculation
	Resorption of seminiferous tubule fluid
	Secretion of molecules into fluid (steroids, carnitine, inositol)
Seminal vesicles, prostate	Production of seminal fluid containing nutrients and enzymes for sperm survival and proteins involved in copulatory plug formation
Coagulating gland	Production of copulatory plug
Preputial gland	Production of pheromones and β-glucuronidase
Pituitary	Secretion of gonadotropins: luteinizing hormone, follicle-stimulating hormone, and prolactin
Hypothalamus/CNS	Secretion of gonadotropin-releasing hormone and dopamine
	Regulation of sexual behavior and performance

Penis and Ejaculation

The penis is composed of three erectile structures: the two corpora cavernosa, which are connected to the ischium by the ischiocavernosus muscle, and the corpus spongiosum, which contains the extrapelvic urethra. The free end of the penis is termed the glans penis and is covered by stratified squamous epithelium. It is contained within a sheath and is partly covered by the prepuce, which is continuous with the inner lining of the sheath. Erection is caused by contraction of the ischiocavernosus muscle, which compresses the penis against the ischium, obstructing the blood flow through the dorsal veins. Consequently, the vascular spaces of the erectile tissue become distended with blood.

Expulsion of the sperm stored in the cauda epididymis is controlled by the sympathetic nervous system that innervates the smooth muscle coat of the epididymis and vas deferens. Contraction of these muscles results in propulsion of the sperm through the vas into the urethra, where the secretions of the accessory sex organs are added to produce semen.

MECHANISMS OF TOXICITY

The diversity of function, combined with the complexity of hormonal regulation of the reproductive tract, provides a vast number of potential sites for the chemical disturbance of fertility (Table 18.4). Toxicity may result in reduced sperm production by the testis, interference with the transport and maturation of sperm in the epididymis, disturbance of sexual behavior or pathways controlling the erection and ejaculation of sperm into the female reproductive tract, or reduced quality of the sperm available for fertilization. The potential target sites are summarized in Figure 18.12.

A small number of reproductive toxicants, such as the phthalate esters, 2,5-hexanedione, and the glycol ethers, have attracted extensive and intensive research activity since the 1980s in an effort to elucidate their mechanism of toxicity. With very few exceptions, the fundamental mechanisms of toxicity have remained elusive. Despite this, the investigations have added greatly to our knowledge and understanding of male reproductive toxicity and have provided a variety of approaches to investigating toxic mechanisms. Mechanistic explanations of toxicity involve a variety of factors, including metabolic and pharmacodynamic considerations, morphological pathogenesis of the lesion, functional disturbances of cell physiology, and identification of the molecular lesion. For risk assessment purposes, such extensive investigations are

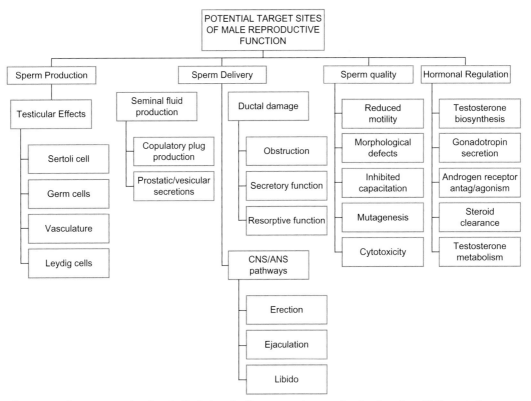

FIGURE 18.12   Potential target sites for chemically induced effects on male reproductive function. CNS, central nervous system; ANS, autonomic nervous system.

generally impractical and too time-consuming. In practice, important, relevant information relating to the mechanism of toxicity can be gained by selective investigation of these factors. For example, the identity of the toxic molecule (metabolite or parent), the site of metabolic activation (testicular or extratesticular), the target tissue and target cell of toxicity, and the reversibility of the lesion are aspects of toxicity that can generally be investigated with relative ease. Identification of the functional disturbances and the molecular biology of a lesion are vastly more difficult goals, partly due to technical difficulties but mostly due to an incomplete and inadequate understanding of normal male reproductive physiology and endocrinology.

Role of Metabolism

The role of metabolism in testicular toxicity is an important consideration not only for risk assessment, but also for the rational design of any *in vitro* investigations. The actively toxic molecule may be the parent compound or a metabolite. Metabolism may occur in extra testicular tissues, e.g., the liver or the intestines, with the toxic metabolite being transported to the testis. Alternatively, metabolic activation may occur within the

testis, either within the target cell or in a neighboring cell, with subsequent transport or diffusion of the toxic metabolite to the target cell (Figure 18.13). Significant levels of xenobiotic metabolizing enzymes are present within the testis. As a consequence of its role in steroid synthesis, the Leydig cell is the major source of these enzymes, but the Sertoli cell also contains a variety of important enzymes, whereas the germ cells mostly contain cytoprotective enzymes. Pharmacokinetic factors can also be an important aspect of toxic mechanisms. The properties of the blood-testis barrier will exclude many potentially toxic molecules. If the toxic species does not gain access to a cell, it cannot have a direct toxic effect. For this reason, most somatic mutagens are not *in vivo* germ cell mutagens. This is also an important consideration for the design of any *in vitro* studies where isolated testicular cells are exposed to a chemical compound. It is important to know whether the cells should be exposed to the parent molecule or to a metabolite and to know what is the physiologically relevant concentration achieved *in vivo*. Pharmacokinetics is also important for risk assessment considerations. Boric acid has been shown to accumulate in the testis, and the nature of the testicular lesion (reversible spermatid retention or irreversible tubular atrophy) is related to the testicular load of boron. There are species

TABLE 18.5   Cell-specific toxicants of the male reproductive tract

Target cell	Toxicant	Effect
Leydig cell	Ethanedimethane sulfonate	Leydig cell necrosis with secondary germ cell death and depletion and atrophy of secondary sex organs
	Lansoprazole	Inhibition of testosterone synthesis with secondary Leydig cell tumor induction
Sertoli cell	Phthalate esters, 2,5-hexanedione	Sertoli cell vacuoles with secondary germ cell death and exfoliation
Spermatogonia	Busulfhan, bleomycin	Spermatogonial death with secondary depletion of postspermatogonial germ cells
Spermatocytes	2-Methoxyethanol, dinitropyrroles	Spermatocyte death with secondary depletion of postspermatocyte germ cells
Round spermatids	Ethylmethane sulfonate, methyl chloride	Spermatid death with secondary depletion of postspermatid germ cells
Elongated spermatids	Boric acid, dibromoacetic acid	Retention and phagocytosis of step 19 spermatids, abnormalities in released sperm
Testicular blood vessels	Cadmium chloride	Endothelial necrosis with secondary ischemic necrosis of all cell types
	5-Hydroxytryptamine, histamine	Reduced blood flow with secondary germ cell death and depletion
Epididymal epithelium	α-Chlorohydrin (high doses)	Inhibits fluid resorption, resulting in sperm granulomas
	Methyl chloride	Epithelial necrosis, resulting in sperm granulomas
Epididymal sperm	α-Chlorohydrin (low doses), deoxychloroglucose	Inhibition of glycolysis, resulting in sperm immotility
Vas deferens	Guanethidine	Inhibition of ejaculation due to adrenergic ganglion blockade, resulting in rupture of vas–epididymal junction and sperm granulomas
Prostate and seminal vesicles	Flutamide	Androgen receptor blockade, resulting in secretory inhibition and atrophy
	Finasteride	Inhibition of dihydrotestosterone production from testosterone, resulting in secretory inhibition and atrophy

differences in the uptake of molecules by the testis and in access of molecules across the blood-testis barrier. Cyclohexylamine, the major metabolite of cyclamate, is toxic to the rat testis but not the mouse testis. This appears to be due to the differential absorption and distribution of cyclohexyamine rather than the different metabolic profile of this compound by the two species.

Cell-specific Toxicity in the Testis

For most testicular toxicants, cell-specific toxicity can be demonstrated when the dose level is reduced and the testis is examined during the initial stages of lesion development (Table 18.5).

Leydig Cell

Toxicity to the Leydig cell is generally manifest as an inhibition of its primary function, the production

of testosterone. This may be brought about by the inhibition of specific enzymes in the biosynthetic pathway, such as inhibitors of 17–20 lyase, which prevent the conversion of 17-hydroxyprogesterone to androstenedione. Such compounds have been used to decrease or eliminate estrogen and androgen production in the treatment of hormonally dependent cancer. Alternatively, a range of steroidogenic enzymes may be affected as with tri-o-cresyl phosphate, which affects enzymes throughout the pathway, or ketoconazole, an antifungal imidazole derivative, which is also used for the treatment of prostatic cancer in man. This inhibits the cytochrome P450 enzymes of the steroid biosynthesis pathway, including the side chain cleavage complex, 17a-hydroxylase, and C17–20 lyase. Less well defined examples include cannabinoids and ethanol, which also inhibit steroidogenesis and decrease the levels of various intermediates in the pregnenolone-testosterone pathway. In the case of ethanol, it is interesting to note that alcohol dehydrogenase appears to be specifically (by immunocytochemical determination) located in the Leydig cells and, in addition to metabolizing ethanol, will metabolize endogenous substrates such as retinol and dihydrotestosterone. Thus competitive inhibition of this enzyme may result in alterations in steroid profiles.

Perhaps the most widely studied Leydig cell toxicant is the sulfonic acid ester, ethane dimethane sulfonate (EDS), which is specifically cytotoxic to the Leydig cell and results in almost complete loss of the Leydig cell population. The mechanism of this cell specific toxicity is unknown, but it is of importance to note that other structurally closely related esters are targeted to other testicular cell types, e.g., spermatogonia in the case of busulfan.

Sertoli Cells

Injury to the Sertoli cell has potentially serious consequences due to its pivotal role in supporting spermatogenesis. Although cell death rarely occurs, the physiological processes of Sertoli cells are easily disturbed and will rapidly result in germ cell degeneration. If the injury is sufficiently severe or prolonged, it is probable that Sertoli cell function will be permanently compromised and recovery of spermatogenesis may not be possible or at best incomplete.

Although a number of toxicants have been categorized as Sertoli cell toxicants, relatively few have been investigated in any detail with regard to their mechanism of action. Even for those that have, such as diethylhexyl phthalate (DEHP), 1,3-dinitrobenzene (DNB), and 2,5-hexanedione, the mechanisms of Sertoli cell injury still remain poorly and incompletely understood. Designation of a chemical as a Sertoli cell toxicant is generally based on morphological or biochemical evidence that this is the earliest cell to be affected. This does not necessarily mean that it is the first cell to be functionally altered. Tri-ocresyl phosphate (TOCP) is toxic to the Sertoli cell on the basis of morphological changes and inhibition of nonspecific esterase (NSE) activity, but LH-induced Leydig cell steroidogenesis is affected at earlier time points, without showing evidence of morphological toxicity. Although molecular mechanisms of toxicity have not been fully elucidated for any toxicants, a number of unique structures and functions of the Sertoli cell are prime targets for toxicity. These include altered protein and fluid secretion (e.g., dinitrobenzene [DNB], phthalate esters [Figure 18.14] and 2,5-hexanedione [HD]), cytoskeletal alterations (colchicines,vinblastine, cytochalasin A), metabolic disturbances (e.g., MEHP, DNB, lead, cadmium, 2-methoxyethanol, 2,5- HD, dibromochloropropane, and gossypol), receptor-mediated cell responses (e.g. MEHP). However the

relationship (if any) of these changes to the mechanism of toxicity is unclear.

Germ Cells
DNA Synthesis

Interference with DNA synthesis can result in the death of a cell as it undergoes mitotic or meiotic division or in a heritable defect in the DNA, which may have consequences if fertilization occurs, resulting in embryo death or paternally mediated congenital defects. The large number of actively proliferating cells in the testis makes it particularly sensitive to agents that damage DNA such as cancer chemotherapeutic drugs or radiation and the intercalating antibiotics such as daunorubicin and adriamycin. These agents bind covalently to the DNA, preventing replication, and may also interfere with RNA synthesis. DNA repair enzymes may be able to repair the damage, but the faster the cell cycle, the less time there is available for repair. Antimetabolites such as cytosine arabinoside, methotrexate, and 5-fluorouracil interfere with nucleotide incorporation, whereas microtubule-disrupting agents, such as colchicine, taxol, vinblastine, and vincristine, prevent spindle formation during division. Radiation and radiomimetic agents such as bleomycin produce reactive-free radicals that interact with DNA, as does 1,3-dimethyl-benzanthracene, which is metabolized to its reactive intermediate by the Sertoli cell but exerts its toxic effect on the adjacent spermatogonia (Figure 18.13). There is differential sensitivity to these toxicants among the various subpopulations of spermatogonia with the slow cycling stem cell spermatogonia proving more resistant to most of the agents than differentiating (committed) spermatogonia. Due to their presence in the basal compartment (outside the blood-tubule barrier), spermatogonia are exposed to any xenobiotic that enters the interstitial fluid, whereas spermatocytes, which also undertake DNA synthesis and meiotic division, are protected by the barrier and are affected far less frequently. The presence of the barrier also restricts the entry of genotoxic chemicals to the sensitive meiotic cells, and although such chemicals have access to the spermatogonia, any damage has time to be repaired or, more frequently, results in death of the cell. However, a number of chemicals, including methyl methane sulfonate and ethyl-methane sulfonate, do gain access to the adluminal germ cells and produce genetic damage in the mid-to late stage spermatids of mice, resulting in pre- and postimplantation loss. In addition, paternal chronic exposure to low doses of cyclophosphamide has been reported to produce congenital abnormalities in offspring as well as implantation losses.

TRI-O-CRESYL PHOSPHATE

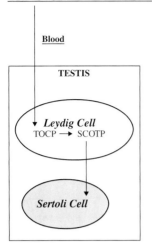

1,3-DINITROBENZENE

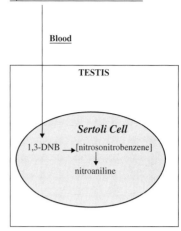

DI-2-ETHYLHEXYL PHTHALATE

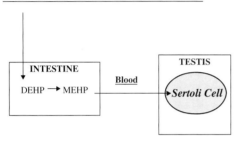

7,12-DIMETHYLBENZ[A]ANTHRACENE

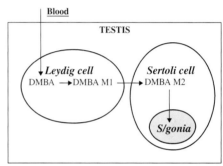

FIGURE 18.13   The role of metabolism in mechanisms of testicular toxicity. Some testicular toxicants (diethylhexyl phthalate) are metabolized to their active metabolite in extratesticular tissues and are transported in the blood to their target cell. Intratesticular-metabolizing enzymes activate other toxicants. In some cases (1,3-dinitrobenzene), the activation occurs within the target cell. In other cases (tri-o-cresyl phosphate), activation occurs within one cell but causes toxicity in an adjacent cell. In the case of dimethylbenzanthracene, different steps in the activation pathway occur in more than one cell type with transportation of the toxic metabolite to a different cell type.

Apoptotic Cell Death

In the testis, apoptosis provides the important physiological function of limiting the size of the germ cell population to numbers that can be adequately supported. The Sertoli cell regulates this function, utilizing the FAS gene system, which has also been implicated in immune regulation. Germ cells express Fas, a transmembrane receptor protein that, when bound by Fas ligand (FasL) expressed by the Sertoli cell, transmits an apoptotic signal within the cell. All chemically induced germ cell death investigated so far also appears to occur through the process of apoptosis. This is true for both direct germ cell toxicity, as occurs with radiation, and indirect germ cell death resulting from Sertoli cell injury. The precise mechanism triggering apoptosis appear to be different in each case. With Sertoli cell toxicants, there is upregulation of Fas and FasL, but with germ cell toxicants there is only upregulation of Fas. Administration of 2-methoxyethanol, or

its active metabolite methoxyacetic acid (MAA), results in apoptosis of the spermatocyte population and, at the lower end of its effective dose range, this toxicity is restricted to very specific stages of pachytene development (Figure 18.15). Although this should provide clues as to the biochemical mechanism involved, this has remained elusive.

Vascular Effects and Indirect Toxicity to the Testis

Indirect mechanisms must also be considered when attempting to establish the mode of action of any male reproductive toxicant. Such effects would range from an effect on the vasculature to interference with the photoperiod of a seasonally breeding animal.

The vascular supply to the testis is relatively poor. Hence, any agent damaging the vascular bed is liable

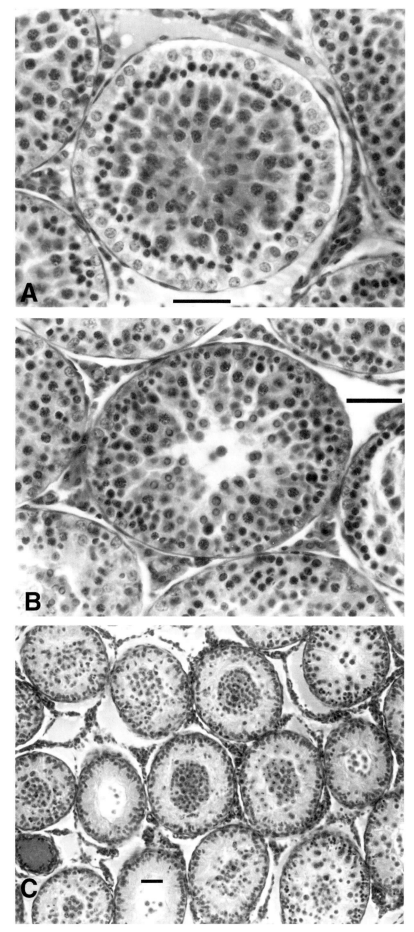

FIGURE 18.14   Effect of di-*n*-pentyl phthalate (DPP) on the testis of the immature rat. (A) Six hours after an oral dose of 2.2 g/kg showing basal Sertoli cell cytoplasmic rarefaction and closure of the tubular lumen. (B) Twenty-four hours after dosing, showing some germ cell
degeneration and sloughing of cells into the lumen. (C) After 3 days of dosing with DPP, showing total exfoliation of germ cells into the tubular lumen. Bar = 50 μm.

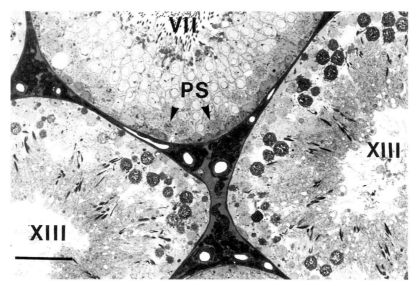

FIGURE 18.15   Stage-specific spermatocyte toxicity 24 hr after an oral dose of 250 mg/kg ethylene glycol monomethyl ether. Late pachytene spermatocytes in stage XIII tubules are necrotic, but the underlying zygotene spermatocytes and the midpachytene spermatocytes (PS) in the adjacent stage VII tubule are unaffected. Bar = 50 μm.

to rapidly produce an anoxic response in the organ and widespread cell death. The most cited example is the heavy metal cadmium. A single ip injection of a salt of this element in the microgram per kilogram range can produce complete necrosis of the testis; it is mediated by an effect on the vascular endothelium.

Certain nutritional deficiencies will also result in a failure of the male reproductive system. For example, zinc and vitamin A deficiencies are known to produce deleterious effects on spermatogenesis. A severe reduction in food intake and body weight can have a detrimental effect on spermatogenesis. In the CD1 mouse, reduced testosterone levels and reduced epididymal sperm and testicular spermatids are seen in mice maintained for 90 days at 70% control body weight (but no effect seen in mice maintained at 80 or 90% of control body weight). In the Sprague-Dawley rat, this level of body weight loss is not associated with any effects on testicular or sperm parameters.

Testicular function in certain species is sensitive to photoperiod. In the hamster, reducing the light period below 14 hr alters the photoperiod and can result in testicular regression and reproductive failure. Similar effects can be observed when a compound induces eye lesions, or perhaps interferes with the pineal gland hormone, melatonin.

Epididymal and Sperm Toxicity

The epididymis plays a major role in the maturation of sperm, and it too can be a target for toxicity. One of the best examples is methyl chloride, which, when administered by inhalation, in addition to producing an effect on the testis, will damage the epididymal epithelium, possibly by the production of leukotrienes. Granulomas form within the epididymis, resulting in obstruction of the passage of sperm because the epididymis is a single tube; hence, infertility results. Infertility arising from methyl chloride administration is associated with preimplanatation loss and postimplantation loss (indicative of genotoxic damage). However, it has been demonstrated that the dominant lethality associated with the administration of methyl chloride is not due to direct genotoxicity of the compound but is a result of oxidative DNA damage to the sperm, caused by the release of oxidative free radicals from the infiltrating leukocytes. The development of sperm granulomas and the dominant lethal effects of methyl chloride can be prevented by the use of anti-inflammatory drugs. Oxidative damage to the sperm is an important potential site of toxicity for any chemical that gains access to the epididymal fluid, as increased lipid peroxidation of the sperm plasma membrane has been linked with defective sperm function in humans. The soil fumigant dibromochloropropane (DBCP) produces testicular damage in a number of species; it is metabolized to epichlorhydrin and in turn to α-chlorhydrin. At high doses, both of these metabolites produce increased capillary permeability in the epididymis, resulting in vascular damage, epithelial necrosis, and sperm granuloma and spermatocoele formation. Cadmium also has a toxic effect on the vasculature of the caput epididymis, resulting in similar effects. Rupture of the duct at the vasoepididymal junction followed by the formation of granulomas and spermatocoeles occurs with the antihypertensive guanethidine, due to ganglion blockade of the sympathetic neural pathways controlling contraction of the vas deferens during ejaculation.

The role of the epididymis in modification of the sperm membrane and the maturation of sperm function is incompletely understood, but the potential for chemicals to enter the epididymal fluid and produce direct effects on the sperm has been demonstrated. A number of compounds, including low doses of α-chlorohydrin, have a specific effect on spermatozoal respiratory function and motility through the inhibition of energy production from the Krebs cycle. Chlorosugars, such as 6-chlorodeoxyglucose, have a similar effect on motility by acting on the glycolytic energy pathway.

Secondary Sex Organs

The importance of the various secondary sex organs for fertility varies with the species. Although a number of chemicals result in decreased size, weight, and secretory activity, through their interference with androgen production or action, there are almost no examples of chemicals that act only on the prostate and seminal vesicles to bring about a reduction in fertility. One exception to this appears to be Finasteride, which inhibits 5α-reductase, and thereby decreases dihydrotestosterone levels.

In the rodent, this reduces fertility by preventing the production of an effective copulatory plug by the coagulating gland, which is necessary in the rodent for retaining the ejaculate in the vagina. Because copulatory plugs are not produced in other species, the general significance of this finding is probably limited.

Hormone Disruption

Hormonal pathways control the functioning of the entire reproductive process. They involve a wide range of endocrine, paracrine, and autocrine hormones, the secretion of which is modified by subtle changes in cell-to-cell interactions or disturbances in any one of a number of tissues. This makes the elucidation of hormonal mechanisms of toxicity difficult, as primary and secondary hormonal changes are almost impossible to separate *in vivo*, and investigations must rely heavily on *in vitro* techniques, which present their own problems for interpretation. The male reproductive system, organ targets, and reported effects of endocrine disrupting chemicals is presented in Table 18.6

Target Sites of Disruption

There are numerous established biochemical mechanisms through which chemicals can affect androgen secretion or androgen action, some of which are species dependent. They include androgen receptor antagonism, 5 α-reductase inhibition, testosterone biosynthesis inhibition, aromatase inhibition, increased dopamine secretion or dopamine receptor agonism, and LHRH receptor agonism and antagonism. Most of the published examples of such compounds have been specifically developed to treat male reproductive disorders or as potential male contraceptives. Whether a disturbance in androgen secretion or action results in adverse effects on male reproduction depends on the dose and the duration of dosing relative to the degree of hormonal disruption and the ability of homeostatic mechanisms to compensate for the disturbance. Effects may also be different in the prepubertal compared with the adult animal, as the hormonal control of reproductive function fundamentally changes with age.

There is no satisfactory way to classify the various hormonally mediated toxicants because most affect more than one site in the reproductive tract, whether it is a primary or secondary event. In addition, many appear to interfere with more than one biochemical target site of hormonal action. With these constraints in mind, toxicants can be loosely divided into agents primarily affecting CNS control pathways, agents affecting gonadotropin release, and agents affecting androgen receptors, androgen biosynthesis, and androgen metabolism (to other active androgens, estrogens, and inactive androgens).

Leydig Cell Neoplasia

Prolonged disruption of the pituitary-gonadal hormone axis in rodents is very likely to result in Leydig cell tumors. In the rat, focal Leydig cell hyperplasia and Leydig cell tumors can be readily induced by a wide range of chemically diverse drugs and chemicals, including dopamine agonists, antiandrogens, LHRH analogs, peroxisome proliferators, and histamine receptor antagonists (Table 18.7). The proposed mechanism of action for these various classes of compounds is through interference with Leydig cell control mechanisms at a variety of points along the hypothalamic/pituitary/testicular axis. A major impetus for Leydig cell tumorigenesis in the rat is considered to be high circulating levels of LH. However, a significant number of Leydig cell tumorigens have no effect on circulating levels of LH, but do alter intratesticular testosterone (and other hormones), thereby affecting the paracrine feedback control of Leydig cell proliferation, presumably through local growth factors.

In contrast, the chemical induction of Leydig cell tumors in the mouse is less common and is generally associated with high circulating levels of estrogen or administration of estrogenic compounds such as diethylstilbestrol. In general, the types of chemicals

TABLE 18.6 The male reproductive system, organ targets, and reported effects of endocrine disrupting chemicals

Male Reproductive Organ	Reported Effects	Chemicals
Primarily developmental effects	Pseudohermaphrodite/vaginal pouch	Procymidone, vinclozolin, DEHP
	Hypospadia	Hydroxyflutamide, procymidone, vinclozolin, finasteride, DEHP
	Microphallus/cleft phallus	DES, procymidone, vinclozolin
	Decreased anogenital distance	Vinclozolin, linuron, p,p' DDE, dibutyl phthalate, procymidone, DEHP
Testis	Cryptorchidism or delayed testicular descent	DES, TCDD, hydroxyflutamide, procymidone, vinclozolin
	Tubular atrophy	TCDD, vinclozolin, linuron, boric acid, dibutyl phthalate
	Decreased testis weight	DES, octyphenol phenoxylate, octylphenol, butyl benzyl phthalate, boric acid, DEHP
	Decreased testosterone	TCDD, heptachlor, boric acid, N-nitroso-N-ethylurea, PCBs, ethane dimethanesulfonate, lindane, dibromoacetic acid, phthalate esters, hexachlorocyclohexane
	Neoplasia	Procymidone, pronamide, lacidipine, lansoprazole, ammonium perfluorooctanoate, acrylamide, gamma-oryzanol
Rete testis	Neoplasia	DES
Efferent ductules	Dilation, decreased epithelial height	Genistein, octylphenol, bisphenol A
Epididymis	Cysts-granulomas/abnormal development/function	DES, linuron, dibutyl phthalate, procymidone, phosphamidon, EDS, epichlorohydrin, TCDD, DEHP, chloroethylmethanesulphonate, alpha-chlorohydrin, cadmium, dibromo-chloropropane, benomyl, carbendazim
Sperm	Decreased sperm production, ejaculated numbers	TCDD, DES, 4-octyphenol, butylbenzyl phthalate, dibutylphthalate, vinclozolin, p,p'DDE
Prostate	Neoplasia/growth or weight changes/abnormal development/absent prostate	Bisphenol A, TCDD, p,p' DDE, coke oven emissions, cadmium, N-hydroxy-3,2'-dimethyl-4-amino biphenyl, procymidone, N-methyl-N-nitrosourea, hydroxyflutamide, 3,2'-dimethyl-4-aminobiphenyl

that produce Leydig cell tumors in the rat are ineffective in mice. Furthermore, estrogen administration to the rat appears to be inhibitory to the development of spontaneous and chemically induced Leydig cell tumors, although, in at least one case (ammonium perfluorooctonate), the major detectable hormonal change leading to Leydig cell tumors is an increase in plasma estradiol levels. Aromatase inhibitors such as formestane and letrozole reduce plasma estradiol levels by inhibiting the conversion of testosterone to estrogen. In the dog, but not rodents, this results in Leydig cell hypertrophy and hyperplasia. This is thought to be due to the differential sensitivity of the pituitary feedback mechanism to estrogens and androgens in the different species. The aromatization of testosterone plays a significant role in the control of gonadotropins in dogs, nonhuman primates, and man, whereas in rodents, testosterone and dihydrotestosterone are the main regulatory molecules.

The testicular tumor profile and the physiology of Leydig cell tumorigenesis in rodents and human

appear to be very different, and on this basis it has been argued that chemical induction of Leydig cell tumors in the rat is a species-specific effect with limited relevance for risk assessment to man. However, such claims need to be supported by careful investigations into the mechanism of hormonal disruption.

Toxicity to the Developing Reproductive Tract

Effects via Estrogen Receptors, the Example of Methoxychlor

Methoxychlor is an insecticide that displays both estrogenic and antiandrogenic activity. If treatment is administered at weaning, methoxychlor will induce a number of effects in male rat offspring, including delays in puberty (preputial separation) and reduced accessory sex gland size. Interestingly, no effects on circulating levels of LH or testosterone were noted in the presence of delayed puberty.

Methoxychlor is metabolized extensively to HPTE [2,2-bis(p-phenylhydroxyphenyl)-1,1,1-trichloroethane],

TABLE 18.7 Examples of drugs and chemicals causing leydig cell hyperplasia and tumors in the rat

Chemical	Class/action	Putative mechanism of tumor induction
Cimetidine	Histamine receptor antagonist	Androgen receptor antagonism, testosterone biosynthesis inhibition
Flutamide	Antiandrogen	Androgen receptor antagonism
Finasteride	5 α-reductase inhibitor	Decreases androgen feedback
Buserelin, leuprolide	GnRH agonists	Bind to Leydig cell LHRH receptors
Mesulergine and norprolac	Dopamine agonists	Decreases prolactin levels (which decreases Leydig cell LH receptors)
Isradipine	Calcium channel antagonist	Testosterone biosynthesis inhibition
Gemfibrozil	Hypolipidemic	Decreases prolactin levels (which decreases Leydig cell LH receptors)
Lansoprazole	Proton pump inhibitor	Testosterone biosynthesis inhibition
Ammonium perfluorooctonate	Plasticizer/lubricant	Increases estradiol levels
Linuron	Herbicide	Androgen receptor antagonism
Procymidone	Systemic plant fungicide	Androgen receptor antagonism

which displays interactions with estrogen receptor α, estrogen receptor β and the androgen receptor (AR). The lack of effect of methoxychlor on LH (estradiol tending to decrease and antiandrogens, such as flutamide, increase these levels) makes it difficult to determine which of these receptor interactions is responsible for biological activity. Methoxychlor does induce effects in females more typical of an estrogen with the induction of lordosis. The lack of an effect on LH is perhaps suggestive that rather than working through the pituitary, the agent may have a direct effect on the reproductive tract. In a study in which methoxychlor was given to pregnant female rats for the week before and the week after birth, and the pups were directly dosed with methoxychlor from postnatal day 7, methoxychlor reduced litter size by approximately 17%. Anogenital distance was unchanged, although male prepuce separation was delayed. Male offspring impregnated fewer untreated

females and had reduced epididymal sperm counts and testis weights.

Effects via the Androgen Receptor, the Example of Vinclozolin

Vinclozolin is a well-characterized fungicide with androgen receptor antagonism. The effects of vinclozolin and its metabolites on male reproductive function and development relate to their ability to interact with AR and disturb androgen-dependent gene expression. A wide variety of antiandrogenic male effects are noted following exposure to vinclozolin during pregnancy in rats, including a female-like anogenital distance (AGD), retained thoracic nipples, cleft phallus with hypospadias, suprainguinal ectopic testes, vaginal pouch, epididymal granulomas and agenesis, small or absent accessory sex glands, and delays in preputial separation. Even though many of these end points (reduced AGD, retained nipples, effects on accessory sex gland weight, hypospadias, epididymal agenesis) are believed to be elicited by interference at the level of the AR, statistically significant changes are seen with a wide variety of effective dose levels, and many do not exhibit an obvious dose-response threshold.

5α-Reductase Inhibition, the Example of Finasteride

Finasteride is a drug developed to inhibit the enzyme 5α-reductase, which normally converts testosterone to 5o-dihydrotestosterone (DHT). The drug has principally been used to combat androgen-dependent prostate cancer but has more recently received attention through its prescription for hair loss in adult men. Because DHT plays such a significant role in the development of the male reproductive tract, it is not surprising that inhibition of the enzyme responsible for its biosynthesis will produce profound effects on male reproductive development, especially the prostate and genitalia. In the rodent, treatment of the dam with finasteride at a dose of 25 mg/kg/day resulted in significant feminization of the external genitalia in male offspring. There was no further feminization of the genitalia at doses up to 300 mg/kg/day. There was also a significant decrease in prostate size at 25 and 50 mg/kg/day, with no further decrease at higher doses. Furthermore, external genital abnormalities can be produced in male monkey fetuses when dams are exposed to a low oral dose (2 mg/kg/day) of finasteride. These studies clearly demonstrate the dependency of both prostate and male external genital differentiation on dihydrotestosterone rather than testosterone. However, unlike androgen receptor blockade with flutamide, finasteride did not totally abolish prostate differentiation or completely feminize the external genitalia, despite increasingly higher dose levels. These results suggest that testosterone can compensate for DHT to some degree at the level of the androgen receptor. Wolffian differentiation, however, was not affected by the inhibition of DHT, demonstrating its testosterone dependency, but seminal vesicle growth was impaired. Androgen receptor blockade can inhibit testicular descent more effectively than inhibition of 5α-reductase activity. It is believed that finasteride causes hypospadias by preventing the formation of the medial mesenchymal plate, which is necessary for assisting the movement of the urogenital sinus from the base to the tip of the genital tubercle. The ability of drugs to elicit such profound changes in male reproductive development must be placed into context with the therapeutic advantage the drug may offer in life-threatening situations. However, there is an increased concern that there may be an environmental impact of pharmaceuticals with endocrine activity once they are excreted from human patients.

Steroid Biosynthesis Inhibition, the Example of Ketoconazole

Ketoconazole is an orally active fungicide that elicits its action by the inhibition of cytochrome P 450-mediated sterol metabolism in fungi. It also has broad activity against cytochrome P450-mediated steroidogenesis in both humans and experimental animals, and effects on Leydig cell function have been demonstrated in human and rodent adult Leydig cells *in vitro*. However, the effects on steroidogenesis are not selective for the testis, as ovary and adrenal steroidogenesis are also affected. In humans the drug has been used therapeutically as an antiandrogen with the production of gynecomastia as a side effect. When administered to rodents, ketoconazole can have dramatic effects on fertility even after a single dose. Due to its effects on ovarian and uterine steroid responses, it is more difficult to determine the role of decreased fetal testicular testosterone production on male reproductive development. That is, treatment of pregnant dams with ketoconazole is more likely to affect the ability to maintain pregnancy due to effects on ovarian progesterone synthesis, resulting in abortion/litter loss, thus precluding the observation of marked effects on the pups.

Other Potential Mechanisms, the Example of Di-*n*-Butyl Phthalate

Di-*n*-butyl phthalate (DBP) is a plasticizer and solvent and has been known to target the rat testis of adults and juveniles for many years. The mode of action of testicular toxicity is mediated by a metabolite (the monoester, monobutyl phthalate) with the target cell in the testis being the Sertoli cell. A multigeneration reproduction study showed very marked effects on the fertility of rats in the F_1 generation in comparison to their parents in the F_0 generation, including fewer and smaller litters and a 50% decrease in sperm count. Furthermore, these F_1 animals showed numerous male reproductive tract malformations at the highest dose level tested that were not observed at comparable dose levels in the standard developmental toxicity studies. When critical differences in the exposure period between the F_0 and the F_1 generations were examined (by the treatment of pregnant and lactating animals followed by an evaluation of their offspring), a high incidence of epididymal malformations and a decreased sperm count, together with delays in preputial separation and decreases in anogenital distance of the male pups, were noted. That is, all of the changes seen in the multigeneration study could be reproduced in this shorter exposure regimen. No effects were noted in the female offspring. By narrowing the exposure window to just late gestation (gestation days 12–21), these findings were essentially reproduced and also showed an increased incidence of retained nipples in the male offspring. When the effects of DBP were compared with those of the AR antagonist flutamide, many similarities in the pattern of effects were noted. However, there were also a number of differences in tissue sensitivity to effects following in utero exposure, with the epididymis being the prime target for DBP malformations, whereas the prostate was the major target for flutamide. Other studies have indicated that neither DBP nor MBP interact directly with the AR. Thus DBP represents a group of chemicals that markedly affect the androgen status of the fetus and disrupt reproductive development via a nonreceptor-mediated mechanism.

RESPONSES TO INJURY

The response of the reproductive tissues to injury is more restricted than most other tissues. Atrophy, resulting from reduced secretory function, and inflammation, resulting from urogenital infection or access of immunocompetent cells to the haploid sperm, are probably the most common responses seen in the transporting ducts and the sex glands. Within the testis, cell death and/or depletion of the germ cells is the most common response to any disturbance, whereas inflammation and repair processes are rarely seen. This is consistent with the fact that most cell death is restricted to the germ cells and this occurs through apoptosis, which does not generally elicit an inflammatory response. The resident interstitial macrophages and the tubular Sertoli cells perform the phagocytic function in the testis. This also serves to protect the testis from the potential to develop autoimmune responses to sperm. With the exception of Leydig cell tumors benign or malignant tumors of the reproductive tract are also very uncommon in laboratory animal species.

Disruption of Spermatogenesis

Most testicular toxicants, if administered at a high dose level over a prolonged period, will produce a similar nonspecific histological appearance regardless of their site of action. This appearance consists of shrunken tubules with generalized germ cell depletion, often leaving only Sertoli cells within the tubules. Leydig cell hyperplasia or hypertrophy, reflecting a secondary endocrine and/or a paracrine response of the Leydig cell to the disturbance of spermatogenesis, frequently accompanies prolonged germ cell depletion. The reason for this nonspecific response lies in the fact that the survival of the germ cells and the maintenance of spermatogenesis are exquisitely sensitive to any perturbation of function of all other cell types within the testis and their degeneration depletion is the major response seen. Although little information regarding the pathogenesis of the toxicity can be obtained from this end stage lesion, examination of the testis at earlier time points and at lower dose levels will frequently identify the target cell. The early changes are often not only restricted to particular cell types, but appear to be specific to particular stages of the spermatogenic cycle. This information can often be useful for providing clues as to the mechanistic etiology of the lesion and a rationale for further investigative studies.

Sertoli Cell Effects

Despite its sensitivity to toxic disturbance, the range of morphological responses shown by the Sertoli cell to injury is small. One of the most commonly reported changes is cytoplasmic vacuolization. In well-fixed plastic-embedded preparations this may be seen at the light microscope level as a generalized fine vacuolization in the basal cytoplasm (Figure 18.16). At the ultrastructural level, the vacuolization appears to originate as dilatation of the smooth endoplasmic reticulum, probably reflecting alterations in cellular permeability. Much larger vacuoles may also be seen, but these must be differentiated from phagocytic vacuoles remaining after the digestion of apoptotic germ

cells. Premature exfoliation or sloughing of germ cells is a frequent finding in testicular toxicity such as that due to phthalate-induced injury (Figure 18.14). The displaced germ cells, which are sometimes apparently normal in morphology, may be present in the tubular lumen or in the epididymal ducts. In such cases their release is presumably due to loss of the tenuous contact between Sertoli and germ cells. In other cases of Sertoli cell injury (e.g., DNB-induced damage), *in situ* germ cell apoptosis and phagocytosis may follow the initial vacuolization of the Sertoli cell cytoplasm. As germ cells are lost from the epithelium, the normal orderly arrangement of Sertoli cell organelles may be lost, the most obvious example being movement of the nucleus away from the basal lamina. With severe or complete loss of the germ cell population, the normal matrical structure of the Sertoli cellular processes is lost and the cytoplasmic extensions retract to form a mass of vacuolated cytoplasm with an irregular outline, containing rounded nuclei with no specific polarity. Death and depletion of the Sertoli cell population are uncommon, except in situations of ischemia.

Germ Cell Apoptosis

Germ cell death is regularly observed during normal spermatogenesis. The most vulnerable cells are type A spermatogonia (stages XI–XIV and I), midpachytene spermatocytes (stage VII), spermatocytes undergoing meiotic division (stage XIV), and step 7 and step 19 spermatids (round and elongate spermatids in stage VII tubules). The number of dying cells varies between individuals and is much higher in the prepubertal than the adult testis. Death and depletion of germ cells are the most frequent manifestations of testicular injury but also the most difficult to interpret due to the dynamic nature of germ cell development. Many chemicals causing germ cell death are cell and stage specific if administered at the right dose; therefore, apoptotic cells may be present only in tubules at specific stages of the cycle (Figure 18.15). Apoptosis of spermatogonia and spermatocytes is very rapid so the early stages of degeneration are rarely seen, even at the ultrastructural level. The cells show nuclear condensation and eosinophilic or PAS positive cytoplasm and are then phagocytized rapidly by the Sertoli cell, leaving no evidence of cell death other than the absence of the affected cell population. Apoptosis and phagocytosis of an entire cell population may be complete within 24 to 48 hr of cell injury (Figure 18.17). If the testis is not observed during the short period of apoptosis, the only change seen will be cell depletion, and the time between cell death and examination of the testis will determine which cell type will be depleted.

Spermatid injury is most easily observed. Degenerating round spermatids sometimes show the

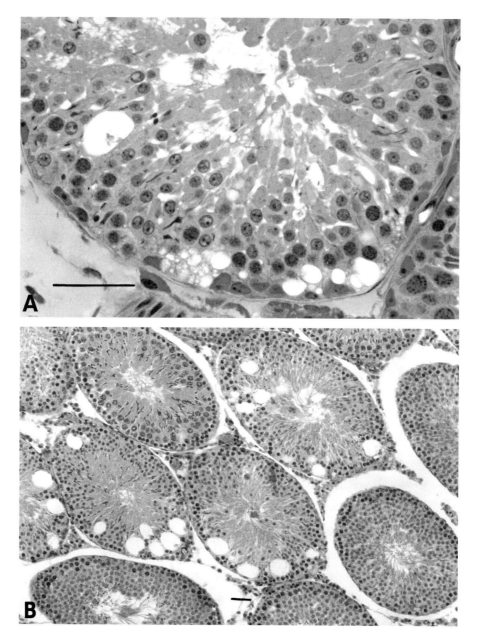

FIGURE 18.16   Vacuolation of the Sertoli cell is a common response to toxicants. (A) Fine vocuolation of the basal Sertoli cell cytoplasm following 7 weeks of dietary administration of cyclohexylamine. (B) Coarse vacuolation of the Sertoli cell cytoplasm produced by the administration of theobromine. Bar = 50 μm.

same pattern of apoptosis but more frequently they show chromatin margination of the nucleus and very often form multicellular aggregates with fused nuclear acrosomes (Figure 18.18). These aggregates are often called multi-nucleate giant cells and are formed by fusion of the syncytial groups of cells that are normally connected by cytoplasmic bridges. Occasionally, but much less frequently, such aggregates are made up of spermatocytes. Death of the elongating spermatids may take the form of cytoplasmic condensation and separation of the head and tail regions, often resulting in the phagocytized remains of the disembodied heads in the basal Sertoli cell cytoplasm. An understanding

of the kinetics of spermatogenesis and an appreciation of the development of germ cell depletion over time are fundamental to the interpretation of the pathogenesis of any testicular lesion. Figure 18.19 illustrates the pattern of germ cell depletion (maturation depletion) that occurs when a spermatocyte toxicant such as 2-methoxyethanol is administered as a single dose or on a daily basis. The term "maturation arrest" is often used to describe the end stage appearance of tubules where only the early germ cell types remain (e.g., spermatogonia and early spermatocytes). However, this is a misleading term because these remaining cells are generally not arrested; they are continuously

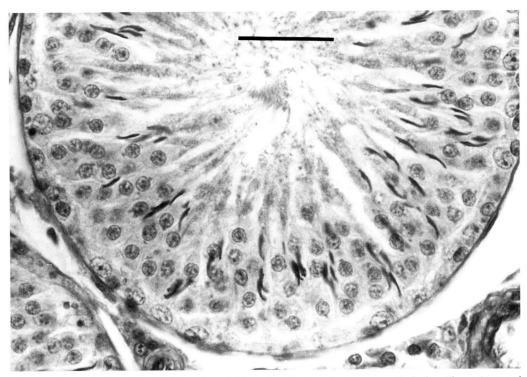

FIGURE 18.17   Stage VI tubule 48 hr after administration of 250 mg/kg ethylene glycol monomethyl ether. The entire population of pachytene spermatocytes (which underwent cell death at 24 hr) has been phagocytized by the Sertoli cells, leaving no trace of their presence. Bar = 50 μm.

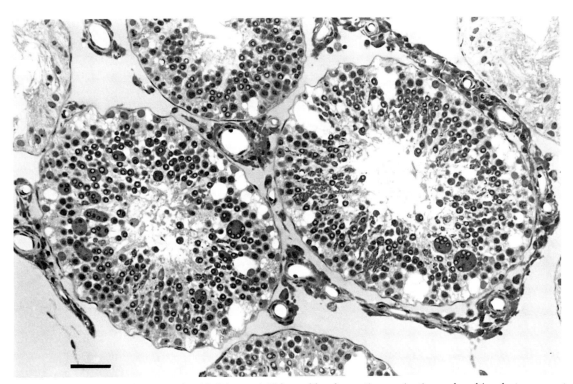

FIGURE 18.18   Degenerate round spermatids with "ring nuclei" formed by chromatin margination and multinucleate aggregates formed by cell fusion. This is a common appearance of degenerating round spermatids. The Sertoli cells also show more severe vacuolization of the basal cytoplasm compared with Fig. 18.16. (Lesion produced by 400 ppm cyclohexylamine given to rats in the diet for 9 weeks.) Bar = 50 μm.

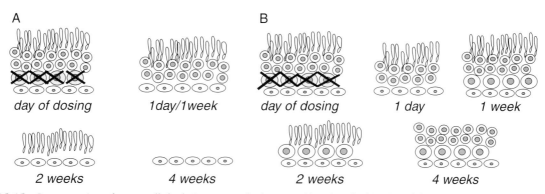

A
day of dosing   1day/1week
2 weeks   4 weeks

B
day of dosing   1 day   1 week
2 weeks   4 weeks

FIGURE 18.19   Interpretation of germ cell depletion must take into consideration the kinetics of the spermatogenic cycle along with the duration of dosing. If a specific cell type is affected, the pattern of cell depletion will depend on the time elapsed since dosing (or toxicity) began. (A) In the case of repeated, daily dosing, the sensitive cell type will be killed with each consecutive dose and the descendent generations will show progressive depletion with each spermatogenic cycle (2 weeks). (B) In the case of a single dose, the sensitive cell will be killed, but will be replaced rapidly by the unaffected preceding cell. However, with each spermatogenic cycle, a window of cell depletion will be seen as the maturation depletion, resulting from the original cell death, moves through each generation of descendent cells.

differentiating but dying once they reach a stage that is sensitive to the toxic effect. An additional facet of maturation depletion is the predictable delay in the onset of infertility following dosing with a specific germ cell toxicant.

Spermatid Retention (Inhibited Spermiation, Delayed Spermiation)

This is a relatively common but subtle histopathological finding where the mature (step 19) spermatids fail to be released during their normal stage VIII, and instead are retained into later stages where many are pulled down to the basal Sertoli cell cytoplasm and are phagocytized (Figure 18.20). The mechanism for this is unknown. It is assumed to be associated with failure of the tubulobulbar complexes between Sertoli cell and spermatid to dissociate normally, but whether this is due to impaired maturation of the spermatid or to impaired function of the Sertoli cell has not been ascertained. It has been observed in association with agents causing hormonal disruption and with several putative Sertoli cell toxicants. It is an early and predominant finding following exposure to boric acid, and mechanistic studies have been carried out in an attempt to elucidate the underlying biochemical changes involved. Measurement of cAMP levels and plasminogen activator activity, both of which are thought to be involved in spermiation, failed to demonstrate any alterations.

Tubular Dilatation and Tubular Shrinkage

Dilatation or closure of the tubular lumen is generally a consequence of an increased or decreased volume of seminiferous tubule fluid (STF). There are a number of possible causes of an increase in volume,

including an inhibition of peritubular cell contraction, leading to failure to expel the tubular contents. Other potential causes include inhibition of reabsorbtion of the STF by the epididymis, obstruction of the flow of STF through the excurrent duct system, or possibly an increase in STF production by the Sertoli cell. Prolonged or severe increases in STF volume and tubular dilatation will lead to germ cell damage and loss due to pressure effects on the seminiferous epithelium. Closure of the tubular lumen (as distinct from reduced tubular diameter due to loss of cells) is due to decreased STF production and secretion. This is commonly associated with the generalized disruption of Sertoli cell function or a reduction in testicular testosterone concentration, as STF secretion is an androgen-dependent Sertoli cell function.

Tubular and Testicular Necrosis

Tubular necrosis is characterized by the cell death of all germ cells and Sertoli cells (Figure 18.21), whereas testicular necrosis may involve all cellular elements, including Leydig cells and peritubular cells. It is a characteristic of ischemic damage brought about by generalized or local reduction in vascular perfusion pressure. It is classically seen with cadmium, which causes testicular and epididymal vascular endothelial damage, causing interstitial edema. It is also seen with vasoactive drugs such as serotonin and histamine. The severity of the lesion depends on the level of anoxia. Severe ischemia, as seen with cadmium or vascular interruption, results in complete infarction of the testis, with oncotic (coagulative) necrosis of all cellular elements and an acute inflammatory infiltrate. Less severe anoxia results in tubular oncotic necrosis of the seminiferous epithelium, whereas mild anoxia may only result in apoptotic necrosis of a proportion

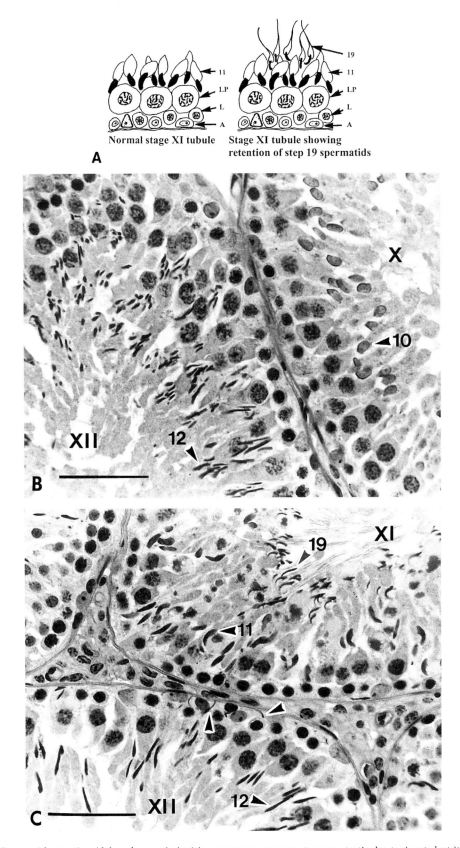

FIGURE 18.20   Spermatid retention (delayed spermiation) is a common response to many testicular toxicants but it is a subtle change to detect. (A) Stage XI tubule in diagrammatic form showing the normal cell association of type A spermatogonia (A), leptotene spermatocytes (L), late pachytene spermatocytes (LP), and step 11 elongating spermatids. When spermatids are retained, there is an additional layer of step 19 spermatids (19), which failed to be released when the tubule was in stage VIII. (B) A normal stage X and stage XII tubule containing step 10 and step 12 spermatids, respectively. (C) A stage XI tubule with retained step 19 spermatids at the lumen and a stage XII tubule where the retained spermatids have been pulled down and phagocytized by the basal Sertoli cell cytoplasm (arrows). Bar = 50 μm.

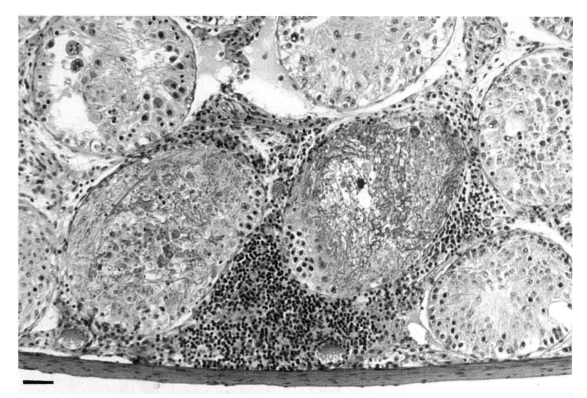

FIGURE 18.21   Tubular necrosis is a characteristic of ischemic injury. The seminiferous epithelium shows oncotic (coagulative) necrosis of germ cells and Sertoli cells and elicits an interstitial inflammatory response, which is largely excluded by the peritubular cell barrier. Bar = 50 μm.

of the germ cells. With the exception of tubular and testicular oncotic necrosis, inflammation in the testis is a rare response to any chemically induced damage. Although the inflammatory infiltrate is directed at the necrotic tubule, it is frequently excluded from reaching the tubular contents by the peritubular cell barrier (Figure 18.21).

Leydig Cell Response

Histopathologic effects on the Leydig cells are often difficult to identify by the qualitative evaluation of wax-embedded tissue. Hypertrophy and/or hyperplasia of the interstitial cells generally reflects increased stimulation by LH, whereas atrophy reflects decreased stimulation and activity. Hypertrophy and hyperplasia may be seen as a primary effect, but more often it reflects a secondary response to spermatogenic disruption. Testosterone is normally secreted as it is synthesized and is not stored in the cytoplasm. However, foamy vacuolation of the Leydig cells is sometimes seen following treatment with hormonally active compounds. Atrophy of the Leydig cells may be seen following the administration of agents that reduce LH secretion. Degeneration and necrosis of the

Leydig cells are rarely seen, but one exception to this is the Leydig cell-specific toxicant ethane di-methane sulfonate. Necrosis and death of the Leydig cell population occur within days of treatment. The subsequent effects on spermatogenesis and on the secondary sex organs provide a well-documented example of the pathogenesis of lesions caused by reduced testosterone levels. Regeneration of the Leydig cell population is mediated through the proliferation and differentiation of fetal-type Leydig cells, which are present in the interstitial tissue.

Disruption of Sperm Maturation

Although most attention is generally given to the effects of chemicals on the testis and on spermatogenesis, the potential for effects on the maturation of sperm within the epididymis exists. Such effects are generally detected by decreases in sperm motility, by decreased numbers of motile sperm, or by increases in the number of morphologically abnormal sperm. These may be the only parameters to show an effect if the toxicant enters the epididymal fluid and has a direct effect on the sperm. The time taken for sperm to be transported through the epididymis may also be affected. TCDD has been shown to alter the epididymal transit time of sperm. This can be measured by comparing the daily sperm production rate (DSP) with the concentration of sperm in the cauda epididymis.

Epididymal Response

The most common chemically induced lesion in the epididymis is inflammation, leading to the formation of sperm granulomas. Although there is a blood-epididymal barrier, formed by occlusive junctions between the apical surfaces of the epididymal epithelium, it is not as robust as the blood-testis barrier. Any damage to the epididymal epithelium is liable to result in the access of immunologically competent cells to the antigenically foreign sperm within the lumen. The result is a progressive granulomatous inflammation, which generally leads to rupture of the epithelial layer to form a sperm granuloma. Vacuolation of the epididymal epithelium is frequently associated with atrophic changes secondary to decreased androgenic stimulation. However, it is also occasionally seen as a primary, chemically induced effect .

Response to Alterations in Hormone Balance

Recognition of patterns of morphological response associated with hormone disruption can be critical for identification of the mechanism of reproductive toxicity. The effect of any compound that disturbs the hormonal balance of the reproductive system will obviously depend on the degree of disturbance and the duration of treatment. Homeostatic mechanisms may be capable of compensating for the altered hormonal status, preventing the development of any detectable morphological effects. However, if morphological effects do ensue, they appear to be relatively predictable and consistent.

Effects on Spermatogenesis

Small to moderate reductions in testicular testosterone concentration may only affect spermatogenesis on a quantitative basis, which may be difficult to detect by routine morphological examination. The most sensitive histopathologic indicator of testosterone insufficiency is the presence of degenerating spermatocytes and round spermatids in stages VII and VIII tubules (Figure 18.22). This occurs within about 4 days of testosterone withdrawal. At later times, spermatocytes and particularly elongating spermatids in later stages (IX–XIV) show degeneration. This reflects the fact that cells have passed through stage, VII–VIII in the absence of testosterone

and have been fatally damaged by so doing, but their degeneration is delayed to a later time when they undergo a critical event, which relies on their previous exposure to testosterone. The endstage lesion for testosterone insufficiency, which is seen after about 2 weeks of treatment, is a slight reduction in the numbers of mid-and late pachytene spermatocytes and round spermatids but an almost complete loss of elongating and maturation phase spermatids (Figure 18.22). This is accompanied by a marked shrinkage of the tubule, which is partly due to a loss of cells but is also caused by a reduction in the secretion of androgen-dependent seminiferous tubule fluid by the Sertoli cell. Testosterone withdrawal also leads to abnormal retention and phagocytosis of step 19 spermatids at stages IX–XII (Figure 18.20). Although this appears to be a common finding with treatments that disturb testosterone levels, it is not unique to this class of compound. Any morphological changes in the Leydig cell will depend on the nature of the hormonal disturbance. Increased LH stimulation of the Leydig cell will result in hypertrophy of the cell due to an increased volume of smooth endoplasmic reticulum and may also lead to diffuse hyperplasia of the cell population. Conversely, reduced stimulation of the Leydig cell by LH or inhibition of the steroidogenic enzymes will lead to a reduction in the size of the cells and the volume of endoplasmic reticulum.

Atrophy of Epididymis and Secondary Sex Organs

Morphological changes in other tissues in response to reduced androgen levels or androgen receptor blockade are less specific than those in the testes. In the epididymis, seminal vesicles, and prostate, the epithelium becomes inactive in terms of secretion and the lumen shrinks in size as the fluid volume decreases (Figure 18.23). There is a dramatic reduction in organelles, particularly rough endoplasmic reticulum, Golgi, and secretory vacuoles, as well as a marked increase in lysosomal content and autophagic vacuoles. Androgen withdrawal, as demonstrated following castration hypophysectomy, results in a loss of viability of epididymal spermatozoa within a few days.

Gonadotroph Hypertrophy and Hyperplasia in the Pituitary

In the pituitary, testosterone withdrawal results in the development of so-called castration cells or signet ring cells. These are hypertrophied gonadotrophs, which contain dilated cisternae of endoplasmic reticulum and extension of the Golgi region, which eventually develops into a large vacuole (Figure 18.24). Secretory granules become smaller. There is also cell

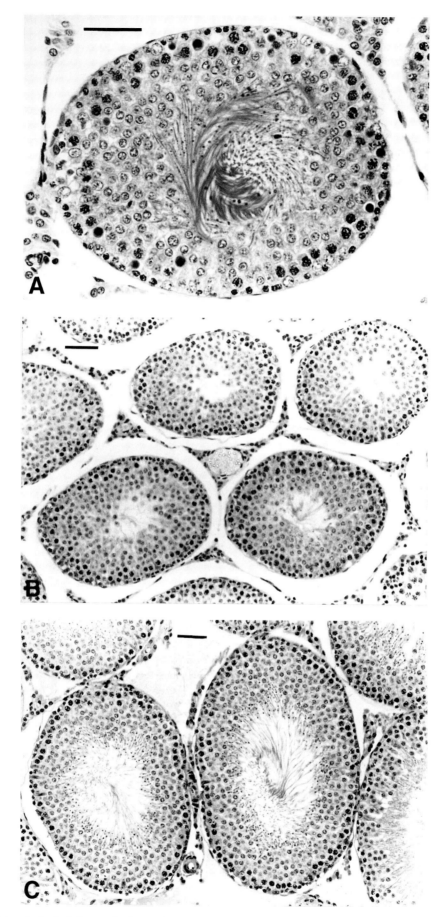

FIGURE 18.22   Histopathological changes in the testis associated with reduced testosterone secretion (produced by a 17–20 lyase inhibitor). (A) Occasional degenerating pachytene spermatocytes and round spermatids in a stage VII tubule. This is the earliest and most sensitive indicator of testosterone insufficiency. (B) Generalized depletion of elongating and maturation phase spermatids in all stages plus decreased lumenal diameter. This appearance develops following longer periods of testosterone insufficiency. (C) Control stage VII tubules at same magnification as B for comparison. Bar = 50 μm.

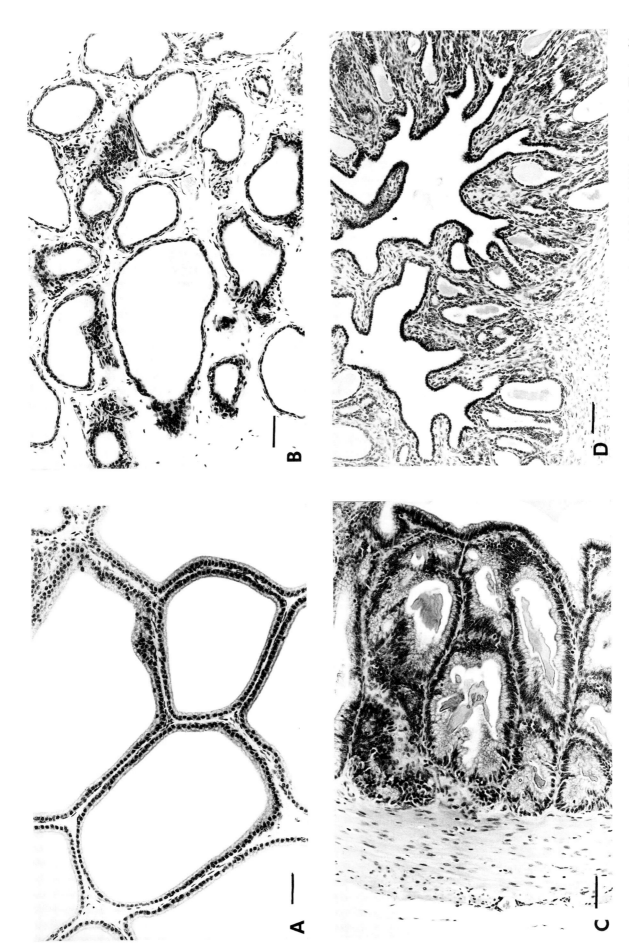

FIGURE 18.23   Histopathological changes in secondary sex organs associated with reduced testosterone secretion (produced by a 17–20 lyase inhibitor): (A) Normal prostate, (B) atrophic prostate, (C) normal seminal vesicle mucosa, and (D) atrophic seminal vesicle mucosa. Bar = 50μm.

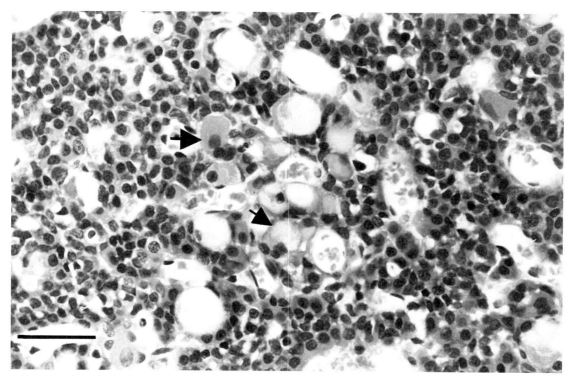

FIGURE 18.24   Pituitary changes associated with decreased circulating testosterone levels are characterized by the presence of castration cells. These gonadotropin-secreting cells have an increased pale cytoplasmic volume, which often contains a large secretory droplet or vacuole (signet ring cells) (arrow). Bar = 50 μm.

proliferation, and most of the cells contain both FSH and LH. Gonadotropin stimulation is an important factor in the proliferation of the cells. Chronic stimulation of gonadotrophs is also associated with a higher incidence of pituitary adenomas.

Neoplasia

Most tumors of the male reproductive tissues are androgen dependent at some stage in their development. In laboratory animals, the most common spontaneous and chemically induced tumor of the reproductive tract is the Leydig cell tumor. The spontaneous incidence is strain specific, but it is relatively common in the rat (up to 100% in aged F344 rats) and less common in the mouse (generally <1%). Although testicular tumors (Sertoli cell and Leydig cell tumors) are a common, spontaneous tumor in aging dogs, they are seen only occasionally in laboratory-maintained dogs, where the life span is normally restricted (Figures 18.25 and 18.26). Chemical induction of Leydig cell tumors in the rat has been reported with a wide variety of compounds many of which disrupt normal hormonal balance. The mouse appears generally less susceptible, but Leydig cell tumors and tumors of the rete testis have been induced in the mouse with estrogens such as DES.

In contrast to man, where prostatic carcinoma is one of the most common tumors seen, spontaneous neoplasia of the prostate in other species is rare. Experimental models of prostate carcinogenesis have been developed in the rat using N-nitrosobis (2-hydroxypropyl)amine, N-methylnitrosourea (MNU), and 3,2′-dimethyl-4-aminobiphenyl (DMAB). Invasive carcinomas are induced when these carcinogens are coadministered with high doses of testosterone. Prostatic carcinoma has also been induced by testosterone administration to a strain of rat (Noble rat) that has a genetic susceptibility to prostate cancer. Neuroendocrine carcinoma is the principal malignancy in the widely used transgenic "adenocarcinoma" of mouse prostate (TRAMP) model.

Reversibility

The reversibility of infertility is a very important consideration for risk assessment in male reproductive toxicology, and the potential for complete recovery is largely dependent on the site and the severity of the toxic insult. This puts additional importance on identifying the target cell of toxicity and the pathogenesis of the lesion.

Repopulation of the Germ Cells and Recovery of Spermatogenesis

Following germ cell damage or depletion, the chances of regeneration of the entire germ cell population and recovery of functional spermatogenesis are good. Although many of the germ cell types are sensitive to physical and chemical disturbances, the renewing stem cell spermatogonial population is relatively resistant. It is often necessary to allow sufficient time for the stem cell population to repeatedly cycle and replenish itself before significant recovery of spermatogenesis can occur.

If the Sertoli cell is injured and the damage is mild, then full recovery may be possible. If Sertoli cells are destroyed or, as more often happens, permanently functionally compromised, regeneration is not possible because these cells are unable to divide in the adult. However, they are remarkably resistant to cell death and are often found as the only remaining cell type in the seminiferous epithelium when all germ cells have been lost.

Most effects of androgen deficiency, including spermatogenic disruption and atrophy of the epididymis and secondary sex organs, are also readily reversible with the reestablishment of normal hormone balance. An obvious exception to this is the Leydig cell tumor, which, once established, is androgen-independent and irreversible. Effects on the epididymis that result in granulomatous inflammation and sperm granulomas are generally progressive and irreversible. The presence of persistent inflammation in close proximity to viable sperm runs the additional risk of leukotriene-induced genotoxic damage to the sperm.

Reproductive Toxicity in Domestic Animals

Although many xenobiotics have been shown to affect the male reproductive system experimentally, there are only a small number of xenobiotics that need to be considered for domestic animals in a diagnostic setting. Table 18.8 lists xenobiotics for which there is reasonable evidence of adverse effects occurring in a clinical/diagnostic setting, however there are few well-controlled experimental studies performed in domestic animals in the literature. Exposure to these xenobiotics can result either in altered spermatogenesis or altered secretory or absorptive functions of the epididymis or accessory sex glands, which can adversely impact sperm maturation and transport.

In large animals, estrogenic effects induced by phytoestrogens and estrogenic mycotoxins present in feed are the most common manifestation (see additional discussion in Chapter 19, Female Reproductive System). Environmental contamination by heavy metals, PCBs and TCDD can also potentially affect male reproductive function. In small animals, inappropriate use/dosage of estrogenic or androgenic type drugs can cause estrogenic effects in the accessory sex glands. Chemotherapeutic drugs, such as adriamycin and cyclophsphamide that target rapidly dividing cells, can adversely affect spermatogenesis. Antimicrobials such as amphotericin B, griseofulvin and gentamycin have also been associated with testicular degenreration.

The major morphologic manifestations of exposure to xenobiotics are testicular degeneration and/or epithelial metaplasia and/or glandular hyperplasia of the epididymus and accessory sex glands. Although a wide variety of factors can cause testicular degeneration in domestic animals, the etiology is seldom established because histologic lesions are nonspecific. These range from decreased number of germ cells, Sertoli cell vacuolation, intratubular multinucleate cells (spermatids), and in more advanced cases interstitial fibrosis. Early stages of degeneration may be difficult to differentiate from hypoplasia. In advanced cases, the increased thickness and waviness of the tubular basement membrane can be used for this differentiation. Sustentacular or Sertoli cells may also be lost followed by loss of interstitial or Leydig cells.

A major manifestation of compounds that have estrogenic activity is squamous metaplasia of the epididymus and accessory sex glands (see Figure 18.26C); testicular degeneration may also occur. Obstruction of the epididymal duct can occur from severe epithelial alterations or sperm granuloma formation. Adenomyosis can occur in the epididymus under estrogenic influence, while prostatic hyperplasia can occur under both androgenic and estrogenic influence. The majority of intact mature (>4 years of age) dogs have benign prostatic hyperplasia (BPH); castration is curative and preventative.

Phytoestrogens

Phytoestrogens are phenolic estrogen analogs (isoflavones, coumestans and lignans) derived from clover (*Trifolium* spp.) and mold damaged alfalfa (*Medicago* sp.). The isoflavones include formononetin, biochanin A and genestin. Estrogenic activity is the result of binding to the estrogen receptor (ER), and induction of specific estrogen-responsive gene products. As discussed in Chapter 19, phytoestrogens can result in exogenous estrogenic activity in sheep and to a lesser extent in cattle leading to infertility of varying severity and permanency, so called "clover disease".

Castrated (wethers) but not intact (rams) sheep that graze on estrogenic pastures for several weeks can have extensive metaplasia, hyperplasia and cystic

TABLE 18.8 Selected toxicants/agents causing male reproductive effects in domestic animals

Category	Toxicant/Agent	Source	Testicular lesion	Other reproductive alterations	Species*	Comment
Plant toxins	Gossypol	Cotton (*Gossypium* spp)	Degeneration		Dog, pig, immature cattle, man	Mitochondrial sheath of sperm is aplastic
	Swainsonine	*Astralgus* spp	Degeneration		Sheep (locoism)	Endocrine disruption
	Phytoestrogens	*Trifolium, Medicago* spp	Degeneration	Accessory sex glands: hyperplasia, squamous metaplasia; gynecomastia	Sheep, castrated (wethers)	Estrogenic effect
	Phytoestrogens	*Glycine max* (soybeans)	Poor fertility		Cat	
Mycotoxins	Zearalenone	*Fusarium* spp (grains)	Degeneration	Accessory sex glands: squamous metaplasia; gynecomastia	Pig, also sheep, cattle	Estrogenic effect
	Trichothecenes	*Fusarium* spp (grains)	Degeneration		All, pig sensitive	Apoptosis of rapidly dividing cells
Environmental	Cadmium	Paint, batteries, industry	Ischemic necrosis			Vascular damage
	Boron (acid salts)	Pesticides, cleaners	Degeneration		Dog	Spermatid retention
Environmental	Chlorinated naphthalenes	Lubricants, oils, flame retardants, etc	Degeneration	Accessory sex glands, epididymus: squamous metaplasia	Cattle (X-disease)	Endocrine disruption
				Accessory sex glands (bulbourethral): hyperplasia	Sheep	
	DES, DDT, PCBs, kepone	Pesticides, industry	Hypoplasia	Male pseudohermaphroditism, hypospadia	Wildlife, especially fetal	Endocrine disruption, xenoestrogens and anti-estrogens
	Heat	Fever, environmental	Degeneration		All susceptible	
	Frostbite		Degeneration	Scrotum: inflammation	Cattle	
Therapeutic	Ionizing radiation		Degeneration		All susceptible	DNA damage
	Adriamycin, cyclophosphamide	Antineoplastics	Degeneration		All susceptible	DNA damage, spermatagonia
	Vinblastine, vincristine	Antineoplastics	Degeneration		All susceptible	Sertoli cell toxicants (cytoskeleton)
	Ketoconazole	Antifungal				Intersitial cell toxicant
	Estrogen	Also Sertoli cell tumor	Degeneration (?)	Accessory sex glands (prostate): squamous metaplasia; epididymus: adenomyosis, sperm granuloma	Dog, pig	
				Accessory sex glands (prostate): hyperplasia	Cat	
	Stilbestrol	Growth promotant		Accessory sex glands: squamous metaplasia	Immature cattle, sheep	Estrogenic effect
	Testosterone and analogs	Anabolic steroids	Degeneration		All susceptible	Endocrine disruption
	Dexamethasone		Degeneration			Endocrine disruption
Diet	Vitamin A	Liver	Degeneration		Cat	

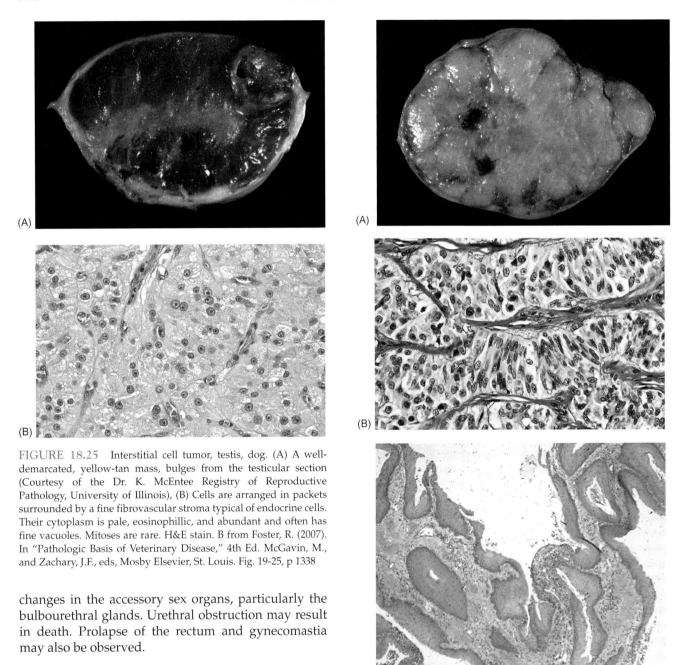

FIGURE 18.25 Interstitial cell tumor, testis, dog. (A) A well-demarcated, yellow-tan mass, bulges from the testicular section (Courtesy of the Dr. K. McEntee Registry of Reproductive Pathology, University of Illinois), (B) Cells are arranged in packets surrounded by a fine fibrovascular stroma typical of endocrine cells. Their cytoplasm is pale, eosinophillic, and abundant and often has fine vacuoles. Mitoses are rare. H&E stain. B from Foster, R. (2007). In "Pathologic Basis of Veterinary Disease," 4th Ed. McGavin, M., and Zachary, J.F., eds, Mosby Elsevier, St. Louis. Fig. 19-25, p 1338

changes in the accessory sex organs, particularly the bulbourethral glands. Urethral obstruction may result in death. Prolapse of the rectum and gynecomastia may also be observed.

Chlorinated Naphthalenes

Exposure of domestic animals to chlorinated naphthalenes in the past occurred from use in lubricants and other oil based product. Today exposure to chlorinated naphthalenes may occur from industrial emissions and landfills. These compounds induce cytochrome P450s and undergo metabolic activation and also act as endocrine disrupters.

The clinical syndrome due to chlorinated naphthalene toxicity in cattle was termed bovine hyperkeratosis or X disease because of thickening of the skin due to hyperkeratosis. The chlorinated naphthalenes cause squamous metaplasia of the accessory sex

FIGURE 18.26 Sertoli cell tumor, testis, dog. (A) A white firm, white and somewhat lobulated mass has virtually effaced the testis (Courtesy of the Dr. K. McEntee Registry of Reproductive Pathology, University of Illinois. (B) Histologically, Sertoli cell tumors have tubular structures lined by cells that resemble Sertoli cells and are surrounded by septa of fibrous tissue. H&E stain. (C) Prostate, squamous metaplasia. Functional Sertoli cell tumors that secrete estrogen can induce hyperplasia and/or squamous metaplasia of the prostate gland. Normal epithelium of the prostatic ducts (transitional) and glandular acini (columnar) is replaced by stratified squamous keratinizing epithelium. H&E stain. B and C from Foster, R. (2007). In "Pathologic Basis of Veterinary Disease," 4th Ed. McGavin, M., and Zachary, J.F., eds, Mosby Elsevier, St. Louis. Fig. 19.26, p 1338.

glands and excretory ducts of the testes in adult cattle (bulls). In the epididymus, the pseudostratified ductal epithelium becomes stratified with keratin plugging of the ducts. Severe testicular degeneration has been reported, with seminiferous tubules lined primarily by Sertoli cells with hyalanized basement membranes. In adult sheep (rams), testicular degeneration was observed but not metaplasia of the excretory ducts or accessory sex glands.

Gossypol.

Gossypol is a polyphenolic compound derived from the seeds, roots, and stems of the cotton plant (*Gossypium* sp.). It is a well known male sterilant, mostly affecting monogastrics, including humans. Dogs are very sensitive, horses are relatively resistant and ruminants (except calves) are resistant. Gossypol blocks spermatogenesis. Considerable evidence points to inhibition of protein synthesis, oxidative stress, formation of reactive oxygen species, and DNA scission. Histologically, there is arrest of spermatogenesis.

EVALUATION OF TOXICITY

The nonspecific morphological response of the testis to a variety of different mechanisms of toxicity, i.e., germ cell loss (generally described as testicular/tubular atrophy), prevents any detailed analysis of cell sites or mechanisms of action. However, in a diagnostic setting, morphological evaluation (see below) is generally the only method that can be used to assess reproductive toxicity in domestic animals.

Testing of compounds for effects on male fertility should aim to show if and where the compound has an effect and whether the damage is reversible. This information can be obtained from a variety of sources ranging from basic histopathology in a standard toxicity test to much more specific assays of functional end points. These data may be useful in the hazard identification of a male reproductive toxicant, but additional information regarding tissue distribution and metabolism, shape of the dose-response curve, target cell, and species affected will be necessary for the proper assessment of the potential risk to man.

In order to characterize the toxicity, different types of studies are needed, and the design of these studies has to be on a case-by-case basis depending on the information gained from the screening studies. Characterization studies may seek additional information from specifically designed fertility studies, morphological studies, biochemical studies, and *in vitro* studies.

Detecting toxicity

Reproductive and fertility studies carried out to regulatory guidelines are all screening studies, designed to detect rather than characterize reproductive toxicants. As such, dosing extends over a prolonged period, and multiple end points of structure and function are measured. Although there are specific guidelines for studies that specifically address effects on reproduction and fertility, it is important to be aware that a conventional repeat dose study of 4 weeks, preferably 13 weeks, dosing duration, using organ weights and histopathology as end points, is often the most effective and easiest method for detecting toxicants affecting the testis. The measurement of multiple end points in fertility studies is extremely important. The reproductive system is made up of a number of different functional units, which are all interdependent on one another for their regulation. No single end point will detect all reproductive toxicants. Histopathology, however detailed, cannot detect any compound that enters the epididymal fluid and causes direct cytotoxicity, metabolic, or oxidative damage to the sperm. This can only be detected by fertility parameters and sperm parameters. Similarly, effects on sexual behavior and performance, which can be caused by agents disrupting hormone balance or automonic or central nervous pathways, can only be determined through measuring specific behavioral/copulatory parameters. In general, fertility per se is not a sensitive method for detecting reproductive toxicants in rodents due to the fecundity of the species. It has been demonstrated that rats can remain fertile with less than 10% of their normal sperm count. However, using a battery of fertility-associated indices, as well as sperm analysis, can provide sensitive and essential information on any post-testicular toxic effects.

Characterization of Reproductive Toxicity

Morphological Characterization

The major objective of morphological characterization should be to establish the earliest site and, if possible, the earliest cell type affected by the toxicant. This has to be carried out using a time course study and careful histological examination. The dose used in this study should be sufficient to cause a consistent effect but not too high that it causes nonspecific toxicity. The time course may range over 1 to 2 days with time points only hours apart (e.g., phthalate esters) or may range over 13 weeks with time points weeks apart (e.g., cyclohexylamine). Preliminary dose and time ranging studies are required to establish the appropriate range.

Gross Examination and Organ Weights

Loss of germ cells from the seminiferous tubules and decreased secretion of seminiferous tubule fluid generally result in a decrease in tubular diameter, a decrease in testis size, and a decrease in testis weight. In scrotal-bearing animals, testis size can be measured "in life" using a pair of calipers. Some toxicants produce a transitory increase in testis size as a result of an increase in interstitial fluid, but degeneration of the seminiferous epithelium will invariably be reflected by a decrease in weight. A consistent increase in size and weight of the testis is likely to be associated with increased production of interstitial fluid or edema, as seen with cadmium. Alternatively, the increased fluid may be seminiferous tubule fluid lying within dilated tubules. Organ weight is therefore a reliable and relatively sensitive indicator of testicular damage. With most tissues, organ weight is proportional to body weight and is generally expressed relative to body weight. Testis weight is more variable and, therefore, is often expressed as an absolute value. Weighing the cauda epididymis will provide a measure of stored sperm reserves, although this will obviously be influenced by the frequency of ejaculation. Seminal vesicle and prostate weight can be used as a crude bioassay of circulating testosterone levels. However, they may also show a weight reduction if there is interference with testosterone binding at the surface receptor. Weight reduction can also occur if body weight decreases.

Preparation of Tissues for Morphological Evaluation

The testis is an organ requiring special fixation procedures for any critical evaluation of morphology. If it is cut or sliced prior to fixation, tubular or interstitial tissue organization is lost. It therefore needs to be fixed whole, but conventional immersion fixation in buffered formalin gives very poor penetration of fixative, resulting in poor nuclear and cytoplasmic definition. Immersion fixation in Bouin's, Davidson's, or Zenker's fluid, together with puncture of the tunica albuginea, gives more rapid penetration and improves cellular definition greatly, though still subject to shrinkage artifacts. Although not always practicable, perfusion fixation vastly improves preservation. Testes perfused with buffered formalin and embedded in paraffin wax show excellent morphology. However, if perfusion fixation is employed, it is worthwhile to embed the tissue in plastic, either methacrylate or epoxy resin, and prepare 1- to 2μm sections for examination by light microscopy. This gives much better resolution of cellular detail and allows more critical evaluation than is possible in wax sections. Methacrylate resin is water soluble and allows special stains to be used, whereas epoxy resin restricts examination to toluidine blue- or methylene blue-stained preparations but does allow subsequent ultrastructural examination. Perfusion fixation of the testis is essential for ultrastructural studies. Interpretation of testis ultrastructure is difficult even in ideally fixed tissue, and minimizing fixation artifacts is essential for the detection of subtle toxicologically induced changes. For ultrastructural studies, a formalin-glutaraldehyde mixture (Karnovsky's fixative) or 5% glutaraldehyde is recommended as the primary fixative. This should be perfused until the testis is firm. The tissue can then be diced and postfixed in 1% osmium tetroxide or a mixture of potassium ferrocyanide and osmium tetroxide, which improves contrast of all cell types but particularly the Leydig cells. If difficulties are encountered with the perfusion technique, it may be necessary to employ a vasodilator (0.1% procaine) or heparin in the saline wash prior to perfusing the fixative or heparinize the animal 15m in prior to perfusion. Whole body perfusion via the heart or local perfusion via the testicular or iliac artery may be used.

Histological Evaluation

A subjective evaluation of testis histology in well-fixed tissue by a trained observer can establish if all cell types are present, if all cell associations are correct, and if spermatogenesis and spermiation are proceeding normally. It is not usually possible to detect subtle reductions in cell numbers. It has been suggested that reductions of less than 25% of a cell population are not readily detectable by qualitative assessment. The purpose of carrying out a sequential time course study is to detect the earliest morphological signs of toxicity. Within the testis these effects are likely to be seen in either the Sertoli cells or the germ cells, but will rapidly be followed by secondary changes in other cell types. Establishing the nature, the sequence, and any stage specificity of such changes and tying them in with the kinetics of the spermatogenic cycle forms the basis of any mechanistic interpretation of toxicity. The ultrastructural evaluation of the testis is extremely complex and not covered in this text.

Quantitative Techniques

Homogenization-Resistant Spermatids

Counting numbers of cells in the testis can be a very labor-intensive and time-consuming exercise if carried out in a thorough manner. However, there is a rapid automated method available for counting the number of elongating spermatids in homogenized testicular tissue (homogenization resistant spermatids) using a computer-assisted sperm analyzer (CASA) or a hemocytometer.

Histological Cell-Counting Techniques

In order to carry out any meaningful quantitation at the histological level, it is necessary to identify the tubular stages of the spermatogenic cycle. This allows accurate identification of the cell type being counted and standardizes the size of the cells in different tubules. It is necessary to take into account alterations in tubular size when counting cells. Only cross-sectional tubular profiles should be counted, but these may vary slightly. In addition, the treatment may have an effect on tubular diameter or length, thus increasing or decreasing the density of cells. Given that Sertoli cell numbers are not affected by the treatment under investigation, these can be used as a standard and the germ cell count expressed as a ratio of Sertoli cell nuclei or nucleoli. Spermatocytes and round spermatids are the easiest cells to count. Elongating spermatids are difficult because they weave in and out of the section. Spermatogonia are difficult to identify into subpopulations and they are a proliferating population. The number of tubules counted must be sufficient to provide a statistically valid comparison at the level of confidence required and with the coefficient of variation for the parameter measured. The complexity of such studies can be tailored to suit the requirements. If the numbers of spermatocytes and round spermatids are counted in every stage of the spermatogenic cycle at varying periods after dosing, then a very comprehensive picture of the precise cell types affected and the progression of the lesion can be acquired. However, a well-designed study that only counts one cell type in one or two selected stages at selected intervals can yield a great deal of useful information with a fraction of the effort.

Flow Cytometry

Another rapid, automated quantitative analysis of spermatogenesis is provided by flow cytometric analysis. Different ploidy subsets provide fractions containing haploid cells (spermatids), tetraploid (primary spermatocytes), and a diploid fraction, which contains all other cells, including spermatogonia, secondary spermatocytes, Sertoli cells, Leydig cells, and connective tissue cells. The different fractions are presented as a percentage of the total of cells counted. This can provide a rapid, quantitative snapshot of the differential depletion of germ cell populations.

Hormone Analysis

Plasma hormone analysis is often carried out as a potentially informative, relatively easy quantitative technique, which will monitor hormone disturbances.

Sampling needs to be controlled carefully with respect to time of day, as gonadotropin secretion is subject to circadian rhythms. In addition the secretions of LHRH, LH, and testosterone are pulsatile, which leads to large variations within and between animals. Ideally, multiple samples should be taken to reduce this variation and measurements should be made of baseline and maximally stimulated values. By comparing baseline versus stimulated hormone release of LHRH, LH, and testosterone (using Naloxone, LHRH, and hCG, respectively), the probable site of an endocrine lesion can be investigated. It should also be appreciated that any disruption of spermatogenesis will be accompanied by hormonal changes, which can make distinguishing primary toxic endocrine disturbance from secondary homeostatic responses more difficult.

Functional Characterization

Once information has been gained on the likely target site and cell of toxicity, functional disturbances may be investigated. The choice of markers of functional disturbance requires a thorough understanding of reproductive physiology and, ideally, information concerning the likely target biochemical processes that might be disturbed by the class of compound under investigation. *In vivo* investigations are possible and potentially informative, e.g., measurement of Sertoli cell functional end points such as protein or fluid secretion, analysis of fluids such as seminiferous tubule fluid, interstitial fluid, epididymal fluid, and seminal fluid, and measurement of plasma or testicular testosterone levels. However, such studies should always be interpreted with caution, taking into consideration the regulation and interdependence of cellular functions within the testis. What may appear to be a primary disturbance in function may be no more than a secondary response to some other disturbance of cellular interaction.

Due to these interdependent interactions it is often necessary to separate the putative target cell from its homeostatic regulatory environment in order to more precisely define the toxicant-induced disturbances in cellular function. A variety of *in vitro* techniques are available for such investigations but again they must be used with caution and with full appreciation of their limitations.

In Vitro Models

Separating the individual cells from the influences of their neighbors is often essential if the primary cell-specific toxicological disturbance is to be identified. Conversely, separation of a cell from its neighbors could represent a major shortcoming by removing important contributing factors in the development of the toxicity. In order to control and minimize these dangers, a certain amount of important information must be known about the *in vivo* toxicity and the metabolism of the compound before *in vitro* models can even be attempted. For an *in vitro* model of the testis to be scientifically valid, it is necessary to expose the appropriate cell to the appropriate molecule (parent or metabolite) at a physiologically relevant concentration and measure a toxicologically relevant end point. As such, most *in vitro* preparations are inappropriate for any basic screening of testicular toxicants.

Separation of the individual cell types within the testis generally provides "enriched cell preparations," which are useful for studying intermediary metabolism, changes in membrane permeability, ion fluxes, and localization of xenobiotic metabolism. Mixed cultures of Sertoli and germ cells can be used to measure germ cell detachment as an indicator of toxicity ("pop-off" assay) which has been used to model the toxicity of the phthalate esters and dinitrobenzene. Isolated seminiferous tubules retain the cell-to-cell interactions between Sertoli and germ cells and their stage-specific cell associations and functions. They have been used to study stage-specific aspects of testicular toxicity, e.g. dinitrobenzene exposure on protein secretion. They can also be used for species comparisons. Other culture systems are also available.

Testing for Toxicity of the Developing Reproductive Tract

Multigeneration and other research studies are able to detect potential effects of endocrine active chemicals on male reproductive development because the critical period of exposure, the late gestational period, is covered. End points such as anogenital distance, retention of thoracic areolae/nipples, and preputial separation are key indicators of pre- and postnatal androgen status, and sensitive to the potential effects of exogenous endocrine active agents In normal reproduction studies, the sexing of rat pups is accomplished by observing the distance between the sex papilla and the anus. In males, this distance is approximately twice that of females and is a function of the androgenic status of the animals. Because the anogenital distance is also related to the size of the pup, it is normal to use pup body weight as a covariate in the analysis of these data (normally the measurement is performed on postnatal day 1). This simply measured end point can therefore be used on a routine basis to detect a variety of treatments that affect androgenic

status. In the normal male rodent pup the anlagen of the thoracic nipples will regress under the influence of dihydrotestosterone. Examination of pups before the hair begins to grow (usually around postnatal day 14) and counting the number of areolae or nipples again provide an indication of the hormonal status of the animals. Thus, for example, the classical antiandrogen, flutamide will result in a female phenotype for male pups with the presence of all thoracic nipples in males. In male rodents, an index of puberty is provided by preputial separation, when the prepuce separates from the glans penis following androgen-induced apoptosis. Significant delays or advances in the timing of this event indicate a change in the androgen status of the animals on test and it is an end point that is relatively insensitive to body weight changes.

CONCLUSIONS

The male reproductive system provides a multitude of potential sites for toxicologic disturbance. Effects on the developing reproductive system must be considered as well as effects on the functional adult system. The two systems are very different in their regulatory control and in their chemical sensitivity. A thorough knowledge of the structure and physiology of the system, as well as the kinetics and organization of spermatogenesis, is essential to the understanding of toxicologic disturbances. Different mechanisms of toxicity generally result in different patterns of histopathologic change, but these are often only apparent during the early stages of lesion development. It is therefore critical that conclusions regarding the target site or cell of toxicity are based on appropriately designed investigations and not only on the results of a 28- or 90-day repeat dose toxicity study.

Elucidation of the critical molecular mechanisms underlying target cell toxicity in the reproductive system is extremely difficult. Despite extensive *in vivo* and *in vitro* investigations, the molecular mechanisms of most toxicants remain elusive. This is partly due to the complexity of intercellular communications and regulation but also due to an incomplete understanding of basic reproductive physiology. However, appropriately designed investigations can yield important information on the target cell of toxicity, the reversibility of the lesion, the functional consequences of the injury, and the metabolic and pharmacokinetic profile of the toxicity. Due to the lack of epidemiological data regarding the relative risk to man of rodent reproductive toxicants, this information provides important data for risk assessment analysis of any chemical shown to alter the structure or function of the rodent male reproductive system.

FURTHER READING

Casteel, S.W. (2007). Reproductive toxicants. In *Current Therapy in Large Animal Theriogenology* (Youngquist, R.S. ed.), 2nd edn, pp. 420–427. Saunders Elsevier, St. Louis.

Cooke, P.S., Peterson, R.E. & Hess, R.A. (2002). Endocrine disruptors. In *Handbook of Toxicologic Pathology* (Haschek, W.M., Rousseaux, C.G. & Wallig, M.A. eds), 2nd edn, Vol. 1, pp. 501–528. Academic Press, San Diego.

Creasy, D.M. (2001). Pathogenesis of male reproductive toxicity. *Toxicol. Pathol.*, 29, 64–76.

Creasy, D.M. (1997). Evaluation of testicular toxicity in safety evaluation studies: the appropriate use of spermatogenic staging. *Toxicol. Pathol.*, 25, 119–131.

Creasy, D.M. & Foster, P.M.D. (2002). Male reproductive system. In *Handbook of Toxicologic Pathology* (Haschek, W.M., Rousseaux, C. G. & Wallig, M.A. eds), 2nd edn, Vol. 2, pp. 785–846. Academic Press, San Diego.

Dreef, H.C., van Esch, E. & De Rijk, E.P.C.T. (2007). Spermatogenesis in the cynomolgus monkey (*Macaca fascicularis*): A practical guide for routine morphological staging. *Toxicol. Pathol.*, 35, 395–404.

Eldridge, J.C. & Stevens, J.T. (eds) (2009). *Endocrine Toxicology*, 3rd edn. Informa Healthcare.

Ellington, J.E. & Wilker, C.E. (2006). Reproductive toxicology in the male companion animal. In *Small Animal Toxicology* (Peterson, M.E. & Talcott, P.A. eds), 2nd edn, pp. 500–518. Elsevier Saunders, St. Louis, MO.

Evans, T.J. (2007). Reproductive toxicity and endocrine disruption. In *Veterinary Toxicology: Basic and Clinical Principles* (Gupta, R.C. ed.), pp. 206–244. Elsevier Academic Press, New York.

Foley, G.W. (2001). Overview of male reproductive pathology. *Toxicol. Pathol.*, 29, 49–63.

Foster, P.M.D. & Gray, L.E. Jr. (2008). Toxic responses of the reproductive system. In *Casarett and Doull's Toxicology* (Klaasen, C.D. ed.), 7th edn, pp. 761–806. McGraw Hill Medical, New York.

Foster, R.A. (2007). Male reproductive system. In *Pathologic Basis of Veterinary Disease* (McGavin, M. & Zachary, J.F. eds), 4th edn, pp. 1317–1348. Mosby Elsevier, St. Louis.

Foster, R.A. & Ladds, P.W. (2007). Male genital system. In *Jubb, Kennedy, and Palmer's Pathology of Domestic Animals* (Maxie, M.E. ed.), 5th edn, Vol. 3, pp. 565–620. Elsevier, New York.

Goedken, M.J., Kerlin, R.L. & Morton, D. (2008). Spontaneous and age-related testicular findings in beagle dogs. *Toxicol. Pathol.*, 36, 465–471.

Golub, M.S. (ed.) (2006). *Metals, Fertility, and Reproductive Toxicity*. CRC Press and Taylor and Francis Group, LLC, Boca Raton, FL.

Hess, R.A. (2003). Estrogen in the adult male reproductive tract: A review. *Reprod Biol Endocrinol.*, 1, 52.

Lanning, L.L., Creasy, D.M., Chapin, R.E., Mann, P.C., Barlow, N.J., Regan, K.S. & Goodman, D.G. (2002). Recommended approaches for the evaluation of testicular and epididymal toxicity. *Toxicol. Pathol.*, 30, 507–520.

McKentee, K. (1990). *Reproductive Pathology of Domestic Mammals*. Academic Press, New York.

Naz, R.K. (ed.) (2004). *Endocrine Disruptors: Effects on Male and Female Reproductive Systems*, 2nd edn. CRC Press and Taylor and Francis Group, LLC, Boca Raton, FL.

Panter, K.E., James, L.F., Stegelmeier, B.L., Ralphs, M.H. & Pfister, J.A. (1999). Locoweeds: effects on reproduction in livestock. *J Nat Toxins.*, 8, 53–62.

Rehm, S., White, T.E., Zahalka, E.A., Stanislaus, D.J., Boyce, R.W. & Wier, P.J. (2008). Effects of food restriction on testis and accessory sex glands in maturing rats. *Toxicol. Pathol.*, 36, 687–694.

Russell, L.D., Ettlin, R.A., Sinha Hikim, A.P. & Clegg, E.D. (1990). *Histological and Histopathological Evaluation of the Testis*. Cache River Press, Clearwater, FL.

Russell, L.D., Ren, H.P., Sinha Hikim, I., Schulze, W. & Sinha Hikim, A.P. (1990). A comparative study in twelve mammalian species of volume densities, volumes, and numerical densities of selected testis components, emphasizing those related to the Sertoli cell. *Am J Anat.*, 188, 21–30.

Suwa, T., Nyska, A., Haseman, J.K., Mahler, J.F. & Maronpot, R.R. (2002). Spontaneous lesions in control B6C3F1 mice and recommended sectioning of male accessory sex organs. *Toxicol. Pathol.*, 30, 228–234.

CHAPTER
19
Female Reproductive System

OUTLINE

INTRODUCTION

Many chemicals in our environment have been shown to interfere with reproductive function Exposure to cigarette smoke and ingestion of large amounts of alcohol can cause infertility. Cigarette smoke contains large numbers of chemicals including known carcinogens and polyaromatic hydrocarbons (PAHs). Cigarette smoke causes infertility, altered hormone levels and early menopause. The follicles within the ovary appear to be the targets of injury. Alcohol in large amounts can cause menstrual disorders, spontaneous abortion and birth defects. Occupational exposure to perchloroethylene, toluene, ethylene oxide, nitrous oxide and organic solvents can have adverse effects on reproductive function. Environmental contaminants affecting female reproduction include polychlorinated biphenyls (PCBs), dioxins, and various pesticides such as kepone and methoxychlor which

target antral follicles. These effects can be caused either through direct injury to the reproductive tract or through endocrine disruption.

Testing for reproductive toxicity is an important component of drug safety evaluation with the rat being the most common test species; dogs and non-human primates are also used. The male is often used to study reproductive toxicity because spermatogenesis is a continuous process. Any interruption of spermatogenesis is manifested as atrophy of the testis or accessory sex glands, which can be easily recognized and assessed both grossly and microscopically. Reproductive toxicity is less often studied in the female because toxicity is more difficult to detect and interpret. Reproductive function in the female is often a noncontinuous cyclic process. The female reproductive tract that ceases to cycle normally due to toxicity can appear similar to one that is in a state of normal diestrus. Consequently, to detect a significant change in female reproductive function, a large number of animals and a long test period may be required. This is especially true in nonrodent species such as the dog and the monkey. Detection of female reproductive changes is further complicated by small group sizes typical in dog and monkey studies (2 to 4 per group) and the use of young (peripubertal) animals. The normal variation of ovarian weight with the formation and regression of follicles and corpora lutea during the estrous cycle also complicates detection of ovarian weight changes. In addition, ovaries do not undergo atrophy as rapidly as testes following toxic insult. The relatively small size of the female gonad in comparison to that of the male makes gross examination more difficult. There are few detailed descriptions of normal cyclic changes of the female reproductive organs available in the literature. The lack of familiarity with normal cyclic changes undoubtedly hinders the study of toxic effects in the female. In this chapter, both the normal morphology and the toxicopathological changes of the female reproductive organs in common laboratory animals will be discussed. Because control of the reproductive cycle in females is complex, safety evaluation should include in its perspective the interaction of the central nervous system with the endocrine system and the reproductive tract. Following input from the cerebral cortex, the hypothalamus secretes gonadotropin-releasing hormone into the hypophyseal portal circulation, which stimulates the anterior lobe of the pituitary to release gonadotropins. Subsequent to gonadotropin stimulation, the ovary synthesizes and releases sex steroid hormones. The levels of circulating sex steroid hormones in turn affect the activity of the hypothalamus and pituitary in the regulation of reproductive function in either a stimulatory (positive) or inhibitory (negative) manner, depending on the stage of the cycle. In addition to steroidogenesis, ovarian tissues are capable of making a large number of growth hormones and cytokines. Ovarian hormones and growth factors exert stimulatory and inhibitory effects both locally (i.e. adjacent follicles) and systemically. For these reasons, it is important to view the ovary and remainder of the reproductive tract as a single unit in order to correctly interpret changes found in toxicologic studies. Accordingly, this approach will be used in our discussion.

Since most toxicologic studies are conducted with young adult animals, findings in sexually immature animals that have been used widely in basic research will not be included in this discussion. It is also the intention of the authors to focus the discussion on the rat, since it is the species most frequently used in toxicologic testing. Brief mention will be made in regard to reproductive toxicity in domestic animals.

STRUCTURE AND FUNCTIONAL PHYSIOLOGY

Structure

The gross and microscopic appearance of female reproductive organs varies with the stage of the reproductive cycle. Discussion of morphological changes will focus on the ovary, uterus, and vagina, since there are very few studies in which toxicologic effects on the uterine (fallopian) tube and cervix have been described.

Ovary

The paired ovaries, suspended from the dorsal abdominal wall by the mesovarium, are globose in the rat, irregularly ellipsoid in the dog, and amygdaloid in the cynomolgus monkey. The ovaries of rodents and dogs are enclosed within the ovarian bursa, which obscures gross examination. In rodents and dogs, which have long and straight uterine horns, the ovaries are located in the caudal portion of the lumbar region posterior to the kidneys. With the short uterine body of primates, the ovaries are located in the pelvic region.

The ovarian surface reflects the stage of the reproductive cycle and may have grossly visible follicles and corpora lutea. In rodents and dogs, several follicles and corpora lutea may develop during each cycle. These structures often protrude from the ovarian surface, thus giving rise to the grape-like appearance of the ovary. In primates, multiple primary follicles develop with each cycle but usually one follicle will be selected to become the preovulatory follicle, resulting in only a few large protrusions from the ovarian surface.

The surface of the ovary is covered by a single layer of mesothelium (previously termed germinal epithelium). Depending on its location, this specialized peritoneal mesothelium may be squamous, cuboidal or columnar. Beneath the mesothelium is a thin layer of dense connective tissue called the tunica albuginea or lamina propria. The parenchyma below the tunica albuginea can be divided into two poorly demarcated zones. The outer zone, or cortex, contains the oocytes, follicles, corpora lutea, interstitial glands, and other glandular structures embedded in a highly cellular compact stroma (Figure 19.1). The inner zone, or medulla, contains larger blood and lymph vessels, interstitial glands, and rudimentary epithelial structures, such as rete ovarii and medullary cords, in loosely arranged connective tissue. Nerves and blood vessels enter the ovarian parenchyma at the center of the median pole or hilus.

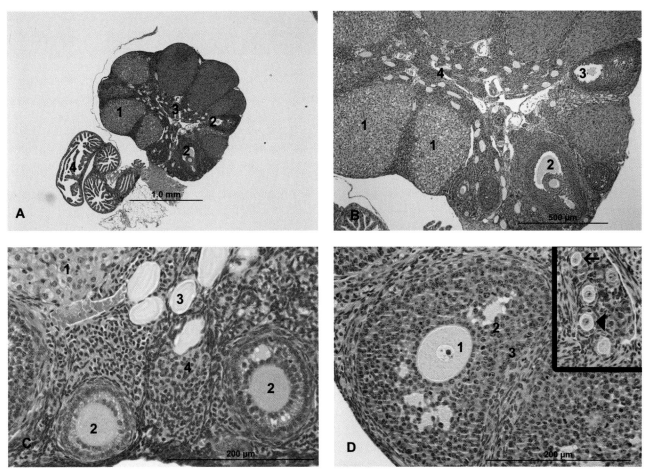

FIGURE 19.1 Ovary, normal mouse. A: The ovary consists of cortex, with corpora lutea (1) and follicles (2), and medulla (3). The uterine (fallopian) tube is present adjacent to the ovary (4). B: Enlarged area from A showing corpora lutea (1), tertiary follicle (2), early atretic follicle (3) and medulla (4). C: Corpus luteum (1), vesicular follicles (2), remnant of zona pellucida (3) and interstitial gland (4). D: Tertiary follicle with oocyte (1), granulosa cells (2) and theca (3). Insert shows primordial follicle (arrow) and primary follicle (arrowhead).

In healthy sexually mature animals, follicles in different stages of development are present. The primordial follicle (Figure 19.1D) is often located immediately beneath the tunica albuginea. It is the least developed follicle and consists of an oocyte surrounded by a single layer of squamous epithelial (follicular) cells. It represents the resting stage of the oocyte and is present during fetal life. The first stage of follicular growth is the recruitment and development of a cohort of primordial follicles into primary follicles (Figures 19.1D). The oocyte rapidly increases in size from approximately 15 μm to 100 μm in diameter and there is a proliferation and transformation, from flattened to columnar, of follicular cells surrounding the oocyte. The next phase of follicular growth consists of further proliferation and differentiation of the single layer of follicular cells into multiple layers of granulosa cells and the formation of the zona pellucida, a glycoprotein coat surrounding the oocyte. The follicle is now designated as a secondary follicle. As the

follicle continues to grow, multiple fluid-filled spaces appear, and it is now called a vesicular follicle. When the cystic spaces become confluent, forming a single large space called an antrum, the follicle is called a tertiary follicle (Figure 19.1C). At this stage, the oocyte with attached granulosa cells becomes eccentrically located in the follicle; the mass of granulosa cells enclosing the oocyte projects into the antrum forming a hillock called the cumulus oophorus. The granulosa cells surrounding the oocyte are called the corona radiata and the fluid in the antrum, the liquor folliculi. The term "Graafian follicle" or preovulatory follicle is used to denote a tertiary follicle during preovulatory growth.

During follicular development, the stromal cells encapsulating the follicle also undergo morphological changes. The elongated fibroblast-like stromal cells which form concentric layers around the developing follicle are called theca cells (Figure 19.1D). Since the granulosa cells of a follicle are avascular, they rely on the vasculature of the theca. At later stages of follicular development, the theca is further divided into the theca interna and theca externa. Cells in the theca interna become polygonal in shape, with vacuolated cytoplasm and vesicular nuclei. These cells further hypertrophy as proestrus approaches and are believed to be the major site of sex steroid production. The cells of the theca externa maintain their fibroblast-like morphology. The theca externa contains contractile elements that are believed to assist in the process of ovulation.

Degeneration of the follicle, known as atresia, occurs most commonly with 200–400 μm diameter follicles (Figure 19.1B). Consequently, the appearance of atretic follicles varies depending on the stage of development at which atresia occurs. The earliest noticeable changes frequently occur in, but are not limited to, the granulosa cells immediately adjacent to the lumen in tertiary follicles and just external to the corona radiata of vesicular follicles. In the tertiary follicle, cells undergo apoptosis and slough from their attachment, resulting in a greatly reduced cumulus oophorus; this sloughing allows the ovum, covered by the zona pellucida, to float in the follicular liquor. The zona pellucida and ovum also undergo degenerative and necrotic changes followed by complete degeneration, necrosis, and disappearance of granulosa cells. In rats and mice, the theca interna persists as the interstitial gland, which often contains the degenerated zona pellucida in the center (Figure 19.1C). The interstitial gland eventually breaks up into small groups of cells that are scattered in the medulla. Dogs also can form interstitial glands or granulosa cell cords derived from atretic follicles and stromal cells. Atresia of follicles at earlier stages of development is not as conspicuous as that of vesicular and tertiary follicles, due to their relatively small size. Degenerating primary oocytes are likely the origin of calcified foci reported as a normal finding in the ovarian cortex of baboons, rhesus and cynomolgus monkeys. The calcified areas may be multiple and/or bilateral.

Only a limited number of developed follicles reaches the stage of preovulatory follicles and ovulates. After ovulation, both the thecal cells and the retained granulosa cells luteinize and become the luteal cells of the newly formed corpus luteum. Histologically, luteinization is characterized by both hyperplasia and hypertrophy of luteal cells and by vascular proliferation. This often results in a corpus luteum larger than the mature follicle. Granulosa cells of canine follicles begin to luteinize with extensive infoldings of the granulosa lining prior to ovulation. Changes observed in the cytoplasm include an initial increased acidophilia, followed by a foamy appearance and, finally, by an accumulation of vacuoles.

It is thus evident that the stage of the reproductive cycle cannot easily be determined by the appearance of follicles in species having a short estrous cycle like the rat. However, the formation, progression, and regression of corpora lutea are somewhat synchronized and their appearance can be used to determine the stage of the cycle in normal cycling animals. Table 19.1 indicates the appearance of the corpus luteum in specimens collected at approximately 9 a.m. from rats with 4-day estrous cycles. The day of the cycle was based on the cytology of vaginal smears that were performed at approximately 8 a.m. These times were selected because most specimens from toxicologic studies are collected during the morning. Detailed description of the cyclic changes can be found in Yuan and Foley, 2002.

With a few exceptions (e.g., hamster), each generation of corpora lutea persists through several estrous cycles before disintegrating and disappearing from the parenchyma. A minimum of three sets of corpora lutea are present in normal cycling rats. This is also the case in most continuous polyestrous animals. As the corpora lutea regress, they decrease in size but increase their content of lipochrome pigment; this is followed by fibrous tissue replacement (corpus albicans) before their final disappearance from the parenchyma. In rats, accumulation of fibrous tissue is negligible and complete resolution is the rule.

Besides follicles and their associated structures, the ovarian cortex also contains interstitial glands. In rats, mice and monkeys, most of the interstitial glands originate from atretic follicles; in dogs, they originate from both atretic follicles and stromal cells. When an interstitial gland is derived from an atretic follicle, the center of the gland often contains hyaline membrane residue from the degenerated zona pellucida (Figure 19.1C). Interstitial glands will become more prominent in response to gonadotrophin stimulation but eventually disintegrate and disappear from the parenchyma.

There are some important species differences in ovarian structure among domestic animals. The size of normal follicles varies widely between species, with the horse (mare) having the largest follicles, up to 7 cm. Polyovulatory follicles (follicles with two or more oocytes) commonly occur in young dogs (bitches), but can be found in all domestic mammals. In the ovaries of dogs and some other carnivores, as well as primates, there are tubular downgrowths of surface epithelium through the tunica albuginea into the superficial cortex. These structures have been termed subsurface epithelial structures (SES) and are most numerous during anestrus. The SES are hormonally responsive and commonly become cystic in aged dogs. Their functional significance is not known. Papillary carcinomas originate from the SES.

TABLE 19.1   Characteristic appearance of the ovary, uterus, and vagina of the 4-day estrous cycling rat

Structure	Estrus	Metestrus	Diestrus	Proestrus
Ovary				
Corpus luteum				
Luteal cells	Small with basophilic cytoplasm	Medium-sized with foamy acidophilic cytoplasm	Very large; may contain tiny cytoplasmic lipid vacuoles	Large; many degenerated and necrotic cells; many contain large cytoplasmic vacuoles
Central cavity	Irregular, filled with fluid and devoid of fibrous tissue	Reduced in size but still devoid of fibrous tissue	Early fibrous tissue proliferation	Further fibrous tissue proliferation
Uterus				
Endometrium				
Epithelial cells	Very large, tall columnar	Large, tall columnar	Small, columnar	Medium-sized, low to high columnar
Cytoplasmic to nuclear ratio	Greater than 2	About 2	Less than 1	About 1.5
Mitotic figures	Rare	Common	Very common	Few
Vacuolar degeneration and necrosis	Very frequent in both luminal and glandular epithelium	Occasional, mostly in luminal epithelium	Rare	Absent
Stromal cell, lamina propria	Spindle-shaped, inactive	Spindle-shaped, inactive	Round to ovoid, active	Spindle-shaped, inactive
Vagina				
Epithelium				
Stratum germinativum	7–8 layers of cells	5–6 layers of cells	8–9 layers of cells	7–9 layers of cells
Stratum granulosum	1–2 layers of cells	Absent	Absent	2–3 layers of cells
Stratum corneum	Present	Absent	Absent	Present
Stratum mucification	Absent	Absent	Absent	2–3 layers of cells
Cytology	Exclusively large cornified epithelial cells	Mostly small polymorphonuclear leucocytes and a few large cornified epithelial cells	Mixture of small polymorphonuclear leukocytes and medium-sized noncornified and large cornified epithelial cells	Mostly medium-sized, noncornified, mucin-containing epithelial cells

In the mare, the cortex is located centrally with medullary tissue and vasculature peripherally. The ovary is kidney shaped with a depressed area called the ovulation fossa. The stroma is very fibroblastic without distinct corticomedullary differentiation. Ectopic adrenocortical tissue is commonly found adjacent to the ovary.

Uterus

Several different configurations of uterus are found in animals; these depend on the degree of fusion of the two mesonephric ducts. The rat has a duplex uterus with two separate uterine bodies joined externally at their cervical ends but with two independent cervical openings. The dog has a bicornuate uterus with two separate uterine horns opening into one common cervical canal. Primates have a simplex uterus with a single uterine body and cervical canal. Most domestic species have a bicornuate uterus. Endometrial caruncles (highly vascularized, non-glandular regions) are only seen in ruminants with caruncular melanosis a normal feature in some sheep breeds.

The gross appearance of the uterus of nonpregnant animals depends on the stage of the reproductive cycle. The uterus is enlarged and hyperemic during proestrus and early estrus, reduced in size at metestrus, and small and pale during diestrus. A grossly distended, fluid-filled uterus is normal for proestrus in rats and the term hydrometra should be avoided.

Histologically, the uterus is composed of an innermost mucosa, the endometrium, a middle muscular layer, the myometrium, and an outer serosal layer, the perimetrium. The endometrium is composed of a surface epithelium, endometrial glands, and the lamina propria. A single layer of columnar epithelial cells lines the lumenal surface and endometrial glands. The lamina propria is composed of abundant small stromal cells, migrating lymphocytes and polymorphonuclear leukocytes, and vascular spaces within a framework of connective tissue. The myometrium is composed of inner circularly and outer longitudinally arranged bundles of smooth muscle cells. The perimetrium is composed of a single layer of mesothelial cells, which overlies a thin layer of connective tissue.

The histological appearance of the uterus also varies with the stage of the reproductive cycle (Figure 19.2, Table 19.1). Detailed description of the cyclic changes can be found in Yuan and Foley, 2002. In dogs, cyclic endometrial changes are more dramatic due to greater cell proliferation resulting from prolonged luteal function. If pregnancy does not occur following estrus, endometrial changes of pseudopregnancy are found. These are characterized by proliferation of the uterine glands and surface epithelium with

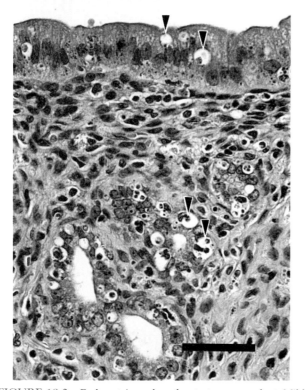

FIGURE 19.2   Endometrium, day of metestrus, normal rat. Mild degeneration is present and often limited to the lumenal epithelium. Regeneration is occurring in the glandular epithelium and mitotic figures (arrows) are frequent. Bar = 50 μm.

folding of the mucosa. Regression is a gradual process which varies greatly in length between bitches.

In cynomolgus and rhesus monkeys, the endometrial changes are similar to those of women, with menstrual discharge toward the end of each reproductive cycle. Endometriosis, ectopic growth of endometrial tissue outside the uterus, and adenomyosis, extension of endometrium into the subjacent myometrium, have been reported across the primate order. Adenomyosis has also been reported to occur in the uteri of aged mice.

Vagina

The vagina consists of an inner layer, the mucosa, a middle layer, the muscularis, and an outer layer, the adventitia. The mucosa is composed of a stratified squamous epithelium and its underlying lamina propria. The muscularis is composed of smooth muscle fibers arranged more or less circularly in the inner layer and longitudinally in the outer layer. The adventitia is composed of a thin layer of connective tissue.

The histological appearance of the vaginal epithelium depends on the stage of the cycle (Figure 19.3). In rats, it is composed of one to four strata of cells with complete cellular renewal in each cycle. The stratum germinativum is the most basal stratum and is the only stratum present throughout the cycle (Table 19.1). It is composed of an inner stratum basale consisting of a single layer of columnar cells with cylindrical nuclei resting on the basement membrane, and an outer stratum spinosum consisting of several layers of polyhedral to elongated cells. The stratum granulosum rests on the stratum germinativum and is composed of one to three layers of flattened epithelial cells which contain many cytoplasmic keratohyalin granules. The stratum corneum covers the outer surface of the stratum granulosum and is composed of closely packed cornified cells with a thickness of 8 to 18 μm. The stratum mucification is composed of two to three layers of cuboidal to ovoid cells which have mucin-containing cytoplasmic vacuoles. This stratum is the outermost tissue lining the lumen during certain stages of the cycle. Histologic sampling of rat vagina should be from the anterior vagina since the posterior third of the vaginal mucosa is always covered by a thick cornified stratified epithelium.

Detailed description of the standard cyclic changes can be found in Yuan and Foley, 2002. However, the progression of cyclic changes may vary greatly among individual animals and regional differences can be found in the same individual. Care must be taken that the process of collecting vaginal cytology does not induce pseudopregnancy in rats.

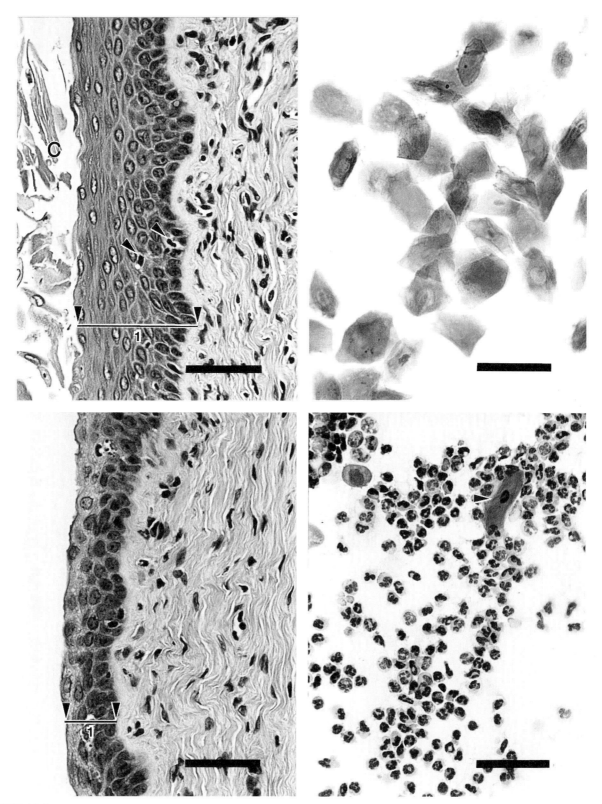

FIGURE 19.3 (Top left) Vagina, day of estrus, normal rat. Stratum corneum undergoes dehiscence with many cornified epithelial cells (C) in the lumen. Early polymorphonuclear leukocyte infiltration (arrows) of the stratum germinativum (1) is present. Bar = 50 μm. (Top right) Vaginal smear, day of estrus, normal rat. The smear consists exclusively of large cornified epithelial cells. Bar = 50 μm. (Bottom left) Vagina, day of metestrus, normal rat. Stratum germinativum (1) is reduced in thickness and consists of 5–6 layers of cells. Bar = 50 μm. (Bottom right) Vaginal smear, day of metestrus, normal rat. The smear consists of numerous polymorphonuclear leukocytes and a few large cornified epithelial cells (arrow). Bar = 50 μm.

In dogs, cyclic changes are well recognized and the stage of the cycle can be identified by cellular components in the vaginal smear. In rhesus monkeys, significant cyclic changes are also noted. In cynomolgus monkeys, the cyclic changes are slight and inconsistent.

Functional Physiology

Hormonal Events during a Given Reproductive Cycle

Between puberty and senescence, the reproductive cycle is manifested by changes of the reproductive organs as described in the previous section. The cyclic changes within the ovary are mainly regulated by luteinizing hormone (LH) and follicle stimulating hormone (FSH), whereas the cyclic changes of the uterus and vagina are dependent on ovarian steroids.

Each cycle begins with follicular growth and maturation, followed by ovulation, and the subsequent formation and regression of the corpus luteum. Although the recruitment and growth of a primordial follicle to the stage of an early tertiary follicle occurs spontaneously and does not require hormonal stimulation, the presence of FSH and LH is necessary for continued follicular maturation to the stage of a preovulatory follicle. It has been estimated that it takes 50 days to develop from a primordial follicle to preovulatory follicle in rats. Selection of follicles to continue on to the preovulatory stage depends on follicles having granulosa cells able to express the necessary gonadotropin receptors at the time of elevated gonadotropin levels. Most follicles undergo atresia and do not reach the preovulatory stage.

LH and FSH are glycoprotein hormones secreted from the anterior pituitary. In polyestrous nonseasonal breeding animals such as the rat, LH and FSH concentrations increase shortly after the end of the preceding cycle. FSH stimulates the proliferation of granulosa cells and induces receptors for LH on these cells. LH stimulates thecal cells to secrete androstenedione, which serves as a precursor for estrogen synthesis by granulosa cells through the catalytic function of aromatase.

The estrogen secreted from growing follicles promotes cell proliferation and maturation in both the uterus and vagina. Under the influence of estradiol, the stromal fibroblasts and epithelial cells of the endometrium proliferate and increase in size. Estrogen also promotes the synthesis of actinomyosin and glycogen in smooth muscle cells, resulting in hypertrophy of the myometrium. In addition, estrogen primes the uterus for its response to progesterone.

Polymorphonuclear leukocyte migration in the uterus, which may be causally related to intercellular edema and hyperemia, is also attributed to the effect of estrogen. In the vagina, estrogen not only stimulates cell proliferation but also induces epithelial cornification.

In the mature preovulatory follicle, a surge of LH results in ovulation with subsequent formation of the corpus luteum. The newly formed corpus luteum incorporates both granulosa and thecal cells and is capable of secreting progesterone for only a certain period of time. Continued function of the corpus luteum requires stimulation by luteotrophic hormones such as LH and prolactin. Prolactin secretion in rats is stimulated by cervical stimulation. The ovarian steroid hormones exert their influence on the uterus and vagina, and other parts of the body, through the circulatory system.

In primates and dogs, ovulation occurs spontaneously. In the rat, ovulation is also spontaneous and coincides with the preovulatory LH surge that is under photoperiod control. In rabbits and other induced ovulators, the LH surge does not occur until cervical neurons are stimulated by mating or other means to activate the release of luteinizing-hormone releasing hormone (LHRH).

In the newly formed corpus luteum, progesterone secretory activity seems to be autonomous and, in most species, does not require luteotropic factors. For continued function, luteotropic hormones from the pituitary are required; LH is considered to be the most important luteotropic factor in most species. However, in rats prolactin has been identified as the luteotropic factor, whereas in rabbits estrogen is the only known luteotropic factor.

The functional life of the corpus luteum varies among animal species. In the rat, it functions only for the first two days after formation. If cervical stimulation takes place, prolactin continues to be secreted by the pituitary gland and the functional life of corpora lutea is prolonged with continued progesterone secretion. If implantation does not take place, the life of corpora lutea is terminated 12 to 14 days after formation. The period during which the corpus luteum is functional is known as pseudopregnancy.

In dogs, luteinization of the preovulatory follicles is accompanied by progesterone secretion prior to ovulation. This is most likely due to the long interval between the LH surge and ovulation. The functional life of corpora lutea in dogs is approximately 60 days and is not affected by mating or implantation, and both LH and prolactin are required for their maintenance. Due to the long luteal lifespan in dogs, pseudopregnancy is common but not always clinically apparent.

In primates, the corpus luteum has a defined functional life span that is unaffected by mating or mechanical stimulation of the cervix. A continuous low level of LH is required to maintain the corpus luteum. If pregnancy occurs, the embryonic trophoblast secretes chorionic gonadotropin as early as 8 to 9 days after fertilization, thus maintaining the corpus luteum throughout early pregnancy.

Progesterone inhibits cell division and maturation but promotes secretion by the endometrial glands. With prior estrogen priming, it can also cause the endometrial stromal cells to change from the small inactive form with fusiform nuclei to large cells with ovoid nuclei. Progesterone causes myometrial cells to become hypertrophic with prominent myofibrils. In the vagina, when estrogen is also present, progesterone induces mucification by increased production and intracytoplasmic accumulation of sialic acid. In primates, corpora lutea secrete estrogen as well as progesterone.

At the end of its functional life, the corpus luteum regresses (luteolysis). The only clearly demonstrated luteolytic factor is prostaglandin $F_{2\alpha}$ produced by the endometrium. Experimental data indicate that this prostaglandin is responsible for luteolysis in large domestic species such as cattle and sheep and in pseudopregnant rodents such as rat and hamster. Prostaglandin $F_{2\alpha}$ has been demonstrated to be luteolytic in rhesus monkeys.

Regulation of Hormonal Secretion

As indicated earlier, the regulation of hormonal secretion is complex and involves many modulators that exert positive (stimulatory) or negative (inhibitory) feedback control. Readers are referred to a standard textbook of endocrinology for a complete discussion. A brief description of the control of gonadotropin secretion is presented as a background for the understanding of toxicologic alterations in reproductive organs (Figure 19.4).

LH and FSH secretion by gonadotrophs in the anterior pituitary is initiated by a rhythmic pulsatile secretion of LHRH from the hypothalamus into hypothalamo-hypophyseal portal vasculature. In this discussion, LHRH is assumed to be the only gonadotropin releasing hormone responsible for the release of both LH and FSH, although some investigators believe a different hormone may specifically control the release of FSH. The pulsatile release of LHRH is essential for normal LH and FSH secretion from the pituitary. The continuous presence of LHRH will at first stimulate and later desensitize secretion of LH and FSH due to a down-regulation of receptors.

Each LH peak is preceded by an LHRH peak, but not every LHRH peak is followed by an LH peak. When LHRH release is not followed by LH release, the pulse may serve as a self-priming signal by increasing the number of LHRH receptors in the pituitary; this requires the presence of a small amount of estrogen in the serum.

Ovarian hormones modulate both the amplitude and frequency of LHRH pulses. Experimental data suggest that estradiol suppresses LH pulse amplitude but not the frequency, while progesterone primarily suppresses frequency. At the beginning of a reproductive cycle, the secretion of LH is inhibited by estrogen secreted from growing follicles. This negative feedback control affects LH release but not LH synthesis, which enables the pituitary to accumulate enough LH for the preovulatory surge.

Similar to their effect on LH secretion, ovarian steroids also affect FSH secretion and this effect depends on the stage of the cycle and the hormonal status of the animal. During late estrus through early proestrus, estradiol has an inhibitory effect on FSH secretion. This inhibition is potentiated by the presence of progesterone. However, this negative feedback changes just prior to the preovulatory surge of LH. Again, it seems that estrogen is the dominant force, acting directly on the hypothalamus, whereas progesterone potentiates the effect by stimulating FSH synthesis. The secretion of FSH is inhibited by the peptide hormone, inhibin, which is produced by the granulosa cells of growing follicles.

When follicles approach their final stage of maturity, the output of steroid hormones increases prior to ovulation. When concentrations of these hormones reach a certain level, their effects on the regulation of LHRH secretion also change from inhibitory to stimulatory. This is the basis of the preovulatory surge of LHRH and subsequent LH and FSH secretion. The preovulatory surge of LHRH induces a cascade of events within the hypothalamus that is necessary for normal ovulation to proceed. The mechanism responsible for this may involve estrogen, which augments the number of pituitary binding sites for LHRH, increases the responses of the pituitary to hormone binding, and directly promotes LHRH secretion from the hypothalamus. An alternative possibility is that estradiol affects norepinephrine activity, which in turn stimulates LHRH secretion. Estradiol may also contribute by inducing and maintaining LHRH receptors in conjunction with LHRH in the pituitary. The effect of progesterone on LHRH secretion is less clear but is believed to be similar to that of estrogen.

Neurons controlling the secretion of LHRH also receive innervation, capable of either stimulation or inhibition, from other neural sites. Accordingly, the

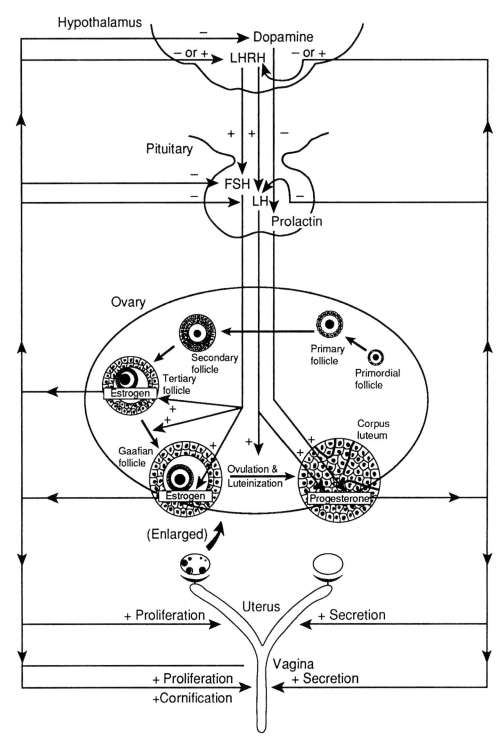

FIGURE 19.4   Schematic drawing of hormonal regulation of reproduction (+: stimulatory, −: inhibitory).

reproductive cycle adjusts to changes in light cycle, seasonal variation, and other physical (cervical stimulation) or olfactory (pheromone) stimuli. LHRH has been found in extrahypothalamic neurons in different regions of the limbic system of the cerebrum and has been implicated in the regulation of reproductive behavior.

Factors involved in termination of the gonadotropin surge may include down regulation of LHRH receptor numbers and subsequent loss of sensitivity of the pituitary gonadotrophs. During the luteal phase, estrogen acts in concert with progesterone to inhibit LH synthesis and release.

Unlike the LH release, prolactin secretion is normally inhibited by the presence of dopamine from the hypothalamus. During the height of prolactin secretion, the level of dopamine is lowest and that of thyroid releasing hormone (TRH) is highest, indicating that TRH may also play a role in the release of prolactin. Estradiol stimulates prolactin release prior to ovulation by acting through the pituitary to decrease the dopamine inhibitory effect. Many growth factors identified in the ovary have a complex interaction with gonadotropins and each other.

MECHANISMS OF TOXICITY

General Toxicity

When considered in the classical toxicology context, reproductive toxicants can act directly or indirectly. Direct acting toxicants can act through structural similarity to endogenous compounds or due to chemical reactivity leading to cellular macromolecular damage. Toxicants with structural similarity are generally agonists or antagonists of endogenous hormones e.g. the estrogenic effects of diethylstilboestrol (DES), zearelanone, DDT, heptachlor, tamoxifen and organochlorines. Those acting through chemical reactivity are generally nonspecific for site of action and induce adverse effects elsewhere. These include drugs, such as chemotherapeutic agents that are alkylating agents; heavy metals such as cadmium; and radiation. Indirect acting toxicants may require metabolic activation which can occur in thecal or granulosa cells of the ovary e.g. polyaromatic hydrocarbons (PAHs), methoxychlor; alter the rate of steroid secretion or clearance, e.g. DDT and PCBs; or affect the hypothalamic-hypophyseal axis, e.g. heroin and methadone.

Most attention has been given to the effect of toxicants on the ovary. Ovotoxicity can result in reproductive abnormalities as well as birth defects and cancer. Reproductive effects include temporary or permanent infertility or sterility, and abnormalities in fertility, cyclicity and hormone levels. Alteration in hormone levels may affect any part of the reproductive tract including the cervix and vagina. For example, decreased hormone levels may increase the risk of cervical infection and promote cervical cancer. Some solvents and pesticides have been shown to affect the uterus.

Ovary, Uterus, and Vagina as a Unit

Control of the female reproductive cycle is complex and comprises a cascade of events emanating from the hypothalamus and extending to the pituitary, ovary, uterus, and vagina, with stimulatory or inhibitory regulation by the ovarian steroids. Any disruption in this cascade of hormonal events may result in functional and structural alterations. Mechanisms of toxicity will be classified into Types I, II, and III, based on the pathological manifestation induced in the reproductive organs. The anticipated hormonal and pathological changes associated with each type of toxicity in rats are listed in Table 19.2. Examples of toxicants causing these changes are listed in Table 19.3.

Type I Toxicity: Factors Which Induce Inactivity in Ovary, Uterus, and Vagina

Atrophy of the ovary can result from reduced gonadotropin secretion, impairment of follicular growth, or enzymatic interference resulting in a reduction of sex steroid hormone synthesis. Atrophy of the uterus and vagina is secondary to a deficiency of ovarian steroid hormones. The underlying mechanism and manifestation of these atrophic changes are similar to those in hypophysectomized animals.

Absence or Reduction of Gonadotropin Secretion

Absence or reduction of gonadotropin is the most commonly observed mechanism of reproductive toxicity. It is often part of a nonspecific general toxicity caused by stress and reduced food intake. Reproduction requires a large amount of energy but is not essential for the survival of the animal. Thus, the reproductive cycle can be easily suspended in order to save energy and will be resumed once general health and energy balance are improved.

Stress induces excessive secretion of epinephrine, which not only stimulates corticosteroid secretion but depresses the frequency and amplitude of LH secretion, thus interfering with the reproductive cycle. Because reduced energy intake is itself stressful, a similar depression of LH release may be seen in the malnourished animal. Reduced body weight gain, increased adrenal weight relative to body weight, and decreased thymus weight relative to body weight in the test animals compared with controls are good indicators of stress; these parameters may be used to determine if ovarian alteration is the result of a primary injury or secondary to stress. Since mitosis is required for both follicular development and luteal proliferation, reduced mitotic activity in the bone marrow indicates that an atrophic ovary may result from a nonspecific toxic effect. Primary and secondary effects may not be easy to distinguish and additional information may be required in order to determine the mechanism of the abnormality.

TABLE 19.2 Hormonal profile and pathological manifestation for each type of reproductive toxicity in the rat[a]

	Type I	Type IIC[b]	Type IIE	Type IIP	Type IIIC	Type IIIE	Type IIIP
Hormonal profile							
Primary effect	↓LHRH	↑E[c] and ↑P[c]	↑E[c]	↑P[c]	↑LHRH[c], ↓LH[c], or ↑HCG[a]	↑FSH[c] or ↑PMSG[c]	↑Prolactin[c] or ↓dopamine
Secondary effect	↓LH, ↓FSH	↓LHRH, ↓LH, ↓FSH	↓LHRH, ↓LH, ↓FSH	↓LHRH, ↓LH	↑LH (from ↑LHRH[b])	↑E, ↑P	↑P
Tertiary effect	↓E, ↓P	↓LH, ↓FSH	↓LH and ↓FSH (from ↓LHRH)	↓LH and ↓FSH (from ↓LHRH)	↑E,↑P	↑E, ↑P	
Ovary	Atrophy with inactive interstitial glands	As Type I	As Type I	As Type I	Moderately[d] enlarged with many[c] corpora lutea and several large follicles; incompletely luteinized and/or cystic corpus luteum may present	Markedly enlarged with numerous corpora lutea and many large follicles; incompletely luteinized and/or cystic corpus luteum may present	Slightly enlarged with several corpora lutea and a few large follicles
Uterus	↑Uterine lumen	↑Pyometra					↑Uterine lumen
Endometrium	↑Endometrial polyp	↑Endometrial polyp					
Epithelium, uterine lumen	Atrophic cells	Moderately hyperplastic and hypertrophic with focal squamous metaplasia	Moderately hyper-plastic and hyper-trophic with focal squamous metaplasia and polymorpho-nuclear leuko-cyte infiltration	Moderately hyper-plastic and slightly hypertrophic with acidophilic foamy cytoplasm	Markedly hyper-plastic and moderately hypertrophic with acidophilic cytoplasm	Markedly hyper-plastic and hypertrophic with acidophilic cytoplasm	Markedly hyper-plastic and very slightly hypertrophic
Endometrial glands	Few, lined by atrophic cells	Moderately hyperplastic and hyper-trophic; cystic glands may be present	Very slightly hyperplastic and hyper-trophic; cystic glands with focal squamous metaplasia may be present	As above	As above	Markedly hyper-plastic and moderately hypertrophic with acidophilic cytoplasm	As above
Stromal cell, zona compacta	Spindle-shaped cells	Spindle-shaped to ovoid cells	Spindle-shaped cells	Spindle-shaped cells	Spindle-shaped to ovoid cells	Spindle-shaped to ovoid cells	Ovoid-shaped to round cells
Vagina epithelium	Atrophic with 2–3 layers of small cells	Hyperplastic and hypertrophic with 5–6 layers of large cells; large cytoplasmic vacuoles in superficial layers	Hyperplastic and hypertrophic with many layers of large cells; squamous metaplasia and incomplete cornification of superficial layers	Four or more layers of medium-sized to large cells; occasional cytoplasmic vacuoles in superficial layers	As Type IIC	As Type IIC	As Type IIP

[a]↑, increase; ↓, decrease; LHRH, luteinizing hormone releasing hormone; LH, luteinizing hormone; FSH, follicular stimulating hormone; E, estrogen; P, progesterone; HCG, human chorionic gonadotropin; PMSG, pregnant mare serum gonadotropin
[b]Subtype designations of E, P and C are induced by compounds that produce changes similar to those of estrogen, progesterone, or a combination of these two steroids, respectively
[c]Exogenous hormone.
[d]Markedly > moderately > slightly > very slightly
[e]Numerous > many > several > a few

TABLE 19.3 Classification of nonneoplastic alterations in the female reproductive tract with selected examples

Toxicity Type	Alteration	Xenobiotic
I	Atrophic ovary, uterus, vagina	Narcotics, cocaine, marijuana, styrene, lead, cadmium, radiation
II	Atrophic ovary with hyperactive uterus, vagina	
IIE*		Estrogen activity: estrogens, tamoxifen, some organochlorines
IIP		Progesterone activity; medroxyprogesterone acetate
IIC		Combined activity: some steroids
III	Hyperplastic or hypertrophic ovary, uterus, vagina	
IIIC		LH activity: LH, LHRH analogs, HCG
IIIE		FSH activity: FSH, PMSG
IIIP		Prolactin activity: prolactin, reserpine, phencyclidine hydrochloride

*Subtype designations of E, P and C are induced by compounds that produce changes similar to those of estrogen, progesterone, or a combination of these two steroids, respectively

Many drugs have either a stimulatory or inhibitory effect on the central nervous system and may therefore disturb the regulation of gonadotropin secretion. Narcotics such as morphine reduce both serum LH and FSH in rodents and humans. Morphine also blocks the proestrous surge of LHRH and subsequent ovulation by decreasing the activity of norepinephrine neurons and the storage of hypothalamic norepinephrine. Norepinephrine is believed to be the neurotransmitter that initiates LHRH secretion by excitation of alpha-adrenergic receptors. Cocaine stimulates LH secretion at low doses and inhibits LH secretion at high doses. This effect is exerted through interference with the catabolism of norepinephrine, which leads to accumulation of this neurotransmitter at the nerve terminals. Cocaine also blocks the uptake of dopamine and thus inhibits the secretion of prolactin. Marijuana, containing tetrahydrocannabinol as its principal psychoactive ingredient, depresses LH, FSH, and prolactin secretion at the level of hypothalamus. Opioid peptides such as β-endorphin also suppress both the amplitude and frequency of the LH pulse and the preovulatory surge of LH, presumably by lowering norepinephrine concentration in the hypothalamus and decreasing the rate of dopamine turnover.

Gasoline by-products such as polystyrene and styrene may alter the secretion of FSH and LH, resulting in decreased estrogen and progesterone output.

Heavy metals may produce multiple adverse effects on reproductive function. Inorganic mercury has been reported to block follicular growth and result in anestrus in laboratory rodents, possibly by altering both pituitary gonadotropin and ovarian steroid secretions. In animals treated with lead, atrophy of the ovary, reduction of serum progesterone concentration, and alteration of uterine hormonal receptors have been observed. These toxicities may result from different effects along the hypothalamic-pituitary-ovarian-endometrial axis. Other metals with the potential to affect reproductive function include manganese, tin, and cadmium.

Impairment of Follicular Development

Maturation of follicles with active proliferation of granulosa cells is an essential part of normal reproductive function. Xenobiotics and radiation have been known to cause direct damage to the oocyte or disrupt granulosa cell proliferation, thus interfering with reproductive function. Many chemicals target follicles of a specific age rather than destroying all the follicles. If follicle development or ovulation is affected, ovarian cysts may result which can secrete high levels of androgens, estradiol or even abnormal products such as insulin. In addition, ovarian cysts may rupture causing abdominal pain

Metabolic transformation of xenobiotics by ovarian enzyme(s) may or may not be required for toxicity. Compounds that do not require metabolic transformation for toxicity are often carcinogenic or mutagenic in other organ systems. These include alkylating agents, chemotherapeutic agents, and some heavy metals. In addition to oocyte injury, these xenobiotics may interfere with granulosa cell proliferation, thecal cell differentiation, and active steroidogenesis. For example, cadmium induces necrosis of preovulatory follicles and damages the microcirculation in the uterus of the rat. Radiation causes abnormal mitosis and death of the oocyte and granulosa cells.

Xenobiotics that require metabolic activation for their toxicity include cyclophosphamide, dibromochloropropane, and the polycyclic aromatic hydrocarbons. Their toxic effects are exerted by highly reactive metabolites formed after oxidation by ovarian microsomal oxygenases.

The result of these processes is a reduction in the total number of oocytes and follicles and an absence of corpora lutea in the ovary. This may result in permanent hormonal imbalance due to the loss of negative feedback control from ovarian steroid hormones. If the insult occurs early in life, neoplasms may develop in the remaining hyperstimulated ovarian components.

Impairment or Alteration of Steroidogenesis

Interference with the production of steroid hormones may affect the appearance of reproductive organs. For example, estrogen is required for proliferation of granulosa cells and maintenance of a healthy follicle. A reduced estrogen level will induce early death of follicles.

Steroidogenesis may be impaired by limiting the supply of precursors or the functional ability of essential enzymes. Malnutrition or reduced food intake may limit cholesterol, which is the precursor for the synthesis of all sex steroids. Chemicals which interfere with enzymatic function required for estrogen synthesis include aminoglutethimide, delta-1-testolactone, 4-hydroxyandrostenedoine, and 10-propargylester-4-ene-3,17-dione. These compounds block the conversion of androgens to estrogens by aromatase, a cytochrome P-450-dependent enzyme, and thus ultimately reduce endogenous estrogen production. They have been used in the treatment of neoplasms derived from estrogen-dependent tissue of the breast and endometrium. Other compounds such as danazol and spironolactone inhibit the synthesis of ovarian steroids by interfering with one or more dehydrogenases.

Metabolic disturbances initiated by interference with enzyme function are likely to induce atrophic ovaries devoid of mature follicles and corpora lutea and secondary atrophy of the uterus and vagina.

Type II Toxicity: Factors Which Induce Inactivity in Ovary but Hyperactivity in Uterus and Vagina

Many naturally occurring and synthetic sex steroid hormones have been developed as contraceptives, fertility drugs, and therapeutic agents for the treatment of cancer. These include both agonists and antagonists of estrogen and progesterone. When sex steroid hormones are given in large nonphysiological quantities in animal toxicity studies, the result is the inhibition of gonadotropin secretion and atrophy of the ovary. However, organs at the bottom of the cascade of control may respond dramatically to the stimulation provided by the massive exogenous doses of these steroids and undergo a high degree of hyperplasia and hypertrophy. Depending on the dominant changes in the uterus and vagina, the type II toxicity can be further classified into three subtypes. Subtypes IIE, IIP, and IIC are induced by compounds that produce changes similar to those of estrogen, progesterone, or a combination of these two steroids, respectively.

Compounds that induce type IIC toxicity include some steroids that possess both estrogen and progesterone activities, although at a low dose they may express their effect mostly as progestational agents. Estrogen at a high dose may express its effect partly as progesterone.

Compounds that induce type IIE toxicity include natural estrogens and synthetic compounds such as diethylstilbestrol, Tamoxifen®, and clomiphene (Clomid®). Organochlorines including chlorophenothane, dichlorophenoxyacetates, hexachlorobenzene, lindane, and toxaphene act as weak estrogens and interfere with estrogen-receptor binding.

Compounds that induce type IIP toxicity include progesterone and synthetic progestins such as ethynerone, norethynodrel, and medroxyprogesterone acetate. Androgens at a high dose may also produce a similar toxicity.

Type III Toxicity: Factors Which Induce Hyperactivity in Ovary, Uterus, and Vagina

Abnormally elevated circulating gonadotropin, unresponsive to negative feedback from ovarian steroid hormones, may be present under certain conditions and result in an abnormal reproductive cycle. The source of excessively high gonadotropin can be either endogenous or exogenous; the result is a hyperactive ovary, uterus, and vagina with hyperplasia or hypertrophy of these organs. Based on the appearance of the ovary, uterus, and vagina, the type III toxicity is also further divided into three subtypes. Subtypes IIIC, IIIE, and IIIP are induced by compounds that produce changes similar to those of LH, FSH, and prolactin, respectively.

Compounds that induce type IIIC toxicity include analogs of LHRH that have been used for the treatment of prostatic cancer and as male contraceptive agents. These agents may also be useful in the treatment of cystic ovaries in cattle and persistent estrus in ferrets by inducing endogenous secretion of LH. Exogenous LH or human chorionic gonadotropin (HCG) can also produce the same effect. HCG has a dominant effect similar to LH and has been used for the treatment of infertility in women. In rats, excessive LH will produce continuous stimulation of the growth and maturation of follicles; the formation of corpora lutea is not overridden by elevated levels of ovarian sex steroid hormones.

Compounds that induce type IIIE toxicity include FSH and pregnant mare serum gonadotropin (PMSG).

PMSG is commonly used in the experimental induction of ovulation. In rats, administration of these exogenous gonadotropins will produce continuous stimulation of the growth and maturation of follicles; the formation of corpora lutea is not overridden by the elevated levels of ovarian sex steroid hormones.

Compounds that induce type IIIP toxicity include prolactin and possibly other luteotropins. Excessive prolactin secretion occurs when dopamine is depleted by compounds such as reserpine or phencyclidine hydrochloride. Elevated prolactin will prolong the functional life of the corpus luteum in rats, thus interrupting the normal reproductive cycle. In rats, the end result is a condition similar to pseudopregnancy.

Local Vaginal Toxicity

The vaginal inflammatory response to an irritant is very similar to the skin, since both are covered by stratified epithelium (see Skin and Oral Mucosa chapter). Toxicity may be caused by irritation alone or by delayed hypersensitivity, with or without irritation.

Irritation

Irritation is the result of direct action of a test formulation on the vaginal mucosa. Acidity and the physicochemical properties of the excipients are the most important factors considered in selecting a vehicle for the preparation of a nonirritating vaginal pharmaceutical formulation. Since vaginal pH in women is slightly acidic due to the fermentation of lactose by the bacterial flora, a slightly acidic formulation is preferred. Extreme acidity or alkalinity will irritate the mucosa. Excipients often consist of surfactants that help the therapeutic agent penetrate the vaginal epithelium. There are three classes of surfactants, namely, nonionic, anionic, and cationic. Cationic surfactants cause the most severe irritation whereas nonionic surfactants are least likely to cause irritation. If the formulation is a suspension that contains insoluble particles, irritation may result when particles become lodged between mucosal folds.

The severity of vaginal inflammation will vary with the nature of the toxic factor and the configuration of the vaginal epithelium. A thick epithelium with a heavily cornified layer will be a more effective barrier and will provide more protection than a thin epithelium lacking a cornified layer.

Delayed Hypersensitivity

Vaginal medications occasionally have been associated with the development of a delayed hypersensitivity reaction in women, resulting in a generalized dermatitis. Delayed hypersensitivity occurs when one or more highly reactive components act as incomplete antigens. These components combine with certain protein constituents of the lamina propria to form a complete antigen. Readers are referred to the Skin and Oral Mucosa chapter, for the mechanism and nature of tissue inflammation in delayed hypersensitivity.

Carcinogenesis

Ovary

Estrogen and progesterone, produced by the growing follicle and corpus luteum, are the main factors involved in the negative feedback control of gonadotropin secretion. When the negative feedback control of gonadotropin secretion is impaired, serum gonadotropin levels may be elevated. Constant stimulation of ovarian tissue by gonadotropins may result in hyperplastic and neoplastic proliferations. Radiation and compounds such as dimethylbenz[α]anthracene destroy oocytes; ovarian tumors may develop from the remaining tissue as a consequence of prolonged gonadotropin stimulation (Table 19.4). Chronic stimulation by estrogenic compounds has also been reported to induce ovarian neoplasia in rats and dogs. In dogs exposed to stilboestrol, metastatic lesions developed and then regressed following withdrawal of treatment. Similar results were observed in rats with the development of granulosa cell tumors and hyperplasia only to see regression following withdrawal of estrogenic treatment. The estrogenic findings may represent hormonally driven hyperplastic responses rather than true neoplasms. Many other carcinogens are also capable of inducing ovarian neoplasia; however, the mechanisms of tumor induction frequently are not understood.

The susceptibility to tumor induction depends on the strain, species, and age of the animal at the time of exposure. Types of tumors induced include granulosa and thecal cell tumors, luteoma, tubular adenoma, Sertoli cell tumor, and fibroma in the ovary, and leiomyoma in the mesovarium.

Uterus

Endometrial cancer has long been associated with estrogen treatment. In humans, unopposed estrogen as hormonal replacement therapy greatly increases the risk of endometrial cancer. Prolonged administration of DES to laboratory animals may produce endometrial polyps, hyperplasia and carcinoma. The uterus is an estrogen-dependent organ, and endometrial cells proliferate as a result of estrogen stimulation. Early neoplastic growth requires the continuous presence of estrogen. However, once neoplastic growth

TABLE 19.4   Selected carcinogenic agents affecting the ovary, uterus, and vagina in animals

Organ	Tumor Type	Factor	Species
Ovary	Granulosa/thecal cell tumor and luteoma	Benzo[a]pyrene	Mouse
		Iodine-131	Hamster
		Progestins	Mouse
		Radiation	Mouse
		7,12-Dimethylbenz[a]anthracene	Mouse
		7,8,12-Trimethylbenz[a]anthracene	Mouse
	Tubular adenoma	Radiation	Mouse
	Sertoli cell tumor	N-Ethyl-N-nitrosourea	Rat
	Fibroma	Mibolerone® (an androgen)	Dog
	Leiomyoma, mesovarium	Soterenol® and Mesuprine® HCl (smooth muscle relaxants)	Rat
Uterus	Adenocarcinoma/adenoacanthoma	Diaminozide	Mouse
		Estrogens	Rabbit
		Intrauterine devices	Rat
		Methylcholanthrene	Mouse
		N,N-Dimethyl-N-nitrosourea	Hamster
		3-Amino-9-ethylcarbazole	Mouse
		4-Methyl-N′-nitro-N-nitrosoguanidine	Mouse
		4-Nitroguaninoline-1-oxide	Mouse
		4,4-Thiodianiline	Mouse
	Deciduosarcoma	Estrogen and progesterone combination	Rabbit
	Fibrosarcoma	2-Acetylaminofluorene	Rat
		3-Methylcholanthrene	Mouse
	Leiomyoma/leiomyosarcoma	Medroxalol® (an antihypertensive agent)	Mouse
	Papillary mesothelioma	Estrogens	Rabbit, dog
	Squamous cell carcinoma	Intrauterine devices	Rat
		7,12-Dimethylbenz[a]anthracene	Mouse
Vagina	Basal cell carcinoma, squamous cell carcinoma, and mucin-secreting tumor	Benzo[a]pyrene	Mouse
		Estrogens	Mouse
		Methylcholanthrene	Mouse
		Phenylmercuric acetate	Mouse
		Polyethylene glycol	Mouse
		Quinine sulfate	Mouse
		7,12-Dimethylbenz[a]anthracene	Mouse
		8-Hydroxyquinoline	Mouse

is established, continuing proliferation or transformation may result in the tumor becoming estrogen independent. Many other compounds are also capable of inducing neoplasms in the uterus (Table 19.4). In some studies, compounds were introduced into the uterine cavity by mechanical means such as a string impregnated with the test compound. The physical presence of a foreign body in the uterine cavity and its effect on the endometrial cells has not been ruled out as a major factor in tumor induction in such cases. The types of neoplasms induced in the uterus include adenocarcinoma/adenoacanthoma, deciduosarcoma, fibrosarcoma, leiomyoma/leiomyosarcoma, papillary mesothelioma, and squamous cell carcinoma.

Vagina

A diverse group of chemicals, which includes chemically inert materials such as urea and propylene glycol, is capable of inducing vaginal neoplasms in laboratory animals (Table 19.4). The mechanism of tumor induction is not understood but the prolonged exposure may induce irritation that stimulates epithelial cell proliferation. Extended proliferation has been postulated to progress to uncontrolled neoplastic growth through a transitional stage characterized by epithelial dysplasia. Basal cell carcinomas, squamous cell carcinomas, and tumors of mucin-secreting cells have been induced in animals. Adenocarcinomas have been reported in a small number of young women whose mothers had been treated with diethylstilbestrol (DES) during pregnancy.

RESPONSE TO INJURY

The response of the reproductive system to insult is similar among different species of laboratory animals because of the similarity of reproductive function control. Responses in the rat will be described as representative of the changes that can be anticipated in toxicologic testing (Table 19.2).

General Responses: Ovary, Uterus, and Vagina as a Unit

Type I Response: Atrophic Ovary, Uterus, and Vagina

The appearance of the reproductive organs following induced atrophy is similar to that observed in hypophysectomized animals. Recognition of an atrophic ovary may be difficult in short-term studies in rats because of continued follicular development. In addition, corpora lutea may not be obviously reduced in number or size due to the orientation of the ovary during tissue preparation. However, ovarian interstitial glands, particularly those located in the medulla, offer valuable information about ovarian activity. Interstitial glands in normal cycling rats are composed of large polygonal cells with round nuclei and a moderate amount of deeply acidophilic foamy cytoplasm (Figure 19.5, left). In atrophic ovaries, these glands are composed of small spindle-shaped cells with dark elongated nuclei and a small amount of lightly acidophilic or basophilic cytoplasm (Figure 19.5, right). In longer term studies, corpora lutea are either reduced in number or absent.

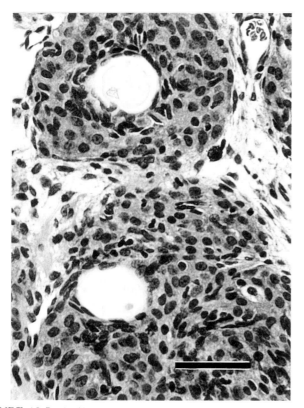 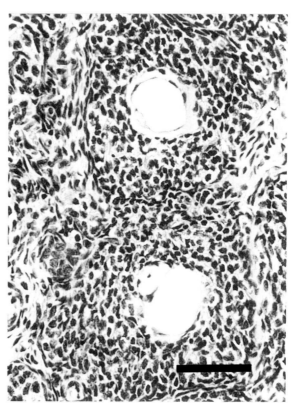

FIGURE 19.5   (Left) Interstitial gland, ovary, normal rat. The glandular cells are large and polygonal in shape with round nuclei and a moderate amount of deeply stained cytoplasm. (Right) Interstitial gland, atrophic ovary from an aged rat (Type I response). The glandular cells are small and spindle shaped with elongated nuclei and a small amount of lightly stained cytoplasm. Bars = 50 μm.

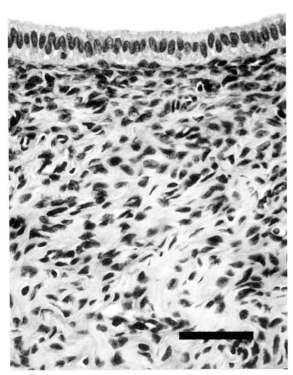

FIGURE 19.6 Atrophic endometrium from a hypophysect-omized rat (Type I response). The lumenal lining epithelial cells are small and the endometrial glands are absent. Bar = 50 μm. Compare with Figure 19.2.

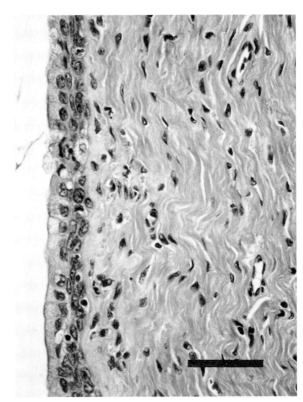

FIGURE 19.7 Atrophic vaginal mucosa from a hypophysect-omized rat (Type I response). The epithelium is composed of two to three layers of cuboidal cells. Bar = 50 μm. Compare with Figure 19.3.

When evaluating ovaries in short-term studies in rats, two principles should be kept in mind. First, the presence of developing follicles should not be interpreted as a sign of normal reproductive function because follicular development, from primordial to early tertiary stage, is intrinsic and does not require hormonal stimulation. Second, the mere presence of corpora lutea should not be regarded as uninterrupted reproductive function since significant regressive changes take place in corpora lutea only on the day of proestrus of the following cycle. If the animal stops cycling, the corpora lutea formed during the last cycle will not regress as rapidly and may retain a healthy appearance for some time. Both of these findings may lead to the impression that reproductive function is not altered.

An atrophic uterus is much easier to identify histologically than an atrophic ovary. Not only is the endometrium thin and lined by small inactive epithelial cells with a cytoplasmic to nuclear ratio of less than 1 and a paucity of endometrial glands (Figure 19.6), but the myometrium is atrophic with small elongated nuclei and scant cytoplasm.

An atrophic vagina is lined by two to three layers of small cuboidal cells (Figure 19.7). Atrophic changes in the vagina are easier to identify histologically in any given short-term study than those in the uterus and ovary.

Type II Response: Atrophic Ovary with Hyperactive Uterus and Vagina

The atrophic ovary appears similar to that described for the type I response in most cases. However, papillary proliferation of the ovarian surface epithelium, in addition to parenchymal atrophy of the ovary, has been observed in both dogs and rabbits treated with estrogenic compounds. In dogs, metastatic implantation of epithelial cells onto the capsule of the spleen, kidney, and other abdominal viscera has been observed. Since continued growth of these cells is estrogen-dependent, they undergo degeneration, necrosis, and mineralization once these estrogenic compounds are removed. The regression of the canine proliferations has posed the questions if they are true neoplasms since they are not autonomous in growth. Similar regression of granulosa cell "tumors" and hyperplasia following withdrawal of Tamoxifen treatment have been described in the literature.

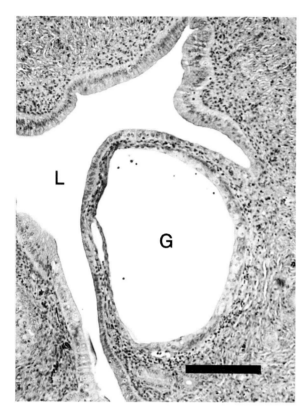

FIGURE 19.8 Hyperplastic endometrium from a rat treated with both estradiol and progesterone (Type IIC response). Uterine lumen (L) is dilated and there is cystic hyperplasia of endometrial glands (G). Bar = 200 μm.

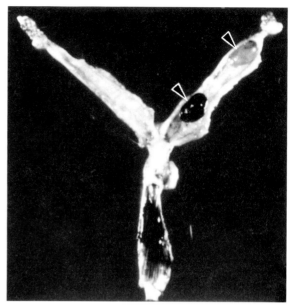

FIGURE 19.9 Uterus from an aged rat. Two endometrial polyps (arrows) are present. The lower one appears as a dark mass due to hemorrhage. Actual size.

The appearance of the uterus and vagina depends on the nature of the compound. Again, subtypes IIE, IIP, and IIC will be used to denote the uterine and vaginal changes resulting from compounds with similar effects to estrogen, progesterone, and a combination of these two steroids, respectively.

In the type IIC response, endometrial hyperplasia with cystic endometrial glands and dilated uterine lumen may be present in mice and rats (Figure 19.8). Focal areas of endometrial squamous metaplasia and large cytoplasmic vacuoles in epithelial cells may also be present in rats. An increased incidence of endometrial polyps has been noted in rats that have received both estrogenic and gestational agents. The polyps often appear as a protrusion of endometrial tissue which forms a pedunculated mass inside the uterine lumen (Figure 19.9). Grossly, endometrial polyps are pink to dark red soft nodules with a glistening surface. Histologically, they consist of spindle-shaped or stellate cells dispersed in an edematous or hemorrhagic stroma covered by a layer of cuboidal to columnar epithelial cells (Figure 19.10). Varying numbers of endometrial glands may also be present within the mass. With the development of selective estrogenic

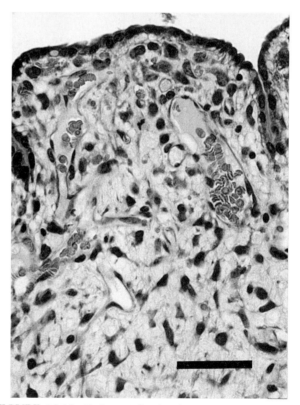

FIGURE 19.10 Endometrial polyp from an aged rat. Beneath the single layer of lumenal epithelial cells, the stroma consists of spindle-shaped cells in an edematous framework of connective tissue. Bar = 50 μm.

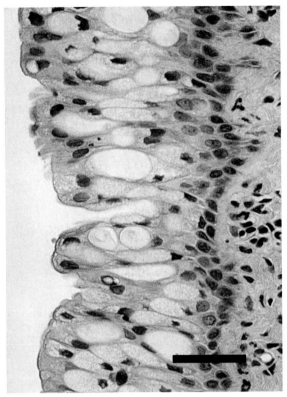

FIGURE 19.11   Hypertrophic vaginal mucosa from a rat treated with both estradiol and progesterone (Type IIC response). The epithelium is composed of 6 layers of cells. Except for the two basal layers, large cells with a single large cytoplasmic vacuole are present frequently. Bar = 50 μm.

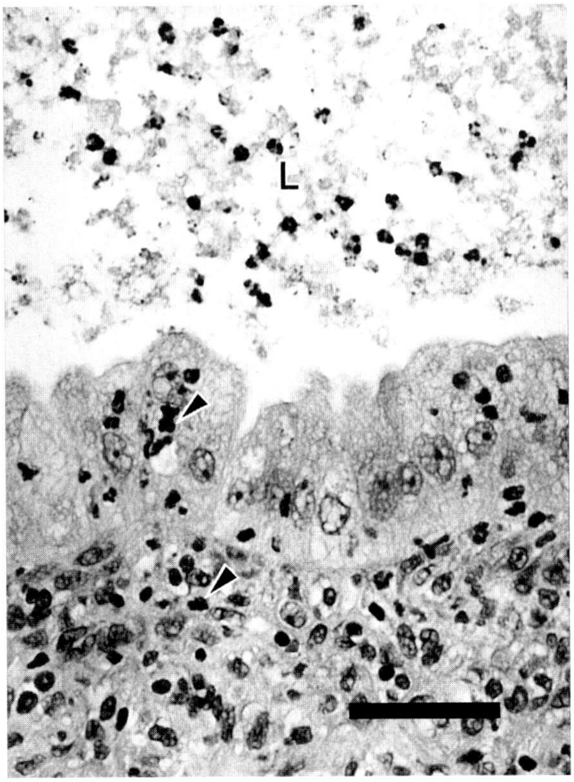

FIGURE 19.12   Pyometra from a rat treated with estradiol alone (Type IIE response). Polymorphonuclear leukocyte infiltration (arrows) in the lamina propria and hyperplastic epithelium. Exudate is present in the uterine lumen (L). Bar = 50 μm.

receptor modulators (SERM), estrogen agonist and antagonist effects may be observed in different tissues. Endometrial polyps were decreased in SERM treated rats compared to concurrent controls in two year carcinogenicity studies.

The vaginal epithelium is hypertrophic and hyperplastic and is composed of five to six layers of large cells; the two basal layers appear to be active, with round nuclei and a moderate amount of cytoplasm (Figure 19.11). The superficial layers are composed of very large epithelial cells with distended cytoplasmic vacuoles filled with mucoid material.

In the type IIE response, the uterus may appear cystic with endometrial hyperplasia and polymorphonuclear leukocyte infiltration that results in pyometra in mice, rats, and rabbits (Figure 19.12). Squamous metaplasia of the endometrium involving both lumenal and glandular epithelium with minimal keratinization may be present in rats (Figure 19.13). An increased incidence of endometrial polyps has been observed in rats after prolonged treatment with a low dose of estrogen, but not with a high dose. In rabbits, adenomyosis, characterized by the invagination of the endometrial glands into the myometrium, and endometriosis, characterized by complete penetration of the endometrial glands through the outer layers of myometrium, may also be present. Hyperplasia of the endometrium, edema of the lamina propria, and hypertrophy of muscular layers have been reported in dogs that received estrogen treatment.

The type IIE response in the vagina of rats and mice includes hyperplasia and hypertrophy of the epithelium with areas of squamous metaplasia (Figure 19.14). Cornification may be incomplete, as indicated by the retention of nuclei in epithelial cells of the vaginal smear. When estrogen is given at a high dose to rats over a long period of time, the vaginal epithelium may be similar in appearance to the type IIC changes described earlier.

In the type IIP response, uterine changes in rats include moderate epithelial hyperplasia and slight hypertrophy of both lumenal lining and endometrial glands. These cells are low columnar with foamy acidophilic cytoplasm and round vesicular nuclei (Figure 19.15). The vaginal epithelium is atrophic and composed of two to three layers of round to ovoid cells in

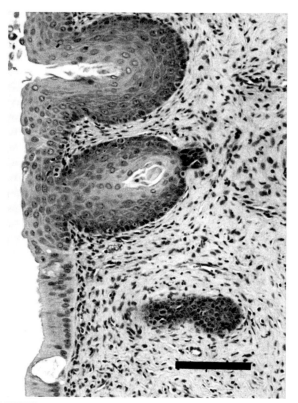

FIGURE 19.13   Endometrium from a rat treated with estradiol alone (Type IIE response). Squamous metaplasia of the endometrial gland and lumenal epithelium is present. Bar = 125 μm.

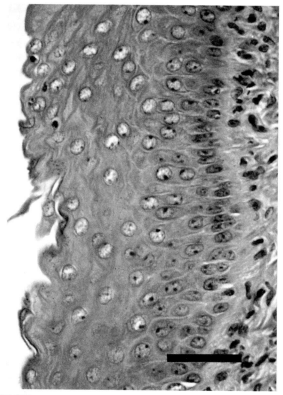

FIGURE 19.14   Hyperplastic vaginal mucosa from a rat treated with estradiol alone (Type IIE response). The epithelium is hyperplastic with squamous metaplasia and cornification at lumenal surface. Bar = 50 μm.

the basal region and two or more layers of moderately hypertrophic cells containing lightly stained foamy cytoplasm with basally displaced nuclei (Figure 19.16). Occasional large intracytoplasmic mucoid vacuoles may be present in focal areas of the epithelium.

Dogs are very sensitive to stimulation by progestins. Papillary proliferation of the surface epithelium of the atrophic ovary with occasional thecal-luteal cell hyperplasia has been reported. The uterus may become uniformly enlarged and the endometrium is lined by hypertrophic epithelial cells with abundant foamy cytoplasm. Endometrial glands may become hyperplastic and cystic, and exudate may accumulate in glandular lumens. The uterine lumen is often filled with mucoid material, which may lead to endometritis and pyometra due to superimposed bacterial infection. Cystic glands may also be present in the vagina.

Type III Response: Hyperplastic or Hypertrophic Ovary, Uterus, and Vagina

The type III response is further divided into subtypes IIIC, IIIE, and IIIP for compounds that induce

an ovarian effect similar to that of LH, FSH, and prolactin, respectively.

In the type IIIC response, the change observed in the hyperactive ovary is similar to excessive LH stimulation while changes in the uterus and vagina are similar to those of combined stimulation by estrogen and progesterone. In rats, the ovary has many corpora lutea and several tertiary follicles (Figure 19.17A). Corpora lutea are formed by luteinization of large follicles without ovulation. Therefore, these corpora lutea may appear cystic or incompletely luteinized. Cystic corpora lutea are characterized by the persistent presence of a central fluid-filled cavity that lacks fibrous tissue invasion (Figure 19.18A). Incomplete luteinization of corpora lutea is characterized by the presence of small cells with condensed nuclei, similar to granulosa cells, in a bed of large luteal cells (Figure 19.18B). In the uterus, endometrial changes resemble those found in estrogen-primed progesterone-stimulated animals. The epithelial cells of the lumenal lining are markedly hyperplastic and moderately hypertrophic with acidophilic cytoplasm (Figure 19.19). In some instances, small supranuclear cytoplasmic vacuoles are also present in the epithelial cells. The endometrial

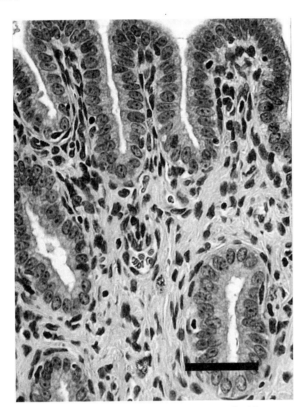

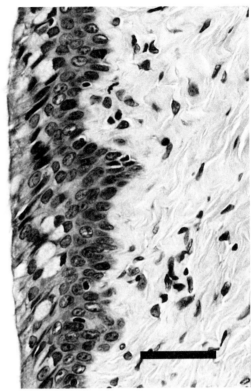

FIGURE 19.15   Endometrium from a rat treated with progesterone alone (Type IIP response). The epithelium is moderately hyperplastic and hypertrophic with low columnar cells. These cells have round vesicular nuclei and foamy cytoplasm. Bar = 50 μm.

FIGURE 19.16   Vaginal mucosa from a rat treated with progesterone alone (Type IIP response). The basal region of the epithelium consists of two to three layers of round to ovoid cells. The surface region consists of 3 layers of moderately hypertrophic cells. Many cytoplasmic vacuoles which displace the nucleus are present superficially. Bar = 50 μm.

glands are well developed and glandular epithelial cells, in most areas, show the same degree of hypertrophy as lumenal lining cells. Papillary folds of endometrium are often present. The vaginal changes are similar to the type IIC response described earlier.

In the type IIIE response, the changes in the hyperactive ovary are similar to those of excessive FSH stimulation while changes in the uterus and vagina are similar to those of estrogen stimulation. In the rat, the ovary has the greatest degree of activity in the type IIIE. Its histological manifestation is similar to type IIIC except that the number of developing follicles and corpora lutea is higher (Figure 19.17C). In the uterus, the lumenal epithelial cells are markedly hypertrophic (Figure 19.20). Endometrial glands are many but the lining cells are only moderately hypertrophic in contrast to the lumenal lining cells. This is quite different from type IIIC, in which both lumenal and glandular epithelial cells have approximately the same degree of hypertrophy. The vaginal changes are similar to the type IIC response described earlier.

In the type IIIP response, the ovarian change is similar to excessive prolactin stimulation while the uterine and vaginal changes are similar to those of

progesterone stimulation. In rats, the ovary may be only slightly enlarged with active corpora lutea. The uterine change is characterized by a marked reduction in the size of the lumen, which is almost nonexistent in many areas. The endometrial lining cells are markedly hyperplastic but only very slightly hypertrophic. The stromal cells of the zona compacta are active, with round nuclei, and are in a stage ready for implantation. In the vagina, the changes are the same as those previously described for type IIP.

Local Vaginal Responses

Irritation

The acute phase of the inflammatory response is similar to that of the squamous epithelium in other locations of the body and may include intracellular edema, intercellular edema (spongiosis), polymorphonuclear leukocyte infiltration, and microabscess formation (Figure 19.21). As the lesion progresses, erosion and ulceration may follow. Repair and recovery are accomplished by the process of regeneration

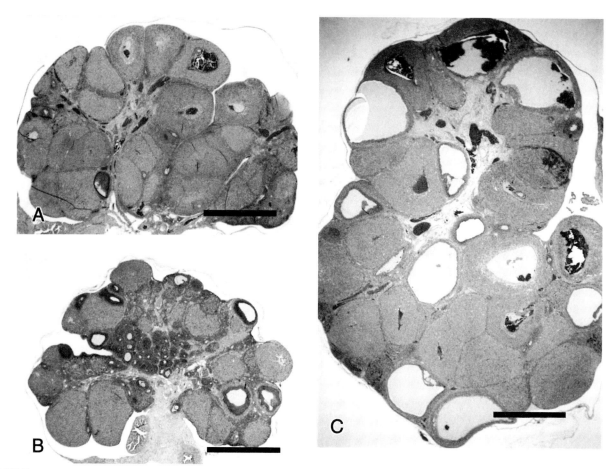

FIGURE 19.17 (A) Hypertrophic and hyperplastic ovary from a rat treated with LH (Type IIIC response). (B) Normal ovary from an untreated rat. (C) Markedly hypertrophic and hyperplastic ovary with many corpora lutea and several developing follicles from a rat treated with FSH (Type IIIE response). Bar = 16 mm.

with accelerated cell proliferation in the stratum germinativum. The number of cell layers increases in the stratum germinativum (acanthosis). This may result in premature migration of epithelial cells with retained nuclei into the stratum corneum (parakeratosis) or an increase in the thickness of the stratum corneum (hyperkeratosis) (Figures 19.21). Once the stratum corneum is formed, the inflammatory response is likely to subside. Since the irritant is usually unevenly distributed on the vaginal mucosa, different areas of the vagina may be affected at different times and the stages of inflammation may differ in the same animal.

Cornification of the vaginal epithelium appears to take place only when the epithelium has reached a certain thickness. If the rate of regeneration does not exceed the rate of loss induced by the irritant, the epithelium will not become cornified and inflammation will continue if treatment with the irritant continues. In this case, the inflammatory process becomes chronic and mononuclear cells become the major component of the exudate.

Delayed Hypersensitivity

Delayed hypersensitivity responses can be observed in the vagina after sensitization by either dermal or vaginal exposure. Since perivascular accumulations of lymphocytes are the hallmark of the lesion, histological examination is necessary to demonstrate the nature of the inflammatory reaction.

When a nonirritating sensitizer is administered, the inflammatory reaction is limited to lymphocytic infiltration. In the case of an irritating sensitizer, the inflammatory response is similar to that induced by any irritant. However, perivascular lymphocytic cuffing is always present. Such vascular cuffs consist of multiple layers of lymphocytes surrounding vessels of the lamina propria, muscularis, and mesometrial attachment.

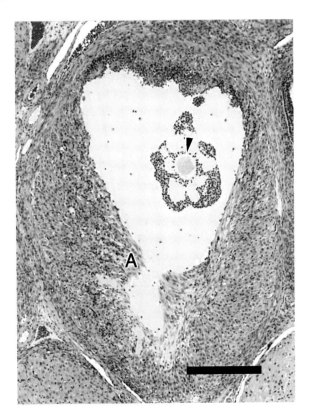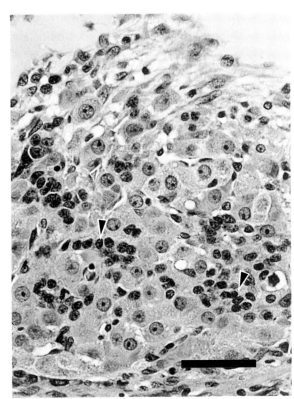

FIGURE 19.18   Corpus luteum from a rat treated with LH (Type IIIC response). (Left) Corpus luteum with a retained ovum. Luteinization proceeds without ovulation as the ovum (arrow) still floats in follicular fluid. Bar = 310 μm. (Right) Incomplete luteinization, corpus luteum (enlarged area from left figure). Many small cells (arrows) with condensed nuclei which have a similar appearance to granulosa cells are present in a bed of large luteal cells. Bar = 50 μm.

Reproductive Toxicity in Domestic Animals

Xenobiotics causing abortion and targeting fetal development are discussed in a separate chapter. Here we focus on the nonpregnant female. Although many xenobiotics have been shown to affect the female reproductive system experimentally, there are only a small number of xenobiotics that need to be considered in a diagnostic setting. In large animals, estrogenic effects induced by phytoestrogens and estrogenic mycotoxins present in feed are the most common manifestation. Environmental contamination by heavy metals, PCBs and TCDD could also potentially affect female reproductive function. In small animals, inappropriate use/dosage of estrogenic or progesterone type drugs can cause endometrial hyperplasia while chemotherapeutic drugs, such as cyclophosphamide and vinblastine that target rapidly dividing cells, can adversely affect primordial follicles within the ovary.

Phytoestrogens

Some pasture legumes produce estrogenic compounds known as phytoestrogens. These can result in exogenous estrogenic activity in sheep and to a lesser extent in cattle leading to infertility of varying severity and permanency, so called "clover disease". Plants found to be a source of estrogenic activity include clovers (*Trifolium* spp), e.g. subterranean (*T. subterraneum*), red *(T. pretense)*, white (*T. repens*) and alsike (*T. hybridum*) clovers, which contain isoflavones, and alfalfa (*Medicago sative*) and barrel medic (*M. truncatula*) which contain coumestans. The isoflavones include formononetin, biochanin A and genestin. They are also found in soybeans (*Glycine max*). Extensive rumenal metabolism of these isoflavones occurs; for example the isoflavone, formononetin, is converted to equol, a potent estrogenic metabolite. Coumestans are primary phytoestrogens.

Infertility associated with abnormal estrus cycles occur in sheep and to a lesser extent in cattle ingesting estrogenic clovers. In sheep, the major changes are cystic hyperplasia of the endometrium and squamous and glandular metaplasia of the cervix (Figure 19.22). Adenomyosis may also be found in the uterus. It is believed that the cervical changes play a major role in infertility due to altered mucin production which decreases sperm penetration. Galactorrhoea

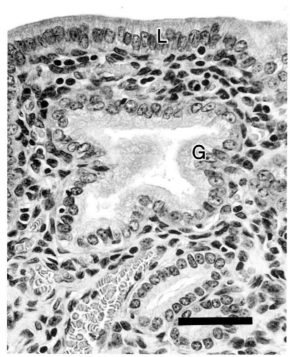

FIGURE 19.19 Hyperplastic and hypertrophic endometrium from a rat treated with LH (Type IIIC response). Lumenal epithelial cells are of medium height with ovoid nuclei and foamy cytoplasm. There is only a minimal difference in size between the lumenal lining (L) and glandular (G) cells. Bar = 50 μm.

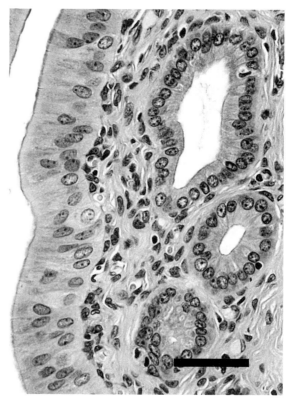

FIGURE 19.20 Hyperplastic and hypertrophic endometrium from a rat treated with FSH (Type IIIE response). Lumenal epithelial cells are very large with round to elongated nuclei and a large amount of cytoplasm while glandular epithelial cells are much smaller with smaller round nuclei and only moderate amounts of cytoplasm. Bar = 50 μm.

and subtle hypothalamic changes have been observed. Additional effects in cattle include cystic ovaries with associated changes. Temporary infertility and suppression of estrus have been reported in sheep exposed to coumestans. The phytoestrogens can also affect LH and FSH release from the hypothalamus.

Zearalenone

Zearalenone and its derivatives are mycotoxins produced by *Fusarium* spp, such as *Fusarium graminearum*, that are often present in grains, especially corn. Because of its structural similarity to estradiol, zearalenone can occupy and stimulate estrogenic receptors with the induced estrogenic response indistinguishable from that caused by estradiol. In addition, zearalenone also acts on the hypothalamus and pituitary similarly to estrogen.

Swine are the most susceptible species to zearalenone toxicity, with prepubertal animals (gilts) the most sensitive. Exposure to the zearalenone (>1–5 ppm) can induce hyperestrogenism characterized by vulval tumefaction (swelling due to edema) and

squamous metaplasia of the cervix and vagina (Figure 19.23). Uterine enlargement due to edema and cellular proliferation and hypertrophy of all uterine layers has been reported. Precocious mammary development with galactorrhoea (milk secretion) and prolapses of the vagina and rectum may also occur.

In adult female swine (sows), anestrus, pseudopregnancy and embryonic death have been reported but higher levels of zearalenone are required. The changes induced depend on the time of administration of zearalenone in relation to the estrus cycle, as well as on the dose administered. Anestrus or nymphomania may be noted. In sows exhibiting nymphomania, ovaries are atrophic and lack corpora lutea and tertiary follicles, indicating follicular atresia. The effects of zearalenone on the uterus, cervix, vagina, and mammary gland are similar to those in prepubertal gilts. Reduced litter size due to fetal resorption (mummification) and/or implantation failure occurs when the effects of dietary zearalenone are present at 7 to 10 days postmating. Pigs may be weak or stillborn, and occasionally exhibit swollen vulvas at or shortly after birth (juvenile hyperestrogenism).

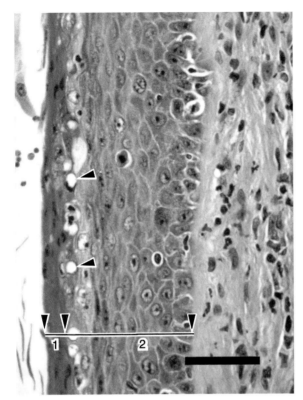

FIGURE 19.21 Vaginal mucosa from a rat treated with a formulation containing an anionic surfactant. Mild parakeratosis (1), intracellular edema (arrows), moderate acanthosis (2), and mild polymorphonuclear leukocyte infiltration (double arrows) are present. Bar = 50 μm.

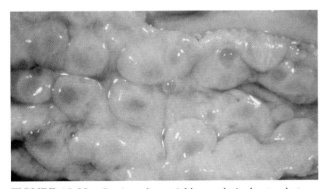

FIGURE 19.22 Cystic endometrial hyperplasia due to phytoestrogens, "clover disease", uterus, sheep. The endometrium is markedly thickened with prominent folds that contain cysts. (Courtesy of the Dr. K. McEntee Registry of Reproductive Pathology, University of Illinois.)

Pseudopregnancy may develop with multiple persistent corpora lutea in the ovary indicating a luteotrophic property of zearalenone. Uterine changes, characterized by both hyperplasia and hypertrophy, are indicative of estrogenic effects from zearalenone as well as a progesterone effect due to the persistent corporalutea. Field observations of zearalenone-induced abortions are now thought to be largely erroneous since estrogens are luteotropic in swine. Instead, it is suspected

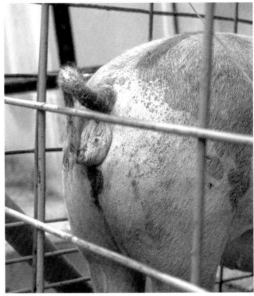

FIGURE 19.23 Vulval hypertrophy and edema, estrogenic effect, sow. Zearalenone, a mycotoxin commonly found in corn, has estrogenic effects that result in vulval edema. (Courtesy Dr. J. Simon, University of Illinois). (From Foster, R.A. (2007). In *Pathologic Basis of Veterinary Disease*, McGavin, M., and Zachary, J.F., eds, 4th edn. Mosby Elsevier, St. Louis. Figure 18-49, p1306.)

that implantation failure followed by pseudopregnancy leads to a diagnosis of abortion.

Cattle and sheep are much less sensitive than pigs to the estrogenic effects of zearalenone. However, similar estrogenic effects have been reported in young cattle (heifers) ingesting 5 to 75 ppm zearalenone in feed. Zearalenone toxicity may be associated with precocious udder development in heifers and reduced fertility in breeding animals.

Chlorinated Naphthalenes

While toxicity due to chlorinated naphthalenes is largely of historic interest, these compounds are still present in many industrial emissions and landfills. These compounds induce cytochrome P450s and undergo metabolic activation, and also act as endocrine disrupters. The toxicity of chlorinated naphthalenes is largely governed by the degree of chlorination.

The clinical syndrome due to chlorinated naphthalene toxicity in cattle, sheep and goats was termed hyperkeratosis or X disease because of skin thickening due to hyperkeratosis. The chlorinated naphthalenes caused squamous metaplasia of the vagina, cervix and uterus, as well as Gartner's ducts leading to cystic enlargement (see Figure 19.13). Metritis, abortion and dystocia have also been reported. Vitamin A deficiency was induced by the chlorinated naphthalene and may be responsible for some of the observed effects.

Synthetic Xenoestrogens and Antiestrogens

In dogs and cats, medroxyprogesterone, used to prevent or shorten estrus, is associated with induction of endometrial hyperplasia. In dogs, the use of DES (diethylstilbestrol) for mismating or pregnancy prevention may result in cystic endometrial hyperplasia. Endometrial hyperplasia predisposes to pyometra.

Neoplasia

Neoplasia can occur in any part of the reproductive tract, particularly in the ovary, uterus, cervix and vagina. In women in the USA, ovarian cancer is the fifth most common form of cancer (excluding skin cancer). Endometrial cancer is less common, occurring mostly in older women, and invasive cervical cancer even less common due to improvement in early detection and eradication. Unopposed estrogen therapy greatly increases the risk of uterine cancer. Some agents capable of inducing neoplastic growth are listed in Table 19.4. The following is a brief description of the characteristic morphological manifestations of some of these tumors focusing on the rodents.

Ovary

There are three main types of primary ovarian neoplasms: germ cell (e.g., teratoma, dysgerminoma), sex-cord stromal (e.g., granulosa cell tumor, Sertoli-stromal cell tumor) and epithelial or epithelial-stromal (e.g. serous cystadenocarcinoma, papillary carcinoma [most common ovarian tumor in dogs], tubulo-stromal adenoma). Mesenchymal tumors such as fibromas, hemangiomas (most common ovarian tumor in swine) and leiomyomas may also occur.

Granulosa and Thecal Tumors and Luteoma

Granulosa cell tumors are uncommon in rats and mice but are the most common spontaneous ovarian tumors in the cow and the mare (Figure 19.24A). However, in certain inbred strains of mice, the incidence may be higher than 60%. Grossly there is enlargement of the ovary with solid to cystic mass formation. Histologically, small cuboidal to polygonal cells grow in anastamosing cords, sheets or strands (Figure 19.24B). In some cases, small gland-like structures filled with eosinophilic material, called Call-Exner bodies, that resemble immature follicles are present. These tumors may be hormonally active and may metastasize.

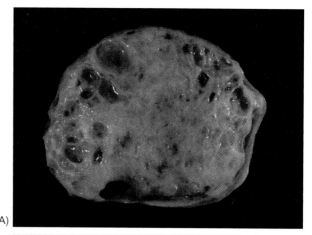

(A)

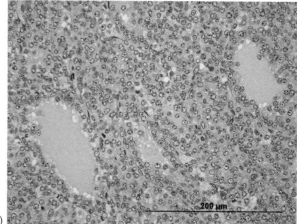

(B)

FIGURE 19.24 Granulosa cell tumor, ovary. A. Cow. The ovary is effaced by a large tumor that is primarily solid but with multiple, variably sized cysts. (Courtesy of the Dr. K. McEntee Registry of Reproductive Pathology, University of Illinois) B. Mouse. Granulosa cells form solid areas and line cystic structures that contain proteinaceous secretory material.

Luteomas appear to arise in atrophic ovaries that have undergone diffuse luteinization. In some strains of mice, such as the CAF1, there is an interim period of luteal proliferation before a luteoma is formed. The luteoma consists of large polygonal cells with abundant eosinophilic cytoplasm and round nuclei with well-dispersed chromatin. Within areas of neoplastic luteal proliferation, progressive change from large cells to smaller cells with compact and dark-staining nuclei may occur. When the neoplasm consists of large numbers of these small cells, they are identified as granulosa cell tumors. In other strains, such as the CNZ hybrids, foci of thecal cell proliferation may arise directly from the atrophic ovary and proceed to form granulosa or thecal cell tumors without the interim period. A more appropriate name for these granulosa cell tumors would be interstitial gland tumor, since they are not truly derived from granulosa cells

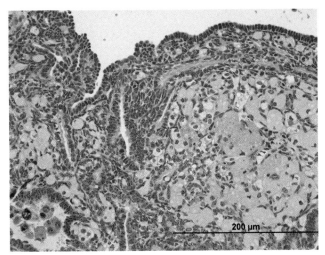 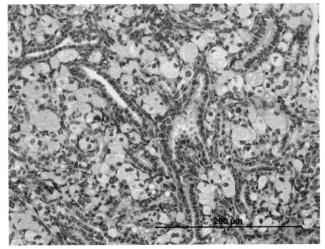

FIGURE 19.25   Tubulo-stromal (tubular) adenoma, ovary, mouse. (Left) The ovarian surface epithelium is columnar and thickened with extension into the subjacent cortex and formation of ramifying tubules. (Right) The tubules are lined by cuboidal epithelium and separated by lipid-laden cells resembling luteal cells.

of the follicles. In male rats with testicular interstitial (Leydig) cell tumors, it is common to find areas of small cells similar to those present in granulosa cell tumors in atrophic ovaries.

Tubular Adenoma (Tubulo-Stromal Adenoma)

Tubular adenomas occur in mice; they vary greatly in size and generally appear as round, firm, tan masses. Development of these tumors has been studied in mice following radiation. The ovarian surface epithelium becomes columnar and thickened, and invaginating folds are formed from the downgrowth of the germinal epithelium with subsequent formation of numerous ramifying crypts (Figure 19.25A). Continuous expansion and proliferation of these tubular down growths may form a large tumor mass that eventually occupies the entire ovary. Histologically, the tumor may appear as papillary, solid, or cystic. The tubules are lined by cuboidal epithelium resembling germinal epithelium. Between these tubular structures, lipid-laden cells resembling granulosa or luteal cells may occur and constitute a major component of these neoplasms (Figure 19.25B).

Depending on the mouse strain, the incidence of spontaneous cases varies from less than 1% (Balb/c) to nearly 100% (C57Bl-Wv/Wv). The latter strain lacks oocytes at birth.

Sertoli Cell Tumor

The development of ovarian tumors composed of cells resembling Sertoli cells is poorly understood yet reported in many species. These tumors in rats are lobulated, solid, white-yellow masses with occasional fluid-filled cysts. They are often unilateral and may become fairly large (up to 5 cm in diameter). Intraperitoneal dissemination with growth on the peritoneal surface is occasionally observed. Histologically, Sertoli cell tumors are characterized by proliferation of tubular or cystic structures lined by large, elongated, or polyhedral cells with basally situated nuclei and abundant cytoplasm. Nests of less differentiated mesenchymal cells may also be found. Spontaneous occurrence of this tumor is rare in rats and mice. Some authors argue that Sertoli cell tumors are a subtype of granulosa cell tumors, however the biological activity of Sertoli cell tumors tends to be more aggressive.

Fibroma

Fibromas may arise from the ovarian parenchyma after prolonged treatment with an androgen. These tumors appear to arise from the ovarian medulla or from the hilar region that lies between the blood vessels and cortex. Grossly the tumor appears as a pale, tan-to-white, very firm nodule up to 1.5 cm in diameter. These unencapsulated tumors grow by expansion and are often poorly delineated from the adjacent compressed tissue. Histologically, small neoplasms are composed of dense fibrous tissue with relatively uniform cellularity, while larger tumors often have a central area of dense collagen deposition with a relatively low cellularity. Spontaneous cases of this tumor have not been reported.

Leiomyoma of Mesovarium

Grossly, leiomyomas appear as circumscribed, tan, firm, and rounded nodules that vary from a few millimeters to a few centimeters in size; they are located closely opposed to the ovary and may extend into the hilar region of the ovary. The neoplastic cells are typical smooth muscle cells arranged in a whorling pattern or forming interwoven bundles with a criss-crossing pattern. Spontaneous occurrence of this tumor has not been described.

Uterus

All uterine neoplasms appear grossly as a segmental enlargement of the uterine body. When multiple tumors are present, irregular regional enlargement can be expected. A brief description of their histological appearance is given here.

Adenocarcinoma and Adenoacanthoma

Adenocarcinomas of the uterus often present as discrete growths involving the entire thickness of the uterine wall. Areas of necrosis and cystic dilatation are often found in the tumor. Histologically, the tumors are composed of large epithelial cells with eosinophilic or amphophilic cytoplasm and large vesicular nuclei with prominent nucleoli. The cells may be arranged in acini, glandular structures, or solid cords. In areas of anaplasia, the cells are smaller with basophilic cytoplasm and a high mitotic index. The term adenoacanthoma is used to describe a uniformly well-differentiated adenocarcinoma limited to the endometrium with a zone of squamous epithelial metaplasia.

Spontaneous adenocarcinoma occurs sporadically in most species and incidence increases with age. In rabbits, the incidence may approach 60% in animals over 4 years old. In domestic animals, uterine adenocarcinomas are rare except in cows.

Deciduosarcoma

Grossly, deciduosarcomas are soft, yellowish-reddish-gray, irregular spherical masses originating from the uterus of rabbits. A necrotic center is a common finding in larger tumors. These tumors usually arise from the endometrium and are often multiple. Large tumors seem to form by coalescence of several smaller tumors. Focal invasion into the myometrium and metastasis by way of lymphatic channels may be observed. Histologically, the tumor is composed of sheets of large pleomorphic polygonal cells. These cells are packed closely together but retain distinct cellular borders. The nuclei are generally small and round with multiple nucleoli. The cytoplasm may vary in stainability depending on the amount and

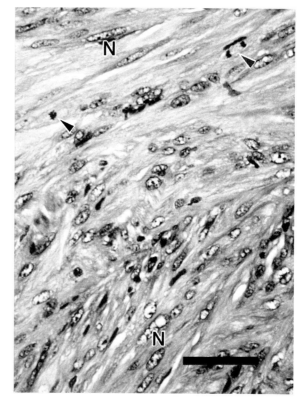

FIGURE 19.26 Uterine leiomyosarcoma from a CD-1 mouse treated with Medroxalol. Cellular pleomorphism with blizzard nuclei (N) and many mitotic figures (arrows) are present. Bar = 50 μm. Slide courtesy of Dr. D. M. Sells of Merrill Dow Pharmaceuticals, Inc., Cincinnati, Ohio.

distribution of glycogen. There are no reported cases of spontaneous occurrence of this tumor in animals.

Decidual reactions have been reported as deciduomas in rats and other laboratory species. Although initial reported as tumors, most current literature regards them as an exaggerated uterine response.

Fibrosarcoma

Fibrosarcoma was induced by 2-acetylaminofluorene in the Buffalo strain of rat. No description of either gross or histological findings was given. Uterine fibromas and fibrosarcomas are rare in domestic animals.

Leiomyoma and Leiomyosarcoma

These tumors originate from smooth muscle cells and can arise from any location in the myometrium. Grossly, they are firm grayish pink nodules. Histologically, leiomyomas are composed of interlacing bundles of smooth muscle cells with long slender vesicular nuclei that are blunted at both ends (Figure 19.26). In leiomyosarcomas, areas of malignancy are characterized by the presence of a high mitotic index, irregular shape and size of the nuclei, cellular pleomorphism, invasive growth, and metastasis.

In rats, these tumors also occur spontaneously with incidences of less than 1–11% for leiomyoma and less than 1–3% for leiomyosarcoma depending on the strain of the animal. In domestic animals, leiomyomas occur in dogs, cats and cattle. Leiomyomas are the counterpart of fibroids in women which occurr in 1 of every 5 women. These can cause irregular and sometimes severe bleeding if large or submucosal.

Papillary Mesothelioma

Papillary mesotheliomas appear as markedly thickened areas of the perimetrium with extensive and complex papillary outgrowths. Although the surface epithelium appears healthy, the underlying tissue may degenerate and become relatively acellular, and may be accompanied by inflammatory changes. Metastasis occurs by direct implantation of sloughed tissue on the peritoneal surface and abdominal organs. Spontaneous occurrence of these tumors is believed to be rare.

Squamous Cell Carcinoma

Squamous cell carcinomas are usually composed of well-differentiated large polygonal cells with prominent vesicular nuclei containing one or more nucleoli. These cells are arranged in nests and cords, infiltrating deep into the myometrium, serosa, and adjacent organs. On the endometrial surface, the epithelium is thickened due to the presence of dysplastic and keratinized areas. Acute inflammation of the lumenal surface may accompany the neoplastic growth. Spontaneous occurrence of this tumor is infrequent in all species of animals.

Vagina and Vulva

Basal Cell Carcinoma

The basal cell carcinoma which occurs in the vagina is composed of compact groups of small darkly staining cells, with hyperchromatic nuclei and scant cytoplasm; intercellular bridges between cells are not observed.

Squamous Cell Carcinoma

All grades of malignancy may be found in squamous cell carcinomas, ranging from slow-growing well-differentiated tumors to fast-growing anaplastic tumors with nuclear pleomorphism and numerous mitotic figures. In domestic animals, squamous cell carcinomas occur predominantly in cattle, sheep and goats.

Mucin-Secreting Tumor

In mucin-secreting tumors of the vagina, the neoplastic epithelial cells are distended with basophilic mucin and most often are located on the surface of the epithelium away from the basal layer. Areas of squamous metaplasia may also be present. As discussed earlier, vaginal epithelial cells become hypertrophic with large amounts of cytoplasmic mucoid material only when they are under sex steroid hormone stimulation. The occurrence of this type of tumor may be partially caused by endogenous prolactin or progesterone stimulation. The incidence of natural occurrence of these vaginal tumors is believed to be very low in all species of animals.

Leiomyoma and Leiomyosarcoma

See description for this tumor above (uterus). Leiomyomas are common neoplasms of the vagina and vestibule in the dog and occurs sporadically in other species.

TESTING FOR TOXICITY

General Toxicity

Design of Animal Study

Rats are the preferred laboratory animal for preliminary study of reproductive toxicity because they are polyestrous, have a relatively short estrous cycle, and can be easily maintained and closely observed in a laboratory setting. They are relatively inexpensive and provide a homogeneous experimental population for testing, thus generating reproducible experimental results. In general, a study length of 14 days is sufficient to detect reproductive abnormalities in the rat. The frequency of dosing should depend on the biological half-life of the test compound. In species that have a long inactive period between cycles, alteration of reproduction may only be detected after a prolonged period of study using relatively large numbers of animals.

Extrapolation of data from rodents to humans has many shortcomings that are frequently overlooked. Through the evolutionary process, rodents have developed a very high reproductive capacity. Rodents are often multiparous and the number of live offspring delivered at the end of the pregnancy is constantly adjusted to the environmental conditions that occur during the gestation period. Early reproductive activities (ovulation, fertilization) are less likely to be affected by adverse environmental conditions in rodents than in primates, simply because a successful pregnancy with delivery of live offspring in rodents is not an all-or-none phenomenon. For uniparous animals such as the monkey and the human, reproductive function is an all-or-none phenomenon. Because of this difference, a conservative approach should be used when extrapolation of data from rodents is truly necessary.

Monitoring during the Live Phase of Animal Studies

Cytological examination of vaginal smears may provide valuable information regarding the status of the reproductive tract. It can provide continuous information regarding the reproductive status of the animal, whereas histological examination can only provide static information, reflecting the condition at the time of terminal sacrifice. In rats, examination of vaginal cytology is easily performed and, thus, should be performed in toxicity studies to determine whether or not there is an effect on reproductive function. The pattern of estrous cycles can also be used as an indicator of the general well being of the animals during the study period as well as an aid in data interpretation. For example, in a chronic carcinogenicity study in rats, the group of animals that receives the maximum tolerated dose may cycle less frequently and show a reduced tumor incidence in their reproductive organs due to less frequent hormonal stimulation.

Monitoring at the Termination of Animal Studies

If abnormal reproductive function is indicated by vaginal cytology, serum may be collected for hormonal assays and bone marrow smears done for examination of mitotic activity. As noted previously, stress and reduced food intake are the most common causes of impairment of reproductive function in animals during toxicity testing. In young animals, reduced body weight gain, a reduced thymus weight relative to body weight, and increased adrenal weight relative to body weight at study termination are good indicators of stress. Weights of ovaries, uterus, and vagina should also be obtained at necropsy and used to aid interpretation of study results when determining whether or not there is a specific adverse effect on reproductive function.

Histological Examination

The morphology of the reproductive tract is age and cycle dependent. In normal animals, the morphology of the ovary, uterus, and vagina should be synchronized and at the same stage of the estrous cycle. Any deviation from this synchrony should be considered potentially abnormal.

Interference with reproductive function is more likely to be detected by histological evaluation of the reproductive organs than by the measurement of serum hormones. When rats are treated with LHRH, the release of LH or FSH is short-lived and peak levels may not differ from those of normal episodic releases. Similarly, subsequent release of estrogen and progesterone may not reach levels as high as those in a normal cycling rat. However, any untimely release of these two steroid hormones will have a lasting imprint on the epithelial cells of both the uterus and vagina.

When interference with reproductive function is present, morphological changes are more apparent and easier to identify in the vagina than in the uterus. The uterine epithelial changes are limited to a single cell layer that lines the lumenal and endometrial glands. Uterine epithelium undergoes only very limited morphological changes under the influence of estrogen and progesterone. The vaginal epithelium, owing to its multilayered structure and high turnover rate, is able to undergo a variety of changes and is a very sensitive indicator of the hormonal status of the animal. When vaginal specimens for histological examination from rats are collected, the posterior one-third should not be sampled because the mucosa in this region is always covered by a thick cornified stratified epithelium.

For routine histological evaluation, specimens fixed in a buffered formalin solution and stained by the hematoxylin and eosin method are satisfactory. Additional approaches, such as histochemistry for steroid synthesizing enzymes (beta-dehydrogenases) and immunohistochemistry for different hormonal receptors, are also available for mechanistic studies. In general, these approaches can provide only qualitative, not quantitative, information and have rarely been used in toxicologic studies.

Quantitative studies of various components, for example, counting the number of follicles at different stages of development by histomorphometry, have been used in the study of reproductive toxicity. This approach is useful when an effect on the less-developed follicles is suspected. However, it is a laborious process and may not be practical, especially in short-term studies, when compared with other avenues in the evaluation of reproductive changes. The use of proliferating cell nuclear antigen (PCNA) as a marker for ovarian follicles has been suggested as a method to facilitate follicle counts.

Serum Hormonal Assay

Radioimmunoassays are available for LHRH, FSH, LH, prolactin, estrogens, and progesterone. Because serum levels of these hormones fluctuate greatly during the reproductive cycle, multiple and timely sampling is required to ascertain the existence of a reproductive disturbance. In rats, a low level of these hormones does not indicate that the animal has defective reproductive function since the highest level only occurs on the day of proestrus. On the other hand, if estrogen or progesterone is high but still within normal range in a large proportion of tested animals, then there are grounds to suspect that reproductive function may be affected. Statistical analyses of hormonal levels may not be fruitful because of the expected high standard deviations in samples collected at different stages of the cycle as would occur when animals are sacrificed on the same day. A significant difference may only be determined if samples are collected at the same stage of the cycle.

In Vitro *Testing*

Once an adverse effect on reproductive function is confirmed, *in vitro* approaches may be employed to further study and identify the possible mechanisms involved. Techniques are available for fractionation and isolation of different ovarian cell types so that the effect of the test compound can be studied on receptor binding and hormonal response in tissue culture. However, because of the complicated interaction in the control of reproductive function and the possible involvement of other growth factors in the regulation of cell function, data generated from *in vitro* studies must be interpreted with caution.

Local Vaginal Toxicity

Animals such as rats, rabbits, dogs, guinea pigs, and monkeys have been used in the testing of vaginal formulations. The macaque monkey is considered the most appropriate animal model for prediction of irritation in women because of the similarity of the vaginal epithelial configuration. The rabbit is believed to be a more sensitive animal model for testing potential for irritation. The response in the rabbit is exaggerated because of its relatively thin vaginal epithelium. The guinea pig has been used to test the delayed hypersensitivity potential of compounds developed for vaginal application.

The duration of treatment is critical in irritation studies. In the rat, a study of less than 7 days, preferably 3 to 4 days, is most desirable since a longer period may be sufficient for epithelial regeneration and cornification to occur. This will act as an effective barrier and may obscure the irritant potential of the test compound.

A potential problem encountered during irritation studies that require multiple dosings over a period of time is the induction of pseudopregnancy in rodent species and guinea pigs, since pseudopregnancy can be induced by mechanical stimulation of the cervix. In order to increase the retention time of the test material in the vagina, it is necessary to deposit the formulation adjacent to the cervix. If the animal struggles during dosing, the cervix may be stimulated and pseudopregnancy induced. Once pseudopregnancy is induced, the vaginal epithelium atrophies, mimicking the progesterone-excessive response. Since the inactive epithelium is much thinner, the response to irritation is exaggerated.

SUMMARY

The study of chemically induced alteration in reproductive organs is a relatively new discipline. Due to species variation and multifactorial control mechanisms, it is often difficult to predict whether reproductive toxicity will occur. Although the information presented in this discussion is far from complete, it provides a background for the identification of most reproductive disturbances and may serve as a guide to understanding pathological changes manifested by animals used in toxicologic testing. During assessment of reproductive toxicity, the general health of the animal should always be considered. Reproductive organs should always be evaluated morphologically as a unit for accurate interpretation. It is hoped that the discussion presented in this chapter will stimulate an interest in the field of reproductive toxicologic pathology for years to come.

FURTHER READING

A monograph on the reproductive system of the female macaque. (2009) *Toxicol. Pathol. Suppl. 36*, 7.

Alison, R.H., Morgan, K.T., Montgomery, C.A. (1990) Ovary. In *Pathology of the Fischer Rat*, (Boorman, G.A., Eustis, S.L., Elwell, M.R., Montgomery Jr., C.A., MacKenzie, W.F. eds), pp. 429–442. Academic Press, San Diego.

Cooke, P.S., Peterson, R.E. & Hess, R.A. (2002). Endocrine disruptors. In *Handbook of Toxicologic Pathology* (Haschek, W.M., Rousseaux, C.G. & Wallig, M.A. eds), 2nd edn, Vol. I, pp. 501–528. Academic Press, San Diego.

Davis, B.J., Dixon, D., Herbert, R.A. (1999) Ovary, oviduct, uterus, cervix and vagina. In *Pathology of the Mouse* (Maronpot, R.R. ed.), pp. 409–444. Cache River Press, Vienna, IL.

Eldridge, J.C. & Stevens, J.T. (eds) (2009). *Endocrine Toxicology*, 3rd edn. Informa Healthcare.

Evans, T.J. (2007). Reproductive toxicity and endocrine disruption. In *Veterinary Toxicology: Basic and Clinical Principles* (Gupta, R.C. ed.), pp. 206–244. Academic Press, Elsevier New York.

Foster, R.A. (2007). Female reproductive system. In *Pathologic Basis of Veterinary Disease* (McGavin, M. & Zachary, J.F. eds), 4th edn, pp. 1263–1316. Mosby Elsevier, St. Louis.

Golub, M.S. (ed.) (2006). *Metals, Fertility, and Reproductive Toxicity.* CRC Press and Taylor and Francis Group, LLC, Boca Raton, FL.

Jones, T.C., Mohr, U. & Hunt, R.D. (eds) (1987). *Monographs on Pathology of Laboratory Animals, Genital System.* Springer-Verlag, Berlin.

Leininger, J.R., Jokinen, M.P. (1990) Oviduct, uterus and vagina. In *Pathology of the Fischer Rat* (Boorman, G.A., Eustis, S.L., Elwell, M.R., Montgomery Jr., C.A., MacKenzie, W.F. eds), (pp. 443–460). Academic Press, San Diego.

McKentee, K. (1990). *Reproductive Pathology of Domestic Mammals.* Academic Press, New York.

Muskhelishvili, L., Wingard, S.K. & Latendresse, J.R. (2005). Proliferating cell nuclear antigen—a marker for ovarian follicle counts. *Toxicol. Pathol.*, 33, 365–368.

Regan, K.S., Cline, J.M., Creasy, D., Davis, B., Foley, G.L., Lanning, L., Latendresse, J.R., Makris, S., Morton, D., Rehm, S. & Stebbins, K. (2005). STP position paper: Ovarian follicular counting in the assessment of rodent reproductive toxicity. *Toxicol. Pathol.*, 33, 409–412.

Schlafer, D.H. & Miller, R.B. (2007). Female genital system. In *Jubb, Kennedy, and Palmer's Pathology of Domestic Animals* (Maxie, M.E. ed.), 5th edn, Vol. III, pp. 429–564. Elsevier, New York.

Witorsch, R.J. (ed.) (1995). *Reproductive Toxicology*, 2nd edn. Raven Press.

Yuan, Y.-D. & Foley, G.L. (2002). Female reproductive system. In *Handbook of Toxicologic Pathology* (Haschek, W.M., Rousseaux, C. G. & Wallig, M.A. eds), 2nd edn, Vol. II, pp. 847–894. Academic Press, San Diego.

CHAPTER

20

Developmental Pathology

INTRODUCTION

Overview of Fetal Toxicologic Pathology

Before the thalidomide tragedy of the late 1950s and early 1960s, it was generally believed that congenital malformations had a genetic cause. Thalidomide showed that this was not the case, and it sensitized both the public and the biomedical community to the hazards of exposing the developing embryo or fetus to foreign substances. This realization was surprising to members of the medical, veterinary, and scientific communities, even though testosterone- and aminopterin-induced human malformations had been reported in the early 1950s. Similarly, anophthalmia and microphthalmia associated with hypovitaminosis A had been reported in pigs in the mid-1930s, and hypervitaminosis A had been experimentally shown to be teratogenic in rodents by the 1950s.

Initially, embryologists used chemicals to alter development, so as to understand the processes of normal development. However, with increasing fetal exposure to environmental contaminants, drugs, and other xenobiotics during pregnancy, the importance of understanding the processes involved in both normal and abnormal development was recognized. This chapter will describe mechanisms of abnormal development and factors that may influence such development, and will give an approach to determining the etiology of fetal anomalies in the field. A glossary of developmental defects can be found at the end of the chapter.

Basic Principles of Developmental Toxicology

Embryonic and fetal toxicologic pathology encompasses the fields of developmental toxicology (the study of the effects of toxic chemicals and physical agents (e.g., ionizing radiation) on the developing offspring), and transplacental carcinogenesis. A related term, teratology, derived from the Greek words "teras" (monster) and "logos" (study), is the study of the causes, mechanisms, and manifestations of developmental anomalies and their prevention. There are six basic principles of teratology:

1. Susceptibility to teratogenesis depends on the genotype of the conceptus, and the manner in which this interacts with adverse environmental factors;
2. Susceptibility to teratogenesis varies with the developmental stage at the time of exposure to an adverse influence;
3. Teratogenic agents act in specific ways (mechanisms) on developing cells and tissues to initiate sequences of abnormal developmental events (pathogenesis);
4. The access of adverse influences to developing tissues depends on the nature of the influence (agent);
5. The four manifestations of deviant development are death, malformation, growth retardation, and functional deficit; and
6. Manifestations of deviant development increase in frequency and degree as dosage increases, from the no-effect to the totally-lethal level.

Incidence of Congenital Anomalies

Congenital defects now rank as a leading cause of perinatal mortality and postnatal morbidity in humans. They are a major cause of human hospital admissions, and one of the leading causes of life potentially lost before the age of 65 in the USA. Their decreased relative importance is largely due to medical intervention, and prevention or treatment of most perinatal infectious diseases.

The overall incidence of abnormal development in humans is quite high. In Western countries, the incidence of human morphologic abnormalities is said to range as high as 7–8% of births per year if defects diagnosed in later years are included, with a 2–4% frequency of major malformations. No more than 30–35% of human birth defects have known etiologies. Adding to the incidence of adverse pregnancy outcome, some 16% of known pregnancies result in miscarriage or stillbirths in the USA, while a significant percentage of additional conceptions fail to survive, but go unnoticed unless highly sensitive methods are used to detect them. Another 8–10% of pregnancies end in premature birth. Furthermore, if one includes CNS anomalies, ranging from mental retardation to minor learning deficits, the incidence is said to be approximately 10–20% of births. Additional functional deficits, such as those of the heart, lungs, kidneys, and immune and endocrine systems, along with biochemical defects, such as untreated maternal phenylketonuria, the Smith–Lemli–Opitz Syndrome (abnormal cholesterol metabolism), or Zellweger Syndrome (a peroxisomal defect) add to the occurrence of anomalies.

Estimates of the incidence of phenotypic anomalies in domestic animals range from 2–12%, depending on the species in question and the survey quoted. Veterinary estimates are likely to be low, as there is no centralized method of recording individual birth data in many species. Data concerning the incidence of spontaneously occurring anomalies can usually be obtained from animal suppliers, and are usually used as historical control data. Morphologic anomalies in laboratory animals have been well-characterized, particularly in those species used for teratology studies.

NORMAL MORPHOLOGIC DEVELOPMENT

The processes involved in the normal development of humans and most animals are well-characterized. Beginning with fertilization, normal morphologic development proceeds through blastocyst formation, gastrulation, organogenesis, histogenesis, and functional maturation, a process that is not complete in some organs until puberty (Figure 20.1). Morphogenesis

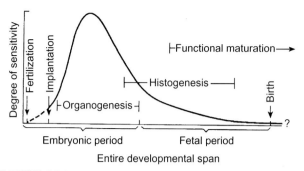

FIGURE 20.1 Sensitivity of the developing mammalian fetus to xenobiotic insults during gestation. (Reprinted with permission from Wilson, J.D. (1973). *Environment and Birth Defects*. Academic Press, New York.)

includes several developmental processes, such as morphogenetic movements, cell contacts, changes in cell shape, tissue interactions (induction), and cell differentiation. An understanding of these processes is essential before alterations caused by prenatal exposure to teratogens can be considered. For a more detailed discussion of embryology and developmental biology, there are several excellent texts available.

Fertilization and Blastocyst Formation

The early stages of development, from fertilization to blastocyst formation, are relatively resistant to toxic insults. Since most of the cells at this time of development are totipotent, the conceptus generally either dies or replenishes its complement of cells following injury by chemicals. Although these scenarios are the norm, exceptions have been recognized.

Gastrulation

The teratogenic susceptibility of the embryo is still relatively low during this period. The expression of an insult during this stage is typically embryonic death and resorption, because not all cells are totipotent (Figure 20.2).

Organogenesis

Organogenesis is the most complex stage of development. It is characterized by cellular and tissue interactions, such as embryonic induction, morphogenetic movements, selective cell proliferation, and programmed cell death. The complexity of this stage of development means that interference by exogenous agents can lead to devastating effects on development.

Induction

Induction is the process of one population of cells (the inducer) influencing another population of cells to differentiate (the induced tissue). Induction is a primary mechanism by which ordered development occurs in the embryo. Primary induction involves establishing the basic embryonic body plan, for example, induction of the neuroectoderm by the primitive streak, and formation of the central nervous system due to the influence of the notochord and paraxial mesoderm. Secondary induction results in a "cascade" of interactions during development of an organ.

The formation of the eye is a good example of primary and secondary induction. The forebrain forms following primary induction of the neuroectoderm. Adjacent mesenchyme secondarily induces the optic vesicle to evaginate from the forebrain to form the optic cup. This evagination induces the surface ectoderm to thicken and form the lens placode, which invaginates to produce the lens vesicle (lens primordium). Finally, the lens vesicle induces the surface epithelium to differentiate as the cornea.

Induction is mediated through direct cell contact, via diffusible substances, or via the extracellular matrix. Cell-adhesion molecules (CAMs), substrate-adhesion molecules (SAMs), and cell-junctional molecules (CJMs) are vital for mammalian form. CAMs determine the place of an embryonic cell with respect to other cells of a "collective" destined to differentiate into a specific structure, whereas CJMs enable communication among cells within a collective. SAMs (particularly their relationship to the integrins) influence collectives and, indirectly, genetic expression. These molecules modulate pattern and form of tissue development. By no coincidence, these molecules are closely related to the immunoglobulin superfamily, indicating that the surface of immunocytes is similar to that of cells important in creating living shape as we know it. Therefore, immunological recognition and response may be very similar to pattern formation in the embryo.

Morphogenic Movements

Morphogenetic movements are a typical response of induced cells. Cell–cell contact affects the direction of movement by contact inhibition of migration, and by eliciting surface changes in cell membranes. The extracellular matrix, in which collagen fibers containing precipitated glycosaminoglycans act as scaffolding or attachment sites for migrating cells, is involved in these movements. Hyaluronic acid may aid movement of the cells through this extracellular matrix, and gradients of SAMs, such as fibronectin and laminin, may provide positional information for migrating cells. Again, it is

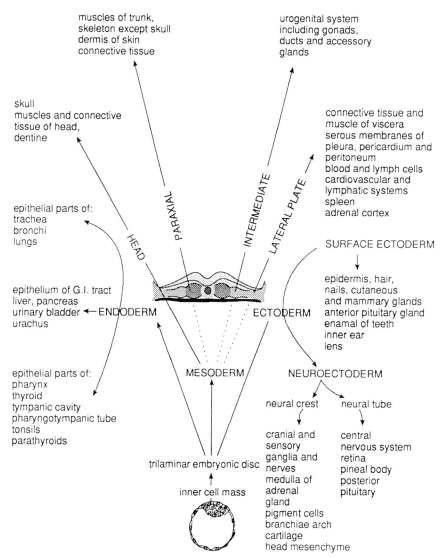

FIGURE 20.2   Schematic diagram of the origin and derivatives of the three germ layers. (Reprinted with permission from Moore, K.L. (1988). *The Developing Human, Clinically Oriented Embryology*, 4th edn. Saunders, Philadelphia.)

unlikely that specific cells are individually-regulated; cell collectives, recognized by their CAM expression, behave as a group. Each cell in a collective passes on information to other members of the collective through the various CAMs. These collectives may then further subdivide into "sub-collectives" as differentiation progresses.

Regardless of the mechanism, when cells differentiate they lose their ability to move. The collectives become more limited in their ability to express a diverse array of tissues. For example, once cells express L-CAM they are committed to being mesenchymal cells, and cannot become epithelium.

Morphogenetic movements depend on the contractile elements of the cytoskeleton, such as actin and tubulin. These elements must move in harmony to cause unified

movement of a cell collective. This coordination relates to the function of various CAMs and CJMs. Here, gap junctions allow passage of macromolecules, tight junctions allow the passage of very small molecules, and desmosomes give an anchor point for the cytoskeleton.

Debate continues concerning the signal that starts a chain of events resulting in morphogenetic movements. One or more morphogens seem to be involved. Morphogen is the term used to describe a compound that has such directional qualities in growth. Critical points of development, e.g., the zone of polarizing activity in the developing limb, may release these morphogens. Presumably, a morphogen acts at the level of integrins and SAMs, thus directing global modulation of movement, in addition to regulating gene expression.

Morphogens

Some chemicals have been suggested as morphogens. For example, retinoids are small molecules with potent effects on development, and they are found endogenously in embryos. The influence of retinoids on development is presumably mediated by specific nuclear receptors of two types, retinoic acid receptors (RAR), and retinoid X receptors (RXR). It is thought that retinoids or similar molecules are responsible for the inductive action of the zone of polarizing activity, an area that induces the apical ectodermal ridge of the developing limb. In fact, retinoids can induce the expression of sonic hedgehog, a gene whose product is a signaling protein involved in dorsal–ventral patterning of the neural tube, the somites, and the anterior–posterior axis of the limb bud.

Morphoregulator Hypothesis

Probably the best model for growth and induction is the morphoregulator hypothesis. This fourpart hypothesis first states that the cells in a collective respond epigenetically to induce cells of another collective in a context set by CAMs. The importance of CJMs has been highlighted by the observation that disturbance of these CJMs relates to chemical carcinogenesis. A network of SAMs acts by global modulation (all cells) that results in a choice of primary processes, such as cell division, movement, or death. In a given signaling situation, such choices direct the response characteristics of the cell collective. SAMs may act through concentration gradients, or through altered physical properties, such as changes in the viscosity of glycosaminoglycans. Thus, CAMs separate collectives, CJMs allow cells within a collective to behave as one, and SAMs modulate the movement of the collectives.

The second part of the hypothesis states that the essential components linking epigenetic mechanochemical events to gene expression are morphoregulatory genes. Morphoregulatory genes are those that are not necessary for the life of the cell, but are necessary for pattern formation. Their action is under the control of historegulatory and selector genes. Historegulatory genes control structural genes involving all other cytodifferentiation events. These structural genes specify general functions necessary for the function of most cells, and also necessary for the emergence of histodifferentiated cells. They are required for life and the specific characteristics of any cell, and make up the largest of the three classes of genes. Selector genes, by affecting certain historegulatory genes, restrict expression of sequences of cytodifferentiation at certain places and developmental times.

Third, it is hypothesized that the link through inductive signal paths arising from adhesion-dominated collectives gives rise to signals between such collectives, so the cells of a collective behave as one. CAMs may affect gene expression by a secondary messenger system; therefore, external influences can influence the genome—the epigenetic phenomenon. CJMs allow simultaneous action of the other cells of the collective. Such signals return from the collectives to the morphoregulatory, historegulatory, and switch genes to change gene expression of morphoregulatory molecules and cytodifferentiation products. Therefore, there is group action of a collective on the genes of each cell.

Finally, the hypothesis concludes that the sequential interactions of morphoregulatory and historegulatory genes provide the basis of pattern via epigenetic paths by controlling temporal sequences of mitosis, movement, death, and further signaling. Therefore, previous temporal–spatial relationships of a cell mass control later events in pattern development. Where the cells are in time and space is probably of more importance than the exact nature of the genes.

Epigenetic Events

Mechanistic studies of cellular signal transduction offer insight into the epigenetic (via transcriptional, translational, or post-translational modification of gene expression) regulation of such embryonic activities as cell proliferation, differentiation, and apoptosis. As previously mentioned, apoptosis, characterized by individual cellular degeneration and death resulting from nuclear-initiated events, is referred to as programmed cell death. Specific toxicants are known to be capable of perturbing intracellular signaling mechanisms via effects on Ca^{2+}, NO, cAMP, protein kinases, etc. Such perturbations can then influence cell adhesion, gap junctions, and cell substrate interactions. It thus seems clear that interference with critical cellular signaling processes by toxicants could result in such unwanted outcomes as abnormal differentiation, excessive or failed apoptosis, and inadequate or excessive cell growth, with resultant abnormal development or death of the conceptus.

Histogenesis and Functional Maturation

Restriction

Restriction is the loss of developmental plasticity that takes place when cells have undergone determination or commitment to a final pathway of differentiation at the completion of organogenesis. When certain structural genes are expressed, differentiation occurs. These genes not only change the cellular structure, but probably also lock out switch genes, so that only specified segments of DNA can be transcribed and translated. Therefore, specialization increases as differentiation occurs, restricting the ability of a cell to move, divide, and diversify. Histogenesis is the maturation of these cells into a fully-functional condition (Figure 20.1).

Biochemical events during histogenesis (cytodifferentiation) include rapid protein synthesis, especially of tertiary or specific proteins characteristic of a particular tissue, with an accompanying increase in the endoplasmic reticulum and Golgi apparatus. This synthesis is regulated either via transcriptional or translational control mechanisms that program the cells to undergo functional maturation. The control of these events is related to internalization of CAMs and growth receptor molecules; thus, the cell surface gives information to the nucleus concerning the outside environment. Intracellular transfer of these maturation messages probably occurs among cells through CJMs.

Functional Maturation

The time of functional maturation of cells depends on the organ system in question. Some organ systems continue development well into the postnatal period (e.g., central nervous, immune, and reproductive systems), whereas the majority of organs become functionally competent during gestation. Development continues throughout life in the immune system (e.g., antigen recognition and antibody production) and in the brain (e.g., synapse formation). Perturbation of these maturation processes will probably not lead to morphologic malformations, but may cause decreased postnatal survival, or functional abnormalities. Subtle behavioral or immunological aberrations may also occur, some of which may be detected by postnatal neurotoxicological or immunotoxicological studies.

MECHANISMS OF TOXICITY

Developmental toxicity depends not only on the nature and dose of the toxicant(s), but also on the stage of embryonic development during which exposure occurs, and on factors that may modify toxicity. Such factors include the fetal and parental genotypes, the maternal environment, and the placenta.

Critical Phases of Intrauterine Development

The critical period of intrauterine development is that time during development at which the conceptus has the greatest sensitivity to noxious influences, most commonly during early organogenesis (Table 20.1). Each organ, or organ system, has its own critical period (Figure 20.3), and complex structures (e.g., the CNS) may have more than one such peak of sensitivity. For this reason, exposure to xenobiotics at different times during development is likely to produce lesions in different organ systems, dependent on their critical periods. Since the critical periods are known for many organs in several species, hypotheses about the cause of a specific defect can be made. Indeed, a malformed organ cannot result from an exposure to a toxic substance if the organ was completely developed at the time of xenobiotic exposure. Nevertheless, fetal organs can be damaged by infectious organisms, such as the syphilis spirochete, and a deformation can occur even in a fully-formed organ, as long as the tissues remain soft and readily deformable.

TABLE 20.1   Gestational milestones for mammals[a]

Species	Gestational milestone[b]				
	Implantation	Primitive streak	Early differentiation	Organogenesis ends	Usual parturition
Rat	5–6	8.5	10	15	21–22
Mouse	5	6.5	9	15	18–20
Rabbit	7.5	7.25	9	18	30–32
Hamster	4.5–5	7	8	13	16
Guinea pig	6	12	14.5	~29	67–68
Monkey	9	17	21	~44–45	166
Human	6–7	13	21	~50–56	266

[a]Adapted from DeSesso (1997), with permission
[b]In gestational days; day of confirmed mating = gestational day 0

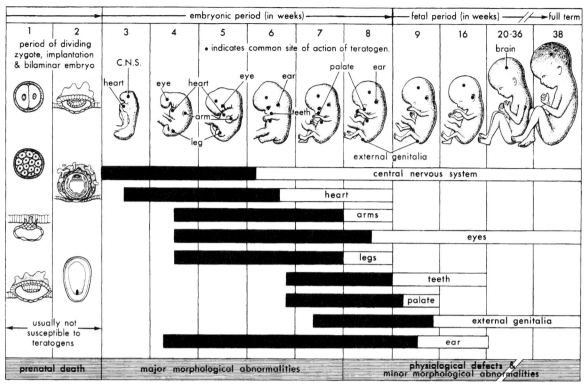

FIGURE 20.3   Schematic diagram of critical periods of human development. (Reprinted with permission from Moore, K.L. (1988). *The Developing Human, Clinically Oriented Embryology*, 4th edn. Saunders, Philadelphia.)

Critical periods begin during organogenesis, when the structures involved are laying the foundations for their ultimate form, i.e., when they are present as organ primordia. Critical periods continue while cell division, differentiation, and morphogenesis are occurring rapidly, and diminish as organogenesis nears completion. If exogenous forces interfere sufficiently with the proper creation of an organ's foundation, the organ's morphology will develop abnormally. Once the foundation is laid, however, only mechanical forces or extensive necrosis can subsequently alter the organ's structure.

Modifying Factors

Embryo and Fetus

Strain and Species

Species differences in expression of defective development following xenobiotic exposure have been clearly shown experimentally. The classic example is thalidomide, which is teratogenic in humans and certain nonhuman primates and rabbit strains, but does not readily cause malformations in rodents or in chick embryos. Species differences in teratogenic response are probably a manifestation of the pharmacokinetic properties of the teratogens, the rate of transplacental teratogen transfer, and species-specific differences in the sensitivity of target cells or their receptors.

Strain differences also occur. They can represent intrinsic differences, such as differences in toxicant interactions with embryonic cell receptors, or they can result from differences in maternal biotransformation rates or products. For example, cortisone induces a higher incidence of cleft palate in A/Jax mice than in CBA or C57Bl/6J mice. Here, the number of genetically-determined glucocorticoid receptors in the developing maxillary processes correlate with the number of observed cortisone-induced cleft palates. Furthermore, A/Jax mice metabolize cortisone differently than CBA mice, thus rendering A/Jax more susceptible to the effects of corticosteroids than are CBA mice. Similar metabolic differences have been observed with 5-fluorouracil in different strains of mice. In one example, SJL/J mice (resistant strain) and C57Bl/6J mice (sensitive strain) differ in the metabolism of uracil by the pyrimidine reductase pathway.

The importance of the embryonic genotype in determining the response of the embryo or fetus to xenobiotics is readily apparent in the discordant defective development that may occur between dizygotic twins exposed to a teratogen during the critical period. This discordance also manifests itself in rodents, since all fetuses in a litter are often not identically affected. Such within-litter discordance may at times arise from other causes, however, such as differences in maternal blood supply to offspring at different locations in the uterine horns.

Multifactorial Threshold Concept

Cleft lip and cleft palate, *spina bifida*, hypertrophic pyloric stenosis, talipes, congenital hip dislocation, and certain cardiac malformations are characteristic of apparent multifactorial types of malformations in humans. Cleft palate is the classical example used in rodents. Essentially, the actions of teratogens require the embryo or fetus to be genetically-predisposed to the malformation and the teratogen causes expression of the genetic predisposition.

For each organ system, a threshold for abnormal organogenesis exists that, if surpassed, will result in a malformation (Figure 20.4). The threshold can be impacted by one or more genes, and by environmental agents. If the genetically-determined normal development is close to the threshold of abnormal development, then only minor noxious stimuli may be necessary to induce abnormality. Thus, as the number of predisposing genes increases, the severity of the teratogenic insult required to overcome the threshold decreases. In fact, it is likely that most, if not all, individuals have one or more "weak points" in their genetically-programmed developmental plans that are especially vulnerable to influences that could result in abnormal development.

Cortisone-induced cleft palate exemplifies the multifactorial threshold concept. The palatal processes of A/Jax mice fuse later in gestation than those of the resistant C57B1/6J strain. As late palatine closure predisposes to the formation of cleft palate, the threshold for teratogenic insult causing the formation of cleft palate is less in A/Jax than in C57B1/6J mice. It is possible that close to 50% of all malformations may involve multifactorial inheritance, with or without added teratogenic insults. Furthermore, embryonic development is highly complex, with many interdependent events that must occur either concurrently or in sequence; thus, it is subject to occasional failure, even in the absence of deleterious outside influences.

Embryonic and Fetal Pharmacokinetics

In addition to phylogenetic differences, variability exists among species in the ontogeny of the monooxygenase system. The biotransforming capability of the embryo (and extraembryonic tissues) during organogenesis is critical. This capacity is likely to be too low to have much, if any, impact on most xenobiotics in both humans and laboratory animals that have not been exposed to potent enzyme inducers. Human fetal liver and adrenal glands possess cytochrome P450, NADPH-cytochrome C reductase, NADPH-cytochrome P450 reductase, cytochrome b_5, and NADH-cytochrome C reductase as early as 6–8 weeks of gestation, but laboratory mammals with short gestation periods typically show little or no such activity until near term, or postnatally. Since these enzymes are capable of affecting side-chain hydroxylation, aromatic hydroxylation, *N*-demethylation, nitroreduction, and, to a limited extent, glucuronic acid conjugation, a human fetus can metabolize many foreign compounds to which it is exposed.

Human fetal hepatic enzyme activities are approximately the same as in the adult on a body weight basis; however, there is considerable variability of these enzyme activities in animals. Therefore, the consequence of fetal drug metabolism is a production of either toxic or nontoxic metabolites. Since these metabolites are water-soluble, they may accumulate in the fetal compartment, due to its higher water content. Fortunately, detoxification reactions tend to predominate over activating reactions; hence, fetal metabolism usually protects the fetus.

Fetal renal excretion also aids elimination of xenobiotics. During the latter stages of gestation, glomerular filtration rate increases, with a concomitant increase in the fetal renal drug clearance. Prenatal exposure to known enzyme-inducing agents increases enzyme activity in laboratory rodents. Both 3-methylcholanthrene and phenobarbital produce similar effects to those seen in mature animals. Again, the risk or benefit of detoxification versus bioactivation as a consequence of enzyme induction depends on the xenobiotic in question.

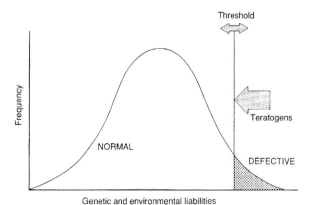

FIGURE 20.4 The multifactorial–threshold concept, in which combinations of genetic and environmental liabilities can cause abnormal development once a threshold has been exceeded.

In rodents, the ability to respond to inducers of phase I and phase II reactions is strain-dependent. For example, aryl hydrocarbon hydroxylase (AHH), which increases the toxicity of benzo[a]pyrene, can be induced with phenobarbital in C57Bl/6J mice, resulting in malformations following benzo[a]pyrene exposure. In contrast, AHH activity cannot be induced in DBA mice, so benzo[a]pyrene is not teratogenic in these mice following similar pretreatment with phenobarbital.

Tissue Binding of Developmental Toxicants

Preferential sequestration of some teratogens, e.g., lead, methyl mercury, and thalidomide, in embryonic or fetal tissues occurs in some species, resulting in higher toxicant concentrations in the offspring than in the maternal blood. Lead accumulates in the fetus by binding to mineralizing fetal bone. The mechanism for sequestration of methyl mercury appears to be the inability of the fetus to convert the methylated form to inorganic mercury, which is more readily eliminated. Fetal sequestration of methyl mercury is so complete that pregnant women are protected from methyl mercury toxicity. Conversely, in the case of thalidomide, hydrophilic metabolites resulting from hydrolysis of the parent compound accumulate in the rabbit embryo, probably due to their inability to readily cross the cell membranes.

Mother

Maternal Physiologic State

Fortunately, alterations in maternal homeostasis must be severe to affect the fetus, since the needs of the fetus are usually met at the expense of the mother. Exceptions do exist, however, since approximately 3.5% of all congenital malformations in humans relate to maternal conditions, such as thyroid disorders (hypothyroidism–cretinism, deafness, and mental retardation), diabetes (sacral agenesis, macrosomia), uncontrolled phenylketonuria (microcephaly, mental retardation, cardiac defects), virilizing tumors (female pseudohermaphroditism), and malnutrition (abortion, stillbirths, neonatal deaths, neural tube defects, hydrocephalus).

Maternal Pharmacokinetics

Absorption from the gut is altered during pregnancy, because of increased gastric emptying time and reduced intestinal motility. This increases residence time in both stomach and small intestine, with the effect on absorption dependent on whether a given xenobiotic is more readily absorbed via the stomach or the intestine. The pulmonary tidal volume also increases during pregnancy, resulting in increased uptake of inhaled xenobiotics. In addition, the volume of distribution markedly increases during pregnancy, because of increased total body water and body fat. This increase in volume leads to decreases in the initial blood concentration of absorbed xenobiotics. There is also a more rapid maternal elimination of water-soluble compounds, because of increased renal plasma flow and glomerular filtration rate.

A progressive gestational decrease in plasma albumin concentration may affect xenobiotic binding by plasma proteins. For example, decreased serum binding of a number of therapeutic drugs has been seen to occur during pregnancy.

Maternal hepatic enzyme activities increase during pregnancy, probably because of the increased need to metabolize fetal wastes. There is also the potential for reduced drug metabolism, because of competitive inhibition of enzymatic pathways by steroid hormones. This assumed competition might be an overgeneralization, since estrogen decreases the efficiency of some metabolic pathways. In contrast, progesterone induces some enzymes. It is probable that the effect of steroids and hormones will depend on the time of gestation, and on the specific xenobiotic.

Father

Direct Effect on the Sperm

Teratospermia is the production of morphologically abnormal sperm, which are often functionally deficient. This alteration can follow exposure to some toxicants. Direct actions of compounds on sperm may reduce ribosomal activity, impair protein synthesis, and reduce their RNA content, in addition to anatomical abnormalities, chromosomal damage, or alterations in sperm motility.

Abnormalities in Seminal Fluid

Xenobiotics dissolved in the seminal fluid can induce secondary morphologic abnormalities in sperm, and impair sperm motility and viability. Dissolved toxins and toxicants may also have some influence on the uterus, either by direct action or through systemic absorption. Subsequent effects on the timing of implantation, distribution of implantation sites, and placentation are possible, and some compounds theoretically may be directly toxic to the developing embryo (Table 20.2).

Placenta

Placental Transfer of Teratogens

Chemical Properties of Teratogens. The rates at which xenobiotics are transported across the placenta determine

TABLE 20.2   Some agents suspected of paternally induced developmental toxicity

Anesthetic gases	Ionizing radiation
Caffeine	Lead
Chlorambucil	Methyl methanesulfonate
Cyclophosphamide	Opiates (e.g., methadone)
Ethanol	Urethane
Ethylnitrosourea	Vinyl chloride

whether toxic levels reach the embryo/fetus. The major factors (lipid solubility, molecular size, ionic charge, formation of complexes, and concentration gradients) affecting transmembrane passage apply to the placenta. However, the placenta produces steroids and peptide hormones, and has diverse and complex functions, thus dispelling the concept that it is just a semipermeable membrane. Since most drugs are absorbed by passive diffusion, the rate of transport tends to increase as lipid solubility increases. Compounds greater in size than 1000 Da do not cross the placenta easily, whereas those less than 600 Da, which includes most drugs, do. Steric hindrance, the process by which the shape and size of a molecule may interfere with molecular binding sites, occasionally plays a part in reducing transport across the placenta. Binding of xenobiotics by plasma proteins is also frequently a major influence, as it decreases the amount of the freely diffusible form.

Physiological Properties of the Placenta. Maturational changes in the placenta are unlikely to influence drug exposure, since the rate of transfer of most drugs correlates with the rate of placental blood flow. If, however, permeability is a rate-limiting step in transfer (e.g., for hydrophilic compounds), physiologic changes in the placenta during development and maturation may cause significant changes in fetal exposure. Some compounds may alter placental blood flow through their pharmacologic activity. For example, epinephrine, 5-hydroxytryptamine, and vasopressin decrease placental blood flow, whereas prostaglandin E_2 increases it.

Fetal blood is relatively more acidic than maternal blood; therefore, "ion-trapping" of basic compounds can occur in the fetal circulation. This trapping can result in a higher concentration of non-ionized drug in the maternal circulation, and a net transfer to the fetus over a prolonged period. Conversely, the blood of organogenesis stage embryos of laboratory rodents is more alkaline than the maternal blood and traps weak acids, such as valproic acid.

Placental Pharmacokinetics

Metabolism. Placental metabolic capabilities may sometimes play a role in the modulation of embryonic/fetal drug exposure, especially when enzyme activities have been enhanced by maternal exposure to inducing agents (e.g., 3-methylcholanthrene).

Sequestration. A generalized decrease in nutrient transport has been observed when xenobiotics, such as cadmium and trypan blue, bind to the placenta. The placenta does not appear to act as a sink for chemicals, but interaction with certain substances can obstruct its function. For example, cortisone exposure decreases glucose transport, and methyl mercury inhibits amino acid transport.

RESPONSE TO INJURY

The ultimate manifestation of cytotoxicity is cell death. Cytotoxicity can lead to death, malformation, or growth retardation in the conceptus, depending on the degree of insult and the time of gestation at which it occurs. Cytotoxicity is not only a property of chemicals. Infectious agents, especially viruses, and physical agents, such as ionizing radiation, can also cause cell-death-mediated abnormal development. Focal or diffuse cell death results in focal or diffuse lesions, respectively. However, an inflammatory response to necrosis is unlikely to occur until the latter half of gestation, since before this time the immune system is immature.

The plasticity of the early embryo allows for compensatory growth after nonlethal exposure. Therefore, some models for teratogenicity testing, such as whole embryo culture, may be overly sensitive to abnormal growth retardation. This abnormal development may not represent teratogenic activity *per se*, but growth retardation that may be compensated for *in vivo* once the insult has been removed. In addition, attempts at repair often follow injury and may result in congenital anomalies; for example, intestinal atresia can result from fibrosis following ischemic injury to the bowel.

Death

Death of the embryo is common in humans. It has been estimated that approximately 50–70% of all conceptuses are lost during the first three weeks of development, and that by the end of pregnancy, 78% will have died. Morphologic abnormalities are often fatal, and ten times more malformed fetuses are born dead than alive. Chromosomal anomalies are apparent in 60% of abortuses occurring at less than 12 weeks of gestation, and have a prevalence of one in 160 live births. These anomalies account for many multi-systemic anomalies in defective fetuses that make it to term. Neural tube defects, cardiovascular malformations, and multiple malformations (non-chromosomal) are commonly seen during early gestation. Although the details of the prevalence of fetal death in domestic animals are less clear, severe injury can result in embryonic or fetal death. The consequences are resorption, expulsion (abortion or stillbirth), or retention with mummification. Important causes of abortion in domestic animals are listed in Table 20.3.

The term "terathanasia" has been used to describe the way nature eliminates nonviable embryos and fetuses. However, mortality does not stop at birth. Approximately 8% of human babies with major malformations die during the neonatal period and early childhood.

Malformations

Excessive Cell Death

Cell populations with a high proliferative rate, and those beginning to differentiate, are the most susceptible to cytotoxicity. This sensitivity may relate to the active "exposed" genome. Such active DNA is susceptible to damage by incorporation of foreign substances which can form adducts. In addition, the internal nutritive requirements of the cell may be higher at such a time than in the G_1 phase.

Selective cytotoxicity has been shown to cause abnormal embryonic development. For example, excessive cell death has a dramatic effect on limb formation. Early cell death may lead to too few cells for induction at a critical stage of development. With a lack of positional information, incorrect temporal-spatial relationships then occur. Limb reduction defects, sometimes seen following cytotoxicity caused by cyclophosphamide exposure, are thought to have this pathogenesis. That the regenerative capacity of tissues can also be important is demonstrated by aminothiadiazole, which causes less severe limb anomalies if digit primordia have sufficient time to restore their cell numbers and orientation.

Interference with Programmed Cell Death (Apoptosis)

As previously mentioned programmed cell death (PCD) by the process of apoptosis is a normal phenomenon during development, and does not damage adjacent cells, as does necrosis. PCD is needed for separation of the digits, limiting size of the digits, decreasing superfluous neurons, cavity formation in solid primordia, and degeneration of primitive structures. PCD can be induced by chemical messages,

such as hormones and/or growth factors. Interference with these signals may prevent cell death, and lead to supernumerary structures. For example, necrotic mesodermal cells of rats release apical ectodermal maintenance factor, following acetyl salicylic acid exposure; this prevents PCD in the apical ectodermal ridge, resulting in pups with polydactyly.

Reduced Proliferation Rate

A reduction in the proliferative rate can occur following a dose of a developmental toxicant lower than the dose that induces cytotoxicity, and may cause growth retardation of specific organs. Growth retardation of an organ can have dramatic effects, since a critical mass of tissue is often necessary to induce secondary structures. For example, if dental anlagen are not of sufficient mass, teeth will fail to develop.

Reduced proliferation of tissues during histogenesis can result in abnormal differential growth rates, with later defective development. This loss in synchrony happens in hypervitaminosis A, folic acid deficiency, and exposure to corticosteroids in some species. For example, corticosteroids reduce palatal shelf size, resulting in cleft palate formation in mice. A more striking example is hypovitaminosis A in pigs, where piglets are born blind because of compression of the optic tracts following premature closure of cranial sutures.

Failed Cellular Interactions

Failed cellular interactions can occur as a result of genetic factors, exogenous agents, or both. For example, in the Weaver mouse mutant, a genetic anomaly of murine cerebellar development results from a decrease in glial processes. These processes act as guides for the migration of granular cells from the molecular layer to the granular layer of the cerebellum. Similarly, a genetic defect has been reported in cattle where anophthalmia or microphthalmia occur following absent or reduced contact between the optic cup and the overlying ectoderm.

Exogenous agents may also prevent cellular interactions. For example, actinomycin D prevents primary induction. Hypovitaminosis A has disruptive effects on the spatial orientation of mesenchymal cell condensations through altered cell adhesion molecule characteristics, so that abnormally-shaped cartilage models form.

Impeded Morphogenetic Movements

Cellular migration can be impeded by factors such as: decreased mobility of the cells; altered quantity or quality of the extracellular matrix (ECM), especially

TABLE 20.3 Selected toxicants with abortifacient or teratogenic potential in domestic animals

Category	Source	Specific toxicant if known	Major species affected	Name	Effect/mechanism
Insect derived	*Malacosoma americanum* (eastern tent caterpillar, ETC)	Caterpillar setae suspected	Horses	Mare reproductive loss syndrome (MRLS)	Abortions
Mycotoxins (fungal metabolites)	*Neophtyphodium coenophialum*, an endophyte of tall fescue (*Festuca arundinacea*)	Ergot alkaloids especially ergovaline	Horses	Fescue toxicoses, reproductive term dysfunction	Dopamine, α-2 adrenergic and serotonergic agonists. Abortions less common than prolonged gestation, thickened placenta, agalactia
	Phomopsis leptostromiformis colonizing lupine stubble	Phomopsins	Sheep, cattle	Lupinosis (Australia)	Abortions
Plants	Ponderosa pine needles (*Pinus* spp e.g., *Pinus ponderosa*, ponderosa pine)	Isocupressic acid (ICA)	Cattle		Vasoconstriction. Last trimester abortions, retained placenta
	Cupressus macrocarpa (Monterey cypress)	Isocupressic acid	Cattle		As above
	Gutierrezia spp, compositae family (Broom snakeweed)	Terpenes, some similar to ICA	Cattle, sheep, goats		Abortions
	Berteroa incana (Hoary alyssum)		Horses		Abortions
	Hybrid Sudan grass		Horses		Abortions, dystocia, arthrogryposis.
	Locoweeds (*Oxytropis, Astralagus* and *Swainsona* spp)	Swainsonine, an indolizidine alkaloid	Multiple	Locoism	Abortions, lysosomal storage disorder. Inhibition of α-mannosidase
	Nitrate accumulating forages e.g., *Sorghum* spp, *Avena sativa* (oat hay), *Zea mays* (cornstalks)	Nitrites (rumenal microorganisms convert nitrates to nitrites)	Cattle		Abortion with fetal methemoglobinemia
	Lupinus sp (lupines)	Alkaloids: anagyrine, ammodendrine	Cattle, sheep	"Crooked calf" syndrome	Arthrogryposis
	Conium maculatum (poison hemlock)	Piperidine alkaloid	Cattle, other ruminants, horses		Arthrogryposis, cleft palate
	Veratrum spp	Steroidal alkaloids: cyclopamine, jervine	Sheep	"Monkey faced" lamb disease	Craniofacial defects, cyclopia a major defect when ingested on day 14 of gestation Inhibition of sonic hedgehog signaling pathway
Gases	Faulty propane heaters as example	Carbon monoxide	Swine		Abortion. Fetal tissues cherry red
Drugs		Griseofulvin	Cats		Skeletal and brain malformations, including cerebellar hypoplasia
		Tetracylines	Dogs		Bone and teeth malformations and discoloration
		Corticosteroids	Dogs		Abortion, cleft palate

altered SAMs; altered quality of cell adhesions through altered CAMs, SAMs, or CJMs; and disruption of microtubules or microfilaments. The ECM is composed of glycosaminoglycans (hyaluronic acid, chondroitin, chondroitin sulfate, heparin sulfate, keratin sulfate, and heparin), and collagen. These and other SAMs interact with the integrins, allowing movement or adhesion among tissues in directional planes.

High levels of hyaluronic acid during early morphogenesis encourage cell migration, by increasing cell proliferation, inhibiting aggregation, and increasing the fluidity of the ECM. During differentiation, hyaluronic acid levels decrease after increased aggregation of cells and chondroitin sulfate production. Similarly, concentrations of fibronectin may vary. Bromodeoxyuridine and 6-diazo-5-exo-l-norleucine inhibit the synthesis of chondroitin sulfate; thus, alteration of the ECM is a possible mechanism for production of limb defects and cleft palate by these teratogens.

Lack of cell adhesion can also result in malformations. Cortisone disrupts glycosaminoglycan and collagen synthesis, resulting in reduction in production and sulfation of ECM components. The decreased adhesive qualities of the ECM may contribute to the inability of the palatine shelves to fuse. In addition, cell surface receptors may be altered, thereby causing faulty recognition of cell collectives and improper induction.

Microtubules and microfilaments are essential contractile elements of cells. Microtubular and microfilamentous function can be affected through alterations in synthesis and turnover of tubulin, number and arrangement of microtubule organizing centers, phosphorylation of tubulin-associated proteins, and tubulin polymerization. For example, colchicine and vincristine disrupt microtubules, whereas cytochalasin B inactivates microfilaments.

Calcium is an essential cation for the function of microtubular and microfilamentous function. Treatment with EDTA induces heart malformations by reducing the movement of pioneer cells through the cardiac jelly. By chelating calcium, EDTA paralyzes the cells during the critical period of organogenesis.

Reduced Biosynthesis of Essential Components

Alterations in the biosynthesis of DNA, RNA, proteins, and energy sources (ATP and NAD/NADP), can have profound effects on normal growth and development. Inhibition of DNA synthesis is not teratogenic *per se*. However, cytotoxicity often accompanies inhibition of DNA synthesis, and can later lead to teratogenesis. The time available for cellular repair by the embryo, and the degree of necrosis, are important factors in the outcome of such inhibition. Further, transient inhibition of DNA synthesis might result in critical populations of cells whose proliferation or differentiation is delayed, to the point of being out of synchrony with the developmental plan of the embryo.

Cytosine arabinoside and hydroxyurea both depress DNA synthesis, the former by inhibition of DNA polymerase, and the latter by inhibition of ribonucleoside diphosphate reductase. Since cytosine arabinoside exerts the more prolonged depression of DNA synthesis, there is less time available for repair before the initiation of anomalous development.

A primary reduction in RNA synthesis may inhibit DNA synthesis, but usually RNA synthesis inhibition results in interference with the synthesis of proteins essential for growth. Actinomycin D, daunomycin, and chromomycin all inhibit RNA synthesis. The degree of reduction correlates well with their cytotoxicity and initiation of abnormal development.

Inhibition of protein synthesis may be affected by a failure of attachment of mRNA to ribosomes, as observed following chloramphenicol administration. This lack of attachment prevents translation of mRNA, and therefore protein synthesis. Other agents interfere with phosphorylation of glucose, as observed following tetracycline administration, which can cause derangement of nucleic acid synthesis. Misreading of mRNA may result in the synthesis of defective proteins, as seen following streptomycin and kanamycin administration. Premature termination of peptide chains interferes with biosynthesis of essential components for cell growth, for example, following puromycin administration. Protein synthesis inhibitors often produce little differential cytotoxicity, but tend to cause embryolethality or growth retardation.

Lack of ATP and NAD/NADP can have serious effects on glycolysis, cellular respiration, and electron transport during the critical periods of organogenesis. Such processes are necessary for many aspects of cellular function. Therefore, it is not surprising that inhibition of ATP synthesis by such compounds as 6-aminonicotinamide, which also forms defective NAD and NADP, has disastrous effects on the developing avian embryo. Similarly, the teratogenic effects of organophosphate and methylcarbamate insecticides in the developing chick lie not only in their ability to inhibit acetylcholinesterase, but also in their ability to reduce NAD pools; hence, interfering with energy pathways in numerous developing cells. Hypoxia, dinitrophenol, and cyanide directly inhibit the electron transport system, thereby causing cell death followed by embryonic or fetal death.

Mechanical Disruption

Mechanical disruption destroys cell interactions, impedes morphogenetic movements, and may cause decreased cell proliferation through pressure necrosis.

Changes in the fluid balance within cells and fluid-filled organs, e.g., eye, brain, and spinal cord, disrupts these structures. In the chick, for example, dimethyl sulfoxide or hypoxia cause increased volume and pressure of the cerebrospinal fluid. This increased volume can result in distention and rupture of the neural structures. In mammals, interference with aortic arch development can cause abnormal cardiac blood flow patterns and pressure changes. Such anomalies may then induce a ventricular septal defect.

Distortion and hypoplasia of external body structures; failure of closure of the lip, palate, neural tube, or abdomen; limb amputation or malposition; and limb reduction anomalies have been linked to mechanical problems of constraint. Oligohydramnios, uterine malformations, amniotic bands, extrinsic pressure, and prolonged severe uterine contractions can lead to mechanical pressure on the developing embryo or fetus.

Decrease in the vascular supply to organs can result in subsequent necrosis of the affected tissue. Amniotomy causes cleft palate in mouse embryos by increasing external uterine pressure. Early embryonic trauma through overzealous manual pregnancy testing of cattle can cause *atresia coli* in calves.

Intracellular pH

Hydrogen ion concentration in developing cells has recently been the subject of attention. Decreased pH interferes with cellular processes, such as proliferation, intracellular communication, enzyme activity, and cytoskeletal protein polymerization. Thus, it is not surprising that alterations in embryonic pH can result in anomalous development. In the mouse, inhalation of 15% CO_2 induces the same limb malformation in C57BL/6J mice, postaxial right forelimb ectrodactyly, as acetazolamide and other carbonic anhydrase inhibitors. This finding indicates that the defect may follow decreased intracellular pH.

Intrauterine Growth Retardation

Children suffering from intrauterine growth retardation are not born prematurely, but are born small for their duration of gestation. Placental insufficiency has often been considered responsible for intrauterine growth retardation, but this is apparently not usually the cause. Because of the placenta's considerable physiological reserve capacity, most pathologic placental lesions appear to be functionally unimportant, and do not result in fetal malnutrition. Fetal exposures to certain drugs, such as aminopterin and busulfan, x-irradiation, and hypoxia cause intrauterine growth retardation in the presence of apparently normal placentation.

Intrauterine growth retardation often occurs with congenital malformations, the severity of which correlates inversely with fetal body weight. Malformations associated with intrauterine growth retardation include microcephaly, macrocephaly, hydrocephalus, ventricular septal defects, renal agenesis, arthrogryposis, *spina bifida*, and intrauterine fractures secondary to *osteogenesis imperfecta*.

Perinatal Toxicology

Functional changes in the offspring may result from exposure to teratogens during the fetal period that cause morphologic or biochemical alterations during organogenesis. Often these functional deficiencies are a result of depletion in the number of cells, without appropriate compensation. Although subtle structural defects may be apparent, functional deficiencies are most often manifested by behavioral or motor deficits, inborn errors in metabolism, and defects in cell functions, for example, abnormal reproductive and immune system function.

Interference with postnatal reproductive functions can follow intrauterine exposure to antineoplastic agents (e.g., procarbazine), alkylating agents (e.g., busulfan), benzo[a]pyrene, dimethylbenz[a]anthracene, DDT, chlordecone, and diethylstilbestrol. Abnormal ontogenetic development of the immune system seen following exposure to xenobiotics *in utero* may lead to immunosuppression or immunostimulation, with resultant immune disregulation, and later neoplasia or autoimmune disease.

The anticonvulsant drugs, diphenylhydantoin and trimethadione, are believed to cause mental retardation and growth retardation, along with a variety of malformations. In addition, prenatal exposure to high levels of alcohol can result in mental retardation, poor coordination, hypotonia, hyperactivity, and growth retardation, in addition to distinctive faces (fetal alcohol syndrome, FAS), and occasional pathologies of various organs.

Environmental contaminants can also have postnatal central nervous system effects, such as cognitive disorders due to lead exposure. Organic mercury can induce sensory and peripheral motor disturbances, although the mechanism is unclear. The developing brain is especially sensitive to methyl mercury, because that compound is lipophilic, and has a high affinity for cysteine residues found in critical proteins in neurons.

Genetically-based inborn errors of metabolism are often not expressed until after birth. In some cases, an environmentally caused "copy" of the genetically-based disease may occur. This copy is termed a phenocopy. For example, α-mannosidosis and locoweed toxicity in cattle are morphologically quite similar; however, in the inherited disorder, accumulation of α-mannoside follows lack of α-mannosidase activity, whereas the environmental phenocopy follows inhibition of α-mannosidase activity after ingestion of the alkaloid swainsonine. Phenocopies highlight the difficulty in determining the etiology of defects. A given developmental anomaly can often occur by more than one pathway; thus, different causes of abnormal development may produce the same defect (e.g., cleft palate). In other words, the potential variety of responses to injury that can be expressed by the conceptus is not unlimited.

Endocrine Disruption

So-called "endocrine disrupters" have received much recent attention (see Further Reading). They are defined as exogenous agents that interfere with the synthesis, secretion, transport, binding, action, or elimination of endogenous hormones.

Most of the interest in xenobiotics that mimic endogenous hormones, enhance their actions, or act as hormone antagonists, has centered on their potential for disruption of reproductive tract development, alteration of sexual behavior, and impairment of fertility. However, compounds that affect the central nervous system, including the pituitary, thyroid, or immune function are also of concern. With few exceptions (e.g., diethylstilbestrol (DES), TCDD, DDT, and DDE), causal relationships between exposure to a specific xenobiotic and endocrine disruption have not yet been established in humans.

Endocrine disruption has occurred in wildlife in some instances, a notable example being the demasculinization of male alligators and "super-feminization" of females in Florida's Lake Apopka. This event has been attributed to a large pesticide spill that occurred in 1980 and contaminated the lake with a mixture of dicofol, DDT, and DDE.

Congenital Neoplasia

Fetal cells are inherently susceptible to carcinogens, because of their high rate of proliferation. The incidence of neonatal tumors in humans up to 15 years of age has been reported as 97.8 to 124.5 per million per year. Leukemia, lymphoma, neuroblastoma, Wilms' tumor, osteosarcoma, and rhabdomyosarcoma are the most common diagnoses made in children. Neonatal tumors occur in other mammals, but the incidence in most species is not known.

Some transplacental carcinogens act directly, usually with intracellular receptors, or with target molecules such as glutathione, while others require bioactivation to reactive intermediates. Some transplacental carcinogens alter DNA, thereby inducing heritable predisposition to carcinogenesis. For example, ethylnitrosourea, methylnitrosourea, and dimethylbenz[a]anthracene produce an increased incidence of tumors in F_1 and F_2 generations of exposed mice and rats.

Metabolism-dependent transplacental carcinogens must be present in the fetus when fetal enzyme levels are sufficient to metabolize the agent to the carcinogen. For example, nitrosamines are metabolized via the mixed-function oxidase system to reactive alkylating intermediates only when the fetal mixed-function oxidase system is operational. Some metabolism-dependent agents become activated through biotransformation by the maternal system. However, circulating concentrations are usually insufficient to begin and promote carcinogenesis in the fetus, unless the metabolite is quite stable and accumulates via a mechanism such as "ion-trapping."

Tumors in the young indicate abnormal embryogenesis. Therefore, it is not uncommon to see tumors in individuals displaying defective development. Some teratogens, such as diethylstilbestrol, can induce both carcinogenesis (uterine clear-cell adenocarcinoma) and teratogenesis (reproductive tract abnormalities). It is probable that permanently-altered DNA causes both the morphologic anomalies and the tumors.

Transplacental carcinogenesis and morphologic abnormalities may be different responses to the same toxic insult. Teratogenesis could result from exposure to the xenobiotic during the early stages of development, and a mixture of teratogenesis and carcinogenesis could occur if the exposure occurred throughout gestation.

Carcinogenesis alone may result after late-gestational or postnatal exposure. An environmental insult could later promote these dysgenic tissues. For example, increased hormonal levels at puberty may stimulate tumors in the dysgenic reproductive tract of diethylstilbestrol-treated females. In addition, postnatal promotion by the same carcinogen to which the fetus has been exposed *in utero* may follow antenatal initiation.

Many teratogens and developmental toxicants, whether human or animal, are not mutagens, and there is no evidence for carcinogenicity of most teratogens, either transplacentally or postnatally. It is true, however, that most carcinogens (and many cancer therapeutic agents) are developmental toxicants. In fact, the known transplacental carcinogens are postnatal carcinogens; therefore, the postulate that teratogenesis and transplacental carcinogenesis may have a common pathway is likely for only a few substances. If one considers that most teratogens do not act by causing mutations, carcinogenic initiation and teratogenesis are unlikely to be different expressions of the same insult. Teratogens are more apt to act by altering the expression of otherwise normal genes, and in fact the genome is more likely to be normal in the lesions of defective offspring than in tumors of neonates showing transplacental carcinogenesis.

How Dose Relates to Manifestation of Abnormal Development

The stage of embryonic or fetal development must be considered before attempting a correlation between dosage and type of abnormal development. Low doses do not necessarily cause functional deficits, and high doses do not always lead to embryonic or fetal death. The result depends on the *stage of development* at which the agent is administered, and the *mechanism* by which it acts.

During early development, moderate exposures to xenobiotics may induce death, but once organogenesis is in progress, similar or lower concentrations of the compound may produce morphologic defects. Toward the end of organogenesis, malformation is less likely, and tends to require doses larger than those effective during the critical period. At this point, moderate xenobiotic concentrations may cause functional deficits and intrauterine growth retardation. During the latter part of the fetal period, larger doses would typically be required to induce functional changes in most organ systems.

The occurrence of transplacental carcinogenesis depends on the nature of the carcinogen. However, exposure of the embryo during organogenesis to small concentrations, or after organogenesis to moderate concentrations, may result in initiation of carcinogenesis, rather than death of developing cells.

SELECTED MALFORMATIONS

The pathogenesis and etiology of selected malformations will be described in the following section, but the list is not complete (Tables 20.4 and 20.5). There is a dearth of data concerning the pathogenesis and etiology of malformations in domestic animals; however, some more common causes are listed in Table 20.3.

Central Nervous System

Neural tube defects result from failure of closure of the neural tube during embryonic development. These include anencephaly, exencephaly and spina bifida.

Anencephaly

Anencephaly (absence of cranial vault with brain missing or greatly reduced), more common in humans than in domestic animals, has prevalence ranging between 0.8 and 18 per 10 000 infants born in different populations. Failed interactions and fusion of the neuroectoderm result in anencephaly. Abnormal vascularization of the exposed tissue results in secondary neural destruction, so only an angiomatous mass remains at birth. In spite of normal development of the optic vesicles, the optic nerves may or may not be present. Populations with a high incidence of one of these defects often have an increased incidence of the other, and dietary folic acid supplementation has been shown to decrease the incidences of both.

Acrania

Although the base of the skull undergoes normal development, acrania (lack of development of the calvarium) occurs in conjunction with anencephaly, as do anomalies of the petrous temporal bones, sphenoid bone, and internal ear. The cranial nerves, cerebellum, and pons are usually abnormal.

Microcephaly

Microcephaly, or small cranium, is a primary defect in cerebral development, with secondary skull involvement. It has a prevalence of 0.6 to 1.6 per 1000 live human births, but the prevalence in domestic animals is not known. The cerebral hemispheres, particularly the frontal lobes, are reduced in size and possess a simplified convoluted pattern; microgyria or macrogyria is seen, with marked asymmetries in the cerebrum. Histologically, there are fewer large neurons in the cortex, with a corresponding increase in undifferentiated neuroblasts and abnormal spindle-shaped cells. Microcephaly has been associated with mental retardation, cleft palate, microphthalmia, and, occasionally, defects in the appendicular skeleton. Microcephaly is the one malformation consistently produced by X-rays in humans, although exposures well above diagnostic levels are required. This morphologic anomaly has not been reliably reproduced in test species. Nonetheless, hyperthermia and spindle toxins, such as vincristine, can induce this defect in rats and guinea pigs.

Hydrocephalus (Hydrocephaly)

Overproduction of cerebrospinal fluid (CSF), or more frequently a block in CSF circulation, causes hydrocephalus, an abnormal accumulation of CSF in the ventricular system (Figure 20.5). Obstruction of the aqueduct of Sylvius, atresia of the foramina of Magendie and Lushka, skeletal malformations at the base of the skull (e.g., platybasia), or obstruction in the

TABLE 20.4   Selected etiologic agents causing congenital malformations in humans or animals

Agent	Effect[a]
Alcohol	Pre- and postnatal growth retardation, MR, unusual facial features, congenital heart defects, CP, diaphragmatic hernia, microphthalmia, urogenital defects, skeletal defects
Aminopterin	Anencephaly, hydrocephalus, CP, meningocele, meningomyelocele, reduced first branchial arch derivatives, talipes, limb and tail defects
Anagyrine (*Lupin* alkaloids)	Crooked calf disease, arthrogryposis, CP, scoliosis
Busulfan	Germ cell depletion (rat)
Cannabis (marijuana, hashish)[b]	IUGR
Carbon monoxide	CNS defects, stillbirth
Wild black cherry	Sirenomelia, rudimentary external genitalia, anal atresia, blindly ending colon (pig)
Cigarette smoking	Spontaneous abortion, prematurity, IUGR, fetal and neonatal death
Coniine (*Conium maculatum*)	Arthrogryposis (rat), scoliosis (cow)
Copper deficiency	"Swayback," enzootic ataxia (sheep)
Coumarin derivatives (dicumarol, warfarin)	Digital and nasal hypoplasia, CNS, choanal atresia, microphthalmia, hearing loss, IUGR, stippled epiphyses
Cyclopamine (*Veratrum californicum*)	Cyclopia, CP, cerebral defects (sheep, rabbit)
Cyclophosphamide	CP, limb reduction, edema (mouse, rat, rabbit)
Danazol (*Danocrine*)	Masculinization of the female fetus
Diabetes	Caudal regression syndrome, macrosomia
Diethylstilbestrol	Genital tract anomalies, vaginal adenocarcinoma
Dioxin (TCDD)	CP, renal anomalies, embryolethality (mouse)
Diphenylhydantoin (phenytoin, hydantoin)	Dysmorphic facies, hypoplasia of nails and distal phalanges, short or webbed neck, abnormalities of growth and mental/and or motor development
Etretinate	Meningomyelocele, meningoencephalocele, multiple synostoses, facial dysmorphia, syndactyly, absence of terminal phalanges, malformations of hip, ankle, and forearm, low-set ears, high palate, decreased cranial volume, alterations of the skull and the cervical vertebrae
Fasting, starvation	Hydrocephalus, meningomyelocele, decreased head circumference
Fluorine	Mottled tooth enamel
Folic acid deficiency	Neural tube defects (humans), heart, kidney, and skeletal defects (rat)
Griseofulvin	CP (cat)
Hypoxia[b]	Decreased birth weight, newborn encephalopathy, motor and cognitive defects, patent ductus arteriosus (may be a postnatal effect)
Iodine deficiency	Endemic cretinism, congenital goiter
Iodine excess	Congenital goiter, hypothyroidism
Isotretinoin (Accutane, 13-*cis*-retinoic acid)	Hydrocephalus, micrognathia, low-set ears, microcephaly, microphthalmia, malformed skull, ventricular septal defect, numerous other CNS, craniofacial, cardiovascular, and other defects
Lathyrism (*Lathyrus*)	Poorly developed muscles and connective tissue, dissecting aneurysms of aorta, spinal malformations, CP (domestic animals, rat)
Lead	Increased stillbirth and spontaneous abortion, MR
Locoweed (*Astragalus, Oxytropis*)	Arthrogryposis
Mercury	Cerebral palsy, microcephaly, MR
Methotrexate	Prenatal mortality, craniosynostosis, oxycephaly
D-Penicillamine[b]	Connective tissue disorders, e.g., lax skin, inguinal hernia
Phenylalanine excess (maternal PKU)	Microcephaly, IUGR, congenital heart defects, dislocation of hips, strabismus
Polychlorinated biphenyls	Cola-colored babies (staining of skin, nails, and gums), IUGR, conjunctivitis, "parchment-like skin"
Primidone[b]	CL/CP and other defects
Propylthiouracil	Congenital goiter
Organic solvents[b]	Spontaneous abortion, "fetal solvent syndrome"
Retinoids (e.g., etretinate, isotretinoin, vitamin A excess)	CNS, head, limb, skeletal, and cardiovascular defects (all species)
Salicylates	Cranial, facial, and skeletal malformations, heart and kidney defects, gastroschisis, diaphragmatic hernia (rodents), cardiovascular, spinal, and skeletal defects (rabbits)

(Continued)

TABLE 20.4 *(Continued)*

Agent	Effect[a]
Streptomycin[b]	Congenital hearing loss
Testosterone, methyltestosterone	Masculinization of the female fetus
Tetracycline	Stained enamel of deciduous teeth, depressed bone growth
Thalidomide	Limb reduction anomalies, external ear defects, facial hemangioma, esophageal and duodenal atresia, tetralogy of Fallot, renal agenesis
Tobacco stalk	Arthrogryposis (pig)
Trimethadione	High-arched palate, cardiac defects, V-shaped eyebrows, developmental delays, low-set ears, irregular teeth, MR, speech disturbances
Vitamin A excess	CP, craniofacial, skeletal, and urogenital anomalies (monkey), exencephaly, CP, eye defects (rat)
Vitamin D excess	Decreased skeletal ossification (rat), microcephaly, skeletal defects (mouse)
X rays	Microcephaly, MR, hypoplastic genitalia, IUGR, microphthalmia, cataracts, strabismus, retinal degeneration and pigment changes, skeletal defects (human)

[a]MR, mental retardation; CNS, central nervous system; CL/CP, cleft lip/cleft palate; IUGR, intrauterine growth retardation
[b]Uncertain association

TABLE 20.5   Examples of specific congenital defects with known etiologic agents in mammals

System	Defect	Etiology	Species
Central nervous/axial skeleton	Anencephaly/exencephaly	Colchicine	Mouse
		Injected inorganic arsenic	Mouse, rat, hamster
		Ethylnitrosourea	Rat
		Methylhydrazine	Rabbit
		Retinoic acid	Hamster
		Thalidomide	Rabbit
	Auditory nerve hypoplasia	Quinine	Human
	Cerebellar hypoplasia	Triamcinolone acetonide	Baboon, monkey
	Encephalocele	Ionizing radiation	Mouse
		Hydroxyurea	Mouse
	Hydrocephalus	Ionizing radiatin	Mouse, rat
		Vitamin A deficiency	Rat, rabbit, pig
	Iniencephaly	Streptonigran	Rat
	Microcephaly	Hyperthermia	Guinea pig, rabbit
		Methylnitrosourea	Rat
		X rays	Rat
	Spina bifida	Actinomycin D	Mouse
		7,12-Dimethyl-benz[a]anthracene	Rat
		Thalidomide	Baboon, monkey
Craniofacial	Agnathia/micrognathia	Injected inorganic arsenic	Mouse
		Pyrimethamine	Rat
		Retinoids	Hamster, monkey
	Anophthalmia/microphthalmia	Ethyl nitrosourea	Rat
		Glycol ethers	Mouse
	Cataracts	Mirex	Rat
	Cleft face	Ochratoxin A	Mouse
	Cleft lip/cleft palate	Dioxin (TCDD)	Mouse
		Diphenylhydantoin	Mouse
		Glucocorticoids	Mouse
		Griseofulvin	Cat

(Continued)

TABLE 20.5 (*Continued*)

System	Defect	Etiology	Species
	Cyclopia	Veratrum californicum	Ruminants
	Microtia and/or synotia	Injected hydroxyurea	Mouse
	Nasal defects	Griseofulvin	Cat
	Open eye	Methyl salicylate	Mouse
	Retinal defects	X rays	Rodents
Cardiovascular	Atrial septal defects	Alcohol	Human
		Dextroamphetamine sulfate	Mouse
	Dextrocardia	Actinomycin D	Rat
	Great vessel and vena cava anomalies	Valproic acid	Rat
	Tricuspid valve anomalies	Methyl chloride	Mouse
	Various defects	Diethylene glycol dimethyl ether	Mouse
	Ventricular septal defects	Alcohol	Human
		Dextroamphetamine sulfate	Mouse
		Thalidomide	Rabbit
Respiratory	Lung agenesis	Vitamin A deficiency	Rat, pig
	Lung hypoplasia	L-Asparaginase	Rabbit
Gastrointestinal	Absent gallbladder	Nitromifene	Dog
		Retinoicacid	Hamster
	Anal atresia	Colchicine	Mouse
	Diaphragmatic hernia	Nitrofen	Mouse, Rat
	Esophageal/duodenal atresia	Thalidomide	Human
	Gastroschisis	Vincristine	Mouse
		6-Azauridine	Rat
	Omphalocele	Actinomycin D	Mouse, rabbit
		Hyperthermia	Rat
Urogenital	Cryptorchidism	Cadmium	Rat
		Vitamin A deficiency	Rat, pig
	Hydronephrosis	Bradykinin	Mouse
	Hydroureter	Vitamin A excess	Rat
	Hypospadias	Chlorambucil	Rat
	Intersexuality	Androstenedione	Rat
		Prunus serotina	Pig
	Ovarian hypoplasia	diethylstilbestrol	Mouse, rat
	Renal agenesis	Chlorambucil	Rat
		Injected sodium arsenate	Rat
		Thalidomide	Human
Musculoskeletal	Arthrogryposis	Anagyrine	Cow, pig, sheep
		Nicotiana glauca	Pig
		Sudan grass	Horse
	Digit malformations	Cyclophosphamide	Human
		Ethylenethiourea	Rat
	Limb reduction defects	Acetazolamide	Mouse, rat
		Caffeine	Mouse
		Hydroxyurea	Rabbit
		N-Methyl-N-nitro-N-nitrosoguanidine	Mouse
		Thalidomide	Rabbit, monkey, human
	Muscular dystrophy	Vitamin E deficiency	Rat, rabbit
	Polydactyly	Cytosine arabinoside	Mouse
	Rib and/or vertebral defects	Ethylene glycol	Mouse, rat
		Injected sodium arsenate	Mouse, rat
		Hydroxyurea	Rabbit
	Tail shortened or malformed	Colchicine	Rabbit
		T-2 toxin	Mouse

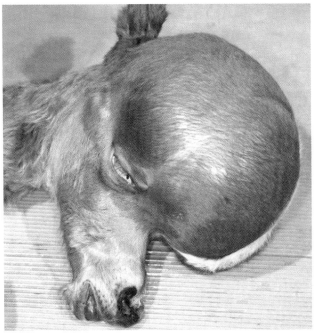

(A)

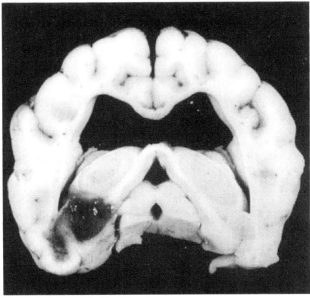

(B)

FIGURE 20.5 (A) Foal with markedly rounded skull due to congenital hydrocephalus. (B) Internal hydrocephalus, in this case caused by an expansile astrocytoma in a dog.

cerebral arachnoid spaces can prevent proper circulation of CSF. Hydrocephalus can occur during development, or at any time during life, if an obstruction of CSF flow occurs, but the congenital incidence typically ranges from about 2 to 7 per 1000 births. Morphologically, this lesion must be differentiated from hydranencephaly.

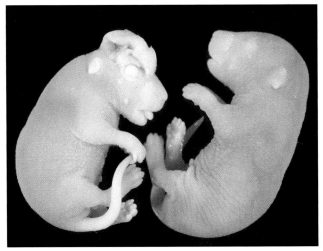

FIGURE 20.6 Exencephaly and open eye in a term CD-1 mouse fetus (left) in comparison with a normal fetus.

Hydranencephaly

Hydranencephaly is an absence of the cerebral hemispheres, with their normal site replaced by fluid, rather than dilation of the CSF-containing spaces. In humans in the USA, the incidence of hydranencephaly averages 0.5 per 1000 births.

Many agents can cause this lesion in some species. Physical agents, such as ionizing radiation; nutritional deficiencies, such as vitamin A, B_2, B_6, or B_{12} deficiency; and foreign substances, such as ethylenethiourea, tellurium, lead nitrate, and methyl mercury, can induce this defect in mice. Hydranencephaly has been associated with viral infections in farm animals.

Dysraphism

In some cases, dysraphism (defective fusion of the neural folds) may occur at the cranial end of the spinal cord (rarely the entire cord may be affected), where it is called craniorachischisis. A rudimentary pituitary gland causes altered development of endocrine glands, i.e., adrenal, gonadal, thymic, and thyroid hypoplasia.

Exencephaly

Exencephaly is a related condition seen in laboratory animals (Figure 20.6). In exencephaly, there is protrusion of the brain outside of the cranial vault, but erosion of the brain tissue does not occur as it does in anencephaly. Numerous experimental agents can cause exencephaly. These include: (1) physical agents, such as x-irradiation in mice; (2) agents that reduce biosynthesis, such as hypoglycemia in BALB/c mice; (3) agents that cause failed tissue interactions, such as

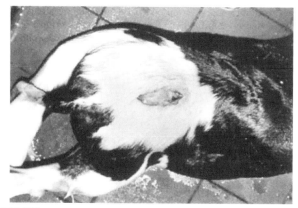

FIGURE 20.7   Spontaneous occurrence of *spina bifida* in a calf.

hypervitaminosis A in several rodent species; (4) agents that inhibit cell division, such as colchicine in mice; and (5) agents that cause general cytotoxicity, such as cyclophosphamide and parenterally-administered inorganic arsenate in rodents.

Neural Tube Defects in the Spinal Region

Spina bifida is a defect of the spine caused by incomplete closure of the neural tube, with consequent failure of union of the neural arches of the vertebrae (Figure 20.7). The least severe form is *spina bifida occulta*, which is not a neural tube defect in the strictest sense, and is most commonly asymptomatic. A sacral dimple or tuft of hair may indicate its presence. It is characterized by a gap in one or more vertebral arches, with no protrusion of spinal cord or meninges outside the vertebral canal, and no break in the skin covering the area. Of more concern are meningocele and myelomeningocele, which are forms of *spina bifida cystica* (so named because of the cyst-like sac characterizing these defects). Meningocele is distinguished by protrusion of the meninges through an osseous defect in the vertebral column; the spinal cord remains *in situ*, but may be abnormal. In the case of myelomeningocele, both neural tissue and meninges are herniated through the vertebral defect. In the most severe form, *spina bifida with myeloschisis*, there is an area of open neural plate, with no covering of meninges or skin. Degeneration of the neural structure results in paralysis of the posterior limbs (paraplegia). In the more severe forms of *spina bifida*, concomitant central nervous system malformations, such as hydrocephalus and cerebellar malformation, may occur.

Spina bifida has been reported to occur in all species, with a worldwide incidence in humans of 0.5 per 1000 live births. There is, however, a wide variation in

frequency, depending on the country (e.g., 0.2 per 1000 in Japan, to 4.1 per 1000 in south Wales). This variation in incidence had raised the question of whether there is an environmental basis for the lesion in humans. That conjecture was subsequently confirmed, in part, by the finding that the recurrence risk can be significantly decreased by maternal folic acid supplementation. Recently, an association with high levels of the mycotoxin, fumonisin B_1, has been identified. Based on experimental data, the mechanism is believed to be via the folic acid pathway.

Arthrogryposis is commonly seen in severe forms of *spina bifida*, because of spinal lesions leading to loss of motor activity. Offspring of rodents given excessive vitamin A, or anticancer drugs, such as vincristine and actinomycin D, often have *spina bifida*, and other spinal cord malformations. Rabbits respond similarly to these agents, and to methyl salicylate.

Craniofacial Structures

Anophthalmia and Microphthalmia

Anophthalmia involves the failure of outgrowth of the optic vesicle, and the subsequent lack of induction of the lens placode. Therefore, the lens, optic nerves, optic chiasma, and optic foramen are absent. Microphthalmia, on the other hand, represents hypoplasia of these structures, due to arrested eye development. Microphthalmia is often accompanied by defects of various eye structures, the extent of which is dependent on the timing of the developmental arrest.

There are three mechanisms by which anophthalmia or microphthalmia may occur: failure of development of the optic outgrowths; suppression of forebrain growth with later failure of eye development; or formation of an optic vesicle that is later destroyed. Both genetic and environmental causes exist. Secondary effects, such as failure of formation of the embryonic blood supply, especially the hyaloid artery to the eye, may result in rodent microphthalmia. Congenital cataract, coloboma of the iris and choroid, pupillary obstruction, corneal scarring, and ocular muscle imbalance are also associated with microphthalmia. The correlation of microphthalmia with facial and cardiovascular defects suggests that this is an anomaly of the first branchial arch.

These defects have been experimentally-induced with numerous chemical substances and physical agents. Anticancer agents, such as actinomycin D, chlorambucil, and methylhydrazine characteristically produce anophthalmia or microphthalmia in rodents. X-irradiation of rats during pregnancy also produces the lesion.

Cyclopia

Cyclopia occurs when the anterior parts of the noto-chord and surrounding mesoderm are deficient. This deficiency leads to aberrant induction of the forebrain tissues, followed by severe derangement of midline facial development. It is part of the cyclopia–arrhin-encephaly series, or holoprosencephaly. Cyclopia may involve complete fusion of the eyes in a single orbit with a proboscis, may be characterized by a single cornea, pupil, and lens without evidence of dupli-cation, or may show two eyes in a single orbit. The cerebral hemispheres are not cleaved, and possess a single ventricle called a holosphere. The olfactory bulbs and tracts are absent. Ocular defects associated with cyclopia include colobomas of the iris, retina, and optic nerve, duplicated or single optic nerve, and absent or abnormal optic chiasma.

Cyclopia is uncommon in humans, but may occur as outbreaks in sheep or cattle grazing on *Veratrum californicum* during day 13.5 of gestation (Figure 20.8). Experimental induction of cyclopia-arrhinencephaly-otocephaly occurs in mouse fetuses after dams are dosed with x-irradiation during pregnancy. The off-spring of mice given cyclophosphamide and vincris-tine may also show this defect.

Agnathia and Micrognathia

Total absence of the maxilla or mandible is extremely rare in mammals. When agnathia occurs, it may be combined with cyclopia or synotia; hence it is seen in fetuses from ruminants grazing on *Veratrum californi-cum*. Again, this defect originates in the first branchial arch. Maxillary micrognathia occurs more often than agnathia. It is an expression of deficient premaxillary tissue during development. Mandibular micrognathia may occur with posterior cleft palate, glossoptosis, microcephaly, and microphthalmia. Actinomycin D, colchicine, and vincristine cause a variety of jaw anom-alies in mice, including agnathia and micrognathia.

Cleft Lip and Cleft Palate

Cleft palate, or palatoschisis, is an important devel-opmental anomaly of mammals, since the neonate cannot nurse properly without an intact palate. A cleft palate usually results in inhalation of milk and aspi-ration pneumonia. In humans, 0.5–1.0 cleft palates without cleft lips occur per 1000 births, while the inci-dence of cleft lip, with or without cleft palate, ranges from 0.5 to 1.6 per 1000 births. The prevalence of pal-atoschisis in animals may be greater than thought at present, since not all animals that die during or after birth undergo a necropsy examination. Grossly, the cleft palate is unilateral when only one side of the tur-binates is visible. However, the lesion is usually bilat-eral, indicating that both palatal shelves did not reach the center of the oral cavity (Figure 20.9).

The pathogenesis of cleft palate is extremely com-plex, and can involve multifactorial inheritance, xeno-biotic effects, or a mixture of both. Cleft palate is an excellent model for demonstrating the mechanisms involved in defect generation. Expression of receptors, programmed cell death, and correct temporal–spatial positioning are essential for correct formation of the palate. Reorientation and fusion of the palatal shelves must occur, and is particularly time-dependent. The

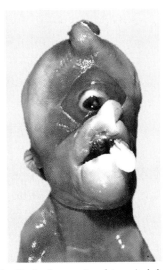

FIGURE 20.8 **Cyclopia, porcine fetus**. A defect of ocular and cranial development has resulted in fusion of the eyes (cyclops) and a proboscis above the eye. Cyclopia can occur in the lambs of ewes that ingest the plant *Veratrum californicum* on the fourteenth day of gestation. (Courtesy of Dr J. King, College of Veterinary Medicine, Cornell University.) (From Foster, R.A. (2007). In *Pathologic Basis of Veterinary Disease*, 4th Ed. McGavin, M., and Zachary, J.F., eds, Mosby Elsevier, St. Louis. Fig. 18-43, p 1302)

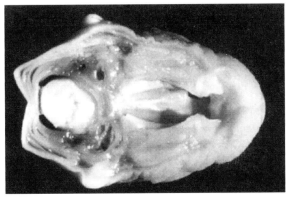

FIGURE 20.9 Cleft palate in a CD-1 mouse fetus from a dam given 2.5 mg/kg dexamethasone on gestation days 9, 10, 11, and 12 and 200 mg/kg all-*trans* retinoic acid on day 10.5 of gestation.

final process of fusion and elimination of the medial edge epithelium requires the formation of cellular junctions, activation or appearance of intracellular contractile elements, synthesis of glycosaminoglycans, and vascularization and innervation of the muscle. Simultaneously, the tongue must descend so that it does not obstruct the reorienting shelves. Obviously, with such an intricate embryology, interference with proper palate formation can occur in many ways. Of children with cleft lip and cleft palate, 14% have diverse malformations in other organ systems. The developmental mechanism of cleft palate differs from that of cleft lip with or without cleft palate. In the latter, it is the abnormal development of the primary palate, which prevents the secondary palate from closing.

As previously mentioned, cortisone-induced cleft palate in mice has often been used to study the pathogenesis of this lesion. The developing palate of mice is particularly sensitive to any agent that may decrease growth of the palatine shelves. These include hypoxia, decreased maternal nutrition, and virtually any chemical that causes cytotoxicity of the palatal processes.

Cardiovascular System

Atrial Septal Defects

Atrial septal defects, which are not fatal malformations, account for approximately 17% of all human heart defects. Four types of clinically-significant atrial septal defects exist. First, an oval fossa defect (a secondary ostium type atrial septal defect) accounts for approximately 70% of human atrial septal defects, and has a female:male occurrence ratio of 3:1. It is characterized by a patent *foramen ovale* with a fenestrated or netlike primary septum, a short primary septum, defective development of the secondary septum, or an abnormally large *foramen ovale* with an exceptionally small primary septum. Second, the relatively uncommon *sinus venosus* type of defect (high interatrial septal defect) results from abnormal absorption of the *sinus venosus* into the right atrium, or from abnormal development of the *septum secundum*. Third, a persistent primary ostium defect results from incomplete fusion of the primary septum and the endocardial cushions, with resultant anomalies in the atrioventricular valves. Finally, complete absence of the interatrial septum results from a failure of development of both the primary and secondary septa, and is the rarest of the four atrial septal defects.

Additional associated cardiac malformations with atrial septal defects include non-cyanotic patent *ductus arteriosus*, coarctation of the aorta, ventricular septal defects, mitral valve anomalies, cyanotic tricuspid atresia, common ventricle, tetralogy of Fallot, pulmonary stenosis or atresia, and transposition of the great vessels. The incidence of atrial septal defects in domestic animals is probably similar to that in humans. Induction of atrial septal defects has been reported in association with fetal alcohol syndrome in humans, and following dextroamphetamine sulfate administration in mice.

Ventricular Septal Defects

Ventricular septal defects occur more commonly than atrial septal defects, and account for 50% of human cardiac anomalies. Some septal defects may close spontaneously. Incomplete fusion of the atrioventricular endocardial cushions with the ventricular muscular septum and *conus* ridges causes the defect. This type of defect is also common in cattle and, to a lesser extent, in other domestic species (Figure 20.10).

Ventricular septal defects can be induced experimentally by agents that delay fusion of the cardiac septae. These include: hypoxia; deficiencies of nutrients, such as vitamin A and folic acid; nutritional excesses, such as vitamin A and copper excess; and various chemicals, including griseofulvin in cats, trypan blue and salicylate in rats, thalidomide in rabbits, and some antineoplastic agents in various laboratory animals.

Tricuspid Valve Anomalies

Tricuspid valve atresia is associated with defective development of the right ventricle, atrial septal defects (patent *foramen ovale* or fenestration of the primary septum), hypoplasia of the left ventricle, hyperplasia of the mitral valve, and an atretic or hypoplastic pulmonary artery. These defects are classified into type I (normal orientation of the great vessels) and type II defects (transposition of the great vessels).

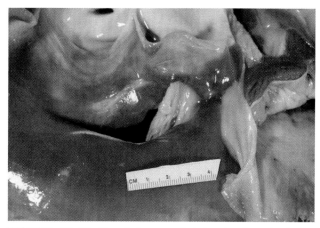

FIGURE 20.10 Ventricular septal defect in the subvalvular region of a horse heart.

Ebstein's anomaly is a rare cardiac malformation linked to human exposure to lithium carbonate. The valve ring is correctly placed, but the tricuspid orifice is displaced into the right ventricle, resulting in a decreased ventricular volume. The posterior and septal leaflets of the valve have an abnormally low attachment. Since excavation of the endocardial outgrowths is incomplete, the upper parts of the posterior and medial cusps remain attached to the wall. Patent *foramen ovale*, and fenestration of the primary septum, commonly occur with Ebstein's anomaly in humans. Experimental production of valvular anomalies in experimental animals is limited to reports of anomalous valves occurring with other cardiac defects.

Transposition of the Great Vessels

The pathogenesis of transposition of the aorta and pulmonary trunk is controversial. It has been thought that the malposition is caused by a lack of spiral twisting of the great vessels around each other, or by abnormal division of the *truncus arteriosus*. When experimentally-induced in the mouse by retinoic acid, however, anomalous cardiac looping, leading to hypoplasia of the conotruncal ridges and aorticopulmonary septum, with delay of fusion of the atrioventricular cushions, appears to be the basis for transposition of the great vessels.

Regardless of the cause, survival requires the presence of additional cardiac anomalies, such as septal defects and persistent *ductus arteriosus* that allow mixing of the two parallel circulations. This disorder appears more prevalent in men; however, in animals it is not recognized as a sex-linked trait. Transposition of the great vessels occurs with numerous other cardiac anomalies in rats exposed to X-rays (100–200 rad).

Respiratory System

Agenesis, Aplasia, or Hypoplasia of the Lungs

Total absence of the lungs, bronchi, and vascular structures—pulmonary agenesis—is usually unilateral. In rodents, it usually affects the left lung. Aplastic lungs have absent pulmonary and vascular structures, with rudimentary bronchi. Both agenesis and aplasia are probably caused by failed interactions between the endodermal components of the tracheobronchial buds and the surrounding mesenchyme. Hypoplastic lungs, commonly associated with renal agenesis, are a more frequent anomaly in which the lung tissue resembles fetal lung tissue. Hypoplasia may be primary (e.g., due to viral infection), or secondary (e.g., the

consequence of a diaphragmatic hernia following nitrofen administration).

Gastrointestinal System

Diaphragmatic Hernia

Failure of fusion or late fusion of the pleuroperitoneal membranes with the *septum transversum* and the dorsal mesentery of the esophagus, premature return of the intestines from the extraembryonic coelom to the abdominal cavity, and weak or abnormal diaphragmatic musculature can all lead to the formation of diaphragmatic hernias. Most herniation is dorsolateral in nature, leaving room for part or all of the abdominal viscera to enter the thorax. Diaphragmatic hernias occur in about 1 in 2200 newborns, and are predominately located on the left side.

Nitrofen and deficiencies of vitamin A or zinc can induce diaphragmatic hernias in rodents. Methallibure, a nonsteroidal pituitary gonadotropin inhibitor, causes the lesion in pigs.

Umbilical Hernia, Omphalocele, and Gastroschisis

Herniation of intestines via an imperfectly closed umbilicus, failure of intestines to return normally to the abdominal cavity, or failure of formation of the lateral folds of the ventral embryonic wall results in protrusion of the intestines or other organs from the abdomen. Such defects are commonly induced in laboratory animals, and are not rare in humans. They range in severity from herniation of intestines at the umbilicus, covered by subcutaneous tissue and skin, (umbilical hernia) to severe eventration of abdominal contents without a sac (gastroschisis). Administration of a number of antineoplastic drugs can produce gastroschisis in rodents, and corticosteroid administration can cause this lesion in rabbits.

Urinary System

Renal Agenesis

Failure of the ureteric bud to form, degeneration of the bud, or lack of contact with the metanephric mesoderm leads to failure of interaction with the metanephric blastema, resulting in renal agenesis. Unilateral renal agenesis is a fairly common finding in humans at postmortem (1–1.8 per 1000), whereas bilateral renal agenesis or severe dysplasia only occurs in 0.02–0.37 per 1000 human births. The remaining kidney in unilateral agenesis is often rotated, hydronephrotic, polycystic, or ectopic. Calculi are frequently found in the pelvis, as are defects in the genitalia, especially in females. Thalidomide treatment in rabbits, hypervitaminosis A or chlorambucil in rodents, and administration of methyl chloride to ferrets can cause renal agenesis.

Hydronephrosis

Transient closure of the ureters occurs during development. If urine secretion by the kidney commences before the reopening of the ureters, hydronephrosis may result. Normal bending and narrowing of the ureter at the ureteropelvic junction predisposes it to fixation against the renal pelvis with obstruction to urine flow, especially when combined with aberrant renal vessels. In 40% of cases of hydronephrosis, concomitant defects, such as agenesis or hypoplasia of the contralateral kidney, cystic kidney, and hypospadias have been reported. Renal pelvic dilation is often noted in rodents during teratologic studies, and may be transient.

Several treatments can reproducibly induce hydronephrosis in rodents; these include aspirin, cadmium, ethylenethiourea, methotrexate, hypervitaminosis A, and rubidomycin. Trypan blue and hypovitaminosis A cause this lesion in pigs.

Hydroureter

Hydroureter is usually a consequence of urethral valvular obstruction, although some unexplained cases may be the result of unduly prolonged preservation of the ureteric membrane, a suggested cause for hydronephrosis. It is a common anomaly in laboratory rodents. Following obstruction, the affected ureter dilates, elongates, bends, and becomes tortuous, before the development of urinary reflux occurs. Ectopic ureter, double ureter, uretocele, dysplastic kidney, uretovesicle strictures, and single kidneys have been seen with hydroureter. Fetal mice and rats irradiated with X-rays often demonstrate obstruction of the ureters. The obstruction frequently leads to hydroureter and hydronephrosis.

Reproductive System

Cryptorchidism

A failure of one or both testes to descend from the inguinal region to the scrotum is called cryptorchidism. It is a common defect seen in many species, and often resolves itself within the first year of life. Fibrous bands that anchor the testes in abnormal positions characterize ectopic testis, an extreme form of cryptorchidism. The failure of correct formation of the gubernaculum and testicular vessels, gonadotropic hormonal deficiency, congenital inguinal hernia, and abnormalities of the *tunica vaginalis* can be contributing factors in the failure of descent of the testes. The persistence of an abdominal testis is associated with an increased risk of testicular cancer.

Cryptorchidism is often produced following exposure to foreign compounds, or nutritional deficiencies. Vitamin A deficiency has been associated with this defect in rodents and swine. Treatment with benzhydrylpiperazines or parenteral sodium arsenate can result in undescended testes in rodents. Endocrine disruptors can also result in cryptorchidism, or delayed testicular descent (Table 20.6).

TABLE 20.6 Selected effects of endocrine distributors on male reproductive tract development

Organ	Reported effects	Chemicals
Developmental effects	Pseudohermaphrodite, vaginal pouch	Procymidone, vinclozolin, di(2-ethylhexyl)phthalate (EDHP)
	Hypospadia	Hydroxyflutamide, procymidone, vinclozolin, finasteride, DEHP
	Microphallus/cleft phallus	DES, procymidone, vinclozolin
	Decreased anogenital distance	Vinclozolin, linuron, *p,p* DDE, dibutyl phthalate, procymidone, DEHP
Testis	Cryptorchidism or delayed testicular descent	DES, TCDD, hydroxyflutamide, procymidone, vinclozolin
	Tubular atrophy	TCDD, vinclozolin, linuron, boric acid, dibutyl phathalate
	Decreased testis weight	DES, octyphenol phenoxylate, octylphenol, butyl benzyl phthalate, boric acid, DEHP
	Decreased testosterone	TCDD, heptachlor, boric acid, *N*-nitroso-*N*-ethylurea, PCBs, ethane dimethanesulfonate, lindane, dibromoacetic acid, phthalate esters, hexachlorocyclohexane

Disorders of Sex Development—Hermaphroditism and Pseudohermaphroditism

Disorders of sex development (DSD), often referred to as intersex, can have a number of causes. The phenotypic sex of mammals (i.e. secondary sexual characteristics and accessory sex organs) is determined by hormones; however, gonadal sex of the individual is purely dependent upon the sex chromosome composition. Aberrations of the sex chromosomes are major reasons for DSD but are not its only cause.

Sex chromosome composition or genetic sex is determined at fertilization. The presence of Y chromosome or the testis-determining gene *SRY* (Sex-determining region of the Y chromosome) then decides the sex of the gonads. In the presence of *SRY*, gonads differentiate into testes. If *SRY* is absent, ovaries form. Mutations of the *SRY* gene in the XY individual or ectopic appearance of *SRY* in the XX individual results in sex reversal. Gonadal sex eventually decides the ability of the fetal gonad to produce hormones (i.e. androgens), which controls the phenotypic sex.

True hermaphroditism refers to the presence of both XX and XY tissues, either as ovary and testis (Figure 20.11) or combined as an ovotestis. Pseudohermaphroditism refers to a mismatch between gonadal sex and phenotypic sex, e.g. a female hermaphrodite will have ovaries but masculinized genitalia.

Androgens induce the male characteristics; hence, a xenobiotic with androgenic function can affect the female fetus by inducing female pseudohermaphroditism. In such a case, the genetic and gonadal sex of the individual is female, but the genitalia and secondary sexual characteristics are male. Prenatal masculinization occurs to varying degrees following exposure of the female fetus to androgens during development, dependent upon the potency of the androgen and the timing of exposure. Alternatively, male pseudohermaphroditism can result from hyposecretion of androgens, defective androgen receptors, or exposure of the male fetus to anti-androgens (such as cyproterone).

Hypospadias

Incomplete fusion of the urethral folds and/or failure of canalization of the glandular plate in male fetuses, possibly as a result of insufficient production of androgens or androgen insensitivity, result in the most common urogenital malformation, hypospadias. The ectopic urethral orifice is usually ventral and proximal to its normal orifice, particularly at the coronal sulci, although penile, penoscrotal, and perineal openings are all possible. The penis is usually underdeveloped

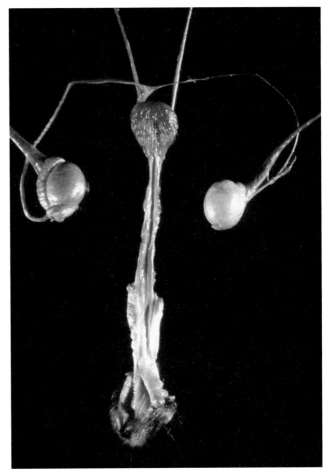

FIGURE 20.11   Male pseudohermaphroditism in a dog. Note testis and epididymus present bilaterally, remnant of paramesonephric (Müllerian) duct (resembling uterus), and poorly developed female external genitalia. (Courtesy of University of Illinois.)

and has a ventral curvature, termed chordee. Exposure of the fetus to exogenous estrogens or endocrine disruptors may produce this lesion (Table 20.6).

Skeletal System

Digit Anomalies

Ectrodactyly, an absence of part or all of a digit, results from interference in normal mesenchymal condensation of digital rays, possibly through failed cell interactions or cytotoxicity. The most common type of ectrodactyly in humans is the split hand or foot, where the middle digits (II and III) are absent. Ectrodactyly is easily induced in rodents following cadmium or acetazolamide administration (Figure 20.12), and in primates thalidomide exposure will repeatedly result in absent digits.

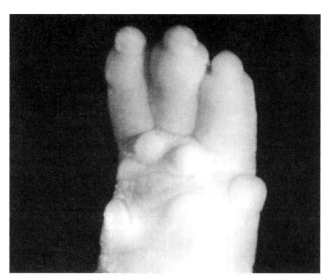

FIGURE 20.12   Ectrodactyly in CD-1 mouse fetus from a dam treated with 9 mg/kg cadmium chloride on gestation day 9. (Courtesy of L.G. MacNabb.)

Syndactyly, a moderately common congenital defect, is due to a lack of differentiation between two digits (interference with programmed cell death that separates digital rays). It is usually cutaneous (webbing), and rarely osseous. In typical split extremities, the remaining digits are syndactylous, and the metacarpals and metatarsals may be reduced. Syndactyly may be associated with other anomalies, such as brachydactyly, ectrodactyly, cleft hand, and angular bands, and is a component of a number of malformation syndromes. Mice receiving hydroxyurea during gestation produce offspring with this defect.

Polydactyly is the name given to the phenomenon of extra fingers or toes. It is a common digital anomaly, resulting from lack of programmed cell death or formation of a supernumerary digital blastema. The extra blastema is formed through changes in the normal composition, configuration, and amount of extracellular matrix of the blastemal cells. The first and fifth digits are most commonly duplicated in humans. X-irradiation, folic acid deficiency, bromodeoxyuridine, cyclophosphamide, and cytosine arabinoside administration can cause murine polydactyly.

Reduction Deformities

Reduction deformities of the extremities vary significantly in severity and frequency. Amelia, absence of the entire upper or lower extremity(ies), has been associated with cleft lip and cleft palate, scoliosis, and

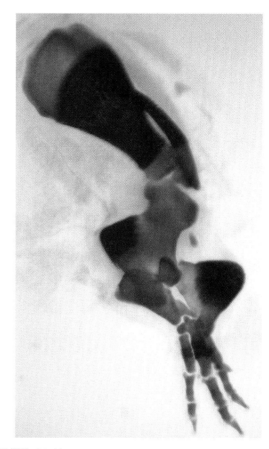

FIGURE 20.13   Forelimb of a CD-1 mouse fetus from a dam treated on gestation day 10.5 with 200 mg/kg all-*trans* retinoic acid. Note the lack of a distinct radius, ulna, and humerus; in their place is a cartilaginous mass, while the digits are essentially normal.

club feet, and may be brachial (absence of the arms), crural (absence of the legs), or both.

Phocomelia, or "seal limbs," characterized by reduction of long-bone development with relatively greater development of the hands or feet, is extremely rare, except in humans and certain primate species following exposure to thalidomide. Rabbits treated with either thalidomide or hydroxyurea can also have this defect. Retinoic acid treatment of mice during pregnancy will produce some offspring with this defect, and others with poorly developed radius and ulna (Figure 20.13).

Hemimelia is the absence of all or part of the distal half of a limb. One of the most common reduction malformations involves the distal forearm and hand. Interference with the development of the limb bud (presumably by disturbance of normal interactions between ectoderm and mesoderm, alteration of morphogen secretion, failed morphogenetic movement, or disturbed inductive processes) produces

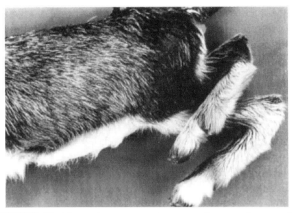

FIGURE 20.14   Arthrogryposis in a goat whose mother was fed lupines throughout gestation.

these reduction deformities. The appearance of normal distal structures and absence of proximal structures, as in phocomelia, suggests an attempt by the limb bud to compensate for the loss of cell mass caused by toxic insult, and to continue with the developmental plan.

Arthrogryposis

Arthrogryposis, persistent flexure or contracture of one or more joints, often accompanied by deformities of the appendicular skeleton, is the most common limb deformity in domestic animals (Figure 20.14). Fibrous ankylosis of the joints, muscular hypoplasia, and denervation atrophy are seen, in conjunction with shortening of the ligaments and lack of loose connective tissue under the skin. When the development of motor neurons and nervous motor pathways in the spinal cord is affected, lack of neuromuscular activation in muscles occurs, with subsequent muscular hypoplasia and arthrogryposis.

Any primary central nervous system lesion affecting axial and appendicular motor pathways may cause arthrogryposis. Both infectious and noninfectious agents can induce the lesion in this manner. Increased intrauterine pressure with mechanical compression of the fetus or paralysis of the fetus may also cause the anomaly.

Although this anomaly is often classified as a skeletal deformity, neurologic, muscular, connective tissue, or skeletal defects or intrauterine crowding can be the cause. It is typically failure of limb movement that produces the abnormal phenotype, not a primary failure of normal skeletal development. *Arthrogryposis multiplex congenita*, multiple joint ankylosis present at birth, is seen in 0.03% of human live births.

A number of plants can induce arthrogryposis in livestock. These plants include *Lupinus sericeus*, *L. caudatus* (calves, lambs, pigs), *Astragalus*, *Lathyrus*,

Oxytropis, *Senecio*, *Sophora*, *Thermopsis*, and *Veratrum* (calves, foals, lambs, pigs). Methallibure and tobacco have caused this problem in pigs. Experimentally-induced arthrogryposis in rodents is rare. Tubocurarine causes this lesion in rats, presumably via fetal paralysis.

DEVELOPMENTAL TOXICITY TESTING AND RISK ASSESSMENT

Hazard Identification and Dose-response Analysis

Hazard identification and dose–response evaluation are the first two steps in the risk assessment process as defined by the National Research Council. The aim of these steps is to assess the adequacy and robustness of the available toxicity data, to determine the degree of confidence that the data warrant. These steps are difficult to separate, as hazard should always be evaluated in the context of the exposure route, dose, timing, and duration.

Default Assumptions

Extrapolation to humans of developmental toxicity data derived from animals is a complex process. General default assumptions that can be made to aid this process have been outlined in the "Guidelines for Developmental Toxicity Risk Assessment" published by the US Environmental Protection Agency in 1991. These default assumptions are as follows:

1. It is assumed that an agent that produces an adverse developmental effect in experimental animal studies will potentially pose a hazard to humans, following sufficient exposure during development;

2. It is assumed that all of the four manifestations of developmental toxicity (death, structural abnormalities, growth alterations, and functional deficits) are of concern;

3. It is assumed that the types of developmental effects seen in animal studies are not necessarily the same as those that may be produced in humans. This assumption is made because it is impossible to determine which will be the most appropriate species in terms of predicting the specific types of effects seen in humans. The fact that every species may not react in the same way could be due to species-specific differences in critical periods, differences in timing of exposure,

metabolism, developmental patterns, placentation, or mechanisms of action;

4. The most appropriate species is used to estimate human risk when data are available (e.g., pharmacokinetics). In the absence of such data, it is assumed that the most sensitive species is appropriate for use, based on observations that humans are as sensitive or more so than the most sensitive animal species tested for the majority of agents known to cause human developmental toxicity; and

5. In general, a threshold is assumed for the dose-response curve for agents that produce developmental toxicity. This is based on the known capacity of the developing organism to compensate for, or to repair, a certain amount of damage at the cellular, tissue, or organ level. In addition, because of the multipotency of cells at certain stages of development, multiple insults at the molecular or cellular level may be required to produce an effect on the whole organism.

Laboratory Animal Studies

Standard prenatal developmental toxicity testing commonly uses one rodent and one non-rodent species, most often the rat and the rabbit, unless other species are deemed more relevant. These animals are treated during the period of organogenesis, although more recent guidelines suggest longer treatment periods, extending until the day of sacrifice (and in some cases starting at the beginning of gestation). Toxicity endpoints are assessed shortly before parturition. Additional studies employing exposure from before mating through gestation, or during late gestation and lactation, are also often employed. Developmental neurotoxicity tests require continuous treatment from implantation through parturition until weaning, and assess abnormal postnatal behavior.

As in any identification procedure in risk assessment, the route of exposure of a test substance should parallel the likely route of exposure in the target species. This is especially true in developmental toxicity tests, because the effects of some compounds are influenced by administration route.

Evaluation of Maternal Toxicity

A variety of endpoints can be employed in assessing the health status of the dam. These include clinical signs, food and water consumption, target organ weights, and histopathology. Maternal weight gain is an important parameter; both weight gain during treatment, and comparison of weight at mating with that at termination (minus the gravid uterus, to avoid bias due to different litter sizes). When treatment begins before mating, fertility endpoints are useful, and if the test includes parturition, changes in its timing can be instructive. Most maternal endpoints are rather crude measures of toxicity, however, and this is especially true of weight gain in rabbits, which often varies greatly for reasons unrelated to treatment.

Evaluation of Developmental Toxicity

The developmental endpoints include litter size, fetal weight, prenatal mortality (as evidenced by the presence of resorptions and dead fetuses), sex ratio, and presence of variations and malformations. In tests that involve parturition and lactation, birth weight, as well as perinatal mortality, weight gain, clinical signs, and histopathology can be added. Since the approved protocol for the prenatal developmental toxicity study calls for dosing throughout organogenesis, the test is a fairly good one for evaluating the potential for developmental toxicity, but it is not efficient at inducing malformations. Malformations are more readily elicited by high-dose, short-term exposures, while effects such as prenatal death and growth retardation tend to predominate following the lower-dose, longer-term exposures used in the required tests.

It is most important to note that the appropriate experimental unit in developmental toxicology experiments is the litter. Not using this experimental unit and combining all defects in a treatment group increases the likelihood of obtaining false positive results, as it increases the likelihood of interference by intra-litter effects. Thus, the dam or litter is most often used as the experimental unit, because of the environment and inheritance shared among littermates. For this reason, if a dosage group contains 1 litter with 10 malformed rodent or rabbit fetuses among 10 normal litters, that occurrence is of less concern than 10 such litters, 5 of which contain 2 defective fetuses each. The total number of abnormal fetuses is the same, but the likelihood of a real treatment effect is much greater in the latter case.

Determination of the significance of teratogenicity test results can be difficult. A substance that causes minor depression in birth weight, or an increase in developmental variants (e.g., extra lumbar ribs, enlarged cerebral ventricles, or dilated renal pelves), is more difficult to assess for potential hazard to the target species than one that induces major malformations at relevant dosage levels. We also recognize that embryolethality may mask teratogenicity; therefore, embryolethality should be considered an important endpoint from that consideration, as well as for prediction of embryonic or fetal wastage.

Examination of the standard teratogenicity testing endpoints, such as gross skeletal and soft tissue malformations, is time-consuming and requires technical expertise. The Chernoff–Kavlock test has been suggested as an alternative. This test originally involved exposure of pregnant mice during the period of organogenesis to test compounds at doses at or near the lowest observable adverse effect level (LOAEL) for maternal toxicity, followed by assessment of viability and growth of offspring to three days of age. Reduced postnatal viability or decreased growth indicates prenatal toxicity. This test has the advantage of being a relatively rapid and simple *in vivo* screen. Later modifications have included use of rats rather than mice, additional dose levels, extended treatment periods, and treatment of both male and female parents. Extending the postnatal observation period can increase the sensitivity of the test, and continuing maternal dosing after parturition can reveal perinatal toxicity, including effects of agents transmitted via the milk.

Animal Models

Rodents

Small size, short gestation, large litter size, ease in breeding, low cost, and ready availability, make rodents particularly useful in initial mammalian screening tests for developmental toxicity. Both mice and rats are used extensively; however, rats have the advantage of producing larger fetuses for evaluation by analytical procedures. Inbred mice have a high incidence of strain-specific malformations (e.g., cCBA/J, C57B/6J, A/J, Ch, and JCl:lCh mouse strains show high incidence of ectrodactyly, an anomaly produced by acetazolamide administration on day 9 or 10 of pregnancy). Other strains, such as the SWV and Crl:CD-1, are very robust. This means that certain inbred strains of mice are available for investigation of specific effects of genotype on susceptibility to some substances. Hamsters are routinely used in some institutions for teratology studies. The golden Syrian hamster is the common type of hamster used for teratogenicity testing. Data are available for rates of spontaneous anomalies in numerous strains and species of rodents.

Rodents and lagomorphs (rabbits and guinea pigs) depend on an "inverted" yolk sac placenta for nutrition until mid-gestation. Therefore, exposure of their embryos to xenobiotics may sometimes give results different from those of other species. Also, if effects of prenatal exposure on functional maturity of certain organ systems (e.g., the central nervous system) must be simulated, postnatal exposure of rodent pups is necessary, since these offspring are more immature at birth than are humans.

Rabbits

Rabbits are the non-rodent species of choice in teratogenicity testing, because of their large size, which provides ample samples for analysis, and accuracy in timing of conception. Although certain rabbit strains manifest malformations similar to those of humans when exposed to thalidomide, they do not appear to be superior to other models in predicting the human response to most developmental toxicants.

Nonhuman Primates

Similarities in maternal metabolism of xenobiotics, placental structure, and reproductive physiology, especially anatomic and temporal aspects of early embryogenesis, suggest that nonhuman primates are an appropriate species for teratogenicity testing. In spite of these similarities, however, differences in sensitivities to teratogens in humans and nonhuman primates are not uncommon, as is seen for methotrexate. The high expense and low availability of certain species of primate, long gestational period, gestation of single offspring, and social issues often preclude the use of nonhuman primates in teratogenicity testing.

Other Mammalian Species

Other species, such as ferrets, guinea pigs, swine, dogs, and cats have been used to a limited extend in developmental toxicity studies. However, characteristics such as size, cost, difficulty in handling, long gestation period, lack of a historical database, lack of any obvious predictive superiority, or relatively lower social acceptability limit their use.

The use of chick embryos for the screening of developmental toxicants has the advantage of a readily available model with a short developmental period, as well as low cost. However, in the strictest sense, chick embryos are not an example of *in vivo* testing, since exposure is *in ovo*, and maternal pharmacokinetic factors play no role in this system.

Although the chick is useful in studying the progression of abnormal development, its relatively high sensitivity to exogenous agents, and significant differences in embryogenesis among avian and mammalian species, preclude the use of chickens in standard developmental toxicity testing. Nevertheless, the chick remains useful for certain types of mechanistic studies.

Human Studies

Epidemiological studies are often used in attempts to identify developmental toxicants, or to confirm or deny evidence from animal studies. In some cases, they have proven very useful in this regard (e.g., anticonvulsants, maternal smoking), but they also have serious limitations.

Unfortunately, human studies cannot prove causality, although they can provide evidence for associations if confounding variables and bias are adequately controlled. Epidemiological studies have poor sensitivity. They can detect only relatively potent developmental toxicants against the normal background of fetal abnormalities, unless the agent in question causes a rather unique effect that is normally relatively rare. They are also limited by the inability to recognize and control all variables. In addition, often the study population must be large to allow detection of an effect, but such populations of exposed and control individuals may be difficult or impossible to obtain. Finally, by the nature of societal living, accurate exposure data are typically difficult or impossible to obtain.

Nevertheless, epidemiological studies have proven valuable in a number of instances in identifying or exonerating putative human developmental toxicants and infectious agents. Examples of detected agents include the aforementioned anticonvulsants and smoking, along with others, such as methyl mercury, maternal alcohol abuse, and rubella infection.

Maternal Versus Developmental Toxicity

The effect of maternal toxicity on the developing fetus is a question that has received much attention. In most test species, maternal toxicity can have profound effects on development of the embryo or fetus. How this effect results in abnormal development is not known. Several hypotheses have been suggested to explain this phenomenon including: failed maternal support of the embryo or fetus (e.g., hypoxia); production of nonspecific toxic material following maternal toxicity (e.g., change in embryonic pH); or modification of the intensity of the effects of the toxicant (e.g., changes in maternal metabolism).

Maternal toxicity can influence the effect of *in vivo* testing for teratogenicity. The question still exists: to what dose should the dam be exposed? Mild embryolethality and nonspecific fetotoxic effects seen with doses at which dams are clinically showing signs of overt toxicity are of problematic significance in extrapolation to low-dose effects in other species.

Maternally-mediated effects on development are adverse effects that occur secondarily, because of some effect on the pregnant mother. They differ from direct effects on the conceptus primarily in their immediate source, rather than their end result. Because the number of mechanisms for maternally-mediated effects is almost certainly lower than the number of direct-acting mechanisms, the range of consequences to the offspring may also be more limited. Nevertheless, maternally-mediated effects can apparently occur by any of several mechanisms, so it is unlikely that they would all result in only a single limited spectrum of effects on the offspring.

The potential for maternally-mediated effects also makes the task of extrapolating from animal data to potential human outcomes more difficult. The conceptus and its maternal support system present a special situation in toxicology and risk assessment. Because of the dependence of the conceptus on the nurturing maternal environment, factors disturbing that environment may adversely affect the offspring's development. It must also be recognized, however, that the maternal organism offers a degree of protection against at least some environmental perturbations.

It is well-known that some fetal disruptions can be maternally-mediated, but questions remain regarding the kinds of effects produced, their prevalence, and their significance. Fetal variations, malformations, functional alterations, and deaths can result from direct effects on the fetus, indirect (maternally-mediated) effects, or a combination of the two. There has sometimes been a lack of concern with regard to the potential of maternally-mediated effects to impact study outcome. The converse can also happen, however, in that some seem to consider any effects on the conceptus that are seen only at maternally toxic doses to be secondary to the maternal toxicity, even in the absence of supporting evidence. A more reasonable approach is to have concern about evidence of developmental toxicity, whether or not there is concurrent maternal toxicity, unless it is known that humans (or other species to be protected) would not be similarly affected.

Short-term Tests

Although so-called *"in vitro* screens" (i.e., tests not using a pregnant mammal) for developmental toxicity may prove useful in prioritizing chemicals for further testing, they are not meant to entirely substitute for *"in vivo"* testing. Also, to date, none have been fully "validated," that is, proven to give reproducible results sufficiently similar to the results of *in vivo* tests and human data.

Effects of possible environmental developmental toxicants on aquatic vertebrates have been assessed by means of a standardized assay using *Xenopus laevis* (South African clawed frog). However, in intra- and inter-laboratory comparisons, this assay (FETAX) has not yet generally shown adequate reproducibility and repeatability. Mammalian *ex vivo* testing for safety of compounds has not gained regulatory acceptance.

Advantages of *in vitro* over *in vivo* teratogenicity testing systems include their rapidity, decreased cost, and decreased numbers of laboratory animals used to obtain initial screening data. Unfortunately, the lack of specific response, altered pharmacokinetics (compared with *in vivo* exposure), and questionable applicability to the target species often render interpretation of their results problematic. Perhaps with the refinement of physiologically-based pharmacokinetic modeling, and selected exposure times relevant to the model, some *in vitro* methods may have more applicability.

Nevertheless, *in vitro* teratogenicity tests can be useful for studying mechanisms of both abnormal and normal development, and for preliminary screens of structurally-related compounds. Excellent control, removal of maternal effects, and the ability to observe developmental changes over time make these methods excellent tools for investigating basic questions in molecular teratology.

Other Considerations

Pharmacokinetics and Pharmacodynamics

Pharmacokinetic parameters are important determinants of developmental toxicity, as is the case with other toxic effects, but are further complicated by the fact that two different organisms are involved, mother and conceptus. Maternal uptake, biotransformation, transfer to and from the embryo/fetus, and elimination are critical parameters influencing effects on the offspring.

Maternal pharmacokinetics follow the same principles as are operative in other adults, with the exception of changes in certain parameters, such as fluid volumes, blood flow to specific organs (e.g., the uterus), and serum protein levels. Rates of transplacental transfer of toxicants and embryo/fetal sequestration or metabolism are possible additional factors, as noted in the earlier section on placental transfer. Regardless of our pharmacokinetic knowledge and abilities, knowledge of the pharmacodynamics (expression of the toxic effect) of specific agents on test species is typically lacking, but would be highly useful in allowing extrapolation from animal models to humans.

Structure-activity Relationships

A limited number of attempts have been made to predict developmental toxicity using the chemical structure of the test compound. Most published studies have compared relative toxicities among closely-related compounds within a chemical class, such as phenols, glycol ethers, or retinoids. Our ability to develop widely applicable predictive models is hampered, however, by several considerations.

A lack of uniform, reliable data that can be used to classify the developmental toxicity status of compounds used as the basis for model development hinders the use of structure-activity predictions. Combined with this lack of data, there is only a modest (though improving) current level of understanding of the mechanisms underlying developmentally toxic effects. This situation is partly due to the complexity of developmental toxicity, with its numerous endpoints and mechanistic bases.

Dose–Response Evaluation

If human dose–response data are available, they should be assessed along with the animal data. Evidence of a dose response is critical for identification of developmental toxicants, especially since sporadic malformations and fluctuations in the incidence of variations and prenatal deaths can occur, even in the absence of treatment effects.

Most known human developmental toxicants affect the conceptus at exposure levels at or near the maternally toxic level. This implies similar sensitivity of mother and offspring, but it could also result from our inability to identify developmental toxicants that cause only modest increases in the incidences of outcomes relatively common in the baseline population. The effects of such weak developmental toxicants would be difficult or impossible to detect against the background level of adverse fetal outcomes, and thus would typically go unnoticed.

Traditionally in animal studies, the no observable adverse effect level (NOAEL) and lowest observable adverse effect level (LOAEL) are identified, usually based on statistical tests. Dose selection is of paramount importance to make these endpoints of use in predicting the risk of developmental toxicity. In addition, the presence of dose-related increases in variations lends support to a finding that an effect may be compound-related.

With regard to developmental toxicity data, it is recognized that biological significance is a critical consideration. The evaluator must exercise judgement, rather than blindly accepting the results of statistical analyses, whether positive or negative.

An apparent improvement over the use of the NOAEL/LOAEL approach is the use of mathematical modeling to calculate the benchmark dose (BMD). The BMD approach makes use of the entirety of the data, and it accounts for data variability. The BMD is defined as the lower confidence limit on a dose that produces a particular level of response, e.g., 1%, 5%, or 10%.

The Reference Dose or Reference Concentration

Because of the assumption that there is an exposure threshold for most developmental toxicity endpoints below which no effect will occur, the types of low-dose extrapolation used for analysis of carcinogenicity data are not typically used. A reference dose or reference concentration for developmental toxicity (RfD_{DT} or RfC_{DT}) can be calculated instead. These are estimates of the daily exposure to the human population that is assumed to be without appreciable risk of deleterious developmental effects. Dividing the NOAEL or the BMD for the most sensitive endpoint by uncertainty factors derives the RfD_{DT} or RfC_{DT}. A drawback of this approach, however, is that it does not estimate risk at any given exposure level above the RfD_{DT} or RfC_{DT}.

Risk Characterization

Developmental toxicity risk characterization must take into account in both toxicity evaluation and exposure assessment. The complexity of the developing system, its interaction with the pregnant mother, and the multiple endpoints evaluated often result in toxicity data that are not easily interpreted. Thus, it is especially important that experienced experts in the field evaluate such data. All available evidence, and the reliability of that evidence, in terms of both quality and quantity (completeness), must be considered in a weight-of-evidence approach. In the future, biologically-based dose-response models, grounded in the knowledge of developmental toxicity mechanisms, may allow for more accurate estimates of low-dose risk to humans or other species of concern.

In summary, fetal toxicologic pathology contributes to the risk assessment process, since the developing conceptus is sometimes the biologic system most sensitive to xenobiotic exposure. The complexity of developmental processes, interactions between genotype and xenobiotic, and functional or morphologic manifestations of such toxicity make assessment of risk to the offspring difficult. To date, hazard identification of new developmentally-toxic xenobiotics, and development of new tests for prenatal toxicity, have predominated in this field of research. However, with our expanding understanding of the mechanistic processes that produce developmental defects, we should be increasingly able to predict, and avoid or ameliorate, such effects of toxic substances.

FIELD INVESTIGATION OF ANOMALIES IN DOMESTIC ANIMALS

Identification of the cause of spontaneous abnormal development can be a problem in domestic animals.

This section provides some guidance in determining the etiology of abnormal development in domestic animals, using the bovine as an example. The method that follows requires examination of one variable at a time, while keeping other variables constant (Figure 20.15). The process starts by defining the developmental anomaly and, in particular, the time of development at which normal development ceased. If an etiology is not evident at this stage, it is necessary to determine the number of affected individuals, so as to evaluate the extent of the problem. If this appears to be a herd or flock problem then genetic analyses, descriptive epidemiology, "natural" experiments, and the experimental methods of epidemiology are used to elucidate the cause. This investigative approach may require interaction between pathologists, geneticists, cytogeneticists, epidemiologists, and statisticians.

Defining the Individual Incident

Clinical Examination and Pathology

Clinical and, if possible, postmortem examination of a defective animal are essential to define the

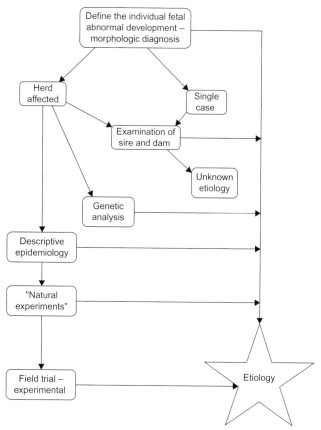

FIGURE 20.15 Flow chart outlining a methodological approach to defining the cause of abnormal fetal development.

abnormality, and to ascertain the time of gestation that normal development ceased. Postmortem examination enables recording these defects in a thorough, standardized fashion.

Characterization of the defects sometimes reveals the etiology immediately, as some defects are pathognomonic for a given defective gene or environmental agent, e.g., periodic acid-Schiff (PAS)-positive accumulations in neurons and other tissues, in conjunction with depression of plasma alpha-mannosidase activity, are characteristic of mannosidosis, an autosomal recessive trait in Angus cattle. Similarly, as has been previously mentioned, cyclopia in a number of lambs indicates probable prior maternal ingestion of *Veratrum californicum* during the sensitive gestational period of 13½ days after conception. Unfortunately, not all defects are associated with a specific etiology, as often the same morphologic defects can arise via a common pathway of abnormal development, even though the initial event of abnormal development was different, e.g., arthrogryposis.

Estimating the time of cessation of normal development may give important clues to whether the anomaly has a genetic or environmental basis. If a teratogen is suspected, knowledge of the time of exposure may help to elucidate a past infection (e.g., bovine viral diarrhea (BVD)), past exposure to a toxic plant, or some other environmental insult that can be traced back to that time.

Ancillary Testing

If the morphology does not indicate the etiology, routine bacteriology, virology, and mycology should be undertaken to eliminate the possibility of infectious agents, such as bovine viral diarrhea (BVD), as the causative agent. Examination of the liver and other organs for trace elements may provide further clues as to etiology, e.g., enzootic ataxia (hypomyelinogenesis) in copper-deficient lambs, and arthrogryposis in manganese-deficient calves. Finally, karyotyping of the fetus can be done using lymphocytes from whole blood, if the fetus is alive, or cultured fibroblasts taken from the pericardial sac or kidney at postmortem.

Defining the Prevalence

Genetic disorders occur in families, whereas teratogens usually affect multiple individuals in the herd or flock in a non-familial pattern, and may have a seasonal occurrence. If more than one abnormal fetus is reported, the crude prevalence of anomalous fetuses, abortions, and stillbirths in the herd or flock should be calculated for the gestational period in question. The prevalence is equal to the number of anomalies, abortions, or stillbirths observed at birth, divided by the total number of births. Percentages make comparison of prevalences between two groups easier.

Prevalence measures anomalies at birth, but does not include defective fetuses that are not carried through to term; thus, the real prevalence of abnormalities is probably higher than reported. A separate calculation of the prevalence of stillbirths and abortions is extremely important, since prevalence at birth calculations do not factor in losses due to preterm abortions. These calculations of prevalence should be combined with the prevalence of anomalies, if the prevalence of abortions and stillbirths is greater than normal. Knowledge of the crude prevalence of anomalies, abortions, and stillbirths not only documents how severe the problem is, but also gives an idea as to whether the anomalies are part of a bigger problem involving early abortions, resorptions, and later stillbirths.

Defining the Maternal Environment

If clinical examination, ancillary testing, and prevalence studies fail to establish a cause, clinical evaluation of the individual may be indicated to identify overt disease during pregnancy, alterations in normal homeostatic functions, or chronic disease. Examination of herd records and production figures may provide clues to subclinical disease in the herd. Reproduction history of the individual that produced the anomalous fetus is particularly important. Such a history should include information on previous abortions, failure to conceive, early abortions, previous malformations, and the sire that produced the malformed offspring.

Ancillary testing of the dam is often limited, but may include serological examination of paired serum samples taken at two-week intervals from members of the herd, as well as microbiological examination of reproductive tracts to evaluate for previous or current infection with a teratogenic infectious agent, such as BVD, akabane virus, blue tongue virus, and hog cholera virus. Karyotyping of the dam to determine the presence of chromosomal aberrations can be done using whole blood. Urine and blood enzyme levels are sometimes useful in making a diagnosis in some inherited storage diseases, whereas serum hormonal levels and trace elements may be of limited use.

Limited examination of the sire can be undertaken, and this should include examination of semen for sperm morphology and abnormalities, karyotyping and, if the epidemiological picture warrants, analysis of the semen for heavy metals, as semen contaminated with some heavy metals has been shown to be teratogenic. In domestic animals, the origin of developmental anomalies can rarely be attributed to the sire.

Genetic Analysis

Genetic analysis of a herd requires enumeration of the normal and defective animals, and each of their relationships. Hence, attempts to develop a pedigree should be undertaken, even if an extended pedigree is not available.

Environmental Analysis: An Epidemiological Approach

If there are no obvious genetic or environmental causes of abnormal development, and the crude prevalence indicates that a herd problem exists, then a more detailed examination of the herd environment, and herd dynamics, is required. Descriptive epidemiology, "natural" experiments (associations between risk factor and effect), and the experimental method are the three basic types of epidemiological investigation which are useful in herds where anomalous development is a problem with moderate prevalence, without obvious etiology.

Descriptive Epidemiology

The purpose of descriptive epidemiology is to portray the herd environment, and to look for patterns of occurrence within the herd. Herd records are used to identify risk factors, and stratified analysis is used to help determine if associations exist among these risk factors, strata, and the occurrence of developmental anomalies.

The herd environment should be carefully described, so that risk factors can be identified following closer inspection. Information gathered should include breed affected, age of parents, geographic region, type of pasture, soil type, water source, feeding and management practices, maternal medication and vaccination records, disease status of the herd, periods of stress, handling procedures, and congenital defects observed in previous years. Time of pregnancy diagnosis should be noted, as *atresia ani* has been associated with this practice. Possible exposure to teratogenic plants or toxicants (e.g., in discarded batteries, chemical dump sites, air or water pollutants) should be established, as any of these factors can be considered a risk factor. Any history of similar congenital defects occurring in neighboring herds is noteworthy.

Examination of these risk factors may lead to identification of the possible etiology.

A stratified analysis of the data involves subdividing risk factors into strata. This stratification allows one to better assess the relevance of each risk factor (e.g., age of dam). The prevalence of anomalies is then calculated for each stratum. Examination of the difference in prevalence of anomalies among strata can help one generate hypotheses about the etiology.

All risk factors are potential candidates for stratification. Construction of simple tables and graphs comparing strata may be all that is necessary to demonstrate obvious differences between strata. To demonstrate whether there are any differences among risk factors, a contingency table approach can be used. If more than one variable or risk factor is implicated by the stratified analysis, e.g., dam age and access to the dumpsite, confounding effects and interactions may be a problem. The use of multivariate analyses is required in such situations.

"Natural" Experiments

During the examination of herd records, one should carefully look for "natural" experiments. Here, the investigator has not actually performed a controlled experiment where all risk factors except one are controlled. Instead, two or more subgroups within the herd can be identified which, by circumstance, were treated identically, except for one risk factor. The prevalence of congenital anomalies is determined for each group. The differences between these calculated prevalences may suggest an association between the risk factor and the congenital defects. John Snow's investigation of a cholera epidemic in London in 1854 is a classic example of a natural experiment. Snow recognized that two randomly-mixed populations, alike in other important respects, could be differentiated by the source of tap water in their individual houses. Two water companies provided water for London: Lambeth Company, with water taken from the Thames River well above London; and Southwark and Vauxhall company, which took water downstream from the sewage-polluted river basin. The mortality associated with cholera was almost ten-fold higher in the houses supplied by Southwark and Vauxhall. Snow's work clearly demonstrated the importance of water supply, even though the precise nature of the disease agent had not yet been established.

A thorough attempt to establish that the two groups defined by the natural experiment were treated similarly except for the risk factor of interest is very important, but often difficult. If a second factor is also identified, examination of the primary and interactive effects of the second factor becomes necessary.

If natural experiments do exist, conclusions regarding cause and effect are risky, as retrospective analysis of herd records only reveals associations. However, recognition of a natural experiment may be the only way that an association between defect and risk factor can be made. In herds where the problem is ongoing, an even more powerful investigative tool exists and should be used: the experimental method.

Experimental Methodology

Descriptive epidemiology, or the recognition of a natural experiment, may provide a hypothesis as to etiology. These methods are retrospective in nature, and cannot be controlled. In addition, records are rarely complete, or if they are, different terminology and data collection can make comparisons between groups in a natural experiment difficult.

The experimental method is the most powerful tool in defining the etiology of recurring developmental anomalies. The basic approach of the applied experimental method is to take one or two of the most likely hypotheses and test them one at a time on part of the herd, using other untreated animals as controls. It is important to randomly select individuals to remove sample bias. If the herd is large, it may be divided into a number of groups, allowing for the simultaneous testing of more than one hypothesis, but this depends on the prevalence of the anomalies. For example, the herd could be divided into four groups: old animals with access to suspected toxicant; young animals with access to suspected toxicant; old animals with no access; and young animals with no access. Developmental anomalies of low prevalence require larger sized groups. Usually, a prevalence of 25% will allow a group size of 50 animals, depending on the variability of expression of the defect.

Records at the termination of the experiment (the next calving season) should include reproductive problems, abortions, stillbirths, and anomalies. Statistical tests to determine if the differences between test and control groups are statistically significant can be used. A statistical difference in the prevalence of anomalies between the two groups is evidence that the risk factor tested is the cause of the anomalies. It should be remembered that lack of statistical significance does not necessarily "disprove" associations among groups, as this often occurs in low prevalence situations with inadequately-sized test and control groups. With proper randomization and care in treating the two groups similarly, a statistical difference in the prevalence of anomalies between two groups is evidence that the risk factor tested is the cause of the anomalies.

In summary, identification of the etiology of developmental anomalies is often extremely difficult, for many reasons. First, defective development alone often does not give clues to a specific cause. Second, specific teratogens such as viruses, plants and toxins, often cannot be demonstrated at the time of expulsion of the defective fetus, or even after intensive pathological and toxicologic investigations. Third, except for certain chromosomal aberrations, hereditary factors are recognized only when they occur in characteristic intra-generational familial frequencies and patterns. Therefore, when a cause cannot be demonstrated, attempts to determine patterns of occurrence must be undertaken. The method described provides a stepwise protocol to determine etiology.

FURTHER READING

Cooke, P.S., Peterson, R.E., and Hess, R.A. (2002). Endocrine disruptors. In *Handbook of Toxicologic Pathology* (Haschek, W.M., Rousseaux, C.G., and Wallig, M.A. eds), Vol. I, pp. 501–528. Academic Press, San Diego, CA.

Edelman, G.M. (1988). *Topobiology: An Introduction to Molecular Embryology*. Basic Books, New York, NY.

Gilbert-Barness, E., Kapur, R., Oligny, L. L. and Siebert, J. (eds) (2007) *Potter's Pathology of the Fetus, Infant and Child*, 2nd edn, Mosby.

Hansen, D.K. and Abbott, B.D. (2009) *Developmental Toxicology*, 3rd Edn, Informa HealthCare.

Homburger, F., and Goldberg, A.M. (1985). *In Vitro Embryotoxicity and Teratogenicity Tests*. Karger, Basel, Switzerland.

Hood, R.D. (ed.) (2006). *Developmental and Reproductive Toxicology: A Practical Approach*. 2nd Edn, CRC Press, Raton, FL.

Hood, R.D., Rousseaux, C.G. and Blakeley, P.M. (2002). Embryo and fetus. In: *Handbook of Toxicologic Pathology*, 2nd edn, (Haschek, W.M., Rousseaux, C.G. and Wallig, M.A. eds.) Vol 2, pp. 895–936. Academic Press, San Diego.

Juchau, M. (ed.) (1981). *The Biochemical Basis of Chemical Teratogenesis*. Elsevier/North Holland, New York, NY.

Kimmel, G.L., and Kochhar, D.M. (eds) (1990). *Vitro Methods in Developmental Toxicology: Use in Defining Mechanisms and Risk Parameters*. CRC Press, Boca Raton, FL.

Korach, K.S. (1998). *Reproductive and Developmental Toxicity*. Marcel Dekker, New York, NY.

Martínez-Frías, M.-L., Frías, J.L., and Opitz, J.M. (1998). Errors of morphogenesis and developmental field theory. *Am. J. Med. Genet.*, 76, 291–296.

Rogers, J.M. and Kavlock, R.J. (2008). Developmental toxicology. In: *Casarett and Doull's Toxicology. The Basic Science of Poisons*, 7th edn, (Klaasen C.D., ed.) pp. 415–451. McGraw-Hill, New York.

Schardein, J. (2000) *Chemically Induced Birth Defects*, 3rd Edn, Informa HealthCare.

Scialli, A.R. (1992). *A Clinical Guide to Reproductive and Developmental Toxicology*. CRC Press, Boca Raton, FL.

Shupe, J.L., and James, J.F. (1983). Teratogenic plants. *Vet. Hum. Toxicol.*, 415–421.

Szabo, K.T. (1989). *Congenital Malformations in Laboratory and Farm Animals*. Academic Press, Toronto, Canada.

US Environmental Protection Agency (1991). Guidelines for developmental toxicity risk assessment; *Notice. Fed. Reg.* 56, 63798–63826.

Wilson, J.G. (1973). *Environment and Birth Defects*. Academic Press, New York, NY.

GLOSSARY

Ablepharia Reduction or absence of the eyelids, with continuous skin covering the eyes.

Abrachia Absence of the arms (**forelimbs**).

Acampsia Rigidity or inflexibility of a joint (**ankylosis**).

Acardia Absence of the heart.

Acaudia, acaudate Without a tail (**anury**).

Acephaly Agenesis of the head (**acephalia**).

Acheiria Congenital absence of one or both hands (**forepaws**).

Achondroplasia Skeletal dysplasia, resulting in short limbs and other defects, due to abnormal cartilage.

Acorea Absence of the pupil of the eye.

Acrania Partial or complete absence of the cranium.

Acystia Absence of the urinary bladder.

Adactyly Absence of digits.

Agenesis Lack of development of an organ.

Aglossia Absence of the tongue.

Agnathia Absence of the lower jaw (**mandible**).

Agyria Small brain lacking the normal convolutions of the cerebral cortex (**lissencephaly**).

Amastia Absence of the mammae (**breasts**).

Amelia Absence of a limb or limbs (**see also ectromelia**).

Ametria Absence of the uterus.

Anasarca Generalized edema.

Anencephaly Absence of cranial vault, with the brain missing or greatly reduced.

Anephrogenesis Absence of kidney(s).

Aniridia Absence of the iris.

Anisomelia Inequality between paired limbs.

Ankyloglossia Partial or complete adhesion of the tongue to the floor of the mouth.

Ankylosis Abnormal fixation of a joint; implies bone fusion.

Anodontia Absence of some or all of the teeth.

Anonchia Absence of some or all of the nails.

Anophthalmia Absent or vestigial eye(s).

Anorchism Uni- or bilateral absence of the testes (**anorchia**).

Anostosis Defective development of bone; failure to ossify.

Anotia Absence of the external ear(s) (**i.e., pinnae, auricles**).

Anovarism Absence of the ovaries (**anovaria**).

Anury see Acaudia.

Aphakia Absence of the eye lens.

Aphalangia Absence of a digit or of one or more phalanges.

Aplasia see Agenesis.

Apodia Absence of one or both of the feet (**paws**).

Aprosopia Partial or complete absence of the face.

Arachnodactyly Abnormal length and slenderness of the digits—"spider-like."

Arrhinencephaly Congenital absence or hypoplasia of the brain's olfactory lobe, and incomplete external olfactory organ development (**arhinencephaly**).

Arrhinia Absence of the nose.

Arthrogryposis Persistent flexure or contracture of a joint.

Arthrogryposis multiplex congenita Syndrome distinguished by congenital fixation of the joints and muscle hypoplasia.

Asplenia Absence of the spleen.

Astomia Absence of the opening of the mouth.

Atelectasis Incomplete expansion of a fetal lung or a portion of the lung at birth.

Athelia Absence of the nipple(s).

Athymism Absence of the thymus (**Athymia**).

Atresia Congenital absence of a normally patent lumen or closure of a normal body opening.

Atresia ani Agenesis or closure of the anal opening (**imperforate anus**).

Atrial septal defect Postnatal communication between the atria.

Bifid tongue Cleft tongue.

Bipartite Division of what is normally a single structure into two parts; usually refers to areas of skeletal ossification.

Brachydactyly Abnormal shortness of digits.

Brachygnathia Abnormal shortness of the mandible.

Brachyury Abnormally short tail.

Buphthalmos Enlargement and distension of the fibrous coats of the eye; congenital glaucoma (**buphthalmia, buphthalmus**).

Camptodactyly Permanent flexion of one or more digits (**camptodactylia**).

Carpal flexure Abnormal flexion of the fetal carpus (**wrist**); most often seen in the rabbit; may be transient or permanent.

Celoschisis Congenital fissure of the abdominal wall.

Celosomia Fissure or absence of the sternum, with visceral herniation.

Cephalocele Protrusion of part of the brain through the cranium.

Cleft face Clefting due to incomplete fusion of the embryonic facial primordia.

Cleft lip Cleft or defect in the upper lip (**hare lip**).

Cleft palate Fissure or cleft in the bony palate (**palatoschisis**).

Clinodactyly Permanent lateral or medial deviation of one or more fingers.

Club foot see Talipes.

Coarctation A stricture or stenosis, usually of the aorta.

Coloboma Fissure or incomplete development of the eye.

Conceptus Everything that develops from the fertilized egg, including the embryo/fetus and the extraembryonic membranes.

Craniorachischisis Fissure of the skull and vertebral column.

Cranioschisis Congenital cranial fissure.

Craniosynostosis Premature ossification of cranial sutures.

Craniostenosis Premature cessation of cranial growth because of craniosynostosis.

Cryptorchidism Failure of one or both testes to enter the scrotum (**cryptorchism**).

Cyclopia Fusion of the orbits into a single orbit, with the nose absent or present as a tubular appendage (**proboscis**) above the orbit.

Delayed ossification Incomplete mineralization of an otherwise normal ossification center.

Dextrocardia Abnormal displacement of the heart to the right.

Diaphragmatic hernia Protrusion of abdominal viscera through a defect in the diaphragm.

Dicephalus Conjoined twins with two heads and one body.

Diplomyelia Complete or incomplete doubling of the spinal cord, due to a longitudinal fissure.

Diplopagus Symmetrically-duplicated conjoined twins, with largely complete bodies that may share some internal organs.

Diprosopus A fetus with partial duplication of the face.

Dysarthrosis Malformation of a joint.

Dysgenesis Defective development.

Dysplasia An abnormal organization of cells into tissue(s) and its morphologic result (s); abnormality of histiogenesis.

Dysraphism Failure of fusion, especially of the neural folds (**dysraphia**).

Dystocia Prolonged, abnormal, or difficult delivery.

Ectopia Displacement or malposition.

Ectopia cordis Displacement of the heart outside of the thoracic cavity.

Ectopic kidney Abnormal position of one or both kidneys.

Ectopic pregnancy Pregnancy occurring outside the uterine cavity.

Ectrodactyly Absence of all or only part of one or more digits.

Ectromelia Hypoplasia or absence of one or more limbs.

Ectropion Abnormal eversion of the margin of the eyelid.

Encephalocele Herniation of part of the brain, encased in meninges, through an opening in the skull (**encephalomeningocele, meningoencephalocele**).

Endocardial cushion defect Heart defects resulting from incomplete fusion of the embryonic endocardial cushions (**AV canal defect**).

Entropion Abnormal inversion of the margin of the eyelid.

Epispadias Absence of the upper wall of the urethra; more common in males, where it opens on the dorsal surface of the penis.

Eventration Protrusion of bowels through the abdominal wall.

Exencephaly Defective development of the cranium resulting in extrusion of the brain through the defective skull.

Exomphalos see Omphalocele (**umbilical hernia**).

Exophthalmos Abnormal protrusion of the eyeball (**exophthalmus**).

Exostosis Abnormal bony growth projecting outward from the surface of a bone.

Exstrophy Congenital eversion of a hollow organ, e.g., of the bladder.

Fetal wastage Postimplantation death of embryo or fetus.

Fetus The developing mammal from the completion of major organogenesis to birth.

Gastroschisis Fissure of the abdominal wall, usually to the right of the umbilicus and involving protrusion of viscera.

Glossoptosis Retraction or downward displacement of the tongue.

Gonadal dysgenesis General term for various abnormalities of gonadal development, e.g., gonadal aplasia, hermaphroditism, "streak gonads."

Hamartoma A benign nodular or tumor-like mass, resulting from faulty embryonal development of cells and tissues natural to the part.

Hemimelia Absence of all or part of the distal half of a limb.

Hemivertebra Incomplete development of one side of a vertebra.

Hermaphrodite An individual with both male and female gonadal tissue (*see also* **pseudohermaphrodite**).

Heterotopia The development of a normal tissue in an abnormal location.

Holocardius A grossly-defective monozygotic twin whose circulation is dependent on the heart of a more perfect twin.

Holoprosencephaly Failure of division of the prosencephalon, resulting in a deficit in midline facial development, with hypotelorism; cyclopia occurs in the severe form, whereas in the mildest form a single central incisor tooth may be present.

Hydramnion, hydramnios see Polyhydramnios.

Hydranencephaly Complete or almost complete absence of cerebral hemispheres, their having been replaced by cerebrospinal fluid.

Hydrocele A collection of fluid in the tunica vaginalis of the testis or along the spermatic cord.

Hydrocephalus Marked dilation of the cerebral ventricles with excessive fluid, usually accompanied by vaulted or dome-shaped head (**hydrocephaly, hydrencephaly, hydrencephalus**).

Hydronephrosis Distension of the pelvis and calyces of the kidney with fluid, as a result of obstruction of urinary outflow.

Hydroureter Distension of the ureter with urine because of obstruction of the ureter.

Hypermastia Presence of one or more supernumerary mammary glands (**polymastia**).

Hypertelorism Abnormally great distance between paired parts or organs, e.g., between the eyes.

Hypoplasia Incomplete development of an organ.

Hypospadias Anomaly in which the urethra opens on the underside of the penis or on the perineum in males, or into the vagina in females.

Ichthyosis Developmental skin disorders characterized by excessive or abnormal keratinization, with dryness and scaling.

Iniencephaly An anomaly of the brain and neck characterized by an occipital bone defect, spina bifida of the cervical vertebrae, and fixed retroflexion of the head on the cervical spine.

Kyphosis Abnormal dorsal convexity in the curvature of the thoracic spine (**humpback, hunchback**).

Lissencephaly see Agyria.

Lordosis Abnormal anterior convexity in the curvature of the spine (**swayback**).

Macroglossia Abnormally large tongue, often protruding.

Macrophthalmia Abnormally large eye(s).

Malformation A permanent morphologic deviation, generally incompatible with or severely detrimental to normal postnatal survival or development; a morphologic defect of an organ, or large region of the body, resulting from an intrinsically abnormal development process. A major malformation is one that has medical, surgical, or cosmetic significance.

Meningocele Herniation of the meninges through a defect in the cranium (**cranial m.**), or spinal column (**spinal m.**).

Meningoencephalocele Herniation of meninges and brain tissue through a defect in the cranium (**encephalocele, encephalomeningocele**).

Meningomyelocele Herniation of meninges and spinal cord through a defect in the spinal column (**myelomeningocele**).

Meromelia Absence of part of a limb.

Micrencephaly Having an abnormally small brain.

Microcephaly Abnormally small head (**microcephalia; microcephalus**).

Microglossia Tongue hypoplasia.

Micrognathia Abnormally small jaw (**usually the mandible**).

Micromelia Having abnormally small or short limb(s).

Microphthalmos Abnormal smallness of one or both eyes (**Microphthalmia**).

Microstomia Hypoplasia of the mouth.

Microtia Hypoplasia of the pinna, with an absent or atretic external auditory meatus.

Misaligned sternebrae When the two ossification centers of each sternebra are not aligned in the transverse plane.

Myelocele Herniation of spinal cord through a vertebral defect.

Myelomeningocele see Meningomyelocele.

Myeloschisis Cleft spinal cord caused by failure of neural tube closure.

Neural tube defect Any malformation (**e.g., anencephaly, exencephaly, spina bifida**) resulting from failure of closure of the neural tube during embryonic development.

Nevus A circumscribed skin malformation, usually hyperpigmented or with abnormal vascularization.

Oligodactyly Having fewer than the normal number of digits.

Oligohydramnios Abnormally reduced quantity of amniotic fluid.

Omphalocele Herniation of intestine covered with peritoneum and amnion through a defect in the abdominal wall at the umbilicus (**exomphalos, umbilical hernia**).

Otocephaly Agnathia or micrognathia plus fusion or approximation of the pinnae inferior to the face.

Overriding aorta Displacement of the aorta to the right, so that it appears to arise from both ventricles.

Pagus Combining form (**suffix**) indicating conjoined twins.

Palatine rugae alteration Misaligned or otherwise abnormal palatal ridges.

Patent ductus arteriosus An open communication between the pulmonary trunk and aorta persisting postnatally.

Patent foramen ovale Failure of adequate postnatal closure of the *foramen ovale*, an atrial septal defect allowing interchange of blood between the atria; a primary atrial septal defect is larger than a patent *foramen ovale*.

Phocomelia Absence of the proximal part of a limb(s), the distal part attached to the trunk by a small, irregularly-shaped bone.

Plagiocephaly An asymmetrical condition of the cranium, resulting from premature closure of cranial sutures on one side, and oblique skull deformation.

Polydactyly Supernumerary digits.

Polyhydramnios Abnormally increased quantity of amniotic fluid.

Polymastia see Hypermastia.

Proboscis A cylindrical protuberance of the face, usually associated with holoprosencephaly.

Pseudohermaphroditism Partial masculinization or partial feminization, with gonadal tissue of only one sex present.

Ptosis Drooping of the upper eyelid, because of abnormal muscle or nerve development.

Rachischisis Congenital fissure of the vertebral column.

Resorption A conceptus that died after implantation and is being, or has been, reabsorbed into the mother's bloodstream.

Runt Normally-developed fetus or newborn significantly smaller than the rest of the litter.

Scoliosis Lateral deviation of the vertebral column.

Sirenomelia Having fused lower limbs (**symmelia**).

Situs inversus Lateral transposition of the viscera.

Spina bifida Localized defective closure of the vertebral arches, through which the spinal cord and/or meninges may protrude; a neural tube defect.

Spina bifida aperta Spina bifida in which the neural tissue is exposed.

Spina bifida cystica Spina bifida with herniation of a cystic swelling containing the meninges (**meningocele**), spinal cord (**myelocele**), or both (**myelomeningocele**).

Spina bifida occulta Spina bifida with intact skin and no herniation.

Stillbirth Birth of a dead fetus.

Sympodia Fusion of the feet.

Syndactyly Webbing or fusion between adjacent digits.

Talipes Congenital deformity of the foot, which is twisted out of shape or position (**clubfoot**).

Teratogen An agent that can cause abnormal development of the embryo or fetus.

Teratogenicity The ability to cause defective development.

Tetralogy of Fallot A combination of cardiac defects, consisting of pulmonary or infundibular stenosis, interventricular septal defect, overriding aorta, and right ventricular hypertrophy.

Tracheoesophageal fistula Abnormal connection between trachea and esophagus.

Umbilical hernia see Omphalocele.

Ventricular septal defect Persistent communication between the ventricles.

Wavy ribs Extra bends in one or more ribs.

Index

immunologic function alterations, 368

localized damage, 368

lysosome alterations, 369

microtubular alterations, 369

myofilament alterations, 369

neurogenic function alterations, 367–368

protein synthesis alterations, 369–370

sarcoplasmic reticulum alterations, 369

toxicity testing

animal models, 376

biochemical evaluation 374, 326

cell cultures, 374

electrophysiology, 374

morphologic evaluation

gross examination, 374–375

microscopic examination, 375–376

Skeleton, see Bone; Joints

Skin

barrier structural components, 139–140

biotransformation, 140–141

cell subpopulations, 138

homeostatic mechanisms, 138–139

injury response

adnexal lesions

alopecia, toxic, 153f, 154

chloracne, 153f, 154f

overview, 152, 153f

sweat gland lesions, 154–155

allergic contact dermatitis, 151, 152f

dermal lesions, 151, 152f

epidermal lesions, 149, 150f, 151f

neoplasms, 155–156, 155f, 156f

microscopic anatomy, 136, 137f, 138

overview, 135–136

percutaneous absorption, 140

toxicants in domestic animals, 148–149t

toxicity evaluation

carcinogenesis bioassays, 157–158

cell and tissue assays, 159

hypersensitivity reactions, 158

irritation tests, 157

morphological assessment, 158

overview, 156–157

photoxicity bioassays, 158

transgenic mice, 158–159

toxicity mechanisms

direct damage

chemical burns, 141, 143f

genotoxic agents, 144

irritation, 143

immune-mediated toxicity

Arthus reaction, 144–145

delayed-type hypersensitivity, 145f

erythema multiforme, 145–146

immunoglobulin E-dependent reactions, 144

overview, 144

photoallergy, 146–147

phototoxicity, 146, 147f

toxic epidermal necrolysis, 145, 146f

overview, 141, 142t

Small intestine

altered blood supply, 178

barrier function, 175–177

carcinogenesis, 184

function, 168

injury response, 190–191

malabsorption, 177

mucosal response to injury, 188, 189f

structure, 168–170

Smooth muscle cell, see Vasculature

Sodium, renal function testing, 56–57

Sodium chloride, neurotoxicity, 402f

Sodium/potassium ATPase, cell swelling modulation, 14

Sorbitol dehydrogenase (SDH), liver function testing, 54, 233

Sound, morphological alteration evaluation effects in laboratory animals, 91

Spermatid

features, 557–558

homogenization-resistant spermatids in toxicity testing, 594

retention, 583

toxicity mechanisms, 574–575

Spermatocyte

features, 559f

toxicity mechanisms, 574–575

Spermatogenesis

hormonal alteration effects, 586

overview, 559f

seminiferous epithelium cycle, 559, 560f

seminiferous epithelium wave, 559

Spermatogonia

features, 556

toxicity mechanisms, 574–575

Spermatozoa, toxicity mechanisms, 574–575

Spina bifida, features, 653

Spleen

anatomy, 463f, 464f

white pulp, 464–465

Squamous cell carcinoma, features, 156f

Stellate cell

alterations, 224–225

features, 200

Stomach

altered blood supply, 177, 178f

carcinogenesis, 183–184

function, 167

injury response

hyperplasia, 190f

mucosal response, 188

ulceration and inflammation, 190

structure, 167–168

Strain A mouse pulmonary tumor test, carcinogen testing, 39

Strychnine, neurotoxicity, 386

Sudan black, lipid staining, 15

Sulfur, neurotoxicity, 402

Sweat glands, lesions, 154–155

Synaptotagmin, botulinum toxin binding, 385

Syndactyly, features, 659

Synovitis, features, 439, 440f

T

T-cell

maturation in thymus, 458

respiratory defense, 101

small intestine, 170

TCDD, see 2,3,7,8-Tetrachlorodibenzo-p-dioxin

Temperature, morphological alteration evaluation effects in laboratory animals, 91

TEN, see Toxic epidermal necrolysis

Terminology, pathology

diagnostic setting influences, 67, 74

Greek and Latin roots

anatomical sites, 69–72t

common prefixes, 73t

common suffixes, 74t

morphological alteration evaluation influences, 91

multiple pathologist problems

diagnostic drift, 75

lesion complexity, 75–76

overview, 67–68

recording of data, 76–77

standardization, 76, 89

suggested practices, 77–78

Testes

gross structure, 554–555

injury response

overview, 579–580

Leydig cell

functional overview, 558

macrophage, 558

necrosis, 583, 585

peritubular cell, 558

Sertoli cell